3/19/88

The
Medical and Health
Encyclopedia

The Medical and Health Encyclopedia

Edited by
Richard J. Wagman, M.D., F.A.C.P.
Associate Clinical Professor of Medicine
Downstate Medical Center
New York, New York

And by the J. G. Ferguson Editorial Staff

J. G. Ferguson Publishing Company/Chicago, Illinois

Portions of this work have been previously published under
the title *The New Complete Medical and Health Encyclopedia*
and under the titles of *The Complete Illustrated Book of Better Health* and *The Illustrated Encyclopedia of Better Health*,
edited by Richard J. Wagman, M.D.

Contributors to The Medical and Health Encyclopedia

Editor

RICHARD J. WAGMAN, M.D., F.A.C.P.
Associate Clinical Professor of Medicine
Downstate Medical Center
New York, New York

Consultant in Surgery

N. HENRY MOSS, M.D., F.A.C.S.
Associate Clinical Professor of Surgery
Temple University Health Sciences Center
and Albert Einstein Medical Center;
Past President, American Medical Writers Association;
Past President, New York Academy of Sciences

Consultant in Gynecology

DOUGLASS S. THOMPSON, M.D.
Clinical Professor of Obstetrics and Gynecology
and Clinical Associate Professor of Community Medicine
University of Pittsburgh School of Medicine
Pittsburgh, Pennsylvania

Consultant in Pediatrics

CHARLES H. BAUER, M.D.
Clinical Associate Professor of Pediatrics
and Chief of Pediatric Gastroenterology
The New York Hospital-Cornell Medical Center
New York, New York

Consultants in Psychiatry

JULIAN J. CLARK, M.D.
Assistant Professor of Psychiatry
and
RITA W. CLARK, M.D.
Clinical Assistant Professor of Psychiatry
Downstate Medical Center
New York, New York

Consulting Editor

KENNETH N. ANDERSON
Formerly Editor
Today's Health

CONTENTS

Illustration Credits

The editors wish to thank the following organizations and individuals for allowing us to use their illustrations in THE MEDICAL AND HEALTH ENCYCLOPEDIA. Abbreviations used include: T (top), B (bottom), C (center), L (left), R (right).

2 American Dental Association
4 Pennsylvania Hospital, Philadelphia
5 Aldus Books
8 Aldus Books
8-9 Aldus Books (B)
11 Peter Karas (T); Martin M. Rotker—Taurus Photos (B)
17 American Heart Association (T); Aldus Books (B)
18 Martin M. Rotker—Taurus
19 National Institutes of Health—Dr. Makio Murayamo
20 Jean-Claude Lejeune (T); Kuntshalle Bremen, Federal Republic of Germany (B)
22 The Francis A. Countway Library of Medicine, Boston; photograph, Eduardo di Ramio
23 Jean-Claude Lejeune
25 Aldus Books
27 Aldus Books
28 Aldus Books
29 British Museum
42-3 Aldus Books
44-5 Aldus Books
51 Ken Tighe
52 Office of Child Development—Richard Swartz
53 Tyrone Hall—Stock, Boston
54 Elizabeth Crews—Stock, Boston (T); Office of Child Development—Richard Swartz (B)
55 Jean-Claude Lejeune (T); Office of Child Development—Richard Swartz (B)
56 Peter Vandermark—Stock, Boston
57 Office of Child Development—Richard Swartz (T); Jean-Claude Lejeune (B)
58 Marty Heitner—Taurus Photos
59 Office of Child Development—Richard Swartz
60 Peter Simon—Black Star
62 Elaine Murray
63 Jean-Claude Lejeune
66 Office of Child Development—Richard Swartz (T); National Council of YMCA's (B)
67 George Bellerose—Stock, Boston
68 Manhattan Eye, Ear and Throat Hospital (T); "The Circumcision" (1599) by Crispin de Passe the Elder, Philadelphia Museum of Art, Charles M. Lea Collection (B)
69 Jean-Claude Lejeune
70 American Podiatry Association
71 Manhattan Eye, Ear and Throat Hospital
72 Office of Child Development—Richard Swartz
73 Manhattan Eye, Ear and Throat Hospital
74 Elizabeth Hamlin—Stock, Boston
76 Paul Fortin—Stock, Boston
78 Jean-Claude Lejeune (T); National Institutes of Health (B)
79-80 Jean-Claude Lejeune
81 Jean-Claude Lejeune
82 Maria College
83 Diane Koos Gentry—Black Star
84 Long Island College Hospital
87 Manhattan Eye, Ear and Throat Hospital
88 Jean-Claude Lejeune
90 Carlsberg Glyptothek, Copenhagen (T); Jean-Claude Lejeune (B)
92 The Francis A. Countway Library of Medicine, Boston; photo, Eduardo di Ramio
93 National Institutes of Health
94 The Council for Exceptional Children; photo, Nanda Ward Hayne
96 Jean-Claude Lejeune
97 Jean-Claude Lejeune
99 Jean-Claude Lejeune
101 National Institute of Allergy and Infectious Diseases
102 Ira Berger—Black Star
103 Merck Sharp and Dohme (T); Jean-Claude Lejeune (B)
105 James Holland—Stock, Boston
107 Erika Stone—Peter Arnold
110 New York University
112 Eric Kroll—Taurus Photos
113 Girl Scouts of the USA
114 Neal Boenzi—The *New York Times*
116 Peter Southwick—Stock, Boston (T); Jean-Claude Lejeune (B)
117 WHO Photo/French National Committee Against Smoking
118 EPA-Documerica—Marc St. Gill
121 Office of Child Development—Richard Swartz
122 Jean-Claude Lejeune
125 Maternity Center Association
128 Uffizi, Florence; photo, Scala/Editorial Photocolor Archives
129 Leo Choplin—Black Star
130 Tim Kelly—Black Star
131 Jean-Claude Lejeune
133 Jean-Claude Lejeune
135 National Institutes of Health
136 James D. Wilson—*Newsweek*
137 National Institutes of Health (T); Long Island College Hospital (B)
138-9 Maternity Center Association
139 Columbia-Presbyterian Medical Center—Lucy B. Lazzopina
140 Aldus Books (T); Lenox Hill Hospital—Herb Levart (B)
141 Mount Sinai Hospital
142 Elizabeth Hamlin—Stock, Boston (T); National Library of Medicine (B)
143 Laimute E. Drukis—Taurus Photos
145 Jean-Claude Lejeune
147 University of Chicago
150 Elaine Murray
151 Jean-Claude Lejeune
153 Dick Dickinson—Black Star
154 Arnold Zann—Black Star
155 National Jogging Association (T); Jean-Claude Lejeune (B)
160 William Hubbell—Woodfin Camp and Associates
162 National Heart, Lung, and Blood Institute
166 Jean-Claude Lejeune
167 Peter Vandermark—Stock, Boston
168 Jean-Claude Lejeune
172 U.S. Census Bureau
173 Robert Goldstein—Black Star
174 Jean-Claude Lejeune
175 UPI
176 George Bellerose—Stock, Boston
177 Owen Franken—Stock, Boston
179 Columbia-Presbyterian Medical Center Fund, Inc.—Bill Ray
180 David Joel
181 Sinai Hospital of Detroit, Wayne State University
184 Shirley Zeiberg—Taurus Photos
185 Bill Grimes—Black Star
186 Jean-Claude Lejeune
187 Eric Kroll—Taurus Photos (T); Jean-Claude Lejeune (B)
188 Dennis Brack—Black Star
190 Natiogal Council on Aging, Inc.
195 David Joel
203-5 National Livestock and Meat Board
207-9 New York State College of Human Ecology at Cornell University (T); Aldus Books (B)
210 Office of Child Development—Richard Swartz
211 National Library of Medicine
217 Center for Disease Control
221 FDA
225 EPA-Documerica—Con Keyes
226 Peter Arnold—Peter Arnold, Inc. (T); Horst Schafer—Peter Arnold, Inc. (B)
227 National Institutes of Health (T); EPA-Documerica—Boyd Norton (B)
228 EPA-Documerica—Bruce McAllister (T); Gerhard E. Gscheidle—Peter Arnold, Inc. (B)
229 UPI
230 Bureau of Sport Fisheries and Wildlife
231 National Library of Medicine
232 Fred Ward—Black Star (T); Peter Arnold—Peter Arnold, Inc. (B)
233 EPA-Documerica—Michael Philip Manheim
234 EPA-Documerica—Eric Calonius
238 Office of Child Development—Richard Swartz
239 The Bettmann Archive
240 Richard Younker
241 The Bettmann Archive
242 Dr. Marvin I. Lepaw (T); The Bettmann Archive (B, L); Library of Congress (B, R)
244 The Bettmann Archive
245 U.S. Department of Agriculture (T); Dermatology Associates, P.C. (B)
246 Dermatology Associates, P.C.
247 *Podiatry News*
249 FDA
250 National Institutes of Health
253 American Dental Association
254 Doug Wilson—Black Star
255 American Dental Assistants Association
256 Jean-Claude Lejeune (L); American Dental Association (R)
258 Naval Dental Research Institute, Greal Lakes, Illinois (T); Yale Medical Library, Yale University (B)
260 American Dental Association (L); National Insitutes of Health (R)
262 The Bettmann Archive
262-3 Columbia University School of Dental and Oral Surgery
266 National Library of Medicine
267 U.S. Department of Agriculture (T); National Library of Medicine (B)
268 Bibliothèque de l'Ancienne Faculté de Médecine, Paris; photo, Jean-Loup Charmet
269 National Library of Medicine
270 Bayer Co.
271 Francis A. Countway Library of Medicine, Boston; photo, Eduardo di Ramio
273 American Podiatry Association
275 National League for Nursing
276-7 National Library of Medicine
277 Center for Disease Control
279 Columbia-Presbyterian Medical Center Fund, Inc. —Bill Ray
281 Jean-Claude Lejeune
283 Metropolitan Life Insurance Co.
284 National Institutes of Health
285 Center for Disease Control
285-6 U.S. Department of Agriculture
287 Medical World News—Ted Russell (R), Charles Hayes (L)
290 Wellcome Institute for the History of Medicine, London
290 Ira Berger—Black Star
293 United Hospital Fund of New York
294 FDA (T); Mandl School for Medical and Dental Assistants (B)
295 Dan McCoy—Rainbow
296 "The Consultation," 1516, Philadelphia Museum of Art, The Smith, Kline and French Laboratories Collection
297 Greater New York Blood Program (T); John Austad, *Chicago Tribune* © 1980 (B)
298 David Powers—Stock, Boston
299 Thomas England
301 Pfizer, Inc.
302 Manhattan Eye, Ear and Throat Hospital
307 Jean-Claude Lejeune (T); Tom England (B)
309 Columbia-Presbyterian Medical Center Fund, Inc.—Bill Ray (T); Cary Wolinsky—Stock, Boston (B)
310 David Joel
311 National Library of Medicine (T); Columbia-Presbyterian Medical Center—Elizabeth Wilcox (B)
315 Columbia-Presbyterian Medical Center—Werner Wolff (T); Tom England (B)
316 Mount Sinai Hospital of Chicago; photo, Richard Younker
317 Children's Memorial Hospital, Chicago; photo, Jean-Claude Lejeune
321 Ellis Herwig—Stock, Boston
330 David Joel
331 Joe Baker for Medical World News (technical assistance by Bellevue Medical Center)
333 Taurus Photos
334 National Institutes of Health (T); *Research Advances*, National Institutes of Health—Herbert E. Kaufman (B)
335 Columbia-Presbyterian Medical Center Fund, Inc. —Bill Ray
341 National Library of Medicine
342 Columbia-Presbyterian Medical Center—Werner Wolff
344-6 Manhattan Eye, Ear and Throat Hospital
350 FDA (All)
351 Columbia-Presbyterian Medical Center—Lucy B. Lazzopina
352 Dr. G. R. Honig, Hematology Division, Children's Memorial Hospital, Chicago (B, L); New York University Medical Center—Robert Grant (T, R); National Institutes of Health—Dr. Mako Murayamo (B, R)
353 National Institutes of Health (T); Smithsonian Institution (B)
354 Jean-Claude Lejeune
356 Peter Karas
357 American Heart Association (T); Goodyear Tire and Rubber Co. (B)
358 NASA (L); Long Island College Hospital (R)
361 National Heart and Lung Institute (T); National Institutes of Health (B)
362 Ted Spiegel—Black Star
363 Columbia-Presbyterian Medical Center—Werner Wolff
365 Mount Sinai Hospital of Chicago; photo, Richard Younker
367 Andy Levin—Black Star
369 WHO—Jerry Hecht
370 Medical Illustration Service, University of Utah School of Medicine—Brad Nelson (T); Wide World (B)
371 Medical Illustration Service, University of Utah School of Medicine—Brad Nelson
372 National Institutes of Health (T); General Electric, Medical Systems Department (B)
375-6 Anthony A. Davis
377 National Library of Medicine
378 National Institute of Allergy and Infectious Diseases
379 Anthony A. Davis
381 University of California at Berkeley
381-2 Center for Disease Control (All)
382 Dr. Steven Arnon, Infant Botulism Research Project, California State Department of Health
383 National Institute of Allergy and Infectious Diseases
384 Anthony A. Davis
385 Columbia-Presbyterian Medical Center Fund, Inc. —Bill Ray
388 National Institute of Allergy and Infectious Diseases (T, L); University of Pennsylvania Medical School—Dr. Robert Austrian (B, L) Aldus Archives
389 Aldus Archives
390 Pfizer, Inc. (T); WHO, photo, J. Mohr (B)
391 American Lung Association (T) and (B, L); Center for Disease Control (B, R)
392 Center for Disease Control
392 GAF Corp.
394 Long Island Jewish Medical Center
395 Jean-Claude Lejeune (B, L); David Joel (T, R)
396 American Cancer Institute
397 American Cancer Society (both)
398 © MacNelly—*Richmond News Leader*
399 Webb-Waring Institute for Medical Research, Denver
400 EPA-Documerica—Bruce McAllister (T); American Lung Association (B)
401 Webb-Waring Institute for Medical Research, Denver
402 National Air Pollution Control Administration (T); Neal Boenzi—The *New York Times* (B)
411 Eli Lilly and Co.
412 WHO; photo, J. Mohr (T); Medic Alert Foundation (B)
413 Joe Senzer—Medical World News
414 WHO—J. Gordon (T), P. Larsen (B)
416 National Eye Institute
417 Aldus Books (T); Long Island College Hospital (B)
418 Manhattan Eye, Ear and Throat Hospital
419 National Institutes of Health (T); Dan McCoy—Black Star (B)
420 Columbia-Presbyterian Medical Center Fund, Inc. —Peter Kaplan (B, L); Bausch & Lomb/Soflens Division (T, R); UPI (B, R)
421 Aldus Books, (T); Long Island College Hospital (B)
422 Columbia-Presbyterian Medical Center Fund, Inc. —Bill Ray (T); Long Island College Hospital (B)
423 Aldus Books (T); FDA (B)
426 South-Eastern Organ Procurement Foundation, Richmond, Va.
427 Stern—Black Star
429 Pfizer, Inc.
431 National Library of Medicine
432 New York City Department of Health
434 American Cancer Society; photo, Arthur Leipzig
435 National Cancer Institute
437 American Cancer Society (T); WHO—Spooner (B)
438 Pfizer, Inc.
440 American Cancer Society (L); Bill Owen—Black Star (R)
441-2 American Cancer Society
445 *Research Advances*, National Institutes of Health (T, L); FDA (T, R); Columbia-Presbyterian Medical Center Fund, Inc. —Bill Ray (B)
446-7 American Cancer Society
451 Fredrik D. Bodin—Stock, Boston (T); Anthony A. Davis (B)
452 Leonard Kamsler—Medical World News
453 Columbia-Presbyterian Medical Center Fund, Inc. —R. P. Sheridan (T); Peter Kaplan (B)
454-5 Arthritis Foundation
455 National Institutes of Health
456 The Bettmann Archive
457 Arthritis Foundation
459 Anthony A. Davis (T); National Institutes of Health (B)
462 Columbia-Presbyterian Medical Center—Lucy B. Lazzopina
463 Anthony A. Davis
464 Columbia-Presbyterian Medical Fund, Inc.—Bill Ray (B)
464-5 Anthony A. Davis
466 Jean-Claude Lejeune
468 Dan McCoy—Rainbow
469 Pfizer, Inc. (T); National Institutes of Health (B)
470 Dan McCoy—Rainbow (T); George Bellerose—Stock, Boston (B)
472 Portrait by Jacques-Louis David, 1812, National Gallery of Art, Washington, D.C., Samuel H. Dress Collection (TL); Oil painting after Thomas Hudson, 1756, National Portrait Gallery, London (TR); National Institutes of Health (B)
475 Columbia-Presbyterian Medical Center—R. Goldstein (T); Medic Alert Foundation (B)
476 Columbia-Presbyterian Medical Center—Lucy B. Lazzopina
477 UPI
478-9 Long Island College Hospital
480 Bruce O. Berg, M.D.
482 *Research Advances*, National Institutes of Health—Dr. Vanda Lennon
483 George Gardner
485 Magee-Women's Hospital —Ronald J. Kubiak
488 National Institutes of Health
490 WHO—Homer Page
494 Magee-Women's Hospital —Ronald J. Kubiak
497 National Library of Medicine
500-1 American Cancer Society
502 George Tames from *Contemporary OB/GYN*, September 1973
503 American Cancer Society
505-8 National Library of Medicine
508 American Cancer Society
509 Jean-Claude Lejeune
512 "Fading Away," by Henry Peach Robinson, George Eastman House Collection
514 ACTION Senior Companion Program
515 Visiting Nurse Service of New York
517 National Library of Medicine
518 Jean-Loup Charmet, Paris
519 Center for Disease Control (L); National Institute of Infectious Diseases (R)
520 WHO—P. Pittet
521 *Research Advances*, National Institutes of Health
522 National Library of Medicine
523 WHO—Homer Page (T); Center for Disease Control (B)
524 Center for Disease Control (T, B); National Institute of Allergy and Infectious Diseases (C)
525 Center for Disease Control
526 National Institute of Allergy and Infectious Diseases (T); Center for Disease Control (C, B)
527 Klaus D. Francke—Peter Arnold, Inc.
528 Center for Disease Control
530 Aldus Books
531 Library of Congress (L); Dr. Siegfried M. Pueschel, Rhode Island Hospital, Providence (R)
533 Museum of Fine Arts, Boston
535 Aldus Books
537 Clark University Archives
538 H. Armstrong Roberts
541 Gary Settle—The *New York Times*
543-4 National Library of Medicine
546 National Highway Traffic Administration
547 Fairfax County (Va.) Police Department
547-8 National Library of Medicine
554 American Institute of the History of Pharmacy
555 Bureau of Narcotics and Dangerous Drugs
558 National Library of Medicine (T); Bureau of Narcotics and Dangerous Drugs (B)
560-1 Bureau of Narcotics and Dangerous Drugs
564 Bruce Hoertel
565 David A. Silva—Wills Eye Hospital, Philadelphia, Pa.
566 Phototake
568 WHO—P. Almasy
569 WHO—P. Larsen
570 Bent Hodge—Phototake
571 John Urban
576-8 American Red Cross
578 Medic Alert Foundation
579 Martin A. Levick—Black Star
579-80 American Red Cross
581 FDA (T); Martin A. Levick—Black Star (B)
586 American Red Cross
588 National Institute of Allergy and Infectious Diseases
591 Michael Malyszko—Stock, Boston
592 National Institutes of Health
593 Dan McCoy—Rainbow
596 National Institutes of Health
597 Dan McCoy—Rainbow
599 AVCO Research Laboratory
603 Peter Karas
604 Pfizer, Inc.
605 National Institute of Allergy and Infectious Diseases (L); U.S. Department of Agriculture (R)

INTRODUCTION

Many questions may run through your mind when you or a family member are ill. Even if you see a physician, you still might have a lot of questions afterward. The doctor was very busy and didn't take time to discuss all the aspects of your condition that you had hoped he would. Or, you did have a good talk with your doctor, but he or she used several terms you didn't understand. You didn't get the details of the diagnosis; surgery was mentioned—what does this kind of operation involve?

The MEDICAL AND HEALTH ENCYCLOPEDIA is designed to give you clear, accurate answers to your questions about health care. Thorough discussions of major diseases like cancer and cardiovascular disease are included, along with facts about many other less serious diseases and physical problems and how they are treated.

Many people today have adopted a consumerist point-of-view and want to take an active part in their own treatment. This usually takes the form of asking your doctor to present the treatment options available to you, then making a decision about which course to follow. Let's assume that your physician agrees to this approach; he is willing to relinquish some of the authority doctors and traditionally have held in telling patients what to do. Still, you need information to ask intelligent questions and also to understand the alternatives presented.

Fortunately, research in medicine is continually advancing. The MEDICAL AND HEALTH ENCYCLOPEDIA has been written to include material on some recent developments—like the portable insulin pump for diabetics—that you may have heard about. In line with the idea of treatment options, the editors have also included information on the many types of surgery now used for breast cancer patients; no longer is the total mastectomy the only choice for women.

Generic drugs have been in the spotlight increasingly in recent years. For your convenience in sorting out which drug is equivalent to which, the editors have included a new chapter on 100 commonly prescribed generic drugs. The chapter includes information on brand names, the action that each drug has in the body, and possible side effects.

Becoming ill and being treated are only part of the picture in health care today. More and more, professionals and lay people are putting the emphasis on preventive medicine, doing everything you possibly can to stay healthy. To help you and your family keep in the best possible condition, the editors have included detailed information on food and nutrition, dieting, care of skin and hair, and dental health.

Families often have questions about children's health. Parents, step-parents, and grandparents want to know what is normal and expected from a child at various ages in terms of physical, mental, and emotional development. Therefore, the editors have included two chapters (one on younger children, another on teenagers) that discuss everything from the common cold to stuttering, and from creativity to sexual maturation.

Older people, too, have special health concerns. Senior citizens or their families will want to read the information on diet, daily habits, mental health, activities to pursue during retirement, nursing homes, and retirement homes for the aging.

These are just a few of the subjects covered in this encyclopedia. How can you make the best possible use of these books? First and foremost, do *not* use this information to treat yourself or anyone else except temporarily in an emergency. If any symptom of disease is present, no one can take the place of a trained professional.

Use the MEDICAL AND HEALTH ENCYCLOPEDIA for background information on a host of topics, as a handy guide to first aid, and as a reference on where to get further information. Throughout the book, the editors have included the names and addresses of organizations that deal with health-related matters, places you can write for further information.

Get acquainted with the encyclopedia by looking through the table of contents. Thumb through the many chapters and familiarize yourself with those new and unusual terms you may be encountering for the first time. An understanding of the material presented in this book could prove to be invaluable to you and your family today, tomorrow, or some time in the future.

                                                                    The Editors

CHAPTER 1

Your Body

THE SKELETON

Say "skeleton" to children and you probably conjure up in their minds a rickety structure of rigid sticks, or, to the more fanciful child, a clickety-clacketing collection of rattling bones cavorting under a Halloween moon. A look at almost any anatomical drawing of the human skeletal system bears out the child's image: dry sticks of bones, stripped of skin and flesh, muscle and tendon —a grotesque caricature of a living human being.

Our living bones are something quite different. They are rigid, yes, but not entirely so: they also may bend a little and grow and repair themselves; and they are shaped and fitted so that—rather than the herky-jerky motions of a wooden puppet—they permit the smooth grace and coordinated power displayed by an accomplished athlete or a prima ballerina.

Our bones do not do just one thing but many things. Some bones, like the collarbone or *clavicle*, mainly give support to other body structures. Others, like the skull and ribs, encase and protect vulnerable organs. Still others, like the *metacarpus* and *phalanges* that make up our hands and fingers, give us mechanical advantages—

leverage and movement. There are even bones, the tiny *ossicles* in the middle ear, whose vibrations enable us to hear.

Finally, to think of bone simply as a structural member, like a solid steel girder in a skyscraper, ignores the fact that bone is living tissue. It is one of the busiest tissues in our bodies, a chemical factory that is continually receiving, processing and shipping a wide variety of mineral salts, blood components, and a host of other vital materials.

How the Bones of the Skeletal System Fit and Work Together

Medical textbooks name a total of 206 bones making up the skeletal system of the normal, adult human being. The words "normal" and "adult" are significant. A newborn baby normally has 33 vertebrae making up its backbone (also called *spinal column* or simply *spine*); but by the time a person reaches adulthood, the number of individual vertebrae has shrunk to 26. The explanation: during the growth process, the nine bottom vertebrae fuse naturally into just two. In like fashion, we "lose" some 60 bones as we

grow up. Some otherwise perfectly normal adults have "extra" bones or "missing" bones. For example, although the normal number of ribs is 12 pairs, some adults may have 11; others may have 13 pairs.

Even a practicing doctor might be hard-pressed to identify each of our 200-plus bones and describe its function. An easier way to gain a general understanding of the various functions, capabilities—and weaknesses, too—of our bones is to visualize the skeletal system as a standing coatrack, say, about six feet high.

Call the central pole the backbone. About ten inches down from its top (the top of your skull) is a horizontal cross-bar (your shoulders—collarbones and shoulder blades), approximately a foot-and-a-half across. Sixteen or so inches below the bottom of the top cross bar is another, shorter cross bar, broader and thicker—the *pelvic girdle*. The coatrack with its two cross bars is now a crude model of the bones of the head and trunk, collectively called the *axial skeleton*. Its basic unit is the backbone, to which are attached the skull at the top, then the bones of the shoulder girdle, the ribs, and at the bottom,

1

the bones of the pelvic girdle.

By hanging down (or appending) members from the two ends of the top cross bar, and doing the same at the lower cross bar, we would simulate what is called the *appendicular skeleton*—arms and hands, legs and feet.

Now, make the coatrack stand on its new legs, cut off the central pole just below the lower bar (if you wish, calling it man's lost tail), and you have the two main components of the skeletal system, joined together before you. Let us look at each more closely.

The Axial Skeleton

Within the framework of the axial skeleton lie all the most vital organs of the body. People have gone on living with the loss of a hand or a leg—indeed, with the loss of any or all of their limbs. But nobody can live without a brain, a heart, a liver, lungs, or kidneys—all of which are carried within the framework of the axial skeleton.

The Skull

The bones of the skull have as their most important function the protection of the brain and sense organs. There are also, of course, the jawbones that support the teeth and gums and which enable us to bite and chew our food.

Most of the skull appears to consist of a single bone—a hard, unbroken dome. Actually, the brain cage or *cranium* consists of eight individual platelike bones which have fused together in the process of growth. At birth, these bones are separated, causing the soft spots or *fontanelles* we can readily feel on a baby's head. As the baby's brain enlarges, the bones grow along their edges to fill in the fontanelles, finally knitting together in what are called *suture lines*, somewhat resembling inexpertly mended clothes seams. Along the suture lines, the skull bones continue to grow until the individual's mature skull size is reached.

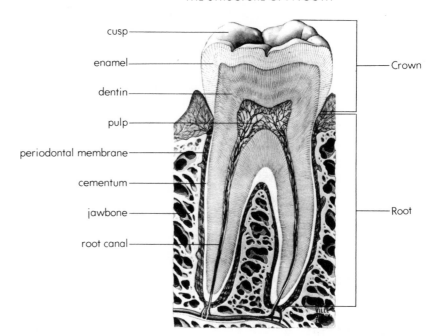

THE STRUCTURE OF A TOOTH

cusp — enamel — dentin — pulp — periodontal membrane — cementum — jawbone — root canal

Crown — Root

TEETH: The hardest substance in the human body is the *enamel* that covers the exposed surface of a tooth. Below the gum, the tooth's outside surface is composed of somewhat softer *cementum*. Beneath enamel and cementum is a bonelike substance, called *dentin*, which covers the soft interior of the tooth, called *pulp*. Pulp is serviced by blood vessels and nerves through the root or roots of the tooth. The passageway of nerves and blood vessels that lead up through the tooth from the gum sockets is called a *root canal*. Tooth and gum are stuck to each other by a tough, adhesive tissue called *periodontal* (or peridental—"surrounding the tooth") *membrane*. See Ch. 10, p. 252, for further information on teeth.

The Backbone

At the base of the skull, the backbone begins. The skull is supported by the topmost *cervical* (neck) vertebra. The curious thing about a backbone is that the word has come to suggest something solid, straight, and unbending. The backbone, however, just isn't like that: it consists of 26 knobby, hollowed-out bones—*vertebrae*, rather

improbably held together by muscles, ligaments, and tendons. It is not straight when we stand, but has definite backward and forward curvatures; and even some of its most important structures (the disks between the vertebrae) aren't made of bone, but of cartilage.

All in all, however, the backbone is a fairly well designed structure in terms of the several different functions it serves—but with some built-in weaknesses. For a discussion of backache, see under *Aches, Pains, Nuisances, Worries*, p. 265.

THE VERTEBRAE: Although they all have features in common, no two of our 26 vertebrae are exactly alike in shape, size, or function. This is hardly surprising if we consider, for example, that the cervical vertebrae do not support ribs, while the *thoracic vertebrae* (upper trunk, or chest) do support them.

But for a sample vertebra, let us pick a rib-carrying vertebra, if for no other reason than that it lies about midway along the backbone. If viewed from above or below, a thoracic vertebra, like most of the others, would look like a roundish piece of bone with roughly scalloped edges on the side facing inward toward the chest and on the side facing outward toward the surface of the back, and would reveal several bony projections. These knobby portions of a vertebra—some of which you can feel as bumps along your backbone—are called *processes*. They serve as the vertebra's points of connection to muscles and tendons, to ribs, and to the other vertebrae above and below.

A further conspicuous feature is a hole, more or less in the middle of the typical vertebra, through which passes the master nerve bundle of our bodies, the spinal cord, running from the base of the skull to the top of the pelvis. Thus, one of the important functions of the backbone is to provide flexible, protective tubing for the spinal cord.

Between the bones of one vertebra and the next is a piece of more resilient cartilage that acts as a cush-ion or shock absorber to prevent two vertebrae from scraping or bumping each other if the backbone gets a sudden jolt, or as the backbone twists and turns and bends. These pieces of cartilage are the intervertebral disks—infamous for pain and misery if they become ruptured or slipped disks.

REGIONS OF THE BACKBONE: The backbone can be divided into five regions, starting with the uppermost, or *cervical* region, which normally has seven vertebrae. Next down is the *thoracic* (chest) section, normally with 12 vertebrae. From each vertebra a rib extends to curl protectively around the chest area. Usually, the top ten ribs come all the way around the trunk and attach to the breastbone (or *sternum*); but the bottom two ribs do not reach the breastbone and are thus called floating ribs. The thoracic section also must support the shoulder girdle, consisting of the collarbones (*clavicles*) and shoulder blades (*scapulas*). At the end of each shoulder blade is a shoulder joint—actually three distinct joints working together—where the arm connects to the axial skeleton.

Below the thoracic vertebrae come the five vertebrae of the *lumbar* section. This area gets a good deal of blame for back miseries: lower back pain often occurs around the area where the bottom thoracic vertebra joins the top lumbar vertebra; furthermore, the lumbar region or small of the back is also a well-known site of back pain; indeed, from the word "lumbar" comes *lumbago,* medically an imprecise term, but popularly used to describe very real back pain.

Below the lumbar region are two vertebrae so completely different from the 24 above them—and even from each other—that it seems strange they are called vertebrae at all: the *sacrum* and the *coccyx*. These two vertebrae are both made up of several distinct vertebrae that are present at birth. The sacrum is a large bone that was once five vertebrae. The coccyx was originally

THE HUMAN SKELETON

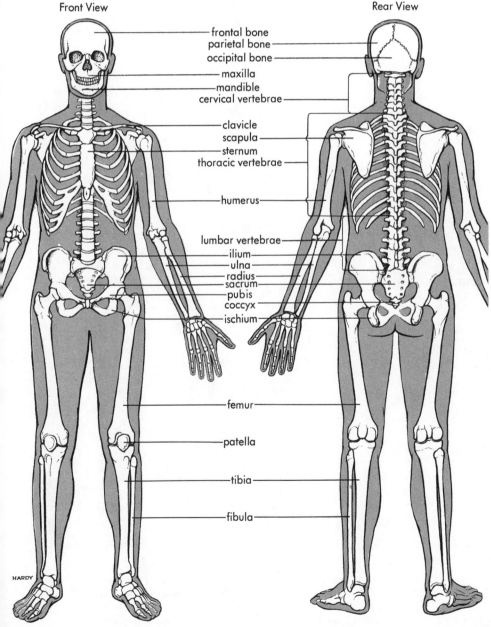

Front View

Rear View

frontal bone
parietal bone
occipital bone
maxilla
mandible
cervical vertebrae
clavicle
scapula
sternum
thoracic vertebrae
humerus
lumbar vertebrae
ilium
ulna
radius
sacrum
pubis
coccyx
ischium
femur
patella
tibia
fibula

HARDY

four vertebrae—and, incidentally, is all that remains of man's tail in his evolution from the primates.

THE PELVIC GIRDLE: The sacrum is the more important of these two strange-looking vertebrae. It is the backbone's connection to the *pelvic girdle,* or pelvis. On each side of the sacrum, connected by the sacroiliac joint, is a very large, curving bone called the *ilium,* tilting (when we stand) slightly forward and downward from the sacrum toward the front of the groin. We feel the top of the ilium as the top of the hip—a place mothers and fathers often find convenient for toting a toddler.

Fused at each side of the ilium and slanting toward the back is the *ischium,* the bone we sit on. The two *pubis* bones, also fused to the ilium, meet in front to complete the pelvic girdle. All the bones of the pelvis—ilium, ischium, and pubis—fuse together so as to form the hip joint *(acetabulum),* a deep socket into which the "ball" or upper end of the thighbone fits.

The Appendicular Skeleton

The bones of the appendages—arms, hands, and fingers; legs, feet, and toes—allow human beings to perform an astonishing array of complex movements, from pushing themselves through the physical rigors of the Olympic decathlon to creating an elaborate piece of needlework. The key points in the appendicular skeleton, as indeed, in the axial skeleton, are where the ends or edges of bones lie together and must work with or against one another in order to achieve coordinated movement. These key points are the *joints*—not really bones at all but the non-bony spaces between bones.

The Joints

A typical joint consists of several different structures. First, there are the bones themselves—two, three, four, or more almost touching in the area of the joint—with their ends or edges shaped to fit in their respec-

tive niches. Between the bones of an appendage joint (as between the vertebrae of the back) is the smooth, resilient material called *cartilage* which allows the bones to move over one another without scraping or catching. At the joint, the bones, with their layer of cartilage between

them, are held together by tough bonds of muscle. *Bursas,* tiny sacs containing a lubricating fluid, are also found at joints; they help to reduce the friction between a joint's moving parts.

THE HIP AND KNEE: The hip joint must not only support the weight of

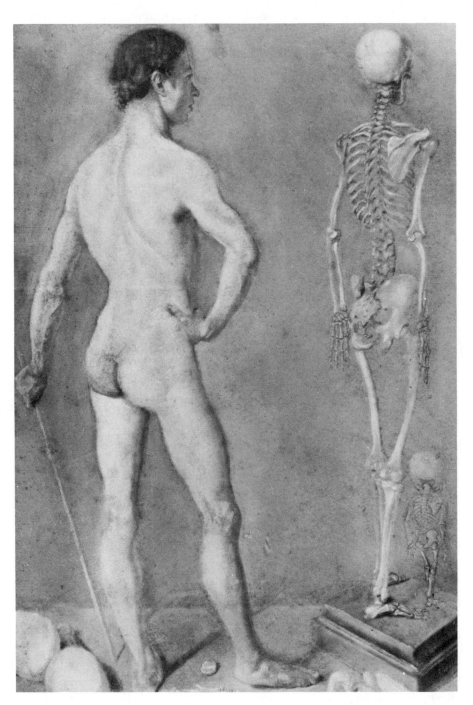

The first medical college in colonial America was founded in 1765 at the College of Pennsylvania in association with Pennsylvania Hospital. The anatomical drawing is one of a series of drawings that was donated to the hospital by an English physician for use in teaching anatomy.

BONES OF THE HAND AND FOOT

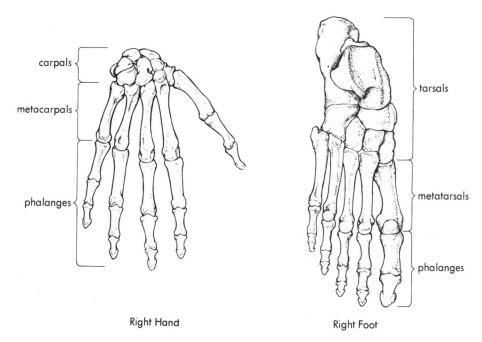

Right Hand

Right Foot

Of all our bony parts, the wrist, hand, and fingers are perhaps the most elegantly and finely jointed—witness the performance of a concert pianist—and our ankles, feet, and toes probably the most subject to everyday misery.

Bone As Living Tissue

Our bones, like all our tissues, change as we grow up, mature, and finally grow old. There are changes in the chemical activity and composition of bone representative of each stage of life.

In young children, the ends and edges of bones are mainly cartilage, forming a growing surface on the bone that is gradually replaced by hard bone as full size is attained. The bones of a child are more pliable and less likely to break than those of a full-grown adult.

Similarly, as an adult ages, the bones turn from a resilient hardness to a more brittle hardness. This accounts for the much greater danger of broken bones in older people.

the head and trunk, but must allow for movement of the leg and also play a part in the constant balancing required to maintain upright posture. Similar stresses and strains, often literally tending to tear the joint apart, are placed on every joint in the body.

The notoriety of athletes' bad knees attests to the forces battering at the knee joint, the largest in the human body. Sports involving leaping or sudden changes in direction, such as basketball, are especially hard on the knee. However, the fact that there are not more disabled sports heroes speaks well for the design of the knee joint. The same can be said of the ankle joint and the joints of the foot and toes.

THE SHOULDER, ELBOW, AND WRIST: The counterpart of the hip joint in the upper trunk is the shoulder joint. Free of weight-bearing responsibilities, the shoulder has a system of three interconnected joints that allow it and the arm far more versatile movements than the hip and leg.

The elbow connects the upper arm bone (*humerus*) with the two bones of the lower arm (*radius* and *ulna*). Like the knee, it is basically a

hinge joint, which allows the lower arm to be raised or lowered. The elbow is also constructed to allow some rotation by the hand; likewise, the knee joint allows us to waggle the foot.

STRUCTURE OF THE FEMUR

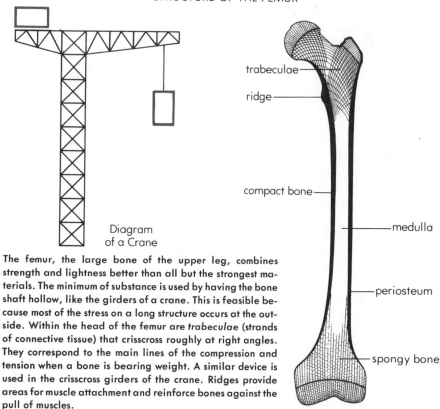

Diagram of a Crane

The femur, the large bone of the upper leg, combines strength and lightness better than all but the strongest materials. The minimum of substance is used by having the bone shaft hollow, like the girders of a crane. This is feasible because most of the stress on a long structure occurs at the outside. Within the head of the femur are *trabeculae* (strands of connective tissue) that crisscross roughly at right angles. They correspond to the main lines of the compression and tension when a bone is bearing weight. A similar device is used in the crisscross girders of the crane. Ridges provide areas for muscle attachment and reinforce bones against the pull of muscles.

These changes with age are an indication of the great amount of chemical activity going on within bone. We sometimes forget that our bones are amply supplied and penetrated by blood vessels. There is a constant building up and breaking down, an interchange of materials between blood and bone.

The Composition of Bone

A living bone does not have a single uniform composition, but instead is composed of several different kinds of tissue. To begin with, there are actually two types of bone tissue in the same bone: compact and spongy. In addition, bone is sheathed in a tough membranous tissue called the *periosteum,* interlaced with blood vessels. Finally, within most of the larger and longer bones of the body, as well as in the interior of the skull bones and vertebrae, are two more kinds of tissue: red marrow and yellow marrow.

MARROW: Within the spongy bone areas, *red marrow* produces enormous numbers of red blood cells, at a rate of millions per minute. These are needed for growth as well as for replacement of red cells, which also die in enormous numbers. Children's bones contain greater proportions of red marrow than adults'. With age, *yellow marrow,* composed mainly of fat cells, begins to fill the interior bone cavities formerly occupied by red marrow.

CALCIUM: Bone also serves as a storage and distribution center for one of the most important elements in our body. Calcium, in the form of calcium phosphate, is the basic chemical of bone tissue, but this element also must always be present in the bloodstream at a certain level to insure normal heartbeat, blood clotting, and muscle contraction. When the calcium level in the blood is deficient, the bones release some calcium into the bloodstream; when the blood has a surplus of calcium, the bones reabsorb it.

Fractures

Like most other tissues, broken bone can repair itself, and it is a remarkable process to observe. It is a process, however, that will proceed even if the ends are not aligned or set—an important reason why any suspected fracture should be checked by a doctor.

A break in a bone causes a sticky material to be deposited by the blood around the broken ends. This material begins the formation of a kind of protective, lumpy sleeve, called a *callus,* around the broken ends. Mainly cartilage, the callus hardens into spongy bone, normally within a month or two. Then, the spongy bone begins to be reduced in size by bone-dissolving cells produced in the marrow, while at the same time the spongy bone in the area of the break is beginning to be replaced by hard bone.

Depending on the particular bone involved and the severity of the fracture, the broken bone can be completely healed within four to ten months.

Potential Trouble Spots

Essentially there are two kinds of things that can go wrong with the skeletal system and cause trouble.

Mechanical Difficulties

A healthy bone's main mechanical functions—support, movement, protection—can be impaired. This can happen as a result of a physical injury resulting in a fracture or dislocation.

The stack of vertebrae called the backbone is vulnerable to a number of painful conditions from top to bottom, especially in the region of the lower back. Unfortunately, man seems to have evolved relatively quickly from a four-footed creature, and his backbone is not ideally suited for standing and walking on two feet. Back troubles become increasingly common with age.

Areas where bones interact are also very susceptible to injury because of the stresses and strains they undergo even in people who are not especially active. Normal wear and tear also takes its toll on our bones and joints; for example, the bones' structure or their alignment at a joint may be altered slightly with age, making one bone or another prone to slipping out of the joint, causing a dislocation. In any case, it is not advisable to make the same demands on our skeletal system at 40 as we did at 20. Joints are also the site of arthritis.

Disease

Second, and generally more serious if untreated, the interior bone tissues themselves may become infected and diseased. This can lead as a secondary effect to impairment of the bones' mechanical functions. *Osteomyelitis,* for example, a bacterial infection of bony tissues, can destroy large portions of bone unless antibiotics are started at once.

Fortunately, disorders of the skeletal system generally reveal themselves early and clearly by pain. Any severe or lingering pain of the joints or bones should be reported to a doctor. For example, some people may feel that aching feet are unavoidable—and a little undignified. But a foot is not meant to hurt, nor is any part of the skeletal system. Consulting a doctor could prevent much present and future misery. See also *Diseases of the Skeletal System,* p. 449

THE MUSCLES

Some 600 muscles of all sizes and shapes are attached to the framework of the skeletal system. Altogether these muscles make up nearly half of a normal adult's weight. They hold the skeleton together and, on signals originating in the brain, empower its various parts to move. Everywhere throughout the skeletal system, muscles work together with bones to protect the body's vital organs and to support and move its parts.

Skeletal Muscle

Such muscles are called, collectively, *skeletal muscle.* They are also called *voluntary muscles* because, for the most part, we can choose when we want them to act and what we want them to do—drive a car, kick a football, turn a page, jump a brook, ride a bicycle. Skeletal muscle also goes by two other names, based on its appearance under a microscope—striped and striated.

Skeletal, voluntary, striped, striated—all refer to the same general type of muscle. To avoid confusion, the term used throughout this section is skeletal muscle.

Smooth Muscle

There are two other general types of muscle. Once is called *smooth muscle* because, under the microscope, it lacks the clearly defined stripes of skeletal muscle. Smooth muscle has another name, *involuntary muscle,* so called because the brain does not voluntarily control its actions. Smooth muscle is responsible for movements such as the muscular action that moves food and waste along the digestive tract, or the contraction and dilation of the pupil of the eye, as well as countless other involuntary movements of the sense and internal organs—with the exception of the heart.

MUSCLES, THEIR LOCATIONS, AND EXERCISES THAT STRENGTHEN THEM

Muscle	Location	Movement
Trapezius	Upper back and each side of neck	Shoulder-shrugging and upward-pulling movements
Deltoids	Shoulders	Arm raising and overhead pressing
Pectorals	Chest	Horizontal pressing and drawing arms across body
Latissimus Dorsi	Wide back muscle stretching over back up to rear Deltoids	Pulling and rowing movements
Serratus	Jagged sawtooth muscles between Pectorals and lattissimus Dorsi	Pullover and Serratus leverage movements
Spinal Erectors	Lower length of spinal column	Raising upper body from a bent-over position
Biceps	Front portion of upper arm	Arm bending and twisting
Forearms	Between wrist and elbow	Reverse-grip arm bending
Triceps	Back of upper arm	Pushing and straightening movements of upper arms
Rectus Abdominals	Muscular area between sternum and pelvis	Sit-up, leg-raising, knee-in movements
Intercostals	Sides of waist, running diagonally to Serratus	Waist twisting
External Oblique Abdominals	Lower sides of waist	Waist twisting and bending
Buttocks	Muscular area covering seat	Lunging, stooping, leg raising
Leg Biceps	Back of thighs	Raising lower leg to buttocks, bending forward and stretching
Frontal Thighs	Front of thighs	Extending lower leg and knee bending
Calves	Lower leg between ankle and knee	Raising and lowering on toes

Cardiac Muscle

The third and last general type of muscle is confined to the heart area, and is called *cardiac muscle.* (Cardiac means having to do with the heart). It is involved in the rhythmic beating and contractions of the heart, which are not under conscious control, and cardiac muscle is therefore termed involuntary.

Structure of the Muscles

Each of the three kinds of muscle shares certain structural similarities with one or both of the others. All are made up of bundles of varying numbers of hair-thin fibers. In skeletal and smooth muscles, these fibers are lined up side by side in the bundle, while in cardiac muscle the fibers tend more to crisscross over one another. Skeletal muscle and cardiac muscle are both striped, that is, they show darker and lighter bands crossing over a group of adjacent fibers, while smooth muscle lacks these distinct cross-bands.

Both involuntary muscle types, smooth and cardiac, are controlled by signals carried by the autonomic nervous system. Signals that result in movements of the skeletal muscles are carried by a different nerve network, the central nervous system. The individual fibers in a muscle bundle with a particular function all react simultaneously to a signal from the nervous system; there is no apparent time lag from fiber to fiber.

How the Skeletal Muscles Work

The great range and variety of func-

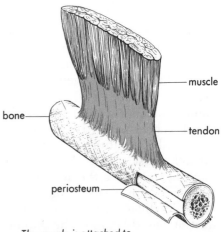

This drawing from one of the notebooks of Leonardo da Vinci (1452–1519) illustrates the anatomy of the shoulder muscles.

tions served by skeletal muscles can be suggested by naming just four: the diaphragm, used in breathing; the muscles that make the eye wink; the deltoid muscle that gives the shoulder its shape; and the tongue.

As with the bones, the body tends to make its greatest demands on muscle tissue in the area of the joints and the backbone. A smoothly functioning joint requires that bone, cartilage, and muscle all be sound and able to work together effectively.

Tendons and Ligaments

We often hear the words tendon and ligament used in the description of the knee or another joint. These are actually two types of skeletal muscles, distinguished as to their function.

A *tendon* can be described as a tight cord of muscle tissue that attaches other skeletal muscle to bone. For example, the Achilles tendon running down the back of the calf, the strongest tendon in the body, connects the muscles of the calf with the bone of the heel. A *ligament* is a somewhat more elastic band of muscle fibers that attaches bone to bone.

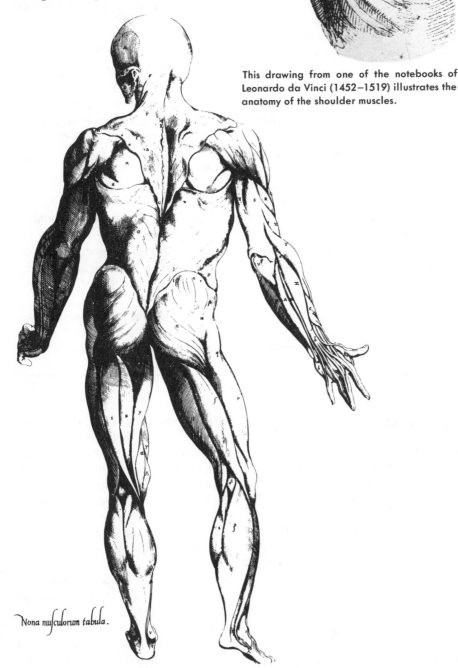

Nona musculorum tabula.

A drawing by Vesalius (1514–1564), the father of modern anatomy.

TENDON

muscle

bone

tendon

periosteum

The muscle is attached to the bone by a tendon. The fibers of the tendon interlace with the fibers of the periosteum, forming a strong bond.

HOW MUSCLES REDUCE STRESS ON BONES

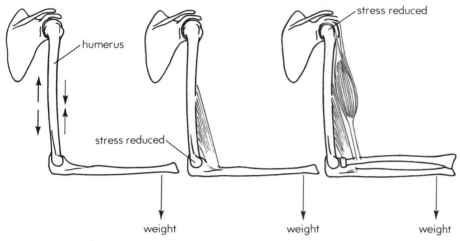

Bones are prevented from bending under normal stress by a system of braces, in which ligaments play an important role. But the main braces are the muscles. The diagrams above show the arm attached to the shoulder blade with the hand supporting a weight. Without muscles *(left)*, the weight would pull unevenly on the humerus, which would bend, thus compressing one side of the bone and stretching the other side. *(Middle)* Addition of a single-jointed muscle (as the brachialis) reduces the stress on the lower end of the humerus. *(Right)* Addition of a two-jointed muscle (as the biceps) also reduces the stress on the upper part of the humerus. There is now no shearing stress that is liable to break the bone, only a compression.

MUSCLE ACTION IN FOREARM MOVEMENT

Muscles usually work in pairs to produce movement of a part of the body.

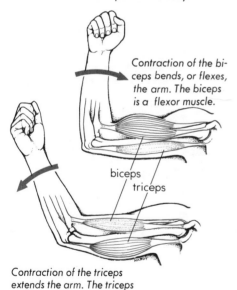

Contraction of the biceps bends, or flexes, the arm. The biceps is a flexor muscle.

biceps
triceps

Contraction of the triceps extends the arm. The triceps is an extensor muscle.

A tendon is not always evident in the connection of muscle to bone. Various groups and shapes of muscle fibers may be similarly employed, forming connective tissue without the formation of a tendon.

Various associated tissues between or around skeletal muscles serve to reduce the wear and tear of friction in areas such as a joint, where muscle, bone, and cartilage may rub against one another. For example, the tendons that pass along the back of the hand from the wrist to the fingertips, as well as many other muscle groups throughout the body, are enclosed in lubricated sheaths. The muscle-sheathed *bursas,* lined inside with lubricating fluid, are also found in areas subject to friction, such as where a tendon passes closely over a bone.

Man's upright posture and two-legged locomotion subject the backbone to heavy stresses. It is buttressed, however, with scores of tightly packed bundles of muscle attached to either side of the spinal column.

Flexors and Extensors

Most of us probably first used the word "muscle" when, as children, we watched an older child or adult flex an arm and proudly display the bump of muscle between the crook of elbow and shoulder. This biceps muscle works together with the triceps muscle on the underside of the arm. The arm is bent at the elbow by contraction of the biceps, which makes this muscle get shorter and thicker; in this position, called *flexion,* the triceps muscle is relaxed. To return the arm to its normal straight position, called *extension,* the biceps relaxes and the triceps contracts. In this bit of muscle teamwork, the biceps, which bends the arm at the elbow joint, is called the *flexor,* while the triceps straightens the arm and is called the *extensor.* Similar flexor-extensor action can be observed at many body joints, including the fingers.

Smooth Muscle

Beginning about midway down the esophagus, layers of smooth muscle line the walls of the 25 feet of digestive tract, extending into the stomach and through the intestines. These muscles keep the stomach and intestinal walls continually in motion, constricting and relaxing to push food along. Smooth muscle also effects the opening and closing of important valves, called *sphincters,* along the digestive tract.

Trouble Spots

The functions and failures of the skeletal muscles are closely allied to those of the skeletal system. The same areas are vulnerable—joints and back—and the same rule holds: severe or persistent muscle pain is a cause to consult your doctor.

HERNIA: One type of disorder associated exclusively with a weakness or abnormality of muscle is a rupture or *hernia.* This is the protrusion of part of another organ through a gap in the protective muscle. A likely area for a hernia to appear is in the muscles lining the abdomen, although hernias may occur in any other part of the body where there is pressure against a muscle wall that is not as strong as it should be. Weight control and a sensible program of exercise—abdominal muscles being particularly liable to slackness—are good preventive measures against hernia.

All our muscles, in fact, benefit from regular exercise; but you don't have to exhaust yourself physically every day in order to reach and maintain the desirable plateau doctors describe as good muscle tone.

ATROPHY OF MUSCLE TISSUE: Muscle tissues are likely to *atrophy* (shrink and weaken) if they are not used for too long a time. Thus, illness or injuries that cause paralysis or an extended period of immobility for the body or a part of it must be followed by a medically supervised program of physical therapy to rebuild the weakened muscles. See also *Diseases of the Muscles and Nervous System*, p. 468

SKIN, HAIR, AND NAILS

Perhaps no other organ of the human body receives so much attention both from its owner and the eyes of others as the skin and its associated structures—hair and nails.

Vanity is hardly the issue. The simple facts are that skin is the last frontier of our internal selves, the final boundary between our inside and outside, and our principal first line of defense against the dangers of the outside world. It shows, not always clearly, evidence of some internal disorders; and it shows, often quite clearly, the evidence of external affronts—a bump, a cut, a chafe, an insect bite, or an angry reaction to the attack of germs.

In personal encounters, the unclothed portion of our skin is one of the first things other people observe, and—if we happen to have some unsightly scratch, rash, or blemish—the last thing by which we wish to be remembered. Of all our organs, the skin is the most likely candidate for a program of self-improvement.

The Organ Called Skin

It is always a little surprising to hear, for the first time, the skin referred to as a single organ. This is not to say it is a simple organ; on the contrary, it is an exceedingly complex and varied one. However, despite variations in appearance from part to part of the body, our entire outer wrapper (the more technical word is *integument*) is similarly constructed.

One might object: "But my nails and hair certainly look different from the skin on my nose!" This is perfectly true, but nails and hair are extensions of the skin, and wherever they occur are composed of similar tissues: the nail on a little toe is made of the same material as the hair.

Functions of the Skin

The skin has three main functions, and its different outward appearance on different parts of the body reflects to some extent which of these functions a certain area of skin primarily serves. The three main functions are protection (from germs or blows), temperature control (e.g., through perspiration, to aid in keeping the body's internal organs near our normal internal temperature of 98.6° F.), and perception. Nerve endings in the skin give us our sensations of touch, pain, heat, and cold. Associated with the skin's important role in temperature regulation is its function as an organ of excretion—the elimination, via perspiration, and subsequent evaporation of water and other substances. Skin is also the site of the body's natural production of vitamin D, stimulated by exposure to sunlight.

ANATOMY OF THE SKIN

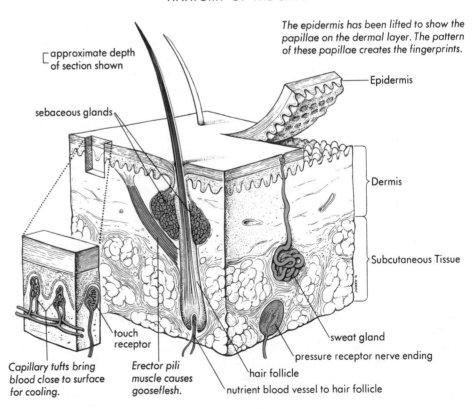

The epidermis has been lifted to show the papillae on the dermal layer. The pattern of these papillae creates the fingerprints.

approximate depth of section shown

sebaceous glands

Epidermis

Dermis

Subcutaneous Tissue

sweat gland

pressure receptor nerve ending

hair follicle

nutrient blood vessel to hair follicle

touch receptor

Capillary tufts bring blood close to surface for cooling.

Erector pili muscle causes gooseflesh.

Anatomy of the Skin

Skin has three more or less distinct layers. The outermost is called the *epidermis;* the middle, the *dermis;* and the innermost, *subcutaneous* (underskin) tissue. The epidermis may also be called *cuticle;* and the dermis either *corium* or *true skin.*

THE SUBCUTANEOUS LAYER: The subcutaneous layer is really a rather vague border zone between muscle and bone tissues on one side, and the dermis on the other, a kind of springy, fatty padding that gives bounce and a look of firmness to the skin above it. With age, the fatty cells of the subcutaneous layer are not continually replaced as they die, and this layer tends to thin out. The result is wrinkles, which form where the outer layers of skin lose their subcutaneous support, much like the slipcover of a cushion that has lost some of its stuffing.

THE DERMIS: The dermis is serviced by the multitude of tiny blood vessels and nerve fibers that reach it through the subcutaneous tissue. In addition, many special structures and tissues that enable the skin to perform its various functions are found in the dermis: *sebaceous* (skin oil) glands and sweat glands; minuscule muscles; and the roots of hairs encased in narrow pits called *follicles.*

The topmost layer of the dermis, interconnecting with the epidermis above it, resembles, under a microscope, nothing so much as a rugged, ridge-crossed landscape carved with valleys, caves, and tunnels. The basic forms of this microscopic terrain are cone-shaped hills called *papillae;* between 100 and 200 million of them are found in the dermis of an adult human being.

Since the dermal papillae serve as the bedrock for the surface layer of skin, the epidermis, we can understand why there is really no such thing as smooth skin; even the smoothest patch of a baby's skin appears ridged and cratered under a magnifying glass.

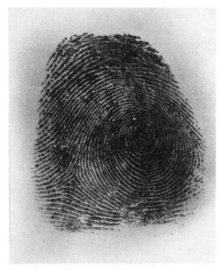

The pattern of ridges in a fingerprint reflects the contours of the papillae (conelike bumps) of the upper layer of the dermis, just below the epidermis.

The distribution of papillae in the skin falls into certain distinctive patterns which are particularly conspicuous on the soles of babies' feet and on the fingertips, and give each of us our unique finger, toe, and foot prints. The mathematical possibility of one person having the same fingerprints as another is thought to be about one in 25 billion. The papillae ridges on the fingertips also make it easier for us to pick up and handle such things as needles or pencils or buttons.

Finally, because there are relatively more papillae concentrated at the fingertips than on most other areas of the body, and because papillae are often associated with dense concentrations of nerve endings, the fingertips tend to be more responsive to touch sensations than other parts of the body.

THE EPIDERMIS: The bottom layer of the epidermis, its papillae fitted into the pockets of the layers of the dermis beneath it, is occupied by new young cells. These cells gradually mature and move upward. As they near the surface of the skin, they die, becoming tough, horny, lifeless tissue. This is the outmost layer of the epidermis, called the *stratum corneum* (horny layer), which we are continually shedding, usually unnoticed, as when we towel off after a bath, but sometimes very noticeably, as when we peel after a sunburn.

A suntan, incidentally, is caused by the presence of tiny grains of pigment, called *melanin,* in the bottom layers of epidermis. Sunlight stimulates the production of melanin, giving the skin a darker color. A suntan fades as the melanin

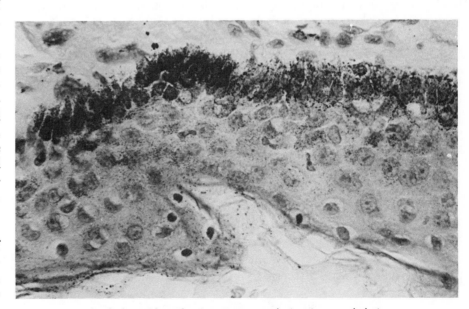

A dark epidermal pigment, or melanin, is revealed in a photomicrograph of the skin, magnified 500 times. Skin color is largely determined by the amount of melanin produced by the skin.

granules move to the surface and are shed with dead skin cells.

Hair and Nails

Certainly the most noticeable of the specialized forms of skin are our hair and nails. What we see of them is really a dead tissue, called *keratin*, similar to the dead skin cells that are continually being shed by our bodies, but much more firmly packed together. However, hair and nails both originate in cells that are very much alive—as anyone who has plucked a group of hairs or suffered the pain of a torn-out nail knows very well. Growth occurs in this living region, with new cells pushing the dead, hard hair and nail stalks upward, then dying themselves and being replaced from below.

The bottom end or root of a hair is lodged, as noted above, in a *follicle,* a hollow resembling a rounded bottle with a long, narrow neck slanting toward the skin's surface. Each follicle is supported by the little hummock of a papilla, and is serviced by tiny oil glands that lubricate the shaft (or neck) through which the hair pushes toward the surface.

The follicles of the long hairs of the scalp, groin, and armpits may be found deep in the subcutaneous layers of the skin; others are no deeper than the top layers of dermis. Attached to a follicle are microscopic muscle fibers that, if stimulated by cold or emotional factors, can contract around the follicle; the result is goose flesh or sometimes even the sensation that our hair is standing on end.

A nail's living, growing part is found beneath the whitish half moon, or *lunula,* at its base. The lunula is sometimes obscured because a layer of epidermis (cuticle) has grown over it. Except at its very top (the part we can trim without pain), the nail is firmly attached to the ridged upper layer of the dermis, a region richly laced with tiny blood vessels.

Oil Glands

The skin's oil-producing (or *sebaceous*) glands are almost always associated with hair follicles, into which they seep their oils (or *sebum*). The oily substance works its way up toward the surface, lubricating both the hair and outer layers of epidermis, which need continual lubrication in order to stay soft and flexible. Also, skin oils serve as a kind of protective coat against painful drying and chapping.

Sweat Glands and Blood Vessels

While everybody is aware that the amount we perspire is related to the temperature around us, not everybody is aware that the countless tiny blood vessels in our skin—some 15 feet of them coursing beneath every square inch of skin—also react to changes in outside temperatures. Working together, and both controlled by an automatic "thermostat" in our brain, sweat glands and blood vessels have the all-important role of keeping our internal organs near their normal 98.6° Fahrenheit temperature.

The trick in maintaining an internal body temperature near normal is to conserve body heat when it is colder outside and to lose heat when it is warmer. Blood circulating near the surface of the skin is warmed (gains heat) or cooled (loses heat) according to the outside temperature.

The skin's myriad blood vessels constrict when the outside temperature is colder. This means that less blood can come into contact with the colder outside air, and therefore the overall temperature level of the blood remains warmer than if the blood vessels had not become constricted. On the other hand, when the body needs to lose heat—for example, during and after a vigorous tennis match—the skin's blood vessels dilate. This accounts for the "heat flush" or reddening of skin that light-skinned people exhibit when very heated.

Sweat glands aid in temperature regulation by secreting moisture, which, evaporating on the skin's surface, cools the skin and therefore the blood flowing beneath it. Moisture that does not evaporate but remains as liquid on the skin or runs off in rivulets is not efficient in cooling. Humid air tends to prevent evaporation, while moving air or wind aids it. Sweat that evaporates as soon as it reaches the skin's surface usually goes unnoticed. Fresh sweat has no odor; but if it remains without evaporating, bacteria begin to give it the odor known medically as *bromidrosis*.

There are some two million sweat glands in the skin. Each consists of a coiled, corkscrewlike tube that tunnels its way up to the surface of the skin from the dermis or from the deeper subcutaneous layer.

Potential Trouble Spots

All of us are very conscious of the condition of our skin and worry when something seems to be wrong with it. The temptations to worry too much, to overtreat, to take the advice of a well-meaning friend, to use the wrong (but heavily advertised) product are very great. Knowing about the properties of the skin and what medical knowledge has to say about skin problems can help to avoid mistakes in caring for it. See *Skin and Hair*, p. 236. For a discussion of adolescent skin problems. See also under *Puberty and Growth*, p. 109.

their tasks, and quite open to improvement.

Advances in heart surgery do, indeed, hold great promise for persons whose hearts had been considered, until now, irreversibly damaged or diseased. But the great attention accorded such miracles of medicine tends to obscure the humdrum, day-in-day-out, low-key drama performed for a lifetime by a healthy, uncomplaining heart.

The Heart and Circulatory Network

Perhaps the best way to put the heart in perspective is to place it where it belongs, at the hub of the body's circulatory system. This hollow, fist-sized lump of sinewy tissue is located behind the breastbone, centered just about at the vertical mid-line of our chest. It is connected into a closed system of flexible tubes, called blood vessels, ranging down from finger-thick to microscopically slender, that reach into every cavern, crevice, and outpost of our body—a network of some 70,000 miles.

The heart has essentially one function—to push blood, by pumping action, through this enormous network of blood vessels. We have about six quarts of blood in our body, pumped at the rate of about five ounces every time the heart beats (normally about 72 times a minute for an adult), which we feel as our pulse. The blood circulates and recirculates through the blood vessels, pushed along by the pumping of the heart.

ARTERIES AND VEINS: The blood vessels are generally described as *arterial*, referring to the *arteries* that carry blood away from the heart; or *venous*, referring to the *veins* through which blood seeps and flows back toward the heart to be repumped. A large artery such as the *aorta* branches into smaller arteries, and these eventually into still smaller vessels called *arterioles*, and the arterioles, finally, into the smallest blood vessels, the *capil-*

laries. These in turn open onto other capillaries, which are the starting point for the return of blood to the heart.

The microscopic capillaries typically form a kind of cat's cradle connection, sometimes called a capillary bed, at the transition zone where arterial blood becomes venous blood. The returning blood moves from the capillaries to small veins called *venules* (the counterparts of arterioles) and through successively larger veins back to the heart.

Blood and Our Internal Fluid Environment

What makes this fairly rudimentary collection of plumbing so absolutely indispensable to life is the fluid it pumps—blood. If any part of the body—cell, tissue, or major organ—is denied circulating blood and the substances it carries with it for longer than a few minutes, that part will fail. It is the job of the heart and the blood vessels to get blood to all the body's far-flung tissues, where it both picks up and deposits substances.

Blood is really a kind of fluid tissue. About 80 percent of its volume is water, and blood's indispensable, life-sustaining power is owed in great part to its watery base, which permits it both to flow and to take up and carry materials in solution. All our tissues and organs have a kind of give-and-take arrangement with the circulating blood.

CARRIER OF OXYGEN: Perhaps the most critical of these give-and-take transactions occurs in the lungs; it is this transaction that if interrupted by heartbeat stoppage for more than a very few minutes causes death by oxygen starvation of vital tissues. Before a unit of blood is pumped out by the heart to the body, it picks up in the lungs the oxygen that we have inhaled and which every cell in the body needs to function. The blood then transports the oxygen, delivering it to other parts of the body. By the time a given unit of blood has made a tour of the blood vessels and

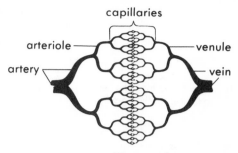

Diagram of
Artery-Capillary-Vein Sequence

returned to the lungs, it has given up most of its oxygen and is laden instead with carbon dioxide, the principal waste product of living processes. The venous blood releases its carbon dioxide, to be exhaled by the lungs.

DISTRIBUTOR OF NUTRIENTS: Food, or more accurately the nutrient molecules needed by cells, are also transported throughout the body by the blood. In the digestive tract, food is broken down into tiny submicroscopic pieces that can pass through the tract's walls (mainly along the small intestine) and be

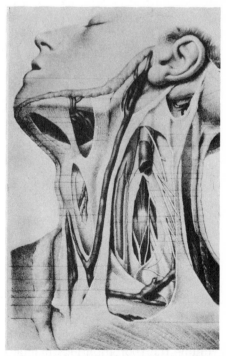

In this anatomical drawing of the major blood vessels of the neck, the long vessel running in front of the ear is the carotid artery. The large vessel in cross-section directly below the ear is the jugular vein.

THE CIRCULATORY SYSTEM

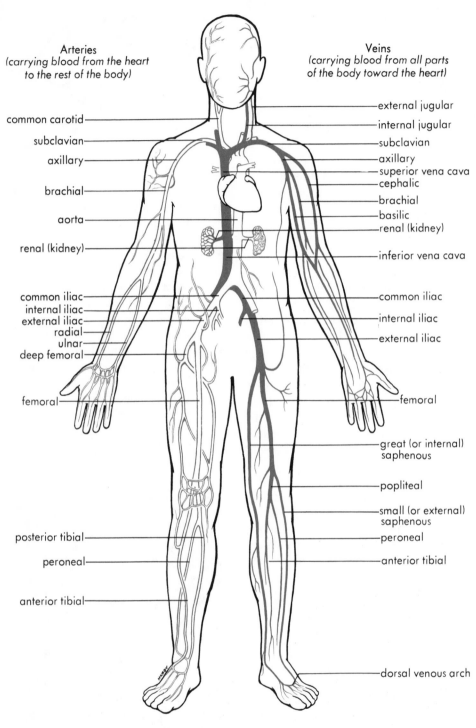

Arteries
(carrying blood from the heart to the rest of the body)

common carotid
subclavian
axillary
brachial
aorta
renal (kidney)
common iliac
internal iliac
external iliac
radial
ulnar
deep femoral
femoral
posterior tibial
peroneal
anterior tibial

Veins
(carrying blood from all parts of the body toward the heart)

external jugular
internal jugular
subclavian
axillary
superior vena cava
cephalic
brachial
basilic
renal (kidney)
inferior vena cava
common iliac
internal iliac
external iliac
femoral
great (or internal) saphenous
popliteal
small (or external) saphenous
peroneal
anterior tibial
dorsal venous arch

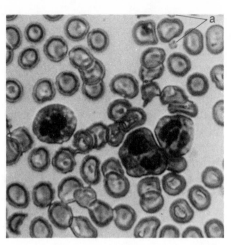

In this normal blood smear, red corpuscles, which are concave on both sides, look like doughnuts. The larger, darker shapes near the center are white blood cells; the smaller shapes (marked with an <u>a</u>) are platelets.

picked up by the blood for distribution around the body.

One of the specialized, small-volume transportation jobs handled by the blood is to pick up hormones from the endocrine glands and present these chemical messengers to the organs they affect.

Composition of Blood

Blood is a distinctive and recognizable type of tissue, but this does not mean it is a stable, uniform substance with a fixed proportion of ingredients. Quite the opposite is true: its composition is ever chang-

ing in response to the demands of other body systems. Other organs are constantly pouring substances into the blood, or removing things from it. Blood in one part of the body at a given moment may be vastly different in chemical make-up from blood in another part of the body.

Despite its changing make-up, blood does have certain basic components. A sample of blood left to stand for an hour or so separates into a clear, watery fluid with a yellowish tinge and a darker, more solid clump. The clear yellow liquid is called *plasma*, and accounts for about 55 percent of the volume of normal blood. The darker clump is made up mainly of the blood's most conspicuous and populous inhabitants, the red cells that give blood its color.

PLASMA: It is the plasma that enables our blood to carry out most of the transportation tasks assigned it. Being over 90 percent water, the plasma has water's property of being able to carry substances both in solution and in suspension. (A substance in solution is one, like salt, that must be removed from water by chemical or physical action, such as boiling; while a substance in suspension—such as red blood cells within whole blood in a standing test tube—separates out more readily, particularly when its watery carrier has been contained and its flow stilled.)

RED BLOOD CELLS: Red blood cells (or *erythrocytes*) numbering in the trillions are carried in suspension by the plasma. In turn, the red blood cells carry the single most important substance needed by the body's cells—oxygen. For such an important task, the red blood cell looks hardly adequate. As it matures, this cell loses its nucleus. Lacking a nucleus, it is sometimes not even called a cell but a red blood *corpuscle*. What gives red blood cells their special oxygen-carrying ability, and also their color, is their possession of a complex iron-protein substance called *hemoglobin*.

HEMOGLOBIN: Molecules of hemoglobin have the property of loosely combining with oxygen where it is plentiful, as in the lungs. They can then hold on to oxygen until they reach an area where oxygen has been depleted by the demands of

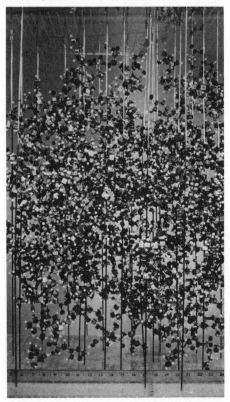

This three-dimensional model of the hemoglobin molecule of the blood is about 127,000,000 times its actual size.

living processes. There—usually in the fine tubes of the capillaries—hemoglobin's hold on oxygen is challenged by the demands of other cells, and the red cells give up their oxygen. The hemoglobin of red cells develops an immediate affinity for carbon dioxide, the waste product of cell metabolism, and the red blood cells then carry this carbon dioxide back to the lungs for exhalation.

Hemoglobin's ability to carry oxygen is not unique. Water, and therefore plasma, also have this ability. Hemoglobin's specialness lies in how much oxygen it can carry. Hemoglobin increases by more than 50 times the oxygen-carrying capacity of our blood.

WHITE BLOOD CELLS: White blood cells have many different shapes and sizes, all going under the general scientific name of *leukocytes*. They are typically larger than red blood cells, but far less numerous. If we accept an estimate of 25 trillion as the number of living red blood cells in our body, then the number of white blood cells might be generously estimated at around 40 billion, a ratio of one white cell to about 600–700 reds.

According to their shape, size, and other characteristics, white blood cells have been divided into various categories such as lymphocytes, monocytes, and granulocytes. But as a group these blood cells are distinguished by their common propensity for attacking foreign bodies that invade our tissues, whether these invaders be sizable splinters or microscopic bacteria. White blood cells move in force to the site of an infection, do battle with the intruding agents, and frequently strew the area with the wreckage of the encounter—a collection of dismantled alien bacteria and dead white cells which we know as pus.

PLATELETS: *Platelets*, also called *thrombocytes*, initiate some of the first steps in the complex biochemical process that leads to the clotting of blood. They thus help to spare us from bleeding to death from a slight

injury. Platelets are the most rudimentary and diminutive of the major blood components. Like mature red blood cells, they lack nuclei, but are only one-quarter as big. By no stretch of the imagination can they be called blood cells. Rather, they are blood elements—bits of cell substance with a recognizable size and shape, circulating with the blood.

THE PROPORTIONS OF BLOOD CELLS: All the several types of blood cells and subcells in a healthy body occur in proportions that, though never precisely fixed and unchanging, are recognized as having normal upper and lower limits. If a particular type of cell shows a sudden increase or decrease in population, so that its proportion relative to other blood cells shows a variation markedly outside its normal range, some infection, disease, or disorder must be suspected.

In adition to occurring in certain normal-range proportions, each type of cellular blood component has a typical shape, appearance, and set of chemical and physical properties. Variations from these norms occur in many diseases.

The analysis of blood samples (usually taken from the finger or arm) and their inspection under a microscope have proved invaluable in diagnosing illness and disease, often before a person feels any symptoms whatsoever. This is why a thorough medical check-up should always include taking a sample of your blood. It is then up to the doctor to decide which of the dozens of tests should be made on your blood in the medical laboratory. One common test is a *blood count*, in which the number of a certain type of cell in a given unit of your blood can be estimated, and then compared to the normal number in the same amount of blood.

BLOOD GROUPS AND RH FACTORS: The identification of *blood groups* and *Rh factors* is another aspect of blood analysis. The four most common blood groups are called A, B, AB, and O, classifications based on

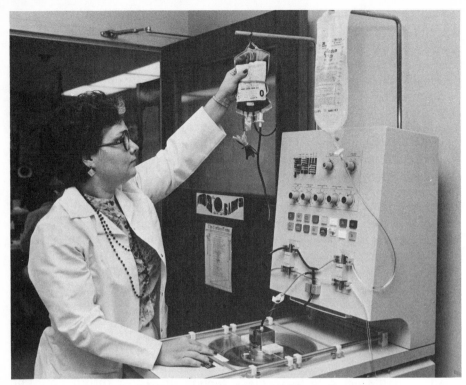

A blood cell processor washes frozen red blood cells, removing glycerol. The glycerol is added to red blood cells to aid freezing for storage but must be removed before the blood is used.

in your body will have died and been replaced with new cells.

THE LIVER AS A PRODUCER OF RED BLOOD CELLS: The red bone marrow is backed up by several other tissues that can, if called upon, turn out blood cells in quantity or serve as specialized producers of certain blood cells and blood elements. One such organ is the liver, which, before and after birth and into childhood, is a site of red blood cell production. In an emergency, such as severe internal hemorrhage, the liver sometimes reverts to its earlier function of manufacturing red cells. The liver also serves as a kind of salvage yard for the iron from dead red cells. It stores the iron for later combination into hemoglobin, and passes off the rest of the red blood cell fragments as part of the bile pigments that empty into the duodenum of the small intestine.

THE SPLEEN AS A PRODUCER OF BLOOD CELLS: Certain white blood cells, in particular the lymphocytes, are produced at a variety of locations in the body—for example, by the lymph nodes, by little clumps of tissue called *Peyer's patches* in the intestinal tract, and by the spleen.

The spleen plays a number of interesting secondary roles in blood cell production. Like the liver, it can be pressed into service as a manufacturer of red blood cells and serve as a salvage yard for iron reclaimed from worn-out red blood cells. A newborn baby is almost totally dependent on its spleen for the production of red blood cells, with a little help from the liver. In an adult, however, a damaged or diseased spleen can be surgically removed, with little or no apparent effect on the health or life span of the person, provided the patient's bone marrow is in good functioning order.

MOVEMENT OF BLOOD CELLS THROUGH THE CAPILLARIES: A blood cell must be able to slip through the microscopic, twisting and turning tunnels of the capillaries that mark the turn-about point in the blood cell's round-trip voyage from the

chemical differences that may be incompatible if one group is mixed with another. Thus, it is absolutely essential before a person receives a blood transfusion to know both his own blood type and the type of the blood he is to be given. Blood group O is considered the safest for transfusion, and people with type O blood are sometimes called "universal donors." It is a wise practice to carry, along with your other important cards, a card giving your own blood type. The blood of a donor, however, is always *cross-matched* (checked for compatibility) with the blood of the person who is to receive it in order to avoid transfusion reactions.

Blood Cell Manufacture and Turnover

Most types of blood cells, both red and white, are manufactured in the red marrow of bones. The rate and quantity of total production is staggering; estimates range from one to five million red blood cells per second. This prodigious output is necessary because blood cells are disintegrating, having served their useful lives, in the same enormous numbers every second. The normal life span of a red blood cell is about four months, which means that four months from now every blood cell

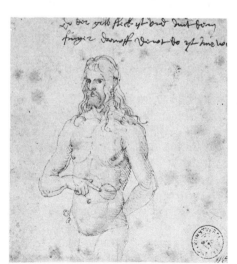

Making practical use of his anatomical studies, the German artist Albrecht Dürer drew a sketch of himself pointing to his spleen and sent the sketch to his doctor to show where his pain was.

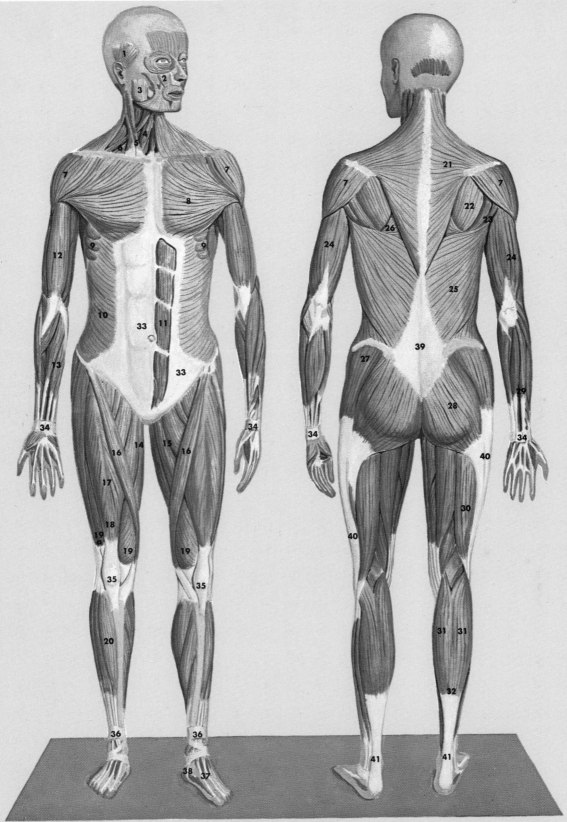

MUSCLES AND TENDONS

MUSCLES
1. Temporal
2. Mimetic muscles
3. Masseter (a muscle of mastication)
4. Infrahyoid muscles
5. Sternomastoid
6. Omohyoid
7. Deltoid
8. Pectoral muscles
9. Serratus anterior
10. External oblique
11. Rectus abdominus
12. Biceps brachii
13. Flexor digitorum superficialis (sublimis)
14. Gracilis

15. Adductor group
16. Sartorius
17. Rectus femoris
18. Quadriceps femoris
19. Vastus medialis
19a. Vastus lateralis
20. Dorsiflexors
21. Trapezius
22. Infraspinatus
23. Teres major
24. Triceps brachii
25. Latissimus dorsi
26. Rhomboideus major
27. Gluteus medius
28. Gluteus maximus

29. Digital extensors
30. Hamstring muscles
31. Gastrocnemius
32. Plantar flexors
TENDONS
33. Rectus sheath
34. Flexor retinaculum of carpal tunnel
35. Patellar tendon
36. Retinaculum of tarsal tunnel
37. Tendons of long digital extensors
38. Tendon of tibialis anterior
39. Lumbodorsal fascia
40. Fascia lata
41. Achilles   © C. S. HAMMOND & Co., N.Y.

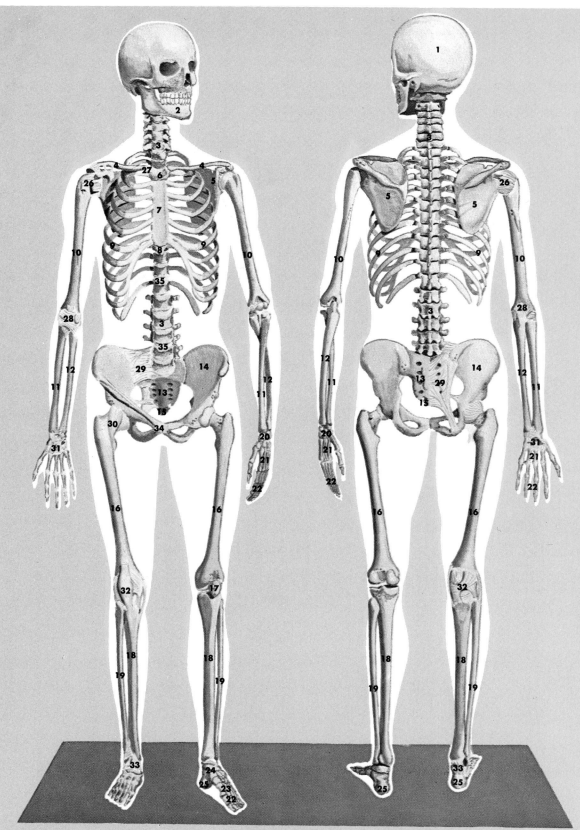

BONES AND LIGAMENTS

BONES
1. Skull
2. Mandible
3. Vertebrae
4. Clavicle
5. Scapula
6. Manubrium
7. Body of sternum
8. Xiphoid process
9. Ribs
10. Humerus
11. Radius
12. Ulna

13. Sacrum
14. Ilium
15. Coccyx
16. Femur
17. Patella
18. Tibia
19. Fibula
20. Carpals
21. Metacarpals
22. Phalanges
23. Metatarsals
24. Tarsals
25. Heel

LIGAMENTS AND JOINTS
26. Capsule of shoulder
27. Sternoclavicular
28. Capsule of elbow
29. Sacroiliac
30. Iliofemoral
31. Wrist
32. Capsule of knee
33. Ankle
34. Pubic symphysis
35. Intervertebral discs

© C. S. HAMMOND & Co., N. Y.

Synapse, Ganglion, and Plexus

When a nerve impulse, traveling away from the neuron's central part, reaches the ends of an axon, it meets a gap which it must jump to get to the tentaclelike dendrites of the next neuron. This gap is called a *synapse.*

At certain points in the body a great many nerve cell bodies and branches are packed closely together, with a resulting profusion of interwoven axons, dendrites, and synapses. Such a concentration of nervous tissue is called a *ganglion,* or *plexus.* A blow or jolt to such an area can be extremely painful and even stupefying—affecting as it does a whole network of nerves—as anyone who has been hit in the solar plexus or learned the pressure points of karate knows.

The Movement of Impulses Along Nerve Fibers

There is really no exact counterpart in the mechanical world for how an impulse moves along a nerve fiber and then jumps across a synapse to the next nerve. Nor is this movement completely understood by scientists. Suffice it to say that it is somewhat like an electrical current moving along in a chemical environment that allows the impulse to travel, in discreet little jumps, at a speed of about 200 miles per hour—quite slowly when we compare it to the speed of light or electricity: 186,000 miles per second. This speed serves us quite well in most situations, but there are times when we wish human beings' nerves could act more quickly—on the highway, for example, or when a cherished vase starts to topple off the mantelpiece.

One of the simplest and quickest kinds of reactions to an outside stimulus is one that bypasses the brain. We don't really think to pull our hand away from a piping hot radiator. This is called a *spinal reflex.* What happens is that the sensory nerve endings in the finger pick up the "too hot" impulse from the radiator; the impulse then travels to the spinal cord where it activates the motor nerve pathway back to the burned finger, carrying the message, "Jerk your finger away!"

When to Suspect Trouble

Our entire existence as human beings depends so much on the normal functioning of our brain and nervous system that any real brain or nervous disorder or disease is a very serious matter. A sprained joint or cut foot can spell doom for an animal that depends on speed and mobility for survival; but the same injury is often not much more than a painful inconvenience to us. Impairment of our brain or nervous system is far more of a threat to our survival.

Multiple sclerosis and meningitis have been mentioned as serious disorders affecting the nerves, others are Parkinsonism, shingles, encephalitis, and brain tumors. The possible presence of one of these disorders is reason enough not to shrug off any of the following signs and symptoms: recurrent headaches, intense pain of unknown cause, tremors, numbness, loss of coordination, dizziness, blackouts, tics, cramps, visual difficulties, and loss of bowel and bladder control. Also, any person who has remained unconscious for more than a few minutes should be taken to a doctor as soon as possible. This applies even when the person has regained consciousness and says he feels fine.

Our complex emotions, of course, are linked to the functioning of our brain and nervous system. A mind free of undue anxiety, guilt, and frustration functions better than a mind racked with worries and conflicts, and is a much more efficient and reliable leader of the body. See also *Diseases of the Muscles and Nervous System,* p. 468. For a discussion of mental and emotional health, see Ch. 30, p. 529.

THE CIRCULATORY SYSTEM, THE HEART, AND BLOOD

When the heart stops beating—that is to say, stops pumping blood—for longer than a couple of minutes, we stop living. But the heart, fortunately, is extremely sturdy. It is also simple in construction, capable of operating at a great many different speeds, in many cases self-repairing if damaged, and probably the one continuously operating automatic pump that we could, with any confidence, expect to last 60 or 70 years or longer.

These simple facts tend to be forgotten today, in what is probably the most heart-conscious era in history. True, heart disease, along with cancer, is statistically one of today's major killers. But we should remember two circumstances: not until about 50 years ago did deaths from heart disease begin to be accurately recognized and reported; second, with longer and longer life spans, it becomes more likely that a nonstop vital organ like the heart will simply wear out. Heart transplants, open heart surgery, and artificial heart parts—often reported sensationally in the public media—have also conditioned us to think of our hearts as terribly vulnerable, rather delicate, a bit inadequate to

Spinal nerves branch out from the spinal cord as it snakes its way through the vertebrae of the spinal column. All the major nerve cords that wrap around the trunk and reach the arms and hands, legs and feet, originate from spinal nerves.

The cranial nerves and the spinal nerves, together with all those nerves lying outside the confines of the brain and spinal cord, are sometimes referred to as the *peripheral nervous system*. This term can be confusing, however, because it is also used to include all the nerves of the autonomic nervous system, next discussed.

The Autonomic Nervous System

The muscles served by the central nervous system are all of one general type (striated), while the muscles served by the autonomic system are called involuntary or smooth. The autonomic nerves regulate body activity without our conscious control—for example, as we sleep. They are rather elegantly divided into two categories: *sympathetic* and *parasympathetic* nervous systems. These are distinguishable primarily by their opposite effects on the body organs. For example, impulses along parasympathetic nerve trunks dilate blood vessels, slow the heartbeat rate, and increase stomach secretions, while the sympathetic system constricts blood vessels, increases rate of heartbeat, and inhibits stomach secretions.

The Neuron— What Nerves Are Made Of

A nerve cell is a grayish blob of tissue from which protrude several short gray fibers, *dendrites,* and one longer whitish fiber, an *axon.* Both the dendrites and the axon resemble ropes with their ends splayed and frayed. Dendrites register impulses coming into the central blob of the neuron (perhaps from a neighboring neuron's axon); an axon picks up the incoming impulses and carries them away.

Both units are equally important for normal nerve functioning, but the axon is far more showy as an anatomical structure. All nerve cords are made up of the single strands of many axons, which may reach lengths of several feet. In other words, if we could stretch out certain neurons in our body—for example, those making up the sciatic nerve that runs from the small of the back to the toes—their axon "tails" would make them three or four feet long.

MYELIN: A normal axon usually has a fatty coating of insulation called *myelin.* An axon severed into two pieces cannot grow together again; but if the myelin sheath is pretty much intact, a surgeon can sometimes restore nerve function by sewing the two ends together, or replace the nerve with one from another part of the body. The part of the severed axon connecting to the central portion usually remains alive in any case—which is why a person can often still retain the sensation of feeling in an amputated part.

Certain serious and progressively disabling diseases involve the gradual loss (*demyelination*) of this coating, causing paralysis, numbness, or other loss of function in an organ; a demyelinated nerve fiber is not able to carry impulses to and from the brain. Two such diseases are multiple sclerosis and "Lou Gehrig's disease" (amyotrophic lateral sclerosis).

EFFECTS OF AGING: Once we reach maturity, the number of our nerve cells begins to decrease, because our bodies cannot manufacture new neurons to replace the ones that die in the normal process of living. (Other kinds of tissue are continually replenished with new cells.) This has some relation to senility, but the loss of a few million out of many billions of brain and nerve cells has little effect on mental powers unless the losses are concentrated in one area.

THE NEURON

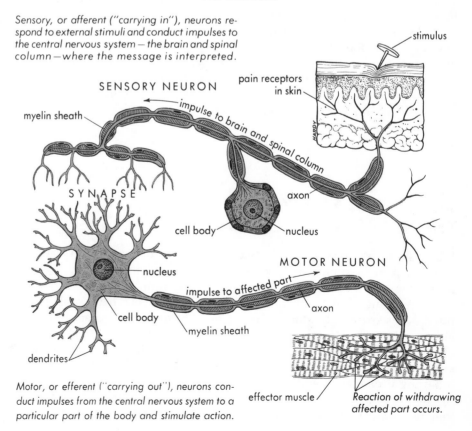

Sensory, or afferent ("carrying in"), neurons respond to external stimuli and conduct impulses to the central nervous system — the brain and spinal column — where the message is interpreted.

SENSORY NEURON

stimulus

pain receptors in skin

myelin sheath

impulse to brain and spinal column

axon

SYNAPSE

cell body

nucleus

nucleus

MOTOR NEURON

impulse to affected part

axon

cell body

myelin sheath

dendrites

effector muscle

Reaction of withdrawing affected part occurs.

Motor, or efferent ("carrying out"), neurons conduct impulses from the central nervous system to a particular part of the body and stimulate action.

THE NERVOUS SYSTEM AND THE BRAIN

Most of us have heard often enough that the brain, acting as control center for a communication network we call our nervous system, is an incredible computer, weighing a mere three pounds. Its form and functions, however, are often described as being so much more intricate and complex than any existing or imagined computer that thorough knowledge of the brain seems very remote. This is certainly true. But it doesn't prevent us from knowing some general things about the brain and nervous system, or what its most significant parts are and how they work.

Basically, the nervous system has just two functions: first, getting information (impulses, signals, messages) from outside or inside the body to where it can be acted upon, usually in the brain; and secondly, feeding back information (for example, to the muscles) so that the indicated action can be taken. Thus, nerves can be divided by their function into two general types, each following a separate pathway: those that receive information—for example, from our senses—and pass it along, are called *sensory*, or *afferent* (inward-traveling). Those that relay information back, with a directive for action, are called *motor*, or *efferent* (outward-traveling).

The brain and the spinal cord can be considered as the basic unit of the *central nervous system*. All sensory and motor information comes or goes from this central core. The spinal cord is the master nerve tract (or nerve trunk) in our body and consists of millions of nerve fibers bundled together, somewhat like many small threads making up a large rope.

Like the spinal cord, all the lesser nerves, shown as single cords in a typical anatomical drawing, are made up of hundreds of thousands of individual fibers. Each fiber is part of a single nerve cell, or *neuron*. Neurons—there are 12 to 15 billion of them in our brain alone—are the basic structural units of the brain and nervous system, the tubes and transistors and circuits of which our personal computer is built.

The Brain

The appearance of the brain within the skull has been described as a huge gray walnut and a cauliflower. The inelegance of such descriptions is the least of many good reasons why we should be happy our brains are not exposed to public view.

Brain tissue—pinkish gray and white—is among the most delicate in our body, and the destruction of even a small part may mean lasting impairment or death. Its protection is vital and begins (if we are so fortunate) with a mat of hair on the top, back, and sides of our skull. Next comes the resilient layer of padding we call the scalp, and then the main line of defense—the rounded, bony helmet of skull.

The brain's armor does not stop with bone. Beneath are three strong, fibrous membranes called *meninges* that encase the brain in protective envelopes. Meninges also overlie the tissue of the spinal cord; infection or inflammation of these membranes by bacteria or viruses is called *cerebrospinal meningitis*.

Between two of the meninges is a region laced with veins and arteries and filled with *cerebrospinal fluid.* This fluid-filled space cushions the brain against sudden blows and collisions. The cerebrospinal fluid circulates not only about the brain but through the entire central nervous system. Incidentally, chemical analysis of this fluid, withdrawn by inserting a hypodermic needle between vertebrae of the spinal column (a spinal tap), can provide clues to the nature of brain and nervous system disorders.

THE CEREBRUM: What we usually mean by "brain" is that part of the brain called the *cerebrum*. It is the cerebrum that permits us all our distinctly human activities—thinking, speaking, reading, writing. Only in man does the cerebrum reach such size, occupying the interior of our entire dome above the level of our eyes.

The surface of the cerebrum is wrinkled, furrowed, folded and infolded, convoluted, fissured—anything but smooth. This lavishly wrinkled outer layer of the cerebrum, about an eighth of an inch thick, is called the *cerebral cortex.* From its grayish color comes the term "gray matter" for brain tissue. There is a pattern among its wrinkles, marked out by wider, or deeper fissures, or furrows, running through the brain tissue. The most conspicuous fissure runs down the middle, front to back, dividing the cerebrum into two halves, the left hemisphere and the right hemisphere. The nerves from the left half of the body are served by the right hemisphere, and the right half of the body by the left hemisphere, so that damage to one side of the brain affects the other side of the body.

THE LOBES OF THE CEREBRUM: Smaller fissures crisscross the cerebrum and mark out various specific areas of function called *lobes.* The frontal lobes, one on the left hemisphere and one on the right in back of our eyes and extending upward behind the forehead, are perhaps the most talked about and the least understood by medical researchers. The specific functions of most other lobes in the cerebrum, such as the two occipital lobes (centers for seeing), the olfactory lobes (centers for smelling), and the temporal lobes (centers for hearing) are much better known.

THE BRAIN STEM: The cerebrum, like a large flower obscuring part of its stalk, droops down around the *brain stem.* Thus, while the brain stem originates just about in the middle of our skull, it does not

THE BRAIN

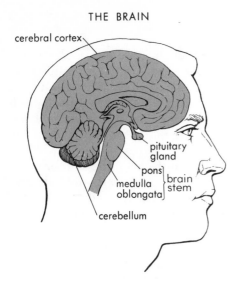

cerebral cortex

pituitary gland
pons
medulla oblongata } brain stem
cerebellum

FUNCTIONAL AREAS OF THE CEREBRAL CORTEX

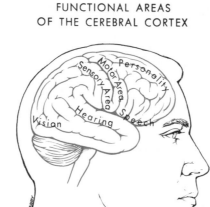

Personality
Motor Area
Sensory Area
Speech
Hearing
Vision

emerge completely from the folds of the cerebral hemispheres until it reaches the back of the neck. Then it soon merges into the spinal cord.

Associated with this portion of the brain—roughly speaking, between the cerebrum and the spinal cord—are centers that take care of the countless necessary details involved in just plain existing, and structures (such as the *medulla oblongata* and the *pons*) that serve also as traffic control points for the billions of nerve impulses traveling to and from the cerebrum. The largest of these "lesser brains" is the *cerebellum,* whose two hemispheres straddle the brain stem at the back of the head.

THE CEREBELLUM: The cerebellum is the site of balance and body and muscle coordination, allowing us, for example, to "rub the tummy and pat the head" simultaneously, or tap the foot and strum a guitar, or steer a car and operate the foot pedals. Such muscle-coordinated movements, though sometimes learned only by long repetition and practice, can become almost automatic—such as reaching for and flicking on the light switch as we move into a darkened room.

But many other activities and kinds of behavior regulated by the part of the brain below the cerebrum are more fully automatic: the control of eye movement and focus-

ing, for example, as well as the timing of heartbeat, sleep, appetite, and metabolism; the arousal and decline of sexual drives; body temperature; the dilation and constriction of blood vessels; swallowing; and breathing. All these are mainly functions of the *autonomic nervous system,* as opposed to the more voluntary actions controlled by the *central nervous system.*

The Body's Nervous Systems

Simply speaking, the human body has only one nervous system, and that is all the nerve cells, nerve cords, nerve centers, voluntary and involuntary, in the body. It is helpful, however, though quite arbitrary, to divide our nerves into the central and autonomic nervous systems. This division tends to obscure the countless interconnections and interplay between the two systems. For example, where do you place the control of breathing, or blinking? Such actions are automatic except when we choose to regulate them.

The Central Nervous System

The central nervous system, as noted above, includes the brain and the spinal cord. It also includes all the nerves of conscious response and voluntary action that link up with the brain and spinal cord.

Twelve pairs of *cranial nerves* originate within the brain and emerge at its base. These include the very important nerves that connect with our sense organs, nerve bundles that control the facial and neck muscles, and the *vagus* (or tenth cranial nerve) that serves the heart, lungs, stomach, intestines, esophagus, larynx, liver, kidneys, spleen, and pancreas. The vagus nerve, although anatomically part of the central nervous system, controls bodily functions that are mainly automatic.

THE BRAIN AND THE CRANIAL NERVES

Cranial Nerves

1. olfactory: smell
2. optic: vision
3. oculomotor: muscle of eyes
4. trochlear: muscle of eyes
5. trigeminal: sense of touch in face
6. abducens: muscle of eyes
7. facial: muscles of face
8. acoustic: hearing and balance
9. glossopharyngeal: taste
10. vagus: heart, lungs, abdomen
11. hypoglossal: tongue muscles
12. accessory: neck muscles, eyeball

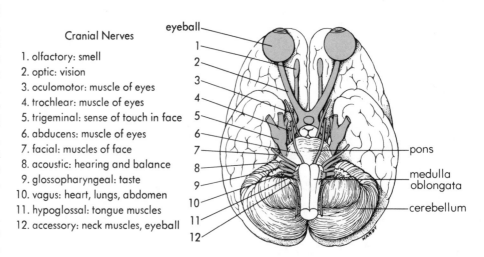

eyeball
pons
medulla oblongata
cerebellum

View of the Underside of the Brain

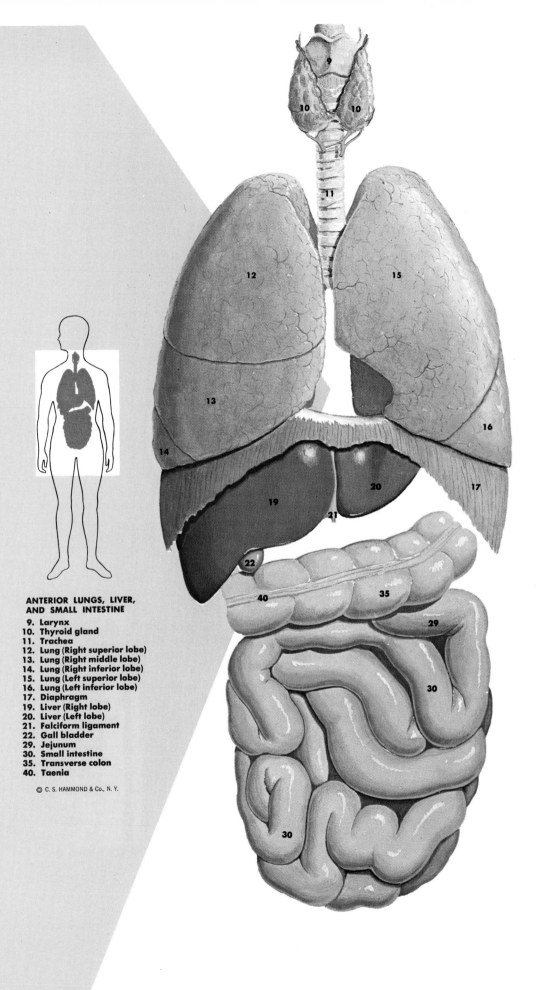

**ANTERIOR LUNGS, LIVER,
AND SMALL INTESTINE**

9. Larynx
10. Thyroid gland
11. Trachea
12. Lung (Right superior lobe)
13. Lung (Right middle lobe)
14. Lung (Right inferior lobe)
15. Lung (Left superior lobe)
16. Lung (Left inferior lobe)
17. Diaphragm
19. Liver (Right lobe)
20. Liver (Left lobe)
21. Falciform ligament
22. Gall bladder
29. Jejunum
30. Small intestine
35. Transverse colon
40. Taenia

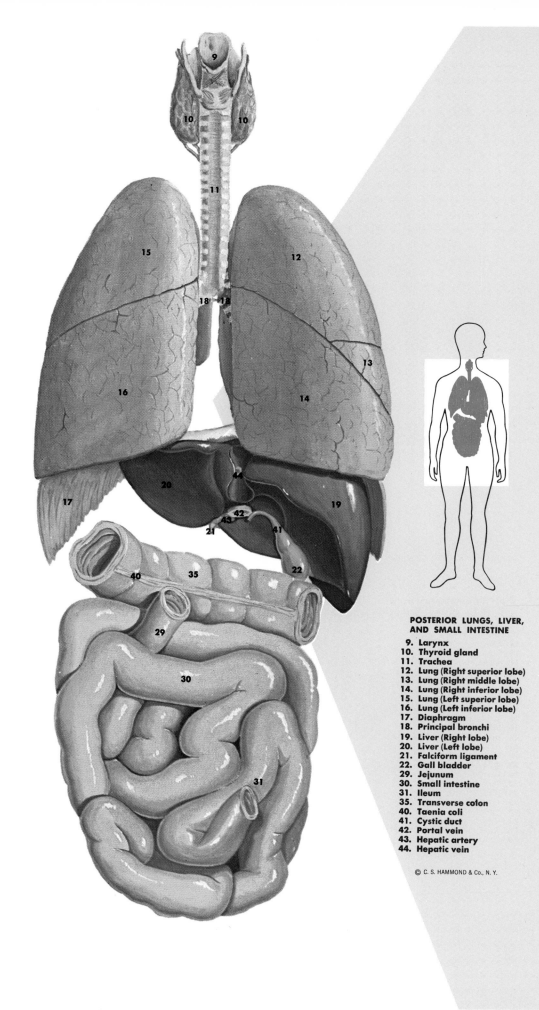

**POSTERIOR LUNGS, LIVER,
AND SMALL INTESTINE**

9. Larynx
10. Thyroid gland
11. Trachea
12. Lung (Right superior lobe)
13. Lung (Right middle lobe)
14. Lung (Right inferior lobe)
15. Lung (Left superior lobe)
16. Lung (Left inferior lobe)
17. Diaphragm
18. Principal bronchi
19. Liver (Right lobe)
20. Liver (Left lobe)
21. Falciform ligament
22. Gall bladder
29. Jejunum
30. Small intestine
31. Ileum
35. Transverse colon
40. Taenia coli
41. Cystic duct
42. Portal vein
43. Hepatic artery
44. Hepatic vein

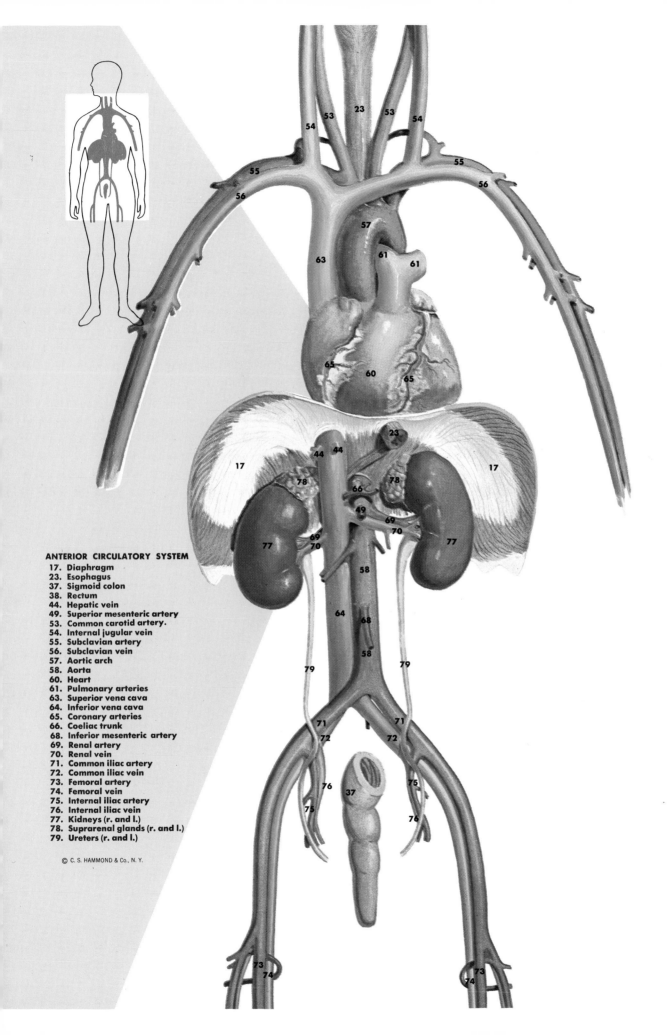

ANTERIOR CIRCULATORY SYSTEM

17. Diaphragm
23. Esophagus
37. Sigmoid colon
38. Rectum
44. Hepatic vein
49. Superior mesenteric artery
53. Common carotid artery.
54. Internal jugular vein
55. Subclavian artery
56. Subclavian vein
57. Aortic arch
58. Aorta
60. Heart
61. Pulmonary arteries
63. Superior vena cava
64. Inferior vena cava
65. Coronary arteries
66. Coeliac trunk
68. Inferior mesenteric artery
69. Renal artery
70. Renal vein
71. Common iliac artery
72. Common iliac vein
73. Femoral artery
74. Femoral vein
75. Internal iliac artery
76. Internal iliac vein
77. Kidneys (r. and l.)
78. Suprarenal glands (r. and l.)
79. Ureters (r. and l.)

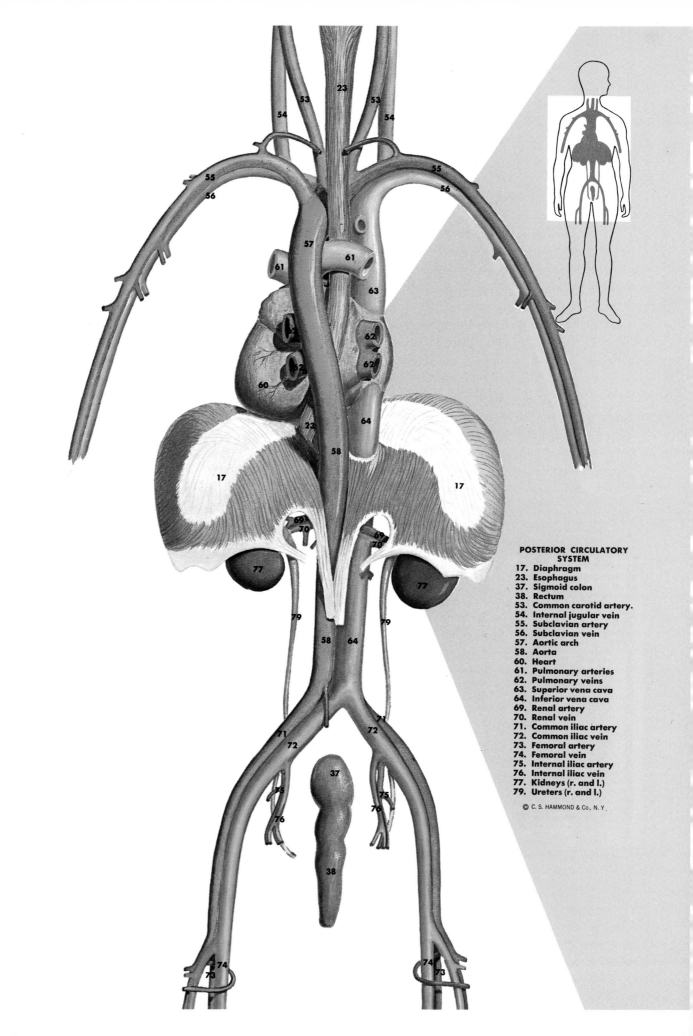

POSTERIOR CIRCULATORY SYSTEM

17. Diaphragm
23. Esophagus
37. Sigmoid colon
38. Rectum
53. Common carotid artery.
54. Internal jugular vein
55. Subclavian artery
56. Subclavian vein
57. Aortic arch
58. Aorta
60. Heart
61. Pulmonary arteries
62. Pulmonary veins
63. Superior vena cava
64. Inferior vena cava
69. Renal artery
70. Renal vein
71. Common iliac artery
72. Common iliac vein
73. Femoral artery
74. Femoral vein
75. Internal iliac artery
76. Internal iliac vein
77. Kidneys (r. and l.)
79. Ureters (r. and l.)

© C. S. HAMMOND & Co., N. Y.

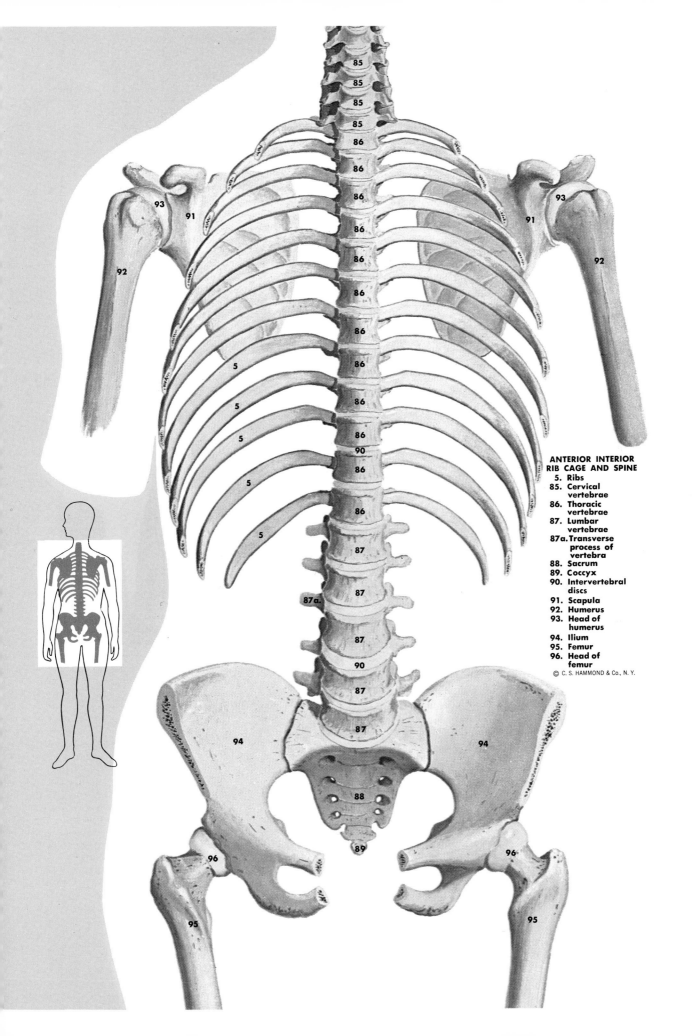

**ANTERIOR INTERIOR
RIB CAGE AND SPINE**

 5. **Ribs**
85. **Cervical
    vertebrae**
86. **Thoracic
    vertebrae**
87. **Lumbar
    vertebrae**
87a. **Transverse
    process of
    vertebra**
88. **Sacrum**
89. **Coccyx**
90. **Intervertebral
    discs**
91. **Scapula**
92. **Humerus**
93. **Head of
    humerus**
94. **Ilium**
95. **Femur**
96. **Head of
    femur**

© C. S. HAMMOND & Co., N. Y.

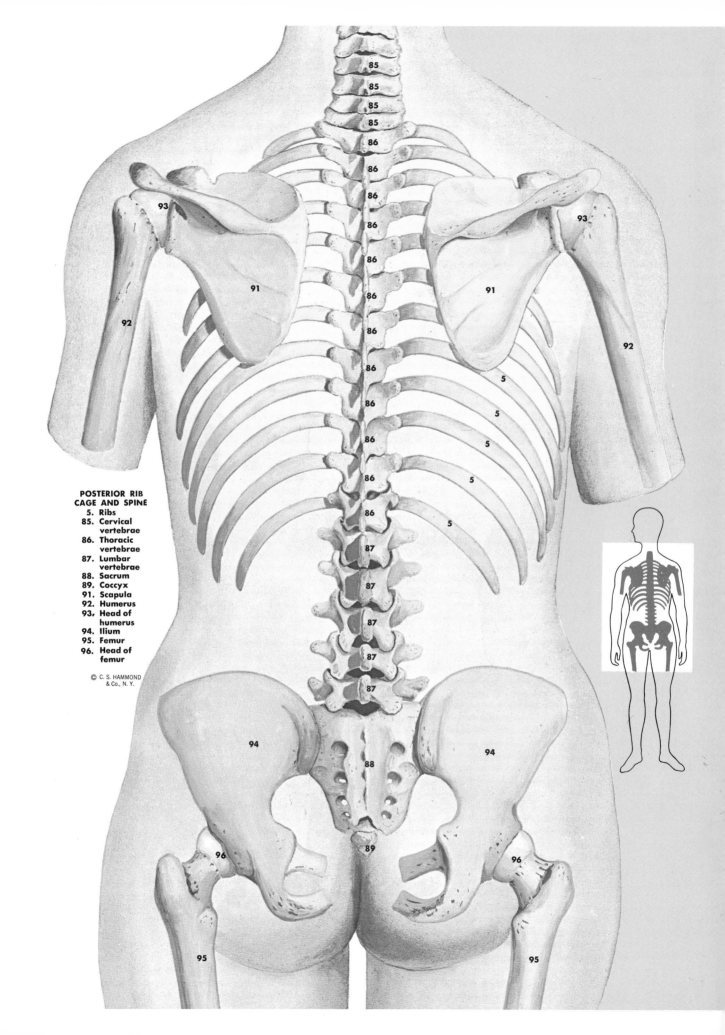

**POSTERIOR RIB
CAGE AND SPINE**
   5. Ribs
  85. Cervical
      vertebrae
  86. Thoracic
      vertebrae
  87. Lumbar
      vertebrae
  88. Sacrum
  89. Coccyx
  91. Scapula
  92. Humerus
  93. Head of
      humerus
  94. Ilium
  95. Femur
  96. Head of
      femur

© C. S. HAMMOND
& Co., N. Y.

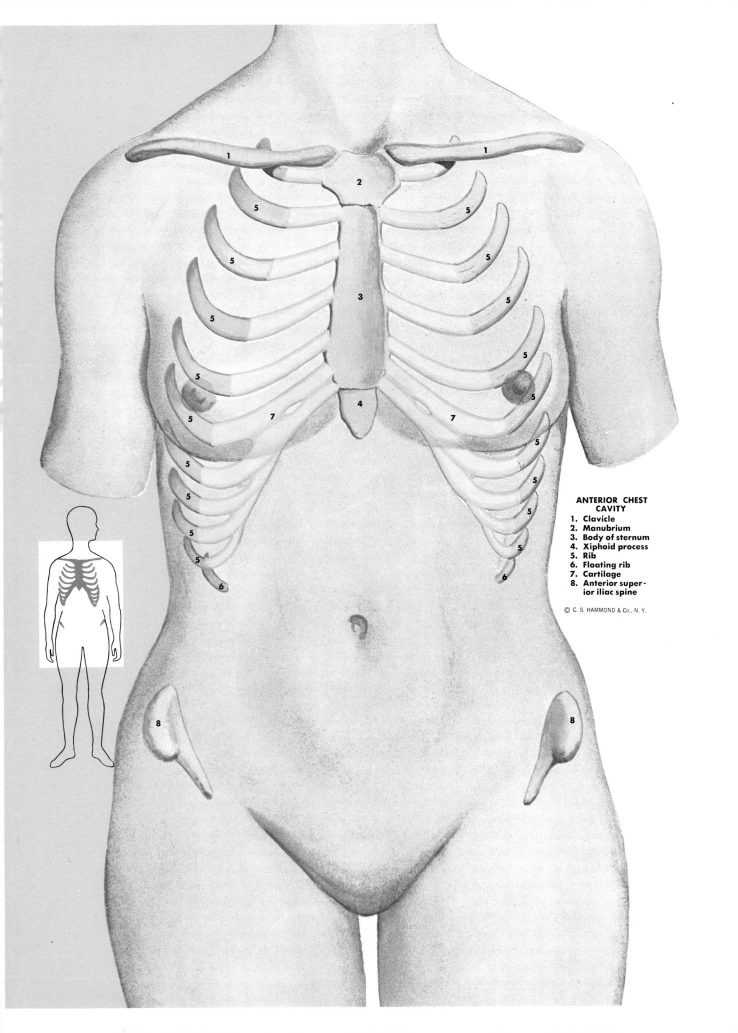

ANTERIOR CHEST CAVITY

1. Clavicle
2. Manubrium
3. Body of sternum
4. Xiphoid process
5. Rib
6. Floating rib
7. Cartilage
8. Anterior super-
   ior iliac spine

© C. S. HAMMOND & Co., N. Y.

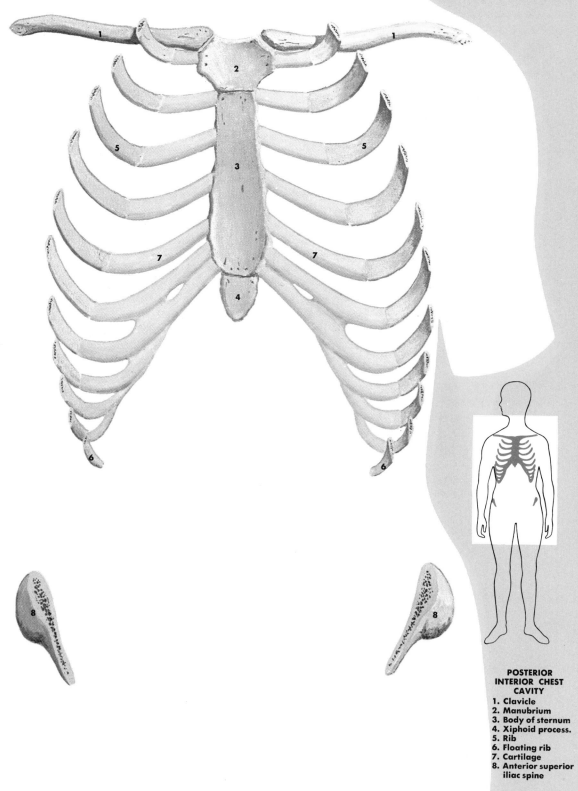

**POSTERIOR
INTERIOR CHEST
CAVITY**

1. Clavicle
2. Manubrium
3. Body of sternum
4. Xiphoid process.
5. Rib
6. Floating rib
7. Cartilage
8. Anterior superior
   iliac spine

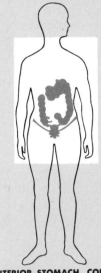

ANTERIOR STOMACH, COLON,
AND
ORGANS OF REPRODUCTION

23. **Esophagus**
24. **Stomach (cardia)**
25. **Stomach (fundus)**
26. **Stomach (body)**
27. **Stomach (pylorus)**
28. **Duodenum**
31. **Ileum**
32. **Ileocolic junction**
33. **Caecum**
34. **Ascending colon**
36. **Descending colon**
37. **Sigmoid colon**
39. **Vermiform appendix**
40. **Taenia coli**
45. **Spleen**
49. **Superior mesenteric artery**
50. **Superior mesenteric vein**
51. **Pancreas (head)**
52. **Pancreas (tail)**
80. **Bladder**
81. **Urachus**
82. **Pubic symphysis**
83. **Inguinal ligament**
100. **Uterus**
102. **Vagina (cross section)**
103. **Fallopian tube**
104. **Ostium of fallopian tube**
105. **Ovary**

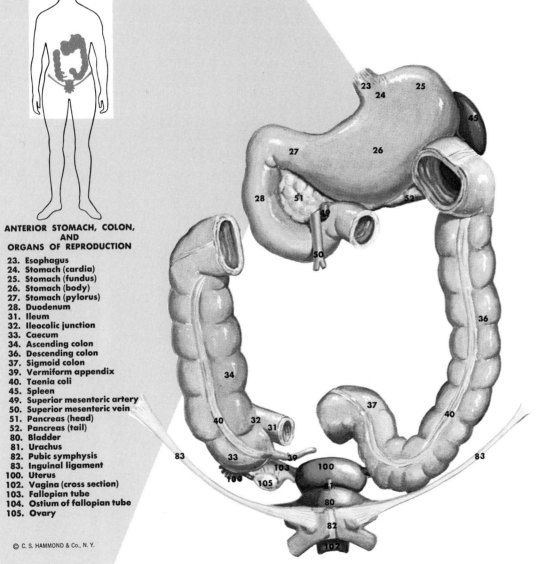

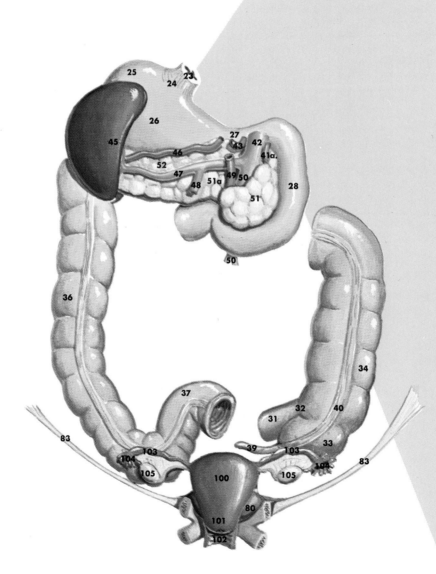
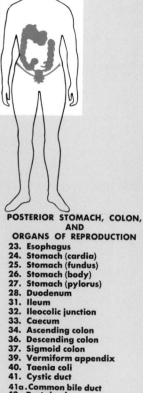

POSTERIOR STOMACH, COLON, AND ORGANS OF REPRODUCTION

23. Esophagus
24. Stomach (cardia)
25. Stomach (fundus)
26. Stomach (body)
27. Stomach (pylorus)
28. Duodenum
31. Ileum
32. Ileocolic junction
33. Caecum
34. Ascending colon
36. Descending colon
37. Sigmoid colon
39. Vermiform appendix
40. Taenia coli
41. Cystic duct
41a. Common bile duct
42. Portal vein
43. Hepatic artery
45. Spleen
46. Splenic artery
47. Splenic vein
48. Inferior mesenteric vein
49. Superior mesenteric artery
50. Superior mesenteric vein
51. Pancreas (head)
51a. Pancreas (body)
52. Pancreas (tail)
80. Bladder
83. Inguinal ligament
100. Uterus
101. Cervix
102. Vagina (cross section)
103. Fallopian tube
104. Ostium of fallopian tube
105. Ovary

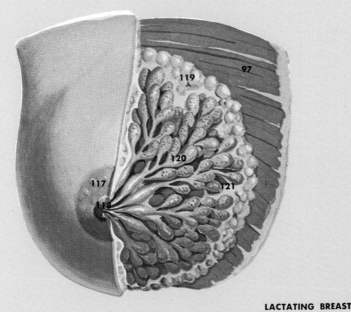

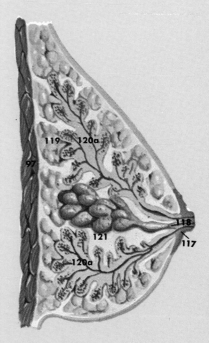

LACTATING BREAST

97. **Pectoralis major muscle**
117. **Areola**
118. **Nipple**
119. **Fat**
120. **Lactiferous (milk producing) glands and ducts**
120a. **Cross section of gland and duct**
121. **Tissue separating and supporting glandular tissue**

STRUCTURE OF THE MAMMARY GLANDS

The mammary glands are composed of three major elements:
1. Their skin covering and special structures (nipple, areola).
2. The lactiferous glands or functional units of the breast.
3. The supporting structures, the connective tissue "ligaments" and the fat tissue that makes up the mass of the breast.

The breast is supported by the "suspensory ligaments." These are anchored to the sheet of connective tissue surrounding the pectoralis major muscle, and extend in a complex network separated by the fat tissue outward to the skin. The lactiferous glands are buried in the supporting tissues and empty outward onto the surface of the nipple. These glands at first are very small and clustered just beneath the nipple and areola. In pregnancy they enlarge and push downward into the mass of the breast causing it to enlarge in turn. The enlargement continues through the period of breast feeding, following which the glands gradually grow smaller and the entire breast returns to normal size.

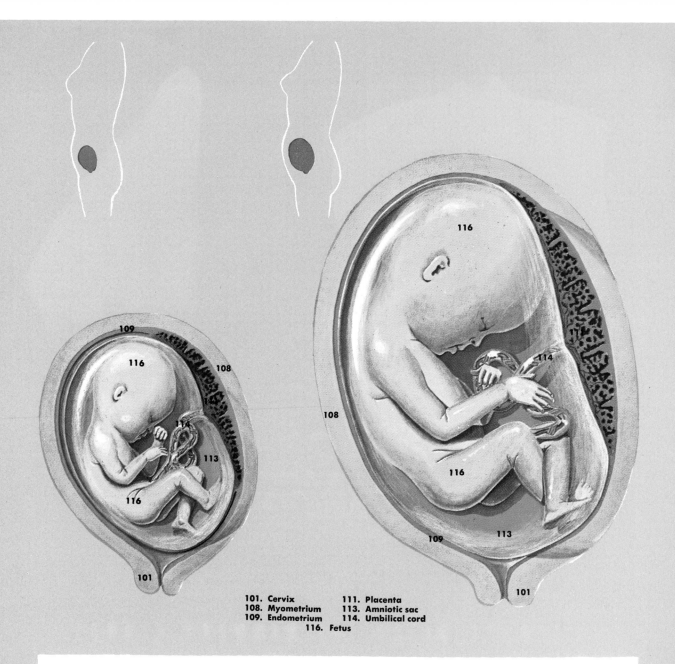

101. Cervix
108. Myometrium
109. Endometrium
111. Placenta
113. Amniotic sac
114. Umbilical cord
116. Fetus

THE FETUS AT 3 1/2 AND 6 MONTHS

Most of the definitive development of the fetus occurs during the first 3½ months, and the remaining 5½ months is primarily concerned with gradual increase in size and maturation of organs already begun. The fetus receives all of its nourishment through the placenta and umbilical cord. There is no direct contact between fetal and maternal blood in the placenta. During its entire development, the fetus floats in a fluid (amniotic fluid) contained within a sac (the amniotic sac) attached to the placenta. This sac is in turn surrounded by the uterine cavity, the endometrium and the muscle or myometrium of the uterus.

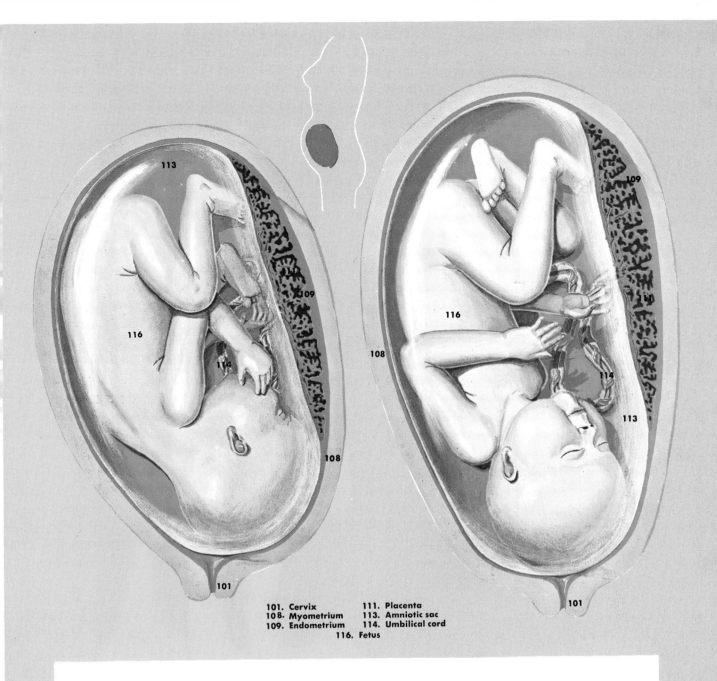

101. Cervix	111. Placenta
108. Myometrium	113. Amniotic sac
109. Endometrium	114. Umbilical cord
116. Fetus	

THE FETUS AT 8 AND 9 MONTHS

Until birth, the fetus is surrounded by the amniotic sac and fluid, and attached to the placenta by the umbilical cord. The fetus continues to increase in size and the uterus stretches to accommodate it. Usually before the eighth month the fetus assumes a head-downward position. At birth, the amniotic sac ruptures, the fluid escapes, and the child is slowly pushed out of the uterine cavity by the contractions of the myometrium. Shortly after birth of the child, the placenta is similarly expelled having been detached from the endometrium.

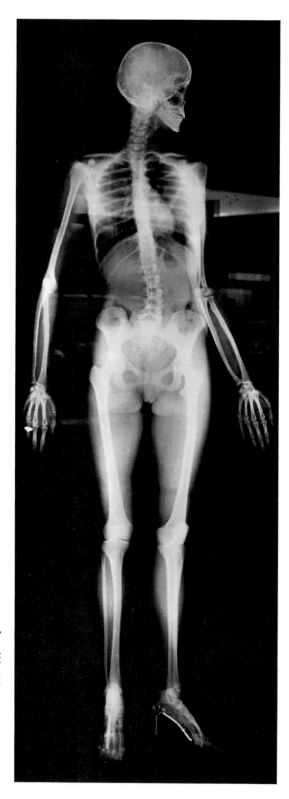

X-RAY OF THE HUMAN BODY
SHOWING THE
BONE STRUCTURE

heart. Blood cells, therefore, must be small (the point of a pin could hold dozens of red blood cells), and they must be jellylike in order to navigate the tight, tortuous, capillary channels without either blocking the channel or breaking apart themselves. A red blood cell is further adapted to sneaking through the capillaries by its concave-disk shape, which allows it to bend and fold around itself. Nevertheless, so narrow are the passageways within some of the capillaries that blood cells must move through them in single file. If a substantial number of the cells are misshapen, as in sickle-cell anemia, they tend to move sluggishly or clog up the passageway—a condition which can have serious consequences. See also p. 352.

Lymph and the Lymphatic System

Of all our body systems, perhaps the most ignored is the lymphatic system, although it forms a network throughout our body comparable to the blood vessels of our circulatory system.

Lymph is a whitish fluid that is derived from blood plasma. As plasma circulates through the body, some of it seeps through the walls of capillaries and other blood vessels. This leakage is of the utmost importance, because the leaked fluid, lymph, supplies the liquid environment around and between individual cells and tissues that is essential for their survival.

The presence of lymph requires a drainage system to keep the fluid moving. If there were no drainage system, two things could happen: the dammed-up lymph could create areas swollen with water in which cells would literally drown, or stagnant pools of lymph could become breeding grounds for infection.

As it moves through the vessels of the lymphatic system, lymph carries away from the tissues the bits and pieces of cells that have died and disintegrated, and also potentially harmful bacteria and viruses.

LYMPH AND LYMPHOCYTES: Confusion often arises about the connection between the white blood cells called *lymphocytes* and the lymph itself. Lymph is not made up of lymphocytes, although it often carries them; lymph is simply a watery vehicle moving through the lymphatic network. At certain points along this network, the vessels enlarge into clumpy structures called *lymph nodes* (or, misleadingly, lymph glands). Lymph nodes are major manufacturing sites for lymphocytes.

LYMPH NODES: Swollen glands are actually swollen lymph nodes, where a small army of lymphocytes is doing battle against invading bacteria or other harmful microscopic organisms. The lymph nodes, more than a hundred of them distributed around the body, serve as defense outposts against germs approaching the interior of the body. Those in the neck, groin, and armpits most frequently exhibit the pain and swelling that may accompany germ-fighting.

CIRCULATION OF LYMPH: Lymph circulates without any help from the heart. From the spaces between cells, it diffuses into lymph capillaries which, like the venous capillaries, merge into larger and larger vessels moving inward toward the heart. The lymph moves—even upward from the legs and lower part of the body—because the muscles and movements of the body are constantly kneading and squeezing the lymph vessels. These vessels are equipped with valves that prevent back-flow. This is not so very different from the way venous blood makes its way back to the heart.

Eventually, master lymph vessels from the head, abdomen, and torso join in the thoracic lymph duct, which then empties into large neck veins that carry lymph and venous blood, mixed together, back to the heart.

The Heart at Work

The structure and performance of

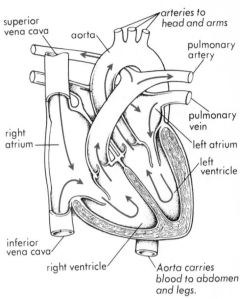

HOW BLOOD CIRCULATES THROUGH THE HEART

superior vena cava · aorta · arteries to head and arms · pulmonary artery · right atrium · pulmonary vein · left atrium · left ventricle · inferior vena cava · right ventricle · Aorta carries blood to abdomen and legs.

Blood from the head and arms enters the right atrium from the superior (i.e. upper) vena cava. Blood from the torso and legs enters from the inferior (i.e. lower) vena cava. The blood, controlled by a valve, passes to the right ventricle. It is then pumped into the pulmonary artery, which divides into two vessels, one leading to each lung. After being enriched with oxygen, the blood is brought back to the left atrium via the pulmonary veins, is admitted by a valve into the left ventricle, and is pumped through the aorta to be distributed to all parts of the body.

Both atria contract at the same time, forcing blood into the ventricles. Then both ventricles contract (while the atria relax), forcing blood into the great arteries. This period of contraction is called systole, and is followed by a period of relaxation called diastole.

the heart, at first glance rather complicated, assume a magnificent simplicity once we observe that this pulsating knot of hollow, intertwining muscle uses only one beat to perform two distinct pumping jobs.

The heart has a right side (your right) and a left side (your left), divided by a tough wall of muscle called a *septum*. Each side has two chambers, an upper one called an *atrium* (or *auricle*), and a lower one called a *ventricle*.

How the Heart Pumps the Blood

Venous blood from the body flows into the right atrium via two large veins called the *superior vena cava* (bringing blood from the upper body) and the *inferior vena cava* (bringing blood from the lower part of the body). Where the blood enters the right atrium are valves that close when the atrium chamber is full.

Then, through a kind of trapdoor valve, blood is released from the right atrium into the right ventricle. When the right ventricle is full, and its outlet valve opens, the heart as a whole contracts—that is, pumps.

TO THE LUNGS: The blood from the right ventricle is pumped to the lungs through the pulmonary artery to pick up oxygen. The trapdoor valve between the right atrium and ventricle has meanwhile closed, and venous blood again fills the right atrium.

Having picked up oxygen in the lungs, blood enters the left atrium through two pulmonary veins. (They are called veins despite the fact that they carry the most oxygen-rich blood, because they lead *to* the heart; just as the pulmonary artery carries the oxygen-poorest blood away from the heart, to the lungs.) Like the right atrium, the left atrium serves as a holding reservoir and, when full, releases its contents into the left ventricle. A valve between left atrium and ventricle closes, and the heart pumps.

TO THE BODY: Blood surges through an opening valve of the left ventricle into the aorta, the major artery that marks the beginning of blood's circulation throughout the body. The left ventricle, because it has the job of pumping blood to the entire body rather than just to the lungs, is slightly larger and more muscular than the right ventricle. It is for this reason, incidentally, that the heart is commonly considered to be on our left. The organ as a whole, as noted earlier, is located at the center of the chest.

The Heart's Own Circulatory System

Heart tissue, like that of every other organ in the body, must be continually supplied with fresh, oxygen-rich blood, and used blood must be returned to the lungs for reoxygenation. The blood inside the heart cannot serve these needs. Thus the heart has its own circulation network, called *coronary arteries* and *veins*, to nourish its muscular tissues. There are two major arteries on the surface of the heart, branching and rebranching eventually into capillaries. Coronary veins then take blood back to the right atrium.

Structure of the Heart

The musculature of the heart is called cardiac muscle because it is different in appearance from the two other major types of muscle. The heart muscle is sometimes considered as one anatomical unit, called the *myocardium*. A tough outer layer of membranous tissue, called the *pericardium*, surrounds the myocardium. Lining the internal chambers and valves of the heart, on the walls of the atria and ventricles, is a tissue called the *endocardium*.

These tissues, like any others, are subject to infections and other dis-

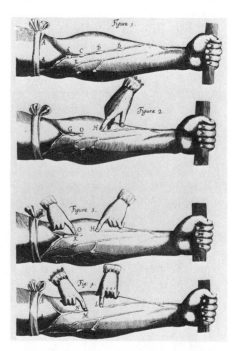

The 17th century physician William Harvey first described how blood circulates. An illustration from one of his classic works shows the circulation of blood in the veins of the forearm.

orders. An infection of the endocardium by bacteria is called *bacterial endocarditis*. (Disease of the valves is also called *endocarditis*, although it is a misnomer.) An interruption of the blood supply to the heart muscle is called a *myocardial infarction*, which results in the weakening or death of the portion of the myocardium whose blood supply is blocked. Fortunately, in many cases, other blood vessels may eventually take over the job of supplying the blood-starved area of heart muscle.

Heartbeat

The rate at which the heart beats is controlled by both the autonomic nervous system and by hormones of the endocrine system. The precise means by which the chambers and valves of the heart are made to work in perfect coordination are not fully understood. It is known, however, that the heart has one or more natural cardiac pacemakers that send electrical waves through the heart, causing the opening and closing of valves and muscular contraction, or pumping, of the ventricles near the normal adult rate of about 72 times per minute.

One particular electrical impulse (there may be others) originates in a small area in the upper part of the right atrium called the *sinus node*. Because it is definitely known that the contraction of the heart is electrically activated, tiny battery-powered devices called *artificial pacemakers* have been developed that can take the place of a natural pacemaker whose function has been impaired by heart injury or disease. Through electrodes implanted in heart tissue, such devices supply the correct beat for a defective heart. The bulk of the device is usually worn outside the body or is implanted just under the skin.

The fact that both ventricles give their push at the same time is very significant. It allows the entire heart muscle to rest between contractions —a rest period that adds up to a little more than half of a person's life-

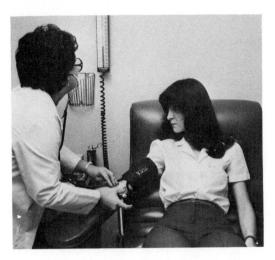

Blood pressure measures the force of the blood circulating through the blood vessels as the heart pumps (systole) and relaxes (diastole).

time. Without this rest period, it is more than likely that our hearts would wear out considerably sooner than they do.

BLOOD PRESSURE: A doctor's taking of blood pressure is based upon the difference between the heart's action at its period of momentary rest and at the moment of maximum work (the contraction or push). The split-second of maximum work, at the peak of the ventricles' contraction, is called the *systole*. The split-

second of peak relaxation, when blood from the atria is draining into and filling up the ventricles, is called the *diastole*.

Blood pressure measures the force with which blood is passing through a major artery, such as one in the arm, and this pressure varies between a higher *systolic* pressure, corresponding to the heart's systole, and a lower *diastolic* pressure, reflecting the heart's diastole, or resting phase. The device with

which a doctor takes your blood pressure, called a *sphygmomanometer*, registers these higher and lower figures in numbers equivalent to the number of millimeters the force of your arterial blood would raise a column of mercury. The higher systolic force (pressure) is given first, then the diastolic figure. For example, 125/80 is within the normal range of blood pressure. Readings that are above the normal range—and stay elevated over a period of time—indicate a person has high blood pressure, or hypertension.

Hypertension has no direct connection with nervous tension, although the two may be associated in the same person. What it does indicate is that a heart is working harder than the average heart to push blood through the system. In turn, this may indicate the presence of a circulatory problem that might eventually endanger health. See also *Diseases of the Circulatory System*, p. 349, and *Heart Disease*, p. 360.

THE DIGESTIVE SYSTEM AND THE LIVER

A doctor once remarked that a great many people seem to spend about half their time getting food into their digestive tracts and the other half worrying about how that food is doing on its travels. The doctor was exaggerating, but he made his point.

The digestive tract has essentially one purpose: to break down food, both solid and fluid, into a form that can be used by the body. The food is used as energy to fuel daily activities or to nourish the various tissues that are always in the process of wearing out and needing replacement.

A normally functioning digestive tract, dealing with a reasonable variety and quantity of food, is designed to extract the maximum ben-

efit from what we eat. Urine and feces are the waste products—things from which our body has selected everything that is of use.

Our digestive system's efficiency and economy in getting food into our bodies, to be utilized in all our living processes, can be attributed basically to three facts.

First, although the straight-line distance from the mouth to the bottom of the trunk is only two or three feet, the distance along the intestinal tract is about 10 times as great —30 feet—a winding, twisting, looping passageway that has more than enough footage to accommodate a number of ingeniously constructed way stations, checkpoints, and traffic-control devices.

Second, from the moment food enters the mouth, it is subjected to both chemical and mechanical actions that begin to break it apart, leading eventually to its reduction to submicroscopic molecules that can be absorbed through the intestinal walls into the circulatory system.

Finally, each of the three main types of food—carbohydrates, fats, and proteins—receives special treatment that results in the body deriving maximum benefit from each.

Sensing the Right Kind of Food

Lips, eyes, and nose are generally given scant notice in discussions of the digestive process. But if we consider digestion to include selection of food and rejection of substances that might do us harm, then all three play very important roles.

The sensitive skin of our lips represents one of our first warning station that food may be harmful if taken into the mouth. It may tell us if a forkful of food is too hot or warn us of a concealed fishbone.

Our eyes, too, are important selection-rejection monitors for food. What else keeps us from sitting down to a crisp salad of poison ivy, or, less facetiously, popping a moldy piece of cake into our mouth?

As mammals' noses go, man's is a very inferior and insensitive organ. Nevertheless, we make good use of our sense of smell in the selection and enjoyment of foods. The nose adds to our enjoyment of favorite food and drink not only before they enter the mouth, but also after, because stimulation of the olfactory cells in the nasal passages combines with the stimulation of the taste cells on the tongue to produce the sensation-and-discrimination gradations of taste.

The Mouth: Saliva, Teeth, and Tongue

By the time food leaves the mouth and is pushed down into the gullet (or esophagus), it has already received a sampling of all the kinds of punishment and prodding that will be provided by the 30-foot tube that lies ahead of it. The chances are slim that any piece of food will end that journey in the same condition it started, but if it did it would have traveled those 30 tortuous feet at the rate of something less than two feet per hour. Normally, the elapsed time is between 17 and 25 hours.

As in the rest of the digestive tract, the mouth puts both chemical and mechanical apparatus to work on a bite of food. Saliva supplies the chemical action. Teeth and tongue, backed up by powerful sets of muscles, are the mashers, crushers, and prodders.

THE DIGESTIVE SYSTEM

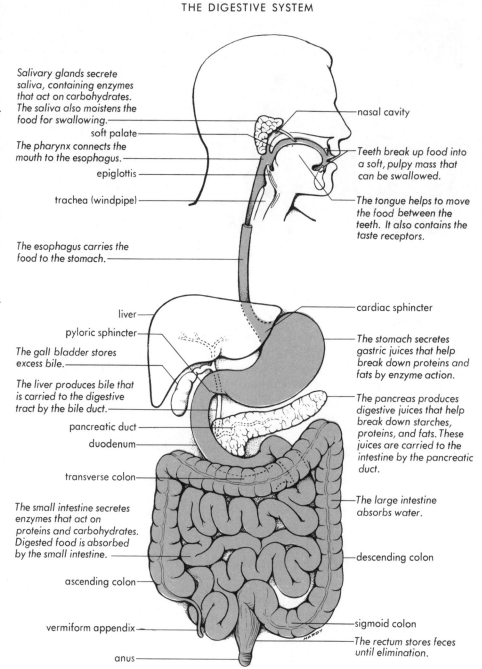

Salivary glands secrete saliva, containing enzymes that act on carbohydrates. The saliva also moistens the food for swallowing.

soft palate

The pharynx connects the mouth to the esophagus.

epiglottis

trachea (windpipe)

The esophagus carries the food to the stomach.

liver

pyloric sphincter

The gall bladder stores excess bile.

The liver produces bile that is carried to the digestive tract by the bile duct.

pancreatic duct

duodenum

transverse colon

The small intestine secretes enzymes that act on proteins and carbohydrates. Digested food is absorbed by the small intestine.

ascending colon

vermiform appendix

anus

nasal cavity

Teeth break up food into a soft, pulpy mass that can be swallowed.

The tongue helps to move the food between the teeth. It also contains the taste receptors.

cardiac sphincter

The stomach secretes gastric juices that help break down proteins and fats by enzyme action.

The pancreas produces digestive juices that help break down starches, proteins, and fats. These juices are carried to the intestine by the pancreatic duct.

The large intestine absorbs water.

descending colon

sigmoid colon

The rectum stores feces until elimination.

Saliva

The mere presence of food in our mouth—or even the smell, memory, or anticipation of it—sends signals to our brain, and our brain in turn sends messages back to a system of six salivary glands: one pair, called the *sublingual glands,* located under the tongue toward the front of the mouth; another pair, the *submaxillary* (or *submandibular*) glands, a bit behind and below

them; and the largest, the *parotid glands,* tucked in the region where jaw meets neck behind the ear lobes.

Saliva is mainly composed of water, and water alone begins to soften up food so that it can pass more smoothly down the esophagus toward encounters with more powerful chemical agents.

There is also a very special substance in saliva, an enzyme called *ptyalin,* whose specific job is to begin the breakdown of one of the toughest kinds of food our digestive system has to handle—starches. Starch is a kind of carbohydrate, the group of foods from which we principally derive energy; but in order for the body to utilize carbohydrate, it must be broken down into simpler forms, which are called simply sugars. Ptyalin, then, begins the simplification of carbohydrate starch into carbohydrate sugar.

Saliva also does a favor or two for the dominating structures of the mouth—the tongue and teeth. Without its bathing action, the tongue's taste cells could not function up to par; and because it has a mild germicidal effect in addition to a simple rinsing action, saliva helps protect our mouth and teeth from bacterial infection.

Teeth

The role of the teeth in digestion can be summed up in one word: destruction. What the wrecker's ball is to a standing building, our teeth are to a lump of solid food. They do the first, dramatic demolishing, leaving smaller fragments to be dealt with and disposed of in other ways.

Starting from the center of the mouth, we have two incisors on either side, top and bottom, followed by a canine, a couple of premolars, and three molars, the most backward of which (it never appears in some people) is the curiously named "wisdom" tooth, so called because it commonly appears as physical maturity is reached, at about 20 years of age.

Our teeth equip us for destroying chunks of food by a gamut of mechanical actions ranging from gripping and puncturing to grinding and pulverizing. The teeth in front—canines and incisors—do most of the gripping, ripping, and tearing, while the premolars and molars at the back of the jaws do the grinding.

The Tongue

The surface of the tongue is not smooth, but has a finely corrugated look and feel. This slightly sandpapery surface is due to the presence of thousands of tiny papillae, little pyramid-shaped bumps. When we are young, the walls of a single papilla may contain up to 300 taste cells, or buds. As we get older, the maximum number of taste buds per papilla may decline to under 100.

There are four kinds of taste cells, distinguished by the type of taste message each sends to the brain: salty, sweet, sour, and bitter. Each of the four types is a narrow specialist in one type of taste. However, simultaneous or successive stimulation of all four types (combined almost always with information picked up by our sense of smell) can produce a tremendous variety of recognizable tastes—although perhaps not so many as some gourmets or wine-tasters might have us believe.

All four types of taste buds—salty, sweet, sour, and bitter—are found associated with papillae in all areas on the surface of the tongue; but there tend to be denser populations of one or the other kinds of taste cells in certain places. For example, salty and sweet cells predominate at the tip of the tongue and about halfway back along its sides; sour cells are more numerous all the way back along the sides; bitter buds are densest at the back of the tongue.

In addition to its tasting abilities, the tongue is a very versatile, flexible, and admirably shaped bundle of muscle. Not only can it flick out to moisten dry lips and ferret out and dislodge food particles in the oral cavity, but it also performs the first mechanical step in the all-important act of swallowing.

Swallowing

Swallow. You'll find that you feel the top of your tongue pressing up against the roof of your mouth *(hard palate)*. You may never have thought about it consciously, but the pressing of the tongue against the hard palate prevents food from slipping to the front of your mouth—and also gives the food a good shove

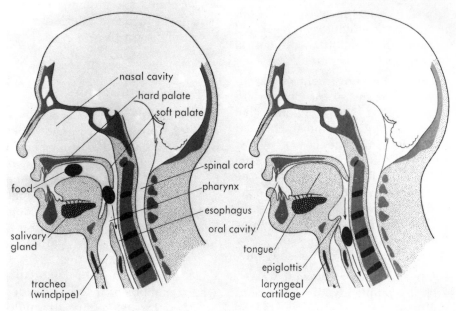

THE TRANSITION FROM BREATHING TO SWALLOWING

nasal cavity
hard palate
soft palate
spinal cord
food
pharynx
esophagus
oral cavity
salivary gland
tongue
epiglottis
laryngeal cartilage
trachea (windpipe)

(Left) The soft palate begins to move upward to close off the nasal cavity, and the epiglottis to move downward to close off the trachea. *(Right)* By the time the food has passed into the esophagus, the trachea and the nasal cavity are completely shut off.

up and to the back of your mouth. At this point, the *soft palate* (from which the teardrop-shaped piece of tissue called the *uvula* hangs down) slips up to cover the passageway between mouth (oral cavity) and nasal cavity, nicely preventing the food from being misdirected toward your nose.

Once past the soft palate, the food is in the *pharynx*, a kind of anatomical traffic circle with two roads entering at the top, those from the mouth and nasal cavity, and two roads leading away from the bottom, the *trachea* (windpipe) and the *esophagus* or food tube.

THE EPIGLOTTIS: A wedge of cartilage called the *epiglottis* protrudes from the trachea side, the side toward the front of the neck. When we are breathing, the epiglottis is flattened up against the front wall of the pharynx, allowing free movement of air up and down the trachea. Simultaneously, the epiglottis helps to close off the entrance to the esophagus; a good part of the esophagus-closing work is done by a bundle of sinewy, elastic tissue we associate primarily with speech—the tissue of the vocal cords, otherwise known as the voice box or *larynx*. The laryngeal tissue is connected to the epiglottis above it, and supplies the epiglottis with most of its muscle for movement.

During the movement of a swallow, the larynx exerts an upward force against the epiglottis that serves to block off the trachea. At the same time, the larynx relaxes some of its pressure on the esophagus. Result: food enters the esophagus, where it is meant to go, and not the windpipe, which as we all know from having had something "go down the wrong way," produces an immediate fit of coughing.

Once we have swallowed, we lose almost completely the conscious ability to control the passage of food along the intestinal tract. Only when wastes reach the point of elimination do we begin to reassert some conscious control.

Peristalsis

The mechanical action called *peristalsis*, affected by muscles in the walls of all the organs of the gastrointestinal tract, first comes into play in the esophagus. Two layers of muscles intermesh in the intestinal walls: the inner layer encircles the esophagus in a series of rings; the outer layer stretches lengthwise along the tube. These two sets of muscles work in tandem to produce the basic action of peristalsis, called a *peristaltic wave*.

The alternate contraction and relaxation of the muscles—closing behind swallowed food and opening in front of it—combine to move both liquid and solid food (medical term, *bolus*) along the digestive tract. Gravity, in a sense, is left behind once food enters the esophagus. Because of peristalsis, we can swallow lying down or even standing on our heads; and astronauts are able to eat in near zero-gravity or under weightless conditions.

Peristalsis has another important function besides moving food through the body. The constricting and relaxing muscles serve also to knead, churn, and pummel the solid remains of food left after our teeth have done their best.

Digestive Sphincters

If you think about it, the gastrointestinal tract has to be equipped with a number of gates that can open or shut, depending on the amount of food that is passing through. Otherwise, the food might push through so fast that little nourishment could be extracted from it: we would feel hungry one minute and glutted the next. The gastrointestinal tract is thus equipped at critical junctures with a number of muscular valves, or *sphincters*, which, usually under the direction of the autonomic nervous system, can regulate the movement of food through the digestive tube. Another function of a sphinc-

ter is to prevent backflow of partially digested food.

The muscles of a sphincter are often described as "pursestring muscles" because the way they draw together the sides of the digestive tube is roughly similar to drawing up the strings of a purse. The first of these pursestring valves occurs at the *cardia*, the opening where the esophagus meets the stomach, and is called the *cardiac sphincter*, from its location almost directly in front of the heart. (But there is no physical connection.)

Another important muscle ring is the *pyloric sphincter*, at the opening called the *pylorus*, located at the other end of the stomach, at the connection between stomach and small intestine. The release of waste from the rectum is controlled, partly voluntarily, by an *anal sphincter*, located at the *anus*, which marks the end of the tract.

The Stomach

About ten inches down the esophagus, the food we swallow must pass the cardiac sphincter. Then the food, by now fairly well diced and mashed, passes into the stomach.

Inelegant as it sounds, the stomach is best described as a rough, leather-skinned balloon. When empty, its skin shrivels around itself like a deflated balloon; but when "pumped up" by a hearty meal, the stomach becomes a plump, J-shaped bag about a foot long and six inches wide, holding about two quarts of food and drink.

The Passage of Food Through the Stomach

Although its food-processing function tends to get more attention, the stomach's role as a storage reservoir is equally important. A moderate, well-rounded meal with a good blend of carbohydrates, proteins, and fats takes usually a minimum of three hours to pass out of the pyloric sphincter into the small intestine—more if the meal is

THE PASSAGE OF FOOD THROUGH THE ALIMENTARY CANAL

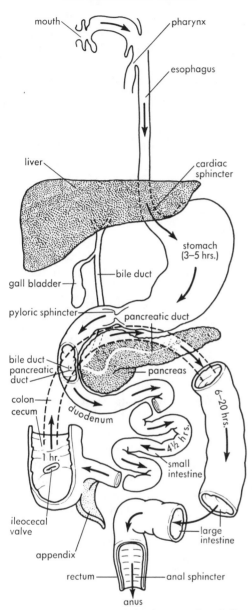

mouth
pharynx
esophagus
liver
cardiac sphincter
stomach (3–5 hrs.)
bile duct
gall bladder
pyloric sphincter
pancreatic duct
bile duct
pancreatic duct
pancreas
colon
cecum
duodenum
6–20 hrs.
4½ hrs.
1 hr.
small intestine
ileocecal valve
large intestine
appendix
rectum
anal sphincter
anus

This drawing indicates the duration of each digestive process. Food enters the mouth and is passed through the pharynx and esophagus into the stomach, where it is partly digested. The small intestine completes digestion and absorbs digested food. The large intestine absorbs excess water. Indigestible residue collects in the rectum for later disposal.

heavy in fats and rich foods. Thus, a meal that might take us 15 minutes to eat, may take up to 20 times as long to pass from the stomach into the small intestine. This decelerating of food's rate of passage has two very significant results: first, it allows time for the food-processing activities within the stomach; and second, it releases food (in a mushy form called *chyme*) in small, well-spaced amounts that can be efficiently handled by the small intestine.

Although the stomach is not an absolutely essential organ—a person can live a full life with part or even all of it removed—it is a tremendous convenience. Without a stomach, frequent, carefully selected, well-chewed small feedings rather than "three square meals a day" are necessary so as not to overburden the small intestine, which can handle only a small quantity of food, well-mashed, at one time. If too much food goes directly to the small intestine, only so much nourishment (carbohydrates, proteins, fats) per meal can be supplied to the body, with the result that we would be weak from hunger after going a few hours without eating.

It will come as no surprise to know that the food processing done in the stomach is both mechanical and chemical. The three layers of crisscrossing muscles in the stomach walls are rarely still. They contract and relax continually, squeezing, pummeling, and mixing the stomach's contents into chyme. So active and relentless is the stomach's muscular activity that it actually "chews up" pieces of food that have been swallowed too hastily.

Stomach Chemicals

The various chemicals found in the stomach are produced and secreted into the stomach cavity by some 40 million gland cells that line the interior stomach walls. The constant wiggling and jouncing of the stomach helps to mix these chemicals thoroughly into the food. Each of the chemicals is secreted by a special type of cell and has a specific function. They include the digestive enzymes pepsin, rennin, and lipase; hydrochloric acid; and watery mucus.

A look at the special assignments of rennin, pepsin, hydrochloric acid, and mucus—and how they interact with and depend upon one another—provides a good glimpse into the elegant and complex chemical events that occur when the stomach encounters a swallow of food.

RENNIN AND PEPSIN: Rennin, well known to cheese-makers, has essentially one task: to turn milk into milk curds. But the curds are not ready to pass on to the small intestine until they are further dismantled by *pepsin*. Pepsin has other duties as well: one of them is to begin the breakdown of proteins. But pepsin can only begin to split up protein foods after they have been worked on by *hydrochloric acid.*

HYDROCHLORIC ACID: Hydrochloric acid is a corrosive substance and, except in very dilute strengths, could quite literally eat away the lining of the stomach. (This is apparently what happens in cases of gastric ulcers.) Mucus secretions, with the help of fluids in the food itself, dilute the hydrochloric acid to a point where (in a normal stomach) it is rendered harmless. Even so, the normal, healthy condition inside our stomach is slightly acid. The slight acidity of the stomach serves to inhibit the growth of organisms such as bacteria.

The Small Intestine

By the time food-turned-chyme gets through the pyloric sphincter, it has already traveled about two-and-a-half feet: about 6 inches from lips to epiglottis; 10 or 12 inches down the esophagus; and about a foot through the stomach. But at this point it has actually traveled less than one-tenth of the gastrointestinal (GI) tract, and the longest stretch lies just ahead: the 20-plus feet of the small intestine, so named because of its relatively small one-to-two inch diameter. The preparation of food particles to pass through the walls of the GI tract is completed in the small intestine—almost completed, in fact, before the chyme has traveled the first foot of the small intestine.

By the time it leaves the small intestine, chyme has given up virtually all its nutrients. In other words, the process called *absorption* or *assimilation* has taken place: the nutrients have left the GI tract for other parts of the body via the circulating blood and lymph. What passes on to the large intestine is principally waste and water.

The small intestine is somewhat arbitrarily divided into three sections: the *duodenum*, the *jejunum*, and the *ileum*.

The Duodenum

Within this horseshoe loop, eight to ten inches long and about two inches in diameter, more chemical interactions are concentrated than in any other section of the GI tract. One of the first jobs in the duodenum is to neutralize the acidity of the chyme. The final steps of digestion, and the absorption of food through the intestinal lining, proceed best in a slightly alkaline environment.

The alkaline juices needed to neutralize the acidity of the chyme come mainly from the liver in the form of bile. Bile produced by the liver but not needed immediately in the duodenum is stored in concentrated form in the gall bladder, a pouchlike, three-inch-long organ. On signal from the autonomic nervous system, the membranous muscular walls of the gall bladder contract, squeezing concentrated, highly alkaline bile into a short duct that leads to the duodenum. Bile components are indispensable for the digestion and absorption of stubborn fatty materials.

Through a duct from the pancreas, a host of pancreatic enzymes, capable of splitting apart large, tough molecules of carbohydrate, protein, and fat, enters the duodenum. These digestive enzymes manufactured by the pancreas are the most powerful in the GI tract.

What triggers the production of bile and pancreatic juice for the duodenum? Apparently, it is a two-step process involving hormones.

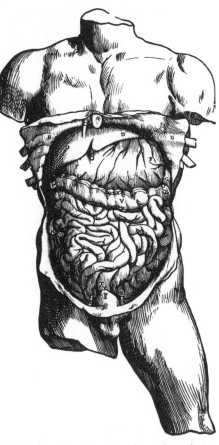

This 16th-century drawing shows the relative positions of the liver (marked D), stomach (F), and intestines.

When the stomach walls secrete hydrochloric acid on the arrival of food, hormones are released; they travel to the liver and pancreas with instructions to step up their production of digestive juices.

Still other strong enzymes are secreted by the walls of the duodenum and join the bile and pancreatic enzymes in the duodenum.

Thus, in the not quite foot-long tube of the duodenum, the final breakdown of food—digestion—reaches a dramatic climax. The nutrients in the food eaten some hours ago have almost all been reduced to molecules small enough to be absorbed through the intestinal walls into the bloodstream. Carbohydrates are reduced to simpler sugars; proteins to amino acids; and fats to fatty acids and glycerol.

Some absorption of these nutrients occurs in the duodenum, but the far greater proportion takes place in the next two, longer sections of the small intestine: the eight- to ten-foot jejunum and the twelve-foot ileum. Likewise, some oversize food molecules that get past the duodenum may be digested further along in their passage through the small intestine.

The Jejunum

As peristalsis pushes the nutrient broth out of the duodenum and into the first reaches of the jejunum, a gradual change in the appearance of the intestinal lining is evident. Greater and greater number of *villi* —microscopic, hairlike structures— sprout from the already bumpy walls of the intestinal lining into the GI tube.

THE VILLI: The villi (singular, *villus*) have the primary responsibility for absorbing amino acids (from protein), sugars (from carbohydrates), and fatty acids and glycerol (from fats) from the digested contents of the small intestine, and starting them on their way to other parts of the body. What the villi do not remove from the chyme—such as the cellulose fragments of fruits and vegetables—passes on to the large intestine in a thin, watery soup almost completely lacking in nutritional value.

Gland cells near the bottom of a villus secrete various enzymes, mucus, and other substances that perform digestive "mop-up operations" along the whole length of the small intestine.

The Ileum

In this third and final 12-foot section of the small intestine, villi line the walls in such profusion that the intestinal lining resembles, under moderate magnification, nothing so much as a plush, velvety carpet. The greatest numbers of the estimated five or six million villi in the small intestine are found along the lining of the ileum, making it the primary absorption site of the GI tract.

Also adding to the ileum's absorption efficiency is its gradually narrowing diameter (just one inch at its junction with the large intestine), which helps to keep the chyme always in close contact with the swishing villi. The end of the ileum is marked by the *ileocecal valve,* beyond which lies the first bulge of the large intestine, the *cecum.*

Principally because of vigorous peristaltic contractions and relaxations, the walls of the small intestine are always moving like the walls within some spasmodically flexing, nightmarish tunnel. Attached to the intestinal walls, the villi, too, are always in restless motion: waving and thrashing, protracting and retracting, even growing thinner or fatter.

Although the entire distance through the small intestine, from the pyloric sphincter to the ileocecal valve at the junction with the large intestine, is only a bit over 20 feet, the villi give the small intestine's internal lining a relatively gigantic surface area—over 100 square feet. This is about five times the surface area of our body's skin. Of course, the greatly enlarged surface area gives the small intestine lining that much more space in which to absorb nutrients.

The small intestine is supported in the abdomen by a fan-shaped web of tissues called the *mesentery.* Attached at the back of the abdomen, the mesentery connects to the small intestine at various points, and yet allows it some freedom to squirm and sway—much like the V network of ropes that attaches either end of a hammock to a tree. Nerve fibers and blood vessels also reach the small intestine via the mesentery.

The Liver, Gall Bladder, and Pancreas

These three organs all share a common function—sending digestive substances to the duodenum—although, except in the case of the gall bladder, it is not their only function. Lying outside the GI tract proper, they nevertheless are indispensable in the processes of digestion and absorption. Digestive fluids from all three converge like tributaries of a river at the common bile duct, and their flow from there into the duodenum is controlled by a sphincter muscle-ring separating the duodenum and common bile duct.

From the liver, bile drips into the *hepatic duct,* which soon meets the *cystic duct* arriving from the gall bladder. Converging, they form one duct, the *common bile duct,* which meets the *pancreatic duct,* carrying enzymatic fluid from the pancreas. Like a smaller river meeting a larger one, the pancreatic duct loses its

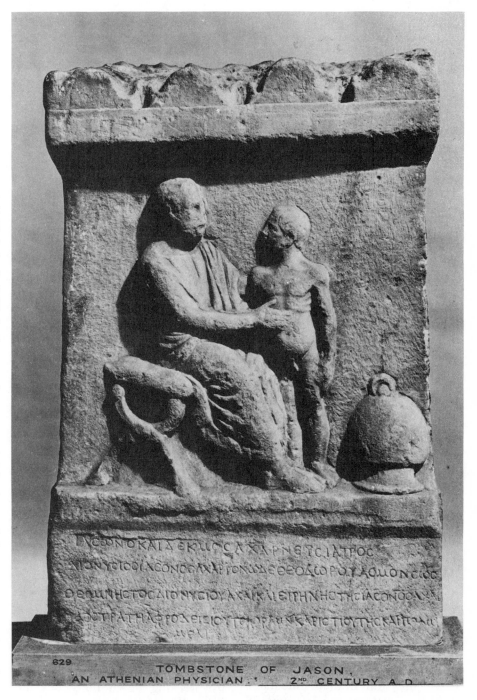

In a Greek sculpture from the 2nd century A.D., a doctor uses his trained sense of touch to examine a patient for a liver ailment. Throughout history, the relationship between doctor and patient has been important.

own name at this confluence and becomes part of the common bile duct, which empties on demand into the duodenum. When the sphincter of the bile duct is closed, bile from the liver is forced to back up into the cystic duct, and eventually into the gall bladder. There it is stored and concentrated until needed, when it flows back down the cystic duct.

The Liver

Four pounds of highly efficient chemical-processing tissues, the liver is the largest solid organ in the body. You can locate it by placing your left hand over your right, lowermost ribs; your hand then just about covers the area of the liver. More than any other organ, the liver enables our bodies to benefit from the food we eat. Without it, digestion would be impossible, and the conversion of food into living cells and energy practically nonexistent. Insofar as they affect our body's handling of food—all the many processes that go by the collective name of nutrition—the liver's functions can be roughly divided into those that break down food molecules and those that build up or reconstitute these nutrients into a form that the body can use or store efficiently.

BREAKING DOWN FOOD MOLECULES: Bile, as we have seen, assists in the destruction of large food molecules in the small intestine, enabling absorption of nutrients by the villi. Bile acts to increase alkalinity, breaking down big fat molecules; stimulates peristalsis; and prevents food from putrefying within the digestive tract. Unusable portions of the bile, destined to be eliminated as waste, include excess cholesterol, fats, and various components of dead disintegrated cells. Pigments from dead cells in bile give feces their normal, dark, yellow-brown color. Other cell fragments in bile, especially iron from disintegrated red blood cells, are reclaimed from the intestines and eventually make their way via the bloodstream to other parts of the body, where they are built into new cells.

RECONSTITUTING NUTRIENTS: Oddly enough, the liver rebuilds some of the proteins and carbohydrates that the bile has just so effectively helped to break down in the digestive tract. But this is really not so strange as it sounds. The types of proteins and carbohydrates that can be used by man for cell-rebuilding and energy are usually somewhat different in fine structure from those in food. Thus, the liver receives the basic building blocks of proteins and carbohydrates—amino acids and sugars—and with them builds up molecules and cells that can be utilized by the human body. The amino acids and sugars reach the liver through the *portal vein,* which is the great collection tube for nutrient-carrying blood returning from capillaries along the stomach and small intestine.

GLYCOGEN AND GLUCOSE: In the liver, sugars from the small intestine are converted into a special substance called *glycogen;* amino acids are made available as needed for building new cells to replace the cells that are always naturally dying in a healthy, normal body. Glycogen, simply speaking, is the liver's solution to a difficult space and storage problem. The form of carbohydrate the body can use best is a sugar called *glucose,* but the liver isn't large enough to store the necessary amount of glucose. The answer is glycogen, a tidy, compact sugar molecule that the liver can store in great quantities. When a call comes from any part of the body for glucose, the liver quickly converts some glycogen to glucose and releases it into the bloodstream. By this mechanism, healthy blood-sugar levels are maintained.

The liver also builds up human fats from fatty acids and glycerol, packs them off to storage, then reverses the process when necessary by breaking down body fats into forms that can serve as fuel to be burned by the body for energy.

OTHER FUNCTIONS: In addition to its functions closely related to digestion and nutrition, the liver also serves as a storehouse and processor of vitamins and minerals—it is, in fact, the manufacturer of vitamin A. It can remove many toxic substances from the blood and render their poisons harmless. It picks up spent red blood cells from the circulation and dismantles them; and it continually manufactures new blood elements.

The liver is also a manufacturing site for *cholesterol,* a substance belonging to the class of body chemicals called steroids. Above-normal levels of cholesterol in the blood have been linked to hardening of the arteries and heart disease; but cholesterol in the proper amounts is needed by almost every tissue in the body. Some brain and spinal tissues, for example, have cholesterol as one of their main structural components.

With all these vital chemical activities and more, the liver might be expected to be a most delicate and fragile organ. In a sense it is: minor liver damage from one cause or another is thought to be fairly common. But what saves our lives (and us) is that we have a great deal more of it than we need for a normal healthy life. Before symptoms of a liver deficiency appear, over 50 percent of the liver cells may be destroyed. Furthermore, the liver has a great capacity for regeneration, rebuilding diseased tissues with new liver cells.

The Gall Bladder

Bile stored in the gall bladder is much more concentrated and thicker than bile that is fresh from the liver. This allows the three-inch gall bladder to store a great deal of bile components. But the thickening process can also create problems in the form of extremely painful gallstones, which are dried, crystallized bile. Fortunately, the entire gall bladder can be removed with little or no lasting ill effect. All that is missing is a small storage sac for bile.

The Pancreas

This manufacturer of powerful digestive enzymes, only six inches long, resembles a branchlet heavily laden with ripe berries. Its important role in digestion is often overshadowed by the fact that it also manufactures the hormone *insulin*. The pancreas cells that manufacture digestive enzymes are completely different from those that manufacture insulin. The latter are grouped into little clusters called the *islets of Langerhans*, which are discussed under *The Endocrine Glands*, p. 36.

The Large Intestine

The large intestine, also called the large bowel, is shaped like a great, lumpy, drooping question mark—arching, from its beginning at the ileocecal valve, over the folds of the small intestine, then curving down and descending past more coiled small intestine to the anus, which marks the end of the GI tract. From ileocecal valve to anus, the large intestine is five to six feet in length.

The junction between the ileum and the *cecum*, the first section of the large intestine, occurs very low in the abdomen, normally on the right-hand side. The cecum is a bowl-like receptacle at the bottom of the colon, the longest section of the large intestine.

Just below the entrance of the ileum, a dead-end tube dangles down from the cecum. This is the *appendix vermiformis* (Latin, "worm-shaped appendage") commonly known as the appendix. Three to six inches long and one-third inch in diameter, the appendix may get jammed with stray pieces of solid food, become infected, swell, and rupture, spewing infection into the abdominal cavity. This is why early diagnosis of *appendicitis* and removal *(appendectomy)* are critically important.

SECTIONS OF THE COLON: The colon is divided into three sections by pronounced *flexures*, or bends, where the colon makes almost right-angle changes of direction. Above the bowl of the cecum, the *ascending colon* rises almost vertically for about a foot and a half.

Then there is a flexure in the colon, after which the *transverse colon* travels horizontally for a couple of feet along a line at navel height. At another flexure, the colon turns vertically down again, giving the name of *descending colon* to this approximately two feet of large intestine. At the end of the descending colon, the large intestine executes an S-shaped curve, the *sigmoid flexure*, after which the remaining several inches of large intestine are known as the *rectum.*

Some people confuse the terms rectum and anus: the rectum refers specifically to the last section of the large intestinal tube, between sigmoid flexure and the anal sphincters, while the anus refers only to the opening controlled by the outlet valves of the large intestine. These valves consist of two ringlike voluntary muscles called anal sphincters.

Any solid materials that pass into the large intestine through the ileocecal valve (which prevents backflow into the small intestine) are usually indigestible, such as cellulose, or substances that have been broken down in the body and blood in the normal process of cell death and renewal, such as some bile components. But what the cecum mainly receives is water.

FUNCTIONS OF THE LARGE INTESTINE: The principal activity of the large intestine—other than as a channel for elimination of body wastes—is as a temporary storage area for water, which is then reabsorbed into the circulation through the walls of the colon. Villi are absent in the large intestine, and peristalsis is much less vigorous than in the small intestine.

As water is absorbed, the contents of the large intestine turn from a watery soup into the semisolid feces. Meanwhile, bacteria—which colonize the normal colon in countless millions—have begun to work on and decompose the remaining solid materials. These bacteria do no harm as long as they remain inside the large intestine, and the eliminated feces is heavily populated with them. Nerve endings in the large intestine signal the brain that it is time for a bowel movement.

THE PERITONEUM: Lining the entire abdominal cavity, as well as the digestive and other abdominal organs, is a thin, tough, lubricated membrane called the *peritoneum*. In addition to protecting and supporting the abdominal organs, the peritoneum permits these organs to slip and slide against each other without any harm from friction. The peritoneum also contains blood and lymph vessels that serve the digestive organs. See *Diseases of the Digestive System*, p. 373.

THE RESPIRATORY SYSTEM AND THE LUNGS

The heart, by its construction and shape, tells us a great deal about the lungs and respiration.

Interaction Between Heart and Lungs

The heart is divided vertically by a wall called a septum into right (your right) and left parts. The right part is smaller than the left: its muscles only have to pump blood a few inches to the lungs, while the muscles of the left half have to pump blood to the whole body.

The function of the right half of our heart is to receive oxygen-poor blood from the veins of the body. Venous blood empties into the top-right chamber, or right atrium, of the heart, and the right ventricle pumps that oxygen-poor blood (via the pulmonary artery) to the lungs, where the blood, passing through minute capillaries, picks up oxygen.

From the lungs, the oxygen-rich blood flows back into the heart's left atrium via the pulmonary veins; and from the left atrium, the oxygen-rich blood drains into the left ventricle, from whence it is pumped via the aorta to the body.

The blood pumped to the lungs by the right ventricle is oxygen-poor blood: it has given up its oxygen to the cells that need it around the body. But this "used blood" is rich in something else—carbon dioxide. As the body's cells have taken oxygen, they have given up carbon dioxide to the circulating blood. For both oxygen and carbon dioxide, the "carrier" has been *hemoglobin,* a complex iron-protein substance that is part of our red blood cells.

CAPILLARIES AND ALVEOLI: The pulmonary artery carrying this lung-bound blood soon branches into smaller and smaller vessels, and eventually into microscopic capillaries which reach into every crook and crevice of the lungs.

In the lungs, the walls of the capillaries touch the walls of equally microscopic structures called

THE ALVEOLI

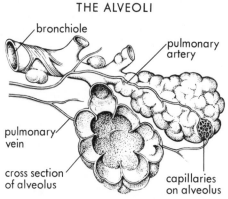

The branches of the pulmonary tree terminate in the alveoli, grapelike clusters of air sacs covered by capillaries, where the gaseous exchange occurs.

alveoli (singular, *alveolus*). The alveoli are the smallest air sacs of the lungs. These tiny, expandable air cells are the destination of every breath of air we take. Estimates of the total number of alveoli in both our lungs vary between 300 million and a billion—in any case, we normally have several hundred million of them.

CARBON DIOXIDE AND OXYGEN EXCHANGE: Where they meet, the membranous walls of both a capillary and an alveolus are both about as thin as any living tissue can be—a thickness that is only the width of one cell. Under such conditions, the carbon dioxide carried by the hemoglobin in our blood to the lungs diffuses (as tiny gaseous "bubbles") across both the wall of a capillary and the wall of an alveolus.

Once inside the sac of the alveolus, carbon dioxide is ready to be exhaled from the body by "breathing out." One indication of just how well this system works is the fact that the air we exhale has roughly 100 times more carbon dioxide than the air we breathe in.

At the same time that hemoglobin dumps carbon dioxide at the interface of the capillary and alveolus walls, it picks up the oxygen made available from inhaled fresh air that has reached the alveoli. The molecular oxygen bubbles cross the

membranes in the same way—but in the opposite direction—as the carbon dioxide.

Hemoglobin in the capillaries picks up the oxygen and carries it via veins leading away from the lungs, to the left atrium of the heart.

ESSENTIAL ROLE OF MOISTURE: The alveolar membranes are supplied with a thin film of moisture that is absolutely indispensable to the exchange of gases in the lungs. As in so many of our body's reactions, our evolutionary descent from water-dwelling ancestors is revealed by the wet environment demanded if our lungs are to supply our body with oxygen.

Respiration at the One-Cell Level

Oxygen molecules, then, are carried to the body's cells by the hemoglobin of the arterial blood pumped by the heart's left ventricle. But how does a cell take oxygen from the blood and use it?

Exchange of Gases

The transfer of oxygen from blood to cell is accomplished in much the same way as the exchanges that take place in the lungs. The circulating arterial blood has a surplus of oxygen; the cells have a surplus of carbon dioxide. When the oxygen-rich blood reaches the finest capillaries, only the very thinnest membranous walls (of cell and capillary) separate it from the carbon-dioxide-rich cells. As in the lungs, both these gases (dissolved in water) diffuse through these thinnest of membranes: the oxygen into the cell, the carbon dioxide into the blood for eventual deposit in the alveoli, and exhalation.

Within the cell, the oxygen is needed so that food, the body's fuel, can be burned to produce energy. At the cellular level, the most convenient and common food is a fairly simple carbohydrate molecule called glucose.

Conversion of Carbohydrates Into Energy

Energy is locked into a carbohydrate molecule such as glucose in the form of chemical bonds between its atoms. If one of these bonds is broken—say, a bond holding together a carbon and a hydrogen atom—a bit of pent-up energy is released as if, in a stalemated tug of war, the rope suddenly broke and both teams went hurtling off a few feet in opposite directions. This is precisely the effect of respiration within a cell: the cell "breaks the ropes" holding together a carbohydrate molecule. The result is the release of energy—either as body heat or to power other activities within the cell.

It is useful—but a somewhat misleading oversimplification—to consider cellular respiration as a type of burning, or combustion. When a typical cell burns food, a carbohydrate molecule (glucose) together with molecules of oxygen are changed into carbon dioxide and water. During this change, chemical energy is released—energy that has been trapped, as we have seen, in the carbohydrate molecule. That complex, energy-rich molecule has been dismantled into the simpler molecules of carbon dioxide (CO_2) and water (H_2O). Oxygen is necessary here just as it is in fiery combustion. But the energy released here, instead of rushing out as heat and flame, is used to power the living activities of the cell.

This description of cellular respiration is all right in principle, but the trouble is this: if it all happened at once—if carbohydrate was so abruptly dismantled, split up at one stroke to water and carbon dioxide—such a great amount of energy would be released that the cell would simply burn itself up. As one biologist has said, the cell would be in exactly the same position as a wood furnace built of wood.

What protects the cell is its army of enzymes. These remarkable protein molecules combine briefly with energy-containing food molecules, causing them to break down bit by bit, so that energy is released gradually rather than all at once.

Carbon Dioxide— Precious Waste

In most of our minds, oxygen tends to be the hero of respiration and carbon dioxide the villain or at least the undesirable waste gas. This isn't really a fair picture. While it is true that too much carbon dioxide would act as a poison in our body, it is also true that we must always have a certain amount of the gas dissolved in our tissues. If we did not, two potentially fatal events could occur. First, our blood chemistry, especially its delicate acid-alkali balance, would get completely out of control. Second—and something of a paradox—the body's whole automatic system of regulating breathing would be knocked out.

It is the level of carbon dioxide in the bloodstream that controls our breathing. This level is continuously being monitored by the autonomic nervous system, specifically by the lower brain's "breathing center" in the medulla at the top of the spinal cord. When the level of carbon dioxide in our body goes above a certain level, signals from the medulla force us to breathe. Almost everybody has played, "How long can you hold your breath?" and knows that, past a certain point, it becomes impossible *not* to breathe. When you are holding your breath, the unexhaled carbon dioxide rapidly builds up in your system until the breathing center is besieged with signals that say "Breathe!" And you do.

Our Big Breathing Muscle: The Diaphragm

What gets air into and out of our lungs? The answer may seem as obvious as breathing in and breathing out. But except for those rare instances when we consciously regulate our breathing pattern—which doctors call "force breathing"—we do not decide when to inhale and when to exhale. And even when we do force-breathe, it is not primarily the action of opening the mouth and gulping in air, then blowing it out, that gets air down the windpipe and into the alveoli of the lungs. The main work of inhaling and exhaling is done by the contraction and relaxation of the big helmet-shaped muscle on which the lungs rest and which marks the "floor" of the chest or thoracic cavity and the "ceiling" of the abdominal cavity. This muscle is the *diaphragm.*

It is the diaphragm that causes the lungs to swell and fill with fresh air, then partially collapse to expel used gases. The muscles and tendons of the sinewy diaphragm are attached at the back to the spinal column, at the front to the breastbone (*sternum*), and at the lower sides to the lower ribs.

The diaphragm contracts and relaxes on orders from the brain's breathing center, orders that are carried along the pathways of the autonomic nervous system. When the medulla sends messages to the breathing muscles to contract, the diaphragm is pulled downward, en-

THE DIAPHRAGM

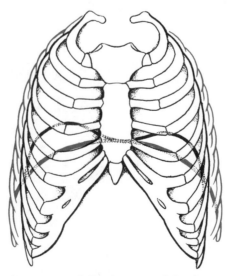

The positions of the rib cage and diaphragm are seen during the inspiration of breath (in color) and during its expiration (in black). Thoracic volume increases during inspiration as the diaphragm is stretched.

larging the space filled by the lungs. This creates a temporary partial vacuum, into which air rushes, inflating and expanding the lungs. When the diaphragm relaxes, the lung space is reduced, pushing air out.

OTHER BREATHING MUSCLES: The diaphragm muscle's leading role in breathing is supported by several other muscles that play minor parts. Among these are the *intercostal muscles* between the ribs that give the rib cage a slight push upward and outward, enlarging the thoracic cavity, and the *serratus muscles*, which are mainly muscular sheaths along the ribs, to which other muscles are attached.

The Trachea and the Lungs

The right lung (your right) is somewhat bigger than the left. The lungs hang in the chest attached to the windpipe or *trachea*.

The Trachea

The trachea itself branches off at the back of the throat, or *pharynx*, where the epiglottis prevents food from entering the trachea and channels swallowed food along its proper route, the esophagus. The top part of the trachea forms the voice box or *larynx*, made up of vocal cords—actually two flaps of cartilage, muscle, and membranous tissue that protrude into the windpipe—whose vibrations in reponse to air exhaled from the lungs give us our voice.

Below the larynx, the trachea descends five or six inches to a spot just about directly behind your breastbone, where the first of many thousands of branchings into *bronchi, bronchioles*, and alveoli occurs. C-shaped rings of cartilage give the trachea both support and flexibility. Running your finger down the front of your neck, you can feel the bumps made by the cartilage rings.

Above the base of the trachea in mid-chest the lungs arch on either side like giant butterfly wings, then fall to fill out the bottom of each side of the thoracic cavity.

The Pleural Membranes

Both lungs are encased in moist, clinging, tissue-thin membrane called the *pleura*, which also lines the inside of the thoracic cavity where it comes into contact with the pleural coating of the lungs. The slippery pleural membranes hold tightly to each other, because there is an air lock or vacuum between them, but at the same time are free to slide over each other. The principle is the same as that illustrated by moistening the surfaces of two pieces of plate glass and placing the moistened surfaces together: the two pieces of glass will slide over each other but will resist being pried apart, because a partial vacuum exists between them.

THE PLEURAL CAVITY: The vacuum space between the pleura of the lung and the pleura of the thoracic cavity—although it is normally not a space at all—is called the *pleural cavity*. Each lung has its own pleural membrane: that of one lung does not interconnect with the other, so that one pleura may be injured without affecting the other.

It is extremely fortunate for us that the pleural linings both stick fast and can slide along each other's surfaces. Although the lungs are virtually without muscle, they are extremely elastic and in their natural condition are stretched fairly taut, held to the sides of the thoracic cavity by the suction of the pleura.

COLLAPSED LUNG: Should this suction be broken and the pleural linings pull apart, the lung would shrink up like a deflated balloon. Such a condition, caused by the rush of outside air into the pleural cavity, is known medically as *pneumothorax* and causes a lung

THE RESPIRATORY SYSTEM

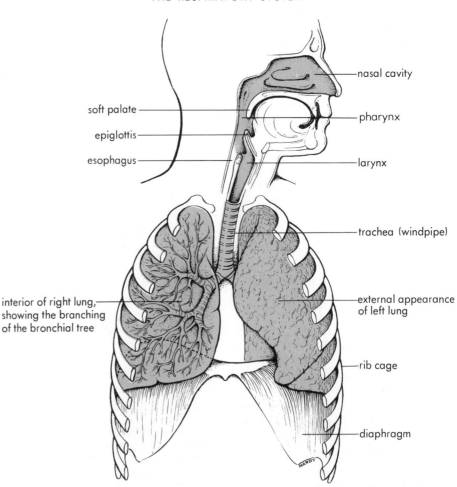

soft palate

epiglottis

esophagus

nasal cavity

pharynx

larynx

trachea (windpipe)

interior of right lung, showing the branching of the bronchial tree

external appearance of left lung

rib cage

diaphragm

collapse. Violent injuries such as gun and stab wounds, various lung diseases, and obstructions of the breathing tubes can cause a lung or portion of a lung to collapse.

In the surgical procedure called *artificial pneumothorax,* a physician deliberately injects air between the pleural linings to collapse a portion of a lung. This is done to rest a lung in severe diseases such as tuberculosis, or to control heavy bleeding within the thoracic cavity.

PLEURISY: The intense chest pains called *pleurisy* are caused by inflammation of the pleura. The pleural linings lose their slipperiness and the increased friction stimulates pain receptors in the pleural lining of the chest. There are, however, no pain receptors in the lungs' pleural linings nor in the lungs themselves: this is why pain is not an early warning signal of lung cancer.

Structure of the Lungs

THE BRONCHI: Just behind the breastbone and just in front of the heart, the trachea divides into the right bronchus and the left bronchus, leading respectively to the right and left lungs. These are the primary two *bronchi* or *bronchial tubes.* Each is the main trunk of a bronchial tree that serves its respective lung.

Soon after leaving the trachea, each bronchus branches repeatedly into smaller tubes called *bronchioles,* which in turn branch into alveolar ducts, which terminate finally with the hundreds of millions of microscopic air sacs called alveoli, discussed at the beginning of this section. The alveoli are the site of the all-important exchange of carbon dioxide and oxygen.

LOBES AND SEGMENTS: The larger right lung has three distinctive sections, or *lobes*—upper, middle, and lower. The left lung has only an upper and lower lobe. The lobes themselves are divided into smaller segments. Medically, these lobes and segments are important because they are somewhat independent of each other and can be damaged or removed surgically, as in operations for lung cancer, usually without damaging the function of adjacent, healthy segments or lobes.

The fact that a lung segment, lobe, or even an entire lung can be removed implies that we have plenty of reserve lung tissue, and this is indeed the case. When we are at rest, we use only about one-tenth of our total lung capacity. The total surface area exposed within our lungs to outside air is, amazingly, 600 square feet. This compares to a mere 20 square feet of skin surface. To appreciate the incredibly intricate, lacelike finery of the lungs' structure, we need only know that those 600 square feet of surface area are contained within two organs that together weigh only two-and-a-half pounds.

Oxygen Requirements

How much air do we breathe, and how much oxygen do we absorb into our body from the air? A normal, moderately active person breathes in and out (a complete respiration or breath cycle) about 18 times a minute; that is, the diaphragm contracts and relaxes 18 times a minute, or something over 25,000 times every day. At about four-fifths of a pint of air per breath cycle, this means that we inhale and exhale about 20,000 pints, or 10,000 quarts, or 2,500 gallons of air every day.

Only a very small proportion of this volume is oxygen that finds its way into our bloodstream: about a pint every minute in normal, quiet breathing, a little over 1,400 pints, or 700 quarts, or 175 gallons of oxygen every day. The amount of oxygen our lungs are capable of delivering to our body, however, varies tremendously: during sleep a person may need only a half-pint of oxygen per minute, half the average, while the lungs of a hard-driving athlete striving to break the mile record can deliver up to five quarts to the bloodstream—ten times the average.

At any given time, there are about two quarts of oxygen circulating in our blood. This is why a stoppage of breathing has an upper time limit of about four minutes before it causes irreversible damage or death. With our body needing about a pint of oxygen every minute for normal functioning, we have about four minutes before we use up the oxygen dissolved in our blood and other tissues.

Pollution Control— Filters, Cleaners, and Traps

Air pollution being what it is these days, it is fortunate that we have several natural devices that serve to filter out and wash away most of the impurities in the air we inhale.

Air gets into the lungs from outside about equally well via the nose or mouth. The mouth offers the advantage of getting more air in at a faster rate—absolutely a must if we have to push our body physically. But the nose has more and better equipment for cleaning air before it reaches the trachea. Via the mouth, air must only pass over a few mucous membranes and the tonsils, which can collect only so many germs and impurities.

NOSE FILTER SYSTEM: Air taken in through the nose, however, first meets the "guard hairs" (*vibrissae*) of the nostrils, and then must circulate through the nasal cavity, a kind of cavern framed by elaborate scroll-shaped bones called *turbinates,* and lined with mucus-secreting membranes and waving, hairlike fibers called *cilia.* Foreign particles are caught by the cilia and carried away by the mucus, which drains slowly down the back of the throat.

It would be nice to be able to ascribe an important function to the eight *paranasal sinuses,* four on either side of the nose: the headache and discomfort of sinusitis might then be more bearable. But these "holes in the head" seem to exist simply to cause us trouble; for example—swelling to close the nasal air passages, making it impossible to breathe, as recommended, through the nose.

FILTER SYSTEM BEYOND THE NOSE: The cleansing and filtering action started in the nose and mouth does not stop there, but is repeated wherever air travels along the air passages of the lungs. Cilia project inward from the walls of even the tiniest bronchioles of the lungs, and impurities are carried from the alveoli on films of mucus that move ever back toward the trachea for expulsion—as when we cough. See also *Diseases of the Respiratory System*, p. 386, and *Lung Disease*, p. 396.

THE ENDOCRINE GLANDS

Technically speaking, a gland is any cell or organ in our bodies that secretes some substance. In this broad sense, our liver is a gland, since one of its many functions is to secrete bile. So too, is the placenta that encloses a developing baby and supplies it with chemicals that assure normal growth. Even the brain has been shown by modern research to secrete special substances. But lymph glands are not considered true glands and are more correctly called lymph nodes.

Doctors divide the glands into two categories. *Endocrine glands* are also known as *ductless glands*, because they release their secretions directly into the bloodstream. *Exocrine glands*, by contrast, usually release their substances through a duct or tube. Exocrine glands include the sebaceous and sweat glands of the skin; the mammary or milk glands; the mucous glands, some of which moisten the digestive and respiratory tract; and the salivary glands, whose secretions soften food after it enters the mouth. The pancreas has both an endocrine and an exocrine function and structure.

Role of the Endocrine Glands

The *endocrine glands* have the all-important role of regulating our body's internal chemistry. The substances they secrete are complex compounds called *hormones,* or chemical messengers.

Together with the brain and nerves, the system of endocrine glands controls the body's activities. The nervous system, however, is tuned for rapid responses, enabling the body to make speedy adjustments to changing circumstances, internal and external. The endocrine glands, with some exceptions, like the adrenal, are more con-

THE ENDOCRINE GLANDS

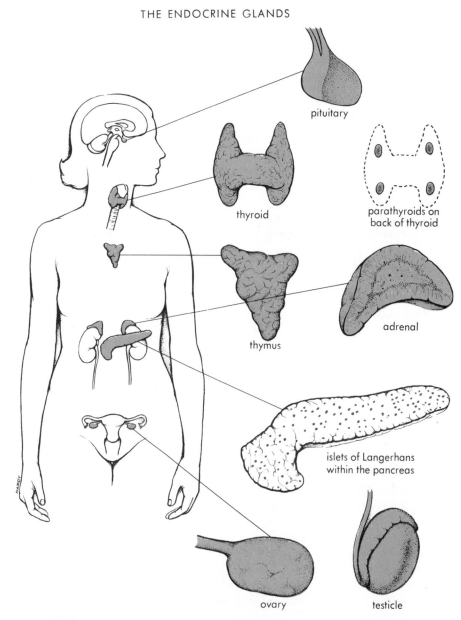

pituitary

thyroid

parathyroids on back of thyroid

thymus

adrenal

islets of Langerhans within the pancreas

ovary

testicle

cerned with the body's reactions over a longer period of time—from season to season, as it were. They regulate such processes as growth, levels of metabolism, fertility, and pregnancy.

For a group of tissues that exercise awesome power over our body's well-being, the endocrine glands are surprisingly small and inconspicuous—all of them together would weigh less than half a pound. Nor are they placed with any particular prominence in our body. They tend to be little lumps of tissue attached to or tucked behind grander bodily structures. Their power comes from the hormones they release into the bloodstream.

Scientists have discovered the exact chemical make-up of a number of these complex substances, have extracted several in pure form from living tissue, and have succeeded in making a few synthetically in the laboratory. This avenue of research, called *endocrinology,* has enabled doctors to treat persons suffering from certain endocrine gland disorders.

Hormones have been aptly described as chemical messengers. Their action, while still not completely understood, is that of catalysts. This means that the presence of a hormone (the name comes from a Greek word meaning "arouse to activity"), even in very small quantities, can affect the rate at which a chemical change occurs or otherwise stimulate a reaction, and without itself being affected. The hormone is a promoter, either of a positive or negative sort; it speeds up a process or slows it down.

The endocrine glands form an interdependent family. The functioning or malfunctioning of one can affect all the others.

The Pituitary—Master Gland

The *pituitary* is often called the master gland because the hormones it secretes play an active part in controlling the activities of all the other endocrine glands. This impressive power is wielded from two little bumps at the base of the brain, about midway between the ears at eye level. The two parts, or lobes, are connected by a tiny bridge of tissue, the three structures together being about the size of a small acorn. The lobe lying toward the front of the head is the *anterior lobe;* the one at the back, the *posterior lobe.* Each lobe is really an independent gland in itself, with its own quite distinct activities.

The Posterior Lobe and the Hypothalamus

The posterior lobe, so far as is known, does not make any of its own hormones, but serves as a storehouse for two hormones manufactured by the *hypothalamus,* located in the brain's cerebellum. The hypothalamus, apart from having a role in controlling the body's autonomic nervous system, also functions as an endocrine gland, secreting its own hormones, and as a connecting link between the brain's cerebral cortex and the pituitary gland.

The posterior lobe of the pituitary releases the two hormones it receives from the hypothalamus, called *vasopressin* and *oxytocin,* into the bloodstream. Vasopressin plays a role in the fluid balance of the body; oxytocin is thought to pace the onset and progress of labor during childbirth.

The Anterior Lobe

The anterior lobe secretes no less than six known hormones, five of which act as stimulators of hormone production by other endocrine glands. The sixth, identified as *somatotrophin* in medical textbooks, is more popularly known as the *growth-stimulating hormone* or simply as the growth hormone. It controls the rate of growth and multiplication of all the cells and tissues in our bodies—muscle, bone, and all our specialized organs.

GIGANTISM: In rare instances, during childhood, the pituitary releases too much or too little somatotrophin.

THE PITUITARY GLAND

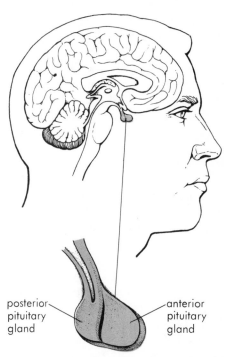

posterior pituitary gland

anterior pituitary gland

Anterior Pituitary Secretes:

Adrenocorticotrophic hormone (ACTH), acting on the adrenal cortex

Follicle-stimulating hormone, acting on the ovaries or the testes

Thyrotrophic hormone, acting on the thyroid gland

Luteotrophin, stimulating milk production in the female

Luteinizing hormone, stimulating testosterone production in the male and estrogen in the female

Growth hormone, stimulating skeletal and visceral growth

Posterior Pituitary Secretes:

Vasopressin, or antidiuretic hormone, raising blood pressure and acting on the kidneys

Oxytocin, causing contractions of the pregnant uterus

If too much is secreted, the result is an overstimulation of growth processes, causing a disorder known as *gigantism.* Victims of this disorder have been known to grow nine feet tall and weigh 500 pounds.

DWARFISM: If too little somatotrophin is secreted, *dwarfism* results. This pituitary-type dwarf, of which Tom Thumb was one, is different from a dwarf suffering from a disorder of the thyroid (another endocrine gland, discussed below). The pituitary dwarf is usually well-proportioned despite a miniature size, while the thyroid dwarf typically has short, deformed limbs.

Neither pituitary gigantism nor dwarfism affects basic intelligence. If oversecretion of somatotrophin occurs after full size has been reached—as, for example, because of a tumor affecting the pituitary, the condition known as *acromegaly* occurs. The bones enlarge abnormally, especially those of the hands, feet, and face.

ANTERIOR PITUITARY HORMONES: Of the five anterior pituitary hormones that regulate other endocrine glands, one affects the adrenal glands, one the thyroid, and the remaining three the sex glands or gonads (the testicles in men and the ovaries in women). Each is identified by a set of initials derived from its full name, as follows:

• *ACTH,* the *a*dreno*c*orti*c*otrophic *h*ormone, affects the production of hormones by the outer "bark" of the adrenal glands, called the *adrenal cortex.*

• *TSH,* the *t*hyroid-*s*timulating *h*ormone, also known as *thyrotrophin,* causes the thyroid gland to step up production of its hormone, *thyroxin.*

• *FSH,* the *f*ollicle-*s*timulating *h*ormone, spurs production in women of estrogen, a sex hormone produced by the ovaries; and in men, of sperm by the testicles. Follicle here refers to the *Graafian follicles* in the ovary, which contain developing female egg cells whose growth is also stimulated by FSH. Graafian follicles have approximate counterparts in the male—tiny pouches (seminal vesicles) on either side of the prostate gland that store mature sperm cells.

• *LH,* the *l*uteinizing *h*ormone, transforms a Graafian follicle, after the follicle has released a ripened egg cell, into a kind of tissue called *corpus luteum.* The corpus luteum, in turn, produces *progesterone,* a hormone that prepares the mucous membrane lining the uterus (the endometrium) to receive a fertilized egg.

• *LTH,* the *l*actogenic *h*ormone, or *luteotrophin,* stimulates the mother's mammary glands to produce milk; LTH also joins with LH in promoting the production of progesterone by the sex glands.

The last three hormones mentioned—follicle-stimulating, luteinizing, and lactogenic—are sometimes called the *gonadotrophic* hormones because they all stimulate activity of the gonads.

The Adrenal Glands

Resting like skull caps on the top of both kidneys are the two identical *adrenal glands.* Each has two distinct parts, secreting different hormones.

Adrenaline

The central internal portion of an adrenal gland is called the *medulla.* Its most potent contribution to our body is the hormone *adrenaline* (also called *epinephrine*). This is the hormone that, almost instantaneously, pours into our bloodsteam when we face a situation that calls for extraordinary physical reaction —or keeps us going past what we think to be our normal limit of endurance.

A surge of adrenaline into the bloodstream stimulates our body to a whole array of alarm reactions— accelerating the conversion of stored foods into quick energy; rais-

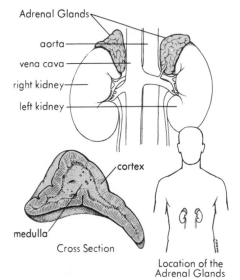

THE ADRENAL GLANDS

Adrenal Glands
aorta
vena cava
right kidney
left kidney
cortex
medulla
Cross Section
Location of the Adrenal Glands

ing the blood pressure; speeding up breathing; dilating the pupils of the eyes for more sensitive vision; and constricting the blood vessels, making them less vulnerable to bleeding.

Adrenaline provides a good example of the interdependence of the endocrine system. Its production stimulates the secretion of ACTH by the pituitary gland. And ACTH, as noted above, causes the adrenal cortex to accelerate production of its hormones. Some of these adrenal cortex hormones enable the body to call up the reserves of energy it does not normally need. For example, body proteins are not usually a source of quick energy, but in an emergency situation, the adrenal cortex hormones can convert them to energy-rich sugar compounds.

The Corticoids

There are some 30 different hormones, called the *corticoids,* manufactured in the adrenal cortex— the outer layer of the adrenal. A few of these influence male and female sexual characteristics, supplementing the hormones produced in the gonads. The others fall into two general categories: those that affect the body's metabolism (rate of energy use), and those that regulate the composition of blood and internal fluids. Without the latter hormones, for example, the kidneys could not maintain the water-salt balance that provides the most suitable environment for our cells and tissues at any given time.

Corticoids also influence the formation of antibodies against viruses, bacteria, and other disease-causing agents.

Extracts or laboratory preparations of corticoids, such as the well-known cortisone compounds, were found in the 1950s to be almost "miracle" medicines. They work dramatically to reduce pain, especially around joints, and hasten the healing of skin inflammations. Prolonged use, however, can cause serious side effects.

THE PANCREAS AND THE ISLETS OF LANGERHANS

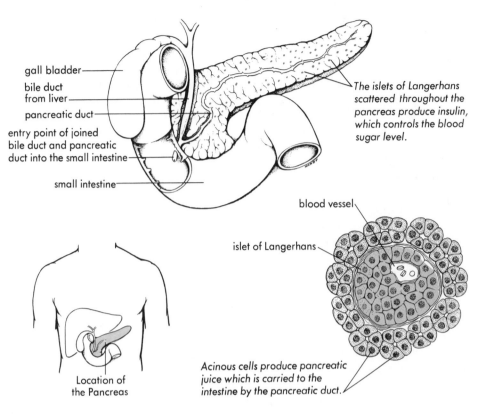

gall bladder

bile duct from liver

pancreatic duct

entry point of joined bile duct and pancreatic duct into the small intestine

small intestine

The islets of Langerhans scattered throughout the pancreas produce insulin, which controls the blood sugar level.

blood vessel

islet of Langerhans

Acinous cells produce pancreatic juice which is carried to the intestine by the pancreatic duct.

Location of the Pancreas

The Islets of Langerhans

Strewn at random throughout the pancreas are hundreds of thousands of tiny clusters of cells. Each of them, when seen under a powerful microscope, forms an "islet" of its own, similar to the other distinct islets, but markedly different from the pancreatic tissue surrounding it. These are the *islets of Langerhans,* named after the German scientist who first reported their existence in 1869. Each of these little cell clumps—up to two million or more of them—is a microscopic endocrine gland.

They secrete the hormone *insulin,* and the disease that occurs if they are not functioning properly is *diabetes mellitus.*

Actually, the islets of Langerhans produce not only insulin, but also a related hormone called *glucagon.* Both regulate the amount of sugar (glucose) that is present in the bloodstream and the rate at which it is used by the body's cells and tis-

sues. Glucose supplies the energy for life and living processes.

When insulin and glucagon are not in sufficient supply, the cells' ability to absorb and use blood sugar is restricted, and much of the sugar passes unutilized out of the body in urine. Since the body's ability to obtain energy from food is one of the very foundations of life, diabetes calls for the most careful treatment.

One of the great advances of 20th century medicine has been the pharmaceutical manufacture of insulin and its wide availability to diabetics. With regulated doses of insulin, a diabetic can now lead a normal life. See *Diabetes Mellitus,* p. 409, for a full discussion of this disease.

The Thyroid Gland

The *thyroid gland* folds around the front and either side of the trachea (windpipe), at the base of the neck, just below the larynx. It resembles a

somewhat large, stocky butterfly facing downward toward the chest. See the illustration of *The Endocrine Glands,* p. 36.

Thyroxin

The thyroid hormone, *thyroxin,* is a complex protein-type chemical containing, along with various other elements, a large percentage of iodine. Like a number of other hormones manufactured by the endocrine glands, thyroxin affects various steps in the body's metabolism—in particular, the rate at which our cells and tissues use inhaled oxygen to burn the food we eat.

HYPOTHYROIDISM: A thyroid that is not producing enough thyroxin tends to make a person feel drowsy and sluggish, put on weight (even though his appetite is poor), and in general make his everyday activities tiresome and wearying. This condition is called *hypothyroidism.*

HYPERTHYROIDISM: Its opposite— caused by too much secretion of thyroxin—is *hyperthyroidism.* A hyperthyroid person is jumpy, restless, and may eat hugely without gaining weight. The difference between the two extremes can be compared to environments regulated by two different thermostats, one set too high and the other set too low.

Although a normally functioning thyroid plays a significant part in making a person feel well, doctors today are less willing than in former years to blame a defective thyroid alone for listlessness or jittery nerves. Thirty or forty years ago it was quite fashionable to prescribe thyroid pills (containing thyroid extract) almost as readily as vitamins or aspirin; but subsequent medical research, revealing the interdependence of many glands and other body systems, made thyroxin's reign as a cure-all a short one.

Of course, where physical discomfort or lethargy can be traced to an underfunctioning thyroid, thyroxin remains an invaluable medicine.

GOITER: One disorder of the thyroid gland—the sometimes massive swelling called *goiter*—is the direct result of a lack of iodine in the diet. The normal thyroid gland, in effect, collects iodine from the bloodstream, which is then synthesized into the chemical makeup of thyroxin. Lacking iodine, the thyroid gland enlarges, creating a goiter. The abnormal growth will stop if iodine is reintroduced into the person's diet. This is the reason why most commercial table salt is iodized—that is, a harmless bit of iodine compound has been added to it.

The Parathyroid Glands

Four small glands, each about the size of a small pea, cling to the base of the thyroid gland, two on each of the thyroid's lobes curving back of the trachea. These are the *parathyroids*, whose main role is to control the level of calcium—as well as other elements needed in carefully regulated amounts by the body—in the bloodstream and tissues. The parathyroids secrete two hormones: *parathormone* when blood calcium is too low; *calcitonin* when the calcium level is too high. These hormones work by controlling the interchange of calcium between bones and blood.

The most common symptom of defective parathyroids is *tetany*—a chronic or acute case of muscle spasms, which can be controlled by administration of synthetic parathyroidlike chemicals or concentrated vitamin D preparations.

The Gonads

The *gonads* refer to both the two male testicles and the two female ovaries. See the illustration of *The Endocrine Glands*, p. 36.

There are four hormones secreted by the gonads: the female sex hormones, *estrogen* and *progesterone;* and the male hormones, *testosterone* and *androsterone*. Each sex merely has a predominance of one or the other pair of hormones. Men have some of the female hormones, and women some of the male hormones.

In both sexes, puberty is signaled by the release of the gonadotrophic hormones (or *gonadotrophins*) of the pituitary gland. These stimulate the production of sex hormones by the sex glands and the subsequent appearance of secondary sexual characteristics. In men, these include the enlargement of testicles and penis, growth of facial, axillary (armpit) and pubic hair, and enlargement of the larynx, resulting in deepening of the voice. Pubescent women also experience pubic and axillary hair growth, in addition to breast growth and changes in the genital tract that give it childbearing capability.

Estrogen and progesterone control the cyclic changes within the uterus that involve the development, ripening, and discharge of the egg (ovulation) to be fertilized; the preparation of the lining of the uterus to receive a fertilized egg; and this lining's subsequent dismantling—all the complex biochemical events that occur as part of every woman's menstrual cycle.

The Thymus and Pineal Glands

These are the least known of the endocrine family; in fact, doctors do not know the function of one of them—the *pineal*—and are not even agreed that it is an endocrine gland. Situated near the hypothalamus, at the base of the brain, this tiny, pinecone-shaped body has follicles that suggest a glandular function and some calcium-containing bits that medical researchers have descriptively dubbed "brain sand."

The *thymus*, only slightly better understood, has the intriguing characteristic of shrinking in size as a person grows up. It is located in the middle of the chest, about midway between the base of the neck and the breast line. There is some evidence that the secretions of the thymus play a role in the body's natural immunity defenses. See also *Diseases of the Endocrine Glands*, p. 404.

THE SENSE ORGANS

Once upon a time, a grade-school teacher would ask, "How many senses do we have?" And his pupils would confidently chorus back, "Five!" People who displayed a knack for predicting future events, or whose quick reactions seemed to give them a jump over most everybody else, were credited with having a "sixth sense."

Scientists now recognize about twice that number—12 or 13 or more. Man, of course, has not grown a number of new senses in addition to the traditional five: sight, hearing, touch, smell, and taste. What has happened is that scientists have discovered many more specific kinds of sense receptor cells. For example, whereas touch was formerly thought of as just one sense, it has now been divided into no less than five different senses, each having its own special kind of receptor cell in the skin.

We can talk with a little more justification of the five sense organs, the five anatomical structures we associate with our senses—the eyes, ears, nose, tongue, and skin. But here, too, it does seem to be oversimplifying things to thus equate the nose—having only a tiny patch of olfactory (sense of smell) receptor cells—with the marvelously complex arrangement of sensing structures that make up the eye. Moreover, the other sense organs are not nearly so specialized as the eye. For example, a good case could be made for the nose being more valuable as an air purifier than as an organ of smell, or for the tongue being more valuable as an aid in digestion than as a source of the taste sensation.

Suppose we accept the proposition that pain is one of the senses of the skin; how then do we explain a pain from inside our bodies—say, a stomach ache or a deep muscle pain? The answer, of course, is that there are pain receptors in many other places besides the skin.

What Is a Sense?

A sense is a nerve pathway, one end of which (the receptor end) responds in a certain way to a certain condition affecting our bodies, and whose other end reaches to a part of our brain that informs our conscious mind of what has happened or is happening. A sense is thus distinguished from the body's countless other nerve pathways by the fact that our brain *consciously* registers its impulses, although the impulses themselves are no different from those of the autonomic nervous system.

While remaining aware of the limitations of the traditional list of five sense organs, let us now analyze what they can do and how they operate:

• The eye (vision): Nerve impulses to the brain are stimulated by light waves, from which the brain forms visual images.

• The ears (hearing): Nerve impulses to the brain are stimulated by sound waves, out of which the brain forms meaningful noise, such as speech. Deep within the ear, also, are structures that give us balance.

• The nose (olfaction): Nerve impulses to the brain are stimulated by airborne chemical substances,

moistened within the nasal cavity, from which the brain elicits distinctive smells.

• The tongue (taste): Nerve impulses to the brain are stimulated (in presence of water) by chemical substances in food, from which the brain forms sensations of sweet, salty, sour, bitter, or combinations of these tastes.

• Skin (touch): Nerve impulses to the brain are stimulated by the presence of outside physical forces and changes in the physical environment, including varying temperatures, which the brain registers as feelings of contact, pressure, cold, heat, and pain. (Some medical texts add traction, as when the skin is pulled or pinched, as well as the sensation of tickle.)

The Eye

Rather than take a name-by-name anatomical tour of the eye, let's instead take just three programed tours of the eye to explore:

• The transformation of light energy into vision

• Focusing, or how the structure of the eye prepares light for transformation into vision

• The supporting structures and service units of the eye.

Transforming Light Energy Into Vision

If you could look through the

opening in the front of your eye (the *pupil*), and see to the very back surface of your eye (as if you could see through the needle valve opening to the inside skin of a basketball), you would see your own *retina*. On your retina are located all the sense receptor cells that enable us to see. There are none anywhere else in the body.

RODS AND CONES: A good argument can be made that man's vision is really *two* senses. For on the paper-thin retina are two quite anatomically distinct sense receptors (nerve endings) named, for their appearance under high magnification, *cones* and *rods*. The cones are concentrated at a tiny spot on the retina called the *fovea*.

If the focusing machinery of the eye (cornea, lens, etc.) is working just right, light rays from the outside have their sharpest focus on the fovea. Surrounding the fovea is a yellowish area called the *macula lutea* (Latin, "yellow spot"). Together, the fovea and macula lutea make a circle not much bigger than the head of a pin.

All our seeing of colors and fine details is accomplished by the cones of the fovea and the macula lutea. Beyond the yellowish circumference of the macula lutea, there are fewer and fewer cones: rods become the dominant structures on the retina. It has been estimated that there are something less than

THE EYE

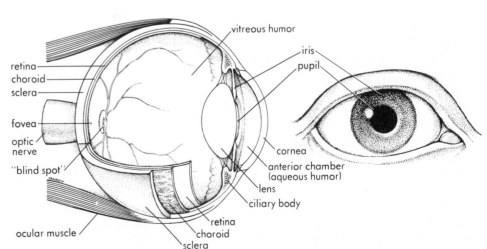

10 million cones on the retina of each eye, but more than 10 times as many rods—100 million of them or more.

Although the tight circle of cones in each eye gives man his ability to do close, detailed work (including reading) and to discriminate colors, the cones are virtually useless in detecting objects that are a bit off center from our direct focus, and furthermore operate only in good lighting conditions or in response to bright light sources.

The rods make up for the specialized limits of the cones. They take over completely in dim light, and also give us the ability to detect peripheral objects and movements—"out of the corner of the eye." Because the rods are not sensitive to colors, our seeing at night is almost completely in black-and-white.

You can give yourself an interesting demonstration of the interacting functions of your own cones and rods if you walk from bright, sunny daylight into a dimly lit theater. In the bright light, your cones have been picking out sharp images and colors. But once in dimness, the cones become inoperative. For a few moments, in fact, you may see almost nothing at all.

VISUAL PURPLE: The momentary interval after the cones stop working but before the rods begin to function is explained by a curious pigment present in the eye called *visual purple*. This substance is manufactured constantly by the rods, and must be present for the rods to respond to dim light—but it is destroyed when exposed to bright light. Thus, after entering a darkened room, it takes a few moments for visual purple to build up in the retina. One of the principal constituents of visual purple is vitamin A, which is why this vitamin (present in carrots and other yellow produce) is said to increase our capacity to see in the dark.

THE OPTIC NERVE: Every nerve ending is part of a larger unit, a neuron or nerve cell, and the sense

THE BLIND SPOT

The blind spot can be demonstrated by holding the book about 5 inches in front of the right eye. Close the left eye. Focus eye on the plus sign and move the book slowly toward or away from the eye until the fly disappears. At this point the image of the fly is falling on the "blind spot." This is the point where the optic nerve enters the eye.

receptors called rods and cones are no exception. Like all nerve cells, each rod and cone sports a long nerve fiber or *axon* leading away from the site of reception. In each eye, fibers serving the hundred-million-plus rods and cones all converge at a certain spot just behind the retina, forming the *optic nerve.* There are no rods and cones at the point where the optic nerve exits from behind the retina at the back of the eyeball: that is why everybody has a "blind spot" at that point. An image passing through that spot completely disappears.

From the retina, both optic nerves set a course almost directly through the middle of the brain. Right and left optic nerves converge, their individual fibers partially intertwining a short distance behind the eyes. Then this joint optic nerve trunk proceeds toward the rear of the head, where the *occipital lobes*, the brain's "centers for seeing," are located. Just before reaching the occipital lobes, the optic nerve splits again into thousands of smaller nerve bundles (called *visual radiations*) that disappear into the visual cortex or "outer bark" of the occipital lobes. Only at this point are the bits of light energy that have stimulated our rods and cones transformed into images that our brain can "see."

Focusing and Light Control

Lacking the structures of the retina and their connection to the brain

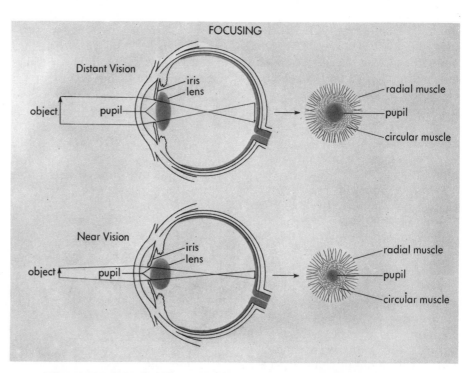

When viewing a distant object (over 20 feet away), the lens flattens and the pupil dilates, allowing more light to enter the eye. The pupil is dilated by the action of the outer radial muscles of the iris, which contract and thus stretch the previously contracted circular muscles. When viewing a near object, the lens becomes more oval and the pupil contracts as more light enters the eye. This prevents overstimulation of the retina. The pupil is reduced in size by the contraction of the inner circular muscles, which serve to stretch the previously contracted radial muscles.

via the optic nerve, we could not see. Lacking reasonably normal functioning of the cornea, lens, and iris, we do not see well.

Good vision depends upon the eye being able to bend incoming light rays in such a way that the image being observed falls directly on the retina—in other words, upon proper focusing. The bending or *refraction* of light rays is the joint work of two curves, transparent slivers of specialized tissue through which light passes on its way to the retina. These are the *cornea* and the *lens*. Broadly speaking, the degree of curvature and thickness of these two structures determines whether we see well or poorly, are nearsighted or farsighted.

THE CORNEA AND LENS: The cornea, which does the major light-bending, has a virtually fixed curvature and thickness. The lens puts the finishing touches on the focusing. Its thickness and curvature are adjustable—more or less without our conscious awareness—depending on whether we wish to focus on something nearer or farther away. The lens is made thicker or thinner, a process called *accommodation*, by the relaxing and contracting of tiny, attached *ciliary muscles*. Normally, these muscles do not have to work at all if we are looking at objects more than 20 feet away: but they often are overworked by a great deal of close work.

THE PUPIL AND IRIS: Effective focusing in various light conditions also depends upon the diameter of the hole through which light enters the eye. This hole is the *pupil*. Its diameter is controlled automatically —wider in dim light, narrower in bright light—by the muscles of the surrounding *iris*. The iris muscle contains pigment that gives our eyes color (brown, blue, green, etc.). The pupil, opening into the dark interior chamber of the eye, is black. A fully dilated (widened) pupil, as would occur in the dimmest light, illuminates over 15 times more retinal surface than the tiny "pinhole" pupil of an eye exposed to very bright light.

Supporting Structures and Service Units of the Eye

STRUCTURAL SUPPORT AND PROTECTION: Two outer layers protect the eye. The tough outermost layer is the *sclera*, the white of the eye. Underlying the sclera is another layer, the *choroid*, which contains numerous tiny blood vessels that service the sclera and other structures on the eyeball. Both sclera and choroid have concentric openings that allow for the hole of the pupil. The cornea

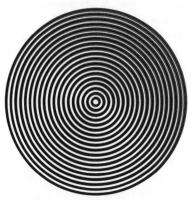

The apparent flickering of the circles is caused by contractions of the ciliary muscles, which control the accommodation (or change in thickness) of the lens for accurate focusing of objects at a variety of distances.

is really a specialized extension of the sclera, and the iris of the choroid.

Two trapped reservoirs of fluid within the eye are important in maintaining the eye's shape as well as the frictionless operation of its moving parts. These two reservoirs contain fluids called the *aqueous humor* and *vitreous humor*. The tiny space between the cornea and lens, corresponding to the pupil, is called the anterior chamber and is filled with the clear, watery, aqueous humor. The larger interior space behind the lens is called the posterior chamber, and is filled with the vitreous humor.

MUSCLES FOR MOVEMENT: In addition to the tiny muscles within the eye that control the opening of the pupil and the shape of the lens, we also have a number of elegant muscles that control the movements of each eyeball, and make both eyeballs move together in unison.

The movements of each eyeball are effected by six muscles attached to its top, bottom, and sides. The teamwork between these muscles —some contracting while others relax—allows the eye to move from side to side, up and down, and at all intermediate angles (obliquely). One of our eyes is always a dominant or leading eye; that is, its movements are always followed by the other eye.

Our protective eyelids, of course, are controlled by opening and closing muscles that lie outside the eye proper. These muscles can function both voluntarily and involuntarily.

LUBRICATION AND HYGIENE: Without the moisture provided by tears, our eyeball would scrape excruciatingly on the inside lining (*conjunctiva*) of the eyelid. In addition to lubrication, tears also have a cleansing action, not only because they supply water for washing and rinsing but also because they contain a mild germicide called *lysozyme* that kills bacteria and other potentially harmful microbes.

Tears are produced by the *lacrimal glands* above the eyeball, just under the eyebrow, a bit further toward the temple side than the nose side. They are discharged from several short ducts and spread over the surface of the eyeball by blinking. The *conjunctival sac* at the bottom inner (nose) side of the eye— visible in the mirror as a pinkish flap of tissue—serves as a collecting pool for tears; from there, they drain down a duct into the nasal cavity. This is why somebody who is crying also snuffles and must blow his nose.

There is another tiny drainage network in the eye, located at the interconnection of the cornea and iris, which serves to keep the fluid pressure of the space filled by the aqueous humor within normal limits. Drainage of this area is through microscopic conduits called the *canals of Schlemm*. Improper drainage can cause build-up of pressure, such as occurs in glaucoma, and impairment or loss of vision.

The Ear

Within the tunnels and chambers of the ear lie the two special types of sense receptors that give us, respectively, the sense of hearing and the sense of balance.

The Outer Ear

The *outer ear* includes that rather oddly shaped and folded piece of flesh and cartilage from which earrings are hung, and more important, the external *auditory canal*, a tunnel leading from the ear's opening to the *tympanic membrane*, or *eardrum*.

The Middle Ear

The *middle ear* includes the inner surface of the eardrum and the three tiny, bony *ossicles*, named long ago for their shape (apparently by some blacksmithing anatomist), *the hammer, the anvil*, and *the stirrup;* or in Latin: *the malleus, the incus*, and *the stapes*. These bones respond to the vibrations in the air that are the basis of sound, vibrate themselves, and transmit their vibrations to the inner ear, where the sense receptors for hearing are located, and the *auditory* (or *acoustic*) *nerve* to the brain begins.

The middle ear is connected to the back of the throat (pharynx) by the Eustachian tube. This tunnel between throat and middle ear makes the pressure on the inside of the eardrum, via the mouth, the same as the pressure of the atmosphere on the outside of the eardrum. (Thus yawning helps to equalize pressure.) Without it, or if the Eustachian tube becomes clogged, the taut membrane of the eardrum would always be in imminent danger of bursting.

The Inner Ear

The chambers of the *inner ear* are completely filled with fluid, which is jostled by the ossicles "knocking" on a thin membrane called the oval window, separating the middle from the inner ear. Another flexible membrane, the round window, serves to restrict the motion of the inner ear fluid when the movement is too stormy.

ORGAN OF HEARING: Within the inner ear is a bony structure coiled like a snail shell about the size of a pea. This is the *cochlea*, the actual Latin word for snail or snail shell. Following the internal spiral of the cochlea is the *organ of Corti*, the true sense receptors for hearing.

The organ of Corti is made up of thousands of specialized nerve endings that are the individual sense receptors for sound. These are in the form of tiny hairs projecting up from the internal membrane lining the cochlea; they wave like stalks of underwater plants in response to the oscillating currents of the inner ear fluid. There are some 20,000 of these hairs within the cochlea, responsive to almost as many degrees of movement of the fluid. These thousands of nerve endings merge at the core of the cochlea and exit from its floor as the nerve bundle of the *auditory nerve*.

ORGAN OF BALANCE: The organ of balance, or equilibrium, is also behind the oval window that marks the beginning of the inner ear. The principal structure consists of three fluid-filled *semicircular canals* arranged, like the wheels of a gyroscope spinning on a perfectly flat plane or surface, at right angles to each other. When we are in a normal, upright position, the fluid in the canals is also in its normal resting state. But when we begin to tilt or turn or wobble, the fluid runs one way or another in one or more of the canals. This fluid movement is picked up by crested, hairlike nerve endings lining the inside of the canals and relayed as nerve impulses along the *vestibular nerve* to the brain. Then, the brain sends messages to the muscles that can restore our equilibrium.

The term *labyrinth* is sometimes used to refer collectively to the cochlea, semicircular canals and associated structures of the inner ear. The space or cavity within the labyrinth is called the *vestibule*, which gives its name to the vestibular nerve.

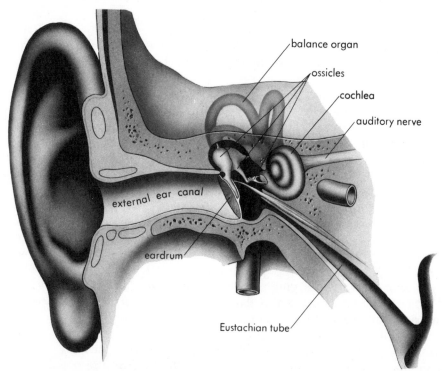

balance organ

ossicles

cochlea

auditory nerve

external ear canal

eardrum

Eustachian tube

The spatial relationships of the parts of the ear are illustrated in this drawing. For a more detailed drawing of the ear and the perception of sound, see page 80.

How We Hear

Just as our eye has certain special equipment—its focusing apparatus—to prepare light for the retina, so our ear has special equipment to prepare vibrations for reception by the organ of Corti.

This equipment consists of structures that amplify the vibrations reaching the ear, or, more rarely, damping (decreasing) the vibrations caused by very loud or very close occurrences.

Sound waves are really vibrations in the air that reach the eardrum at the narrow end of the funnel-shaped auditory canal. These vibrations set the membrane of the eardrum vibrating ever so slightly. Behind the eardrum, the first ossicle encountered is the hammer, which is attached to the eardrum by a projection descriptively called the hammer-handle.

From the eardrum, vibrations travel up the handle and set the hammer vibrating. The hammer, in turn, sets the anvil vibrating; and

THE EAR AND THE PERCEPTION OF SOUND

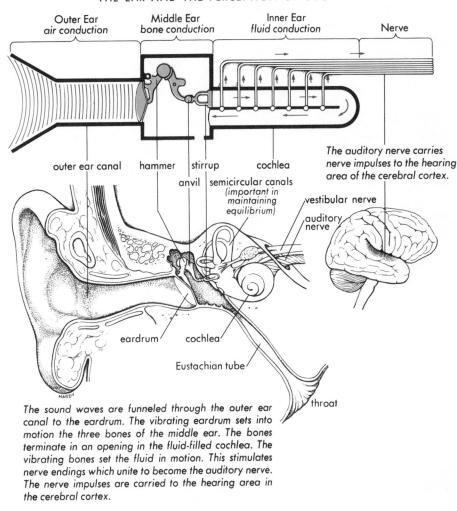

The sound waves are funneled through the outer ear canal to the eardrum. The vibrating eardrum sets into motion the three bones of the middle ear. The bones terminate in an opening in the fluid-filled cochlea. The vibrating bones set the fluid in motion. This stimulates nerve endings which unite to become the auditory nerve. The nerve impulses are carried to the hearing area in the cerebral cortex.

THE SEMICIRCULAR CANALS

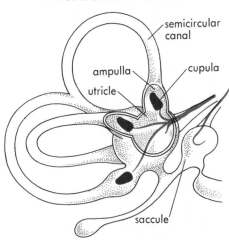

The semicircular canals are swollen at their bases into three ampullae in which receptors are located. When the head moves or accelerates, the fluid within the canals (endolymph), tends to move slower than the head, and the cupula is displaced. This is communicated to the hairlike nerve receptors. Soon the endolymph catches up to the head movement and the cupula returns to its normal position. When movement stops, the endolymph continues to move, the cupula is again displaced, and the nerve receptors are activated until the endolymph ceases to move.

the anvil, the stirrup. The stirrup then knocks like an impatient caller on the oval window of the inner ear, and the then vibrating oval window stirs the fluids within the cochlea. This chain of events can account for a tremendous amplification of vibrations—so that we are literally able to "hear a pin drop."

Tiny muscles in the middle ear relax or tighten the eardrum and adjust to changing volumes of sound. For example, a muscle connecting the stirrup and the eardrum relaxes when the stirrup is vibrating violently in the presence of very loud noises. A lax eardrum is less likely to rupture and transmits fewer vibrations to the delicate mechanisms of the middle and inner ear than a taut one. Thus we have to some degree built-in, automatic protection against the assaults of noise

pollution—but not nearly enough, according to doctors who are convinced that more and more cases of deafness are caused by the incessant battering of the modern world against our eardrums. Human eardrums are not made to withstand the sound of jet planes taking off, for example. See *Noise Pollution* under *The Environment and Health*, p. 232.

The Nose and Tongue

TASTE: The sense receptors on the tongue and within the nasal cavity work very closely together to give us our sense of taste. These five kinds of receptors—the olfactory cell in the nose and the four special cells or taste buds on the tongue for discriminating salty, sweet, sour, and bitter tastes—also have a functional similarity. All are chemical detectors, and all require moisture in order to function. In the nose, airborne substances must first be moistened by mucus (from the olfactory glands) before they can stimulate olfactory cells. In the mouth, the saliva does the wetting.

The general number and distribution of the four types of taste receptors are described under *The Digestive System and the Liver*, p. 23 These nerve endings, numbering in the hundreds of thousands, merge into two nerve bundles traveling away from the tongue to the brain's "taste center." The receptors toward the rear of the tongue collect into the *glossopharyngeal nerve;* those at the front and middle are directed along the *lingual nerve.*

THE SENSE OF SMELL: Our smell receptors are clustered in an area about a half-inch wide on the ceiling of the nasal cavity. This is called, appropriately enough, the smell patch. The nerve endings pass upward through the sievelike *ethmoid bone,* separating the nasal cavity from the brain, and connect to the olfactory bulb, which is the "nose end" of the *olfactory nerve.* At the other end of the olfactory nerve is the "nose brain" or *rhinencephalon*—a tiny part of the cerebrum in man, but quite large in dogs and other mammals whose sense of smell is keener than man's.

Although man's sense of smell is probably his least used sense, it still has a quite remarkable sensitivity. With it we can detect some chemicals in concentrations as diluted as one part in 30 billion—for example, the active ingredient in skunk spray. Also, man's ability to smell smoke and to detect gas leaks and other warning scents has prevented many a tragedy.

Skin

The sensations stimulated by the various types of sense receptors in the skin are described at the outset of this section. It is worth noting, however, at the end of our tour of the sense organs that the senses associated with the skin are really in a class by themselves. Perhaps the most telling indication of their unique place in the hierarchy of senses is the fact that practically our entire central nervous system (see *The Nervous System and the Brain,* p. 13) is given over to handling the impulses transmitted by these receptors. See also *Diseases of the Eye and Ear,* p. 417.

THE URINOGENITAL SYSTEM AND THE KIDNEYS

In large part our good health depends on the quality of the body's internal environment. There is a kind of ecological principle at work within us—if one chain threatens to break, one system becomes polluted, one balance is tilted, then the whole environment is in imminent danger of collapsing. The major responsibility for keeping our internal environment clean and unclogged lies with our two kidneys. They are the filters and purifiers of body fluids: the body's pollution-control stations, its recycling plants, and its waste-disposal units.

The Kidneys

The kidneys are located just behind our abdominal cavity on either side of the spinal cord, their tops usually tucked just under the bottommost rib. Each of our kidneys is four to five inches long and weighs about half a pound. The right kidney is normally placed a bit below the left, to accommodate the bulky liver lying also on the right side above it. Neither kidney is fixed rigidly; both can shift position slightly. Lying outside the muscular sheath of the abdominal cavity, the kidneys are more vulnerable than most internal organs to outside blows, but good protection against all but the severest jolts is afforded by surrounding fatty cushions, the big back muscles, and the bone and musculature associated with the spinal column.

As it has with the lungs, the liver, and most other vital organs, nature has supplied us with a large reserve capacity of kidney tissue—a life-giving overabundance in the event of kidney disease or injury. Indeed, normal function of only one-half of one kidney can sustain a person's life.

The kidneys' task of purifying our internal environment—that is, our circulating blood—is really a double task. Each kidney must purify the blood that passes through it, sending back into circulation only "clean blood"; and it must dispose of the impurities it has taken from the blood. The latter is accomplished by the urine draining down a tube, or *ureter,* leading from each of the two kidneys to one common urinary *bladder.* Urine is discharged from the bladder down another tube called the *urethra* to the external opening for urination.

How the Kidneys Process Body Fluids

Blood is brought to the kidney by a renal artery, is treated in the kidney's unique microscopic structures, and exits via the renal vein. (*Renal* means associated with the kidneys.) The sheer volume of blood processed by both our kidneys is prodigious: between 40 and 50 gallons are processed every day.

INTERNAL STRUCTURE: Within each kidney are over a million micro-

THE ANATOMY OF THE KIDNEY

The cortex is the darker, outer part of the kidney. The medulla, the inner part, includes the renal pyramids and the straight tubules associated with them.

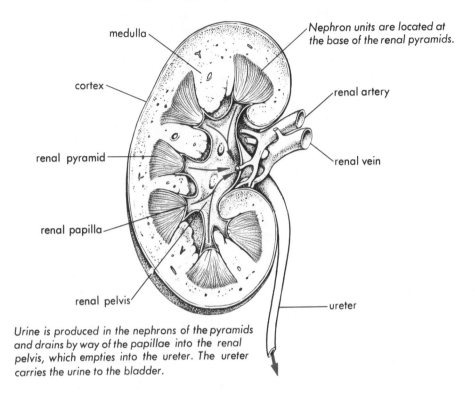

Nephron units are located at the base of the renal pyramids.

renal artery

renal vein

ureter

medulla

cortex

renal pyramid

renal papilla

renal pelvis

Urine is produced in the nephrons of the pyramids and drains by way of the papillae into the renal pelvis, which empties into the ureter. The ureter carries the urine to the bladder.

SULE: The fluids and dissolved materials filtering into Bowman's capsule are by no means all wastes and impurities. In fact, some of the substances must soon be reclaimed. Among the waste substances captured by Bowman's capsule and destined for excretion in urine are various nitrogen salts and other waste products of cellular metabolism, as well as actual or potential poisons that have entered or accumulated in the bloodstream. Nonwaste substances include needed sugars and salts, and water.

RECLAIMING ESSENTIAL SUBSTANCES: Before we leave the glomerulus altogether behind, it should be noted that like any capillary bed, this small ball of blood vessels has not only an inflow from the renal artery but also outflow vessels leading eventually back to the renal vein.

From the cupped lips of Bowman's capsule, fluid and dissolved substances from the blood trickle into a single tube called a kidney *tubule.* The outflow vessels from

scopic units called *nephrons.* The nephron is the basic functional unit of the kidney—a little kidney in itself—and is really a superbly engineered and coordinated arrangement of many smaller structures, all working together.

Blood arriving at the kidney from the renal artery is quickly channeled into finer and finer vessels, until finally it flows into a kind of cat's cradle or "ball of wool" structure called a *glomerulus* (composed of intertwining, microscopic vessels called glomerular capillaries). The entire structure of the nephron is built around the microscopic glomerulus (Latin, "tiny ball"). Surrounding the glomerulus, like a hand lightly cupping a ball of wool, is another structure called *Bowman's capsule.* Fluid and dissolved materials filter out of the blood from the glomerular capillaries through the membranes into Bowman's capsule.

SUBSTANCES IN BOWMAN'S CAP-

THE NEPHRON

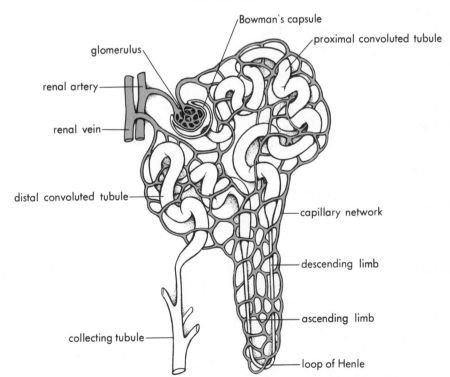

Bowman's capsule

proximal convoluted tubule

glomerulus

renal artery

renal vein

distal convoluted tubule

capillary network

descending limb

ascending limb

collecting tubule

loop of Henle

The nephron is a microscopic unit that filters out certain products from the blood. Useful products are reabsorbed by the capillary network. The waste product (urine) is carried to the collecting tubule and emptied into the renal pelvis.

the glomerulus wind closely over and around the tubule, forming a capillary network around it. By this means the nonwaste substances are reclaimed and returned to refresh the blood moving away from the nephron.

The tubule itself makes many twists and turns—including one hairpin turn so stunning that it has its own medical name—*Henle's loop.* So much twisting and turning gives the tubule a great deal more surface area than a simple, straight tube would have within the same space, thus increasing the amount of water and dissolved substances that can be recaptured by the encircling capillaries.

If there were no recapturing system in the kidneys, death would probably result from dehydration. Even if that could be avoided, the loss of essential salts and other substances would prove fatal in a short time.

The arithmetic of the situation goes something like this: every day, an estimated 42 gallons of fluid filter out of the glomeruli and into the two kidneys' approximately two and a half million tubules. Dissolved in this 42 gallons—representing about three times the body's weight—are about two-and-a-half pounds of common salt, just one of the many substances in the fluid that our body needs in sufficient amounts. The loss of either water or common salt at a rapid rate would prove fatal in a matter of hours.

But so efficient is the tubule-capillary recapturing system that only an average of less than two quarts of fluid, containing just one-third ounce of salt, pass daily out of the kidneys into the ureter and are excreted as urine. In other words, over 99 percent of both the water and common salt removed from the blood at Bowman's capsules is returned to the blood.

The Kidneys and Blood Pressure

A surprising insight into the critical role played by our kidneys in almost every body function is provided by the relation of blood pressure to kidney function. The blood in the glomerular capillaries must be at higher pressure than the fluid around them, so that the fluid and its dissolved substances can push through the capillary membranes toward Bowman's capsule. If blood pressure in the body falls too low (severe *hypotension*) the formation of urine ceases.

On the other hand, if a portion of the kidney is suffering from anemia due to some disorder, kidney cells secrete *pressor hormones,* which serve to elevate the blood pressure. Thus, high blood pressure (*hypertension*) may be a sign of kidney disorder.

The Urinary Tract

From the ends of the million or so tubules in each kidney, urine drains into larger and larger collecting basins (called *calyces,* singular *calyx*) which drain in turn into the kidney's master urine reservoir, the *kidney pelvis.* Then, drop by drop, urine slides down each ureter to the

THE FEMALE URINARY SYSTEM

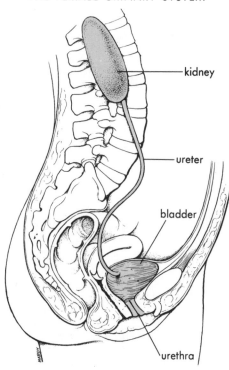

kidney

ureter

bladder

urethra

urinary bladder.

Urine is held in the bladder by the contraction of two muscle rings, or *sphincters,* one located just inside the bladder before it meets the urethra, and the other encircling the urethra itself. When about a half-pint has accumulated, nerves convey the urge to urinate to the brain, and the person voluntarily causes the sphincters to relax, emptying the bladder. (In exceptional circumstances, the elastic-walled bladder can hold two or three quarts of urine.) Up to the point where the bladder drains, the male and female urinary tracts are very similar, but after the bladder, any similarity stops.

FEMALE URETHRA: The female's urethra, normally about one and a half inches long, is not much more than a short channel by which urine is eliminated from the bladder. Its very shortness often gives it an undesired significance, because it represents an easy upward invasion route for bacteria and other infection-causing microbes from the outside. Acute and painful inflammations of the urethra (*urethritis*) and bladder (*cystitis*) are thus common in women. These lower urinary tract infections, however, can usually be halted before spreading further up the urinary tract by the administration of any of several antimicrobial drugs. See *Disorders of the Urinary System,* p. 494, for more information on these disorders.

MALE URETHRA: In contrast to the female, the male's urethra is involved with reproductive functions. So closely connected are the male's lower urinary tract and genital organs that his urethra (from bladder to the outside) is properly called the urinogenital (or genito-urinary) tract. This is the reason why the medical specialty known as *urology* deals with both the urinary and genital apparatus of men; but with only the urinary tract of women. The urologist's specialty does not extend to the female genital and childbearing organs, which are the concern of

THE MALE URINARY SYSTEM

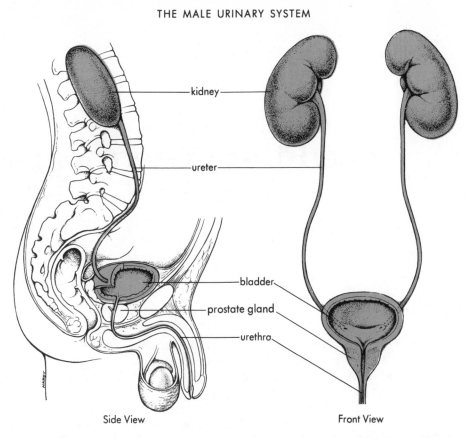

Side View

Front View

called the *scrotum*. Although the vulnerable position of the testicles remains something of an evolutionary mystery, one clue is that the optimum production of spermatozoa takes place at a temperature some degrees lower than the normal internal body temperature.

Spermatozoa produced in the testicles travel upward toward the urethra through a seminal duct or tube called the *vas deferens* (one from each testicle). (These are the ducts, incidentally, that are tied and cut in the male sterilization procedure known as a vasectomy.) The sperm cells are then stored, until ejaculation, in little reservoirs called *seminal vesicles* which are situated on either side of the urethra in the area just above the prostate gland.

The portion of the male urethra from the bladder to where it emerges from the encircling prostate, having received the emission of both the prostate and the testicles, is called the prostatic or posterior urethra. The remainder, mainly consisting of the conduit running down the middle of the shaft of the penis, ending in the external opening called the *meatus,* is known as the anterior urethra. See also *Diseases of the Urinogenital System,* p. 424.

the *gynecologist* and *obstetrician.*

However, all the distinctly male sex glands and organs are linked more or less directly into the eight- or nine-inch length of the male urethra.

The Genitals

The Female Reproductive System

As indicated above, the urinary and genital systems of women are dealt with by two different medical specialties. For this reason, the female genitals are discussed elsewhere. For a description and illustration of the female reproductive system, see p. 124 under *Social and Sexual Maturation.* For a description of infections of the female reproductive tract, see p. 487 under *Women's Health.*

The Male Reproductive System

From its emergence below the bladder, the male urethra serves as a conduit for all the male sexual secretions.

PROSTATE GLAND: Directly below the bladder outlet, the *prostate gland* completely enwraps the

urethra. The prostate secretes substances into the urethra through ejaculatory ducts; these substances are essential in keeping alive the spermatozoa that arrive from their manufacturing sites in the *testicles* (or *testes*).

TESTICLES: The two testicles hang down within a wrinkled bag of skin

THE MALE REPRODUCTIVE SYSTEM

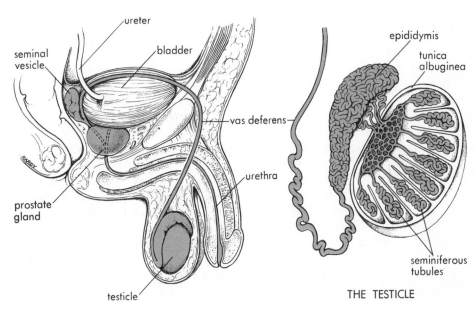

THE TESTICLE

CHAPTER 2

The First Dozen Years

BIRTH, INFANCY, AND MATURATION

Before the Baby Arrives

When a husband and wife decide to have a baby they should both undergo complete physical examinations. This will make it possible to detect and treat abnormalities like diabetes and anemia that might affect the future pregnancy. A pregnant woman should have periodic checkups so that her physician can observe both her progress and that of the growing fetus. Such observation will help to assure a pregnancy and delivery which are free from troublesome complications.

What the Newborn Baby Looks Like

At birth the baby's skin is wrinkled or scaly, and may be covered by a cheesy substance called *vernix caseosa*. During the first two weeks the skin will become quite dry to the touch. The skin of white newborns is red, and sometimes turns yellow during the first few days. Black newborns often are not as dark as they might be later. Their skin becomes just as yellow as that of white babies, but the change is more difficult to observe.

The newborn's head is large in proportion to the rest of its body. The genitals too may seem large,

especially in girls. Newborn girls may have swollen genitalia due to *edema* (fluid in the tissues, causing puffiness), but the swelling is usually present for only a few days after birth.

The eyes, slate blue in color, can open and react to light, but are unable to focus. Noises produce a *startle response*, a complex involuntary reaction marked by a sudden, jerky, arm and leg movement. The newborn cries a great deal, sucks, and may sneeze.

The infant's stomach may look rather large and protuberant, and, of course, it has the stump of the umbilical cord dangling from it. The umbilical cord has been cut and tied near the navel, and will eventually fall off.

If you feel the front and back of the baby's head, you will notice one or two soft spots, called the *anterior* and *posterior fontanels*. The posterior fontanel usually closes at the baby's second month of life, and the anterior at 18 months or earlier.

You also may feel many different ridges in the baby's head. These are the borders of the different skull bones, which fuse as the baby gets older. They are present so that the skull can grow as the baby's brain and head continue to grow.

Soon after birth, you may detect a

swelling on the baby's head just under the scalp. This is called *caput succedaneum*. It is nothing to worry about, as it dissolves a day or two after birth. Occasionally, another swelling known as *cephalhematoma* may also be present. This, too, disappears, within a few weeks.

The baby's weight will, of course, vary. Most full-term babies weigh between six and eight pounds. Babies of diabetic mothers are often heavier, and may weigh up to twelve pounds.

Some Advice to New Mothers

Unless the new father and mother are really prepared to change some of the conditioned patterns of their relationship, both can be in for a very difficult time. The father suddenly finds himself taking second place in his wife's attentions and affection. The new mother is tired physically and mentally. In-laws and other relatives may infringe on the couple's privacy and interfere with their right to make their own decisions. The new mother may find it hard to reconcile her maternal instinct with her desires as a woman and wife.

All of these problems can be

The feet look more complete than they are. Xray would show only one real bone at the heel. Other bones are now cartilage. The skin is quite commonly loose and wrinkly.

A deep flush spreads over the entire body if the baby cries hard. Veins on the head swell and throb. You will notice no tears, because the tear ducts do not function yet.

The legs are most often seen drawn up against the abdomen in prebirth position. Extended legs measure shorter than you'd expect compared to the arms. The knees stay slightly bent and legs are somewhat bowed.

Weight unless well above the average of six or seven pounds will not prepare you for how really tiny newborn is. Top to toe measure: anywhere between 18 inches to 21 inches.

Genitals of both sexes will seem too large (especially the scrotum) in comparison with the scale of the hands, for example, to adult size.

On the skull you will see or feel the two most obvious soft spots, or fontanels. One is above the brow; the other is close to the crown in the back.

The hands, if you open them out flat from their characteristic fist position, have finely lined palms, tissue-paper-thin nails, dry, loose-fitting skin, and deep bracelet creases at the wrist.

The skin is thin and dry. You may see veins through it. Fair skin may be rosy red temporarily. Downy hair is not unusual. Some *vernix caseosa* (white, prenatal covering) remains.

Eyes appear dark blue and have a blank stary gaze. You may catch one or both of them turning or turned to a crossed or wall-eyed position. The lids are characteristically puffy.

Head usually strikes you as being too big for the body. It may be temporarily out of shape—lopsided or elongated—due to pressure before birth or during the birth process.

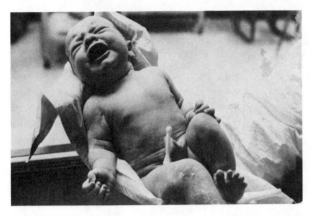

The trunk may startle you in some ways: short neck, small sloping shoulders, swollen breasts, large rounded abdomen, umbilical stump (future navel), slender, narrow pelvis and hips.

The face will disappoint you unless you expect to see pudgy cheeks, a broad, flat nose with only the merest hint of a bridge, a receding chin, and an undersized lower jaw.

the baby, it is more important that family and friends be made to follow a "hands off" policy except at your discretion. A new baby should not be subjected to excessive stimulation. For example, you may notice that if you pick her up and put her back in her crib, and then let someone else hold her a few minutes later, the baby may cry. If you slam a door, the baby's body reacts in the startle reflex, the involuntary reaction previously described. A baby needs a quiet, organized home, free from the kind of upsetting distraction that comes from being surrounded and fussed over by too many people. You and your husband must decide when you want the baby to have visitors and how those visitors are to behave. You must do this even if it causes hurt feelings among your friends and relatives. When the baby is a little older there will be time enough for friends and relatives to admire and play with her.

Feeding the Baby

One of the first questions a mother-to-be must ask herself is how she will feed her baby.

Breast feeding is certainly the simplest method, and many women believe that both mother and child get more emotional satisfaction from it than from bottle feeding. It is also, obviously, less expensive.

Breast Feeding

Almost any healthy woman who wants to breast-feed her baby can do so. All she needs is the desire and motivation. No special preparation is necessary except, perhaps, some stimulation of the breasts, as prescribed by her doctor during pregnancy.

On the other hand, a variety of different factors might necessitate a change from breast to bottle feeding. Although breast feeding may be discontinued at any time, some mothers may feel a sense of failure or frustration at being unable to continue having the intimate relationship that so many other mothers en-

minimized if the mother follows a few common-sense guidelines:

• The new baby is a shared responsibility. Do not shut your husband out of the experience of parenthood. Let him learn to feed the baby, diaper the baby, hold him, get acquainted with him. Make your husband feel just as important to the baby as you are, and just as important to you as he was before the baby was born.

• Arrange for some kind of assistance in your home, and don't wait until the day you bring the baby home to do it. Plan ahead. You will be physically and emotionally tired after childbirth, no matter how marvelous you may feel when you leave the hospital. During the hospital stay the baby was cared for by a trained staff. At home the burden will fall mainly on you, unless you take steps to get help. If you cannot get your mother or another relative to stay with you, engage a housekeeper or some other trained person. The investment will pay off for

you, the baby, and your husband.

• If it is at all possible, arrange to have a separate area for the baby. It is best for a baby not to be kept in the parents' room. Parents must have privacy. If you do not have a bedroom for the baby, section off some spot where you can put a crib and a dressing table to hold the supplies you will need when you feed, change, bathe, and dress him or her.

• Don't make the baby the focus of attention 24 hours a day. If she fidgets and fusses at times, try not to get nervous. Don't run to her at every whimper so long as you know she has been fed, is dry, and nothing is really wrong. Relax. The baby will be very sensitive to your emotional responses, particularly when you hold her. Through your physical contact you will develop a kind of communication with your baby which she will sense when you pick her up or feed her.

• As important as it is for you and your husband to avoid overhandling

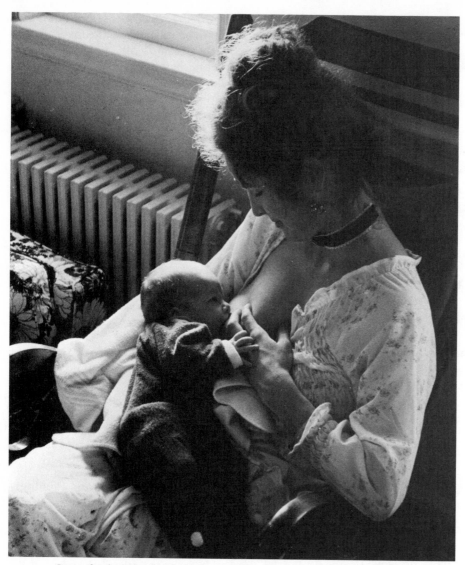

Breast feeding should be begun gradually. The baby should be allowed to suck for only a few minutes on each breast until the nipples have toughened.

joy. No harm will come to the baby by being switched to a formula. Once started on a formula, however, it may be difficult to go back to breast feeding on a regular basis. For a while, at least, the mother will have to stimulate her breasts artifically to increase their milk-producing capacity.

THE FIRST FEW DAYS: When a mother first starts to breast-feed, she may be worried that she won't have sufficient milk for the baby. Her breasts are just beginning to fill up with a creamy, yellowish substance called *colostrum*. Transitional and then regular breast milk will not come in for three to five days or

longer. Colostrum contains more protein and less fat than breast milk. Secretions of colostrum are small, but during this time the baby does not need very much fluid, and the colostrum will give her adequate nutrition.

Actually, it is important that the milk does not fill the breasts right away because engorgement would be so severe that the baby would not be able to suck well or strongly enough to empty them. During engorgement, the mother's breasts feel extremely tender and full. A good nursing brassiere will lift and support the breasts and alleviate the tender sensation during the day-or-two period of the engorgement.

SOME ADVICE TO NURSING MOTHERS: If you do not have enough milk for the first few days, don't worry about it. Let the baby suck on your nipples for three, five, or even ten minutes. Don't keep her on your breasts for twenty or thirty minutes right from the beginning. Start with three minutes the first day, five minutes the second, and so on until you work up to fifteen or twenty minutes. In this way you will toughen your nipples so that your breasts will become accustomed to the baby's sucking. A bland cream may be used to massage the nipple area, particularly if the nipples become sore or cracked.

Be sure to use both breasts. By emptying the breasts, milk production is stimulated; thus an adequate milk supply is dependent upon using both breasts. To avoid any soreness or tenderness, use one breast longer than the other during each nursing period.

Let us assume, for example, that at the first feeding of the day you nurse the baby on the left breast for a long period, then on the right for a short period. During the next feeding the right breast will become the first one on which the baby nurses (for the long period), and the left will be nursed second (for the short period). After a few weeks you should be nursing the baby on the first breast for twenty minutes and on the other for ten minutes.

THE FEEDING SCHEDULE: Depending on how often the baby wants to feed, you will be wise to adhere to a modified demand schedule. Don't watch the clock and feed the baby every four hours on the dot. You might feed at approximately every fourth hour, which means that you could start a second feeding early—at a three-hour interval—or late—at a five-hour interval. And, needless to say, never wake your baby up at night. She will awaken you.

Bottle Feeding

New parents nowadays have a choice between prepackaged formulas and the homemade variety. Either provides the same basic nutritional requirements.

The basic homemade formula for newborns consists of evaporated milk, water, and sugar or one of the sugar derivatives. Twice as much water as evaporated milk is used with one to two tablespoons of sweetening. A similar formula can be made with whole milk in somewhat different proportions. As the baby gets older, the formula will be changed from time to time by your physician.

If one formula does not agree with the baby, it will not help to put her on a similar formula; its ingredients are likely to be virtually the same. You must switch to a radically different formula, such as one containing no milk at all or no carbohydrates. It is up to your doctor to advise you which modified formula to try.

As to how much formula should be given at each feeding, let the baby decide. If she is satisfied with two-and-a-half ounces, she is probably getting enough. If she wants up to four-and-a-half ounces, give it to her. The amount is not important as long as your doctor feels the baby is in good health.

A final thing to remember about feeding is this: whether you use breast or bottle, you must give your baby the love, warmth, and body contact that she needs. As you feed her, you are not only providing nutritional nourishment for her growing body but giving her emotional and mental food for her evolving personality.

The First Six Months

It is extremely important that the baby have regular health supervision. Your baby's doctor—whether pediatrician or general practitioner —will check the baby's height and weight on each visit, and make certain he is growing and gaining at a satisfactory rate. Often, the first sign of illness in a baby is a change in his height and weight pattern.

Although no two children develop at the same rate, it is possible to make certain generalizations about their development. See the charts on pp. 85–86 showing the growth rates for boys and girls.

By two months a baby often holds his head up when he lies on his stomach or when he is being held up. He recognizes large objects, and he knows his bottle or feeding position. He can probably smile.

Sometime during the second or third month, your physician will start a series of injections against diphtheria, whooping cough, and tetanus (called *DPT*), as well as oral immunizing agents against polio— the *Sabin vaccine.* See the chart on p. 89.

THE THREE-MONTH MARK: By three months most babies are eating some solids specially processed for babies—fruits, cereals, vegetables, meats—in addition to having formula. They may, of course, still be entirely on breast milk. Your doctor will also suggest the use of vitamin supplements, in the form of drops, which can be added to the baby's milk or solid food. All babies need vitamins A, C, and D. Occasionally, vitamin B is also prescribed. If fluorides are not present in your drinking water, they are often added to the baby's vitamins to retard tooth decay.

AT FOUR MONTHS: By four months the baby will look at moving objects. Do not be surprised if his eyes cross. This is a normal condition during early infancy, and may even persist for a year.

At about this time, the baby may also learn to turn over from front

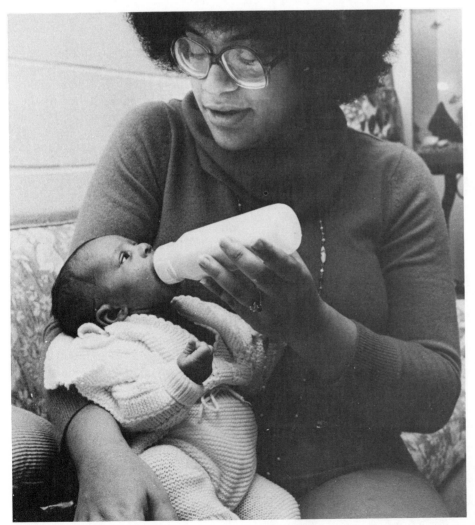

Just how much the bottle-fed infant needs varies from child to child. As long as the baby is healthy, let her decide when she's had enough.

to back—an important milestone. Some babies may have developed bald or flat places on the back of the head from lying more or less in one position. At about this time the condition should begin to disappear.

The Second Six Months

At six months most babies smile when they are brought to the doctor's office. At one year of age a visit to the doctor is more likely to produce tears and screams. The friendly, sociable attitude of the six-month-old gives way to one in which strangers are shunned or mistrusted, and everyone other than mother may qualify as a stranger.

By the sixth month the baby may roll over when placed on her back. She may learn to crawl, sit, pull herself up, and even stand. By a year she may start to walk, although walking unaided does not often occur so soon.

At this stage the baby is full of life and activity. She won't lie still when you change her diaper, and often needs distraction. She cries if you put her down or leave her alone. Unless you are firm and resist running to her at her first whimper, you may set the stage for spoiling her as she gets older. Of course, if

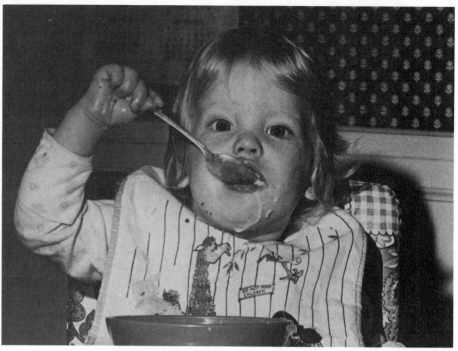

This baby has mastered the art of keeping the spoon right-side up and has even gotten almost half of its contents into his mouth.

she continues to cry for any considerable length of time—not more than half an hour—make sure there is nothing wrong with her besides her displeasure at your not appearing like a genie because she screams and fusses.

OTHER CHANGES: Other changes occur at this age. Where before she had been a good sleeper, she may now not want to go to sleep or she may awaken at night. Let her know that you are near by, but don't make a habit of playing with her in the middle of the night—not if you value your sleep.

If you should notice, as many parents do at about this time, that your baby seems to be left-handed, do not try to make her right-handed. Each of us inherits a preference for one hand or the other, and it is harmful to try to change it. In any case, you are not likely to know for sure which hand your child prefers until the second year of her life.

In this second six-month period, the baby will probably take some of her milk from a cup. Don't be surprised if she takes juices out of a cup but insists on taking milk from a bottle. If she tries to hold the bottle or cup herself, let her. Of course, it may be wise to keep a mop handy at first, but after a few months her skills will improve. In any case, nonbreakable cups are recommended.

DIET AND TEETH: The baby's diet is soon expanded to include pureed baby foods. You might even want to try the somewhat lumpier junior

By the time that baby is eight months old, he is usually proficient at crawling around the house.

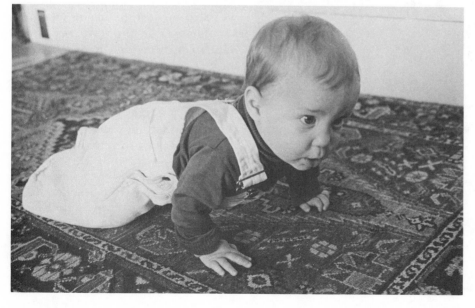

foods; as more of her teeth erupt, the baby will enjoy the lumpier food more and more. Teething biscuits can be added to the diet, too. By the time she is one year old she will usually have six teeth (incisors), although, since no two children are alike, she may have none at all. By the end of the first year she will have lost some of her appetite, and her rapid weight gain will cease. This is entirely natural in a period when the outside world is taking on more and more interest.

As she starts to move around she wants to investigate everything. Keep dangerous objects—detergents, poisons, and medicines, especially baby aspirin—out of her reach. Tell her "No" to emphasize the seriousness of certain prohibitions. She should understand what "No" means by the time she is one-year-old, and will also probably respond to other simple commands.

It is essential that your baby's health supervision be continued without interruption. During the second six months of life she will complete her protection against diphtheria, whooping cough, tetanus (DPT), and polio (Sabin), and be tested for exposure to tuberculosis (the tuberculin test).

Behavioral Development During Infancy

During a child's first year she needs a warm and loving emotional environment in the home. It is during this time that a child establishes what psychiatrists and psychologists call basic trust. That is, she learns to be a trusting individual who feels that her important needs—those of being cared for, fed, and comforted—will be met by other human beings, initially by her mother.

EMOTIONAL NEEDS: Such activities as holding and cuddling the infant, talking to her, and playing with her in an affectionate, relaxed way are important for her emotional growth. Experiments with animals have shown that if the infant animal does not get sufficient cuddling and physical contact from its mother

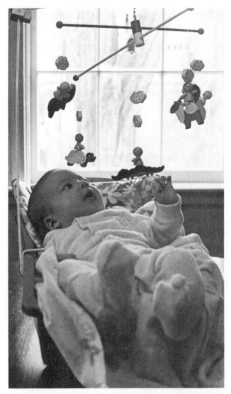

Providing a baby with visual stimulation helps to keep her occupied at the same time as it develops coordinated eyesight.

during its early development, it is unable to perform adequately as an adult later in life. It has also been shown that infants growing up in an environment lacking warm, loving, close physical and emotional contact with a mother or a mother-substitute often fail to thrive and may even die.

Fondling and Sucking

During the first year, most of an infant's satisfactions and gratifications are through the skin's perception of being touched—through physical contact with her mother and other caring adults—and through the mouth, especially sucking. Infants have a great need to suck even when they are not hungry, and this sucking should be both allowed and encouraged.

Parents frequently worry that if they respond to a baby's crying by picking her up they will spoil her, and the baby will cry often in order to get attention. In general, it could be said that during its first year an infant cannot be spoiled. When an

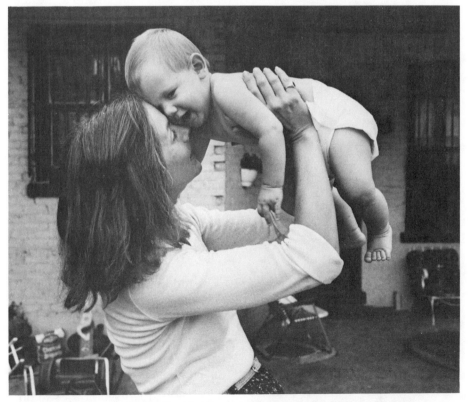

A warm, loving environment is important for a child's emotional growth. Babies deprived of affectionate physical contact do not develop normally.

infant cries she usually does so because she is uncomfortable, hungry, sick, or needs some physical attention.

Social Responses

As she matures, one of a child's tasks is to begin to see herself as separate from the world around her. During early infancy, the infant does not see herself as an individual who is separate from her mother, from other adults, and from the rest of the world. But, gradually, some time within the first year of life, this feeling of separateness and individuality begins to emerge in the developing infant.

One of the important and gratifying events in the early months of a child's life is the smiling responses. For the first time the infant can respond in a social way to other human beings. It is often at this time that the infant's mother and father begin to think of her as a real person and an individual. Thus the smile could be considered one of the infant's first social communications.

Suspicion of Strangers

Somewhere around the age of eight months, an infant who has in the past without complaint allowed anyone to pick her up begins to distinguish her mother from other individuals. When picked up by another the infant usually cries, acts frightened, and, in general, looks unhappy. This response indicates that she can now tell her mother and other individuals apart—an important and normal step in an infant's development.

FEAR OF SEPARATION: Some time later, usually around the age of one year, the infant begins to become fearful upon separation from her mother. When her mother walks out of the room or leaves the baby with a sitter, the child may respond with crying, fear, and anger. This again indicates that the infant can now tell her mother from strangers and does not like being separated from her. Although the response is normal and usually subsides within three to

four months, parents should learn to leave the child in the hands of a competent sitter, and walk out without guilt or anger. The child must learn that separations are temporary and that parents do return.

The Second Year: The Toddler Stage

It is during the second year of a child's life that he begins to develop independence and separateness from his mother. Beginning with his growing ability to walk, usually some time early in the second year (age 12–16 months), an infant starts to explore the world around him more actively. He experiments with greater and greater distances and

A baby first learns to walk with assistance from her parents or by holding onto things. Many children begin their walking between the ages of 12 months to 16 months.

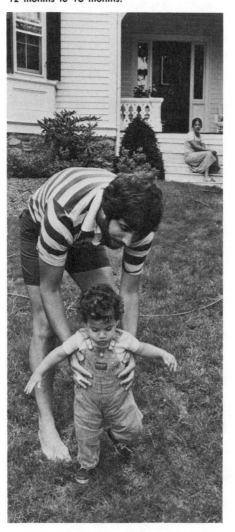

increasing independence from his mother.

Towards the end of the second year, children frequently become quite independent, trying to do many things for themselves, and resenting their parents or other well-meaning adults doing things for them. Even if the child is not yet capable of performing the tasks he attempts, he should be encouraged in these early moves toward independence. It is also during the second year that speech begins to develop, with the child's first words usually being "ma ma," "da da," "milk," and the ever-present "no."

Developing Relationships With Mother and Father

It is in this phase of the child's life that he develops a real relationship with his mother. In most homes, mother is the loving, warm, secure comforter in his life, the giver of rewards and disciplinarian of his daily activities, the center of his life. During this period it is imperative that the child's father spend as much time with his son or daughter as he is able to, so that the child begins to recognize the difference between his relationship to his mother and father.

In some cases the father, because of the demands of business, may find it impossible to spend enough time with his family. This is an unfortunate fact, but one that can be dealt with positively, since it is the quality of the time a father spends with his child, rather than the quantity, that is most important.

Testing Himself and the World Around Him

The toddler is insatiably curious. He wants to explore and investigate everything. Take him outdoors as much as possible. Let him meet children of his own age so that he can play and learn the beginnings of social contact.

Physically, the toddler tries to do many things apart from walking, running, and climbing—including

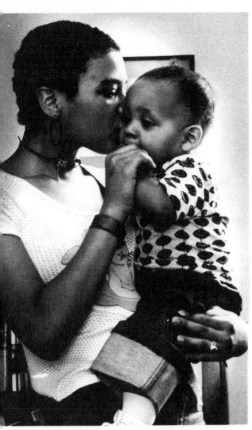

During the second year the child becomes devotedly attached to his mother.

quite a few things that he can't do. He is easily frustrated and may have a short attention span. (Girls are better than boys in this respect.) Don't be impatient with your toddler; don't punish him for his clumsiness. He has a great many experiences ahead of him, and many skills to learn and develop.

You can now expect a negative reaction to your control. Obviously, you must set limits on your child's behavior—on what is acceptable and what is not, while still giving him the freedom to express his emotions and energies in vigorous physical play.

Make the rules easy to understand so that the child will not become confused about what is expected of him. And do not set up impossible standards.

The Third Year

The third year is extremely important. Children are usually toilet trained, show marked growth in their language abilities, and demonstrate a continuing and growing independence.

Negativism

From two to about three and perhaps beyond, a child is extremely negative. When asked to do anything or when asked about anything, he often responds by saying, "No, no, no, no, no." This saying of the word "no" on the slightest provocation indicates a child's wish to become separate and independent from parents, to do what he wants to do when he wants to do it, and to be free from the control of others.

The child's desire for independence can be respected and encouraged by parents within limits, but this does not mean that a parent must give in to a child on every issue. A parent should try to determine what is really important and not make an issue over petty matters that can best be handled with relaxed good humor.

Language Development and Play

A rapid spurt in language development takes place at this time. A child may increase his vocabulary from about 50 words at the beginning of the third year to an almost countless vocabulary at the end of the third year. It is during this year, too, that children first show marked interest in imaginative play activities. Play, including making up stories, using toy trucks and cars, blocks, dolls, and toy furniture, is vital activity for children and should be encouraged by parents. It is through play that children express their feelings, often feelings that cannot be expressed in ordinary ways. The child also experiences what it feels like to be an adult by playing the role of doctor, fireman, policeman, teacher, mother or father. In addition, during play children discharge tensions and learn to use their muscles and bodies.

Exploring the Body

From very early infancy, all children show a strong interest in their own and in other's bodies. During infancy this takes the form of playing with his own and his mother's body. A baby puts his fingers in his own mouth, in his mother's mouth, ears, eyes, and pats her on the tummy or on the breast. An infant also explores and touches his own body, including the genital region.

Encouraged by his father, a child develops coordination and spatial concepts as he matches block shapes to openings in a cube.

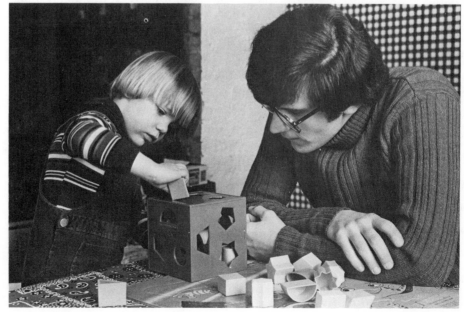

This interest is normal and need not be discouraged.

Dental Development

The roots of all 20 primary teeth are complete at the child's third year of life. These teeth, which began erupting between 6 and 7 months of age, are called the *central incisors*. The primary teeth, the last of which usually fall out between the eleventh and thirteenth year, are smaller and whiter than the permanent teeth, of which there are 32. The first permanent tooth erupts between 7 and 8 years of age, while the last, the third molars, or *wisdom teeth,* erupt between the seventeenth and twenty-first year.

The Preschooler

This is the age when many children go to school for part of the day and begin learning how to get along with

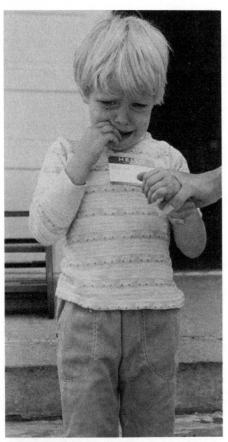

A child's first separation from mother can be a painful experience. Parents can ease the child's anxiety by openly discussing her fears and reassuring her long before the first day of school.

other children in play and in organized activities. They also begin to meet adults other than their parents.

First Separation From Mother

During the ages of three and four, the preschooler develops increasing interest in the world around him, in children his own age, and in himself. One of the key problems that the preschooler has to deal with is his impending separation from his mother when he becomes old enough to go to school. This can often be made less painful by arranging for the child to spend at first short and then increasingly longer periods of time away from his mother. By using baby-sitters both in the evening and during the day, by later having the child spend three or more half-days a week at a preschool, and lastly by enrolling him in kindergarten for either all day or half a day, five days a week, the mother can ease the child's adjustment to the world outside the home.

Although his first nearly full-time separation from mother is difficult for the child, it may be difficult for the mother as well. Mothers often feel that this initial separation from their child will eventually lead to their child's growing up and leaving home. Parents are often nostalgic and somewhat regretful about their children's first going off full time to school. The child's fearful anticipation of a strange situation can be eased by a mother's anticipating school with the child, talking with him about it and reassuring him regarding his fears of abandonment or separation.

Differences Between Boys and Girls

A word might be mentioned here concerning differences between boys and girls. At the age of five most girls are ready to attend kindergarten; they can sit in their seats for long periods of time, pay attention to a teacher, and be interested in a task. Boys, because of their

somewhat slower rate of maturity, are often less ready than girls for coping with a classroom situation at the age of five.

A child of five grows at a slower rate than in earlier years, but his body is nonetheless changing. The protruding abdomen and knock-knees of the toddler begin to disappear.

Television

Now that television is a part of nearly every family's life, it may absorb a good part of the child's time. Television is an advantage if it does not usurp the time the child would ordinarily spend in vigorous outdoor play or in some quiet indoor activity—working with construction toys, playing house with dolls, playing doctor with a makeshift stethoscope, or just leafing through picture books. A child seldom sticks to television if there is something better going on.

Personal Hygiene

Good habits of cleanliness should be established. The child should know that hand-washing before meals is essential even when the hands look clean. He will learn this only if he sees parents do it. As he gets older he should select his own clean clothing and know that dirty clothing should be washed. A daily routine of washing or bathing should be set up, and the child should be encouraged to observe it.

School-Age Children: Parent-Child Relationships

Beginning around the age of four, boys show a decided preference for their mothers. A boy may, for example, tell his mother that when he grows up he would like to marry her and kick father out of the house. At times he may even suggest that he would work to support her and that life would be much nicer if daddy were not around.

This interest in his mother is often expressed in what may be thought of as sexual ways. That is,

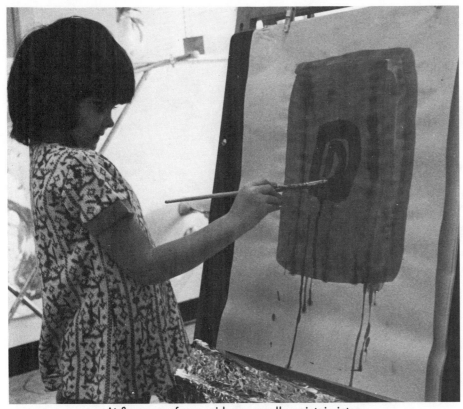

At five years of age, girls can usually maintain interest in an activity for a longer period of time than boys.

the child of this age enjoys his mother's affection, including kissing, hugging, and close bodily contact. This wish to have mother all to himself and to have father out of the picture is called by psychiatrists and psychologists the *Oedipal complex*, after the ancient Greek tragedy, *Oedipus Rex*, in which Oedipus kills his father and marries a woman whom he later discovers to be his mother.

At about this same age, similar emotional developments take place in a girl. She will likely be somewhat seductive, coy, and coquettish with her father, and may talk about marrying father (or a man like father) and having mother out of the picture. This phase of emotional attachment between a girl and her father is called the *Electra complex* after the Greek play, *Electra*.

At these times, both the girl and the boy have a strong, although not always conscious, wish to displace the parent of the same sex and have the opposite-sexed parent all to

themselves. Strong conflicts disturb children in this phase of development, for they also realize that they love and need the same-sexed parent to instruct them, to guide them, to provide for them, and to love them.

Identification

Both males and females eventually resolve these conflicts by abandoning their so-called sexual attachment to the opposite-sexed parent, forming a closer attachment to the same-sexed parent and trying to be like that parent. This is not a conscious decision, but one that a child makes without realizing it. This process of *identification* with the parent of the same sex starts very early, perhaps as early as the second year, and continues through adolescence, but it is especially noticeable from five to ten.

Much of the energy that had previously been utilized in loving the parent of the opposite sex is now spent in loving the parent of the

same sex. The boy follows father around, wants to do whatever he does, and holds as his greatest ambition to be exactly like father when he grows up—even to marrying a woman like the one father did.

The girl during this same period spends the energy that was once expended in love for her father in an attempt to learn to be like mother and perhaps eventually to marry a man resembling in some way her father. This, however, does not mean that children do not continue to love the opposite-sexed parent; it means only that their primary attachment during these years is to the same-sexed parent. It is this process of identification with the same-sexed parent that facilitates the chief task of the school-age child from 5 or 6 to 11: the task of learning.

Six Years to Adolescence

The years from 6 to 11 have generally been regarded as quiet years as far as emotional development is concerned. Many of the tasks of earlier childhood have been completed, and the relatively stormy years of adolescence have not yet begun. A child's interests begin to turn more and more away from his family and to other children his own age, usually children of the same sex. At this stage, a child's interest in learning is broad and intense.

During this period children begin to be more and more individualistic. Some are solitary, others sociable; some are athletic, others not. One likes only other children, another prefers the company of adults. Some children have imaginary fears which disappear with age or when the fears are discussed with an adult who can explain how or why they originated.

CURIOSITY ABOUT SEX: The child's earlier curiosity about naked people may change to a concern about being clothed and being with people who are clothed. Questions about sex should be answered simply and truthfully.

Adolescence

Adolescence arrives anywhere from 9 to 14 years of age. A girl usually enters adolescence at 10, a boy at about 12.

In female children, there is growth of the breasts and nipples; the pelvis matures, and the external genitalia develop. Axillary (underarm) and pubic hair appear. On the average, girls have their first menstrual period around age thirteen, but it can occur between 10 and 16 years of age. Be sure to explain menstruation to your daughter before the beginning of adolescence.

In male children, the penis and testes develop. Facial, axillary, and pubic hair appear. The voice begins to deepen.

In both boys and girls, there is a rapid growth in height and weight which is related to sexual development. In general, the average height of the adolescent is double what it was at age two. See *Puberty and Growth*, p. 109.

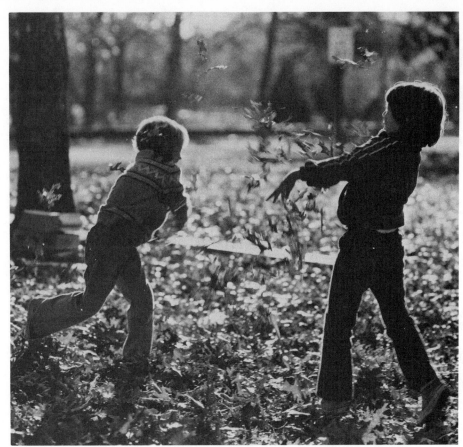

As children become older, they become more interested in developing friendships and participating in activities outside the family.

ALPHABETIC GUIDE TO CHILD CARE

The following Guide is an alphabetically arranged list of articles dealing with many of the problems that confront parents. It includes articles on physical disorders and ailments of childhood; behavioral and emotional problems; and on situations that occur normally in the life of almost every child which may cause tension or distress for parents, child, or both. It is hoped that having information about such normal developmental tensions will help to minimize them.

A NOTE ON THE CROSS-REFERENCES: Where a particular subject is covered elsewhere within this Guide, the reference is printed in small capital letters. (For example: See also TONSILLITIS.) References to sections in other chapters are printed in italic type followed by a page number. (For example: See *Tonsils and Adenoids*, p. 330.)

Abilities and aptitudes

In families that place a high value on "performance," a child who has a special aptitude for dealing with animals may get less recognition than a sibling who is an athletic whiz; a mother who never went to college and wishes she had may encourage her daughter's intellectual gifts at the expense of any others.

Parents should make every effort not to foist their own unrealized fantasies onto their children. They should try to keep in mind that each child differs in aptitudes and abilities, and that these individual differences should be fostered, respected, and allowed to find expression.

PRECOCITY: The emphasis on the competitive—not to mention showoff—aspects of any special talent rather than on the satisfaction of accomplishment for its own sake, is a tendency that some parents have to guard against. The most satisfactory approach to outstanding abilities of no matter what category is to recognize their existence as a fact and to keep them for becoming a burden to the child and an ego trip for the parent.

SIBLING RIVALRY: In large families, the relationship between brothers and sisters is sufficiently complicated by tensions between the oldest and next oldest and so on without introducing additional reasons for competitiveness. Sibling rivalry should not be further fostered by parents who favor the offspring with special abilities. Here is the defensive remark of a middle child (often neglected) in a family with four children: "Tommy is the smartest and Ann is the best swimmer and Jesse is the best at chess, but I'm the goodest." Is the ability to be good a special ability?

Accidents

See *Medical Emergencies*, p. 573, and *The Emergency Room*, p. 305.

Adenoidectomy

See *Tonsils and Adenoids*, p. 330.

Adenoids, swollen

The adenoids are clusters of lymph tissue located behind the soft palate where the nasal passages join the throat. Along with the tonsils and lymphoid tissues elsewhere in the body, the adenoids are involved in warding off infection. When they themselves become inflamed because of bacterial or viral invasion, they become swollen. Swelling may also occur because of allergy.

Swollen adenoids may block the air passages sufficiently to cause mouth breathing, which in turn will not only give the child an "adenoidal" look, but will lead to more frequent upper respiratory infection, as well as to eventual malformation of the lower jawbone. Chronic swelling may also block the Eustachian tube, causing pain in the ear and increasing the possibility of ear infection as well as of intermittent hearing loss. The child's doctor can keep track of the severity of such symptoms during periodic checkups and can evaluate the need for surgery. See also TONSILLITIS. For a description of adenoidectomy, see *Tonsils and Adenoids*, p. 330.

Adopted children

No matter what their individual differences about child rearing, all specialists agree that an adopted child should be told that she was adopted. It doesn't matter that the adoptive parents have come to feel that the child is completely their own. Biologically, she isn't, and it is her human right to find this out not from a neighbor or schoolmate but from the people she trusts as her parents. The fact of her adoption should be talked about naturally in the child's presence even before she can understand what it means. If she is being raised in a loving atmosphere and feels secure in the acceptance of her adoptive parents, she isn't likely to be upset by the reality of her situation.

When the child becomes curious about the circumstances of her adoption, or if she wants to know about her "real" mother and father, she should be given no more—and no less—information than the adoption agency provided originally. It isn't unusual for a couple to adopt a baby because they can't have one of their own, and then, because of some hormonal magic, for the woman to become pregnant. In families where this has occurred, the adopted child can be given the feeling that, whatever the advantages of the "natural" child, she was the chosen one.

A widow or divorcee who remarries when her children are still very young may be faced with the possibility that her second husband wants to legally adopt the offspring of her first marriage. Far-reaching consequences are involved in such a decision, and it should not be undertaken lightly. The problem should be discussed with a lawyer who can present the facts in a detached way so that the decision will cause the least anguish and fewest unpleasant consequences.

Aggressiveness

In the rough and tumble of play, some puppies are obviously more aggressive than others, and one of them is clearly determined to be top dog. The same is true of children, especially in any society where energy and enterprise are rewarded.

Aggressive tendencies are natural; the form they take is up to the civilizing efforts of the parents. It is they who have the responsibility of helping a child understand that bullying and bossiness are unacceptable. It seems that because of inheritance, body build, or temperament, some youngsters, whether male or female, are more clearly aggressive than others. It is especially for such children that healthy outlets must be provided for aggression—in the form of toys and playground activities when they are little, and in suitable physical and intellectual endeavors when they get older.

GUILT FEELINGS: Making a child feel guilty about the strength of his aggressive feelings or thwarting them constantly won't wipe out or destroy the feelings; they'll simply be turned inward, or take the form of nail-biting, or express themselves in some sneaky and antisocial way. Parents who are upset by children's play that simulates violence and who disapprove of toy guns should make their feelings clear without making the youngster feel like a monster because he enjoys them. Aggressiveness that expresses itself

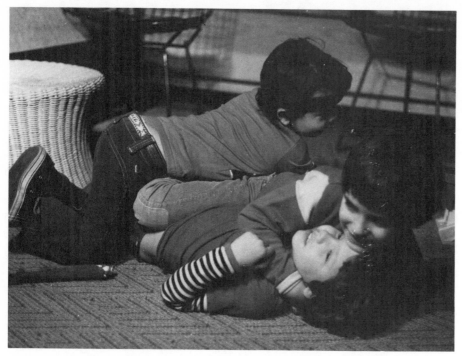

Some aggression is often expressed in play—by children of both sexes
—and need not be discouraged unless it endangers other children.

in violence and bloodshed—as it so often does in Westerns and in TV programs—should not be the day-in-day-out entertainment to which children are exposed no matter what the parental feelings are.

BOY/GIRL DIFFERENCES: As for a boy who doesn't seem aggressive enough to suit a parent's idea of what a boy should be, or a girl who seems too aggressive to conform to family notions about what "feminine" is all about: these stereotypes are being reexamined and discarded by many people because they are too confining and too rigid to permit the full development of a child's personality. It's no disgrace for a boy to cry, and it should be a source of pride to have a daughter who's determined to be the best math student in the fourth grade.

Allergies

See *Allergies and Hypersensitivities*, p. 283.

Allowance

See MONEY.

Ambitions

No matter how grandiose and un-realistic a child's ambitions might seem to parents who pride themselves on being practical, they should be taken seriously and permitted to thrive if the child is working to achieve them. Sometimes the clumsy little girl does become a ballet dancer against all odds, and the boy whose father was a day laborer does become a doctor. Ambitions needn't be that exalted. The youngster who goes down to the firehouse with his father may indeed dream of being a fireman; the girl who loves looking after babies should be encouraged in her goal to be a pediatric nurse.

LACK OF AMBITION: What about the youngster who isn't ambitious about anything and who seems to have no goals, not even small ones? This passivity may be a reaction to over-ambitious parents who have given him the feeling that nothing he aspires to is good enough for them. Or it might result from his never having been made to feel worthwhile enough to have his thoughts about his future taken seriously. Many children who suffer from parental neglect or inadequate educational facilities may need some extra atten-

tion from an older person before ambition plays a role in their lives. No matter what the limitations of circumstance, it's rare to find a child who doesn't have some special skill, aptitude, or interest that can become the basis of ambitions for his future as an adult.

Anger

Anger is a feeling that everyone is familiar with. There are moments when even the most controlled and civilized adult experiences the kind of anger that might become blind rage. A child whose bike has been stolen has a right to her anger; a child whose baby brother has broken a valuable doll is justifiably angry. Some youngsters seem to be angry all the time because they feel they're always being pushed around by adults. (Many adults are always angry because they feel they're being pushed around by other adults.) Almost continuous anger seems especially common among some children of six, seven, and eight. Their theme song is "It isn't fair" and they get to be known as injustice-collectors, angry at their friends, siblings, teachers.

MEANS OF EXPRESSING ANGER: When parents know that a child's anger comes from a healthy feeling of outrage or because of confusion, they should allow the anger to be expressed—in words or tears. But it does have to be made clear that smashing things in a fit of rage or having a tantrum is unacceptable. A child at the mercy of powerful feelings of rage can be frightened by them and should be helped to understand and control them. It's also a comfort to children to know that grown-ups get terribly angry from time to time, but that part of growing up consists in being able to handle one's feelings and in learning how to express them in the right way at the right time. Thus, a father who is in a rage with his boss will find ways of letting him know that he feels an injustice has been done rather than swallow his anger at work and let it out against his wife or children as soon as he comes home.

Animal bites

See *Animal Bites*, p. 586.

Anxiety

Children become chronically anxious when their parents constantly criticize them for failing to measure up to some unachievable standard of perfection. Likewise, parents become anxious about being parents when they criticize themselves for failing to measure up to some unachievable standard of perfection.

Anxiety is one of the most widespread and most debilitating stresses from which people of all ages suffer in the United States, chiefly because many Americans have been victimized by the notion that everybody can be everything. Thus, a parent will expect a little child to be good, bright, neat, polite, aggressive enough to compete adequately but not so aggressive that the other children don't like him, relaxed and cheerful at the same time that he's supposed to do all his chores and the homework and remember to be nice to his baby sister. What child

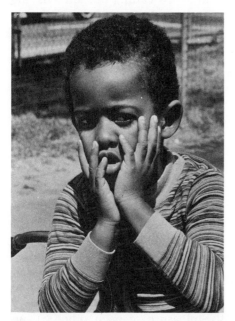

Chronic anxiety in children can be very harmful. Parents can keep their children emotionally healthy by setting realistic goals for each child and not expecting too much.

burdened with such expectations isn't going to feel anxious about fulfilling them so that he can gain his parents' love and approval?

Parents may waste emotional energy feeling anxiety because they think they're inadequate mothers or fathers, perhaps because they lose their tempers from time to time or because they're often too tired to play with their toddler and stick him in the playpen just to keep him out of trouble. A child will also be made chronically anxious if he's always being threatened with punishment, or if he's made to feel that he's bad when he's trying to be good but doesn't know how. The way to keep anxiety at a minimum is to have achievable goals. Is the child healthy, moderately well-behaved, cheerful, and inspiring no complaints from his teachers? Are you as a parent helping him to be healthy, moderately well-behaved, cheerful, and cause no trouble at school? No reason for anybody to be anxious.

Aptitudes

See ABILITIES AND APTITUDES.

Asthma

Asthma, also known as *bronchial asthma*, is a respiratory disturbance in which breathing becomes difficult and labored and is accompanied by a wheezing sound. It is a chronic disorder in which the bronchial tubes suddenly contract or go into spasm, thus cutting off the passage of air from the windpipe to the lungs. Spasms are accompanied by secretion of mucus into the air passages and a swelling of the bronchial tubes, causing the intake and outflow of air to be further obstructed. The disorder may be triggered by a variety of factors; in children it is associated chiefly with allergy and emotional stress. In some cases, asthma may accompany a bacterial or viral infection of the nose or throat.

THE ASTHMA ATTACK: It can be very frightening to witness a child's first asthma attack, since judging from the sounds and the effort involved

in breathing, the child seems to be suffocating. Call the child's doctor promptly. Until the doctor can be consulted for emergency treatment, parents should try to be calm and reassuring. Immediate symptoms can be alleviated by prescribed medicines given orally or by injection, or by placing the child in a moist environment, such as in the bathroom with the shower turned on (but not *in* the shower). Otherwise, the child should be kept in bed in a humidified room. The condition itself should be carefully assessed by the doctor to decide whether desensitization to a particular food or pollen is necessary, whether a pet has to be given away, or whether the child's emotional needs are being neglected. Chronic asthma should not go untreated since frequent and acute attacks can affect general health. Medicines now available can sometimes prevent acute attacks if taken daily by inhalation when one is well.

Autism

See under MENTAL ILLNESS.

Baby sitters

Families who can always count on a grandparent or an older child to look after the little ones in their absence are spared the complications and expense of hiring baby sitters. However, many parents must rely on their own resources, especially when both parents work. In such situations the sitter has become an indispensable adjunct of the family.

INSTRUCTION IN BABY SITTING: In some communities, parents have found it worthwhile to offer a free, informal course in baby sitting to groups of teen-age girls and boys. The course need consist of no more than two or three sessions and can be given by the parents themselves at a local community center. All aspects of the sitter's responsibilities and privileges should be covered. Does the sitter do the dinner dishes? May local phone calls be made? May the refrigerator be raided? The potential employees should be encouraged to ask all the questions they feel uncertain about, and after the course is over, a single sheet of paper summarizing the most important material can be prepared, reproduced in quantity, and distributed to everyone taking the course. The sheet should include a list of hourly rates with all variants: base rate per hour; increase in rate after midnight; increase per number of children to be looked after, and so on. It might also be a good idea to include the names and telephone numbers of places where sitters can be obtained, such as nursing schools and coed colleges.

COOPERATIVE SITTING: For families who want to get out occasionally but can't afford the extra expense of a sitter, a cooperative parents' pool is a good solution. Each month, one participating parent is responsible for keeping track of who has been sitting for whom, how many hours are owed and how many have been "paid for," and so on. The advantage of this arrangement is that mothers or fathers sit for each others' children and no money changes hands. If such a cooperative pool is worked out, remember that the more accurately the records of time asked for and given are kept, and the more businesslike the arrangements, the longer the system will work and the less friction there will be. Each group should decide for itself what the maximum number of participants should be, and as the group becomes too large to function efficiently, it can split into two separate pools.

PROVIDE INFORMATION FOR EMERGENCIES: Parents should always leave clear and explicit instructions about possible emergencies with baby sitters and if possible should leave a telephone number where they can be reached. As the children become opinionated about hired sitters, their wishes should be taken into account. When your own youngsters begin to be hired as sitters themselves, you might keep track of where they're working and when they'll be escorted home. See also p. 150.

Battered child

In 1962, the chief pediatrician at the University of Colorado Medical Center, Dr. C. Henry Kempe, coined the term *battered child syndrome* in a report published in the Journal of the American Medical Association describing his nationwide survey of child abuse. According to his definition, the victim is "any child who received *nonaccidental* injury or injuries as a result of acts or omissions on the part of his parents or guardians."

Medical authorities now consider child battering the most common cause of childhood death, outnumbering fatalities caused by disease and accident. The more obvious forms of battering include severe beatings, head-crackings, burnings, scaldings, and stompings. Children are kicked to death; crying infants are shaken so violently that whiplash injuries either kill them or irreversibly damage the brain. Sexual maltreatment, gross neglect, starvation, and abandonment are common.

The only solution to such tragedies is to protect the battered child and simultaneously treat the abusive parent. Many professions are and must be involved in dealing with this challenge: doctors, lawyers, judges, social workers, lawmakers, psychotherapists, teachers, and community leaders. On the most immediate level, friends, relatives, or neighbors of a family in need of counseling or of a child in need of protection should contact a local child welfare agency. If at all possible, the disturbed parent should be directed towards some form of therapy.

PARENTS ANONYMOUS: Parents Anonymous is a growing organization where abusive parents who essentially have a low opinion of themselves can meet in therapy sessions to help themselves and each other. This nation-wide organization, similar to Alcoholics Anonymous, has chapters in many parts of the United States. Information is available from Parents Anonymous, 2810 Artesia Blvd., Suite F, Redondo Beach, California 90278. See also CHILD ABUSE.

Bedtime

From babyhood on, the routine of bedtime should be as relaxed as possible for both parent and child. Little babies love to be chanted to (even off-key) or talked to in a gentle tone of voice (even though they don't understand the words) or rocked a bit in their crib. Some little ones seem to resist and fight falling asleep: they fuss and whimper, and then, as though they had been bewitched in the middle of a cry—off they go, all of a sudden. Toddlers may want to hear the same story every night for months, or may cling to the bedtime bottle for quite a while after they've begun to use a cup in the daytime.

Keeping things peaceful at bedtime doesn't mean giving in to the child's pressures or whims. It generally involves keeping one's voice calm, pleasant, and firm: "It's bedtime, and you tell me which story to read to you tonight." The youngster who keeps calling out after having been tucked in—for water, for a last hug, for a last question, for a last trip to the bathroom—isn't determined to make a nuisance of herself; she's just a little scared and wants to make absolutely sure that you're still there. If the family tradition calls for prayers at bedtime, the tone should be cheerful. No child can be expected to relish, "And if I die before I wake I pray the Lord my soul to take" as an accompaniment to sleep.

In a crowded family where siblings share a bedroom, compromises have to be made about the bedtime hour: the younger ones may stay up a little later than they otherwise would, and the older ones may go to bed a little earlier—but they have the pleasure of each other's company. Adjustments in the bedtime hour should be made from time to time not because of a child's wheedling, but because you decide that the occasion calls for it.

Bedwetting

See *Bedwetting*, p. 430.

Behavior problems

See AGGRESSIVENESS, ANGER, DELINQUENCY, DESTRUCTIVENESS, DISHONESTY, DISOBEDIENCE.

Birthmarks

See p. 250.

Blindness

See HANDICAPPED CHILD.

Booster shots

See IMMUNIZATION.

Boredom

Babies are usually too hungry or too sleepy—or too cranky—to be bored. Toddlers have so much to investigate around the house that boredom is not likely to be one of their problems. As a child gets older and complains about having nothing to do, you might get him involved in a household chore by saying, "Let's . . ." rather than "Why don't you" or "How would you like to." "Let's tidy the cans on the pantry shelf" or "Let's make some cookies" can make a three-year-old feel useful and interested.

RAINY DAYS: If you're too busy for a cooperative effort and there's a long rainy day ahead, provide for it in advance by keeping a "boredom box" in the closet and renewing its contents from time to time: wrappings saved from gifts; bits of material; boxes of various sizes; discarded magazines to be cut up; old clothes for dress-up activities, and the like.

COPING WITH BOREDOM CAN BE PRODUCTIVE: A child who is never allowed to be bored because his parents or older siblings feel that they have to entertain him or play with him is deprived of the possibility of calling on his own resources and learning how to amuse himself. The fact that an only child may have to live through stretches of boredom often contributes to his exploring his own abilities in a creative way. Sometimes just asking a child to "Tell *me* a story" can work wonders. Some parents solve the recurrent problem of boredom by organizing informal play groups of three or four children; others find a nursery school the best solution.

CONVALESCENCE: An older child who is recovering from an illness that has kept him out of school and isolated him from his friends may require some special project to work on in addition to catching up on his homework. A period of protracted convalescence is a good time to introduce a new hobby or craft such as model-making or clay sculpture that may solve the boredom problem for years to come.

Brain damage

Brain damage refers to an organic defect of the brain—that is, tissue destruction—caused by an injury to the nervous system occurring before, during, or after birth. Such injury can be caused by toxic chemicals as well as by physical trauma. It can result in any of a variety of neurological disorders, such as cerebral palsy or other impairment of motor coordination, mental retardation, convulsive seizures, hyperkinesis, or perceptual difficulties.

MINIMAL BRAIN DAMAGE: Minimal brain damage (or, more formally, *minimal brain dysfunction*) refers to a condition of some children who suffer from a motor or perceptual impairment that may affect their ability to learn or use language, interfere with memory, or make it difficult for them to control their attention. Some learning disabilities are attributed to minimal brain damage. See also DYSLEXIA.

Bribes

No child should be bribed into behaving properly except in an emergency. If she's given an ice-cream cone so that she'll stop having a tantrum in public, or if she gets a toy instead of a spanking when she carries on in a store, it will surely occur to her that she can blackmail her parents into getting whatever she wants—which ends up by her being rewarded for being naughty.

A child should not be bribed with money for doing the things that should be expected of her as a matter of course. As a member of the family, she can be counted on to help set and clear the table, and when she's a little older, to help with the dishes without being paid to do so. She should be expected to do as well as she can at school without being told that her allowance will be increased if her grades are better than her best friend's.

The line between a bribe and a reward is a delicate one and should be kept somewhat flexible if it is to be realistic. Certainly a youngster who has made extra efforts should be rewarded, but in some way that doesn't involve the handing over of money. Treating her and her friends to a special outing, or spending some extra time with her in a pursuit of her own choice is a way of showing that you appreciate the good job she's done—whether it's taking the responsibility for cleaning up the garage or doing a series of complicated errands without complaining about them. See also MONEY.

Brothers and sisters

Rivalry and jealousy and bickering are inevitable among brothers and sisters; companionship, a helping hand, and good times together are part of the picture too. Parents can keep resentments and quarrels at a minimum by not playing one child off against the other or by refraining from holding up one child as an example of virtue to another. In an atmosphere of equal recognition, brothers and sisters will love and respect each other most of the time and fight only occasionally. Special privileges granted on the basis of such distinctions as "Well, he's the oldest" or "She's the youngest" or exceptions made because "He's a boy" or "She's only a girl" can cause resentments that last a lifetime.

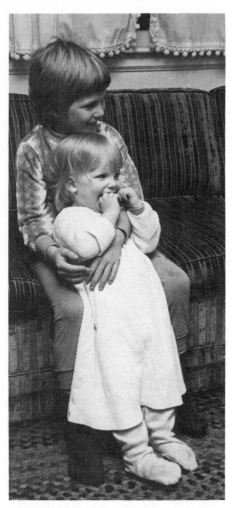

In families where all the children are treated with love and respect, brothers and sisters find it easy to show affection for one another.

Burns

See *Burns*, p. 590.

Camps

There seems to be no end to the diversity of camps available for summer enrollment. Most urban and suburban communities have day camps in which children may be accepted for certain minimum periods. They range from expensive groups that offer sightseeing trips, swimming instruction, and other special attractions to groups that cost very little and function more or less like day care centers. "Sleepaway" camps run by organizations such as the Scouts and the 4-H Clubs are comparatively cheap and will register a child for a week rather than for a month or for the entire summer. Camps subsidized by community funds or private endowment are available for urban children from poor families.

SPECIAL CAMPS: The proliferation of special camps has been a blessing to the parents of handicapped children: those with diabetes, muscular dystrophy, learning disabilities, obesity, and other problems need no longer be deprived of a camping experience with their peers. In many cases, particularly for overweight youngsters, the summer experience can be a major health contribution.

In general, an effort should be made to choose a camp that suits the tastes and temperament of the child. A youngster who hates competitive sports is likely to have a miserable time in a camp that emphasizes team spirit. He may enjoy a place that offers lots of nature study, hiking, and animal care. A child eager to improve his swimming should go to a camp with better-than-average water sport facilities rather than one that concentrates on arts and crafts and offers only a nearby pond for all water activities. Information about camps that have official standing can be obtained by writing to The American Camping Association, 225 Park Avenue South, New York, New York 10003.

Cancer

Rare as it may be and affecting only one child in about 7,000 each year, cancer still claims the lives of more children between the ages of one and fourteen than any other single disease. Among the cancers that more commonly affect children in their early years are the following: *acute lymphocytic leukemia*, in which white blood cells proliferate in the bone marrow in such great quantities that they disrupt normal blood production; *neuroblastoma*, which may occur in any part of the body but characteristically involves a tumorous growth in the sympathetic nerve tissues of the adrenal glands; *brain or spinal cord tumor*; *Hodgkin's disease*, or cancer of the lymph nodes; *Wilm's tumor*, a rare kidney cancer that accounts for about one-fifth of all childhood can-

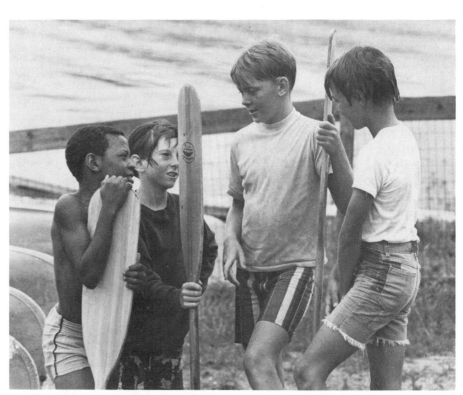

The best camp for a child is one that emphasizes his special interest, whether it be water sports, tennis, crafts, or music.

cers; *retinoblastoma,* an eye tumor that is probably hereditary and is most frequently encountered in children under four; and *bone cancer* that may attack the long bones of the forearm and leg during the growing years. Many of these cancers can now be arrested, and some can be cured if symptoms are detected early enough. See Ch. 24, p. 434, for further information about cancer.

EARLY SYMPTOMS: Early detection is best accomplished by calling to a doctor's attention any of these symptoms that last for more than a few days: continued crying or pain for which there appears to be no explanation; intermittent nausea and vomiting; the development of lumps or swellings in or on any part of the child's body; stumbling or walking unsteadily; a loss of appetite and general lassitude; any marked change in bowel or bladder habits; any unexplained discharge of blood, whether in the stool or urine, or in heavy nosebleeds, or any marked slowness of bleeding to stop after an injury.

Celiac disease

Celiac disease, officially known as *malabsorption syndrome,* is the designation for a group of congenital enzyme deficiencies in which certain nutriments are not properly absorbed from the intestinal tract. *Celiac* means having to do with the abdomen. Celiac disease is characterized by frothy, bulky, and foul-smelling stools containing undigested fats. Diarrhea may alternate with constipation, the child has severe stomach cramps, and the abdomen becomes conspicuously bloated. If the disease is untreated, anemia results, and the child's growth is impaired. Early symptoms should be brought to a doctor's attention so that a correct diagnosis can be made based on laboratory investigation of the stools. Treatment consists of a special, gluten-free diet under a doctor's continuing supervision. *Gluten* is a protein component of wheat and rye; special

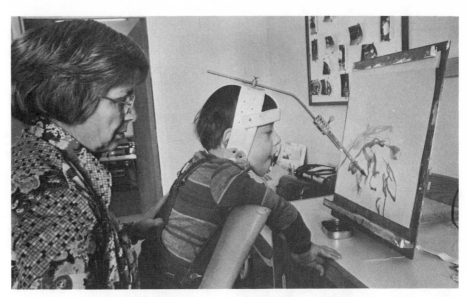

In a special training program, an occupational therapist teaches motor coordination to a child with cerebral palsy.

breads, cookies, etc., must therefore be used. If the diet is strictly adhered to, full recovery can be expected, although it may take over a year.

Cerebral palsy

Cerebral palsy is the general term for a group of abnormal conditions commonly associated with a brain disorder that causes the loss or impairment of muscle control. Approximately one child in about 7,000 suffers from some degree of this disability. Damage to the nervous system that results in cerebral palsy may have occurred before birth, during delivery, or in rare cases, as a consequence of accident, injury, or severe illness during infancy or childhood. Since symptoms vary widely, each individual case is assessed for proper treatment by a team of therapists under the supervision of a specialist, usually a pediatrician. One of the most important aspects of treatment involves parental understanding of the fact that it is essential that they help the child to help himself as much as possible. Guiding the youngster towards self-acceptance and independence requires the patience, persistence, and resourcefulness of

the entire family, and may require a certain amount of group therapy and counseling. For a discussion of symptoms and treatment, see *Cerebral Palsy,* p. 470.

Cheating

See DISHONESTY.

Checkups

Medical and dental checkups are essential to everyone's health, but they are especially important for the growing child. An infant should be examined by a doctor every month for the first six months, and less frequently after that. The doctor usually recommends a schedule for immunization and future checkups. If possible, parents should try to maintain continuity with the same physician so that when an illness occurs, the child sees the doctor as an old friend rather than a threatening stranger. Continuity also gives the doctor a total picture of the child in sickness and in health, and enables him to diagnose variations from the normal with more accuracy. Parents who cannot afford the services of a private physician can be assured of good infant and child care at a local child-health station or at the well-baby clinic of a nearby

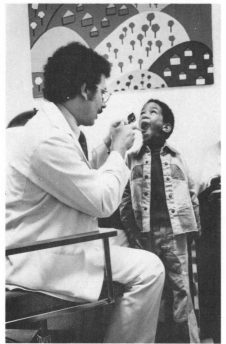

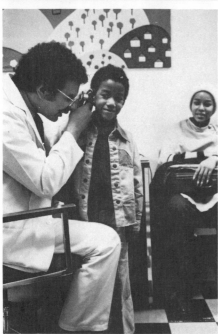

Regular checkups monitor a child's growth and alert the doctor and the parents to any problems. This boy's checkup includes an examination of the throat and ears, as well as recording of his height and weight.

hospital. Between checkups, it's a good idea for parents to keep a running list of questions or problems they would like to discuss with the doctor at the next visit.

Chicken pox

Chicken pox cannot be prevented at this time. It does not usually cause any severe complications in a child, but it can be serious in an adult. It is highly infectious and spreads rapidly.

Chicken pox is caused by a virus. Its incubation period is two to three weeks. Symptoms include those of the common cold, a fever, general malaise, and a rash.

The rash, which may be either mild or severe, is different from that produced by measles or by rubella. The measles rash is red and blotchy. Chicken pox look like bunches of blisters close together. These blisters are filled with fluid, and there is a reddened area around each lesion. As new blisters appear, the older ones become encrusted. The rash may affect the mouth, nose, ears, vagina, penis, or scrotum. In an older child the symptoms may be more severe than in a younger one, and may be accompanied by headache and vomiting.

TREATMENT: The only way to treat chicken pox is symptomatically. The rash is very itchy, and an affected child must be prevented from scratching. Otherwise, he may develop a secondary infection and be left pitted and scarred.

Treatment involves the use of lotions, such as calamine, which is applied locally to the pox to relieve the itching. If the child is old enough, it's a good idea to let him paint it on himself. Your physician may also prescribe medicine to be taken orally to help the child stop scratching the blisters. In a few days, the rash clears up, the lesions dry, and the crusts fall off.

Child abuse

Although the present-day emphasis on problems of child abuse is on the rehabilitation of parents, it is still essential to safeguard the victimized child. In 1974, a National Center on Child Abuse and Neglect was established by federal law as part of the Children's Bureau of the Office of Child Development. It has been heavily funded to provide protective services for the short-term care of endangered children outside the home, as well as counseling for parents, foster-care payments, and other services. Information about local services provided by private and public agencies can be obtained by writing to the National Center on Child Abuse and Neglect, Department of Health, Education, and Welfare, Office of Child Development, Box 1182, Washington, D.C. 20013. The national organization that sets the standards for voluntary child welfare agencies and that provides information about programs throughout the United States is the Child Welfare League of America, 67 Irving Place, New York, New York 10003. See also BATTERED CHILD.

Circumcision

Circumcision is a minor surgical procedure in which the foreskin that covers the cone-shaped tip of the penis is removed, usually a few days after birth. It is spoken of in the Book of Genesis as a religious rite, but in many parts of the world circumcision is now routinely per-

Circumcision is an important religious rite in many parts of the world, as shown in this 16th-century engraving. Religious reasons aside, the operation is done to promote good hygiene.

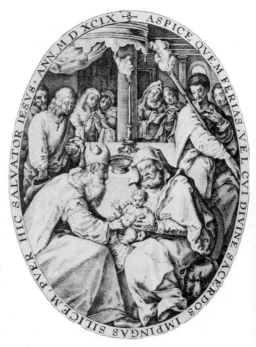

formed to facilitate male personal hygiene. Since the operation can be upsetting to a baby who is several months old and terrifying to a little boy of three or four, circumcision is best performed by a doctor or by a qualified person with the doctor's approval before the newborn leaves the hospital. If the operation is recommended as a necessity because the boy's foreskin is so long or so tight that it interferes with urination or encourages infection, it is likely to involve hospitalization and general anesthesia. In that event, it should be postponed until the child is old enough to accept the surgery as a health measure. If circumcision is not performed, the foreskin should be pushed back to minimize the risk of infection.

Cleanliness and neatness

Most healthy youngsters are too busy exploring the world or are too involved in what they're doing at the moment to be concerned about being neat and clean.

What is cleanliness all about anyway? Parents used to talk a lot about germs, and the germs are certainly still all around us in spite of the success of antibiotics in dealing with a large number of them. But there are the unconquerable viruses, and parasites, and worms, and children should thus be told in a factual way that habits of personal cleanliness are important for reasons of their own health and the health of the people around them. Coming to the table with freshly washed hands, keeping their bodies clean, washing their hands after using the toilet, covering their coughs and sneezes—these minimal practices should be instilled until they become habitual and no longer need to be discussed. Children do get dirty, but TV commercials have taught practically every one of them that getting their clothes clean is no big deal, so it's futile for parents to get worked up over stains.

As for neatness, the point of put-ting things where they belong is not merely for the sake of appearances, but for the more important reason that time won't be wasted and tempers lost in trying to find them when they're needed. The aesthetics of tidiness doesn't interest most children, but a functional reason that makes sense to them usually does. When it comes to looking neat, some children seem to accomplish that with no effort at all; others look like slobs until adolescence begins, when parents deprived of the use of the bathroom mirror may yearn for the good old untidy days of childhood.

Cleft palate and cleft lip

A *cleft palate* is a split in the roof of the mouth sometimes extending to the lip and into the nose. The split is caused by the failure of the two sides of the face to unite properly during prenatal development. The condition occurs in about 1 out of 1,000 births and is sometimes associated with a foot or spine deformity. It is in no way related to mental retardation.

An infant born with a cleft palate cannot suck properly unless a special device, called an *obturator*, is inserted into the split to close it against the flow of air. Where this is undesirable, feeding may be done with a spoon or a dropper.

Since the condition eventually causes speech distortion, it should be corrected at about 18 months of age, before the child begins to talk. The surgery consists of reconstructing the tissue. Sometimes, even at this early age, the child may need some corrective speech therapy following the operation.

If the split occurs only in the lip, commonly called a *harelip*, surgery may be recommended when the infant weighs about 15 pounds, usually at the age of 12 to 15 months. When the operation is performed this early, there is no danger of speech impairment, and the result is only a thin scar.

Clothing

Children's clothing should fit comfortably so that it doesn't chafe or bind, especially in hot weather. In addition to allowing for freedom of movement, it should be sturdy and washable. In most communities, blue jeans and shirts seem to serve both sexes in all stages of growing up, starting with nursery school. In some few places, schools have more formal clothing codes, but it's a rare

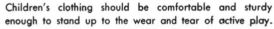

Children's clothing should be comfortable and sturdy enough to stand up to the wear and tear of active play.

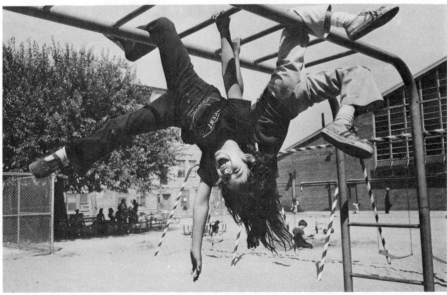

institution that still insists on white shirts and ties for elementary students. A youngster who occasionally enjoys wearing a dress shirt or a party dress can usually find one that's drip-dry and doesn't require ironing.

Many families economize on children's clothing by buying at rummage sales or thrift shops. (Not shoes!) If parents are proud of having found bargains, children will be pleased to wear them. Parental attitude also affects a child's feelings about hand-me-downs from within the family or from friends. There's no reason why children's clothing—and especially such expensive items as heavy outer coats—shouldn't be successively used as long as they fit properly.

FASHIONS AND STATUS: Even sensible clothing can present problems of status that require tactful handling. Your eight-year-old son may announce that everyone in his class is wearing those fancy imported sneakers that cost as much as a pair of good shoes; or your ten-year-old daughter brings you the news that all her friends have expensive coats with a suede look or fur-trimmed collars. For families that can't afford or don't believe in acquiring such luxuries—and the majority can't—the facts are probably these: a few privileged youngsters may indeed be wearing such sneakers or such coats, and the majority have embarked on a concerted campaign of pressuring their parents into making the same expenditures. If your child is really conspicuous because he doesn't own an expensive garment that all his friends have, you must decide whether to make it clear to him that you spend money in different ways—say on family vacations or good dental care. On the other hand, you may decide to capitulate about the item of clothing and deprive the child (not yourself) of something else—perhaps his birthday present for the coming year. That's one way to teach a child a basic lesson about the inevitability of choice-making.

Clubfoot

Clubfoot is a bone deformity characterized by an inturning or outturning of the foot. An orthopedist must put the clubfoot and part of the leg into a cast in order to correct the condition. If casting does not cure the abnormality, orthopedic surgery may be necessary.

Occasionally, a benign and easily correctable condition involving a child's legs may have been produced by the position the baby was in while still in the uterus.

The mother can help to correct the condition by daily passive exercises of the baby's feet. She does this by turning the feet correctly for a few minutes every day. To maintain the corrected position, the application of plaster is sometimes necessary. Such a procedure requires the attention of an orthopedic surgeon.

Colic

During the first three or four months, many babies have occasional attacks of *colic*, a general term applied to infantile digestive discomfort. After feeding, the baby may cry out in pain and draw up her arms and legs. Her abdomen may feel hard. Apart from making sure the baby is as comfortable as can be, there's not much that can be done for colic. You must try not to let the baby's crying make you a nervous wreck, for your nervousness will be communicated to the baby, which will only create a vicious circle of increasing tension. Usually colic tapers off at about the third month. If the baby's colic attacks are very frequent or persistent, consult your doctor.

Color blindness

Color blindness is a congenital inability to distinguish between certain colors, most commonly between red and green. This defect, which is characteristically male, is inherited through the mother. That is, a woman whose father was color-blind can pass the trait to her son without herself suffering the defect. About 8 million people in the U.S. have the red/green form of color blindness which can neither be cured nor corrected. Many of them are scarcely aware of their deficiency. Parents who suspect that their child may have this minor disability can arrange for simple testing.

Common cold

By recent count, there are about 150 different viruses that cause common cold symptoms, and since not a single one of them can be treated effectively by medicines, coping

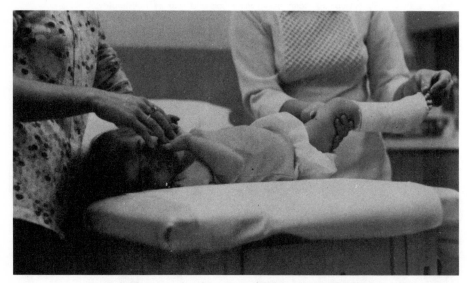

A clubfoot can often be corrected without surgery if a plaster cast is applied to the foot and leg early in childhood.

with a cold seems to be part of the human condition. Parents who are sniveling, sneezing, and coughing should ask the doctor what precautions to take when handling the baby.

Young children with stuffy noses and breathing difficulties should be kept indoors, near a humidifier or steam kettle if the air is especially dry. Nose drops should not be given unless the doctor says so. Older children may not want to miss school because of a cold. If they do go, they should be given lots of liquid when they get home and steered in the direction of an afternoon nap. Colds in and of themselves are unavoidable and not serious, but the proper precautions should be taken to prevent complications, such as an ear infection or a sore throat.

Competitiveness

See AGGRESSIVENESS.

Conscience

See GUILT AND CONSCIENCE.

Constipation

Parents who are anxious about the frequency of their own bowel movements or who are excessively refined in their attitudes towards defecation are pretty sure to transmit these feelings to their children unless they make some effort not to. Concerns of this kind are one sure way of constipating a child. Actually, if a child is eating a proper diet, getting enough exercise, and drinking a sufficiency of liquids, constipation is not likely to be a problem.
FREQUENCY OF BOWEL MOVEMENTS: Not everyone has a bowel movement every day. On the other hand, some people routinely have more than one movement a day. There is considerable variation among normal patterns of bowel movements. This should be borne in mind before parents conclude that their child is constipated. Children need to be reassured that they are not necessarily abnormal if they deviate from the one-a-day pattern.

However, any abrupt change in the normal pattern of bowel movements should be noted, and if it persists the doctor should be informed. Frequent small movements can be a sign of constipation.

A youngster on a light diet because of illness, or one who is dehydrated because of a fever, may suffer from mild constipation which will clear up when he recovers. If constipation becomes chronic, don't resort to enemas or laxatives on your own; discuss the problem with your doctor who will want to check on other symptoms that might indicate an intestinal disorder.

Cradle cap

This condition is marked by yellowish crusts on the baby's scalp. It is usually harmless, and can be taken care of by regular shampooing. Occasionally, a special soap as well as a very fine comb may be helpful.

Crib death

See SUDDEN INFANT DEATH SYNDROME.

Crossed eyes (strabismus)

Do not be alarmed if your baby's eyes do not focus. Crossed eyes are a common condition that usually corrects itself somewhere between the ages of six and twelve months. If crossing of the eyes persists after one year, an ophthalmologist (eye specialist) should evaluate the baby's vision.

If a real problem does develop, one eye—or each eye alternately—may cross, turn outward, or focus below or above the other. Frequently the reason for "turning" is that there is a larger refractive error in one eye than in the other. Eyeglasses will often correct this condition.

Occasionally, eye muscle weakness is the cause of crossed eyes. This is most often true of premature children. The weakness of some muscles causes overaction of other muscles.

Eyeglasses will often prevent the need for eye surgery. Sometimes, however, surgery will be necessary to straighten the eyes. Either before

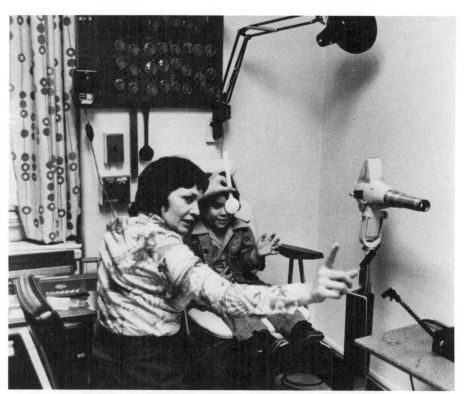

An *orthoptist*, a specialist in diagnosing and correcting muscular defects of the eyes, tests a child's vision to see if his eyes are working together correctly.

or after surgery the eyes may need further attention in the form of eye drops, a patch to cover one eye, or glasses.

Croup

Croup, a most harassing and terrifying experience for new parents, is a spasm of the windpipe or trachea, especially involving the larynx. When such a spasm occurs, an affected child has great trouble in breathing and produces a cough that sounds like the bark of a dog. In some cases, the child can't breathe at all.

An attack of croup is an emergency. The younger the child, the more dangerous it is. You must get the baby's airway open. The best thing to do is to take the child into the bathroom, shut the door, and turn on the hot water of the shower full force, or of the bathtub and sink if you don't have a shower. The idea is to fill the room with hot steam in order to loosen the mucus plug in the baby's trachea, thus enabling him to cough up the mucus.

Get to your physician as soon as possible so that more effective treatment can begin. If the croup is viral in origin, antibiotics may not help; but when the infection is caused by bacteria, your physician will put the child on one of the antimicrobial agents. If your child is subject to croup, it is a good idea to invest in a hot or cold air vaporizer and use it whenever he has congestion due to a cold.

In a really severe emergency, when the windpipe closes completely, a *tracheostomy* must be performed so that the throat can be opened and an airway inserted. A tracheostomy should be performed in a hospital, but if for some reason it is performed elsewhere, the child should be hospitalized as quickly as possible.

Curiosity

If we weren't born curious, we'd never learn a thing. Even before a

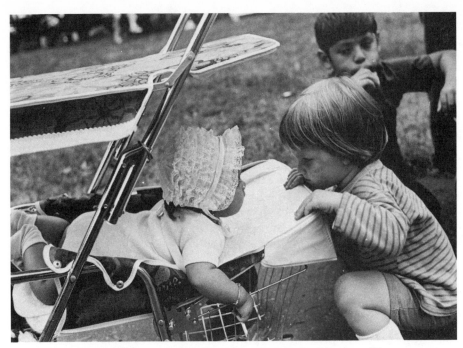

Young children are naturally curious about each other. A stroll in the park provides a fine opportunity to strike up a new friendship.

child can walk and talk, curiosity motivates a good part of her behavior: putting things into her mouth, poking at things, pointing at people, and as the natural urge to speak becomes stronger, holding things up or bringing them to mother or father in order to find out what they're called.

RESPECTING CURIOSITY: A parent who respects the child's curiosity will be attentive to it and satisfy it as part of the ongoing learning experience. It doesn't take any extra time when a toddler is sitting in your lap to say the words for the parts of your face (and hers) as she touches them, or the words for her articles of clothing as she tries to help put them on. Dealing with the "why" stage of curiosity is more complicated, especially because in many instances, the child is asking "Why?" for the sheer joy and sense of power of being able to do so.

Many parents who don't know anything about mechanics or astronomy have developed a sense of security by heading for the children's shelves at the local library and reading the simplest books on the subject that interest their pre-

school children so that they can answer some of their questions. Of course, no one can answer all the questions that a child might ask during an average day. Some should be answered by mother, some by father, and some will have to wait. There's no harm in telling a four-year-old child who wants to know why the wind makes a whistling sound that she'll find out about such things when she goes to school. That's a much better answer than "Don't ask so many questions." Questions should always be listened to even if the answers aren't readily available.

As the child reaches the age of eight and can do a certain amount of reading, it's a good idea to invest in a fairly simple encyclopedia. With such a source of information available, it's possible to respond to some questions with "Let's go find the answer together."

Each family must decide for itself where the line is to be drawn between legitimate curiosity and unacceptable snoopiness or nosiness as children get older and become interested in such matters as how rich the neighbors are, or "What were you and mommy fighting about when I was falling asleep last night?"

Cystic fibrosis

Cystic fibrosis is an inherited disease in which the child cannot handle the normal secretions of the respiratory tract. There is a lack of ciliary action—the beating movement by the hairs of the cells lining the bronchial tubes of the lungs. Thick mucus collects at the base of the lungs, obstructing the smaller air passages and causing labored breathing and chronic cough.

RESPIRATORY COMPLICATIONS: Bacteria multiply in the accumulated lung secretions, predisposing the patient to chronic bronchitis and other respiratory infections, such as pneumonia. Lung tissue changes can result eventually in severe, permanent damage to the lungs.

DIGESTIVE COMPLICATIONS: The abnormally thick, viscous mucus produced by the cystic fibrosis patient tends to obstruct the ducts or openings of the mucus-secreting glands. When such mucus obstructs the pancreas, it interferes with its ability to supply important digestive enzymes to the intestinal tract, thus leading to poor digestion and malabsorption of a number of important nutrients. A child with cystic fibrosis may therefore be poorly nourished in spite of an adequate diet.

OTHER COMPLICATIONS: Tissue changes in the lungs can restrict blood flow to the heart, leading to increased blood pressure and chronic heart strain. Loss of large amounts of salt through malfunctioning sweat glands can become a very serious problem for youngsters in hot weather, causing dehydration and heat exhaustion. Laboratory tests usually find an abnormally high concentration of salt in the sweat of cystic fibrosis patients. (Indeed, the skin of a cystic fibrosis patient is apt to taste salty.) Some tissues may show three times the normal concentration of sodium and twice the normal levels of potassium.

TREATMENT: There is no known cure for cystic fibrosis. Treatment includes the use of humidifiers and inhalation medication in the form of aerosols to loosen secretions. Another method used is *postural drainage*—lying face down with the head lower than the feet to let gravity help loosen secretions. Antibiotics are used to control infections; special diets with reduced fat intake and added nutrients are prescribed to compensate for abnormal digestive function. Other medical techniques are utilized in individual cases to maintain normal heart and lung function.

Once considered strictly a disease of early childhood, an increasing number of cases of cystic fibrosis have been detected in recent years among adolescents and adults. Symptoms of the disease, including respiratory difficulty with chronic coughing, may resemble those of an allergic reaction.

HOW THE DISEASE IS INHERITED: Cystic fibrosis is transmitted to a child only when both parents are carriers of the trait. When only one parent carries the trait, however, some of the children can become carriers. Through marriage with other carriers, they may then become the parents of a child afflicted with the disorder.

Information on new treatment techniques, the location of treatment centers, and genetic counseling may be obtained from the national headquarters of the Cystic Fibrosis Foundation, 3379 Peachtree Road, N.E., Atlanta, Georgia 30326.

Daydreaming

See FANTASIES.

Deafness

Major advances have been made in recent years in educating and socializing incurably deaf children who are normal in all other ways. Starting with a proper assessment of the child's degree of deafness at the earliest possible time and the fitting of a hearing aid are two crucial considerations. The child's instruction in lip-reading and the use of her own vocal equipment are professionally supervised, and the rest of the family is very much involved in

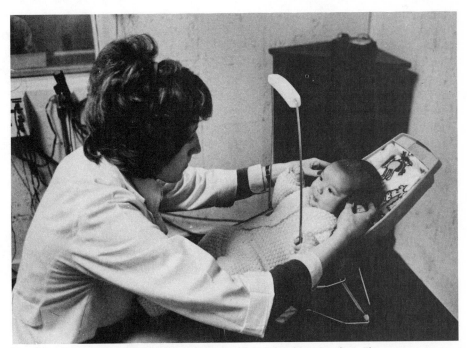

Even very young babies can be tested for signs of hearing loss. The sooner therapy is begun, the better a child's chances of developing normal speech.

the whole process. Nowadays an important advance in speech therapy is the use of a feedback system that make it possible for the youngster to be self-corrective. Parents seeking information about special schools and services, summer camps, and other facilities can write to the following agencies: Alexander Graham Bell Association for the Deaf, 3417 Volta Place, N.W., Washington, D.C. 20007; the American Speech and Hearing Association, 9030 Old Georgetown Road, Bethesda, Maryland 20014. See also HEARING.

Death

Some children's first experience of death is the loss of a grandparent; others may have to confront the fact of death for the first time when a beloved pet dies. A child wants to know where people or animals go when they die. Parents should be as honest as possible in answering such questions and tell their offspring what they themselves truly believe. Those parents who believe that there is life after death should say so; those who do not should say that they do not. Whatever one's beliefs, there are better ways to phrase them than "Grandma is in heaven watching you" or "People who are naughty go to hell when they die."

DEATH OF A PARENT: A child who has to cope with the death of a parent may be so disoriented that his behavior will seem odd to the adults around him. He may pretend that the death never happened; others may protect themselves from the shock by burying their feelings and never talking about the dead parent. Still others may feel rage at having been abandoned. Many youngsters are overwhelmed by guilt, feeling that in some magic way they caused the death because from time to time they secretly wished it. In cases where the bereft child cannot cope with the loss, it may be advisable to provide some help in the form of psychiatric therapy.

Delinquency

Juvenile delinquents are minors who are guilty of breaking the law or who are engaged in associations and activities considered harmful to children's morals, such as running errands for gamblers, acting as a lookout during a robbery, or sniffing glue for kicks. Swiping a candy bar or a comic book at the age of ten doesn't define a child as a hardened delinquent, but where such behavior becomes chronic, it's a sign that something is wrong that needs to be corrected. With the guidance of a therapist, it may turn out that the child alone is not entirely responsible for his delinquent tendencies. See also DESTRUCTIVENESS, DISCIPLINE, DISHONESTY, DISOBEDIENCE.

Dental care

The proper attitude toward dental care is best instilled not by lectures or warnings, but by example. Parents who themselves go regularly to the dentist for checkups, who take care of their teeth by keeping them clean with routine brushing and the use of dental floss, can do more for their child's dental health than those who depend on stern warnings to shape the attitudes of their children. Parents can hardly expect their offspring to be heroic about dental visits when they themselves scarcely ever go unless they have a toothache.

START EARLY: Dental care can begin by having the toddler accompany the parent to the dentist so that his baby teeth can be inspected and he can be given a special toothbrush of his own with instructions about how to use it. In communities where the water supply is not fluoridated, the dentist may recommend an ongoing program of fluoride application to the teeth themselves. Some families find that a pediatric dentist who specializes in children's dentistry can deal with a frightened or anxious child more expertly than the family dentist. Other families use the services of the dental clinics that are part of the dental schools of large universities.

No matter who is in charge of the family's dental health, it is important that professional attention is

Good dental hygiene, proper nutrition, and regular trips to the dentist are necessary for the maintenance of good dental health.

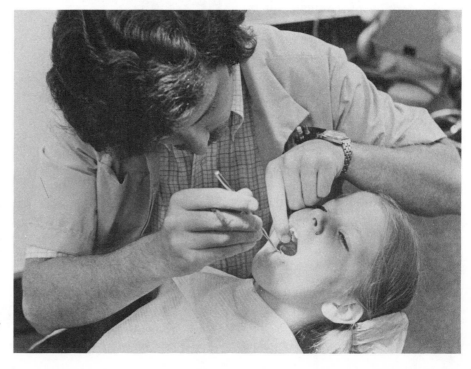

given to the child's dental development at every stage: fillings for decay in the first teeth, routine cleanings and checkups, and preventive orthodontics where advisable. Another aspect of dental care involves keeping the consumption of sweets to a minimum, and making sure that the child's daily diet contains the proper nutrients for building healthy teeth. See also ORTHODONTICS. For full discussion of the teeth and gums, see Ch. 10, p. 252.

Destructiveness

"It was an accident!" is a common cry when a child destroys a valuable object because of carelessness. And it probably was an accident. Parents who don't want precious bric-a-brac or other delicate possessions broken had better put them out of the reach of curious and clumsy little fingers. Young children should not be punished because their toys always seem to be destroyed; better to give them playthings that are sturdy and comparatively indestructible.

The child who is destructive unwittingly should not be spoken to in the same way as one would speak to a boy who willfully breaks his sister's doll or a girl who spitefully tears her brother's model-making manual. Destructiveness born of anger ("I was so furious, I smashed a dish") may happen rarely, but when it does, it should be commented on as an unsuitable way of dealing with the problem that caused the anger in the first place. When destructiveness gets out of hand or involves group activities amounting to vandalism, parental action should be taken with the guidance of a professional counselor.

Developmental disability

Any disability that interferes with a child's normal development is a *developmental disability*. The term has been used more specifically, however, to refer to mental retardation, cerebral palsy, epilepsy, and autism.

Diabetes

No one knows why some children develop diabetes. Diabetes is a noncontagious disease that results from the body's inability to produce enough insulin for the normal metabolism of sugar. The diabetic child is thus improperly nourished because the sugar which should be incorporated into the tissues is excreted in the urine. Finding sugar in the urine facilitates early diagnosis. Also, because this disorder causes a disturbance in the metabolism of fat, there is an increase of fat in the blood, detectable in a routine blood count.

EARLY SIGNS: Parents who are themselves diabetic will be alert to any symptoms in their offspring. The disease occurs more frequently in children where there is a family history of diabetes. However, since the disorder may occur in children where there is no previous family history of diabetes, alertness to the following signs is advisable: an abnormally frequent need to urinate; an excessive desire for fluids; itching of the genitals; general listlessness; frequent boils and carbuncles; slow healing of cuts and bruises.

If a diagnosis of diabetes is made by the doctor, the child may be hospitalized for a few days for a series of definitive tests, and all the members of the family will be educated in the best way to supervise the child's diet and daily routine so that serious complications can be avoided. Professional guidance is also available to ensure that the youngster's emotional adjustment is a healthy one. For a full discussion of diabetes, see Ch. 21, p. 409.

Diaper rash

See RASHES.

Diarrhea

Diarrhea, or loose and watery bowel movements, is common in babies because they are more sensitive to certain intestinal germs than older children. They may also be reacting to a change in their formula or to the roughage in a newly introduced fruit or vegetable. In older children, diarrhea may occur not only as a symptom of bacterial or viral infection, or because of food poisoning, but also as an allergic response, or because of overexcitement or anxiety.

Diarrhea in an infant should always be brought to a doctor's attention if it continues for more than 24 hours. The same holds true for an older child, especially when there are also symptoms of cramps, fever, or aches and pains in the joints. Persistent diarrhea from any cause, since it can lead to serious dehydration, especially in infants, requires prompt medical attention.

Diphtheria

Diphtheria is a severe and contagious bacterial infection, often fatal if untreated. Once one of the most threatening of all childhood diseases, there are now fewer than 1,000 cases a year in the United States because of widespread and effective immunization.

The first symptoms—fever, headache, nausea, and sore throat—may be confused with the onset of other disorders. However, there is a manifestation of diphtheria that is uniquely its own: patches of grayish yellow membrane form in the throat and grow together into one large membrane that interferes with swallowing and breathing. The diphtheria bacteria also produce a powerful toxin that can eventually cause irreversible damage to the heart and nerves. Diagnosis is usually verified by laboratory identification of the bacteria in a throat culture.

If diphtheria does occur, it is best treated in a hospital. The prompt prescription of antitoxin serum and antibiotics results in recovery in practically all cases. See IMMUNIZATION.

Discipline

There are no easy answers or sure guides to the discipline of children; but there are some basic principles that, if followed, can make life together more enjoyable and tolerable for parents and children alike. All children, whether they be normal, retarded, geniuses, sick or well, need and want discipline in their daily lives, even though they will say, when asked, that they would rather do as they please. From time to time most parents have been jolted to realize that their only interactions with their children seem to be when they are nagging them to do something or reprimanding them for doing something wrong.

THE EFFECT OF PRAISE: One of the most important principles of discipline is that praise is more effective than punishment. As has been noted by many students of human behavior, children crave attention from their parents. In order to gain this attention, they will behave in any way necessary; if misbehavior is the only action that receives attention, the child misbehaves. Parents should make a point of being attentive to their children when they are behaving properly and should reinforce good behavior with praise. The result will usually be an in-

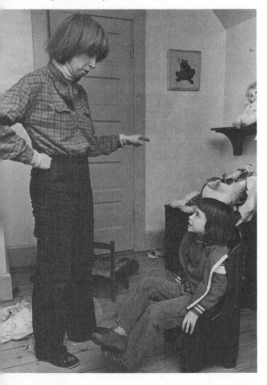

All children require discipline to learn what is expected from them. To be effective in disciplining children, parents should be consistent.

crease in good behavior and a decrease in misbehavior.

NEED FOR CONSISTENCY: Consistent discipline is important. Children should know what is expected of them and should know what the consequences of their misbehavior will be. Once a promise or threat is made, it should be carried out. Failure to carry out a threat encourages a repetition of the undesirable behavior. Failure to carry out a promise may cause the child to lose faith in the parent. See also p. 151.

Discrimination

See PREJUDICE.

Dishonesty

Nobody is honest about everything all the time, and that goes for children as well as adults. It's unrealistic to expect a child never to lie about anything.

PARENTS LIE, TOO: Many parents will lie in the presence of their children without realizing that they're doing it. "No, Mrs. Clark, I won't be able to pick the children up today because I have a bad cold." Your five-year-old girl looks you in the eye and says "Are you really sick, mommy?" Well, your explanation is likely to be just as lame as hers would be if you caught her out in a similar duplicity.

Little children like to make things up and can't be held strictly accountable for some of their tall stories when they're still at an age at which fact and fantasy are not clearly distinguished. A colorful exaggeration needn't call for an accusation of lying. It's better to respond with, "That's an interesting story," or "You're just imagining."

LYING AND PUNISHMENT: As youngsters get older, they should feel secure enough to tell the truth about having been naughty, knowing that although they may be punished, they will get approval for having told the truth. Children shouldn't be so fearful of their parents that dishonesty is their only protection against a beating.

CHEATING: Children who are pres-

sured beyond their ability to perform are the ones likeliest to cheat; so are those for whom winning has been held up constantly as a transcendent value. A child who has been caught cheating at school is usually punished by the authorities. If the incident is discussed at home, the parents might reexamine their values before adding to the child's burdens. A youngster who cheats regularly at games will suffer the natural punishment of exclusion by his peers.

STEALING: Young children who embark on group enterprises of stealing "for fun"—whether it's taking candy from the corner market or shoplifting from a department store—needn't be viewed as case-hardened criminals unless the stealing becomes habitual. A nine-year-old who swipes a candy bar once or twice and regrets it belongs in a different category from one who is hired as a lookout for older delinquents. Children usually have respect for other people's property when they have property of their own that they value and don't want anyone else to take.

Disobedience

Father gets a parking ticket because he forgot about alternate sides of the street on Wednesdays; mother has a whipped cream dessert in spite of her doctor's orders not to. Are mother and father disobedient? When Junior comes home from the playground at five instead of obeying orders to come home at four, is his disobedience any worse than theirs? Genuine forgetfulness, negligence, or occasional breaking of a rule is only human. Willful chronic disobedience is another matter.

Some children with a strong urge toward independence may test out many parental rules by disobeying them on purpose. A child who has been ordered not to spend any time with another child because the families are feuding, may, by flouting the order, be telling his parents that he has a right to choose his own friends. Where disobedience affects a youngster's health or safety or morals, it's time for parental action, not necessarily in the form of punishment, but in taking stock of the situation in order to find out why the child won't obey.

Divorced parents

See. p. 168.

Dreams and nightmares

Children go through periods of having "bad dreams" or nightmares that wake them up in the middle of the night in a state of terror and bewilderment. It won't do to say, "It's just a dream." To a young child who is just beginning to grasp the difference between what's real and what isn't, a nightmare can be extremely threatening. If the child wants to describe the dream after she collects herself, she should be allowed to do so even at 3 A.M. She may amplify and exaggerate a little bit, but that's only to let you know that she's been very brave through it all. Parental patience is called for; with a certain amount of reassurance, the child can usually be led back to bed and to sleep.

Youngsters whose sleep is regularly interrupted by nightmares or who are in the grip of the same nightmare may be feeling anxious about a daytime activity or may be feeling guilty about some undiscovered naughtiness. A tactful chat can sometimes reveal what the trouble is so that it can be disposed of during waking hours.

NIGHT TERRORS: Some children may have occasional nightmares—often called *night terrors*—in which they scream or tremble in terror. They may sit up in bed while still asleep, or even walk around. Their terror is certainly real, but the parents should remember that the cause of it is purely imaginary. Accordingly, they have no reason to be alarmed; in spite of the child's appearance, she is not in any danger, and no drastic action is called for.

Simply comfort the child, who frequently will be disoriented and confused in a half-awake state, until she can go back to sleep. She will probably have no recollection of the episode the next morning.

If night terrors occur only occasionally, there is no cause for concern, although it might be a good idea to check on the television shows your child is watching before bedtime. If there is a great deal of tension in the household, that could be a contributing cause. If night terrors are persistent or frequent, however, a physician should be consulted. See also SLEEPWALKING.

Dyslexia

Dyslexia is a condition in which an otherwise average or intelligent child suffers from a complex of motor-perceptual disabilities that interfere with the orderly processing and acquisition of language. The disability that results in an inhibition of symbol recognition essential for learning how to read, write, and spell is thought to originate in some form of brain circuitry malfunction that may have been caused by injury or by genetic defect. Recent researchers have established some connection between dyslexia and a faulty pathway between the lower brain—the cerebellum—and the inner ear, causing the dyslexic child to suffer from a mild and permanent form of motion sickness that interferes with learning.

SYMPTOMS: The symptoms of dyslexia vary considerably and may include: garbled or disordered development of speech during the early years; an inability to learn the relationship between sounds and symbols for purposes of reading aloud; an inability to learn how to spell or how to organize written expression; confusion about serial order, as in naming the days of the week or in number concepts; unusual difficulty in doing simple repetitive tasks.

If a parent suspects that a child is suffering from dyslexia, a diagnosis should be made on the basis of tests administered by trained professionals. The child's pediatrician or the school guidance counselor should be consulted about where such tests are best given and assessed. Should the child be diagnosed as dyslexic, an appropriate remedial program or an accredited special school can help surmount some of the learning difficulties.

Earache

Earache is one of the most common complaints of childhood.

AS SECONDARY INFECTION: Earache is often attributable to bacterial infection of the middle ear and should be treated promptly by a doctor. Because the Eustachian tube that connects the back of the throat with the middle ear is shorter and wider in a child than in an adult, it affords easier entry to bacteria. Infections of the ear may thus occur as the result of a sore throat or a postnasal drip. Infectious mucus from the nose is often forced into the middle ear by way of the Eustachian tube because young children are inclined to sniff it back rather than to blow it out. And when a child is mastering the technique of nose-blowing, he should be told that neither one nor both of the nostrils should be pressed closed in the process. Rather, both nostrils should be blown out gently at the same time, and with the mouth open. If gentle blowing doesn't clear the nostrils, the nose should be wiped as necessary.

RECOGNIZING EARACHE IN AN INFANT: Earache in an infant may be combined with fever and the kind of crying associated with sharp pain. A toddler may indicate the source of discomfort by pulling at the earlobe. Until the doctor can prescribe proper medication, discomfort can be relieved by applying a heating pad to the involved ear and with aspirin.

OTHER CAUSES: Earache may also accompany teething or tooth infection, or it may be the result of pressure caused by water that has been trapped in the ear after swimming or bathing. In small children, an earache may be a sign that the

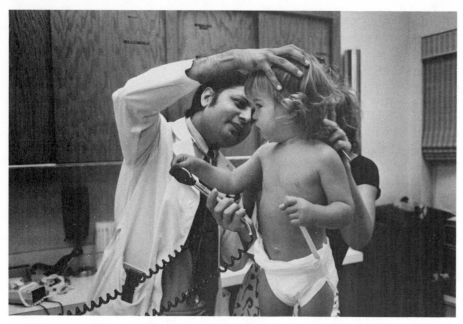

A child's complaints about earaches should not be ignored because serious ear infections in childhood can cause a hearing loss.

youngster has stuffed a bean or a tiny plastic object so far into his ear that it won't come out as easily as it went in. If you suspect such an occurrence, avoid poking and prodding in an attempt to remove the object. The child should be taken to the doctor or to a hospital so that the object can be removed with the proper instruments and the ear examined and treated for possible injury.

CONSEQUENCES OF NEGLECT OF EARACHE: An earache should always be brought to a doctor's attention without delay since untreated middle ear infections can lead to irreversible hearing loss. The leading cause of mild hearing loss in toddlers is believed to be *serous otitis media,* or serous infection of the middle ear. This condition is specifically an inflammation of the middle ear with an accumulation of fluid behind the eardrum. When the condition is chronic or improperly treated during the first three years, it may impair hearing permanently and as a consequence lead to a failure to develop normal language skills. Occasionally the physician may have to make a small opening in the eardrum to drain the fluid, a procedure known as a *myringotomy.* See also HEARING.

Eczema
See under RASHES.

Education
See SCHOOL.

Epilepsy
Epilepsy in childhood most commonly takes the form of petit mal or psychomotor episodes.

PETIT MAL SEIZURES: Petit mal episodes are characterized by brief lapses of consciousness, sometimes occurring many times a day. The child does not fall down but simply stops what he is doing and may appear to stare absently.

PSYCHOMOTOR SEIZURES: Psychomotor episodes are characterized by the performance of some activity during a brief lapse of consciousness. The child may walk around in circles, or sit down and get up in a purposeless way. During this type of seizure the child may babble nonsensically or chant the same word over and over. Such an attack may last no more than a few minutes, and when the child recovers he is likely to have no memory of its occurrence.

In many instances, parents who expect a certain amount of bizarre behavior from their youngsters may not realize that a form of epilepsy is the cause. Should such incidents

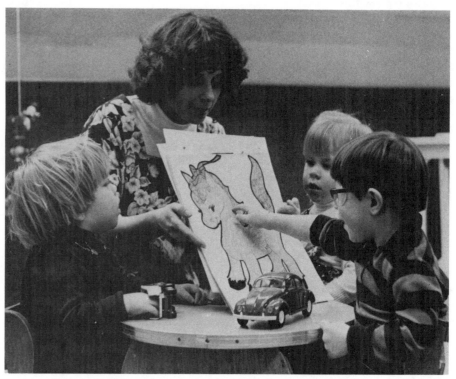

Preschool children with epilepsy and other neurological disorders learn language skills at a special clinic.

occur frequently, they should be called to the attention of the doctor who may think it advisable to have the child examined by a neurologist.

A parent witnessing a *grand mal* or convulsive epileptic seizure for the first time may be unduly alarmed and take measures that may harm the child rather than help. For a description of emergency measures during a grand mal seizure, see p. 595. For a full discussion of epilepsy, see p. 472.

Exercise

Some children seem to sit around a great deal; others are on the move from morning until bedtime. A youngster might be listless or lethargic because there's something the matter that needs to be investigated by a doctor. This type of sitting around is quite different from playing with dolls for hours at a time or looking at picture books instead of running around. A young child who really cannot sit still at all may have a problem that needs diagnosing by a doctor, too. Practically all children are found between these extremes.

EXERCISE AS A DEVELOPMENTAL NEED: Toddlers must be allowed to get the exercise necessary for the development of their bodies. They shouldn't be confined in a playpen for most of the day. Three- and four-year-olds who don't go to a nursery school and have no play equipment in their back yard (if they have a back yard), should be taken whenever possible to a local park or playground that has swings, slides, seesaws, jungle gyms, or other devices that are safely designed and installed. Most schools have some kind of supervised gym activity or a free time for yard play, and if they don't, they should. If this scheduled exercise is insufficient for a nine- or ten-year-old, inquiries can be made about athletic facilities at a local YMCA, settlement house, church, or fraternal organization.

CHOICE OF ACTIVITIES: As children get a little older, they should be permitted to choose the exercise

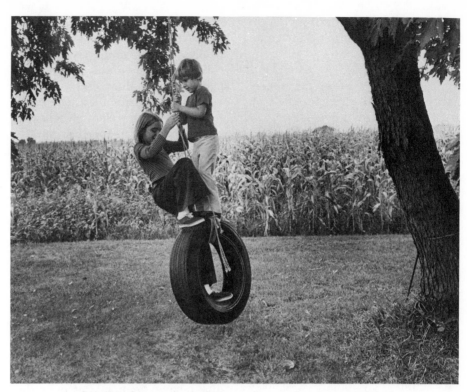

Sometimes homemade playthings are the most fun. A rope and tire hung from a tree can give children hours of pleasure.

that appeals to them unless there's a good reason for its being forbidden. A girl who wants to join a sandlot baseball team shouldn't be forced to go to a ballet class, and a boy inspired by the dancing he's seen on TV shouldn't be discouraged if the family can afford the lessons. Exercise needn't be synonymous wtih competition unless the youngster wants it to be. Riding a bicycle regularly may be sufficient exercise until a child is attracted to a particular sport. See also p. 115.

Eyeglasses

Now that infants and youngsters have periodic eye checkups with their physicians, and regular tests are given to all students, more children are wearing glasses than in former years. In addition to *strabismus* (crossed eyes), the three major eye problems encountered in children are *myopia* (nearsightedness), *hyperopia* (farsightedness), and *astigmatism*.

MYOPIA: The *myopic* or nearsighted child cannot see distant objects well but can see close objects clearly. A very young child so afflicted may stumble and fall easily. An older child attending school may make errors in copying because she has difficulty in making out the words and figures written on the chalkboard. She may be called a behavior problem or may even be said to be mentally retarded. Most cases of myopia can be helped with glasses.

HYPEROPIA: The *hyperopic* (also called *hypermetropic*) or farsighted eye is shorter from front to rear than the normal eye, and if not corrected will often hinder close work like reading. When a farsighted child reads she often complains of blurring of the printed page, sleepiness, and headache. Farsightedness is often associated with crossed eyes and is usually correctable with glasses.

ASTIGMATISM: In *astigmatism* or distorted vision, there is an uneven curvature of the cornea or lens surface of the eye. This condition causes some light rays to focus further back than others and produces a blurred, distorted image on the retina.

Either a farsighted or nearsighted eye can be *astigmatic;* the abnormality can usually be corrected by properly prescribed eyeglasses.

Fantasies

Every normal child has fantasies, some highly pleasurable, some fearful and frightening. Young children sometimes have a hard time sorting out what they imagine from what's real; this may be especially true when a nightmare interferes with sleep. Many children quite consciously say, "Let's pretend" or "Let's make believe" when they embark on a dress-up activity; others simply and straightforwardly act out their fantasies by playing games of violence with toy guns. An only child may create a fantasy companion with whom she has conversations; a child who is encouraged to draw may give shape to her fantasies in pictures that mean a lot to her but not much to anyone else.

DAYDREAMING: Some children infuriate their energetic parents by sitting around and daydreaming (with one sock on and one off) instead of doing their chores. Whatever form fantasies may take, they are an inevitable part of growing up and should be respected, unless they become the equivalent of a narcotic escape from reality rather than a means of enriching it. When a child's fantasy life appears to be turning into a substitute for his real one, the time has come to consult a psychiatric authority.

Fatherhood

More and more fathers are finding themselves involved in child raising on an active basis rather than a passive one. As an increasing number of women take part- or full-time jobs even when children are very young, fathers have been taking over the care and feeding of their children on prearranged mornings, evenings, and weekends. Some men resent the responsibility; others enjoy it. But all who undertake it for the first time are surprised to discover how much time, energy, patience, resourcefulness, and thought are required in order to be a good mother. If the woman of the house is expected to be an attractive wife as well as a good mother, she needs some time to herself for her own development as a person.

Where child care is shared more than it used to be, mothers and fathers should agree on a consistent set of values: what's permitted and what isn't; what's expected and what's unacceptable, etc. Otherwise the child may be confused by the demands of two conflicting authorities.

ESTRANGED PARENTS: The part-time father who sees his child or children on a prearranged schedule following a separation or divorce shouldn't pack too many exciting experiences—and too many feelings—into every meeting with them. He, like the mother, should scrupulously avoid any disparagement of the other parent. He and the child will enjoy each other more, no matter what their age, if the hours together are comparatively calm and unhurried, and the projects for their time together are not overstimulating.

Fears and phobias

Babies are fearful about being dropped, and they're frightened by a sudden loud noise. (You *can* make babies cry by saying, "Boo!" When they get older and catch on, they'll think it's fun to be scared.) Toddlers are taught to be afraid of a hot stove, and as children get a little older, they develop night fears that become bad dreams. Many parents transmit, deliberately or unknowingly, some of their fears to their children: fear of dogs, or thunder and lightning, or infection by germs.

Only a thin line separates sensible caution from anxiety. Where a threat of punishment is involved, an anxiety may develop that can last a lifetime. Parents should control the impulse to say such things as, "Don't eat that, it's going to make you sick" or "Don't climb so high, you're going to fall" or "Don't play

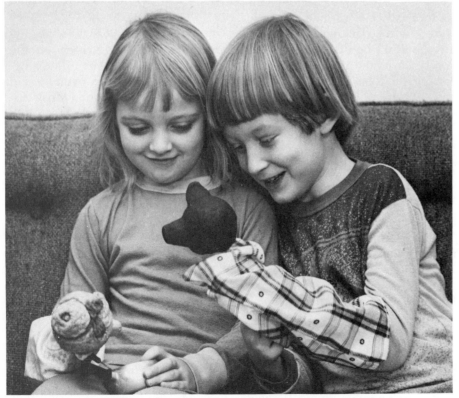

"Let's make believe!" Puppets can provide a wonderful outlet for acting out children's fantasies.

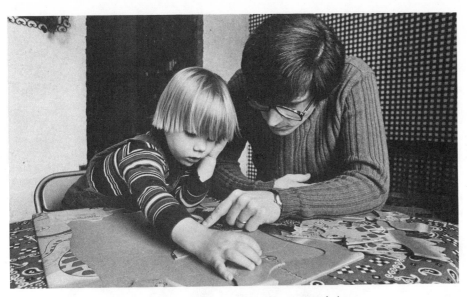

As more mothers enter the job market, many fathers take a more active role in raising their children.

in the mud; the germs will make you sick." Or, worse yet, "If you do that, the bogey man will get you" or "God will punish you."

PHOBIAS: If fears are often legitimate and usually outgrown through reassuring experiences, phobias are deep-seated unconquerable fears. Many adults suffer from them; two of the most common are *claustrophobia*, the fear of being in an enclosed place, and *acrophobia*, the fear of heights. *Phobia* is a clinical term and shouldn't be used to describe a youngster's aversion to school at a particular time, or his apprehension about elevators and escalators. If parental reassurance can help a child overcome fears of this type, they need not be classed as phobias.

Fever

As every parent knows, babies can run very high fevers. In itself, a rectal temperature of 103° or 104° is not necessarily cause for alarm. (Normal rectal temperature is about ½° to 1° higher than the oral norm of 98.6°F.) Of course, you should take the immediate step of calling your doctor to find out what's causing the fever.

If a baby's fever climbs over 104°, the baby may experience convulsions. To avoid this possibility, he may be bathed with cool water or with equal parts of water and alcohol. (The alcohol is not necessary.) If convulsions do occur, protect the baby from injuring himself by seeing that his head and body don't strike anything hard. The convulsion, though frightening, is usually brief and ends of its own accord. Get in touch with your doctor without delay.

Although the mechanism that results in fever is not precisely understood, the elevation in temperature is almost always a sign that the child's normal body processes are being disturbed. A child old enough to talk can let you know that his throat is sore or that he has an earache.

POSSIBLE CAUSES: Fever is often the sign of the onset of an infectious disease such as measles or influenza; it usually accompanies severe sunburn; it may be a warning that the infection of a local cut is spreading through the rest of the body. When it comes suddenly and rises quickly, along with cramps or diarrhea, it may indicate a gastrointestinal infection or food poisoning. No matter what a child's age, if temperature by mouth rises above 101°, the doctor should be informed of the fever and accompanying symptoms.

TREATMENT: Until a diagnosis is made and treatment prescribed, the feverish youngster should be put to bed and kept on a diet of light foods and lots of liquids. If the elevated temperature is combined with stiff neck, aching joints, or headache, aspirin can be given for relief according to dose instructions indicated.

Fluoridation

Although it has been unequivocally established that fluoridated drinking water is the best safeguard

A child's fears can often be calmed by a sympathetic adult who encourages the child to talk about what is bothering her.

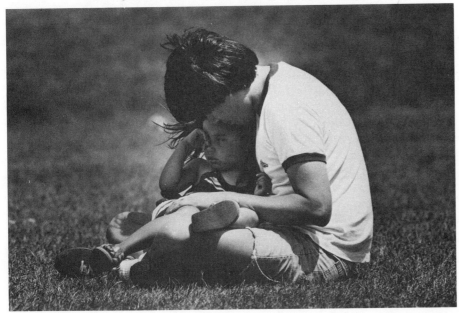

against tooth decay, many parts of the United States continue to resist this public health measure, thus placing a special burden on the parents of preschool children. Families in such communities are strongly urged to consult their dentist or the closest dental clinic connected with a university's college of dentistry for advice on the appropriate measures to be taken to protect their children's teeth. A consultation of this nature is advisable as soon as the baby shows signs of teething, since the fluoride treatments should begin as early as possible.

In many areas where the water supply remains unfluoridated, programs in the public schools supply youngsters with fluoride tablets every day. Although this method of applying the chemical is less effective than its availability in the drinking water, it is a step in the right direction. Concerned parents can make an effort to initiate such programs where none exists by contacting state public health officials.

Foot care

Unless the child's doctor indicates the need for corrective or orthopedic shoes, parents need have little concern for pigeon toes or bowed legs or flat feet. If a shoe salesman suggests remedial footwear, his suggestions should be discussed with the doctor before complying with them. A good general rule to follow about the fit of shoes is that they should be about three-quarters of an inch longer than the foot itself. For a child whose feet have a tendency to perspire heavily, sweat socks made of cotton or wool are to be preferred to those made of synthetics. Blisters that form on the instep, heel, or any other part of the foot because of ill-fitting footwear must be treated promptly to avoid serious infection.

Friends

Everyone needs friends. Some children need only one; others seem to enjoy having several. A three-year-old who is just beginning to learn

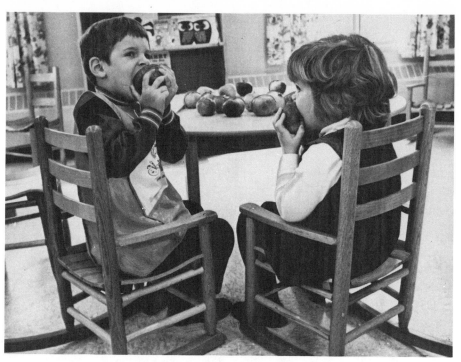

A special treat at nursery school tastes even better when a special friend is there to share it with you.

about sharing may be more relaxed playing with just one other child; a ten-year-old may like the hurly-burly of a group of friends to get together with when school is out.

PARENTS PLEASE STAY OUT: Parents should try to steer clear of squabbles between children. One day, Nancy and Harriet are best friends, the next, bitter enemies, because of some real or imagined outrage. Left to their own devices, the children will probably patch things up. If parents get involved, the situation gets magnified out of all proportion. It's not unusual in such situations for the two sets of parents to stop speaking to each other and the two little girls to go back to being best friends again.

KEEPING BAD COMPANY: What's to be done about "unsuitable" friends? Some parents may think a particular child is unacceptable because she's too aggressive or too foul-mouthed. If your child seems fond of her nonetheless, voice your opinions, but don't forbid the youngster from coming to the house. Any attempt to break up the friendship is likely to be resisted until your child learns from experience that

your judgment was the right one. Children who are discouraged from bringing their friends home because they make a mess or make too much noise are actually deprived of feeling at home in their own house.

Friendships between girls and boys may begin in nursery school and continue for years afterward. Although the tone of the friendship may change, the closeness can be very valuable if it doesn't exclude other relationships.

Frostbite

See *Frostbite*, p. 596.

Frustration

When infants want food, they want it now. Since frustration isn't something they can deal with, they cry until they get what they want. A toddler whose desire to stay in the playground is frustrated when his mother firmly leads him out may have a temper tantrum. A five-year-old who can't put a particular puzzle together may be so frustrated that he destroys it.

Practically all situations involving frustration are those in which a child (or person of any age) is trying to transcend arbitrary limitations, either his own or those imposed by circumstance. Parents can't eliminate the frustration factor from a child's life, but they can help him to cope with it. Suitable simple clothing is much less frustrating than garments with lots of buttons and buttonholes. Playthings can be a challenge, but not so complicated that they defeat a child's desire to learn. Too many strict rules frustrate a child's impulse to exercise his own judgment and to grow up by learning from his own mistakes.

AN ONLY CHILD: An only child may be frustrated in his desire for attention when he starts to go to school. In this case, he may actually be spurred on to superior achievement so that he continues to get the attention he's been accustomed to at home. Or he may behave like a spoiled brat and get attention, but for the wrong reasons.

Some children learn that the desire for instant gratification is one of the chief characteristics of an infant, and so, with parental help and approval, develop the character traits of patience and self-discipline. Others become the kind of adult for whom frustration is so intolerable that it becomes an excuse for escape into drugs.

German measles

See RUBELLA.

Gifted child

See ABILITIES AND APTITUDES.

Grades

Many schools don't use a grading system for children under the age of ten. But no matter what the nature of the report and how elaborate it is, evaluation of the child is involved, and the evaluation is based on values, so the child is in fact being graded in a way after all. Some children are called more cooperative than others; some are said to try harder; some get along better with their peer group.

With or without grades, children usually know whether they're doing well or badly at school. If a youngster's accomplishments are falling short of her abilities, there may be temporary reasons for her underachievement. In some cases, underachievement is a child's way of saying "no" to too much pressure about grades; in other cases, something about the teacher or the classroom situation is interfering with the child's performance. If parents suspect such a case, they should arrange a parent-teacher conference to try to get to the bottom of the problem.

Grandparents

Children are fortunate when both sets of grandparents are easily accessible for visiting, treats, vacation trips, playing checkers, and babysitting. Parents and grandparents are lucky too, for family continuity is important to young and old alike.

Relationships between the generations have their difficulties, though. Tact may be essential in keeping a grandparent from spoiling a child, and a grandmother should resist the impulse to show how competent she is with the baby compared to her inexperienced daughter or daughter-in-law. Parents who are still working out some of their own problems may take a rebellious tone toward the grandparent who moves into the household as a matter of economic necessity. Under these circumstances, the older generation should certainly expect consideration and politeness but should try not to impose its attitudes or child-rearing methods on its adult offspring—especially not in the presence of the children.

Growth rates in boys and girls

See pp. 85–86.

Guilt and conscience

Children often feel as guilty about bad thoughts as they do about bad deeds. After being angry, a child may feel as badly about having had a fleeting wish to hurt his mother as he would have felt had he actually hurt her. A child should be helped to understand that his thoughts are his own, that his thoughts cannot harm anybody, and that he will not be punished for his thoughts. He should understand that it is only actions of certain kinds that cannot be allowed and that will result in a reprimand or punishment. In other words, a child should not be made to feel guilty for angry or aggressive thoughts toward other members of his family, but only for angry and aggressive acts.

A parent might say to a child, "I understand that you really disliked your brother when you hit him, in fact, even hated him and would have liked to hurt him. It's okay for you to be angry with him, but I am not going to let you hurt him." A clear distinction should be made between hostile feelings and hostile behavior.

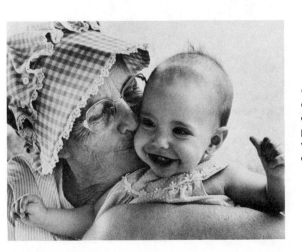

Children are fortunate when they are able to see their grandparents on a regular basis. Grandparents provide a special kind of love, as well as a sense of family continuity.

Handicapped child

Whether a handicap is hereditary or acquired, mental or physical, temporary or permanent, it is always a condition that prevents a child from participating fully on an equal footing in the activities of her own age group. But how fully she can participate and her attitude toward her disability are usually a reflection of the attitudes of her parents, teachers, and the community. Of primary importance is an assessment at the earliest possible age of the extent to which the handicap can be decreased or corrected.

Exactly how deaf is the deaf child? Can surgery repair a rheumatic heart? Is a defect of vision operable? Is the child with cerebral palsy mentally retarded or is the seeming mental malfunction a reversible effect of the physical condition? Parents should investigate all the available services offered by voluntary organizations and community groups that might help them and their child.

One promising development in recent years is the attempt to integrate handicapped children, whenever possible, into the mainstream of education rather than segregate them in special classes. School systems in various parts of the United States are placing deaf, blind, physically disabled, and emotionally disturbed youngsters into classrooms with their nonhandicapped peers and providing them with essential supportive services at various times during the school day. The experience of dealing with nonhandicapped children will provide them with a more realistic preparation for their adult lives.

Health records

It may seem somewhat troublesome to keep orderly health records for every member of the family, but the accumulated information can be extremely helpful if it can be supplied at a moment's notice to a doctor or a hospital. Chronologically arranged facts can also provide the material eventually needed by summer camps and school applications and insurance policies.

A notebook containing essential data about past illnesses, accidents, allergies, surgery, and other facts can be extraordinarily helpful and time-saving in supplying a doctor with a medical history that simplifies diagnosis and treatment. Such a notebook should have separate sections for immunizations and booster shots and their dates; annual weight and height progress; illnesses with dates and special notations; accidents with dates and any permanent consequences; hospitalization and reason; individual problems relating to allergies, hearing, vision, speech, and the like. Visits to the doctor and dentist should be recorded, and the blood type entered in a conspicuous place. If possible, parents should also provide a summary at the back of the notebook of their own major illnesses, disabilities, and surgical history.

Hearing

Approximately half of all adult hearing problems are thought to have originated in childhood. About five out of every hundred children reveal some hearing disability when screening tests are given. Total deafness among children is uncommon, and where it does exist, its symptoms become manifest to parents and doctors alike during infancy.

PARTIAL HEARING LOSS: Partial hearing disability, on the other hand, is common, and is likely to be overlooked until it may be too late

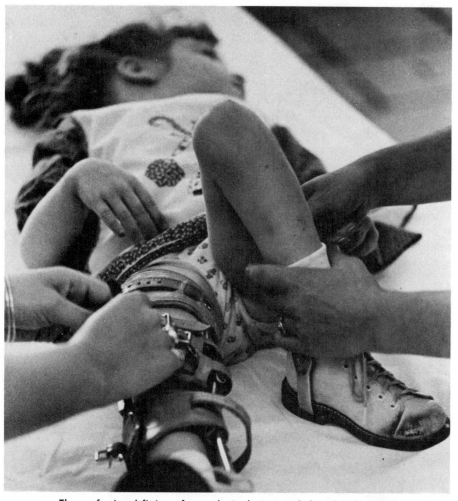

The professional fitting of an orthotic device can help a handicapped child to participate more fully in the normal activities of her age group.

GROWTH RATES IN BOYS*

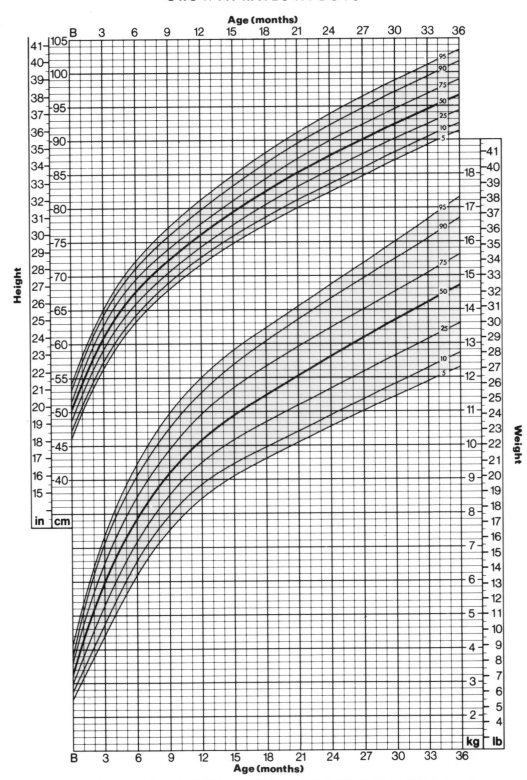

*Adapted from National Center for Health Statistics *NCHS Growth Charts*, 1976. Monthly Vital Statistics Report. Vol. 25, No. 3, Supp. (HRA) 76-1120. Health Resources Administration, Rockville, Maryland, June, 1976. Data from The Fels Research Institute, Yellow Springs, Ohio. © 1976 Ross Laboratories

These charts indicate the rate of growth of boys and girls from birth to 36 months in the United States. In each chart the upper gray area indicates the range of growth in height from the 5th to 95th percentile, and the lower gray area indicates a similar range in weight. (If a boy or girl is in the 95th percentile in height, 95% of all other boys and girls are not as tall as he or she. If someone is in the 50th percentile in weight, half of other children weigh more and half weigh less. If one is in the 25th

GROWTH RATES IN GIRLS*

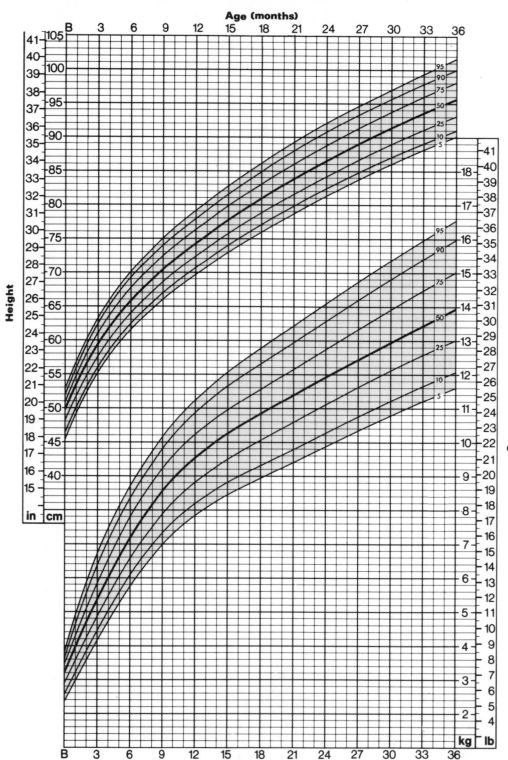

*Adapted from National Center for Health Statistics *NCHS Growth Charts*, 1976. Monthly Vital Statistics Report. Vol. 25, No. 3, Supp. (HRA) 76-1120. Health Resources Administration, Rockville, Maryland, June, 1976. Data from The Fels Research Institute, Yellow Springs, Ohio. © 1976 Ross Laboratories

percentile of weight, 75% of other children weigh more and 25% weigh less. Thus, the percentile indicates how your child compares in height or weight with other children of the same sex and age in the United States.) Height, indicated at the left-hand side of each chart, is shown in inches and in centimeters. Weight, indicated at the right-hand side of each chart, is shown in kilograms and in pounds. The bottom and top lines of each chart indicate age in months.

to correct its consequences.

The doctor begins to suspect a hearing problem when the mother of a young baby tells him that the child does not react to her voice, to noises, or to other auditory stimuli. As the child gets older, he may not speak properly. Since he has never heard speech, he cannot imitate its

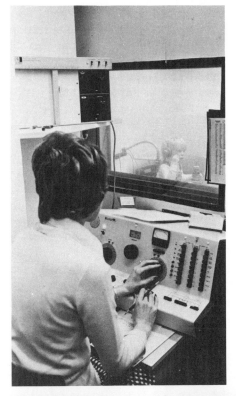

sound and may fail to develop normal language skills. Sometimes these children, like visually handicapped children, are mistakenly called mentally retarded or are classified as suffering from hyperkinesis or brain dysfunction. Often the undetected hearing disability stemmed from a middle ear infection that was treated inadequately or not treated at all.

LANGUAGE PROBLEMS: A hearing loss of 15 decibels is considered sufficiently large to produce language problems for a very young child, causing a major handicap in the acquisition of language skills. Specialists therefore recommend that parents ask that their doctor test a baby's hearing, especially during and after an ear infection. If a compensatory hearing aid is necessary, the baby should be supplied with one immediately. Speech will not develop normally—that is, the langauge function of the brain will be impaired—unless the essential sounds of language can be perceived during the first two years of life.

Just as glasses or surgery can help eye problems, simple hearing aids, the surgical removal of excessive

Two audiologists, working together, test the hearing of a two-year-old boy. One controls the transmission of sounds (top), while the other (bottom) works directly with the child.

lymphoid tissue blocking the Eustachian tube, or special instruction in lip reading can often help a hearing problem and open up a new world for the child afflicted with a hearing disability.

Heart disease

See RHEUMATIC FEVER. See also *Congenital Heart Disease*, p. 370.

Hernia

A *hernia* is a condition in which part of an organ protrudes through a weak spot or other abnormal opening in the wall of a body cavity. There are three types of hernias that may occur in children.

UMBILICAL HERNIA: The most common is an *umbilical hernia*, in which there is a protrusion of some of the contents of the abdomen through an opening in the abdominal wall at the navel where the umbilical cord was attached. When the baby cries or strains, the protrusion becomes more obvious, and when the baby is at rest, the bulge recedes. An umbilical hernia usually disappears by the time a child reaches the second year. Since it represents no danger to any of the body functions, the condition need be no cause for concern. It is very common in non-Caucasian children.

INGUINAL HERNIA: The second most common type of hernia in childhood is known as an *indirect inguinal hernia*, occurring frequently in boys. At birth it may have the appearance of a marble located under the skin at the groin. In time, it may descend into the scrotum that encloses the testicles. This type of hernia is usually corrected by simple surgery that repairs the weakened musculature. The weak muscles are often present on both sides.

HIATUS HERNIA: Another congenital hernia is known as a *hiatus hernia* (or *diaphragmatic hernia*) in which part of the stomach protrudes upward through the part of the esophagus that opens into the diaphragm. In some cases, this structural defect is self-healing. Surgical correction is advised only if the hernia interferes with respiration. See also p. 380.

Hobbies

Since hobbies are considered leisure-time activities, they don't usually develop until a child begins to go to school. His day is then separated into doing what he has to do—homework, household chores—and doing what he wants to do. Some youngsters get ideas about hobbies from their school friends, especially in the earlier grades where some form of "show and tell" is likely to be part of the group's activities.

COLLECTING: Such hobbies are often based on collecting: foreign stamps, seashells, baseball cards, minerals, dolls—the list is endless and often involves little expense. Whatever the trivia that's being collected, parents should refrain from criticism. Many children have had the last word when their masses of comic books turned out to be valuable properties as the years went by.

Some youngsters choose their hobbies from among the pursuits that give pleasure to their parents or older siblings: crafts, boating, reading, sewing, fishing, drawing, tennis, chess. There are those children who don't seem to be able to settle on a hobby until they've tried and discarded several. Although parents should be patient about this, they certainly needn't rush out for a telescope or a chemistry set—or a silver flute!—at the slightest suggestion of their ten-year-old's enthusiasm. A child who thinks he'd like to try some experiments should be encouraged to use materials that are close at hand. A child who expresses interest in astronomy can be told to identify the constellations he can make out with the naked eye and with the help of a library book.

Homework

See RESPONSIBILITIES.

Hospitalization

Most children at some time in their first 15 years of life require at least one hospitalization, ranging in time from a few days to many months. This can be a frightening experience and may leave permanent emotional scars on a child. Parents can do many things to make the experience less harmful.

Preparing the child for the hospital stay may be the most important task for the parent. Authorities generally agree that parents should:

• Try to answer all the questions the child asks. If you have no answer, try to find one.

• Be as honest as you can. The child will want to know why he or she has to go to the hospital, what will be done there, how long it will take, and whether it will hurt.

• Be reassuring. The child should know that he or she will receive good care and that the hospital visit will be temporary.

• Explain what the hospital is and what it is like—with wheeled carts, people in uniform, and so on.

• Using sheets as gowns, role-play to make it clear that under the gowns will be helping people.

• Let your child know when you will be in the hospital and how long you will stay.

Most hospitals today try to work with parents to make the child feel at home and to allay the child's fears. Many hospitals offer rooms so that parents can "room in"—and stay near the young patient. A playroom may be available. Hospital staff members may hold parent–nurse sessions to introduce mothers and fathers to the hospital's schedule, locations of facilities, and other details. As the parent of a child who has to be hospitalized, you can, by learning as much as possible and cooperating with the staff, help alleviate your child's natural fears of separation, of mutilation, and of the strange new situation.

FEAR OF SEPARATION: Hospitalization for an operation or an illness affects different children at different stages of their development in different ways. Very young children may be particularly worried about separations from their mothers. Parents can help with this fear by assuring the child that separation will not be permanent.

If at all possible, the child's mother or another member of the family should stay with the child during much of the hospital stay. During an extended hospitalization, of course, this may become difficult or imposible. Barring accidents, children should always be forewarned of a hospitalization; if they are not, they may feel they were deceived by their parents and lose trust in them.

FEAR OF MUTILATION: Children of about 4 to 10 or 11 may be more worried about possible damage or mutilation of their bodies than about separations from their families. They often have fears that parts of their bodies may be cut out or that in some way they may be permanently harmed. They may feel that when they come back from the hospital they will not be the same as they were when they went in. Matter-of-fact reassurance by the parents can be most helpful in alleviating these fears.

FEAR OF THE STRANGE: Both younger children and older children aged 10, 11, or 12 may fear the new or strange, such as the anesthetic that goes with an operation. The child should be allowed to talk out fears. Simple explanations usually help. A child can, for example, understand that when you get sick taking medicine can sometimes make you better. At other times an operation, or surgery, is the only thing that will help. In the hospital, doctors or nurses may have to make tests to find out what is wrong. One such test is the X ray, which is simply a "picture" of a part of the child's body.

The parent can prepare the child for the operating room and for the operation. Everything in this special place, for example, must be kept perfectly clean, so nurses and doc-

THE FIRST DOZEN YEARS   89

tors wear long-sleeved gowns. They also wash carefully before the operation begins. They wear sterile gloves so that they can touch patients without passing on germs. They also wear masks, shoe coverings, and caps. They may make a small opening in the patient's skin so that they can take out or get rid of whatever is making the child sick. The doctors and nurses use stitches, or sutures, to pull the skin edges together and allow healing to begin. Some stitches may be under the skin; these simply melt, or dissolve, by themselves.

A dressing may be placed over the part of the child's body that was opened up. These pieces of soft cloth protect the skin opening and keep out germs. When the dressing comes off, a white scar may remain. The scar will not open up and it will not hurt. It will be a sign that the child was sick, got well, and came home.

Hostility

See ANGER.

Hyaline membrane disease

Hyaline membrane disease, now technically called the *respiratory distress syndrome,* is a disorder that affects approximately 50,000 newborn babies each year, and until recently was fatal for about half of them. The disorder occurs especially among premature infants, those born by Caesarian section, and those with diabetic mothers. In premature infants, the immaturity of the lungs may result in a collapse of the air space within the lungs themselves when the first breath is exhaled. Each new breath then becomes a greater struggle, and with the spread of lung collapse, exhaustion and asphyxiation may occur.

A treatment known as *continuous positive airway pressure* is now being successfully used in many of the special hospital units equipped for newborns with disabilities. The therapy involves a pressure chamber that forces high-oxygen air into the lungs and keeps these air spaces open. The method has already prevented thousands of infant deaths. Newborns who need this assistance acquire the ability to breathe normally in about a week.

Hyperkinesis

Hyperkinesis is a behavioral disorder diagnosed in a large number of school children—more often boys than girls—who are unable to concentrate and who are overactive and excitable. These characteristics cause them to become disruptive in the classroom as well as disturbing to their families. There are indications that this disorder manifests itself in infancy, when the doctor might describe an excessively fretful and restless baby as *hypertonic,* and prescribe medication to calm him down.

For reasons not yet understood, it has been found that the symptoms of hyperkinesis often respond to antidepressants or stimulants, and as a result, a significant number of otherwise unmanageable youngsters are being treated medically. Although the medication enables them to conform to classroom situations, it may have the negative effect of appetite loss; to avoid sleep difficulties, the medication is never given in the evening.

Hyperkinesis appears to run in families, although there is some evidence that imperceptible brain damage may be one of its causes. Parents of a clinically hyperkinetic child—not one who is simply rambunctious—should seek advice about proper treatment from the psychiatric and neurological staffs of the nearest teaching hospital or from specialists recommended by the family doctor.

Imagination

See FANTASIES.

Immunization

Recently developed vaccines against measles, mumps, and rubella (German measles) should eventually wipe out these diseases in the same way that smallpox has been eliminated practically everywhere in the world. Routine immunization follows a schedule of shots administered with minor variations by most pediatricians and child care clinics. Severe reactions are rare, but should they occur, they should be reported to the doctor promptly.

KEEPING RECORDS: Records should be kept of the child's immunization history so that booster shots can be given at proper intervals. Since families move from one place to another, changing doctors as they relocate, it saves a great deal of time and trouble if immunization data is written down rather than committed to memory. See HEALTH RECORDS.

DPT INJECTIONS: DPT stands for diphtheria, pertussis (or whooping cough), and tetanus. DPT injections are usually given in the muscles of the mid-thigh or upper arm, at intervals of one month, sometimes longer. To prevent fever or other severe reactions, the two-to-five month old baby should receive one grain of baby aspirin within a few hours after the injection. If she nevertheless develops fever or has other severe reactions, your doctor may have to give lower doses, and therefore give more than three injections. Very rarely is a severe reaction reported with smaller doses of the vaccine. If there is such a reaction, no further injections of pertussis vaccine will be given.

Occasionally, redness or a lump appears at the site of the injection. This is a local reaction. It is harmless and will disappear within a few weeks. If it does not, consult your physician.

It is recommended that a booster or recall shot be given at one-and-a-half and at three years of age. Another recall injection of only TD (tetanus-diphtheria toxoid) is given at six years and at twelve years.

Following is a chart listing the recommended schedule for active immunization and tuberculin testing of normal infants and children:

IMMUNIZATION AND TESTING SCHEDULE

2–3 months	DPT, Sabin Type 3 or Trivalent
3–4 months	DPT, Sabin Type 1 or Trivalent
4–5 months	DPT, Sabin Type 2 or Trivalent
9–11 months	Tuberculin Test
12 months	Measles Vaccine*
12–24 months	Mumps Vaccine* Rubella Vaccine*
15–18 months	DPT, Trivalent Sabin
2 years	Tuberculin Test
3 years	DPT, Tuberculin Test
4 years	Tuberculin Test
6 years	TD, Tuberculin Test, Trivalent Sabin
8 years	Tuberculin Test, Mumps Vaccine (if not given earlier or if child did not have mumps)
12 years	TD, Tuberculin Test
14 years	Tuberculin Test
16 years	Tuberculin Test

*Measles, Mumps, and Rubella Vaccine can now be given in one injection, or two of the three can be combined in one injection.

Smallpox vaccination is no longer required any place in the United States before entry into school. There are now other immunization requirements, and since they may differ from place to place, families should find out about them through their doctor. In planning a trip abroad with children, sufficient time should be allowed for recovery from any possible adverse reactions to immunizations.

Independence

Many parents feel that the most memorable moment in a child's progress towards independence comes when he takes his first steps alone. Upright and walking! Most children accomplish this by going independently from the secure arms of one adult to the waiting arms of another. As youngsters move toward greater independence, they will do so with confidence if they can start out from a secure foundation of

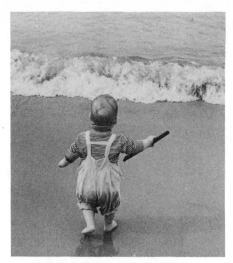

As a child begins to walk, he begins to get a sense of independence.

rules and limits, and return to the security of acceptance and understanding should they come to grief.

THE TODDLER STAGE: The toddler relishes the independence of being able to explore the house or the playground but he won't go very far before he returns to check in with the person in charge of him so that he can start out all over again. He voices his independence, too: "No" to naps; "No" to outings; "No" to a bath. This is the phase during which parents must be wary of asking "Would you like to" or "Do you want to" instead of just proceeding with the business at hand. Patience is required for the self-assertive fumblings and clumsy efforts at self-feeding and putting clothes on. Assistance should be subtle and tactful, not hurried and bossy: "Baby do, daddy help," is the general idea.

SCHOOL AGE: As the child moves into the larger arena of school and friendships, "I'm not a baby any more" may become a complaint if he wants more freedom than he's permitted to have. At this stage, he begins to learn that responsibility goes hand-in-hand with freedom and independence Old enough to ride the bike farther and farther from home means taking on the responsibility of keeping it in good repair and obeying all the traffic rules.

Influenza

See *The Common Cold, Influenza, and Other Viral Infections*, p. 387.

Insect stings and bites

When a child is bitten or stung by an insect, he often complains about the pain or the itching, but with the application of a lotion or salve to relieve discomfort and a bandage to prevent infection, the incident is soon forgotten. There are times, however, when a sting or a bite may require emergency treatment.

It has been estimated that about four children out of every 1,000 have serious allergic reactions to the sting of a hornet, wasp, bee, yellow jacket, or the fire ant. A child who has sustained multiple stings, or whose body, tongue, or face begins to swell because of a single sting should be taken to the hospital immediately. Tests can clearly distinguish between those children who are highly sensitive to stings and those who are not.

PREVENTIVE MEASURES: A doctor should be consulted about the advisability of testing youngsters who are going off to camp for the first time or who are planning long hikes. Rather than curtail the activities of a child who turns out to have an acute sensitivity, it may make sense to plan a series of desensitization treatments against the particular venom. For children who are very allergic to insect stings, an emergency kit containing adrenaline is now available and should always be carried.

MOSQUITOS: Every effort should be made to eradicate mosquitoes by eliminating their breeding places. A mosquito bite can be a serious threat to a child's health, since these insects transmit several diseases. Where mosquitoes are a problem, infants and children should be protected against them by screens, netting, and the application of repellents.

TICKS: Families with pets should guard against the possibility of disease-bearing parasites, especially the tick that transmits Rocky Mountain spotted fever. A child who has been bitten and is harboring a tick carrying this disease will develop a characteristic rash on the palms of the hands and the soles of the feet. Prompt medical attention is essential to prevent possible complications. See ROCKY MOUNTAIN SPOTTED FEVER under RASHES.

Intelligence and IQ

Intelligence is a quality, not a quantity. It therefore cannot be measured as precisely as height or weight; nor can it be exemplified as definitely as mechanical skill or athletic ability or musical talent. Although child development authorities and educators may disagree about how to assess intelligence, they generally agree on the following premise: no matter what is inherited and what is instilled by experience, children function best in later life if their earliest years of nurture bring out and develop their inborn capacities.

ENCOURAGEMENT AND ENRICHMENT: Beginning with proper prenatal diet and care, a healthy baby is born, and from then on, her intellectual capacities are shaped by experience. Loving and attentive parents give her the self-confidence to explore and learn. She is encouraged to express herself in language. She is exposed to a variety of experiences that will stimulate her curiosity and interest: plants, drawing materials, pets, picture books, outings to the beach. Her efforts to use her intelligence by asking questions are respected and encouraged rather than minimized and ignored.

IQ TESTS: Once a child gets to school her capabilities may or may not be measured by a standard IQ test. Such tests, which have been abandoned in some states, assess specific areas of intelligence and are graded according to a statistical norm. Newer techniques for measuring intelligence are designed to compensate for a cultural bias that some authorities believe exists in the standard tests.

Jealousy

See ABILITIES AND APTITUDES, BROTHERS AND SISTERS, NEW BABY.

Kidney diseases

For a discussion of kidney diseases, see under *Diseases of the Urinogenital System*, p. 424, and *Cancer of the Kidney*, p. 443.

Learning

See CURIOSITY, INTELLIGENCE AND IQ, READING, SCHOOLS.

Lead poisoning

Lead poisoning in children is usually associated with the ingestion of paint and plaster flakes containing high levels of lead. This is a problem in city slums where old buildings are being leveled, or in cases where youngsters manage to gnaw on repainted cribs and other furniture originally covered with lead-base paint. In addition to this traditional source of poisoning, however, the daily exposure to exhaust fumes of leaded gasoline is causing an increasing number of children to have an excessively high level of lead in their blood. Suburban areas adjacent to heavily traveled superhighways are particularly susceptible to this problem. Those parts of the city regularly jammed with buses and cars are also unhealthy.

Lead poisoning is a serious danger to the health of approximately half a million children in the United States. Irreversible brain damage and anemia can occur if the condition becomes chronic; convulsions and death may occur in an acute case. To lessen such hazards, legislation now requires new cars to use only lead-free gasoline.

Learning disability

A child with a learning disability is one who, though otherwise normal, cannot acquire certain skills or assimilate certain kinds of knowledge at the same rate as most other children. Obviously, almost every child lags behind her peers at one time or another in certain subjects; but the difficulties of a learning disabled child are far more severe. A sixteen-year-old who suffers from a learning disability may, for example, be capable only of third or fourth-grade math while functioning at her own grade level in other subjects. Some learning disabilities are attributed to minimal brain damage, but in most cases the cause is unknown. See also DYSLEXIA.

Leukemia

See CANCER.

Lying

See DISHONESTY.

Malnutrition

Poor nutrition or undernourishment can occur not only as a result of a faulty diet, but also because a child may have a metabolic defect that prevents her body from making proper use of a particular essential nutrient. Temporary malnutrition may also accompany a long illness in which the child's appetite wanes.

Although malnutrition is usually associated with poverty and child neglect, it can also occur because of ignorance, carelessness, or fanaticism. Children have been found to be malnourished by parents following a macrobiotic diet or a faddish type of vegetarianism. Using vitamins as a substitute for food can also cause certain types of undernourishment.

Older children, especially girls approaching puberty, may embark on starvation diets in an attempt to ward off inevitable body changes and end up seriously malnourished. The general signs of malnutrition are increasing physical weakness, vague and unfocused behavior, as well as the particular symptoms associated with anemia and vitamin deficiencies. See also p. 202.

Manners

Decent manners are most easily instilled in children not by scoldings, lectures, nagging, or punishments, but by setting a good example. In a family where consideration of each person's feelings is naturally taken into account, adults say "Please" and "Thank you" to each other and to their children. Thus even the youngest child gets the idea that part of growing up is to be polite to the people around him. If good manners begin at home, they're less likely to be forgotten in public.

Measles

Measles is by far the most dangerous of the common childhood diseases because of its possible complications, such as meningitis, encephalitis, and severe secondary staphylococcus infection. Fortunately, widespread protection is available in the live measles vaccine, which should be given to every child over one year of age.

SYMPTOMS: Measles, a highly contagious disease caused by a virus, has an incubation period of one to two weeks. The most noticeable symptom is the rash which begins on the head and face within a few days after the onset of the disease, and gradually erupts all over the body, blending into big red patches. Other symptoms include fever up to 104° or higher, a severe cough, sore throat, stuffy nose, inflammation of the *conjunctiva* (the mucous membrane on the inner part of the eyelid and extending over the front of the eyeball), sensitivity of the eyes to light, enlarged lymph nodes, and a generalized sick feeling.

Any child who has contracted measles should be seen by a physician and watched carefully for possible complications. Moreover, if he is of school age, the school should be promptly notified. This, of course, is true for any contagious disease.

TREATMENT: Measles can be treated only symptomatically. During the incubation period, an injection of gamma globulin will lessen the severity of the disease, or occasionally prevent it. If there are other children at home besides the af-

fected one, they should also receive gamma globulin injections. Antibiotics are of no help unless there is a secondary bacterial infection.

All parents should make certain that their children are vaccinated against this potentially serious disease. See IMMUNIZATION.

Medication

New parents can save themselves time and trouble by getting into the habit of writing down the doctor's instructions about medication when the child requires it. Although dosages are usually clearly indicated on labels prepared by the pharmacist according to the prescription, the doctor may add comments about how or when to change the dosage.

HOW TO GIVE MEDICINES TO CHILDREN: As for administering medication, a calm and assured approach and a minimum of fuss are more effective than wheedling and urging. A very young child may need to be distracted by cheerful conversation as the spoon goes into her mouth; an older child can be given some factual information about the medica-

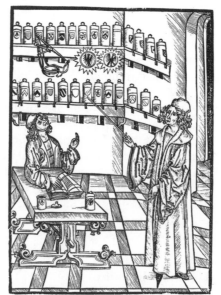

In a 16th-century engraving, a doctor personally visits a pharmacy to select the medicine he wants to give to his patient.

tion and what it will do. No matter what the youngster's age, parents should never trick or fool her about what she's being given, nor should candied medicine be used under any circumstances. Setting up this type of confusion in a young mind can lead to an overdose of "candy" serious enough to require emergency hospitalization.

OVERUSING MEDICATION: As a child gets older, she will become increasingly conscious of the medication her parents take. Families that are constantly swallowing one or another kind of pill—diet pills, sleeping pills, tranquilizers—might give some thought to their attitude towards drugs and how these attitudes are affecting their children. Generally, it's a good idea to refrain from medicating a child unless the doctor recommends it.

OLD MEDICINES: Once the illness for which a particular medication has been prescribed is definitely over, the remains of the bottle or the left-over capsules should be flushed down the toilet. Old, outdated pills can be dangerous. For safety's sake, parents should review the contents of the medicine cabinet on a regular basis and get rid of any medications left over from a previous illness. Basic medications that are essential for occasional emergencies should be reviewed for continuing effectiveness. Some of these might have a limited shelf life and be completely ineffective should they be needed.

Meningitis

Meningitis is an inflammation of the *meninges*, the thin membranes that cover the spinal cord and the brain. The inflammation, which may be caused by a virus or by bacteria, is more common among children than adults, and may occur in epidemics. This is especially true if the infectious agent is meningococcal (*meningococcal meningitis*), since the meningococcal bacteria are also found in the throat and are transmitted by coughing, sneezing, and talking. This type occurs mostly in young adults. Another type of meningitis which commonly occurs among young children during the spring and summer is caused by such organisms as the mumps virus and the Coxsackie virus.

SYMPTOMS: Whatever the cause, the symptoms are generally the same: headache, fever, vomiting, and stiff neck. If untreated, the child may go into delirium and convulsions. Drowsiness and blurred vision may also occur, and if the disease develops in an infant, the pressure on the brain caused by the inflamed meninges will create a bulge on the soft spot (fontanel) of the baby's head. No time should be lost in calling the doctor about any of these symptoms.

Meningitis was almost always fatal before the availability of antibiotics, and although it is no longer the threat it once was, it must be treated promptly if irreversible consequences are to be avoided.

Mental illness

Behind the search for the causes and treatment of mental illness in children is the current research in the relationship between that mysterious entity called the mind and that palpable physical organism called the brain. Parents of children diagnosed as mentally ill are themselves caught up in this distinction, often preferring to call their youngsters "emotionally disturbed." It is now estimated that about 1½ million youngsters under 18 require some kind of treatment for mental illness, and this figure does not include the one million children diagnosed as hyperkinetic. The two most serious forms of childhood mental illness are autism and schizophrenia.

AUTISM: The term "early infantile autism" was coined in the 1940s to describe babies and young children who show unpredictable deviations in development. Some never learn to speak; others refuse to look anyone directly in the eye. Autistic children may have one or two extraordinary skills and be incapable of remembering their own names. In spite of a tendency on the part of a few specialists to ascribe autism to a rejecting mother's refusal to love the infant, most authorities now describe this mysterious disorder as an organic condition caused by neurological rather than by psychological abnormalities. The same conclusions are more or less being reached about schizophrenia.

SCHIZOPHRENIA: In schizophrenia, a child is likely to exhibit any of the following symptoms: confused speech and thinking; lack of emotional responsiveness; withdrawal into fantasy; and occasionally, hallucinations. There are indications that genetic inheritance plays some role in this disorder, and that environmental influences are also involved.

Studies suggest that symptoms originate in abnormalities of brain chemistry that may be corrected by the proper medication. Over the past twenty years, many special schools, both day schools and residential ones, have been established for training autistic and schizophrenic children. The most successful enlist the cooperation of parents as co-therapists. The National Society for Autistic Children was organized to initiate schools, offer counseling to parents, and foster research. The Society operates a National Information and Referral Service which can be addressed at 306 31st Street, Huntington, West Virginia 25702. See also HYPERKINESIS.

Mental retardation

An estimated six million people in the United States are in some degree mentally retarded—almost three percent of the population. Mental retardation occurs among all nationalities, races, and religions, and among the children of those in the highest social and economic groups as well as the lowest.

WHAT IS MENTAL RETARDATION? Mental retardation is a developmental disability in which the individual's rate of development as a child is consistently slower than average.

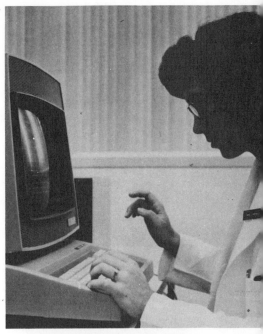

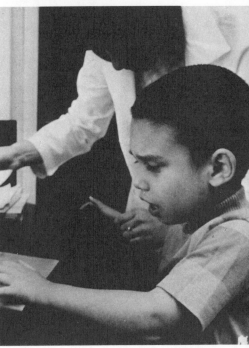

A specialist in autism research uses the Health Sciences Computing Facility *(top)* and works with an autistic child *(bottom)* in an effort to locate new genetic factors involved in the disorder.

Learning cannot be acquired at the usual rate, and the child encounters difficulties in social adjustment.

DEGREES OF MENTAL RETARDATION: Mentally retarded children (and adults) are classified into four categories depending upon the degree of retardation.

Mildly retarded children—those with IQs roughly between 50 and 70—belong to by far the largest category; nearly 90% of all retarded people fall into this group. IQ scores by themselves can be misleading, but they are a convenient guide to probable learning and development patterns if understood properly—that is, simply as one of the criteria by which the degree of a child's disability can be estimated. The retardation of mildly retarded children is usually not apparent until they are of school age. With special educational help, such children can achieve satisfying progress in school and, as adults, will be capable with proper training of handling any of a wide variety of regular jobs. They may be indistinguishable from nonretarded people and can be expected to take their places in the life of their community.

Moderately retarded children —those with IQs somewhat below 50—belong to a group that comprises about 6% of all retarded people in the United States. The retardation of these children is usually apparent before they begin school, often during the child's first year, in the form of delayed developmental landmarks—for example, late sitting, late standing, late

walking, and delayed talking. Many children with Down's syndrome (Mongolism) fall into this group. These children require a more sheltered environment than the mildly retarded, but can be trained as adults to do productive, satisfying work.

Severely and profoundly retarded children often have other handicaps, such as impaired motor coordination or defective vision or hearing. The great majority of these children can be taught to care for their basic needs, and many can do useful work under supervision.

CAUSES: There are numerous causes of mental retardation. Some cases are specifically caused by congenital factors (conditions existing at or before birth). Among these are the following: deprivation of oxygen to the brain of a baby during the birth process; the mother's contraction of rubella (German measles) during the first three months of pregnancy; complications resulting from Rh-factor blood incompatibility between mother and baby; a grossly inadequate prenatal diet of the mother; syphilis; hydrocephalus (accumulation of spinal fluid in the brain); or any other pressure or injury to the brain of the fetus.

Some forms of retardation result from hereditary factors, the genetic

makeup of the parents. Down's syndrome and phenylketonuria (PKU) fall in this category.

Mental retardation can also occur as a result of disease. Inflammation of the brain is a possible complication of measles—now wholly preventable by the administration of the measles vaccine. Other causes are brain injuries due to a severe blow to the head, as from a fall. Some of these injuries are deliberately inflicted, usually by parents. (See BATTERED CHILD.) Among environmental hazards, lead and mercury poisoning are of particular importance. Lead-based paint chips have been eaten by unattended children. (See LEAD POISONING.)

If retardation is suspected by parents, medical advice should be sought immediately and a thorough evaluation of the child conducted. Some types of retardation can be greatly benefited by medical and educational treatment. It should be emphasized that all retarded children can learn and that many can be helped to the extent that they can become productive citizens. Parents would like further information about mental retardation or who are in need of counseling should write to the National Association for Retarded Citizens, 2709 Avenue E East, Arlington, Texas 76011. See also HANDICAPPED CHILD.

Minimal brain damage

See under BRAIN DAMAGE.

Money

Money may not be the root of all evil, but it certainly is the cause of a lot of family quarrels. In order to communicate to children the value of money and how to use it, spend it, save it, borrow it, lend it, and earn it, parents should try to clarify their own attitudes and settle their own differences.

Young children hear money talked about all the time: "We can't afford it," "That's a bargain," "That's a waste of money." What does it all mean to a preschooler?

Special education programs can help children with Down's syndrome develop to their maximum potential.

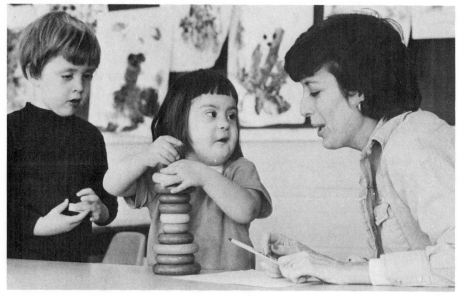

THE WEEKLY ALLOWANCE: The best way for a child to get first-hand experience in dealing with "I need" and "I want" in terms of cash on hand is to give her a weekly allowance. There isn't any point in doing this until she has mastered addition and subtraction. If the prospect of getting an allowance is motivation for improving her number skills at school, so much the better. The amount of the allowance should be calculated in terms of what it's supposed to cover. These details should be spelled out so that there's no confusion about who is responsible for paying for what. As the child gets older, the amount is adjusted for increasing needs—social occasions such as a ten-year-old might enjoy when she and her friends stop off for an ice-cream cone on the way home from school.

SAVING: If the family feels that a child should be required to save part of her allowance, a piggy bank and a brief talk about the virtues of saving are essential. Some children get so anxious about money that they turn into misers. When this occurs, it may be advisable to point out that the money is not meant to be hoarded but to be spent on needs and treats. Children who receive birthday or other special presents in the form of money from relatives can open a bank account and learn about interest accrual. Although the money is rightfully theirs, they might be encouraged to consult the family before they spend it all on a passing enthusiasm.

Mumps

Mumps, a mild disorder in most children, is caused by a virus and has an incubation period of from two to three weeks. The most familiar symptom is swollen glands involving the jaw. The glands usually affected are the *parotid glands*—large salivary glands below and slightly in front of the ear—although other glands may be affected, too. Other symptoms include fever and a general sick feeling. No rash is present. Mumps lasts about five days; then the swelling disappears.

In an adolescent boy, the disease sometimes causes an inflammation of the testes (called *orchitis*) and may be very painful. In addition, if it involves both testes, there is a possibility—fortunately only a very slight one—that sterility will result.

In older children mumps occasionally produces the complication called *mumps meningoencephalitis*. The signs of this more serious disease are headache, fever, and extreme debilitation. Finally, there may be an inflammation of the pancreas which can cause severe abdominal pain and vomiting.

Since mumps is now preventable, it is important that every boy and girl be given the mumps vaccine. Boys should be given the vaccine before puberty.

Muscular dystrophy
See p. 480.

Nausea and vomiting

Nausea, the signal that vomiting may occur, is often described as feeling sick to the stomach. The feeling is experienced when irritated nerve endings in the stomach and elsewhere send messages to the vomiting reflex in the brain. When the nerve irritation is acute, vomiting occurs.

PHYSICAL CAUSES: Although nausea and vomiting are usually associated with a child's upset stomach or the sudden onset of a high fever and an acute infection, many youngsters feel nauseated and throw up because of motion sickness in a car or plane, or as the result of severe pain occasioned by a bad fall or other accident. A doctor should always be consulted when nausea and vomiting are accompanied by fever, cramps, or diarrhea. For the child who feels sick in a moving vehicle, the doctor can prescribe suitable medication. For a youngster who has swallowed a toxic substance, vomiting must often be induced. See p. 578 for further information on poisoning.

EMOTIONAL STRESS: Chronic nausea may result from emotional stress. A child who doesn't want to go to school because of some threatening situation, or who is always too anxious before a test because of pressures to do well, or who is fearful about some athletic challenge but ashamed to admit it—children under these pressures are likely to develop symptoms of nausea. However, instead of dismissing the recurrence of nausea and vomiting as typical of an oversensitive child, parents should try to find out the source of the problem and, if necessary, arrange some family therapy sessions with the child.

Nervous habits

Nervous habits both express and release inner tension, and since growing up isn't an easy process, it's inevitable that most children have one or another way of dealing with their fears, anxieties, and emotional pressures. There's no point in parental scolding or ridicule or punishment, since any of these approaches simply adds yet another pressure to those that exist already. After all, most adults have nervous habits too—whether it's smoking, or picking at a cuticle, or tooth-grinding—and no amount of nagging is likely to put a stop to any of them.

Some nervous habits can be unhealthy, and some can be socially unacceptable but essentially harmless. All are unconscious, and most eventually disappear with age. Among the habits that may need looking into in order to decide that they have no basis in a physical disorder are squinting and throat-clearing. Hair-twirling and foot-shaking can be entirely ignored. Nail-biting may persist for years, or it may yield to vanity or the comments of friends.

Thumb-sucking, abandoned at two, may recur at three because of the arrival of a new baby or because of the stresses of going to nursery school. Many school-age children continue to suck their thumbs when they're going to sleep. There's no need to worry about this habit unless the dentist notices the beginning of an orthodontic problem, in which case, the dentist and not you should discuss it with the child. Nose-picking in public is almost always abandoned when a child enters school. If a big fuss has been made about it, he may continue the habit at home as a gesture of defiance—or because it really is unconscious. When done in private, it's completely harmless.

Masturbation is a nervous habit that bothers many parents more than it should. In and of itself, there's no harm in it, but as a chronic expression of anxiety, it might be dealt with tactfully and indirectly by trying to get to the source of the tension rather than by punishing or humiliating the child.

New baby

It's a good idea for parents to talk about the anticipated arrival of a new baby with their child or children before the pregnancy is really obvious. Conversations can be ca-

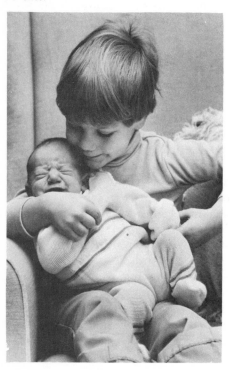

The birth of a family's second child can be an exciting, positive experience for the older child if he is prepared for the new arrival well in advance.

sual, and questions should be answered simply and factually. If any basic changes are to be made—especially if a child is to be shifted to a bed so that the new arrival can have the crib—this transition should be accomplished before the infant appears. Adults should refrain from asking such questions as "Would you like a little brother or a little sister?" or "Isn't it wonderful that there's going to be a new baby in the family?" Preparations made in advance of going to the hospital should, if possible, consider whether the child would prefer to stay at home or with a relative during mother's absence. When the baby is brought home and well-wishers arrive with presents, it's comforting for the first-born to sit in mother's or daddy's lap while visitors coo over the infant in the crib. Thoughtful baby-present givers will always include a little present for the baby's older siblings, too. Parents should do their best to make baby's big brother or sister feel that the new baby is his or hers no less than mother's or father's. See also ABILITIES AND APTITUDES, BROTHERS AND SISTERS.

Nightmares

See DREAMS AND NIGHTMARES.

Night terrors

See DREAMS AND NIGHTMARES.

Nosebleeds

Children are likely to have nosebleeds more often than adults, and they are usually no cause for alarm. A small blood vessel near the nostril may be injured by energetic nose-blowing, the presence of a foreign object, or by an accidental blow or an intentional wallop.

APPLY PRESSURE: A minor nosebleed is most effectively stopped by applying pressure over the bleeding area. A child old enough to follow instructions should be told to sit down, hold the head slightly forward, and compress the soft portion of the nose between thumb and

forefinger, maintaining the pressure for about five minutes and breathing through the mouth. Application of an ice pack to the outside of the nose is usually helpful. Fingers should be withdrawn very slowly in order not to disturb the clot that should have formed.

PACKING THE NOSTRIL: If this method doesn't stop the bleeding, a small twist of sterile cotton can be inserted gently into the nostril so that some of it protrudes. Light pressure should be applied once again for five minutes and the cotton allowed to remain in place for a while. Should the bleeding continue in spite of these measures, the child should be taken to a hospital emergency clinic.

Orthodontics

Orthodontics is the branch of dentistry that specializes in the correction of *malocclusion* (an improper alignment of the upper and lower teeth at the point where they meet) or to irregularity of tooth positioning. Emphasis is now being placed on the prevention of malocclusion before it can occur. General practitioners of dentistry, *pedodontists* (specialists in children's dentistry), and orthodontists now believe that the need for expensive, time-consuming, and emotionally unsettling orthodontics can sometimes be avoided by beginning treatment as early as the age of four.

The positioning of the permanent teeth is the result not only of inheritance, but of other variables, such as lip-biting and thumb-sucking. Premature loss or partial disintegration of primary teeth also has a strong influence on whether the permanent teeth will be properly positioned.

PREVENTIVE ORTHODONTICS: By the time the child is five, an X ray will show exactly how all the permanent teeth are situated in the gums. In some cases, it may be possible to guide these teeth as they erupt. If potential overcrowding and eventual crookedness are indicated, some baby teeth may be pulled to make room for the permanent ones. Normal positioning may also be accomplished by establishing a different balance of muscular forces.

CORRECTIVE APPLIANCES: Corrective orthodontics uses many different types of appliances for the repositioning of permanent teeth, all of which operate on the same principle of applying pressure to the bone. Widening the arch of the upper jaw, for example, is accomplished by the use of a screw appliance fixed to the upper teeth so that the two halves of the hard palate are slightly separated along the middle suture, permitting new bone to fill in the space. Specialists point out that a bonus of this orthodontic correction is increased respiratory ease for youngsters who were formerly mouth-breathers.

Parents who have been advised by the family dentist that an orthodontic consultation is advisable for a child, and who are concerned about the eventual economic burden that prolonged treatment might represent, should get a second opinion from the clinical staff of a dental school associated with a university. See also DENTAL CARE.

Overeating

It's simple enough to define overeating as putting more food into the stomach than the body needs for good nutrition, but that doesn't shed much light on why certain children do so. Parents need only indulge in some honest introspection and they are likely to remember times when they overate—or drank too much —because they were anxious about something or because they felt lonely or neglected or angry. These feelings may lead to compulsive overeating in children, too.

There are also those parents for whom plumpness is a sign of well-being. Without thinking of the permanent harm they might be doing, they overfeed their children; from an early age such children get in the habit of eating too much as a way of gaining parental approval. It's not unusual for girls about to enter pu-

berty either to starve themselves or to stuff themselves; either impulse is an expression of fears about sexuality that are gradually eased if the family atmosphere is relaxed and understanding.

WHAT TO DO AND WHAT NOT TO DO: The least effective way of dealing with chronic overeating is parental nagging or teasing. Punishment in the form of cutting down a child's allowance or withholding permission to attend a birthday party will very likely only make the child more anxious and angrier. In most cases, a pattern of overeating has to be changed by the child and not by the parent. However, where the problem is the result of overt or hidden pressure on the child to overeat, parents will have to change their notions of good eating habits, health, and attractive appearance. See also *Nutrition and Weight Control*, p. 194.

Pacifiers

Some parents can't stand the sound of a baby's crying; others can't stand the sight of a baby sucking on a pacifier. Whatever the perference, what the baby needs during the early months is satisfaction for the sucking impulse. For most babies, this need seems to taper off at about six months; with those babies in whom

the need remains strong, the thumb seems to be a convenient substitute for the pacifier. Whatever decision is arrived at between you and your doctor, the important thing to keep in mind is that the pacifier is no substitute for holding and cuddling the baby when she wants comforting, and that sometimes a parent is more dependent on a pacifier than the baby is.

If pacifiers are used regularly, more than one should be available, and they should be inspected periodically to make sure that bits and pieces of rubber haven't been chewed so loose that they may be swallowed and lodge in the windpipe.

Pets

Rural children usually have their own pet animals even if the animals aren't allowed in the house. Suburban families are likely to own a dog that's a pet as well as a discouragement to prowlers. It's the city child who may have to wage a persistent campaign before his parents capitulate to the idea of a pet. Yet even the smallest apartment can accommodate a pet bird or a small fish tank; a cat and a litter box won't cause extra crowding. Of course, dogs offer the greatest companionship but also impose the greatest responsibility;

Pets provide wonderful companionship and give children the responsibility of caring for another living creature.

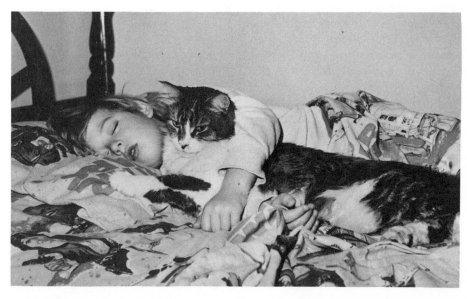

they do have to be housebroken and walked in all weathers at least twice a day. If a child brings a stray animal home, the dog or cat must be checked by a vet before it becomes a household member. Once a youngster can read, the acquisition of a pet hamster or a guinea pig or a pair of gerbils will provide the incentive for trips to the library for books on care and feeding.

CHOOSING A DOG: When a dog is to be the choice, it's often cheaper and more satisfactory to select one from the litter of a healthy dog you know than to buy one in a pet shop or from a commercial kennel. The breed chosen should be suitable in terms of size, temperament, and cost of feeding. Relative advantages and disadvantages should be checked out at the library by the child whose responsibility the pet will be.

For an only child, a pet animal is almost a must, not only for companionship, but so that there's a being in the house who's smaller and more helpless than she is. In families where allergies are a problem, the doctor should be consulted about the type of pet that will cause the least discomfort to a vulnerable member of the household.

Pica

Pica is the technical term for an abnormal desire to eat substances that are not fit for food, such as clay, earth, plaster and the like. This tendency is not to be confused with the tendency of babies and toddlers to put unsuitable things into their mouth. Pica is habitual and compulsive, and may result in serious disabilities. Since the phenomenon is especially conspicuous among poor and neglected children, some authorities associate it with nutritional deficiency, others with unsatisfied emotional needs. Signs of pica should be brought to the attention of a doctor or a social service agency that can provide guidance on how the child's circumstances should be altered even if the total environment cannot be changed. See also LEAD POISONING.

Pills

See MEDICATION.

Pinworms or threadworms

See p. 382.

PKU

PKU stands for *phenylketonuria,* an inherited metabolic defect. Approximately one baby in 10,000 is born with this disease, in which the body is incapable of producing certain enzymes that are essential for the metabolic conversion of the amino acid phenylalanine. The disorder causes the amino acid and some of its by-products to accumulate in the bloodstream to a dangerous degree. If the condition goes undetected and untreated, irreversible brain damage and mental retardation are the result.

PKU babies are characteristically blond and blue-eyed, with sensitive skin and faulty muscle coordination. In many parts of the United States, state laws require that three days after birth, all babies be given the blood test that detects the presence of PKU so that treatment can begin at once if necessary. Supervised treatment usually continues for several years, and in some communities is available at special therapy centers. Parents or prospective parents who would like to find out whether any member of the family is a carrier of the recessive gene that transmits the PKU disorder can arrange for diagnostic testing and genetic counseling based on the results.

Play

See FANTASIES. TOYS.

Pneumonia

See *Pneumonia,* p. 389.

Poisons and poisoning

Every year, hundreds of thousands of children swallow some poisonous substance—in too many cases with fatal results—because of parental carelessness, or because the child hasn't been given clear and unequivocal instructions about the difference between "candy" and medicine. Poisoning because of the ingestion of sugar-coated aspirin is a continuing problem; iron-containing multiple vitamins that seem to be a gourmet treat to some children also present a problem because iron in excess doses is a stomach irritant.

SAFETY MEASURES: Toddlers can do themselves damage because they're curious about everything, and their sense of taste isn't all that discriminating. Thus it's an absolute necessity to see that all household cleansers and strong chemicals are kept on high shelves rather than on the floor. Many bottles containing medicines come with safety caps that presumably cannot be opened by children—for instance, because pressure must be applied—but can be opened by adults. The experience of many parents, however, is that whereas their children can often open such caps, *they* frequently have a great deal of difficulty. Suffice it to say that the perfect childproof bottle cap has yet to be designed.

Since it's practically impossible for anyone except an expert to know what substances are poisonous to children in what amounts, or which seeds of which plants are harmful if swallowed, many authorities feel strongly that parents should immediately call the closest Poison Control Center for first-aid information rather than try to cope with antidotes or emetics on their own. The Centers are available by phone on a 24-hour-a-day basis. See p. 580 to find the Poison Control Center nearest you. Make a note of the telephone number and make sure it's available to baby-sitters as well as to all responsible family members.

Poliomyelitis

Until the Salk vaccine was developed in the 1950s, there was no protection against polio (or, as it was then popularly called, *infantile paralysis*). The disease caused paralysis of the extremities and could cause death by paralyzing the muscles used in breathing.

The Salk vaccine utilizes doses of killed virus and is given by injection. Although it is still widely used in many parts of the world, in the United States the Sabin live virus vaccine, which is given orally, has virtually supplanted it. Repeated series of booster shots are unnecessary because the immunity persists for years.

It is advisable that a child receive three doses of the Sabin vaccine, six to eight weeks apart, starting at about the age of two months. One method employs *trivalent* vaccine, in which each dose contains three kinds of vaccine—to give protection against three strains of polio. Three separate doses are necessary, however, to insure full protection. The other method employs *monovalent* vaccines, in which each dose insures protection against a different type of polio.

Posture

"Stand up straight" is an order that many parents issue to their children with the regularity of drill sergeants. Actually, most youngsters tend to slump and have a potbellied look until they're about nine years old. This inelegant posture is not necessarily the sign of any disorder.

Youngsters who are regularly checked by a doctor and given a good bill of health are not in any danger of developing a permanent curvature of the spine because they slouch. However, certain kinds of chronically poor posture may be an expression of some disorder that should be checked. Among these are flat feet, near-sightedness or astigmatism, or a hearing loss.

Emotional problems may also be expressed in a child's bearing. Anxiety can lead to carrying one shoulder higher than the other as if warding off a blow. Shyness or insecurity may cause a hangdog stance. For pubescent girls, embarrassment about burgeoning breasts may result in a round-shouldered slump. Some of these causes of poor posture should be discussed with a doctor;

others may be temporary and shouldn't be turned into major problems by incessant and unproductive nagging. A better corrective is participation in a dancing class or an exercise class. Sports such as ice-skating and bicycle-riding are good posture correctives, too.

Prejudice

The A student (female) who avoids studying mathematics because "girls aren't supposed to be good in math" and the black boy who goes out for the track team even though he'd rather be in the science club "because blacks are better at sports than at brainwork" have unconsciously accepted the prejudiced views of other people about them. What a waste for themselves and society!

Children who are raised in an atmosphere of contempt for and fear and mistrust of Catholics, Jews, Italians, blacks, women, men, are likely to spend the better part of their lives alternating between apprehension and arrogance. It's difficult to believe that adults can have a

prejudice such as, "All Orientals are sneaky," which is supposed to describe millions of human beings, or "She's only a girl," which makes a judgment about one-half of the human race.

BEING THE OBJECT OF DISCRIMINATION: Parents who have themselves been discriminated against have to prepare their children for the reality of discrimination and how to cope with it. A child raised in an atmosphere of love and respect will have enough self-esteem to refuse to accept anyone else's false notions about him.

Privacy

Every child has a right to a certain amount of privacy even when he's very young. If, for instance, a parent or older child doesn't allow anyone into the bathroom when he's using it, a four- or five-year-old should be given the same option. When children share the same room, or even the same furniture, each one should have a drawer of his own and a shelf of his own for his things. Respecting

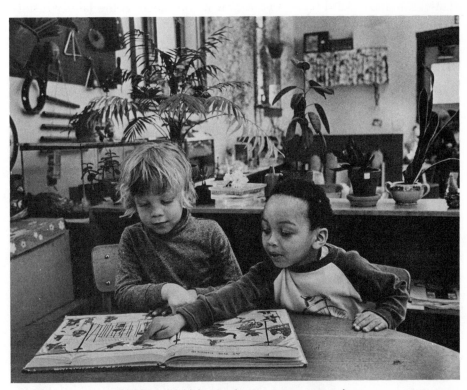

Children should be taught to respect one another
regardless of racial, religious, or ethnic differences.

his private property will lead him to respect other people's. A youngster does like the privacy of playing with his friends without having a parent hovering around all the time, and he certainly doesn't want anyone listening in on his phone conversations by the time he's nine or ten.

Parents have a right to privacy, too! Children should be led to understand—pleasantly but firmly—that some adult conversations are private and not meant for their ears. They should also be educated to the fact that when an older member of the family is behind a closed door, it's rude to barge in without knocking.

Puberty

See *Puberty and Growth*, p. 109.

Punishment

Severe physical punishment should be avoided. Ideally, punishment should be carried out because it has an instructional value for the child rather than because it helps a parent relieve his or her feelings of anger or frustration. Severe physical punishments—for example, the use of sticks, belts, or hard blows to the body—are extremely frightening and may even be permanently injurious to the child. Frequently, this kind of discipline can evoke even further anger on the part of the child and lead to further misbehavior.

DURATION: Punishments should not be long and drawn out, but should be as immediate as possible and last only a reasonable length of time. For example, withdrawal of television privileges for a month for a seven-year-old's misbehavior would be excessively long, because at the end of the month it would be difficult for her to remember what she had done that was wrong. Excessively long punishments are also difficult to enforce. If possible, a punishment should be related to the misbehavior for which the child is receiving the punishment.

IMMEDIACY: Punishment "when father gets home" or a day later frequently has little meaning for the child and is unlikely to help her stop misbehaving. Rewards for good behavior should also be immediate; affection and approval for most children are often more powerful rewards than candy and money. See also DISCIPLINE.

Radio, record player, and TV

Music hath charms not only to soothe the savage beast but also to lift the spirits and provide entertainment.

However, children who have their own transistor radios should be informed that playing them in public at a level audible to another person is against the law in most places, and if they're listening to music with ear plugs, the sound should be kept low enough not to damage their ears. Countless young people of the 60s have grown to adulthood with a permanent hearing disability because of chronic exposure to dangerously high sound levels.

The child who has a record player or a cassette deck of his own should be permitted to express his own tastes in the music he buys with his own allowance. If the family installation is an expensive one, a young child should be permitted to use it only when he demonstrates the proper respect for the delicacy of the mechanism.

TELEVISION TIME: As for the problem of how much time should be spent watching television: if as soon as the toddler's eyes can focus on the screen, TV is used as a pacifier, the child is likely to get the idea that the way to please mommy is to be glued to the screen as often as possible.

Rashes

Rashes of one kind of another are among the most common occurrences of childhood. Whether it's the discomfort of diaper rash soon after birth, the childhood markings of chicken pox, or a case of poison ivy, most skin eruptions aren't too serious and are usually of brief duration.

THE FIRST SIX MONTHS: Skin rashes are especially common during the first six months. They may be due to overheating or overdressing, or to the use of detergents, powders, perfumes, and oils which cause *contact dermatitis*. In addition, certain foods may make the baby break out in facial rashes. Prolonged contact with wet diapers causes *diaper rash*, from the ammonia produced by urine.

Skin rashes can usually be prevented or controlled by:
- Control of temperature
- Proper clothing
- Avoidance of irritating perfumes, powders, and detergents in laundering baby clothes
- Avoidance, in certain circumstances, of milk or other foods, as suggested by your physician
- Avoidance of rubber pants over diapers
- Applications of ointments to rashy areas.

If a disturbing skin condition persists or gets worse, your physician will check for special infections like impetigo or fungus, and, should they exist, recommend proper treatment. During the early years, most children develop the characteristic rashes of the contagious childhood diseases, and at these times, a doctor's care is usually essential for the prevention of complications.

ECZEMA: Some children suffer from intermittent eczema which has a tendency to run in families. Eczema can be extremely uncomfortable, because the more it itches, the more it is scratched, and the more it's scratched, the more it itches. This cycle may be triggered by an allergy to a particular food or pollen; it may be a contact dermatitis caused by a particular fabric, or it might flare up because of emotional tension created by family arguments or anxiety about schoolwork. Eczema should be treated by the family doctor who may be able to discover its source and prevent further attacks.

OTHER ALLERGIC RASHES: Other

rashes that are essentially allergic in origin are those resulting from contact with poison ivy, oak, or sumac. For information about these and other skin conditions, including hives, see *Disorders of the Skin*, p. 245.

The discomfort of many rashes can be eased by ointments or salves. Plain cornstarch is helpful for prickly heat. Rashes that are bacterial in origin, such as impetigo, or parasitic, have to be treated by a doctor with antibiotic or fungicidal preparations.

ROSEOLA: Among the more common rashes of early childhood is the one known as *roseola infantum*. It is believed to be caused by a virus. It begins with a high fever that subsides in a few days. There are no other specific signs of illness, and the end of the disorder—when the fever is usually gone—is signaled by the appearance of a body rash of red spots that disappear overnight. The one aspect of roseola that requires medical attention is the fever. Since high temperature can produce convulsions in infants and babies, efforts should be made to reduce it by sponging and aspirin. Antibiotics are not indicated unless there's some sign of a secondary infection.

PITYRIASIS ROSEA: A long-lasting rash thought to be viral in origin is *pityriasis rosea*, easily identifiable because the onset of this infection is preceded by one large raised red scaly eruption known as the herald patch. The rash itself appears symmetrically and in clusters on the trunk, arms, and legs, and in some children on the hands and feet as well as the face. Unfortunately, this rash may last for more than a month. There is no treatment for it, and although it leaves without a trace and almost never recurs, it can cause severe itching that should be eased with a salve or ointment. Soap is very irritating and should be avoided.

ROCKY MOUNTAIN SPOTTED FEVER: Among the diseases caused by organisms known as rickettsiae and

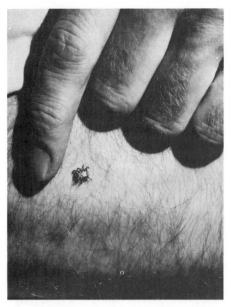
Proper clothing can help to protect children against the bite of this wood tick which causes Rocky Mountain spotted fever.

transmitted to people by the animal ticks that are infected with them is *Rocky Mountain spotted fever,* also called *tick fever.* In addition to rising temperature, headache, nausea, and malaise, this disease produces a characteristic rash that starts on the ankles, lower legs, and wrists, and then spreads to the rest of the body. Children who wander about in the woods during the summer or whose pets run loose in tick-infested areas should be watched for the presence of a tick on the skin and the ensuing rash. Rocky Mountain spotted fever is a serious disease against which youngsters should be protected by wearing the proper clothing.

Reading

Children who see their parents reading or who've heard an older sibling say, "Don't interrupt me when I'm reading" are much more likely to want to learn how to read than those who have never seen an older person absorbed in a book or magazine.

READING DIFFICULTIES: No matter how much the world changes, the child who can't read easily is handicapped. Where a true reading problem exists, parents should confer with the school about a practical solution. If a learning disability appears to be the explanation, tutoring or a special class may be essential. (See DYSLEXIA.)

READING FOR INFORMATION: Many youngsters who don't see the point in reading for pleasure when there are so many other things they'd prefer to do may dash off to the library if they want information about horses or sailing ships or sewing. Families who would like their youngsters to read more than they do have the responsibility of providing a quiet corner, a decent reading light, and an occasional hour of uninterrupted leisure and privacy. Parents who object to their ten-year-old daughter's habit of "always having her nose in a book" instead of "getting some fresh air and exercise" should withhold their criticism unless the doctor recommends a change in the child's activities.

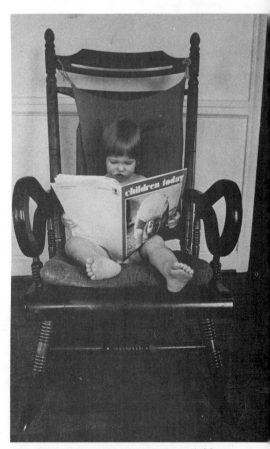
If reading matter of high interest to children is available, children will be highly motivated to learn to read.

Responsibility

Most young children enjoy being given responsibilities suitable to their age and capabilities because it makes them feel grown up. Too few responsibilities and they think they're being treated like babies; too many, and they're likely to look for ways of shirking them.

The style and tone with which responsibilities are assigned have a lot to do with how cheerfully they're executed. A three-year-old can be assigned the responsibility of putting his toys away; a four-year-old can be trusted to help clear the table after dinner, and a five-year-old can be allowed to help with the new baby. Parents can provide a good example by shouldering their own responsibilities cheerfully. See also INDEPENDENCE.

Retardation

See MENTAL RETARDATION.

Rheumatic fever

Once called growing pains, rheumatic fever is actually a disease of the connective tissues, a secondary manifestation of a primary infection by streptococcus bacteria of the throat or tonsils. Its chief symptoms are pains and tenderness in the joints and sore throat.

Rheumatic fever may be mild enough to escape attention or it may be disabling for a period of months. The insidious aspect of the disease is that it may damage the child's heart in such a way that tissue is permanently scarred and function is impaired in the form of a heart murmur. Acuteness of symptoms varies. Any time from a week to a month after the occurrence of a strep throat, the child may complain of feeling tired and achy. Fever usually accompanies the fatigue, and pains in the joints may precede swelling and the development of nodules under the skin in the areas of the wrists, elbows, knees, and vertebrae. The doctor can usually detect an abnormal heart finding. The sooner treatment begins, however, the less likely the risk of permanent heart damage.

Close supervision of the affected child may be essential over a long period. Antibiotics, aspirin, hormones (cortisone), and other medicines control the course of the disease and protect the child from its potentially disabling effects. See also *Rheumatic Fever and Rheumatic Heart Disease* p. 368.

Roseola infantum

See under RASHES.

Rubella (German measles)

Rubella once used to be thought of as a benign disease. Then it was discovered that it could have serious consequences if it were contracted by a woman during the first three months of her pregnancy. The virus that causes rubella is transmitted from the infected woman to her unborn baby, and has been linked to birth defects of the heart, eye, ear, and liver, and to mental retardation.

In addition, a baby who has been exposed to the disease in utero may infect others even though he himself is not affected by it and shows no symptoms. (In fact, most babies are immune to rubella during their first year.) The rubella virus is highly contagious and spreads rapidly.

The incubation period for rubella is two to three weeks. Symptoms include earache, swollen glands be-

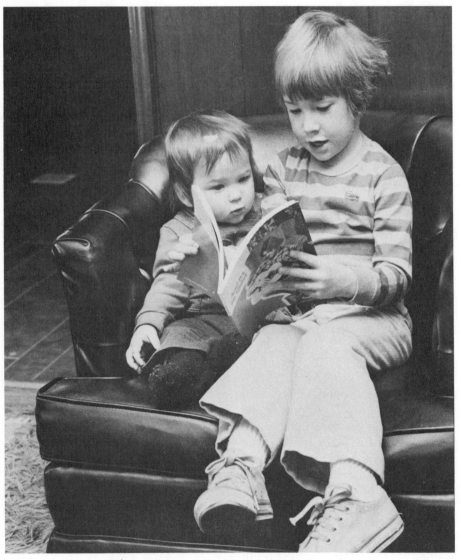

Helping one's parents by taking care of a baby brother or sister can be a proud responsibility for the older child.

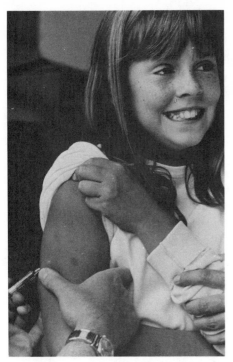

Vaccine for rubella will protect this girl from contracting it in child-bearing years and prevent its spread to pregnant women.

hind the ears, a low-grade fever, and a usually mild, blotchy rash which erupts over the body but lasts only a few days.

Most children are only mildly affected by rubella and require little treatment except rest. However, a pregnant woman who comes in contact with the child can contract it. It is, therefore, of great importance that all children over one year of age be immunized with the vaccine that prevents rubella. Any woman of childbearing age who might be pregnant should *not* be given the vaccine, since the effects of the vaccine on an unborn fetus are not known.

Scarlet fever

Scarlet fever used to be a disease which everyone dreaded. It is highly contagious, and can result in severe aftereffects like rheumatic fever, or the kidney disease known as nephritis.

It is now known that scarlet fever is simply a streptococcal infection —a strain of a specific organism that also causes a diffuse red rash. It can be dealt with quite simply by your physician, the usual treatment being a ten-day course of penicillin, which cures the streptococcal infection and prevents most complications.

Schizophrenia

See under MENTAL ILLNESS.

School

In the United States, an elementary school is a place where children are taught not only how to read, write, handle numbers, and correlate sets of facts; they are also taught how to get along with children different from themselves, how to express themselves creatively, and how to become responsible citizens of a democratic society. If the reality of education falls short of these goals, parents are supposed to exert influence on the proper authorities to see that they are in fact accomplished.

NURSERY SCHOOL: For a child, leaving the protection of the family if only for a half-day in a nearby nursery school is a big step forward. The step is likely to be taken with eagerness if parents present the school as a pleasurable place to be, and not as a dumping ground for a youngster who's in the way of a new baby or a working mother.

ELEMENTARY SCHOOL: The elementary grades represent a major change in many different ways, but most importantly because new authority figures begin to displace parents as the source of all wisdom. Adults and older siblings can help a child make a happy and productive adjustment to school by talking about it with interest and respect. Wherever possible, one or another parent should be present at parent-teacher meetings and participate in the activities of the child's group, such as class trips, visiting days, and the like.

HOMEWORK: When youngsters come home with school assignments that they find baffling, parents should feel free to ask the teacher for clearer instructions. If the child is at fault through inattention or ignorance, it might be pointed out to her that whether or not she gets a good education depends on how hard she's ready to work and not how efficiently the teacher can spoon-feed her.

PRIVATE SCHOOLS: Some families feel that the local public school is not the best place for their children to learn during the lower grades. Alternative private schools, whether denominational, discriminatory, or for gifted children, may have advantages that are less apparent to the

Going to school brings about many changes for a child. One of them is the necessity of dealing with new authority figures—teachers.

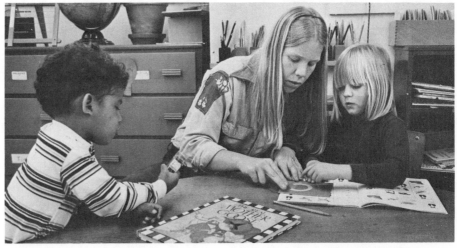

child than to the parents, especially if attendance isolates the youngster from her friends in the neighborhood.

STAYING HOME FROM SCHOOL: It's not unusual for a child to avoid going to school once in a while by saying she's sick. She may actually need a rest from the routine every few months. This is quite different from truly getting sick at the thought of facing school. A child who is nauseated in the morning, or who throws up, or who has a bellyache at breakfast, is probably experiencing feelings of anger, resentment, or anxiety beyond her ability to cope with them. Whatever it is in the school situation that's worrying her, she should be given the opportunity to talk about what's going on and the reassurance that efforts will be made to help straighten things out.

For children with disabilities, special facilities are often provided within the structure of the local school so that they can spend at least part of their day with their own age group.

Sex education

Children need and deserve to have access to correct information about sexual functioning. If there is a natural openness in a family about questions of all types, children first start asking questions about sex when they are three or four; it is then that parents can begin describing sexual functioning to their children.

QUESTIONS ABOUT BODY PARTS: The first questions about sex usually have to do with the functioning of body parts. For example, children want to know where urine comes from, what happens to food when they eat it, where feces come from, and where babies come from. Explanations should be given in a straightforward, unembarrassed manner. Children should not be overloaded with information that they do not understand, but parents should be willing to answer questions to the best of their ability.

With older children, particularly 11- and 12-year-olds, it is often helpful for sexual questions to be answered by the parent of the same sex. Reading a book on sexual development together with the child can be a good experience for both parent and child. Parents frequently wonder if sex education may not lead children to engage in experimentation. Most of the evidence on this question indicates that children are more likely to experiment sexually when they are ignorant than when their questions about sex are reasonably and accurately answered.

Sibling rivalry

See ABILITIES AND APTITUDES, BROTHERS AND SISTERS, NEW BABY.

Sickle-cell anemia

See p. 352.

Sisters and brothers

See BROTHERS AND SISTERS.

Sleep

See BEDTIME, DREAMS AND NIGHTMARES, SLEEPWALKING.

Sleepwalking

Sleepwalking may be distressing to the parent who witnesses it, but it usually does the child no harm. If the child seems to be about to do something dangerous, it's a good idea to wake her up with a few reassuring remarks and guide her back to bed. In most sleepwalking incidents, the child goes back to bed by herself and gets up the next day without the slightest recollection of her nighttime prowl. Parents shouldn't tease or scold or make the child feel peculiar about walking in her sleep. It can be ignored unless it continues over a long period, and then it might be mentioned to the doctor.

Smallpox

Smallpox has been eradicated everywhere in the world except for a very few places, such as Somalia, in east Africa, where the disease persists. Vaccination against small-pox has therefore been discontinued in the United States.

Smoking

Young children who see older children in the family or at home smoking cigarettes are going to equate smoking with being grown up even if their parents don't smoke. A ten-year-old who sneaks off to experiment with a cigarette shouldn't be treated like a criminal, but he should be told that he is harming himself. Parents who smoke and wish they didn't should concentrate on their own efforts to stop and hope that their offspring get the message. In any event, it might help to emphasize how hard it is to stop smoking once one has acquired the habit.

Sore throat

"It hurts when I swallow" is a common complaint of childhood. It may be connected with a cold or tonsillitis, but if there is tenderness at the sides of the neck and a rise in temperature, the doctor should be called promptly so that tests can be made to see whether the child has a strep throat. Often a throat culture is necessary. A steptococcus throat infection that is undiagnosed and untreated can have serious consequences. See also TONSILLITIS.

Speech defects

Among the more common speech defects are *lisping* (the substitution of *th* for *s* and *z* sounds); *lallation* (the inability to pronounce *l* or *r* correctly), and stuttering. Although many children do outgrow their speech disabilities, a considerable number do not. There are about 2 million adult stutterers in the United States.

THERAPY: Corrective therapy should be undertaken without too much delay. In the case of stuttering, it is generally agreed that psychological factors play a considerable role in creating and perpetuating the problem. When professional efforts are made to correct it, they almost always involve some family therapy sessions. There have been many advances in the techniques used by speech pathologists, including the audio-visual devices and feed-back systems that promote self-correction. A list of certified speech pathologists can be obtained from the American Speech and Hearing Association, 9030 Old Georgetown Road, Washington D.C. 20014.

Stealing

See DISHONESTY.

Stepchildren

See p. 169. See also ADOPTED CHILDREN.

Stomach ache

A wide variety of disorders begins with some kind of abdominal pain, but in most cases, a stomach ache is temporary and unaccompanied by any other symptoms. Digestive upsets are frequent in infancy, becoming rarer as the baby approaches the fourth month. See COLIC.

After the baby's first year, a stomach ache may signal the onset of a cold or some other infection. The doctor should be called if any of the following conditions occurs.

• When the stomach pain is accompanied by fever, vomiting, or diarrhea

• If moderate pain lasts for a considerable time—several hours, for example

• If the pain is obviously acute—the child is doubled over

• If the location of the pain shifts from one place to another.

Never give a child a laxative or an enema except on the doctor's orders.

A youngster who complains regularly of stomach aches without any other symptoms, and who might also complain of headaches or constipation shouldn't be dismissed as a worrier. The problem should be discussed with the doctor so that an investigation can be made of possible causes. In many cases, constipation is the source of stomach pain. When the constipation is cleared up, the stomach pains cease.

Stomach pain may also be of psychosomatic origin, in children as well as in adults. If the pain cannot be explained after a physical examination and tests have been made, parents should consider how they can lighten some of the stresses and tensions in the child's life.

Strabismus

See CROSSED EYES.

Stuttering

See SPEECH DEFECTS.

Sudden infant death syndrome

Sudden Infant Death Syndrome, sometimes referred to as SIDS and generally known as *crib death,* claims about 10,000 babies every year. It is the chief single cause of fatalities in infants, usually occurring between the ages of one month and six months. Although there are a number of plausible theories being investigated, its cause remains unknown. In some cases, autopsies indicate a hidden infection or an unsuspected abnormality, but in 80% of the deaths, no obvious explanation can be found. One cause appears to be an inherited heart irregularity, and another is respiratory distress, discussed under HYALINE MEMBRANE DISEASE. Improved hospital facilities for the care of premature babies who are considered to be at higher risk than those born at full term, as well as prenatal tests and ultrasonic alarm systems that monitor breathing are expected to reduce the number of SIDS victims.

Parents of infant SIDS victims often suffer intensely, apart from their natural grief, from feelings of guilt, as if they were somehow careless or negligent. They must be reassured that they could not possibly have foreseen the susceptibility of their child to this affliction and that there is therefore no way they could have averted its tragic result. They will have suffered enough without the wholly unwarranted feeling that they were somehow responsible.

Swallowed objects

Babies in a crib or playpen can certainly be depended on to put anything within reach into their mouths, so it's a good idea to make sure that surfaces are cleared of anything that would cause a crisis if it were swallowed. Plastic toys and rattles should be inspected for loose parts. Pins, buttons, and small change should be kept in drawers. It's no serious matter if a child swallows a cherry stone or a plum pit or a small button, since these are not likely to cause problems in their passage through the digestive system. They will be disposed of in regular bowel movements.

EMERGENCIES: Emergencies occur when the object is stuck in the windpipe or when it goes into the bronchial passage. If it is in the windpipe and isn't coughed up right away, use the first aid maneuver for *Obstruction in the Windpipe,* p. 577, without delay. If it doesn't work the first time, do it again—

Small objects that can be swallowed should be placed out of baby's reach—even if that means she chews on her hand or foot instead.

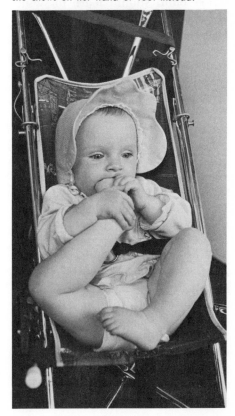

and again. You must clear the windpipe. If all efforts fail, rush the child to a hospital.

Swearing

Sooner or later most children learn swearwords, either from hearing their parents use them or from their peers. Young children may use curse words without knowing what they mean or without appreciating how offensive they may be.

Nowadays it is virtually impossible for children to avoid hearing words in everyday use that were strictly taboo when their parents were growing up. However jolting it may be to hear foul words issuing from their angelic-looking children, parents should be neither surprised nor unduly upset if this happens occasionally, especially if they themselves use curse words. They might well point out to the child, however, that many people object strongly to such language, and if they want to be treated courteously by adults, they had better watch their language.

Swimming

Every child should learn to swim, and the earlier the better. Families fortunate enough to have their own large pools can accomplish this in their own back yards; others may spend summers near a suitable body of water.

Although there's nothing like the ocean for water play, it's not a good place to try to teach a small child how to swim. There are too many extraneous hazards, such as undertow, waves, and unexpected depths. Many communities have outdoor public pools; most large cities have indoor and outdoor pools where professional instruction is available. Even when a child can swim moderately well, it's not advisable to allow her to do so alone, and she shouldn't be allowed to go out in a boat by herself either. Rubber floats, rafts, and the like shouldn't be made available to youngsters until they can swim. A nonswimmer depending on such a device is in trouble if it should drift away from her in deep water.

Talking

The ability to speak is part of the human heritage. How soon and how clearly a child begins to do so depends on several factors. First and foremost is the ability to hear.

HEARING AND SPEECH: Any illness or infection in infancy that has caused even a small hearing loss will interfere with the baby's perception of sounds. This in turn will prevent the normal development of those parts of the brain that govern the imitative aspect of speech.

A STIMULATING ENVIRONMENT: How much attention and stimulation the baby gets from his environment and the people around him will have a great effect on how much he tries to say and the age at which he begins to say it. Being listened to and automatically corrected instead of being ignored or teased is the indispensable feedback process that enriches the learning of language. The clarity of the child's speech depends to a large extent on the examples before him; what his ears hear his brain will order his vocal equipment to imitate. Parents who want a child to outgrow baby talk should avoid responding to the baby in kind. Normal adult speech should become the norm toward which the child is constantly striving. See also HEARING, SPEECH DEFECTS, SWEARING.

Tantrums

See ANGER, FRUSTRATION.

Teething

Babies of four to six months drool a great deal and put their fingers in their mouth. These habits, and the telltale small bumps you may detect on the baby's gums, are the signs of teething. But they don't necessarily mean that the first tooth is about to erupt. That may not happen until he is nearly one year old, although it usually happens earlier.

Teething may or may not be painful. If the baby does fret, medication is available to alleviate the pain. (A little whisky rubbed on the gums is a home remedy that often helps.)

Television

See RADIO, RECORD PLAYER, AND TV.

Tetanus

Tetanus (also called *lockjaw* because it causes spasms of the jaw) can occur at any age as the result of contamination of a simple wound. The causative organism is usually found in soil, street dust, or feces.

The disease is preventable by immunization. The triple vaccine DPT should be started at two to three months of age. See the chart on p. 89.

When a child suffers a puncture wound, dog bite, or other wound that may be contaminated, ask your doctor to give the child a booster dose of tetanus toxoid if she has not had a shot within one year.

Tick fever

See ROCKY MOUNTAIN SPOTTED FEVER under RASHES.

Toilet training

It is during the toddler stage that you will begin to teach your child how to control his bowel and urinary functions.

WHEN TO START: A simple question parents always ask is, "How do I know when my child is ready to be toilet trained?"

Generally, children do not have muscular control over their bowel movements and urination until about the age of two, so attempting to toilet-train a child much before this is usually wasted effort. If it is accomplished, the result is usually a training of the parents rather than of the infant. Toilet training should usually take place some time between the age of two and three and one-half.

A child is emotionally ready when he understands what is meant by toilet training and is willing to perform toilet functions without expressing fear of them. This may occur at any age, but is perhaps most apt to start between the ages of 18 and 24 months. With a first child it is usually later than with a second or third child, because the first child has no siblings to emulate. But a first child should be trained, usually, by the time he is three. Training the child to stay dry through the long night hours may take even longer.

RESISTANCE TO TOILET TRAINING: Early toilet training—training that is begun during a child's first year—may work, but as a child develops and asserts his personality and independence, he will resent any insistence on manipulating the control of his bodily functions. He may get even by refusing to empty his bowels when put on the potty. Worse yet, if another baby has entered the scene, the early-trained child may develop constipation, or may revert to wetting and having bowel movements in his training pants.

When you feel the child is ready for training, establish the fact that

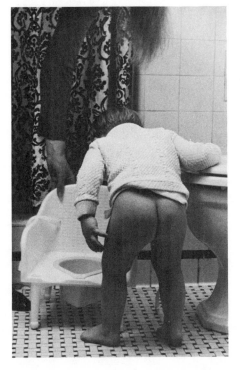

Praise should be used instead of blame while a child is being toilet trained. Strict punishment will only delay training and may cause future emotional problems.

going to the bathroom is a normal part of daily life. If the child expresses fear, don't struggle with him. Don't fight about it. Take him right off the potty and let him know that you are not concerned or displeased. A genuine complication can arise if the child connects his fear of toilet functions with your displeasure at his failures.

Training can usually be facilitated by praise from the parents for putting the bowel movement and the urine in the proper place, rather than by punishment. Excessive punishment or the threat of it usually results in anger on the child's part and increasing stubbornness and resistances to toilet training. Praise immediately following the proper performance of the act is far more effective in encouraging compliance with the parents' goals.

Tonsillectomy

See *Tonsils and Adenoids*, p. 330.

Tonsillitis

The tonsils are two masses of soft spongy tissue that are partly embedded in the mucous membrane of the back of the throat. Bacterial or viral infection of this tissue is known as tonsillitis. It used to be considered advisable to remove the tonsils if they became enlarged— which they normally do in the process of filtering out mild infections.

Nowadays, an occasional bout of tonsillitis isn't considered sufficient reason for surgical removal of the tonsils, especially since they're likely to be less prone to infection as the child gets older. However, even a mild case of tonsillitis should be called to a doctor's attention. Acute symptoms such as swollen tonsils, sudden high fever, swollen neck glands, and severe pain when swallowing must be treated promptly since they might be an indication of a strep throat. The proper antibiotics are always effective in controlling this infection so that it doesn't turn into rheumatic fever or involve the kidneys. Tonsillitis caused by a virus usually responds to aspirin,

bed rest, and a soft diet. See also ADENOIDS. For a description of tonsillectomy, see *Tonsils and Adenoids*, p. 330.

Toys

Grandma is put out because the beautiful doll she brought to her 2-year-old granddaughter has been promptly discarded in favor of the parts of the percolator. Those parts are something to put together and separate; they have interesting shapes; they clink when they touch and make a nice sound. That's what toys are about, especially to younger children. In selecting them, look for sturdiness and versatility. Smoothly sanded wooden blocks are wonderful toys that stimulate the imagination, encourage putting things together creatively, and can last not only from older to younger child but from one generation to another.

SIMPLICITY AND SUITABILITY: Suitability of a toy is important: the right object for the age and circumstance. A good strong pail and shovel and a few cookie molds taken to the beach make more sense than a complicated plastic toy with parts that will get lost in the sand. Water toys that float in the tub make the bath that much more interesting and less threatening to very little children.

USE YOUR IMAGINATION: Where there's not much money available for spending on playthings, the results can be more satisfactory to the child if you use your imagination—you can be sure she'll use hers. Pots and pans are great toys for toddlers, especially if there's a collection of smaller items, such as lids and little plastic containers to go with them. A roasting pan with a cord tied to the handle at one end becomes a sturdy pull-toy.

Never throw anything away until you've considered its adaptability as a toy: empty spools of thread, large buttons, plastic juice containers or milk cartons with the tops cut off, bits of twine, and especially the corrugated cardboard cartons that groceries are delivered in. As children get older, toys can be con-

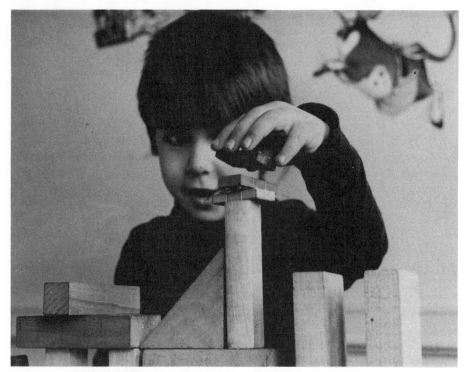

Wooden blocks make wonderful toys. They encourage creativity, and they're sturdy enough to provide enjoyment for many more than one child.

structed of odds and ends according to instruction books available in the local library. The communal effort of putting them together can be a special rainy-day activity.

Tuberculosis

See *Tuberculosis*, p. 390.

Twins and triplets

Multiple births may be *identical*— that is, the result of the splitting of a single egg fertilized by a single sperm— or they may be *fraternal*, which means that they developed from different eggs fertilized by different sperm. Most multiple births are fraternal; except for their birthdays, most twins and triplets are no more alike than other brothers and sisters of the same family.

Although there is no ready explanation for the occurrence of multiple births, the tendency is thought to be genetically determined through the mother. Twins occur about once in every 86 births, triplets once in every 8,000. Multiple births can be anticipated by the doctor at least a month before delivery.

They usually arrive about two weeks early, and if they give any indications of prematurity, they receive special hospital attention.

Typhoid fever

See *Typhoid*, p. 377

Urinary infections

Urinary infections of either viral or bacterial origin are more common among girls than boys, especially during the preschool years. Such an infection is sometimes the explanation for a fever unaccompanied by other symptoms. Any inflammation that creates a burning sensation during urination should be cultured and treated promptly since it can spread from the bladder to the kidneys and create a major problem.

Girls can be spared frequent infection if tactful suggestions are made at an early age about their toilet routines. Since fecal matter is high in bacterial content, little girls should learn to wipe their bottoms from front to back so that there is no possibility of contaminating the urethra after a bowel movement.

Vaporizer

A vaporizer is a device similar to a humidifier that moistens the air with steam and thus alleviates some of the discomfort of respiratory congestion. During the winter months when heated interiors are likely to be especially dry and when colds are more common, children and grownups can benefit from moist air that keeps the throat and nasal and bronchial passages from feeling like sandpaper. Medication shouldn't be added to a vaporizer except at the doctor's recommendation. If the device is used near a child's bed throughout the night, it should be placed on a surface high enough to prevent bumping into it accidentally should the child wake up in the middle of the night to go to the bathroom.

Vomiting

See NAUSEA AND VOMITING.

Warts

See p. 249.

Whooping cough

Whooping cough (also called *pertussis*), like diphtheria a bacterial disease, occurs more frequently than diphtheria because immunity to it wears off, especially in the older child in whom the disease may appear as a severe bronchitis.

Whooping cough can be very serious in young babies because it can cause them to choke and be unable to catch their breath. If your child does contract whooping cough, call your physician immediately. The doctor may give a specific drug against the organism that causes the disease as well as a specific antitoxin against the poison which the bacillus releases.

It is advisable to immunize children against whooping cough as early as possible. The effective triple vaccine known as DPT provides immunization not only against whooping cough, but against diphtheria and tetanus as well.

Worms and parasites

See p. 381.

CHAPTER 3

The Teens

PUBERTY AND GROWTH

The bridge between childhood and adulthood is a period of growth and change called puberty. There seems to be no standard pattern for the physical changes of puberty. Two boys of the same age who have been nearly identical throughout childhood may appear to set off along entirely different paths of physical development as they enter the teenage years. One may quickly shoot up to a height of 5 feet 8 inches within a couple of years while his companion lags for a while at preteen size, then begins growing into a six-footer. One may develop a heavy beard in his early high school years while the other boy will have no use for a razor until he is in college. However, both boys are normal youngsters, and each will eventually attain all of the physical attributes of adulthood.

Similarly, one girl may begin menstruating in her 11th year while a classmate will not experience her first menstruation until she is 16. One girl may need a bra while still in grammar school but her friend will fret about a small bustline for many years. But both girls can look forward to normal womanhood. Each has an individual pattern of development, and if there is any rule of thumb about puberty it is that each youngster has his or her own time schedule for the transformation into a mature man or woman.

Puberty: Changes in Girls

The physical changes that occur in the female body during puberty probably are more dramatic than those associated with a boy progressing into manhood. One definite milestone for the girl is her first *menstruation,* commonly regarded as the first sign of puberty. Actually, the first menstruation, known as the *menarche,* is only one of several signs of puberty, along with the slimming of the waist, gradual broadening of the hips, the development of breasts, the appearance of hair about the genitals and in the armpits, and a change in the rate of growth.

The Menarche

The age at which a girl first experiences menstruation generally varies over a period of ten years and depends upon the structural development of the youngster, her physical condition, the environment, and hereditary factors. Menarche can occur as early as the age of 7, and most doctors would not be overly concerned if a girl did not begin to menstruate until she was approaching 17. The age range of 9 to 16 usually is considered normal. The median age for the start of menstruation is around 13½ years, which means that 50 percent of all females are younger than 13 years and 6 months when they reach the menarche, and half are on the older side of that age when they first menstruate. In general, the pubertal experiences of a girl follow a pattern like that of her mother and sisters; if the mother began menstruating at an early age, the chances are that her daughters will also.

If the girl has not reached the menarche by the age of 18, she should be examined by a *gynecologist,* a doctor who specializes in problems related to the female reproductive system. A medical examination also should be arranged for any girl who experiences menstruation before she reaches the age of 8 or 9 years.

When menarche occurs on the early side of childhood, the condition is sometimes called *precocious puberty.* The child may suddenly begin menstruating before her mother has told her what to expect, a situation which can prove embarrassing to both child and parents. It may first be detected by a teacher at school; occasionally, a young girl may be aware of bleeding from the vagina but because of fear or false modesty does not report the event to her mother or teacher. For this reason, parents should be alert for changes associated with early puberty and be prepared to explain the facts of life to their children. Also, in the case of precocious puberty, parents should arrange for medical consultation to be certain the bleeding actually is the result of first menstruation and not the effects of an injury or tumor.

Growth Spurt Before Menarche

During the year or two preceding the menarche there is a growth spurt of two or three inches. This is because of the hormone changes of puberty. The *hormones* are chemical messengers secreted by glands in various parts of the body and carried rapidly through the bloodstream to organs or other glands where they trigger reactions. The spurt in growth preceding menarche is due to the secretion of a growth hormone which is produced by the pituitary gland, and androgen, a hormone secreted by the adrenal glands. They produce rapid growth of the bones and muscles during puberty. The girl who is first among her classmates to menstruate often is larger than those who are of the same age but have not yet reached the menarche.

From numerous research studies of the menarche, it has been learned that poor nutrition and psychological stress sometimes delay the onset of menstruation, that girls reared in cities tend to menstruate earlier, and that climate is a factor, although both tropical and arctic climates seem to be related to early menarche. The first menstrual periods also are likely to occur during the school year, September to June, rather than during the summer vacation.

The First Menstrual Cycles

The first menstrual cycles tend to be very irregular and have been known to be as short as 7 days and as long as 37 weeks. Even when regularity becomes established, the ado-lescent menstrual cycle usually is longer than the average for adult women. The typical menstrual cycle of a young girl may be about 33 days, compared to an average of 28 days for an adult woman. About three years elapse before the menstrual cycles become regular. In the meantime, irregular menstrual patterns can be considered as normal for girls during puberty.

The first menstrual cycles also are *anovulatory*. In other words, the young girl's ovaries have not matured sufficiently to produce an *ovum,* or egg cell, that can be fertilized by the sperm of a male. There are, of course, the exceptions which make newspaper headlines when a little girl gives birth to a baby. But anovulatory menstruation generally is the rule for the first few months after the menarche.

Delayed Puberty

Delayed puberty probably causes as much anguish as precocious puberty. The last girl in a group of childhood chums to develop breasts and experience the menarche may feel more self-conscious than the first girl in the class to menstruate. If the signs that usually precede menarche have not appeared by the age of 17 or 18, a medical examination should be considered, even though the girl may be a late-late-bloomer at the other end of the spectrum from the 7- or 8-year-old child who has menstruated.

The absence of menstruation after a girl is 18 can be the result of a wide variety of factors. The cause sometimes can be as simple as an *imperforate hymen,* a membrane that blocks the opening of the vagina. It can be the result of a congenital malformation of the reproductive organs, such as imperfect development of the ovaries. Accidents, exposure to carbon monoxide gas, or diseases like rheumatic fever or encephalitis in earlier years can result in brain damage that would inhibit the start of menstruation. The relationship between emotional upset and delayed menarche was vividly demonstrated during World War II when some girls who suffered psychological traumas also experienced very late signs of puberty.

Preparing Your Daughter for Menstruation

A mother's main responsibility is to convince her daughter at the beginning of puberty that menstruation is a perfectly normal body function. The mother should explain the proper use of sanitary napkins or tampons and encourage her daughter to keep records of her menstrual periods on a calendar.

The mother also should explain that menstruation usually is not a valid reason to stay in bed or avoid school or work. The girl should be advised that bathing and swimming should not be postponed because of menstruation. There are many old wives' tales about menstruation which are not true. But there may be some truth to stories that loss of menstrual blood can be weakening, particularly if the girl's diet does not replace the body stores of iron which may be lowered during menstrual flow. Iron is a key element of the red blood cell, and if iron-rich foods are not included in the meals of women during their years of menstruation they can eventually suffer a form of iron-deficiency anemia.

Hormone Activity: Becoming a Woman

Although the sex hormones are the key to what makes girls grow into women and boys into men, both sexes appear to receive secretions of male and female sex hormones in approximately equal amounts for about the first ten years of life. But as puberty approaches, the adrenal glands of girls seem to increase production of a female sex hormone, *estrogen.* Meanwhile, a nerve center in the hypothalamus area of the brain stimulates the pituitary gland, the master gland of the body, to secrete another kind of hormone, *gonadotropin.* Gonadotropin in turn activates a *follicle-stimulating hormone* which causes a maturation of the ovaries, which are part of the original equipment girls are born with but which remain dormant until the start of puberty.

During the second decade of life, the hormone activity stimulates the development of body tissues which not only grow in size but give a girl more womanly contours. However, the fully mature contours of a woman usually do not appear until after the ovaries are functioning and still another female sex hormone, *progesterone*, has been introduced in the system. The ovaries, uterus, Fallopian tubes, and vagina gradually mature as the menarche draws near.

Puberty: Changes in Boys

The appearance of male sexual characteristics during puberty is also influenced by hormonal changes. But the manifestation of male puberty is somewhat more subtle. The pituitary gland in a boy also secretes a gonadotropic hormone which stimulates maturation of *gonads*. In the male, the gonads are the *testicles*, the source of *sperm*. But whereas maturation of the ovaries in females leads to the menarche, there is no obvious sign in the boy that *spermatozoa* are being produced.

However, the secondary sexual characteristics, such as the growth of a beard and pubic hair, the spurt of growth of bones and muscles, the increase in size of the sex organs, and the deepening of the voice are all indications of puberty. The changes in a boy's characteristics during puberty are usually spread over a period of two years, beginning with an increase in the size of the penis and testicles and reaching completion with the production of spermatozoa in the testicles. During the two-year period there usually is a noticeable increase in the chest size of a boy, with the broad shoulders of manhood appearing during the peak of bone and muscle growth. Generally, the appearance

of pubic and facial hair, as well as hair in the armpits, follows the growth of the shoulder and chest area and precedes the change in voice.

THE TESTICLES: The testicles are contained in a walnut-size sac of skin called the *scrotum*. It is held outside the body by a design of nature in order to maintain a temperature for spermatozoa production which is less than internal body temperature. Muscle fibers in the scrotum hold the testicles closer to the body for warmth in cold weather and relax to allow the sperm-producing organ to be farther away from the body when surrounding temperatures are warm.

As the young man passes through puberty, he should be advised that tight clothing which holds the scrotum close to the body can result in sterility because of degeneration of the sperm-developing tubules from body heat. In some cases, the testicles do not descend from the abdomen during development of the male child. The result is the same as that of wearing clothing that holds the scrotum against the body; the boy will be sterile. Other variations are the descent of one testis while the other is retained in the abdomen; or they may descend only as far as the *inguinal* area, at the junction of the thigh and the lower part of the abdomen.

Although undescended testicles usually do not cause any medical problems other than sterility, the danger of malignant change may be sufficient to warrant surgical correction of this disorder. If the testicles become trapped in the inguinal region, they may become inflamed because of the pressure of larger body parts in that area. In many cases, however, the testes descend spontaneously during the second decade of life after being trapped in the abdomen during the early years. Doctors frequently are able to assist the descent by administration of hormones as well as by surgery. At some point during puberty, a medical examination should include the

condition of the testicles.

GENITAL SIZE: Many boys are as sensitive about the size of their genitals as girls are about breast size. In the case of an empty scrotum because of undescended testicles, it is possible to have the scrotum injected with silicone plastic for cosmetic or psychological reasons so the sac appears less flaccid or larger. The size of the penis may become the subject of discussion in the school shower room. If a boy appears sensitive about the subject, he should be assured that there is a wide variation in normal sizes and that like ears, noses, and other body parts the dimensions have little to do with function.

NOCTURNAL EMISSION: Another cause for concern by adolescent boys is the *nocturnal emission*. The nocturnal emission, sometimes called a *wet dream*, is the automatic expulsion of *semen* through the penis while the young man is asleep. The semen is secreted by the *prostate gland*, the *seminal vesicle*, and other glands which open into the *urethra*. The opalescent white fluid carries spermatozoa during intercourse and if the young male does not engage in sexual intercourse or does not masturbate, the semen simply accumulates until it overflows during a nocturnal emission. It is a harmless, normal occurrence.

Bone Growth

As the growth spurt subsides in the late teens, the *cartilage plates*, or *epiphyses*, in the long bones of the body close. Until the growth plates become filled in with calcium deposits, each long bone is in effect three bones—a central shaft separated from the ends by the cartilage growth plates. The growth plates are not completely replaced by bone until a female is about 20 and a male 23 years old. But the rate of growth begins to taper off as sexual maturity is achieved. After that, young women tend to retain fatty tissue and young men gain in mus-

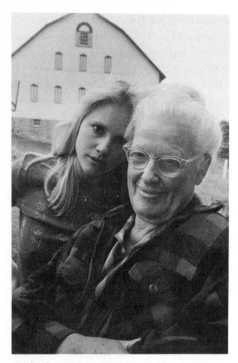

Each of us inherits physical traits from our ancestors, because of various combinations of chromosomes and genes. This girl inherited her facial shape from her grandmother.

cle mass. It is a time to begin weight watching so that the hazards of obese adult life can be avoided. But the ravenous appetites developed during the period of rapid body growth and intense physical activity can easily evolve into bad eating habits during the teen years.

Skin and Hair Problems

Hereditary influences may determine many of the physical and psychological traits that an individual first becomes aware of in the teen years. Because of the various crossovers of the 23 sets of *chromosomes* and the nearly infinite combinations of *genes,* it is not always easy to predict how a child is going to appear as a young adult. But some features, such as hair color and eye color, usually can be identified with one or both parents; other traits may seem to be those of uncles, aunts, or grandparents. Heredity and hormones frequently are involved in the distribution of hair on the body and the oiliness of the skin, both of which can cause concern to teen-

agers who are plagued by an overabundance or lack of these cosmetic traits. An example of hereditary influences on hair patterns can be seen in early baldness. A receding hairline is not a trait of the parents but rather an influence of the genetic makeup of a grandparent—the trait skips a generation.

Removal of Excess Hair

While not much can be done about baldness that is hereditary, there are ways of handling the problems of excess hair. If a woman has excess hair on her face, arms, and legs, it can be removed by shaving, with wax, by electrolysis, or depilatories. Shaving is the most direct but not always the most satisfactory method of hair removal, since it is intended only as a temporary measure. An alternate shortcut is bleaching with diluted hydrogen peroxide; the hair is still there but it is not as noticeable. Another method involves the use of hot wax spread on the skin and allowed to harden. When it is removed quickly, the hair is pulled away.

Depilatories are chemicals that destroy the hair at the skin line. Both hot wax and depilatories have longer-lasting effects than shaving, but they must be repeated at intervals of several weeks.

Depilatories, too, can produce unpleasant allergenic reactions. The only permanent method of removing excess hair is *electrolysis,* which is a time-consuming technique. Each hair root has to be burned out individually with an electric current. Electrolysis is recommended only for small areas and because of the time and expense involved would not be feasible for removing excess hair from regions other than the face.

Acne

There is some evidence that *acne* is partly hereditary. But it is such a common problem among teenagers—it has been estimated that up to 90 percent of all youngsters endure some degree of acne—that

it must have been inherited from a mutual ancestor like Adam or Eve. In fact, one of the deterrents to effective control of the skin disorder is that acne is so common that it is neglected by many youngsters. Waiting to outgrow acne can be a serious mistake, because the pimples, blemishes, blackheads, and boils that make life miserable for so many teen-agers can be eliminated or considerably reduced. They can also cause scarring. A doctor should be consulted in cases of severe or especially persistent acne.

OVERACTIVE OIL GLANDS: Acne is not a serious threat to the life of a youngster, but it can be seriously disfiguring at a time of life when most young people are sensitive about their appearance. It can occur at any time from puberty into early adulthood, and it is caused by poor adjustment of the skin to secretions of sebaceous glands. The imbalance resulting from hormones in the bloodstream will correct itself eventually. But to prevent permanent scarring, a program of simple skin care must be followed faithfully.

Acne is caused by oil glands in the skin that become overly active at puberty. The glands become clogged, with the result that blackheads or pimples appear. The solution is to wash the skin frequently and thoroughly to remove the oils and to clear the plugged oil glands. The color of blackheads, by the way, is not caused by dirt but rather by a chemical change in the secretions of the oil glands.

SKIN CARE: The face should be washed several times a day with hot water and soap. The skin should be rinsed twice after washing, first with warm water, then with cold. Each time the face should be dried thoroughly with a clean towel. At bedtime, the face should be given a massage with soapsuds and water, rinsed, and patted dry with a clean towel. Any medication prescribed by the doctor should be applied after the final washing of the day. Careless handling of blemishes, such as squeezing blackheads or picking pimples, can result in scarring. Teen-agers also should avoid such habits as supporting the face with the hands or unconsciously rubbing the face.

OTHER PRECAUTIONS: Young women should not use cold creams or cosmetics unless they have been approved by a physician. Young men who shave must be careful to avoid cutting pimples. The doctor also should be consulted about how diet can help control acne. Although the skin disorder is not a dietary disease, there is some evidence that certain foods tend to aggravate it. However, there is a lack of agreement among doctors as to whether chocolate, carbonated beverages, nuts, sweets, and other specific snack items may be the culprits. And there always is the possibility that since each youngster develops along an individual path, a food item that causes one teen-ager's face to break out with blemishes will not affect a sibling or classmate in the same way.

Diet

A survey by the Food and Nutrition Board of the National Research Council recently showed that 40 percent of boys between 13 and 19 years of age and 60 percent of the girls in the same age group subsisted on diets that were substandard. Generally, the young people surveyed had abandoned the eating routines of their families. They habitually skipped breakfast and failed to make up the nutritional loss during other meals.

Perhaps in rebellion against parental control and to assert their independence, they tended to gather with their friends at candy stores and snack shops. They purchased items that could be held in the hand during informal rap sessions— chocolate bars and cans of soda. The economic standards for the quickie street-corner meals were based on what could be obtained with money from allowances and after-school jobs. The snack habit persisted through the potato chip and carbonated beverage evening routine before a TV set. Their idea of a good meal included a side dish of French fries, a food lacking in almost everything except calories.

Calories and Nutrition

Calories are not all bad. Young people burn hundreds of them daily through dancing, working, athletic competition, and other activities. A typical male teen-ager may burn up to 3,600 calories a day; a teen-age girl can easily handle 2,500 calories daily—and calories are easy to come by in snack foods. For example, a chocolate milk shake at 520 calories, two doughnuts, totaling 270 calories, a chocolate candy bar at 150 calories, a can of soda at 100 calories, and a handful of potato chips at 10 calories each will easily provide half the daily energy requirements for a busy high school girl. Adding French fries, at 15 calories each, and more cans of soda plus other snacks will bring the total up close to the 2,500-calorie level.

However, there is more to nutrition than snacking on calorie-rich foods. An individual obviously can fill up on high-energy goodies but suffer from malnutrition by disregarding the body's normal requirements of proteins, vitamins, and minerals. Also, calories have an insidious way of becoming excess weight. A calorie is a unit of energy, and the human body requires a certain amount of energy each day in order to sustain life and permit the muscle activity of work or play. To maintain the proper balance between foods consumed and energy used in work and play, the teen-ager, like the adult, must estimate the calories in his meals and check the results regularly by stepping on the bathroom scale.

People in their teens should develop the habit of weighing themselves at least once a week, recording the weight so it can be compared with previous readings. The weight check should occur at the same hour each time, and the same scale should be used. Also, the same

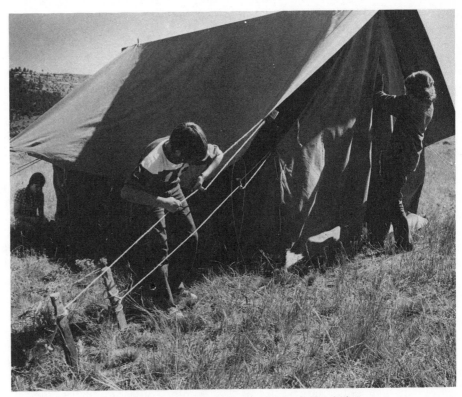

Teen-agers can burn up thousands of calories daily in vigorous outdoor activities such as camping and hiking.

type of clothing should be worn each time the weight is checked. If an overweight or underweight youngster can find a companion to challenge in a race toward optimum weight, the competition will be an added inducement.

CALCIUM AND PHOSPHORUS: Among the important minerals in teen-age diets are calcium and phosphorus. Milk is the most easily available source of calcium and phosphorus, which are required for the development of strong bones during the period of life in which the body is still growing. Calcium also is required for the effective contraction of muscle tissues and is vital for normal heart function. The recommended daily intake of milk for teen-agers is four eight-ounce glasses. It can be served as fluid whole milk, as skim milk, buttermilk, evaporated milk, or as nonfat dry milk. Cheese or ice cream can be substituted for part of the fluid milk allowance. One cup of ice cream is equivalent in calcium to one-half cup of milk. A one-inch cube of cheddar cheese is equal to two-thirds of a cup of milk, which also is equivalent in calcium to one cup, or eight ounces, or cottage cheese. Cream cheese can be substituted for milk in a two-to-one ratio; that is, two ounces of cream cheese are equal to one ounce of milk.

IRON: Iron is needed for the formation of *hemoglobin*, the substance that gives red blood cells their red coloration and is responsible for the transport of oxygen and carbon dioxide in the bloodstream. Hemoglobin has such an affinity for oxygen that without it humans would require 60 times as much blood to transport oxygen from the lungs to tissues throughout the body. Studies indicate that girls are five times as likely to need additional supplies of iron in their diets because of blood loss through menstruation. Recommended sources of iron are liver, heart, kidney, liver sausage, meat, shellfish, egg yolk, dark molasses, bread, beans and other legumes. If

basic food lists seem drab and boring, the teen-ager might think of the iron sources in terms of a peanut butter sandwich or two hamburgers; either choice would provide the daily iron needs for a girl. Other minerals which are important to a teen-ager's diet include the following:

• Sulfur is needed by the body for hair, skin, nails, and cartilage, and is available by eating nearly any protein-rich foods.

• Sodium is required for muscle activity and normal body fluid balance, and can be obtained by using ordinary table salt on foods.

• Iodine is needed for normal thyroid control of body metabolism, and is supplied in the form of iodized table salt.

• Potassium is a tonic for the nervous system and the muscles, and is available in adequate amounts in most kinds of meats, as well as bananas, orange juice, and milk.

• Magnesium collaborates chemically with calcium and phosphorus for normal muscle and nerve function, and is found in most forms of protein.

Weight Problems

Teens who are seriously overweight or who are contemplating radical weight reduction programs should be examined by a physician. Otherwise, unfair comparisons with other persons of the same age and height may lead to wrong conclusions about the need to gain or lose weight. The weight-height standards are based on averages, and there are many youngsters who are above or below the average but quite healthy and normal. Good examples of misinterpretation of weight-height tables can be found among beefy football players who have been rejected by military recruiters because they weighed more than other fellows of the same height.

Another reason for a medical exam is to check the possibility of

disease as the cause of the weight problem. The exam will also indicate whether the youngster has some other disorder that could be aggravated by a sudden weight loss.

Achieving optimum weight is only one step toward proper physical conditioning. A youngster who has been able to avoid physical activity by living in an elevator apartment, riding a bus to school, and watching TV after school hours instead of working or playing, could be right on the button as far as weight for his age and height are concerned, but his muscular development and heart and lung

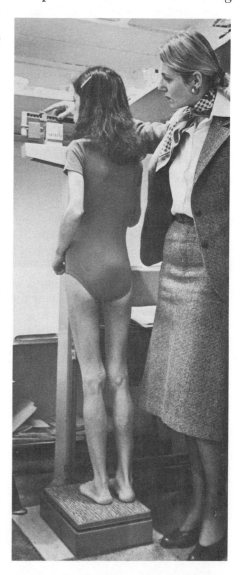

A victim of anorexia nervosa willfully starves herself until she deteriorates into a dangerously emaciated state. The disease occurs primarily in adolescent girls and has deep-rooted psychological causes.

capacity could be at the same time at a very low ebb.

ANOREXIA NERVOSA: A psychological disorder that in extreme cases results in death, anorexia nervosa appears most commonly among teenage girls. The victims starve themselves in an exaggerated effort to lose weight. Medical experts believe that true anorectics weigh 25 percent or more less than the norm for their height and weight.

Anorectics may show other common symptoms. Many have been high achievers in school, and many are sports enthusiasts. An anorectic may alternate periods of strict fasting and periods of food binges, or develop rituals around eating. Where binges become "gorge and purge" sessions—stretches of overeating followed by self-induced vomiting—anorectics may also have a disorder called *bulimia*. But bulimia may afflict otherwise normal persons. Anorectics may weigh themselves several times a day and avoid eating even when they are hungry. Some avoid social situations that may call for eating. Most, according to experts, are unusually preoccupied with their appearance or bodily "image" as a result of personality or ego problems or deficiencies. Adolescent girls who are anorectic frequently suffer from amenorrhea, cessation or delay of menstruation.

Treatment of anorexia nervosa may be a lengthy, costly process. Psychiatric counseling is usually a part of such treatment. Physically, treatment seeks to build a normal relationship between *norepinephrine*, a body chemical that carries messages about food, and the *hypothalamus*, the part of the brain that directs eating behavior.

Physical Fitness

Good physical conditioning is as important as weight control during the teen years. Everybody cannot be an athletic champion, but almost anyone can improve his heart, lungs, and muscles so that he can cope more effectively with the stresses of young adult life. Physical conditioning can be accomplished with little or no exercise equipment. It can be programed for city living or country living, in a gymnasium or in an apartment. All that really is required is a little time each day plus a great deal of determination and patience. It is important for young people to understand the major health role of daily exercise. Although many school physical education programs are excellent, some still remain inadequate, and in many cases students are only going through the motions of calisthenic routines and are not really benefiting from the effort.

Exercise Goals for Teen-Age Boys

One of the goals of physical conditioning for teen-age boys is muscle development. When muscles are not used they atrophy, or shrink in size. A muscle that has been immobilized because of an injury may shrivel to one-fourth its normal size. Some of the muscle fibers are replaced by nonelastic fibrous tissue. On the other hand, muscles that are exercised regularly and vigorously will grow in size and strength. Exercise causes an increase in the number of individual muscle fibers as well as an increase in the number of blood capillaries supplying the muscle tissue. A fringe benefit is

A favorite fantasy of teen-aged boys is making it as a pro basketball star, but even though few will achieve that goal, regular play keeps them physically fit.

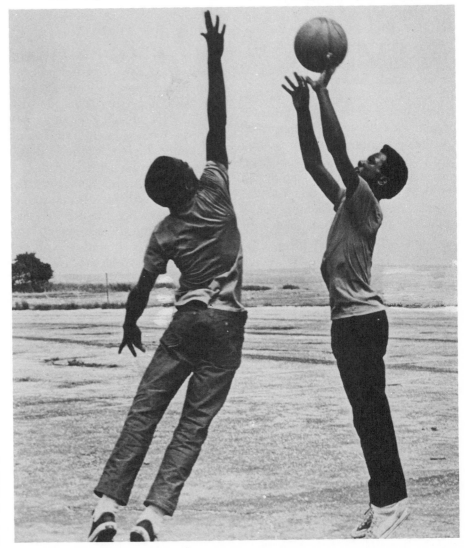

that muscles become more efficient as they grow in size from exercise. In other words, the muscles can perform more work with less wasted effort.

In addition to muscle development, which every exercise program should provide, physical conditioning should include optimum cardiopulmonary development. This means increased heart activity and greater oxygen consumption and is the basis for the popular aerobics workouts. *Aerobic* means, literally, with oxygen. A goal of aerobics training is to achieve a steady state of exercising in which breathing is heavier than normal. In the steady state, the heart, lungs, and muscles work together as an efficient machine at an activity level that is more demanding of the body than the resting state. Jogging, running, and rapid walking are examples of aerobic exercises. They can be practiced with no special equipment.

The individual goals for physical fitness should be kept within sensible limits to avoid injury or impaired health. The maximum level of performance can be determined by the appearance of the panting and puffing that occurs when exercise exceeds the normal ability of the lungs to supply oxygen to the muscles. A youngster who is not in good physical condition may huff and puff after walking up a flight of stairs, whereas a classmate in top condition might run a mile without showing signs of excessive breathing.

There are many fine exercise programs which teen-agers can follow, such as those published by the U.S. Air Force and the President's Council on Physical Fitness.

Exercise Goals for Teen-Age Girls

The young girl of today can be as involved in sports and the working world as the male, and the general guidelines for masculine conditioning apply to young women as well.

Girls should follow exercise programs which develop muscular strength and the endurance provided by a sound cardiovascular system. Regular exercise causes the heartbeat to grow stronger and steadier and breathing to become deeper. As the flow of blood through the tissues is improved, waste products of the cells are removed more efficiently and complexion problems are reduced. Another benefit is that the body uses energy more efficiently in both physical and mental tasks; coordination is improved. Girls should not worry about developing bulging muscles when they follow a regular, well-balanced exercise routine which includes workouts for the hips and thighs, waist, bustline, calves, and ankles.

Care of the Teeth

During the teen years, careful supervision by the dentist and cooperation from the teen-ager are especially necessary. The poor eating habits of many teen-agers are reflected in their cavity rate, which is usually higher during adolescence than in later life.

If a young person is conscientious about oral care, he can avoid not only a high cavity rate, but also bad breath and the unpleasant appearance of food particles left on the teeth. These problems are really caused by the same thing—*dental plaque*. For more information on this subject, see *Tooth Decay*, p. 257.

Need for Frequent Checkups

During the adolescent period, the dentist will often recommend more frequent checkups than in the past. Small cavities are treated before they become deeper and infect the pulp, the inner chamber of the tooth, containing nerves and blood vessels. Should the pulp become infected, the tooth must have special treatment, usually a root canal process, or be extracted.

The dentist also treats tooth decay, or *caries*, more popularly known as cavities, to prevent their spread. While they are not thought to be contagious, cavities begin as a break in the tooth surface, which later enlarges. Food debris can become lodged in the cavity, be attacked by bacteria, and cause a cavity on the next tooth. The only way to avoid such a problem is to have the affected tooth treated immediately.

Front teeth often decay for the first time during this period. They are restored with a silicate or plastic filling close in color to the tooth rather than silver or gold, which would be unattractive. Unfortunately, these materials are not permanent and will need to be replaced in time. As a result, neglect of diet and oral cleanliness by an adolescent may mean that he may need many replacement fillings in the same cavity over his lifetime.

Orthodontic Treatment

The development and growth of teeth is completed during the adolescent period. When oral growth is improper, the adolescent needs treatment by an *orthodontist*, a dental specialist who treats abnormalities of the bite and alignment of teeth and jaws. Correction of such conditions as buck teeth, which mar a person's appearance, is a major reason for orthodontic treatment. But there are also major health reasons for orthodontic care. If teeth, for example, come together improperly, efficient chewing of food is impossible. The digestive system is strained because chunks of improperly chewed food pass through it. Orthodontic treatment will, therefore, result in lifelong better health and appearance. For more information, see *Orthodontics*, p. 262.

Stimulants and Alcohol

Initial exposure to caffeine, tobacco, drugs, and alcohol usually occurs during adolescence. Teen-agers should be fully educated regarding their physical effects and potential danger. They should learn how to use them, if at all, sensibly and in moderation, and to resist peer-group pressures.

Caffeine

Caffeine, which is naturally present in coffee and tea and is used in many carbonated beverages and medications, stimulates the central nervous system to overcome fatigue and drowsiness. It also affects a part of the nervous system that controls respiration so that more oxygen is pumped through the lungs. In large amounts, caffeine can increase the pulse rate, but there are few long-range effects because the substance is broken down by the body tissues within a few hours and excreted. Because of the action of caffeine in stimulating an increased intake of oxygen, it sometimes is used to combat the effects of such nervous system depressants as alcohol.

Nicotine

Nicotine is one of nearly 200 substances in tobacco. It affects the human physiology by stimulating the adrenal glands to increase the flow of adrenaline. The blood vessels become constricted and the skin temperature drops, producing effects not unlike exposure to cold temperatures. When comparatively large amounts of nicotine are absorbed by the body, the pulse becomes rapid and the smoker has symptoms of dizziness, faintness, and sometimes nausea and diarrhea. The release of adrenaline, triggered by nicotine, will produce temporary relief from fatigue by increasing the flow of sugar in the blood. However, the effect is transient, and the feeling of fatigue will return again after the increased blood sugar has been expended.

OTHER PROPERTIES OF TOBACCO: The nicotine in tobacco can be absorbed simply by contact with the mucous membranes of the mouth; the tobacco does not have to be smoked to get the nicotine effects. Burning tobacco produces a myriad of substances found in the smoke of many plant materials when they are dried and burned. More than 50 different compounds are known to occur in concentrations of one microgram or more in each puff of tobacco smoke. Again, laboratory tests have demonstrated that the substances in burning tobacco do not have to be inhaled; most of the chemical compounds can be absorbed through the mucous membranes while a puff of smoke is held in the mouth for a few seconds. At least ten of the substances in tobacco smoke have been shown to produce cancer in animals. Other chemicals in tobacco tars are known as *co-carcinogens*; although they do not produce cancer themselves, they react with other substances to produce cancers.

Smoking and Disease

The relationship between tobacco smoking and cancer, heart disease, and emphysema-bronchitis are well established, even if some of the cause and effect links are missing. Large-scale studies of the death rates of smokers and nonsmokers have been carried on for the past 20 years. One group, consisting of nearly a quarter-million war veterans, yielded results indicating that smokers are from 10 to 16 times as likely to die of lung cancer as nonsmokers. (The higher ratio is for heavy smokers.) Similar results have been obtained from studies of smokers and nonsmokers with heart disease and lung ailments.

BUERGER'S DISEASE: One of the possible, although rare, effects of smoking is the aggravation of symptoms of a particularly insidious circulatory disorder known as *Buerger's disease*. As noted above, one of the effects of nicotine is a drop in skin temperatures. Smoking a single cigarette can cause the temperature of the fingers and toes to drop as much as 15 degrees Fahrenheit; the average is a little more than a five degree drop. The temperature change results from constriction of the blood vessels at the extremities. Blood clots may develop in the vessels that have been constricted, cutting off the flow of blood to the tissues of the area. When there is numbness or pain in the extremities, the condition should receive swift medical attention to prevent serious consequences.

CARBON MONOXIDE ACCUMULATION: Another little publicized effect of smoking is the accumulation of carbon monoxide in the blood. Carbon monoxide is one of the lethal gases emitted in automobile exhaust. It is also produced by burning plant materials such as tobacco. It is a dangerous gas because of its strong affinity for the hemoglobin of red blood cells. Unlike oxygen and carbon dioxide, which become temporarily attached, then released, from the hemoglobin molecule, carbon monoxide becomes permanently locked into the red blood cell chemistry so that the cells are no longer effective for their normal function of transporting oxygen to the body tissues. With the oxygen-carrying capacity of part of the red blood cells wiped out, brain cells and other tissues suffer a mild oxy-

A French poster encourages people to quit smoking and cut down on alcohol.

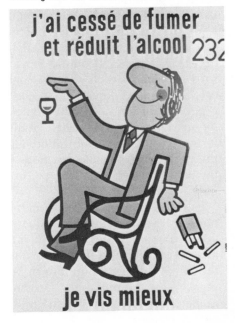

j'ai cessé de fumer et réduit l'alcool

je vis mieux

gen starvation and the results are a form of intoxication.

A strong whiff of carbon monoxide can be fatal. Smokers, of course, do not get that much of the substance into their blood, but they do pick up enough carbon monoxide to render up to eight percent of their red blood cells ineffective. Experiments at Indiana University show that pack-a-day smokers have the same level of carbon monoxide in their blood as subjects who inhale an atmosphere of one-fourth of one percent carbon monoxide. That level of carbon monoxide increases the shortness of breath during exercise by approximately 15 percent, and, the study shows, about three weeks of abstinence from smoking are required to permit the oxygen-carrying capacity of the blood to return to normal. It is the carbon monoxide of burning plant materials that produces most of the "high" associated with the smoking of many substances.

Alcohol

Alcohol usually is not considered as a potentially dangerous drug because it is easily available at cocktail lounges and liquor stores, and is served generously at parties. Alcohol has been used by man for thousands of years, at times as a sedative and anesthetic, and when used in moderation has the effect of a mild tranquilizer and appetite stimulant. But when consumed in excess amounts, alcoholic beverages can produce both psychological and physical dependence. It can produce illusions of being a pick-me-up, but studies indicate that this is due to a letdown of inhibitions and the weakening of some functions of the central nervous system, particularly in the cerebral cortex.

Parents and teachers share an important responsibility to educate young people about the use and misuse of alcohol. Like marihuana, the effects of alcohol on human beings are not thoroughly understood. Some users develop a tissue toler-ance for alcohol so that their body tissues require increasing amounts. When alcohol is withdrawn from such users, they develop tremors, convulsions, and even hallucinations. However, there are many varied reactions to the use of alcohol, and an individual may react differently to alcoholic drinks at different times. See *Alcohol*, p. 540.

Drugs

During the 1960s there was an alarming increase in drug-use among teen-agers—a problem which deservedly received nation-wide attention. Education concerning the hazards and occasional tragedies accompanying drug use is imperative.

Marihuana

Marihuana affects the central nervous system, including the brain, after it enters the blood-stream. According to some researchers, the substance accumulates in the liver. Some of the effects of marihuana are not unlike those of tobacco. The rate of the heartbeat is increased, body temperature drops, and blood sugar levels are altered. The drug user also feels dehydrated, the appetite is stimulated, coordination of movements becomes difficult, there are feelings of drowsi-ness or unsteadiness, and the eyes may become reddish. Taken in higher strengths, marihuana can cause hallucinations or distortions of perception.

VARYING EFFECTS: Scientists are uncertain about the pathways of the drug in the central nervous system and its effects on other body systems. The drug's effects seem to vary widely, not only among individual users but also according to the social setting and the amount and strength of the marihuana used. The effects, which usually begin within 15 minutes after the smoke is inhaled and may continue for several hours, vary from depression to excitement and talkativeness. Some users claim to experience time distortions and errors in distance perception. But others sharing the same marihuana cigarette may experience no effects at all.

Although marihuana is not addictive, in that users do not develop a physical dependence upon the substance and withdrawal of the drug produces no ill effects, there are dangerous results from the use of marihuana. Marihuana users find it hard to make decisions that require clear thinking, some users develop psychotic reactions or an emotional disorder called "acute marihuana panic," and there is some evidence

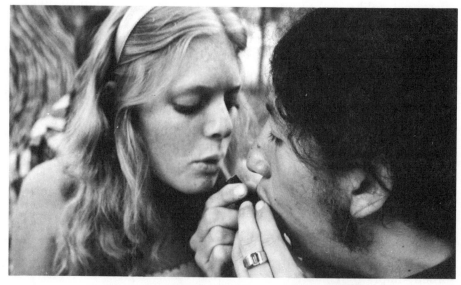

Although not addictive, marihuana distorts the perception of time and distance and, like alcohol, impairs judgment.

that the active ingredient is transmitted by expectant mothers to their unborn children.

Hallucinogens

Marihuana sometimes is described as a *hallucinogen* because of visual hallucinations, illusions, and delusions reported by users after they have inhaled the smoke from a large number of "joints" or "sticks" of the drug. But marihuana should not be confused with the true hallucinogenic drugs such as *mescaline* and *LSD* (lysergic acid diethylamide) which are known by doctors as *psychomimetic* drugs because they mimic psychoses.

LSD AND MESCALINE: LSD and mescaline have marked effects on perception and thought processes. Teen-agers usually become involved with the use of LSD because they are curious about its effects; they may have heard about its purported "mind-bending" properties and expect to gain great personal insights from its use. Instead of great insight, however, the user finds anxiety, depression, confusion, and frightening hallucinations. The use of LSD is complicated by the reappearance of hallucinations after the individual has quit using the drug; the very possibility of repeated hallucinations causes a sense of terror.

Morphine and Heroin

Besides the hallucinogenic drugs, there are *opium* derivatives, *morphine* and *heroin*. Morphine is one of the most effective pain relievers known and is one of the most valuable drugs available to the physician. Morphine and heroin depress the body systems to produce drowsiness, sleep, and a reduction in physical activity. They are true narcotics, and their appeal is in their ability to produce a sense of euphoria by reducing the individual's sensitivity to both psychological and physical stimuli.

ADDICTIVE PROPERTIES: A great danger lies in the ability of the body tissues to develop a physical dependence on morphine, and its de-

rivative cousin, heroin. The degree to which heroin's "desirable" effects are felt depends in part on how the user takes it. *Sniffing* is the mildest form of abuse, followed by skin-popping—subcutaneous injection—and then by *mainlining*—injecting directly into a vein, which is the method used by almost all those dependent on heroin.

The body adjusts to the level of the first doses so that increasingly larger injections of the drug are required to produce the same feelings of euphoria. The ability of the body to adjust to the increasingly larger doses is called *tolerance*. And with tolerance goes *physical dependence*, which means that when heroin or morphine is withdrawn from the user he experiences a violent sickness marked by tremors, sweating and chills, vomiting and diarrhea, and sharp abdominal pains. Another shot of heroin or morphine temporarily ends the withdrawal symptoms. But the user, now dependent upon the drug, must continue regular doses or face another bout of the withdrawal sickness. Heroin has no value as a medicine and is available only through illicit channels at a high price. The heroin addict usually is unable to hold a job because of effects of the drug and often turns to crime in order to finance his daily supply of the narcotic.

SHORTENED LIFE SPAN: The health of a narcotics addict declines so that his life span is shortened by 15 to 20 years. He usually is in continual trouble with the law because of the severe penalties for illegal possession of narcotics. If he sells narcotics, as many heroin addicts are driven to do to get enough money to support their habit, the punishment is even more severe.

Amphetamines and Barbiturates

Other commonly abused drugs are *amphetamines*, also known as *uppers* or *pep pills*, and *barbiturates*, sometimes called *downers* or *goof balls*. Amphetamines are used by doctors to curb the appetite when weight reduction of patients

is needed and to relieve mild cases of depression. However, some doctors doubt that amphetamines should be used as a weight-control medication because of the risks involved; other experts have questioned whether the drugs are actually effective for that purpose.

Amphetamines stimulate the heart rate, increase the blood pressure, cause rapid breathing, dilate the pupils of the eyes, and produce other effects such as dryness of the mouth, sweating, headache, and diarrhea. Ordinarily, amphetamines are swallowed as tablets, but a more extreme form of amphetamine abuse involves the injection of the drug, usually Methedrine, directly into the vein.

DANGERS OF AMPHETAMINES: The danger in the use of amphetamines is that they induce a person to do things beyond his physical endurance, cause mental disorders that require hospitalization, and, in large doses, can result in death. Although they do not produce the kind of physical dependence observed in the use of narcotics, amphetamine withdrawal for a heavy user can result in a deep and suicidal depression.

BARBITURATES: Barbiturates are sedatives used by doctors to treat high blood pressure, epilepsy, and insomnia, and to relax patients being prepared for surgery. They slow the heart rate and breathing, lower blood pressure, and mildly depress the action of nerves and muscles.

DANGERS OF BARBITURATES: Barbiturates are highly dangerous when taken without medical advice. They distort perception and slow down reaction and response time, contributing to the chances of accidents. Barbiturates are a leading cause of accidental poison deaths because they make the mind foggy and the user forgets how many pills he has taken, thus leading to overdosage. They also cause physical dependence with withdrawal symptoms that range from cramps and nausea to convulsions and death. See also *Drugs*, p. 552.

SOCIAL AND SEXUAL MATURATION

The Prospect of Adulthood

As a youngster passes from childhood into adolescence, it is the psychological adjustments rather than the physical changes that are most likely to produce difficulties. The emotional problems, of course, are related to the hormonal activity of the developing body. However, the conflicts which frequently are upsetting to both the adolescent and other members of his family are the result of adjustments which must be made between the young person and the society in which he must live.

In certain primitive cultures, for example, the boy becomes an "instant adult" by undergoing puberty rites. There may be no restrictions on sex play between boys and girls; the girl does not have to be concerned about dating procedures because her parents select her husband. There is no question about economic independence; the young couple becomes a part of the economic unit of the parents.

In our own culture, the teen-ager must continually adjust to a complex set of rules and regulations. He frequently may feel that he must accept the responsibilities of adulthood before he is entitled to the privileges of being treated as an adult. Childhood is only a step behind, but he has learned to suppress or ignore childhood relationships. He can easily forget the point of view of children and even resent the ability of his parents to recall the "cute" incidents of his earlier years. At the same time, he may be startled by the suggestion that within a few short years he and his teen-age friends will face the selection of a career, marriage, establishment of a home, and a lifetime of responsibilities he may feel ill-prepared to assume.

Future Outlook for Girls

For a girl, the future is somewhat more complex than it was for her mother at the same stage of life. In her mother's day, a teen-age girl might look forward to a brief period of work as a secretary, store clerk, or factory hand between the day of her high school graduation and her wedding day. After the wedding, there followed a couple of decades or more of being a housewife and mother. Today's teen-age girl can still follow the pattern of her mother's life. Or she can plan a lifetime professional career as a doctor, lawyer, or scientist. She can compete with men as a business executive, writer, or politician, and she can schedule marriage and motherhood to complement rather than compete with career goals.

Future Outlook for Boys

The adolescent boy also has a wider choice of goals. He may or may not follow in his father's footsteps. If he decides to join a family business venture, the chances are that he will go to college and contribute a working knowledge of computer techniques or tax laws to the accumulated experience and business contacts his father acquired by starting as an apprentice and working for many years.

Advanced Education

The educational requirements for the jobs of tomorrow place an added strain on the pace of growing into adulthood. Although going steady may begin at an earlier age for both sexes, marriage may have to be postponed until the boy and girl have completed college or even gone to a university in pursuit of an advanced degree. An alternative is marriage and the start of a family while the boy and girl are still in college and dependent economically upon their parents.

Need for Independence

Just as natural as the boy-girl relationships of the teen years are the needs for independence and privacy. Sometimes a youngster feels it necessary to demonstrate a mind of his own by taking independent action, although such action could be considered as rebellion against parental authority. A recent survey showed that a girl may go steady with a boy not because she really likes the boy that much but to prove she is capable of handling a relationship which her parents have criticized. Carried to a sometimes tragic extreme is the compulsion of a boy or girl to marry a person the parents dislike in order to demonstrate so-called independence. The wise parent will avoid efforts to force a young person into a position in which the alternatives are a surrender to the will of the parents or an action such as a premature marriage that might have unfortunate consequences.

Conflicts Between Parent and Teen-ager

Some conflicts between the generations are avoidable. The parents may be protective and slow to cut the apron strings because they love their children and want to prevent them from becoming involved in unhappy situations. The teen-ager resents the overprotective actions of the parents, regarding them as evidence that they do not trust their own children.

What parents should try to make clear to their children is that they are offering their years of experience as guidelines. Teen-agers should value the counsel of more experienced members of the family; they should cooperate by listening to the adult viewpoint. If, after serious consideration of the parents' point of view the youngster still wants to make his own decision in the matter, it should be understood that he may have to accept the responsibility for the consequences. A keystone in the training for adulthood is the concept that being an adult entails more than just privileges and the authority to make decisions; along with decision-making

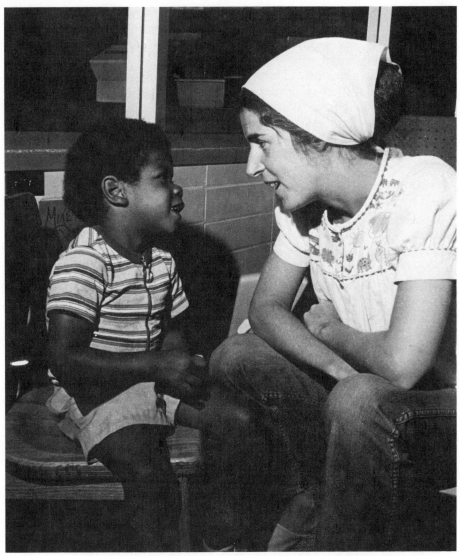

Young people who get along well with children may find the experience of working in a nursery school or day-care center rewarding.

ethnic backgrounds, they may become aware of parental prejudices in addition to new rules of propriety as they grow into their teen-age years.

Decisions of the teen years can involve the use of tobacco, alcohol, owning an automobile, handling of money, overnight trips with friends, association with friends who use drugs illegally, and relationships with members of the opposite sex. The consequences of all alternatives should be outlined for the adolescent.

Search for Identity

Part of the youngster's struggle for independence will involve what sometimes is described as a search for identity. A child accepts without much questioning that he is a member of a certain family and lives in a certain neighborhood. But as he grows older, he becomes aware of his status in the family as well as the status of his family in society. A seven-year-old could not care less about the background of his family or that of his second-grade friends. As he becomes a teen-ager he learns that such subjects may be matters of concern to parents and their circle of friends. He may imitate the attitudes of his family or disregard them, perhaps inviting criticism that he is rebellious.

More important to the youngster, however, is a growing concern about his position and role in life and where it may lead. He is still in the so-called formative years and is sensitive to countless influences in the world about him. Teen-agers become concerned with approaching education and career decisions. It is natural for them to identify with older members in the family, teachers, and celebrities.

Need for Privacy

For the teen-age girl, party invitations, dances, and diaries are important and an increasing amount of privacy is required. Even if she must share a room with a sister, there should be a part of the room

goes a responsibility to the family and society for the consequences of one's decisions.

Few parents, of course, would refuse to bail out a teen-age son or daughter in real trouble. And even when a youngster is rebellious enough to leave home, he should know that the door will always be open to him when he decides to return. Again, limiting the options available to a teen-ager can lead to a snowballing of bad decisions and resulting complications.

In many cases, the conflicts between parents and teen-agers derive from the illusion that a younger child has more freedom of choice. A small child may actually seem to

have a freer choice of friends he can bring into his home and the games he can play with them. But there are always limitations to a child's choices, and parents are more understanding of the bad choices by attributing mistakes to the fact that "he's only a child."

Older youngsters become involved in situations in which the decisions are more important. A boy and girl at the age of five can "play house" together in an atmosphere of innocence. However, the same boy and girl could hardly suggest to their parents that they intended to play house at the age of 15. If the boy and girl, although next-door neighbors, are of different social or

which is her territory. She should have personal belongings which are not shared by a parent or sibling. If she has her own room, everything in the room probably will be regarded as her property. Even her mother should respect her privacy by knocking on the door and getting permission to enter her private world.

Although sometimes less sensitive about such matters, boys also are likely to insist on a certain amount of privacy as they grow older. They may share a room with a brother but they need trunks or other containers with locks in which they can keep personal possessions. Proof that such desire for privacy is not a passing fad for young men is found in their adult compulsion for private offices and a den or workshop area at home.

Contacts With Older Friends

Young teen-agers, through part-time jobs as baby-sitters or errand boys, usually come in contact with young adults outside the family circle for the first time. The young adults may accept the teen-agers as peers, which is flattering to the youngsters, who may in turn admire and imitate the young adults. If the teen-ager has been able to identify closely with his family's sense of propriety, the contacts can be a good social experience. But if the youngster has not been able to identify effectively with his parents and family members, he may be vulnerable to misguiding influences. Because of the urge for adult status, the teen-ager may find a premature outlet for testing his abilities to live the adult life in the company of young adults. He (or she) can absorb a lot of information—and misinformation—about sex, alcohol, drugs, and other subjects.

Teen-agers certainly should not be cautioned against contacts with all young adults, but they should also have a reliable older person aside from their parents with whom they can discuss matters they would not discuss with a mother or father.

The alternate adult might be a clergyman, the family doctor, a teacher, or even a favorite aunt or uncle. Such an arrangement provides the youngster with a means of learning a bit more about life in an independent manner and from a different point of view than could be obtained within his own immediate family circle.

Relationships With the Opposite Sex

First teen-age contacts with the opposite sex tend to be awkward and sometimes embarrassing despite the best efforts and intentions of parents. The meetings may be at school dances or movie dates, perhaps in the presence of a chaperon who is a teacher or parent.

OVERCOMING INSECURITY: Some youngsters will feel more secure than others in social gatherings; those who feel insecure may not participate at all when such opportunities first arise. As the youngsters grow older, however, they find that more and more of their friends are dating or going to dances or parties to meet members of the opposite sex.

Some boys or girls who feel insecure may find that they are more gregarious or less ill-at-ease if they fortify themselves with a couple of drinks of an alcoholic beverage, or with drugs, before they join their friends. Youngsters who feel the need for stimulants or depressants in order to enjoy parties usually can be helped with psychological counseling to overcome their fears of inadequacy.

Young people should be assured that getting together at parties of mixed sexes is a natural thing to do. It has been going on for generations and although an individual youngster may feel ill-at-ease at his first few dances or parties, he probably will survive. As the boy or girl attends more parties the chances increase that he or she will meet a person of the opposite sex who is particularly attractive. If the feeling is mutual, the acquaintanceship may develop into more or less steady dating.

GOING STEADY: Steady dating, which leads to a formal engagement and marriage in many cases, should not be encouraged at an early age or before a young person has had an opportunity to date a number of prospective partners. At the same time, it should not be discouraged to the point of producing a rebellious

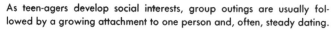

As teen-agers develop social interests, group outings are usually followed by a growing attachment to one person and, often, steady dating.

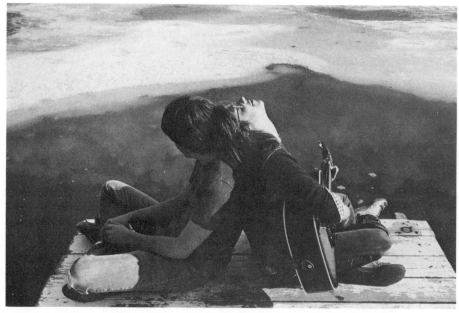

reaction. As was pointed out earlier, some girls admit going steady with a boy for no other reason than to demonstrate their independence of judgment.

Controlling the Sexual Impulse

Teen-agers who spend a lot of time together at parties, in their homes, or at recreational meetings such as beach outings, are likely to be physically attracted to each other. It may begin with kissing, dancing, holding hands, or simply a natural urge to neck or pet. In more primitive societies, the couple might simply indulge in sexual intercourse without any concern for the possible consequences. But in our own society, young people are expected to control their natural urges.

INFLUENCE OF THE MASS MEDIA: Complicating sincere efforts of a teen-ager to make the right decisions in relations with the opposite sex is the constant exposure of youngsters to movies, magazine articles, books, and other media suggesting that sexual relations between unmarried couples are not only acceptable but a common practice. Compared to the image of young love as displayed in movie promotion advertising, a teen-age boy and girl may believe that a few ardent hugs and kisses in a secluded spot may be as innocent as making a plate of fudge together in the girl's kitchen.

Some girls, but not all, are as easily aroused as boys by close bodily contact with the opposite sex. Physical contact for most boys arouses sexual desire, partly because of the physiological makeup of the male.

THE SEX DRIVE IN BOYS: Males are so constituted that during periods of abstinence from intercourse, their sperm builds up. During periods of sperm buildup, the male sex drive increases in strength. There are no standards or averages for the male sex drive; instead there is a wide variety of sexual appetites and abilities.

A girl who cuddles too closely to a boy may trigger a response she did not expect and may not want. Depending upon the boy and the status of his sex drive at that time, he might accept the girl's approaches as a suggestion that she is willing to have intercourse or is at least interested in petting. If the girl is simply being friendly, the results can be embarrassing to one or both of the youngsters. If the boy is the type who likes to discuss the details of his dates with friends, the girl may discover a sudden and unwelcome change in attitude by other boys of the group.

Walking hand-in-hand, or with an arm around the waist, and kissing which is not too passionate, usually are acceptable ways for young teen-agers to display affection. And there are activities such as hiking or bicycle riding which afford a boy and girl a chance to be together and apart from the rest of the world. There also are picnics, ball games, movies, and concerts which permit togetherness without setting the stage for hard-to-control sexual impulses.

Masturbation

Another manifestation of the natural sex drives of young persons is masturbation. Prohibited by the rules and regulations of modern society from fulfilling sex urges in the same manner as married couples, teen-agers discover they can find sexual satisfaction in masturbation. Despite the stories that warn of physical or mental decay for youngsters who masturbate, there is no evidence that the practice is harmful unless the parents make an issue of it.

If there are dangers in masturbation, they are likely to be the isolation and loneliness associated with the practice and the confusion and anxiety which can result if the youngster feels guilty or is punished or criticized for masturbating. Masturbation is such a natural reaction that most youngsters discover it by themselves even if the subject is

never discussed by friends or family members. Like many other matters that seem important during the teen-age years, masturbation usually diminishes as a matter of concern as adulthood is reached.

Sex Education

Since boys and girls in their teens may be capable of producing children and are known to have strong sexual urges, they should be provided with authoritative information about human reproduction and birth control. It is up to the parents to make decisions regarding the proper sources of such information, how much information should be given, and at what age.

One of the reasons for the popularity of sex education in the schools is that teachers can get the parents off the hook by explaining the facts of life to youngsters. However, by forfeiting their prerogative to explain sex and human reproduction to their own children, parents must depend upon the teacher to make an acceptable presentation to the youngsters. The likely alternative is that youngsters will obtain a considerable amount of misinformation from friends and acquaintances at street-corner seminars or by experimentation.

In the days when the majority of the population lived on farms or near rural areas, children learned a few things about sex and reproduction simply by working with farm animals. They learned that cats produced kittens, dogs produced puppies, cows produced calves, and so on. This on-the-job type of sex education also provided farm youngsters with a smattering of genetics, because cross-breeding strains of animals frequently had economic consequences. It was not too difficult for the rural youngsters to relate their barnyard education to human experience.

Children enrolled in sex education classes in the urban areas of America today receive similar information—dogs have puppies, cats have kittens, etc.—by watching movies and reading books. However, the lessons may be superficial or incomplete, depending upon the teacher and the prescribed curriculum. For example, the children in one eastern school were taught that the baby develops in the mother's abdomen, which led some youngsters to believe the baby lived in the mother's stomach until born. "Why isn't the baby digested by the stomach acid?" asked one confused girl. And when asked how the baby gets out when it's time to be born, the teacher told the students that such questions should be answered by their parents. The point here is that parents should establish some rapport with their children to be sure they are learning a practical set of facts about adult love, sex, and reproduction, including the possible emotional and physical consequences of premarital sexual intercourse.

Although parents may find it difficult or embarrassing to explain the facts of life to their own children, it is one of the most important contributions that can be made to a maturing youngster. At the present time, at least one out of six teen-age girls in the United States will have an unwanted pregnancy. Obviously, thousands of parents and teachers are not providing adequate instruction in sex education subjects.

The Male Reproductive System

Any instruction in the facts of life should begin by use of the proper names for the body parts involved. In the male, the external sex organs are the *penis* and the *testicles*, or *testes*. The penis contains a tiny tube, the *urethra*, through which urine is eliminated. Much of the fleshy part of the penis is composed of spongy tissue. When the penis is stimulated sexually, the spongy areas become filled with blood which makes the penis larger and firm, a condition called an *erection*. The testicles contain male *sperm cells*, also called *spermatozoa*.

The sperm travel up tubules inside the abdomen to a storage organ,

THE MALE REPRODUCTIVE SYSTEM

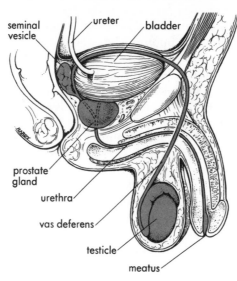

or reservoir, the *seminal vesicle*. The sperm storage area also contains a thick white fluid called *semen* which is secreted by glands which open into the urethra. One of the glands, the *prostate*, serves partly as a control valve to prevent urine from mixing with the semen, since both are discharged through the urethra. The semen, containing millions of sperm, empties periodically in a more or less automatic action, being squeezed out of the seminal vesicle by pulsating contractions. The contractions and ejection of semen are called *ejaculation*. During the sex act, or *intercourse*, with a female, the semen is ejaculated into the woman's vagina.

The Female Reproductive System

The *vagina* is the proper name for the tubular female sex organ. At the end of the vagina is an opening, called the *cervix*, which leads into the *uterus*. The uterus, or *womb*, is shaped somewhat like an upside-down pear. When a baby develops within the mother's abdomen, it grows inside the uterus. The uterus also is the source of the bloody discharge which occurs periodically during the fertile years of women. When the blood is discharged it is called *menstruation*, or the menstrual period. The menstrual blood passes out through the vagina, which stretches to become the *birth canal* when a baby is being born. The urethra of a female empties outside the vagina.

THE MENSTRUAL CYCLE AND CONCEPTION: Unlike the male reproductive organs, which produce perhaps millions of spermatozoa each day, the female reproductive system ordinarily releases only one germ cell, called an *ovum* or egg, at a time. An ovum is released at an average frequency of once every 28 days. It should always be remembered that the 28-day figure is only an average; the actual time may vary considerably for reasons that are only partly known. The cycles are more likely to be irregular for teen-age girls than for mature women. An ovum is released from one of the two

THE FEMALE REPRODUCTIVE SYSTEM

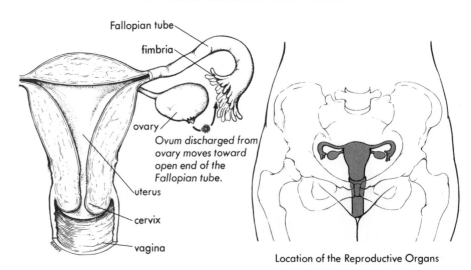

Ovum discharged from ovary moves toward open end of the Fallopian tube.

Location of the Reproductive Organs

ovaries, or sex glands, comparable in function to the male testicles, located on either side of the uterus. The ovum or egg is transported from the ovary to the uterus through a *Fallopian tube.*

If the ovum encounters male sperm during its passage from the ovary to the uterus, there is a good chance that fertilization, or *conception,* will occur through a union of a spermatozoon and the egg. The fertilized ovum, called a *zygote,* soon divides into a cluster of human tissue cells which become the embryo of a baby. For further information about pregnancy, see under *Infertility, Pregnancy, and Childbirth,* p. 127.

During the time that the egg is maturing in the ovary and passing into the uterus after its release, the membrane lining of the uterus becomes thicker because it accumulates blood and nutrients. If the ovum is fertilized, it finds a spot in the membrane where it becomes attached and develops rapidly into an embryo, gaining its nourishment from the blood and nutrient-enriched lining of the uterus. If the ovum is not fertilized, it passes through the uterus, and the blood-rich membrane sloughs off. The blood and some of the cells of the membrane become the discharged material of menstruation. The unfertilized ovum could pass through undetected since it is nearly microscopic.

After menstruation has begun, the female reproductive cycle starts over again. The lining of the uterus once more builds up its supply of blood and nutrients to support a fertilized ovum. Ordinarily, the next ovum will be released about 14 days after a menstrual period begins. If a female does not have intercourse, or avoids intercourse during the time the ovum is released, or in some other manner is able to prevent sperm from reaching an ovum, she will not become pregnant but will experience a menstrual period at intervals which average around 28 days.

When fertilization of an ovum occurs, menstruation ceases and no further egg cells are released until the outcome of the pregnancy has been determined. In other words, the cycles of ovulation and menstruation start anew after the baby is born or the pregnancy has been terminated.

Contraception

The first rule of birth control is that no method is guaranteed to be 100 percent effective. Sexual intercourse nearly always is accompanied by some risk of pregnancy, and the teen-agers who try to beat

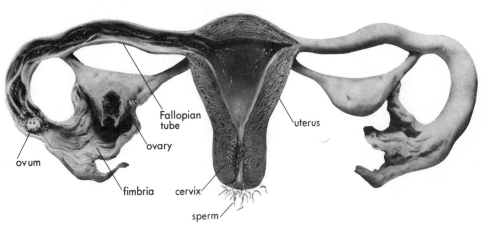

If ovum, released from left ovary (shown in cross section), meets sperm in passage through Fallopian tube to uterus, fertilization is likely.

the odds should be willing to take the responsibility for the results. Teen-agers should be provided with the basic facts of birth control as soon as they are capable of producing children themselves. But the emphasis should be on the relative unreliability of the techniques which do not require a visit to a physician's office. There are many birth control devices and substances that can be purchased without a doctor's prescription. But if young men and women were aware of their chances of effecting a pregnancy while using such methods, they probably would have second thoughts about taking the risk. See under *Marriage and Parenthood,* p. 144, for a full discussion of birth control methods.

Venereal Disease

Equally important in the education of teen-agers is a knowledge of the hazards of venereal disease. A poster prepared for a New York campaign against venereal disease carried the words "If your son is old enough to shave, he's old enough to get syphilis." The American Social Health Association estimates that 300,000 teen-agers each year become infected with one or more forms of venereal disease. Most insidious has been the recent increase in gonorrhea, partly because girls who carry the infection may show no symptoms. A girl may have a

slight but seemingly unimportant vaginal discharge. She may not be aware that she has gonorrhea until she is contacted by health officials after her boyfriend has reported to a doctor for treatment. For more information on venereal disease in relation to women, see p. 489.

Two reasons for the rising incidence of gonorrhea after it was once thought to be virtually eliminated by antibiotics are that condoms, once used as a mechanical barrier by males, have become less popular since teen-age girls have obtained the use of oral contraceptives, and that new strains of the bacteria are resistant to the antibiotics. Some boys delay treatment when they realize they are infected with VD; they believe it makes them appear "tough" to be able to go without medical treatment even when it endangers their health. Because of rebelliousness, youngsters may have a venereal disease and either refuse to tell their parents or boast about it, depending upon which approach they think will make them appear independent.

It is a bitter irony for many parents to realize that their children might carry the spirit of independence and privacy into areas which could endanger their health, for untreated syphilis can result in blindness, insanity, and heart disease. Such grave consequences can be avoided in most cases by establishing effective channels of communi-cation between parents and teen-agers, or between teen-agers and another responsible adult.

The Generation Gap

Despite the attention devoted in recent years to the so-called generation gap, the gap is nothing new to the process of evolving from childhood to adulthood. Every generation has had its generation gap—a period in which the fledgling adult tests his ability to make his own way in the world. In previous eras youngsters were considered old enough to take on an adult role when they were big enough physically. A boy left home to become a farm hand or a factory apprentice. A girl would leave home to become a live-in maid with another family. Sometimes the generation gap was masked by great social upheavals such as a war or a wave of emigration. The fictional hero of many romantic stories was a young man who left home to make his own way in the world, discovering in the process a girl who wanted to be rescued from her environment. With a few jet-age variations the adolescent boys and girls of today experience the same emotional struggles as nature develops their minds and bodies toward becoming another generation of adults.

CHAPTER 4

The Beginning of a Family

INFERTILITY, PREGNANCY, AND CHILDBIRTH

The decision of a young couple to begin a family is usually a happy event, with overtones of great responsibility for the parents-to-be. Although parenthood does bring fulfillment, happiness, and great rewards, it can also involve anxiety and heavy responsibility. Therefore, the decision to have a child should not be made lightly. Before increasing the family unit and thereby complicating it, the husband and wife should have a strong, good marriage, one based on love, understanding, and the ability to compromise and share.

Infertility

Once the decision to have a child has been made, a new set of problems can arise. Though the majority of women are able to conceive within a year after ceasing all methods of birth control, a large number of couples are faced with the problem of infertility. Old census reports and records show that in the early 1800s about one in six marriages was childless—the same proportion as today. However, because of improved medical and sur-

gical techniques, the modern woman has a much better chance of overcoming a condition of infertility. For a description of the female reproductive organs and of the processes of conception and fertilization, see under *Social and Sexual Maturation*, p. 120. For a full treatment of women's health concerns other than those relating to pregnancy and childbirth, see *Women's Health*, p. 483.

STRAIN AND FATIGUE: There are many causes of infertility, and an equal number of cures. Nervous strain and mental fatigue can interfere with reproductive capacity, as can fatigue from physical work. If a woman has worries or fears about financial security or other matters, she may fail to conceive. It is believed that nervous tension can suppress human ovulation cycles through the relationship of the hypothalamus, a part of the brain, and the pituitary gland, which controls the flow of sex hormones. Recommended treatment for a wife under strain might include a vacation, a temporary interruption in her business or professional goals, or a reorganization of her living pattern

to relieve tension.

A similar tension problem can challenge the potential fatherhood of the husband. He may appear to lose his sex drive or suffer from impotency because of stress related to his job. The solution may be a second honeymoon to remove the couple from a stressful environment, or a willingness to accept a lower standard of living until financial security is truly established. Keeping up with the Joneses may put an extra car in the garage, but the penalty might be an empty crib in the nursery.

TIMING OVULATION: Occasionally, the reason for infertility may be something as basic as timing. Because of misinformation or misapplication of the correct information, husbands and wives may time their intercourse so the husband's sperm does not enter the female reproductive organs during the 24 hours or so of the menstrual cycle in which the ovum is most likely to become fertilized. The wife's menstrual cycle must be watched with extreme care so that the time of ovulation can be judged. Ovulation takes place 14 days before menstruation. In women with a 28-day cycle, ovulation would occur approximately 14 days after the previous period. Women with longer cycles ovulate later in the cycle.

If the couple is in the habit of having rather frequent intercourse, including at the time of ovulation, they should abstain for a few days before the expected day of ovulation so the sperm count in the husband can build up to a higher level. Then, at the time of ovulation, the couple should have intercourse at least twice with an interval of six to eight hours between. For further assurance of success, the wife should lie on her back with her legs flexed following intercourse so that a pool of sperm will remain near the cervix.

REPRODUCTIVE INCOMPATIBILITY: Still another factor that can interfere with normal fertility is that of reproductive incompatibility, or an immune reaction, between sperm and ovum. This reaction between the male and female cells is similar to an allergic one, and may happen in one or two ways. In the more complicated case of reaction between the sperm and the egg cell, the ovum may treat the sperm as a bit of foreign tissue which it will reject. There is at present no foolproof remedy for this problem, but medical scientists are investigating it.

In the second type of situation, there can be an incompatible reaction between the acid environment of the female reproductive tract and the alkaline male sperm. Although the lining of the vagina usually is acid, it normally becomes alkaline at the time of ovulation to facilitate the survival of the sperm on its way to the cervix. But in some cases, the vagina remains acid enough to kill or immobilize the sperm. In cases of couples unable to have children for this reason, chemicals can be introduced into the vagina to neutralize its acidity.

The Fertility Examination

Although it has been popular for centuries to hold the female partner responsible for childless marriages, the male is just as likely to be the infertile one. But the ego of the man is often such that he may refuse to admit that he is infertile until it has been proved that the wife is indeed capable of bearing children. The easiest way to check out the causes of infertility is to submit to a series of tests by a physician.

The physician giving the tests may be a general practitioner or a specialist. There are two types of specialists who concentrate on the female reproductive system—the *gynecologist* and the *obstetrician.* The gynecologist is a physician who specializes in the care and treatment of women, especially of the reproductive organs; an obstetrician specializes in the birth process. Since the areas of responsibility frequently overlap, the same doctor often handles both specialties and is referred to as an *Ob-Gyn* doctor.

Fertility examinations usually require a series of at least four visits by the wife over a period of about three months, and a similar series of visits by the husband. Both husband and wife usually attend the first meeting, when the doctor explains some of the common causes of infertility and outlines the rules for the tests to be performed.

Next, the physician schedules separate conferences with the marital partners so that he can obtain information which husband and wife might be reluctant to discuss in each other's presence. This discussion might touch upon possible venereal diseases of earlier years, previous marital experiences, possible illegitimate pregnancies, and so on. The medical records also will include information about general health, diet, surgery, or diseases such as mumps (which might affect fertility), sex interests and practices, family histories of miscarriages or abnormal children, and contraceptive methods used.

BASAL BODY TEMPERATURE: The doctor will often suggest that the wife begin the BBT, or Basal Body Temperature charts. Using a special thermometer, the BBT is taken each morning at the same hour, before getting out of bed or having a first cigarette, which would alter the results. The BBT record is a remarkably accurate way of determining the day of ovulation, because ovulation causes a sudden rise in temperature. If there is no sudden rise in temperature during the menstrual cycle, it is an indication that no ovum was released by the ovary. If the temperature rises to indicate ovulation and remains elevated for over two weeks, it suggests that a pregnancy has begun. There are factors that can distort the readings, such as a fever or a mistake in reading the thermometer, but in general the BBT charts provide a reliable guide to the fertility cycles of the female partner.

SEMEN EXAM: On the second visit to the doctor, the husband is usually asked to bring a sample of semen in a corked bottle. The husband is generally advised to avoid intercourse for at least 48 hours before collecting the semen. The glass container of semen must be protected from heat and cold, and for this reason should be carried in a paper bag to help insulate it from external temperature variations. A condom should not be used to collect or carry the semen because most rubber prophylactics contain chemicals that are harmful to spermatozoa.

The sperm examination should be made within an hour or so after it is collected so the spermatozoa will be nearly as alive and healthy as they are at the time of intercourse. If for some reason the results are not conclusive, the husband will be asked to bring another sample of semen when he accompanies his wife on her third visit, which will be scheduled about four weeks later.

During the second visit, both husband and wife may be given physical examinations, with emphasis on the pelvic and genital areas. Laboratory tests of blood and urine are made, and the examining physician may decide to make a study of thyroid function.

TUBAL INSUFFLATION: The doctor generally tries to schedule the third visit to coincide with the 12th day of the wife's menstrual cycle. The examination at that time may include a *tubal insufflation* test. Also known as *Rubin's test*, tubal insufflation involves the injection of carbon dioxide gas, or sometimes ordinary air, into the uterus. Normally, the gas passes up through the uterus and Fallopian tubes and exits into the abdominal cavity. This would be a sign that the tubes are not obstructed. A pressure gauge shows a drop in pressure as the gas passes into the abdominal cavity, and the doctor may listen through a stethoscope for sounds of gas escaping through the tubes. The tubes are very narrow, and even a mild infection or scar tissue from a past infection can block them. Sometimes, forcing gas through the tubes is all that is needed to open them again so that chances of pregnancy will be enhanced.

A fourth visit, scheduled about four weeks after the third, should occur just before normal ovulation

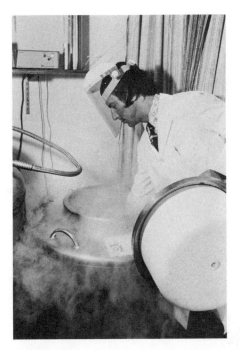

Vials of semen intended for artificial insemination are frozen and stored until ready for use. The donor's semen will be introduced into the female recipient's reproductive tract during ovulation.

time. The couple may be instructed to perform intercourse about six hours before the visit. The tubal insufflation test may be repeated if the results of the earlier test were not satisfactory. In addition, a study of the cervical mucus may be made. In this study, the mucus is stretched into thin fibers or strands, which is possible only at the time of ovulation. During most of the reproductive cycle, the mucus is thick, dense, and jellylike. But the presence of estrogen hormones at the time of ovulation changes the mucus so that it makes a fibrous, fernlike pattern when placed on a glass slide.

The cervical mucus is also studied for the presence of active sperm. By using a high-power microscope, the examining physician can tell whether the cervical secretions are hostile to sperm. This would be the case if an adequate number of sperm are present, but are inactive or dead. The tests can be verified by placing a bit of semen on a microscope slide next to a sample of cervical mucus.

HYSTEROGRAM: If the tests up to this point have not revealed the cause of infertility, the doctor (or a recommended radiologist) can inject a special oil into the uterus and tubes and follow its path through the reproductive organs by an X-ray procedure called a *hysterogram*. If there is an obstruction or even a kink in the tubes that might interfere with the movement of an ovum, it should appear in the X-ray photographs, and the doctor can then treat the problem accordingly.

FIBROIDS: The hysterogram may also reveal the presence of *fibroids*, benign tumors composed of fibrous tissue which usually attach themselves to the walls of the uterus. Fibroids come in varying sizes—from smaller than a pea to larger than a fist—and are present in varying degrees in about 30 percent of all women. Depending on where they occur, they may block conception, in which case they can be removed by surgery.

OTHER PROCEDURES: Depending on what cause of infertility is suspected, the physician may recommend that the wife undergo a *culdoscopy, peritoneoscopy,* or *laparotomy*. The culdoscopy and peritoneoscopy require only a local anesthetic and a brief hospital stay. In the culdoscopy procedure, tubes are used to examine the pelvic organs without making a surgical incision. In the peritoneoscopy, a small incision is made just below the umbilicus. A laparotomy refers to any procedure involving an incision in the abdominal wall. Depending on the nature of the problem, a laparotomy and, to a lesser extent, the other two procedures, allow the gynecologist latitude to make some on-the-spot corrections.

The physician may also decide to do an examination of tissue cells from the vagina or the testicles of the husband in an effort to find out what is causing infertility.

In general, the chances of success in the treatment of infertility vary with the severity of the abnormality and the length of time the disorder has gone untreated. Most minor problems can be treated by surgery, restoring normal hormone balance, proper diet, psychotherapy, or other methods, such as a change in the techniques or frequency of intercourse.

REPRODUCTIVE   TECHNOLOGY: The science of *reproductive technology* offers other ways of achieving fertilization and parenthood. In all cases, the new methods require that a third party enter, at least indirectly, into the reproductive relationship. The following techniques range from the very simple to the very complex:

In vitro fertilization (IVF) is the process that produces test-tube babies. A doctor removes an egg from the woman's ovary and places it in a shallow dish filled with a special nutritional "bath." Some of the husband's sperm is added to the bath. If the egg becomes fertilized it is allowed to grow for a few days, then implanted in the woman's uterus to

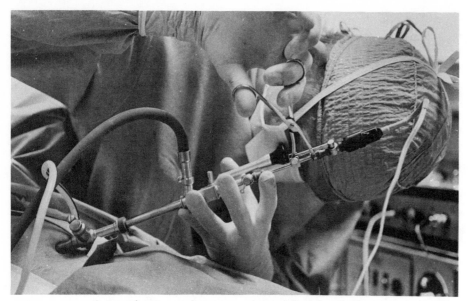

A gynecologist uses a laparoscope, inserted through an incision, to view a woman's reproductive system and pinpoint problems.

nor, not that of the husband, is used to fertilize the volunteer "mother." Again the embryo is flushed out after a few days; the embryo is then implanted in the wife for gestation and delivery.

Many couples have specific personal reasons for using one of these methods of reproducing. The wife may, for a variety of physical reasons, be unable to conceive or carry a child. One spouse or the other may have inherited genetic defects that the couple do not want to pass on to their children. Two such defects are Huntington's chorea and hemophilia, for example.

complete the gestation process.

Artificial insemination by donor (AID) is the injection by syringe of a donor's sperm into the woman's vagina. Injection takes place shortly before the woman is scheduled to ovulate. In such cases the husband's sperm, for one reason or another, cannot be used.

Surrogate motherhood occurs when a woman carries to term and delivers a child for another woman. The surrogate mother is first inseminated with the sperm of a husband whose wife cannot, for health or physical reasons, conceive and bear the child. After delivery, the surrogate mother signs for adoption by the husband and wife.

Egg donation involves removal of an egg from one woman for implantation in another. In some cases the transferred egg can be fertilized by the husband's sperm in natural intercourse. Following gestation, the baby is delivered through normal childbirth or caesarian section.

In *artificial embryonation* (AE) an infertile wife agrees to carry to term the embryo developed briefly in another woman's womb. In artificial embryonation, the childless couple form an agreement with the second woman, who is then inseminated with the husband's sperm. The em-

bryo is allowed to develop for four or five days; doctors then try to flush out the growing embryo for implantation in the wife.

Embryo adoption (EA) is a procedure similar to artificial embryonation. But in EA the sperm of a do-

The Expectant Mother

In most marriages there is no problem of infertility. A majority of women between the ages of 20 and 25 become pregnant during the first year of marriage. And that includes a substantial number who have tried to prevent conception with various

THE FETAL ENVIRONMENT IN THE UTERUS

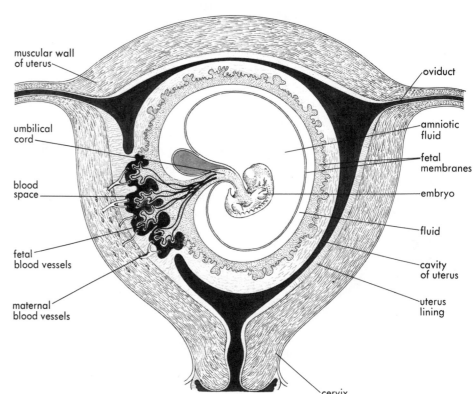

birth control methods. The fertility prospects usually continue to be satisfactory for women up to the age of 35, but the chances decline for women in their late 30s.

When pregnancy does occur, it should be regarded as a natural process rather than a confining illness. Although some of the bodily functions are altered by approaching motherhood, it should be remembered that women have been bearing children for thousands of years, and the chances for a safe and successful delivery were never better than today.

The expectant mother can look forward to hearing a variety of old wives' tales about the hazards of pregnancy from well-meaning friends. But unless there are complications, there is no reason for anxiety. And many of the complications can be prevented or corrected with good medical care. The woman preparing for motherhood generally can relax and enjoy the state of pregnancy if she follows basic rules of health and hygiene.

Drugs and Cigarettes

Many obstetricians recommend that women refrain from taking any medications, including patent medicines such as cold remedies, during the first three months of pregnancy unless the medicine is essential for the preservation of the mother's health. There are a number of chemical substances in drugs which may or may not affect the development of the embryo. An example of the unfortunate results of drug use during the early months of pregnancy was that of thalidomide, used by a number of women in 1961–1962. The drug was one of the safest sedatives ever developed. But when used by pregnant women, thalidomide caused physically deformed babies.

Should an expectant mother smoke? A study of more than 16,000 pregnancies shows that mothers who smoke cigarettes are more likely to have stillborn babies, premature babies, and babies who are below average in weight than non-smoking mothers. Other researchers have found that cigarette smoking stimulates contractions of the uterus, which could lead to premature birth. Mothers who smoke are also more likely to have spontaneous abortions or miscarriages.

Diet and Digestion

Acute dietary deficiencies also can affect the development of an unborn child. As the fetus develops, its growth rate is tremendous—the weight gain is as high as 650 percent per month after the unborn child has passed the third month in its mother's uterus. All of the nutrients needed for fetal growth must be taken from the mother's own diet and transmitted through the placenta. If the food eaten by the mother is not sufficient to sustain both mother and child, it is frequently the child who suffers.

This does not mean, however, that an expectant mother should eat double-sized meals because she has to feed two bodies. Obesity can be nearly as great a hazard to normal pregnancy as not eating enough. Overweight women should curb their food intake with such dietary shortcuts as drinking skim milk and eliminating as many fats and carbohydrates as possible. Meals should include a high level of proteins and all the essential minerals and vitamins. The number of total calories should not be less than 1,800 per day, unless the doctor recommends otherwise.

The rule of thumb on weight gain for a pregnant woman is that she should be about 20 pounds heavier at the end of the nine months than she was before conception. The rate of gain is important. It should be held to around one pound per month during the first three months, and between two and three pounds per month during the last six months.

Throughout the pregnancy, cravings for such foods as strawberries, ice cream, pickles, or whatever, are usually caused by psychological reasons rather than physical ones. However, if the food items craved are nutritious and low in calories, there is nothing wrong with satisfying the whim. Pickles, incidentally, are lower in calories and richer in vitamin C, iron, and other nutrients than most other snack foods.

HEARTBURN: Many mothers experience heartburn during pregnancy, and investigators have found that the treatment should be related to the length of time the mother has been carrying the unborn child. Heartburn during the first trimester, or three-month period, is usually due to anxiety and tension. If the symptoms are severe, the doctor may prescribe antacids or tranquilizers. Heartburn during the last six months is usually due to the crowding of the enlarged uterus within the abdomen, which lessens stomach capacity. The solution in such cases is to eat a number of smaller meals during the day rather than three large ones. Expectant mothers with heartburn should also use additional pillows so they sleep with the head and shoulders higher than the rest of the body, avoid tight clothing that squeezes the abdominal area, and not stoop or bend over after eating.

MORNING SICKNESS: Morning sickness, characterized by nausea and vomiting, is one of the most common complaints of mothers-to-be. Although it is unpleasant, morning sickness rarely becomes so serious that special medical treatment is needed. While friends and relatives may try to convince the expectant mother that the sick feeling is all in her mind—and she certainly may feel some anxiety about her pregnancy—there is good evidence that there is also a physical cause. The level of gastric acid in the pregnant woman's stomach declines during the first trimester of pregnancy. Also, stomach activity during that period is at a low ebb, and digestion is one to two hours slower after a meal than before pregnancy.

In most cases of morning sickness, the mother is unable to hold down her breakfast. The feeling of nausea usually subsides by lunch time, and does not appear again until the following morning. For the majority of women, the feeling fades away entirely by the 12th week. If it continues into the last two trimesters, the condition may not be related to the pregnancy.

Food for periods of morning sickness should include crackers and dry toast, lemonade or soft drinks served at cold temperatures, and hot soup, tea, or coffee. Items to be avoided are greasy foods and liquids that are only lukewarm.

Toxemia of Pregnancy

The expectant mother should visit her doctor as often as recommended and follow instructions carefully. She should report to her doctor any signs of puffiness of the hands and face, headaches, or visual disturbances that she experiences. Such signs and symptoms, especially in the last trimester of pregnancy, suggest *toxemia*. It is one of the most serious complications of pregnancy, and it affects about five percent of all expectant mothers.

Toxemia of pregnancy is a catch-all term that covers *hypertension*, or abnormally high blood pressure, and *edema*, or swelling of tissues due to fluid accumulation. Other symptoms are weight gain, *proteinuria*, or excretion of protein, and, in severe cases—when the disorder is sometimes called *eclampsia*—convulsions and loss of consciousness. Toxemia in late pregnancy is called *preeclampsia*.

Weight gain can amount to over two pounds a week and may be due almost entirely to fluid retention. Proteinuria usually does not appear until after high blood pressure and weight gain have appeared. But even these clinical signs may develop before the mother-to-be knows that she has toxemia. As the problem progresses, she may have visual disturbances, puffy eyelids, headaches, and abdominal pains. When the latter symptoms occur the disease is rather well established.

The cause of toxemia is believed to be a failure of the mother's body to adjust to the metabolic and physiological stresses of pregnancy. With careful management, toxemia can be controlled with the help of drugs, regulation of weight gain and fluid intake, bed rest, and in some cases by early delivery of the baby. The fact that delivery of the child seems to resolve the problem of toxemia reinforces the theory of metabolic-physiologic relationships in the stresses of pregnancy in some women.

During pregnancy a number of complex changes take place in the mother's body—a different pattern of hormone activity, alterations in the glands secreting hormones, increased blood supply with greater demands on the heart, and a rapidly growing parasitic human in the uterus, which also grows and presses against other organs within the body. Each woman reacts somewhat differently to these changes, and toxemia is one of the reactions.

Backaches and Other Disorders

Some expectant mothers are concerned about whether the baby should be carried high or low. There is a belief among some women that a baby carried high will be a boy. The truth is that no single pregnancy is either high or low for the entire nine months. Some babies seem to be carried higher at certain stages of pregnancy while at other times they seem to be carried low. The position has nothing to do with the sex of the child.

Where the baby is carried also has nothing to do with a common complaint associated with pregnancy—backache. Backache in pregnant women is usually caused by changes in posture, and only rarely by abnormality of the organs within the pelvis. Usually it is due to bending, lifting, or walking without properly compensating for the added strain of the weight of the child, especially in the later stages of pregnancy. Generally, backache responds to rest, heat, and drugs,

which relax the muscles—although the drugs should be used only on a doctor's recommendation. The physician also may recommend that a lightweight maternity girdle be worn to help minimize the strain.

Improper posture in the final weeks may also be responsible for numbness and tingling or crawling sensations in the hands and arms. The hand-and-arm complaints frequently are related to what is called the *lordotic posture*, where shoulders are slumped, the spine curved forward, and the neck bent forward. The tingling sensations usually vanish when the posture is corrected. Exercises are used to help change the lordotic positioning of the spine and shoulders.

The mother-to-be must be careful about the use of seat belts when traveling by automobile or airplane. In the final months of pregnancy the belt should be fitted snugly around the lower third of the abdomen to protect the uterus from the steering wheel or dashboard in the event of an accident or sudden stop.

PELVIC X RAY: Occasionally, a doctor will want to have X rays made of the pelvis of the mother to determine whether it is adequate to permit an uncomplicated childbirth. There is little hazard in a brief diagnostic X ray if modern equipment is used. Nevertheless, the mother should avoid exposure to unnecessary X rays, particularly during the first three months of pregnancy. Embryonic tissue is highly sensitive to radiation because the cells have not reached the degree of differentiation found in the fetus in the later months of pregnancy. In other words, the embryo's tissues are much more likely to be adversely affected by radiation.

INFECTION OF THE URINARY TRACT: Urinary tract disturbances are not unusual during pregnancy, and may be recurrent in women who were treated for kidney or bladder infections before pregnancy. It is not unusual for women to void as frequently as once an hour or oftener, and half a dozen times during the

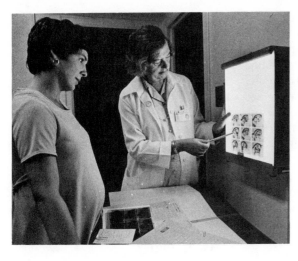

A doctor uses pelvic X-rays to explain fetal development to a pregnant woman.

night. The disorder may be accompanied by fever and a burning sensation while voiding the urine. But most cases respond to the medications and special hygiene instructions prescribed by the doctor.

Leg Cramps and Varicose Veins

Leg cramps and varicose veins affect a significant number of pregnant women. Leg cramps are the most common problem, and probably 85 percent of expectant mothers experience an occasional spasm of the calf muscles while carrying a child. The leg cramps may occur suddenly and be quite painful; at other times, the cramp may feel more like a simple kink in the muscles. The cramps occur more frequently in the last three months of pregnancy and are more likely to be experienced during a second or third pregnancy than during the first. Sluggish blood circulation and a dietary deficiency of calcium are thought to be the causes of leg cramps. The treatment consists of applying heat to the legs, massaging them, and sitting or lying down with the legs elevated. Drinking fortified milk will add calcium and vitamin D to the diet. In severe cases, muscle-relaxing drugs may be prescribed.

Varicose veins are more likely to appear during the second or third pregnancy, and tend to disappear after the birth of the baby. They are caused by a pooling of blood in the veins of the legs. Normally, the contraction of the leg muscles during walking has the effect of pumping blood from the legs back up toward the heart. But just the strain of standing can produce varicose veins even in normally active people who are on their feet for long periods. The strain of pregnancy also can upset the normal return flow of blood in the legs, so the veins become dilated. As with leg cramps, some relief can be had by sitting or lying with the feet raised. Additional relief can be obtained by wearing elastic stockings. If the varicosities remain after pregnancy, they can be treated by drugs or surgery.

Immunization

There are certain facts about immunization that a woman should know if she contemplates pregnancy. One is that the mother's reaction to smallpox vaccine can be transmitted through the placenta to the fetus. The disease can be fatal to an unborn child. Fortunately, smallpox has been eradicated from almost all areas in the world, and vaccination is no longer routinely required for travel abroad.

If the mother plans to be pregnant during the winter months, she should arrange to receive a series of influenza shots beginning in September and ending by mid-December. If she has been immunized against influenza within the past two years, a booster shot should be sufficient.

Rubella, or German measles, can be a serious threat to the normal development of a baby if contracted during the first 12 weeks of pregnancy. The rubella vaccine normally given to children should be given to women of childbearing age only with caution. Some medical scientists believe that the virus can be transmitted by the vaccine to the fetus if conception occurs within two months after the vaccine is given. If the virus infects the unborn child, particularly during the first trimester, the child may be afflicted with cataracts, deafness, or damage to the heart and nervous system.

Immunizations should also be obtained for diphtheria, malaria (if in an area where this is common), and mumps. If these diseases occur during pregnancy they result in spontaneous abortion in about one-third of the cases.

Tetanus is regarded as one of the most serious complications of pregnancy. The period of incubation for tetanus is shorter in pregnant than in nonpregnant women. It is particularly hazardous during the period immediately after abortion or childbirth. But the threat can be avoided by receiving proper tetanus immunization before pregnancy.

The Rh Factor

Blood incompatibilities between the mother and father can be another complication of pregnancy. The condition is caused by a blood protein known as the *Rh factor*. A person whose blood contains the protein is called *Rh-positive; Rh-negative* people lack the blood factor. Approximately 85 percent of the population is Rh-positive. The term *Rh* is derived from the first two letters of the name of the Rhesus monkey, a laboratory animal which was used for much of the basic research on the blood incompatibility problem.

About ten percent of all marriages in the United States involve an Rh conflict. If both husband and wife are either Rh-positive or Rh-negative, there is no problem. But if the wife has Rh-negative blood and her husband Rh-positive, the child of such a union may be threatened by death or mental retardation, particularly after the first pregnancy.

The Rh factor is inherited, and if the unborn offspring inherits the Rh-positive factor from its father while the mother has Rh-negative blood, the mother's blood may develop antibodies that destroy the baby's blood. The threat to the unborn child can be modified by a blood transfusion to the newborn infant or to the fetus before birth. The mother can also in effect be immunized against the development of antibodies by the injection of a gamma globulin blood fraction rich in passive Rh antibodies.

Usually, the first child is not affected by Rh blood conflicts. The red blood cells of the fetus can cross the placenta and trigger the reaction in the mother's blood system. But they do not reach their peak of entry into the mother's blood supply until the time of delivery. Thus, to prevent sensitization of the mother, doctors must eliminate the fetal red cells around the time of delivery— before the buildup of antibodies can begin. Once the antibodies have developed in the mother's blood, all future Rh-positive babies will be threatened unless preventive steps are taken.

If the husband of an Rh-negative woman has Rh-negative blood, or if he carries genes for both Rh-negative and Rh-positive, the baby will probably inherit the Rh-negative factor, and there will be no blood conflict. In nearly every case of Rh conflict today the baby can be saved and the production of antibodies suppressed in the mother. But the blood of both parents should be checked at the start of pregnancy plans, and arrangements made to protect the fetus if there is a threat of blood incompatibility.

Genetic Counseling

The genetic background of each marital partner has an influence on the fetus, since hereditary factors have a tendency to show up in the offspring. In addition to desirable hereditary traits, over 1,200 congenital defects have been catalogued. However, genetic factors do not always appear in a new generation, and environmental influences do not always affect mothers in the same manner. During the thalidomide episode of the 1960s, for example, only 20 percent of the pregnant women who used the drug had deformed babies; the other 80 percent had normal offspring.

While the expectant mother should take all normal precautions and follow her doctor's orders faithfully with regard to diet, hygiene, and exercise, if she and her husband have normal family histories she should not be concerned with congenital birth defects. However, there are cases where there is cause for legitimate worry about the chances of an inherited disorder. If there are cases of cystic fibrosis, phenylketonuria (PKU), sickle-cell anemia, or other genetic diseases in the background of either prospective parent; if the prospective mother is over 40 (at which age there is an increased chance of giving birth to a child afflicted with Down's syndrome or Mongolism); or if the parents or others in the family have previously given birth to a mentally retarded child, then it is recommended that the couple seek the advice of a genetic counselor.

Genetic counseling is available through a network of genetic counseling and treatment centers which were set up to help couples who are planning a family but are troubled by the possibility that their children may be born with a genetic disorder. When the wife gets pregnant a prenatal diagnosis is made. This procedure, known as amniocentesis, involves obtaining a small sample of the amniotic fluid that surrounds the fetus by inserting a hypodermic needle through the abdominal wall. The sex of the fetus can also be determined by this method, and since many inherited disorders are sex-linked (for example, transmitted only from mother to son), this information can be critically important. If the fetus is found to be affected with the suspected disorder a therapeutic abortion is performed, if so desired by the parents. Those interested in consulting a genetic counselor should write to the National Genetics Foundation, Inc., 250 West 57th Street, New York, New York 10019.

Miscarriage

About ten percent of all pregnancies end in a miscarriage, often called a spontaneous abortion. A miscarriage can occur for a variety of reasons, many of which are related. Some of the reasons may be hormone malfunction or deficiency; a faulty sperm or ovum, which would, in the vast majority of cases, result in a cruelly malformed child or one incapable of staying alive if the pregnancy were carried to term; a poor endometrium, or lining of the uterus, in which the ovum is implanted; changes in the mother's body chemistry; or other factors that interfere with normal development of the child within the uterus.

Hormone Deficiency

Hormone malfunction is responsible for many spontaneous abortions. Once the placenta is established on the inner wall of the uterus, it ordinarily produces sufficient hormones to maintain the pregnancy. But the condition of the endometrium at the time the embryo becomes implanted in the uterine wall affects the later development of the placenta. That situation, in turn, may affect the secretion of the hormones needed to continue the pregnancy. The level of one hormone, called the human chorionic gonadotropic hormone, is frequently used as a barometer of the condition of the uterus. When the amount of that hormone excreted in the urine suddenly decreases, it is a warning signal that

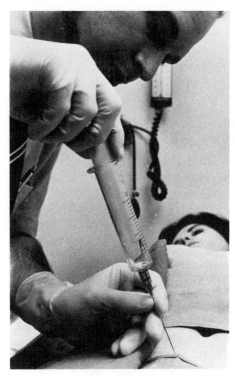
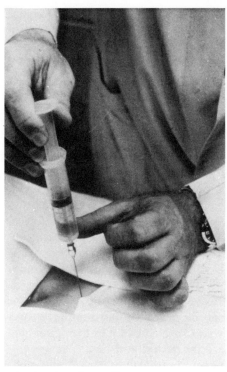

Amniocentesis, shown here, refers to the drawing of a small amount of amniotic fluid from a pregnant woman. Examination of fetal cells in the fluid can tell whether the fetus is genetically defective.

spontaneous abortion may be imminent.

Other physiological barometers are thyroid function and the rate of excretion of a substance known as sodium pregnanediol. Normally, there is a rise in thyroid activity when a woman becomes pregnant. The level remains elevated as long as the pregnancy continues, declining when the pregnancy is terminated either by delivery of a child or abortion. The expectant mother who has an underactive or overactive thyroid gland needs special medical attention because the hormone secreted by the gland seems to influence both the ovaries and the pituitary gland. Thyroid dysfunction is associated with infertility and the tendency toward spontaneous abortions.

Hormone deficiencies can contribute to the failure of the ovaries to produce thriving ova. In younger girls, the ovaries may be too immature to yield ova that are capable of continuing life after they are fertilized. In older women, the egg cells may be faulty because of approaching menopause. Even if the egg cell is perfect, defective sperm from the husband may be responsible for failure of the egg cell to develop into a healthy embryo after fertilization.

Still another cause of spontaneous abortion related to unfavorable hormone levels is the infantile or underdeveloped uterus, which may not have the capacity to maintain the fetus as it grows toward normal size for delivery. The undersized uterus can be treated with a hormone, estrin, to make it large enough to sustain a full-term pregnancy.

Other Causes of Miscarriage

Fibroid tumors or polyps in the uterus can interfere with both conception and pregnancy. Congenital malformations, such as a divided uterus, may also result in miscarriage. These problems can usually be corrected by surgery. A retroverted, malpositioned or tipped uterus can also be corrected to make carrying to term possible if this situation has caused a spontaneous abortion. An abnormality of the uterus called incompetent cervix used to be the cause of many spontaneous abortions in the last half of pregnancy, but in recent years a simple operation has been devised to correct the defect. See *Women's Health,* p. 483, for further information on gynecological problems.

Symptoms of Miscarriage

Spontaneous abortions usually are classified as threatened or inevitable. Generally, an abortion is considered to be of the threatened type when there is bleeding or cramps or both. Even when bleeding and cramps seem to be severe, it is possible that they will stop, or can be stopped, and the pregnancy will continue. If the bleeding and cramps become progressive and there is dilation of the cervix with the passage of tissue, the abortion is considered inevitable. Doctors sometimes can estimate the length of time that a spontaneous abortion has been progressing by examining the blood. If the blood is dark brown rather than bright red, it suggests that bleeding may have started at some time in the past. The longer the bleeding continues, the less chance there is that the fetus will survive.

Ectopic Pregnancy

Bleeding and cramping are not always signs of spontaneous abortion. Bleeding may be caused by a polyp or a malignant growth on the cervix. Cramps or bleeding can also occur if there is an *ectopic pregnancy,* a pregnancy outside the uterus. For example, the fertilized egg may become implanted in a Fallopian tube or even in the abdominal cavity instead of in the uterus. Many cases of ectopic pregnancy go undiagnosed because the symptoms are quite similar to those of a threatened abortion. Most ectopic pregnancies end in miscarriage when the pressure of the growing fetus causes the tube to rupture. In rare cases, the fetus may lodge in the abdominal cavity after rupture and continue to grow and develop. Such a fetus can be delivered by Caesarian techniques, but is thought to be extremely dangerous for the mother. Most physicians prefer to perform a therapeutic abortion if this situation occurs.

Trophoblastic Disease

In about one of every 1,500 to 2,000 pregnancies in the United States, the placenta degenerates into a *hydatidiform mole,* a benign tumor consisting of a mass of grapelike cysts. This condition is known as *trophoblastic disease,* in reference to the *trophoblast,* a layer of cells that develops around the fertilized ovum and contributes to the formation of the placenta.

Signs and symptoms of a hydatidiform mole generally appear one to two months after conception. They include nausea and vomiting, persistent bleeding from the uterus, and an increase in uterine size more rapid than normal. X rays fail to show a developing skeleton and there is no fetal heartbeat perceptible at the usual stage of pregnancy. X-ray arteriograms and ultrasound scanning of the uterus also reveal signs of the mole. Spontaneous

abortion commonly threatens and often occurs. Laboratory analysis of chorionic gonadotropic hormone levels in serum and vaginal smears are among other tests used to verify the presence of a hydatidiform mole.

The mole must be removed as soon as feasible after it has been identified, to decrease the chances of its invading the uterine wall and becoming cancerous. It is removed by surgical methods, such as suction curettage, or occasionally surgical excision. In those few cases in which the mole invades the uterus, the uterus is removed. Following a molar pregnancy that is neither invasive nor cancerous, a woman should be examined regularly for a year or so. Subsequent pregnancies are permitted and have every prospect of being successful. If the mole is invasive or cancerous, antitumor chemotherapy is essential. Occasionally, radiation therapy also is used.

Habitual Abortion

Among some women, spontaneous abortion occurs repeatedly and is known as habitual abortion. Habitual abortion usually threatens

at the same stage of each pregnancy, and the measures needed to prevent a repetition of the miscarriage should be started as soon as the expectant mother knows she is pregnant. The usual prenatal care should be followed conscientiously, including the rules about nutrition and exercise. Cigarette smoking should be curtailed or eliminated because, among other reasons, tobacco use seems to affect the carbohydrate metabolism of smokers, and pregnant women are particularly sensitive to changes in carbohydrate balance. The cells which form the placenta and fetal membranes require large amounts of carbohydrates that can be assimilated easily. Even before the fertilized egg cell becomes implanted in the lining of the uterus, the cells of the endometrium demand unusually large quantities of glycogen, or body starch, that has been converted to simple sugar molecules. Other nutrients are also needed, of course, but the demand for them is not as critical as that for carbohydrates.

Induced Abortion

Not all abortions are involuntary. The induced abortion is a deliberate interruption of the development of an embryo or fetus because of therapeutic or nonmedical reasons. Such an abortion, usually performed in a hospital or clinic, requires antiseptic conditions. Local anesthetics are used if needed. In the procedure called *dilation and curettage,* or *D and C,* the doctor enlarges the opening of the uterus to permit entry of the surgical tools used to scrape the lining of the uterus. The tissue is removed from the lining with a *curette,* a surgical instrument resembling a scoop with sharpened edges. Another method often used, called *vacuum aspiration,* employs suction to pull the embryonic tissue from inside the uterus. These techniques —the D and C and vacuum aspiration—can be used only during the first trimester of pregnancy.

If the abortion is delayed beyond

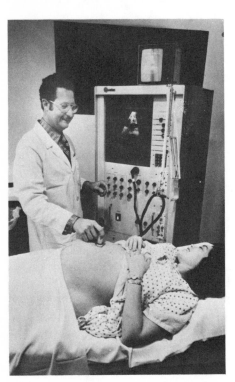

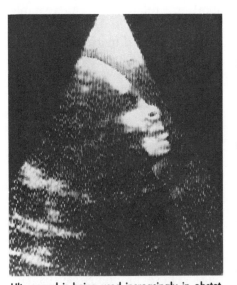

Ultrasound is being used increasingly in obstetrics and gynecology. The image of the fetus appears on the screen of an oscilloscope revealing stage of development and fetal position. Ultrasonic diagnosis can detect such irregularities as multiple births, breech presentation, tumors, and foreign matter in the uterine cavity.

the first three months, more complicated surgery may be required. An alternative method called *salting out* (medically, *saline amniocentesis*) involves the injection of a saline solution into the amniotic fluid. The salt water kills the fetus and induces labor, and the fetus is delivered, thus terminating the pregnancy. This method involves somewhat greater risk of complications than the other methods.

If an induced abortion is performed by a doctor in a hospital or clinic equipped with facilities to cope with possible complications—standard in states where induced abortion is legal—the procedure is safe, with very low risk of complications. The notion that women are rendered sterile or more likely to have spontaneous abortions or premature deliveries of wanted children in later years can be true; but this is so only in those cases where women went to illegal abortion mills and had the procedure performed under unsanitary conditions or by someone who was medically incompetent.

Approaching Delivery

When all is going well with a pregnancy—and it does in the vast majority of cases—a favorite guessing game becomes the prediction of delivery day. There are several ways in which to estimate the approximate birth date of the new addition to the family. One is to calculate 267 days from the date of conception. Another approach is to count 280 days from the first day of the last menstrual period. This method is easier, since women are more likely to know the date of the last menstrual period than the last time they ovulated. Still another method commonly used is to count back three months from the first day of the last menstrual period and add seven days. No matter what method is used it will probably be wrong, since surveys show that fewer than five percent of all babies arrive on the day they were expected. How-

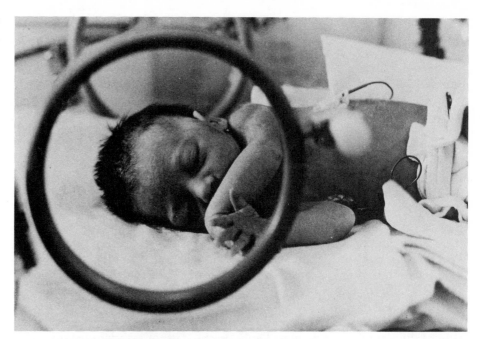

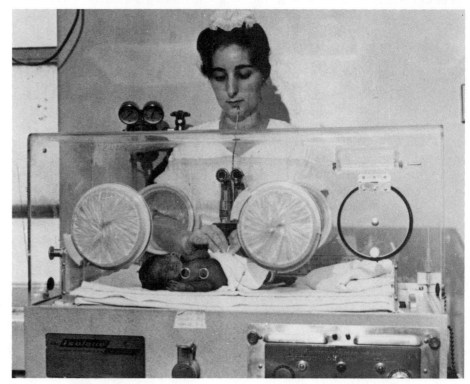

Premature babies need the specially controlled environment of an incubator *(bottom)* to regulate oxygen and reduce the risk of infection. Electronic monitors *(top)* keep a constant watch as the baby sleeps.

ever, the majority of babies are born within five days of the anticipated date.

As delivery day approaches, the doctor usually wants to make some last-minute studies of the position of the child and its general condition. He may also want to check the size of the bony area of the mother's pelvis in an effort to determine in advance whether there will be any complications in delivery. During the examination, the doctor usually looks for varicose veins around the vulva and vagina; they are a common occurrence among pregnant women, and some women claim they can tell when they are pregnant—even before a period is missed—by the appearance of these varicose veins.

By pressing the abdomen with the palms of his hands and his fingers, the doctor can determine the position of the unborn child in the uterus. He also can get a fair idea of the size of the fetus and can tell how low it is in the pelvic region. The doctor listens to the heartbeat of the fetus and, if labor is near, he may mark the position of the fetus on the skin of the mother's abdomen so that he can tell later if it has moved and in which direction.

In about half of all pregnant women, reddish streaks appear on the skin of the stretched abdomen. The streaks sometimes have the appearance of broken skin fibers due to stretching, but most doctors agree that the streaks are the result of hormone activity. It is another sign of a successful pregnancy.

In the final days before delivery, the doctor usually makes an estimate of the space through which the baby must move to reach the outside world. He also must make a rough guess about the weight of the baby at birth. If the baby weighs less than five pounds at birth it is *premature* by definition and may require special care which the doctor would want to schedule.

Lightening

The phenomenon of *lightening* is a sign that pregnancy is approaching an end and that birth can be expected within about three weeks. When lightening occurs, the mother feels less pressure on the upper part of the abdomen and more discomfort in the pelvic region as the head of the fetus descends toward the birth canal. Lightening may be accompanied by strong contractions of the uterus, which may be mistaken for labor pains. If lightening does not occur during the final weeks, the doctor may conduct further examinations to learn if the delay is due to a large fetus, twins (though a possible multiple birth is usually discovered earlier in the pregnancy), or another reason such as an unfavorable fetal position. When lightening does occur on schedule, the doctor usually assumes that the head of the fetus is low in the pelvic region and can pass through the birth canal without difficulty, since it has already completed the first part of the obstacle course to the outside world.

Fetal Position

With X rays and fetal electrocardiograms, it can be determined whether the unborn baby is upside down or in some other position in the uterus. A fetal electrocardiogram is made by placing electrodes on the mother's abdomen while she is lying on an examination table. The electrical impulses of the fetal heart muscle will produce a pattern revealing the direction of the heart which, in turn, tells which way the head is positioned. If the pattern indicates the head is toward the top of the abdomen rather than the bottom, a *breech presentation* can be expected in the delivery room.

Although 95 percent of all babies are in the head-downward position when labor begins, about three percent are in the more difficult breech presentation. Some doctors believe that a breech presentation is more likely if the fetus is delivered before term, since nearly 40 percent of the fetuses are in the breech presentation at the 20th week of pregnancy. However, this percentage declines as delivery day approaches, because the growing fetus finds it more comfortable to move its feet and bottom into the widest part of the pear-shaped uterus while the head fits into the narrow lower part.

Labor

The contractions of labor pains are something of a mystery. They are independent of the will of the mother. Women who are paralyzed or who feel no labor pains because of severed nerves can have a normal delivery. The uterus may even continue contractions automatically after it has been removed from the body.

First Stage of Labor

The first stage of labor is characterized by regular pains which may occur at intervals of 5 to 15 minutes.

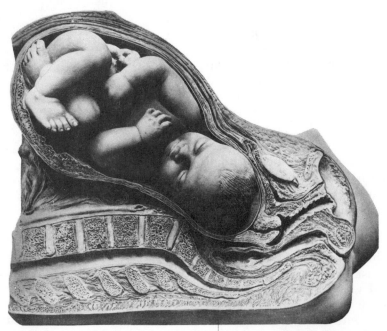

When labor begins, 95 percent of all babies are in the head-downward position. About three percent are in the more difficult breech presentation.

During this stage the cervix becomes dilated and forms a passageway into the vagina. There is a rest period between the labor pains which lasts at least a minute and gives the mother a brief respite while permitting the flow of oxygen to the fetus by way of the placenta. (If the uterine contractions were continuous they would cut off the baby's oxygen supply.) During uterine contractions, the uterus rises in the abdomen; the change in shape can be observed at the start and end of each labor pain.

The so-called *bag of waters*, which actually is the *amniotic fluid* within the membrane, may be discharged at almost any time during labor. Sometimes the bag of waters ruptures before the labor pains begin, but this usually occurs during one of the strong contractions. The fluid generally comes out with a gush, but it may also be discharged in small amounts with each contraction. The term dry labor is used to describe contractions that begin after the bag of waters has ruptured. Ordinarily, the contractions become stronger and more frequent and the cervix dilates more rapidly after the amniotic fluid has been discharged.

Occasionally, the baby is delivered with the amniotic membrane still intact about its head. The membrane in such a case is known

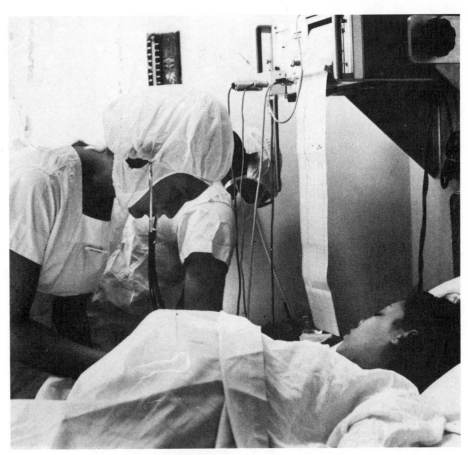

Fetal monitoring checks the baby's heartbeat so that potentially dangerous changes can be detected immediately and corrective measures taken.

as a *caul*. At one time, a caul was regarded as a symbol of great superstitious value; midwives sold cauls to sailors who carried them for good luck on voyages.

Second Stage of Labor

Rupture of the bag of waters frequently climaxes the first stage of labor, which may last over 12 hours if it is the first pregnancy. The second stage of labor is considerably shorter and can be expected to last around 2 hours in a first pregnancy, 30 minutes for a woman who has had children previously. The second stage may begin with rupture of the bag of waters if the amniotic fluid was not released earlier. The contractions are more intense and frequent, occurring at intervals of 2 to 3 minutes rather than the 5- to 15-minute intervals of the first stage. There also is a conscious desire on the part of the mother to help expel the fetus. She may feel additional pains, pressures, or irritations because of the presence of the fetus in the lower pelvic area.

During this series of labor pains the baby gradually makes it appear-

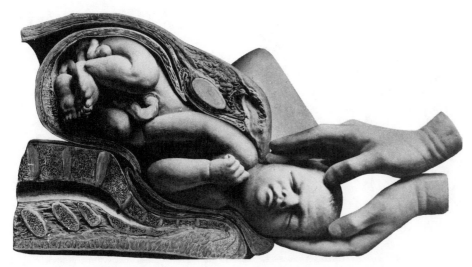

A representation of a baby in a normal delivery—showing the usual head position after it has squeezed through the birth canal.

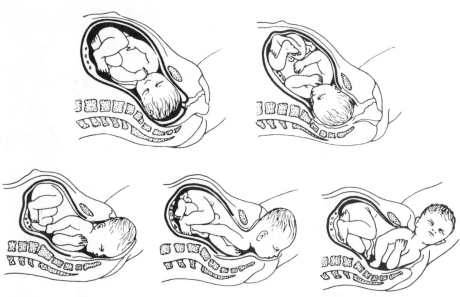

This sequence of drawings illustrates how a baby's head must squeeze through the narrow birth canal. Usually there is little danger of deformity, for the skull has not yet calcified, i.e., it is still soft.

ally one that affects only the part of the nervous system associated with pain. If the substance also affected the motor nerves, the delivery would become stalemated. On the other hand, it would be very simple to handle the childbirth in a satisfactory manner as far as the baby is concerned if the mother were given no relief from pain.

Drugs used as aids in childbirth include analgesics, tranquilizers, barbiturates, and the type of drugs used in so-called twilight sleep— scopolamine and morphine. They can be given orally or by injection. In nearly all cases the drugs are used with caution, and they are frequently administered in combination with a gas anesthetic.

The gases frequently used during delivery are nitrous oxide, which provides intermittent relief from pain during the second stage of labor, and cyclopropane, which may be administered for Caesarian sec-

ance outside the mother's womb. At first a bit of the scalp shows, then recedes as the labor pain subsides. With the next labor pain more of the head appears. Finally, the entire head is outside the mother's body, followed by the shoulders, trunk, and lower extremities.

Anesthetics and Drugs

Although it is standard practice to refer to the uterine contractions as labor pains, the amount of actual pain varies, and there are numerous methods for reducing the pain. True painless labor is rare, and when it occurs it is sometimes attributed to an abnormality of the nervous system.

The doctor is as concerned about the welfare of the mother and baby as the mother herself, and this concern is reflected in the approach taken to provide relief from labor pains. The drug or anesthetic the doctor chooses to use will be one that gives optimum relief to the mother without creating an environment in the womb that would threaten the life of the baby. A number of rather common drugs that could be used to relieve pain without harm to the mother could very easily be fatal to the infant, who would share through the

placenta substances injected into the mother's bloodstream.

The type of anesthetic or drug administered to the mother is usu-

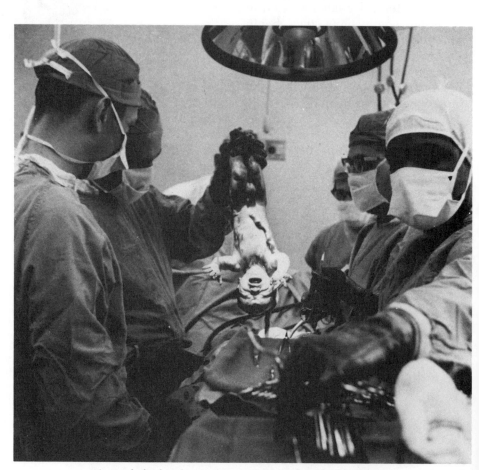

A new baby boy has just entered the world. The attending surgeon holds the baby upside down as it takes its first breath.

of specially trained personnel.

When delivery can be timed rather precisely, a spinal anesthetic, sometimes called a *saddle block*, is injected into the region of the spinal cord in the lumbar area while the mother is in a sitting position. After the injection, the mother lies on her back and, in most cases, is free of pain for the remainder of labor and delivery.

Natural Childbirth

Natural childbirth methods are preferred by some women who want to participate as consciously as possible in the act of bringing a child into the world. Others, by contrast, want to go into the delivery room completely anesthetized—to enter a pregnant woman and awaken as a mother. In natural childbirth, most women receive a local anesthetic for the *episiotomy* incision, to make the vaginal area large enough for passage of the baby, drugs to relieve tension when requested, and *oxytocin*. Oxytocin is a hormone naturally secreted by the pituitary gland to help the muscles of the uterus contract normally.

LAMAZE METHOD: A woman who chooses the natural childbirth technique developed by Dr. Ferdinand Lamaze conditions herself for labor pains by substituting a different response. Instead of crying out, for example, her response is a pattern of rapid, shallow breathing which she begins at the first sign of a uterine contraction. The conditioning exercises take about 30 minutes a day and should be started two months before the expected delivery date. Although some women who start natural childbirth training lessons are not able to complete the course for various reasons, most agree that they were better prepared for labor because of what they learned about the control of muscles and breathing.

Fathers-to-be are encouraged to participate in preparations for natural childbirth by coaching their spouses in breathing exercises and timing their contractions. Many

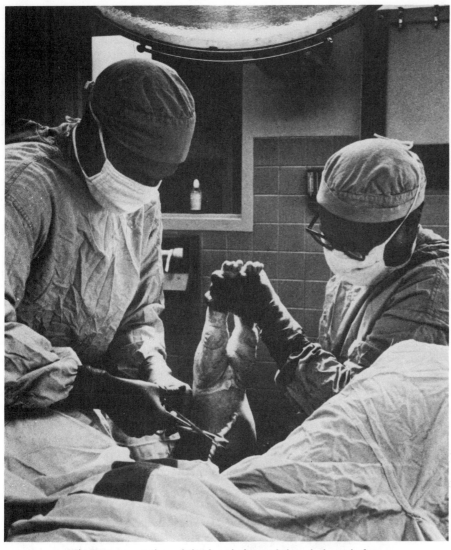

The surgeon cuts the umbilical cord of a newly born baby girl after the blood from the placenta has drained into the baby's body.

tion or cases of delivery in which there are complications requiring unconsciousness or deep analgesia (incapacity to feel pain). Nitrous oxide sometimes is provided during labor pains on signal from the mother. When she wants relief for a few moments or when she feels a pain starting, the mother signals the anesthetist, who places the mask over her face so she can take a few deep whiffs. The procedure is repeated when the next labor pain begins. Nitrous oxide may also be used in conjunction with ether or one of the other standard anesthetic gases. When properly administered, ether is safe and reliable for producing deep anesthesia or relaxation.

Still another anesthetic commonly used during delivery is a drug injected either for local anesthesia or for putting the mother to sleep for the period of delivery. Sodium pentothal is injected intravenously in many cases, particularly when forceps are used to assist in delivery. However, the doctor has to work fast in these cases, because this is one of the drugs that can be transmitted through the placenta in a short time.

A caudal anesthetic can be used to block pain in the entire pelvic area. In this case, a drug is injected into the area at the bottom of the spinal column. Most women who have had a caudal anesthesia like it as a means of obtaining relief from labor pains, but it requires the presence

hospitals now permit husbands to be with their wives during the second stage of labor in the hospital and even to be present in the delivery room.

Hypnosis sometimes is used instead of drugs or anesthetics for childbirth. But only a minority of women are able to accept the long period of training for the effective deep trance required, some applicants are not susceptible to hypnosis, and few obstetricians are adequately trained to control the hypnotic situation during delivery. Many doctors feel that the type of woman who would be a good subject for child delivery while hypnotized would get along just as well with the natural childbirth method.

LEBOYER METHOD: "The infant is like one possessed," writes Dr. Frederick LeBoyer of the moment preceding birth. "Mad with agony and misery, alone, abandoned, it fights with the strength of despair. The monster drives the baby lower still... The baby is now at the height of its travail. The effort required is too great. The end is surely near. Death seems certain. The monster bears down one more time, and it is then that...

"Then that everything explodes! The whole world bursts open. No more tunnel, no prison, no monster. The child is born."

In such terms Dr. LeBoyer focuses on the trauma that the child experiences at birth. The LeBoyer method seeks to train the mother to concentrate on that trauma while delivering her child. A form of natural childbirth, the technique also requires that silence or near-silence be maintained in the delivery room—to protect the newborn infant's ears and sensitivities.

"Relaxing, accepting the slow pace (of birth), letting it take command"—these responses on the mother's part lie at the heart of the LeBoyer method. When birth proceeds in this way, Dr. LeBoyer notes, the child enters the world

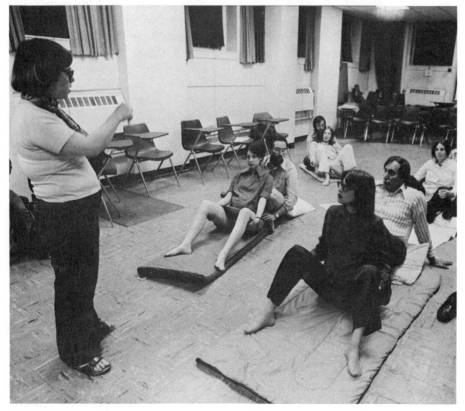

A baby being delivered by Caesarian section is shown here in a woodcut by an early 17th-century Venetian artist.

relaxed and already adjusted. The painful aspects of birth have been eliminated; both mother and child enter on the new relationship outside the womb with calm acceptance.

Like other approaches to natural childbirth, the LeBoyer method requires the full understanding and cooperation of the mother-to-be. The benefits of natural methods are said to be shorter periods of labor and reduced birth trauma. Natural childbirth is also said to reduce morbidity and mortality rates among newborn babies.

Caesarian Section

A Caesarian section may be performed in cases of diabetic mothers with rapidly growing fetuses, when delivery is complicated by breech or shoulder presentation, if the uterus is weak due to previous surgery or other reasons, or when the mother has a history of losing the child after carrying it to the time of delivery. There are several variations in Caesarian techniques, some requiring a general anesthetic and others using local anesthetics and other medications. But all approaches are

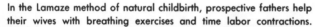

In the Lamaze method of natural childbirth, prospective fathers help their wives with breathing exercises and time labor contractions.

directed toward the same goal of saving the lives of both mother and baby. In nearly all instances, the uterus is closed after the baby and placental material are removed. Only in extremely rare cases is it necessary to remove the uterus. Most mothers who have Caesarians can have more children in the future if they so desire.

Third Stage of Labor

After the baby is delivered through the normal birth canal, the placenta is expelled by the same route. This is called the third, or placental, stage of labor. The placenta, also known as the *after-birth*, is connected to the baby by the umbilical cord. The cord is not cut until the blood has drained from the placenta into the baby's body; to help the flow the placenta is held above the level of the baby to get an assist from gravity.

Before the infant leaves the delivery room, it is examined for a normal heartbeat, possible abdominal distention or evidence of fluid in the abdominal region, possible abnormalities of the ears, and possible deformities of the mouth area, such as cleft palate or lip. The health of newborn babies is scored by the *Apgar system* when the baby is 60 seconds old. Five items of physical condition are noted and scored on a scale of 0 to 2. They are heart rate, muscle tone, respiration, nerve reflexes, and skin color. Babies that score 8 to 10 points are considered in excellent condition and are given routine postnatal care. If they score 7 points or less, additional measures are taken to get the infants off to a normal start in life. Since the system was started, nearly three-fourths of all newborn babies tested have passed with 8 points or more.

Breast and Bottle Feeding

Whether the infant is to be breast fed or bottle fed is usually a personal matter to be decided by

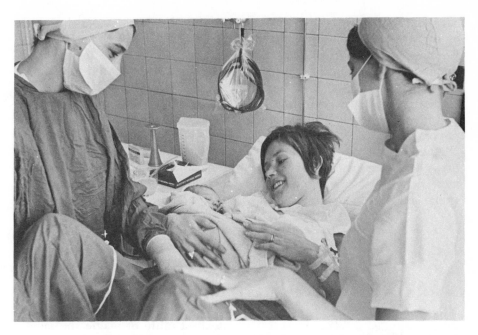

Few satisfactions equal that of a mother with her newborn. The long ordeal of labor is over, and at last she can turn her attention to the baby.

the new mother. For the average healthy baby, there are no obstacles to breast feeding if the mother desires it and is able to produce and deliver milk. A few women are unable to produce a sufficient supply of milk and most supplement their output with bottle feedings. In a few cases, babies are allergic to mother's milk, but in such instances the allergen can be identified and removed from the mother's diet.

Feeding problems are sometimes fewer and less serious among breast-fed babies. The mother's milk contains most of the necessary nutrients and is available when needed at the proper temperature. It also is more likely to be fresh and free of infectious bacteria than bottled milk.

The mother's milk during the first few days after birth is yellowish in color and rich in proteins and minerals. It is called *colostrum*, and is replaced gradually by regular human milk by the fourth week. Mother's milk is low in iron and may lack vitamins C and D. However, the baby arrives in the world with enough stores of iron in its tissues to last through the first few months of life. Compared to cow's

milk, human milk is richer in carbohydrates, but cow's milk has a greater proportion of proteins and minerals. The vitamin content of both mother's milk and cow's milk varies with the vitamin intake of each.

Mother's milk generally is more easily digestible in the baby's stomach than cow's milk, since the curd of mother's milk is fine and more rapidly metabolized. On the other hand, mothers who breast-feed sometimes suffer from fissuring or cracking of the nipples, *mastitis* (breast inflammation), or diseases which require temporary or permanent discontinuance of breast feeding.

Surveys indicate that more than three-fourths of babies today are bottle fed. Many mothers avoid breast feeding because they feel it is socially unacceptable, that it interferes with employment or social life, that it will affect their physical attractiveness, or because of fear of failure. For mothers who select bottle feeding over breast feeding, the procedure is much simpler today than in previous years. Many of the differences in nutritional values of mother's milk and cow's milk have been reduced or eliminated by improved formula development. Equipment for preparing the bottled meals is superior to that used in previous generations. And there is less danger today of bacterial infection from cow's milk because of improved dairy sanitation methods. New mothers who choose not to breast-feed are usually given hormones, along with ice packs and analgesics, to relieve any breast discomfort that may appear during the first few days.

If the mother wants to breast-feed the baby, plans should be made in advance of delivery. The first feeding can be started as soon after delivery as is feasible for both mother and child, usually within hours after birth. Although the first breast feeding can be delayed for several days, because of the stimulation of milk secretion immediately after delivery, the first ten days to two weeks are crucial in the establishment of a breast feeding program. The sucking reflex of the baby at the mother's breast triggers release of the hormone oxytocin, which in turn influences the release of another substance of the pituitary gland, prolactin, needed for the production of milk in the mother's breast. See also *Birth, Infancy, and Maturation*, especially, pp. 51–52.

MARRIAGE AND PARENTHOOD

Early Marriage

Although young newlyweds are ready physically for marriage, and can prove it by having babies, they are not always ready for the responsibilities of marriage. Often, the parents of the newlyweds have to contribute to the support of the family in one way or another. If the older generation can afford it, they may help the young couple to purchase a home or help them finance an apartment that would not otherwise be available to them. Sometimes the newlyweds will move into the home of the parents of the bride or the groom.

In the view of some experts, a number of teen-agers enter marriage as a kind of initiation into adulthood. These young couples marry not for sexual reasons but to satisfy a desire to have the status of adulthood. Although the average age of marriage for men and women has been rising in recent years, a substantial number of young people are still marrying before the age of 21. About 50 percent of teen-age marriages end in divorce within five years. The couples find that marriage and adult status do not offer the magic they had expected, and the bride and groom find themselves locked into a life which can be quite mundane and dull.

When the wife realizes that instead of a life of magic she faces a life of pots and pans and diapers, and the husband discovers that two cannot live as cheaply as one, arguments may evolve. Not all marriages of young couples are destined for failure, of course, and millions of unions that are threatened by divorce survive the rocky first years to develop into well-adjusted and realistic lifetime partnerships.

Marriage Counseling

At some point in the early years of marriage, the couple may decide to consult with someone outside their inner circle of friends and family when personal problems arise which defy an amicable solution. An outside point of view can be more objective, and the conflict may involve matters the couple would not want to discuss with family, friends, or a clergyman.

Rather than face separation or divorce, they can take their problems to someone professionally trained, such as a psychiatrist, psychologist, or a marriage counselor. However, they should be forewarned that solutions are not quick and easy. Several sessions, at least, may be needed. If the problems are serious enough to warrant professional help, the couple can expect that it will take time for a stranger to separate facts from emotions and develop a future course acceptable to both parties.

Selecting the right counselor can be a problem in itself, since not all counselors are equally qualified. A family doctor or a psychiatrist may be asked to give direct help or to make a referral. A counselor who uses systems or formulas, such as astrology charts or computer analysis, or who communicates by mail or telephone, should be avoided. Marital problems require a personal approach; it is unlikely that a marriage counselor could have simple solutions that might be applied to any couple who come to him with questions ranging from sexual incompatibility to the handling of family finances. The couple should also be suspicious of a counselor who offers a contract for his services or who suggests that a certain set number of sessions will be required.

Sexual Compatibility

According to a study made by the American Psychiatric Association, the typical newly-married American woman is not the mate-swapping, cocktail circuit, jet-set female portrayed in some movies and television dramas. She is emotionally well adjusted, average or above-average in physical attractiveness, content with her lot in life, and realistic about her social aspirations. She tends to idealize her husband and is confident of his fidelity. She does not try to dominate her husband; if she has children, they tend to be emotionally healthy.

Her husband is a well-adjusted, normal male whose responses to social and psychological tests are so similar to her own that psychiatrists are convinced that "like marries like." The couples experience deep, meaningful pleasures in stable relationships with each other and in raising their children.

Most of the wives, according to the study, married with full parental consent; more than 80 percent had a religious ceremony. The wives had reached approximately the same level of education as their husbands, tended to be of the same religious faith, and usually were of the same age or slightly younger than their husbands.

The Honeymoon

During the first weeks or months of marriage, the husband and wife have an opportunity to become better acquainted on an intimate basis. The honeymoon period usually provides ideal settings for intimate living, away from the daily pressures of earning a living and the social pressures of well-meaning friends and relatives. Even so, honeymoons frequently are disappointing, perhaps because of the disproportionate emotional investment in them. This does not, by any means, indicate that the marriage is doomed to fail.

Fatigue

After the honeymoon, both partners may suffer a bit from mental and physical fatigue in the evenings, particularly if both are employed; sexual intimacies might be fewer and less frequent than the couple had anticipated. The wife may be in the mood for sex play but the husband might be tired or distracted by financial worries. Or the husband may be in the mood, but

the wife may be too tired physically or emotionally upset. However, if fatigue serves as a frequent excuse for not having sexual relations, it may be rationalization, and the attitudes of both partners toward sex should be examined. One of the best ways to get the marriage off to a pleasant beginning is to make sure that the husband and wife can retire in the evening and leave the cares of the day for tomorrow.

Importance of Foreplay

Despite the seemingly open attitude toward sex among today's young people, many marital partners can be rather inept in the bedroom. If the sex act were a complicated procedure, the human race

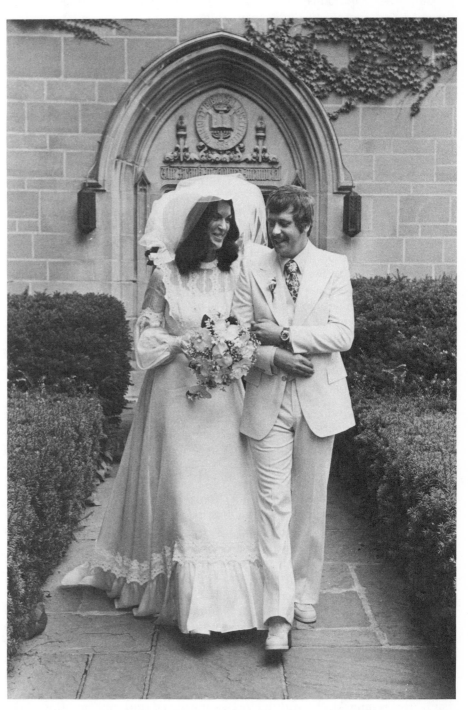

Despite changing social patterns and family roles, a picture of a bride and groom still evokes thoughts of love and hope for the future.

would not be around today. However, the many superstitions, fears, and restrictions superimposed upon a normal function almost from the time of birth until marriage can lead to emotional conflicts and frustrations when the young man and woman are face to face in a double bed.

If the husband does not take into account the importance of sexual foreplay and timing, the wife may not respond in the manner he expected, and he may reject her as frigid. Or the husband may experience premature ejaculation in his sexual excitement and complete the sex act before the wife has had time to respond. Premature ejaculation is one form of impotence. In another form, because of shyness or other psychological reasons, the man may not be able to sustain an erection.

The wife may not experience a true orgasm until after several months of marriage, and it may take the same amount of time for the husband to develop his techniques to the point where the wife is satisfied. The idea that practice makes perfect in *coitus*, or the sex act, may seem facetious, but it is nevertheless true. Patience and consideration for each other's preferences should result in a mutually pleasurable sexual adjustment.

Frigidity and Impotence

Only a small percentage of women fail to achieve orgasm eventually, and probably a smaller percentage of men remain impotent for an extended period of time. The most frequent cause of frigidity and impotency is psychological. For those who do feel frustrated in the sex act after many weeks or months of serious effort, advice should be sought from a psychotherapist, or the family doctor may make a referral to a doctor who specializes in this area of medicine. In some cases, impotence can be treated with drugs or medication. On the other hand, the wrong kinds of drugs or alcohol may interfere with normal sex functions.

Birth Control

Female frigidity can be caused by nothing more serious than fear of an unwanted pregnancy. If the couple has agreed to postpone starting a family or adding to it, the wife might feel insecure about her birth control method, especially if she depends upon a technique known to be less effective than the oral contraceptive.

Oral Contraceptives

Although "the pill," or *oral contraceptive*, has received a bad press in recent years, it probably ranks second only to sterilization as a birth control method. Oral contraceptives are composed of synthetic sex hormones; they are manufactured by pharmaceutical companies from substances found in plant materials such as Mexican yams. The hormones are chemical cousins of the hormones naturally secreted in the female body during a normal reproductive cycle. They work by "fooling" the woman's reproductive system with a simulated pregnancy.

HOW "THE PILL" WORKS: Normally, an ovum is released from the ovaries once during each menstrual cycle. If the ovum becomes fertilized by male sperm and implanted in the uterus, the hormones send back chemical signals that tell the ovaries to suppress ovulation until further notice. If this natural defense did not occur, a woman could find herself carrying several embryos and fetuses of different ages at the same time.

In other words, when an ovum is fertilized, the mother's reproductive machinery is mobilized to protect and encourage the development of the newly created life, and the monthly release of ova is halted until the birth of the baby. The synthetic hormones in the pill are of the type that signal the body that a pregnancy has been started, even though it is not true. Ovulation is suppressed and menstruation is delayed as long as the pills are taken.

At the end of a series of approxi-

mately 20 pills, one per day, menstruation is allowed to occur. The periods of women using oral contraceptives usually are only of two to three days' duration, and the menstrual flow is considerably lighter than in women not taking the pill. Then the series of pills is resumed for another menstrual cycle, but the hormones again suppress ovulation with a false pregnancy message. Since no ovum is released, there is very little chance that pregnancy will result from intercourse while the pills are used. Oral contraceptives are almost 100 percent effective, but errors occur from time to time, usually human errors in which the woman forgets to take a pill each day.

SIDE EFFECTS: Some women who use the pill have experienced undesirable side effects, which may range from break-through bleeding or cramps to hypertension, neurologic disorders, or *thromboembolism* (the blocking of a vein or artery by a blood clot). However, the most unpleasant side effects, such as blood clots and hypertension, usually occur when the woman taking the pill has high blood pressure. Therefore, women with this condition should not take the pill unless under strict medical supervision.

Although there is a danger of circulatory disorders and other side effects from the use of oral contraceptives, many doctors agree that the hazards of pregnancy are a greater threat to possibly millions of women. However, it is advisable for women using the pill to have periodic checkups. This is particularly important for women over 40 and from families with a tendency toward cancer. The Food and Drug Administration has recommended that all women over the age of 40 be made aware of the increased risk to their health of oral contraceptives and that doctors urge them to use other forms of contraception.

The IUD

Next in popularity after the pill is

the IUD, or *intrauterine contraceptive device,* a plastic or metal coil inserted in the uterus. A plastic coil can be produced at a cost of about 10 cents and inserted easily by a doctor with a syringelike device. However, the costs usually run much higher for the patient because of follow-up examinations and related care.

IUD's come in a variety of shapes and sizes. One is a plastic spiral, another has a double-S loop, still another looks like a tiny hour-glass. Each is about an inch and a half in length, and most have a tail that extends through the cervix.

HOW IT WORKS: Once the IUD is inserted, the woman can make her own examination, usually once a week, to determine whether it is still in place. If, by feeling the tail of the IUD, the woman suspects it has slipped out of place, she notifies her physician immediately. Otherwise, if there are no side effects, the IUD remains in place indefinitely, to be removed only when the woman wants to become pregnant. The IUD apparently functions by interfering with the natural implantation of a fertilized ovum in the wall of the uterus.

SIDE EFFECTS: Side effects might include pelvic pain, irregular bleeding, occasional perforation of the uterus, or pelvic infection. Because of minor problems sometimes encountered in fitting IUD's through the cervix, some doctors feel that the devices are better suited for the woman who has already had one or more children.

The Vaginal Sponge

The vaginal sponge, another kind of sperm barrier that also contains a spermicide, requires no visit to the doctor or clinic. Made of a soft polyurethane that is permeated with nonoxynol-9, the spermicide used in many jellies, creams, gels, and foams, the sponge is inserted manually into the vagina. There it blocks the opening to the cervic and absorbs and traps semen.

HOW IT WORKS: The sponge has to be dampened with water before insertion. A few tablespoons will do. When damp, it should feel slightly soapy. About the size of a collapsed golf ball, the sponge's sides are folded together, with the removal loop underneath. It is then inserted into the vagina as far as it will go—until it covers the cervix.

The sponge offers protection against conception for 24 hours. No additional spermicide, other than that already contained in the sponge, is necessary. But the sponge has to remain in place for at least six hours after the last act of coitus.

To remove the sponge, the woman hooks a finger into the removal loop or simply pulls the device out with two fingers. A new sponge can be inserted hours before intercourse. Each package of sponges contained detailed, printed instructions. Even though the sponge does not have to be fitted, as does the IUD, many women check with their doctors when first using the contraceptive to make sure they are inserting it properly. Many are also advised to avoid using the sponge during their periods.

Diaphragms and Cervical Caps

The oral contraceptive, the intrauterine contraceptive device, and two kinds of mechanical sperm barriers, the *cervical cap* and *diaphragm,* require a visit to the doctor's office or birth control clinic. The diaphragm or cervical cap must be fitted to the size and shape of the female reproductive organs at the opening of the uterus.

HOW THEY WORK: The main difference between the diaphragm and the cervical cap is that the diaphragm is placed at the back of the vagina in such a way that it serves as a barrier against spermatozoa that would be ejaculated during intercourse. The cervical cap, as the name suggests, is a cap that fits over the cervix to prevent the passage of spermatozoa.

The diaphragm must be coated on both surfaces as well as along the rim with a contraceptive jelly or cream. The soft rubber cup is placed at the back of the vagina and over the cervix before intercourse and should be left in place for at least 6 hours but not more than 16 hours after coitus. When removed, it should be cleaned according to directions and not used again for a period of 6 to 8 hours. Because of changes in weight and other factors, the diaphragm should be refitted at least once every two years. It should be replaced periodically, regardless of changes in size, because, being made of rubber, it does deteriorate with use, and the flaws are not always obvious to the naked eye.

A cervical cap may be made of rubber, plastic, or metal. It is carefully fitted over the cervix by a physician. During use, it is filled with contraceptive cream or jelly. The metal variety can be left in place from the end of one menstrual period to the beginning of the next, but other types should not remain in place for more than 24 hours. The cervical cap should be checked from time to time, since it can slip out of position during intercourse.

Condoms

Among birth control devices that do not require a visit to the doctor is the *condom,* usually made of soft rubber and shaped to fit as a sheath over the penis. They are inexpensive and are the preferred method of contraception for many couples, since they require the least advance preparation of all the methods except the oral contraceptive and the IUD.

Although condoms manufactured in the United States for the past 35 years have been subjected to quality control tests and are checked by federal inspectors, they are not immune to failure. For this reason, many women insert a spermicidal jelly or cream in the vagina when the man uses a condom.

The condom frequently is used by newlyweds as a birth control device while the wife waits to be fitted with a diaphragm after the first weeks of marriage. It also permits intercourse when one of the partners has an infectious disease affecting the genitals.

Because the condom dulls the sensation of intercourse somewhat, it is recommended for men who experience premature ejaculation. On the other hand, some men object to the lessened coital sensation associated with the wearing of a condom.

The Rhythm Method

In the *rhythm method,* the couple schedules intercourse before or after ovulation. In order for this method to be effective, a woman must keep extremely accurate charts of her basal temperature with a basal body thermometer in order to determine exactly when she ovulates. One problem with the rhythm method is that few women, especially newly married, have had experience keeping careful records of this kind and often misinterpret the results without a doctor's counsel. About one in five women simply does not have regular menstrual cycles, which is the key to avoiding days of peak fertility.

Spermicides

Spermicides in the form of jellies, creams, foaming tablets, gels, aerosol foams, and suppositories are available in nearly any drugstore and can be obtained without a prescription. The chemical substances are inserted with special applicators and form a film over the vaginal lining. The tablets and suppositories melt inside the vagina to spread a film over the lining.

The main objection to the use of chemical contraceptives is that coitus must take place within an hour after the substances are applied. When tablets are used, up to 15 minutes must elapse before coitus can begin. Generally, the chemicals should remain in the vagina for at least six hours after intercourse. If coitus is repeated during that period, another dose of chemicals must be inserted in advance.

Coitus Interruptus and Douching

Two of the least reliable birth control methods are *coitus interruptus* and *douching.* Coitus interruptus requires that the man withdraw his penis from the vagina before ejaculation. If carried out to its ideal conclusion, the technique requires a lot of self-control and split-second timing. Ejaculation is triggered by an automatic nerve reflex after the seminal vesicles are filled with semen; once the message gets through the nervous system, there is little the man can do to prevent ejaculation. Needless to say, the coitus interruptus technique has a high rate of failure. Beyond that, it is psychologically bad because it places undue anxiety on both partners during coitus.

Douching with water or special solutions works on occasion, but it is rated only as better than no birth control method at all. The douching, or flushing, of the vagina seems to have some effect in that it reduces the number of spermatozoa in the female reproductive system. Water alone is sufficient to kill sperm, although special preparations are available. The important factor with a douche is timing. The douche must be used immediately after intercourse, since spermatozoa can be moving through the cervix within in a couple of minutes after ejaculation and are normally able to reach the Fallopian tubes within 45 minutes.

Sterilization

About ten percent of the married couples in the United States have chosen to have one of the partners sterilized as a permanent form of contraception. A rather quick and simple operation called a *vasectomy,* performed on the male, has become increasingly common in recent years. By the mid-1970s more than half a million men were being sterilized each year by this operation. A vasectomy consists of the removal of a portion of the *vas deferens,* or sperm ducts, thus preventing semen from reaching the seminal vesicles, where it would ordinarily be discharged during intercourse. A vasectomy can be performed in a doctor's office with no more than a day or two lost from work.

The operation to sterilize a female is more involved; the abdomen is opened and the Fallopian tubes are cut or tied. A general anesthetic is employed and the operation is performed in a hosptial. It is a safe and almost bloodless operation requiring hospitalization for only a few days. One variation of this procedure utilizes a *peritoneoscope* (or *laparoscope*) for viewing the Fallopian tubes through a small incision below the navel while the tubes are cut through a second incision. With this method the average hospital stay is reduced to one or two days.

The problem with sterilization is that it is generally not reversible. It does not interfere with sex activity once the patient has recovered, but if the couple decides later to have more children, or if the sterilized partner remarries and wants to have children, the odds are against success in patching together the Fallopian tubes or the sperm ducts so that normal reproductive function can be restored.

Research on Other Methods

There are other birth control methods in the research and testing stage, such as oral contraceptives for men, morning-after contraceptives, and once-a-month shots. Eventually, some scientists speculate, foods in the supermarket will be treated with harmless substances that prevent conception. They will be similar to the iodine in iodized salt or the vitamin D added to homogenized milk. When the wife wants a baby, she will merely change the menu for a few days to exclude birth-control foods or switch to the foods in a special grocery store.

The Working Mother

A woman's place is in the home—and in the office, laboratory, factory, classroom, or any other place where she is qualified to fill a position that will pay her for her talents and help her fulfill her own needs and achieve professional goals. Since World War II, when women took over the assembly lines and women in uniform released military men from office tasks, the role of the working mother has been generally accepted as an integral part of the modern social scene. More than half of all mothers in the U.S. with children over six years old are employed; almost a third with children under the age of six also work.

Just as a wife does not mind the amount of time a husband must devote to his job as long as he does not neglect his family, psychologists have found that men are happy and content with working wives and mothers, as long as they do not neglect their husbands or the needs of their children.

Agreement on Priorities

Managing a home and a job and trying to raise a family at the same time can be a frenzied routine beset with tension and emotional strain. The strain is frequently related to the priorities a working wife and mother assigns to her various responsibilities. If the family really cannot subsist adequately on the husband's income, most women can devote a considerable amount of time to an outside job without feeling they are neglecting other duties. Also, mothers who pursue a career for the sake of self-fulfillment have probably calculated the assorted risks and feel little or no anguish about the goals they have chosen.

The women most likely to suffer are the ones who believe that total, full-time devotion to home and family is necessary. These women may have intense guilt feelings if they take an outside job in order to improve the standard of living in the home.

The decision of a mother to take on a full- or part-time job should be based on mutual understanding and a thorough discussion between husband and wife. It is most important that both husband and wife realize each other's feelings and the changes a job can bring about. For example, the husband should realize that if his wife agrees to remain at home despite her desire to get a job, her frustrations will undoubtedly be transmitted to her children. He must also realize that if the couple cannot afford the services of a maid to help with the housework, he himself must help with the housework or care of the children.

On the other hand, the wife must realize that her husband's position may require him to work occasional evenings—at which time he cannot also help her with housework—and that she may have to entertain clients or other people for him, even on days when she has worked a full day and is tired. The important thing is to weigh all aspects of the problem and base the decision on whatever brings the most satisfaction to everyone concerned. When both husband and wife are satisfied with the home-and-job decision, the children will be in a more secure position, regardless of which choice was made.

Age of Children

The age of the children should also be considered. Although many experts feel that the mother should postpone working outside the home if possible until the children are about six years of age, others maintain that this is not necessary if the children are well cared for in her absence and are given ample love and attention by both parents. A child of six or younger is particularly vulnerable, and his emotional needs must be served just as completely as are his physical needs.

Parents' Division of Labor

The roles of both parents are often subjected to revisions and modifications in a family where both parents work. The father usually assumes more responsibility for the care of a child at the end of a workday, while the working mother gets dinner ready. This may actually enable father and child to know one another more intimately and may also result in the father's feeling more sympathy and understanding toward the problems involved in child care.

LIMITATIONS ON THE MOTHER'S TIME: One recent study revealed that working mothers spend an average of 34 hours a week at housework, compared to about 56 hours a week for mothers who stay at home. Since the 34 hours are in addition to the time spent on her job plus commuting time, the working mother obviously has little time for recreation or community activities.

However, many women drive themselves to exhaustion by trying to prove they can hold a job and be perfect housekeepers and community leaders. The working mother must be able to accept limitations and decide what is most important; otherwise, she may feel guilty and insecure as well as continually tired. At some point the couple might consider alternatives; perhaps the mother should give up all extracurricular activities in favor of a career, or she might drop out of the work force for a few years, resume community activities, and return to work when the children are old enough to be more self-sufficient.

She also might consider a part-time job until the children are older. Even when the children are in the early years of grammar school, the mother may want to find employment that allows her to be at home when they are dismissed from class in the afternoon.

Economic and Other Factors

If economic factors are the prime motive for the mother's outside job, her take-home pay should be considerably greater than the costs of a baby sitter, maid, or housekeeper, nursery school or day care center, clothing needed for the job, transportation, lunches, and so on. The economics of the situation may be complex. For example, the couple may decide that even though the wife's earnings are not that sizable to begin with, she will be a far better wage earner in the long run if she continues working now rather than tries to return to a career at some later date when her skills will be rusty or completely outdated. Besides, economic considerations are not the only criteria; the woman's emotional needs to be productive or challenged intellectually must also be considered.

Care of the Child

The baby sitter must be a person responsible enough to assume the role of the parents in their absence, although the sitter does not have the authority to treat the child as she might her own. Because of the many gray areas, such as whether the sitter is authorized to punish the child, some firm ground rules should be established by the parents before the sitter begins work. Even if the sitter is a close relative, such as a grandmother or aunt of the child, there should be an understanding about what the child can and cannot do in the absence of the parents and what the sitter can and cannot do.

TEEN-AGE SITTERS: If the sitter is a teenager, she should be instructed as to whether she can let her friends visit her at the home where she is baby-sitting, whether she can chat with her friends on the telephone while she is sitting, and so on. She should have the telephone numbers where the parents can be reached if a problem arises, as well as the telephone numbers of doctors, friends, and neighbors who could assist in an emergency.

Usually, the main job of the baby sitter is the safety and welfare of the child. But when a sitter is expected to spend as much as a full working day with a child, five days a week, parents should try to find a sitter who is emotionally compatible with the child and can provide

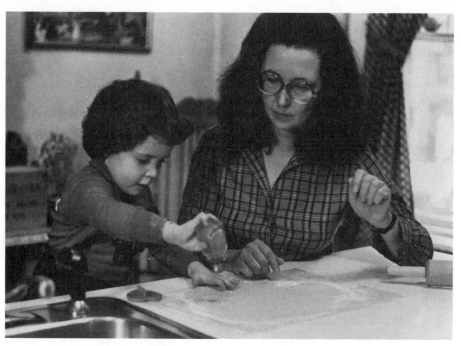

An imaginative baby sitter can plan activities for a child that engage his interest and stimulate his intellectual growth.

warmth and companionship, particularly for the preschool-aged child.

If the sitter is a close relative, she probably will know all about changing diapers, bottle feeding, minor first aid for bumps and bruises, and so on. A teen-ager, however, may not be experienced in these areas. Just because she has never changed a diaper doesn't mean the girl is unqualified for the job of sitter. But the parents should learn in advance how experienced the sitter is. She may need only a brief lesson in formula preparation or diaper changing to make the grade.

Nursery Schools

There are good nursery schools and not-so-good nursery schools, as well as children who do and those who do not benefit from a nursery-school experience. The facilities should supplement rather than substitute for home care of a child. Although the child may at first be reluctant to leave his home, he should be mature enough to spend part of each day away from home. The staff, physical setting, and equipment should be appropriate for the needs of the individual child.

Many states have strict licensing requirements for nursery schools, while others do not, so it is up to the parents to investigate thoroughly. Under no circumstances should a child be parked for the day in any facility in order to solve emotional conflicts of the child or the parents or because it is cheaper than others.

Nursery school can be a rewarding and enriching experience for the preschool youngster. Perhaps the most important purpose of nursery school is the opportunity it provides for children to experience peer relationships. This is particularly necessary if children lack frequent opportunities to play with other children. For most preschoolers, nursery school is the first time they experience a group situation, and what they learn in nursery school in terms of cooperation with others prepares them for the dynamics of the more formal learning situations to come.

The programs for nursery school children may include excursions, exposure to music, story books, creative work with clay and paints, and organized games. It is wise to investigate several schools in terms of staff, facilities, and professional standards before making a decision.

Parental Responsibilities

Parents who are separated from their children because of the demands of their jobs should not abdicate their responsibilities as mother and father either to baby sitters or nursery school staff members.

Need for Strong Father

The father, particularly, must not avoid his responsibilities in the child-raising department. Too often in the past the father made himself unavailable for guidance by telling a child to "ask your mother," when what the youngster wanted was a decision from the father. The trend in recent years for the father to assume a greater share of the responsibility for the children is a wholesome one. Families need a male authority who can command the respect of the children, but the father cannot expect to have much of a voice in family affairs if he passes the responsibility to the mother.

Agreement on Discipline

Many children learn at an early age that they can play the parents against each other to gain their objectives. If the father continually tells a child to ask his mother for a

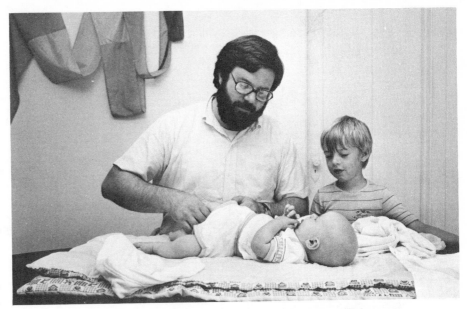

Fathers who actively participate in child raising are more likely to command their children's respect than fathers who abdicate this responsibility.

decision, the youngster may learn to work the game into a "yes" from the mother whenever he wants his own way. This should not be interpreted to mean that the father should be harsh or stern, but rather that he be actively concerned and involved in all phases of his child's growth, particularly in guiding his behavior.

If parents cannot agree on a course of discipline, the effect on a child can be as bad as no direction at all. In such a home the growing child has difficulty in learning to discipline himself because of uncertainty as to whom to model himself after. Although the female influence in child raising may seem more immediate because it is the mother who nurtures the baby during his first few months, growing children need two loving and attentive parents to give them support and provide them with behavioral models.

For more information on child care and parental responsibilities, see the *Alphabetic Guide to Child Care,* p. 60.

CHAPTER 5

The Middle Years

Maintaining good health over the years is far simpler, less expensive, and more comfortable than restoring health that has become poor. Since some diseases cannot be cured after they are contracted, it is only logical to try to prevent all possible health problems. The techniques of modern preventive medicine are available to Americans of every age.

All people are not beautiful or handsome, but nearly everyone can have the kind of attractiveness and vitality that comes from good health. The health of an individual depends upon the kind of body he inherits and the care he gives it. Good health can be thought of as a state of social, physical, and mental well-being, a goal virtually everybody can attain—if the responsibility for maintaining one's own health, with occasional help from the health experts, is accepted.

KEEPING FIT

Physical Changes

Physically, middle age should be a pleasant plateau—a time to look back on a vigorous youth, enjoy an active present, and prepare for a ripe old age.

Middle age should not be measured by chronological age but by biological age, the condition of various parts of the body. You might say that the middle-aged body is like a car that has been driven a certain number of miles. It should be well broken in and running smoothly, but with plenty of reserve power for emergencies, and lots of mileage left.

Biological age should be measured by the state of the heart, arteries and other essential organs, the length of life and comparative health of parents and grandparents, temperament and outlook on life, and outward appearance. The way you have fed or treated yourself is important. Eating the wrong kinds of food, being overweight, smoking too much, or worrying too much can add years to biological age.

However, no one should be surprised if he is not in quite the shape he was when he was 25 to 30 years old. At age 40 to 50 it is perfectly normal to have only 80 percent of the maximum breathing capacity, 85 percent of the resting cardiac output, 95 percent of the total body water, and 96 percent of the basal metabolic rate. These factors, however, should not slow anyone down very much.

There is one difference, though, that can be anticipated in middle age. Reaction time and decision-making processes may be a bit slower. This is because the nervous system is one of the most vulnerable to aging. The cells of the central nervous system begin to die early in life and are not replaced, while other organs are still growing and producing new cells. Specific response to input is delayed because it takes a greater length of time for an impulse to travel across the connections linking nerve fibers.

Thus, though you may function as usual under normal conditions, you may find it a little harder to respond to physical or emotional stress. However, if you have followed a sound health maintenance program, including good nutrition, enough mental and physical exercise and rest, and moderate living habits, you should respond to unusual physiological or emotional stress quite adequately.

The Importance of Checkups

Physical disabilities associated with

chronic disease increase sharply with age, starting with the middle years. While more than half (54 percent) of the 86 million persons who have one or more chronic conditions are under age 45, the prevalence of disability from illness is greatest in the 45 and older age group. Of those under 45 who have chronic conditions, only 14 percent are limited in activity as compared with almost 30 percent of the 45 to 64 age group. And only 1 percent of those under 45 with chronic illness are completely disabled, as compared with 4 percent in the 45 to 64 age group.

These figures suggest that it is wise to have an annual checkup so that any disease process or condition can be nipped in the bud. Further evidence of the value of medical checkups comes from the Aetna Life Insurance Company, which compared two groups of policyhold-ers over a five-year period. Those who did not have checkups and health counseling had a death rate 44 percent higher than the group who did. Regular checkups will not only help prolong life, they will also help you to live it more comfortably.

Here are some other good reasons for having a physical checkup:

• If an organ has been attacked by serious disease in youth, it may deteriorate at an early adult age.

• Heredity may play an important role in determining the speed at which various organs age. If your parents and grandparents had arteriosclerosis, there is a chance you might develop this condition in your middle years.

• Your environment (smog, poor climate, etc.) might affect the rate at which your body ages, particularly the skin.

• Individual stresses and strains, or abuses or overuse (of alcohol, for example) may create a health problem in middle age.

• The endocrine glands (pituitary, thyroid, parathyroids, adrenals, ovaries, testicles) play important roles in aging. Serious disease of one or more of these glands may lead to premature aging of an organ dependent upon its secretions.

• At middle age you are more likely to be beset by emotional strains at work or at home that could make you an early candidate for heart disease, arteriosclerosis, and other degenerative disorders.

• The earlier a chronic disease is detected, the better the chance that it can be arrested before permanent damage is done. This is especially true in the case of glaucoma, diabetes, heart disease, cancer of the lung or breast or other cancers—all of which could have their onset in middle age.

To help detect disease and other debilitating conditions, many physicians utilize automated medical screening, which combines medical history with selected physiological measurements and laboratory tests to give the doctor a complete health profile of the patient. This profile should indicate the probability of any chronic condition, which the physician could then pinpoint with more thorough tests.

Also, annual checkups enable the doctor to observe changes taking place over a period of time. For example, he is able to observe gradually changing blood chemistry levels or a progressive increase in eye pressure that could signal the onset of disease.

Don't Try To Be Your Own Doctor

A panel of medical specialists from the University of California at Los Angeles recently found that many men of 40 years and older were dosing themselves with unnecessary pills and "conserving" their energy by increasing bed rest to the point that it actually became enervating.

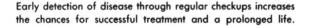
Early detection of disease through regular checkups increases the chances for successful treatment and a prolonged life.

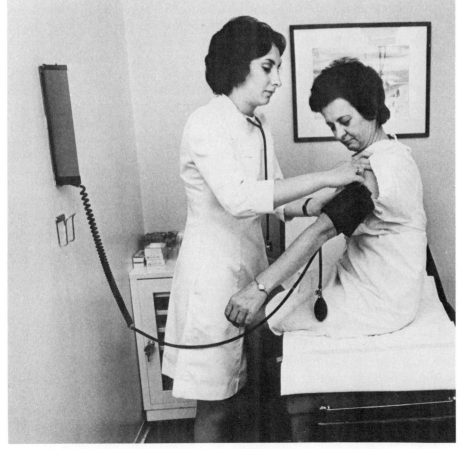

These doctors point out that increasing dependence on pills can be harmful as well as expensive. Laxatives are a good example of a popular commercial medicine taken unnecessarily by large numbers of people. Perhaps only one person in 100,000 may have an actual motor disability of the bowels, and most constipation can be easily corrected through proper foods and exercise, without resorting to laxatives. Also, taking vitamin pills or avoiding all high-cholesterol foods is unnecessary—unless recommended by a physician.

But, most important, "conserving" energy through prolonged bed rest or avoiding exercise can be fatal. The panel members pointed out that before age 40, a person exercises to improve his performance, but that after age 40 he exercises to improve his chances of survival.

Physical Fitness and Exercise
In middle age most of us stop performing most forms of exercise other than those that we enjoy doing. In other words, we find it easier to bend

The Multiple Risk Factor Intervention Trial tests those who risk the likelihood of having a heart attack. The purpose of the study is to determine whether a reduction in the risks can decrease the incidence of heart attacks.

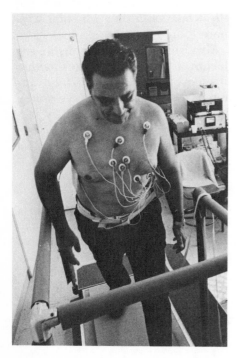

an elbow than lift weights. This is unfortunate, because in middle age most of us need regular exercise to maintain both mental and physical fitness and to increase endurance, strength, and agility.

As noted earlier, in middle age there is some decrease in breathing capacity, cardiac output, and metabolic rate; yet exercise can improve these functions. The more often the normal heart and circulatory system are required to move blood to active regions of the body through exercise or movement, the more efficient they become. Protracted exercise also improves the work of the lungs by increasing their ability to expand more fully, take in more air, and utilize a greater proportion of the oxygen in the inhaled air.

While exercise alone cannot eliminate obesity, it can help prevent it by improving digestion and bowel movements and by burning up excess calories. Exercise can also make you feel, look, and think better. Some traditional formal exercises, however, like touching the toes while keeping your knees stiff, or doing deep knee bends, are potentially harmful in middle age; they put too much stress on weak parts of the back and legs.

Despite protests about not having enough time, everyone has time to exercise, particularly if it is worked into the daily routine—for example, walking instead of riding to the train, office, store, or bus stop. You might find you'll get there faster, especially in traffic-clogged metropolitan areas, and you'll save money as well. More important, those minutes of "stolen" exercise accrue over the years in the form of improved health.

Sports and Games

If you don't like formal exercise, you can get exercise informally—through a favorite sport, whether it be golf, tennis, swimming, jogging, skiing, cycling, or whatever. Many sports and games are stop-and-go activities that do not provide helpful, rhythmic exercise, but here's how

you can make them more beneficial.

GOLF: Instead of riding in a golf cart between shots, walk—in fact, stride vigorously, lifting your head and chest. And don't make golf a cut-throat competition or business pursuit. Relax and enjoy it—count your blessings rather than your bogeys.

TENNIS: Like golf, tennis can be a cut-throat competitive sport or a pleasant pursuit. If it's played with muscles tied in knots from nervous tension, it will not provide any fun or healthful exercise. Also, players over 30 are well-advised to play more doubles than singles, and to avoid exhausting themselves in the heat of competition.

SWIMMING: Along with fast walking and jogging, swimming is one of the best all-around exercises. When swimming, most of the muscles are exercised and lung capacity and cardiac output are improved. The exercise potential can be increased by doing pull-ups with the diving board or ladder and by bobbing up and down in the water.

JOGGING: This popular sport can be combined with walking, done in a group or alone, either outdoors or indoors, and alternated with other exercises. Moreover, it doesn't require any special equipment and has been recognized by fitness experts as one of the best exercises for the heart and circulation. However, it is wise to get your doctor's advice and approval before embarking on a jogging program.

SKIING: Skiing is healthful as well as fun. You can get in shape for skiing and improve your ability by jogging and by practicing some of the techniques needed in skiing—such as the rhythmic left-right-left-right twist of foot, knee, and leg in short turns. To do this exercise, stand up straight with your feet quite close together and flex your knees forward so that the weight goes onto the balls of the feet. Now, arms apart for balance, twist your feet and knees to the left without twisting your upper body. As you do this, try the modified half-bends of

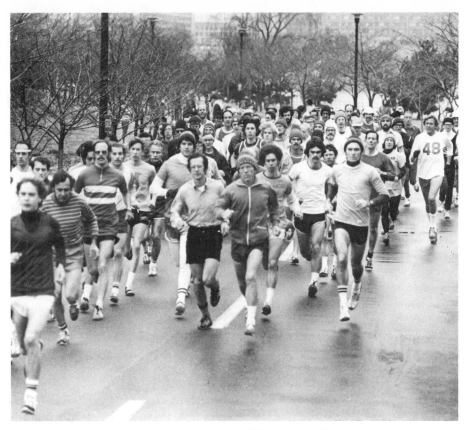

Many people in recent years have discovered the benefits of jogging, a sport that requires no special equipment and can be practiced at all ages.

that help to improve circulation. You can also try exercises that will relieve tense muscles and improve breathing. The exercises described below were developed by Dr. Josephine L. Rathbone of Columbia University.

BREATHING TO RELAX: Lie on your back on the floor with knees bent and feet resting on the floor. Take a deep breath, letting both the abdominal wall and chest rise. Hold the air for a few seconds, then expel it through your mouth with a gasp. Repeat four or five times at regular intervals.

FOR TENSE ARMS: Standing erectly, swing both arms forward, then to the side, letting them drop during the swings so that your hands brush your thighs with each motion. Keep your shoulders low. Repeat a few times. Then, sit on the edge of a chair and clench one hand tightly. Swing your arm vigorously in large circles, keeping your hand clenched. Then repeat with other arm.

FOR TENSE LEGS: Sit on the edge of a table with lower legs hanging free. Then, alternately, swing them backward and forward. Try to keep your legs moving in rhythm.

FOR STOMACH TENSION: Kneel with your feet under your hips and swing

the traversing position that all ski schools teach. Then reverse the position to the right, and keep repeating.

OTHER SPORTS: Other worthwhile sports for healthful exercise include badminton, bicycling, canoeing, rowing, table tennis, skating, and squash. However, they should be sustained for at least 30 minutes at a time, and ideally four times a week, and should be combined with supplemental exercises.

A WORD OF WARNING: Everyone should beware of becoming a weekend athlete and punishing himself with an overdose of exercise or sports only on weekends. It makes as much sense as stuffing yourself on weekends and starving the rest of the week. It's far more sensible— and healthful—to engage in sports activities for an hour or so at a time on a daily basis.

Exercises

Participating in sports activities is

not the only way to keep fit. Special exercises can help reduce tension and build muscles. For instance, one way to relax is to do rhythmic exercises, particularly for the trunk,

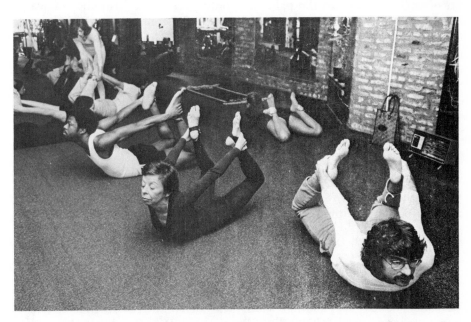

Yoga exercises have become increasingly popular in the western world. The exercises build muscle tone and help produce a relaxed body and state of mind.

your trunk down to one side and around, sweeping your arms in a wide circle, coming up again on the opposite side. Or stand with your hips supported against the wall, feet apart and a few inches from the wall. Bend your body forward, arms drooping, and let your body sway from side to side, with your arms and head loose.

RELAXING AT WORK OR HOME: Relieve tension while sitting by holding the spine erect, shoulders low. Turn your head so that the chin touches first one collarbone, then the other. Move slowly and rhythmically.

YOGA: You can also relax and become revitalized through various Yoga exercises. Courses are taught at many recreational centers. Some of the exercises require only a minimum of time, and can be done not only before and after the workday but in the office during the lunch hour.

ISOMETRICS: Isometric exercises —pitting one muscle against another without moving—can also be practiced at odd moments. These exercises should, however, be done only by healthy persons, and not by anyone with a cardiac problem. To strengthen arm and shoulder muscles through isometrics, put the fist of one hand against the palm of the other and push without moving. Or push up with your arms from a chair or the edge of a table. Strengthen arm and neck muscles by grasping the back of the neck with laced fingers and pulling forward—again, without movement.

All of the above exercises and sports can put you on the road to physical fitness. Just remember, whatever form of exercise or sport you choose, make it fun and do not strain yourself unduly.

Rest and Sleep

Rest and sleep adequate for one's personal needs are another vital component of good health and good appearance. They also influence human relationships and mental alertness. Scientists believe that during sleep the body replaces tissue cells and eliminates waste products created by fatigue at a faster rate than when awake.

Sleep also rests the heart and blood system, since heart muscle contractions and blood pressure are slower then. Excessive fatigue from lack of sleep increases susceptibility to a number of ailments, including the common cold. If an individual gets an adequate amount of sleep (usually seven to eight hours for an adult), he will feel ready to meet the day's activities. If not, his memory may not be sharp, and he may be irritable because his nervous system has had inadequate rest.

A quiet, dark, ventilated room, a fairly firm mattress, and performance of a moderate amount of exercise during the day will aid sleep. When worry, frustration, or anxiety make it difficult to sleep, a conscious attempt to relax will help. Sedatives or sleeping pills should not be taken unless they are prescribed or recommended by a physician.

Personal Hygiene

Disease germs can enter the body only in a limited number of ways. One of the major ways is through the skin. The skin is a protective covering which, when broken, can admit harmful bacteria or viruses easily.

Simple precautions are very effective. The hands come into contact with disease germs more than any other part of the body. Therefore, they should be washed whenever they are dirty, prior to preparing food or eating, and after using the lavatory.

The rest of the body must also be kept clean, since adequate bodily cleanliness will remove substances which, by irritating the skin, make it more susceptible to infection. Bathing also improves the muscle tone of the skin. Hair should also be washed frequently enough to prevent accumulation of dust and dead skin cells.

Openings in the body are also paths by which disease germs can enter the body. The nose and ears should be carefully cleaned only with something soft, for instance, a cotton swab. Genital orifices should be kept clean by frequent bathing. Any unusual discharge from a body opening should be promptly reported to a physician. The problem can then be treated at its earliest stage—the easiest time to solve the problem.

Personal hygiene includes care of the nails. They should always be kept clean and fairly short. Hangnails can be avoided by gently pushing back the cuticle with a towel after washing the hands.

Care of the Feet

"My feet are killing me!" is a complaint heard more frequently in middle age, especially from women. The devil in this case usually takes the shape of fashionable shoes, where the foot is frequently squeezed into shapes and positions it was never designed to tolerate. Particularly unhealthy for the foot was the formerly fashionable spike heel and pointed toe.

Any heel two inches or higher will force the full weight of the body onto the smaller bones in the front of the foot and squeeze the toes into the forepart of the shoes. This hurts the arch, causes calluses on the sole of the foot, and can lead to various bone deformities.

The major solution to this problem is to buy good shoes that really fit. The shoes should be moderately broad across the instep, have a straight inner border, and a moderately low heel. To fit properly, shoes should extend one-half inch to three-fourths inch beyond the longest toe.

Avoid wearing shoes that have no support; also, avoid wearing high heels for long periods of time. Extremely high heels worn constantly force the foot forward and upset body balance. Changing heel height several times a day will rest the feet and give the muscles in the back of the legs a chance to return to their normal position. It's highly desirable to wear different shoes each day, or at least alternate two pairs. This gives the shoes a chance to dry out completely. Dust shoes with a mild powder when removed.

Shoes should not be bought in the morning. They should be tried on near the end of the day, when the feet have broadened from standing and walking, and tightness or rubbing can be more easily detected.

As to hosiery, socks and stockings should extend a half-inch beyond the longest toe. Stretch socks are fine in many cases, but plain wool or cotton socks help if your feet perspire a lot.

Foot Exercises

Exercise your feet by trying these simple steps recommended by leading podiatrists:

• Extend the toes and flex rapidly for a minute or two. Rotate the feet in circles at the ankles. Try picking up a marble or pencil with your toes; this will give them agility and strength.

• Stand on a book with your toes extended over the edge. Then curl your toes down as far as possible, grasping the cover.

• After an unusually active day, refresh the feet with an alcohol rub. Follow this with a foot massage, squeezing the feet between your hands. When you are tired, rest with your feet up. Try lying down for about a half-hour with your feet higher than your head, using pillows to prop up your legs.

• Walk barefoot on uneven sandy beaches and thick grass. This limbers up the feet and makes the toes work. Walking anywhere is one of the best exercises for the feet if you learn to walk properly and cultivate good posture. Keep toes pointed ahead, and lift rather than push the foot, letting it come down flat on the ground, placing little weight on the heel. Your toes will come alive, and

your feet will become more active.

Foot Ailments

Doing foot exercises is particularly important in middle age, because the foot is especially vulnerable to the following problems:

BUNIONS: A bunion is a thickening and swelling of the big joint of the big toe, forcing it toward the other toes. There is also a protuberance on the inner side of the foot. Unless treated, this condition usually gets progressively worse. Surgery is not always necessary or successful. Often, special shoes to fit the deformed foot must be worn.

STIFF TOE: People suffering from this problem find that the big joint of the big toe becomes painful and stiff, possibly due to a major accident or repeated minor trauma. This condition usually corrects itself if the joint is protected for a few weeks, usually by a small steel plate within the sole of the shoe.

HAMMER TOE: This clawlike deformity is usually caused by cramping the toes with too small shoes. The pressure can be eased with padding and, in some cases, the deformity can be corrected by surgery.

INGROWN TOENAIL: Cutting the nail short and wearing shoes that are too tight are major causes of ingrown toenails; the edge of the nail of the toe—usually the big toe—is forced into the soft outer tissues. In some cases the tissues can be peeled back after soaking the foot in hot water, and the offending part of the nail can be removed. To prevent ingrown toenails, the nails should be kept carefully trimmed and cut straight across the nail rather than trimmed into curves at the corners. For severe or chronic cases of ingrown toenails it is best to seek professional treatment.

MORTON'S TOE: This is the common name for a form of *metatarsalgia*, a painful inflammation of a sheath of small nerves that pass between the toes near the ball of the foot. The ailment is most likely to occur in an area between the third and fourth toe, counting from the

large toe, and usually is due to irritation produced by pressure that makes the toes rub against each other. In most instances, the pressure results from wearing improperly fitted shoes, shoes with pointed toes, or high heel shoes, which restrict normal flexing of the metatarsals (the bones at the base of the toes) while walking.

Temporary relief usually is possible through removal of the shoes and massaging of the toes, or by application of moist, warm heat to the afflicted area. In cases of very severe pain, a doctor may inject a local anesthetic into the foot. Additional relief sometimes can be obtained by wearing metatarsal arch supports in the shoes. However, continued irritation of the nerves can result in the growth of a tumor that may require surgical removal.

Care of the Teeth

An attractive smile is often the first thing that one notices about others. In addition to creating an attractive appearance, healthy teeth and gums are a basic requirement for good overall health. One cannot have a healthy body without a healthy mouth, and vice versa. The dentist should be visited at whatever intervals he recommends, usually every six months.

Neglect of oral hygiene and the forgoing of dental checkups are commonplace in the middle years. An often-heard excuse is that the eventual loss of teeth is inevitable. Years ago, loss of teeth really was unavoidable. Today, however, thanks to modern dental practices, it is possible for nearly everyone to enjoy the benefits of natural teeth for a lifetime. For more information on dental care, see Ch. 10, p. 252.

Problems of Aging

When the human body reaches middle age, a number of problems and conditions which are the result of advancing years begin to make themselves felt. These include wrinkling of the skin, baldness, varicose veins, menopause and the male climacteric, and the body's decreased ability to deal with nicotine, caffeine, alcohol, and excess calories.

Skin

The skin usually starts to show its age in the mid to late 30s. At that time it starts to lose its elasticity and flexibility, and becomes somewhat thinner. Little lines—not yet wrinkles—start to show up, usually crow's feet around the eyes.

Wrinkling takes place at different times with different people, and sometimes in different areas of the skin. Heredity may play a part. For instance, one family may have the trait of wrinkling around the mouth rather than the eyes. In another family, wrinkling or crow's feet may start early and then stop.

TREATMENT FOR WRINKLES: While wrinkles do not hurt, many people want to do something about them. Experienced physicians and dermatologists have a number of techniques for removing or minimizing wrinkles. One accepted method is *dermabrasion*, or planing of the skin. The doctor sprays on a local anesthetic, then scrapes the skin with a motor-driven wire brush or some other abrasive tool. The treatment usually takes one session, and no hospital stay is required. There will be some swelling and scab formation, but this should clear up in a week to ten days.

Another method is called *cryotherapy*, in which the doctor freezes the skin with carbon dioxide. This induces peeling, which improves the appearance of flat acne scars and shallow wrinkles.

Still another procedure involves the application of chemicals, which are neutralized when they have obtained the desired action.

SKIN TEXTURE CHANGE: Besides wrinkling, the skin has a tendency in some people to become thinner, leathery, and darkened as they move towards the 40s and 50s. This effect can be minimized if the skin is toned up with cold cream and other emollients that provide the moisture and oil the skin needs. Also, overexposure to the sun—one of the prime agers of the skin—should be avoided.

In fact, most doctors feel that the sun is a lethal agent, and that exposing the face to too much sun is like putting it in a hot oven. Many say that the sun destroys some inherent good qualities of facial skin, and ruins any chance of improving the appearance through cosmetic surgery.

Cosmetic Surgery

Cosmetic surgery for both men and women is becoming increasingly popular and sophisticated. Cosmetic surgery procedures include *rhinoplasty* (nose); *facial plasty* or *rhytidoplasty* (face lift); *blepharoplasty* (upper eyelids and bags under the eyes); breast augmentation and reduction; as well as the dermabrasion and other methods mentioned earlier. See *Plastic and Cosmetic Surgery*, p. 345.

Baldness

While cosmetic surgery for men is relatively new, the problem of baldness has its roots in ancient history. Men were worried about baldness 4,000 years ago—and they were just about as successful as they are today in finding a cure. Dr. Eugene Van Scott, head of the Dermatology Service of the National Cancer Institute, expressed the opinion of most authorities when he said: "Baldness is caused by three factors: sex, age, and heredity. And we can't do a thing about any of these."

Other causes of baldness include infections, systemic diseases, drugs which have a toxic effect, mechanical stress, friction, and radiation. Diet does not usually affect baldness, but chronic starvation or vitamin deficiencies can contribute to dryness, lack of luster, and hair loss. Also, excessive intake of vitamin A can cause hair loss.

In women, loss of hair is quite common toward the end of pregnancy, after delivery, and during menopause. In these cases, most hair eventually grows back.

There are two common types of baldness in men: *male pattern baldness* and *patchy baldness*.

MALE PATTERN BALDNESS: Male pattern baldness (*alopecia*) usually begins in the late twenties or early thirties. Hair falls out from the crown until a fringe of hair remains at the sides and along the back of the head from ear to ear. At the onset, a bald spot may appear on the crown of the head, and balding spots in other areas may merge to form the fringe pattern. There is little one can do to prevent or retard hair loss through typical male pattern baldness.

PATCHY BALDNESS: In patchy baldness (*alopecia areata*) hair might fall out suddenly in patches. In this case, hair eventually returns after going through three growth periods. The new hair may be thinner than the original hair. Although patchy baldness is self-limiting and usually self-curing, therapy is indicated in some patients. This usually consists of injections of insoluble steroid suspensions directly into the scalp. Regrowth generally begins in three to four weeks, but remains localized at the site of injection.

Treatment for other types of scalp disorders varies. Dermatologists can usually diagnose a disorder caused by a toxic agent, and they can usually clear up scalp infections with antibiotics. But there is no effective cure, treatment, or drug for male pattern baldness.

In some cases, *hair transplantation* can help. Using a skin biopsy punch and a local anesthetic, a doctor can remove small grafts from the sides and back of the scalp and transplant them to bald areas. As many as 60 transplants can be made in one hour. However, this procedure works only if there is sufficiently dense hair on the sides and back to provide donor sites to the bald areas without noticeably changing the appearance of the "fringe" areas.

WIGS: Some men who wish to hide their baldness find it easier and less expensive to buy a wig. Not surprisingly, wig shops exclusively for men are opening throughout the country. Men can buy synthetic stretch wigs in many natural colors for as little as $25. They are made with tapered back and sideburns, and it's reported that they can even be worn when swimming.

Of course, wigs for women are even more prevalent and fashionable. Some women own a wardrobe of wigs in a variety of colors and styles to match their moods, clothes, and the climate.

EXCESS HAIR: For some middle-aged women, the problem is too much hair in the wrong place, instead of too little. Excess hair can grow on the face, chest, arms, and legs. In some instances, unwanted hair may be a sign of an endocrine disorder that can be detected by a doctor. In other cases, it can be caused by chronic irritation, such as prolonged use of a cast, bandage, or hot-water bottle; it can also be due to excess exposure to the sun, iodine or mercury irritation, or localized rubbing.

Excess hair can be bleached, shaved, tweezed, waxed, or removed by chemical depilatories and electrolysis. Only electrolysis is permanent. See *Hair Removal*, p. 242.

Varicose Veins

Another complaint of middle-aged men and women is *varicose veins*. About half the women over 50 years of age have these enlarged veins with damaged valves in their thighs and calves.

Varicose veins are usually caused by years of downward pressure on the veins, causing the valves to break down. This often happens to people who must stand for many hours at a time. The large, bluish irregularities are plainly visible beneath the skin of the thighs and calves, and they cause a heavy dragging sensation in the legs and a general feeling of tiredness and lack of energy.

TREATMENT: In most instances, the best treatment involves surgery to tie off the main veins and remove all superficial veins that lend themselves to this procedure (called *stripping*). In other cases, varicose veins can be relieved by wearing elastic stockings or compression bandages.

Varicose veins that remain untreated can cause *varicose ulcers*, which usually form on the inner side of the leg above the ankle. Treatment calls for prolonged bed rest, warm applications, and surgical ligation and stripping of the varicose veins responsible for the ulcers. Thus, it is wise to consult a doctor if varicose veins appear.

Menopause

At some point during middle age, women go through what is often called the *change of life,* when the capacity to bear children comes to an end. The start of the menopause usually comes between ages 40 and 50. However, about 12 percent of women reach the menopause between ages 36 and 40; 15 percent between ages 51 and 55; and another 6 percent earlier or later. As a general rule, it may be said that the later in a girl's life menstruation begins, the sooner menopause starts.

While menopause is sometimes abrupt, the onset is usually gradual, and the process normally lasts several years. The ovaries gradually reduce their ovulation and hormone secretion. Menstruation becomes irregular and finally ceases.

The periods between, during, and after the menopause are called *premenopausal, menopausal,* and *postmenopausal.* Premenopausal symptoms include skipped menstrual periods and scanty or lessened menstrual flow. During the menopausal period, menstruation ceases, and there are sometimes various systemic disturbances. The postmenopausal period is characterized by the return of bodily equilibrium and a renewed feeling of good health.

SYMPTOMS OF MENOPAUSE: Physical symptoms of the menopause are believed to be caused by an estrogen deficiency which upsets the hypothalamic control of the autonomic nervous system. While many women go through menopause with little or no distress, about one out of five may feel hot flashes and chills, nervousness, insomnia, heart palpitation, dizzy spells, or increased or diminished appetite. Generally, most women suffer from only a few of these symptoms, sudden hot flashes and dizziness being the most common.

SURGICAL MENOPAUSE: Many women develop benign uterine tumors called *fibroids*, and these tumors may cause irregular bleeding, prolonged menstrual periods, massive hemorrhages, or pain and discomfort due to pressure on other organs. In these cases a *hysterectomy*, or surgical removal of the uterus, may be performed. In cases where the cervix is also removed, the procedure is called total hysterectomy. It is only when the complete removal of the ovaries and tubes, called radical hysterectomy, is also necessary, that the production of ova and the normal menstrual cycle are stopped abruptly and surgical menopause occurs. See under *Benign Tumors*, p. 499, for further information about fibroids.

Though more abrupt and severe than menopause that occurs naturally, surgical menopause is treated in much the same manner as natural menopause. Tranquilizers or sedatives may be prescribed. In some cases, the doctor may prescribe hormone replacement therapy to supplement the body's reduced supply of estrogen. This can be especially beneficial in the relief of hot flashes.

Emotional Aspects of Menopause

In addition to physical symptoms, a woman often has a pronounced psychological reaction to menopause. Though there is no medical basis for believing that menopause adversely affects her sex life or appearance, a woman may feel this is true. Common emotional problems may include the following: the feeling that she has lost her beauty, sex appeal, or sexual desire; a fear of cancer; the idea that the onset of menopause means the loss of her husband's love; fears that her job may be lost because of illness, bad nerves, or general debility; or a feeling that menopause means that she has lost youthful energy and spirit and is becoming old.

It is only normal to feel sad occasionally about growing older, but there is no need to identify the menopause with loss of attractiveness, an end to sexual desire, or a so-called nervous breakdown. For anyone who is emotionally unstable, this transition may be especially hard to weather, but for such a personality, any time of change—such as marriage or motherhood—might also be accompanied by emotional turbulence.

Probably those women who see their total identity in terms of motherhood are the ones hardest hit when faced with the loss of their child-bearing functions. A woman who has a more complete sense of herself can accept the menopause with equanimity and can also face the tapering off of her child-rearing activities without feeling useless and discarded.

The most satisfying way to continue to express a strong maternal instinct after the menopause is in the role of grandmother, and if there are no grandchildren, in the role of occasional babysitter. Volunteer work in the children's ward of a local hospital or as a helper in a day-care nursery has also brought satisfaction to women who miss mothering as their own children leave them.

A HEALTHY ATTITUDE TOWARD CHANGE: "Change of life," the old-fashioned term for the menopause, really isn't accurate, since change is a rule of life at all times. It is the ability to adjust to different circumstances and to find contentment in new outlets that marks the happy woman of any age.

Instead of feeling frustrated, or wallowing in self-pity, or hunting for sexual adventures, a woman whose emotions are disturbed during the menopause should set herself the goal of finding better ways to cope with them.

If depression and anxiety are deep enough to result in a loss of interest in daily affairs, the wisest thing to do is to have an honest conversation with the family doctor or gynecologist. He may be able to alleviate these symptoms by such temporary measures as prescribing hormones or tranquilizers. Or he may feel that a few sessions with a psychiatrist would be helpful. It is no sign of personal failure or weakness of will to need professional guidance, and no woman should feel guilty if she seeks it out.

ADVICE TO THE HUSBAND: A husband can help his wife through this difficult period if he makes an effort to be especially considerate. For example, he can take special care to show her that she is appreciated and still physically attractive. When she is in a bad humor or moody and depressed, he can sympathize with her moods and remain tolerant. He can pamper her and show his interest by remembering anniversaries and birthdays and by taking her out more

often. Instead of hiding behind a newspaper or watching television in the evening, he can talk to his wife and show an interest in what she is doing.

By taking a realistic view of menopause as a natural process of life, and with the aid of an understanding husband, friends, and family, most women can get through the menopause without frequent visits to a family doctor. However, if a woman experiences any unusual symptoms—abnormal vaginal discharge, spotting between periods, excessive or too frequent periods, periods that last too long, or unusual irritation of the genitals—she should by all means see a doctor.

PAP TEST: Cancer may be a major fear during the menopause, especially cancer of the cervix. Such fears can easily be allayed by having a simple diagnostic test called the *Papanicolaou* (or *Pap*) *smear*. This is a painless process in which the cervix is exposed by an instrument which dilates the cavity to make it more visible. The doctor can then take samples of the cells, which are examined for the possible presence of cancer. All women should have a pelvic examination and Pap test at least once a year.

A number of other forms of

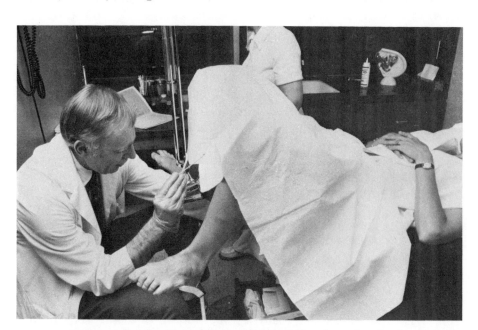

During an annual pelvic examination a gynecologist takes a sample of cells from the cervix for a Pap test, a diagnostic test for detecting cancer.

cancer, including cancer of the lining of the uterus, cancer of the ovaries, cancer of the breast, and cancer of the vulva and other sexual organs, appear more frequently in women over 50. However, these conditions can be detected before they do much, if any, damage by having regular examinations during and after the menopause. If such cancers are caught in an early stage, they are much easier to treat and cure. See also *Women's Health*, p. 483.

Male Climacteric

Many men go through a psychological equivalent of the menopause, which may be called the "foolish forties," the "frenzied fifties," or the *male climacteric.*

According to Dr. Charles Wahl, a psychiatrist at the University of California (Los Angeles), some men tend to blame all sorts of symptoms —forgetfulness, self-doubt, worry, depression, and a declining sexual interest—on this mythical male menopause. "These symptoms are of psychic origin," says Dr. Wahl, "when found in a middle-aged man who is not afflicted by a specific disease. The body undergoes no organic or functional changes that might account for such complaints."

This may be of small comfort to the man who—for whatever emotional reasons—goes through this period of psychological upset. But there is some help in this remark from Dr. John F. Briggs, Associate Professor of Clinical Medicine at the University of Minnesota: "The best way to steer a successful course through the hazards of the frenzied fifties is to assay your assets and liabilities dispassionately, and adapt to the circumstances and changes they dictate."

ADVICE TO THE WIFE: Just as a husband can help his wife through her menopause, so can a wife help her husband. The thoughtful wife can bolster her husband's ego by being aware of what deflates him and what builds him up. Concentrate on building up his self-confidence and avoid nagging criticisms and arguments. Show your husband how much you need him and depend on him; sustain his sense of self-importance. Be affectionate and give him tender loving care, especially if you feel that he is worried or tense. He may want more company than usual, or he may prefer not to go out socially. Whatever the case, give in to him. He will assume his normal pace after a while.

There can be a physical reason for the male change of life, called primary testicular failure. In such cases, the testes fade out earlier in life than might be expected. Since it is an illness, like diabetes or kidney trouble, testicular failure can happen at any age. When it does occur, the physical discomforts may be surprisingly similar to a woman's symptoms in menopause.

Any man who suspects he may be really ill should see a doctor who can make a thorough examination. This is necessary because any treatment with hormones (androgen) could hurt as much as it could help if the case is not a true testicular failure. Androgen could also be harmful in the case of prostate trouble, which becomes more prevalent after the age of 40. See under Ch. 23 p. 424, for a fuller discussion of prostate trouble.

Other than testicular failure, which is rare, there is no physical reason why a man should be impotent in middle age. As the late Dr. Kinsey reported: "Only a slight portion of the male population ever becomes impotent before death."

If a man thinks that he needs "one last fling" before his virility is curtailed by glandular deterioration, he will not find support for this idea from Dr. Josiah Brown, an endocrinologist with the University of California (Los Angeles). Says Dr. Brown: "There is no significant change in the endocrine function between the ages of 40 and 55."

Also, if a man looks for a sex stimulator for flagging interests, he need look no further than this statement by the late Dr. Kinsey: ". . . good health, sufficient exercise, and plenty of sleep still remain the most effective of the aphrodisiacs known to man."

Nicotine

Used in moderation, nicotine is not harmful, and according to some researchers may be helpful, improving memory and learning ability, perhaps by stimulating the flow of adrenaline. Nicotine also stimulates the adrenal glands, causing blood vessels to constrict and skin temperatures to drop.

Interestingly enough, nicotine is thought to get into the system through the membranes of the mouth and related areas. Thus, a person who holds an unlighted cigar in his mouth may absorb nicotine.

While a little nicotine is not harmful, most steady smokers absorb too much nicotine for their own good. Lung cancer kills over 85,000 persons a year, about 80 percent of whom are cigarette smokers. Also, cigarette smoking is believed to be a primary cause of *emphysema* (a disease that decreases efficiency of the lungs) which kills over 15,000 persons a year. Approximately 100,000 cigarette smokers die from heart attacks each year.

In their book *Vigor for Men Over 30*, the authors, Drs. Warren R. Guild, Stuart Cowan and Samm Baker suggest these tips on giving up smoking:

• *Try a program of enjoyable physical activity.* They suggest that if the urge to smoke becomes overpowering, the smoker should take a brisk walk, do a set of invigorating exercises at home or in the office, or engage in an enjoyable sport.

• *Don't use antismoking drugs or other nostrums without a doctor's advice.* Such devices may do more harm than good. Your doctor is the one who can advise you on the best way to cut down on smoking, and he can help you cope with any withdrawal symptoms such as nervous-

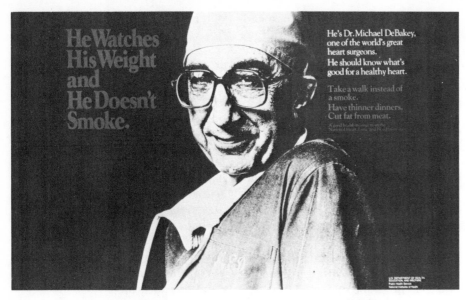

He Watches His Weight and He Doesn't Smoke.

He's Dr. Michael DeBakey, one of the world's great heart surgeons. He should know what's good for a healthy heart.

Take a walk instead of a smoke. Have thinner dinners. Cut fat from meat.

The esteemed cardiologist Michael DeBakey speaks up for good health habits in an advertising campaign sponsored by the U.S. government.

ness, dizziness, or insomnia.

• *Don't try to cut down on too many things at the same time.* Concentrate on cutting down on your smoking, and relax about cutting down on diet and drinking, too. One reduction at a time is best.

• *You've got to quit completely.* Like the alcoholic, you've got to say, "This is my *last* cigarette"—and mean it.

• *Quit when there's a major break in your routine.* The recovery from an operation or illness is a good time to stop. After you have established the habit of *not* smoking, make that habit a part of your daily life.

• *Try something different to throw desire off the track.* Take a shower—you can't light a match under water. Also, you can't hold a cigarette if you're playing table tennis or practicing your golf swing.

Caffeine

Like nicotine, *caffeine* can be a pleasant stimulant if used in moderation. Laboratory studies show that caffeine appears to work on the central nervous system: fatigue and drowsiness fade while mental activities quicken. But too much caffeine can produce headaches, irritability, and confusion.

Although tea leaves contain almost twice as much caffeine as an equal weight of coffee, smaller amounts of tea are used to make a cup of tea, thus lessening the per-cup intake rate. Cola and chocolate also contain caffeine. Although these drinks are not addictive, abstaining from them is no easy matter, as anyone who has tried to give up coffee drinking can attest.

Ordinarily, drinking a few cups of coffee or other caffeine beverage is not harmful—unless your doctor tells you to cut down for some reason. But if you find that you need a caffeine beverage to keep going, you might be better off taking a rest instead.

Alcohol

Many doctors feel that a person's capacity to handle liquor diminishes after age 40, and that alcohol intake should be cut down after this age. Also, some people seem to develop an allergic reaction to alcohol—an allergy that can be fatal. One doctor described the extra dry martini as "the quick blow to the back of the neck."

Drinking too much and too fast can jar the whole system. It tends to make the drinker nervous and on edge instead of providing calming

relief from tensions. The hard-pressed executive is especially vulnerable to the quick, fast drink he takes to provide instant relaxation when he is fatigued.

"The key to the real value of alcohol is intelligent drinking," says Dr. Harry J. Johnson, of the Life Extension Institute. Dr. Johnson says that he sometimes recommends a drink or two before dinner, which he says is the best time to indulge. However, Dr. Johnson suggests a tall, well-diluted highball taken in a peaceful, quiet setting.

How to Avoid Drinking

If you find that drinking is a problem at business luncheons, conventions, and cocktail parties, Dr. Warren R. Guild recommends the following commonsense ways to pass up drinks:

• Say "no thanks" if you do not like the taste or effect of alcohol. Order a juice or nonalcoholic beverage just to have something to sip. Actually, many more jobs and clients have been lost through drinking too much than by not drinking at all.

• Wait for others to order drinks. If someone else refuses a drink, you can decline too. Or, you could say, "I'm not having one but you go ahead." This usually sets the pace for drinking.

• Instead of a powerhouse martini, try vermouth on the rocks, beer, wine, or a well-diluted highball.

• Use dieting as a reason to cut down or out on drinking. You have a good excuse—a drink has 100 or more calories.

• Make arrangements with your favorite restaurant or bar to serve you "your usual." You could make this a nonalcoholic drink.

Remember that alcohol definitely decreases your ability to concentrate, absorb, or produce thoughts or ideas. After drinking you will not be as efficient at writing, drawing, handling objects, or driving. If the level of alcohol in your blood exceeds 0.05 percent—which, depending on weight, is approximately the equivalent of two ounces of hard liquor or two bottles of beer at one session—*you are not a safe driver.*

Treating a Hangover

What if you do drink too much and have a hangover? Is there anything you can do about it? Dr. Harold T. Hyman, formerly of the Columbia University College of Physicians and Surgeons, recommends calling a physician if the case is particularly bad. He will probably prescribe a large dose of paraldehyde or a tranquilizer such as Librium or Thorazine, and put the patient to bed.

Less acute sufferers should, on awakening after a binge, take warmed fluids (tea, consommé, clam broth). As soon as your stomach feels in shape, eat warm, soft foods at frequent intervals—poached egg, milk toast, pureed soup, mashed potatoes. Despite your craving for cold, carbonated fluids, avoid them; they may cause stomach cramps.

To prevent a hangover as you drink, Dr. Guild recommends taking *fructose.* Fructose, or *levulose,* is a crystalline sugar, the sweetest of the sugars. It increases the rate at which the body metabolizes and eliminates alcohol. It seems to work best when the alcohol is combined with something naturally high in fructose, as the tomato juice in a Bloody Mary, for example. Or just sip tomato juice between drinks.

Looking for quick panaceas in the medicine cabinet to cure a hangover or any other condition seems to become increasingly popular after age 40. Panaceas are all right up to a point, but indiscriminate self-treatment can do a great deal of harm, since it may mask a more serious illness or may prevent a condition from clearing up if left alone. In drinking, as in eating, the key is moderation.

Proper Diet

Proper diet is an important contribution an individual can make to his good health, because foods build body tissues and provide energy for the body to work. Adequate diet planning is not difficult. The basic rules of good nutrition must be learned. See under Ch. 7, p. 194, for a full treatment of diet and nutrition. Applying these rules to a daily diet will take only a few minutes of planning when the menu is decided upon, and will reap enormous rewards in good health and appearance. The hardest part of planning a balanced diet is to avoid selecting food solely on the basis of taste or convenience, and ignoring nutritional value.

VITAMINS: Eating a proper, balanced diet will fulfill vitamin and other nutritional requirements. Therefore, there is no need for a healthy person who eats nutritious foods to take vitamin pills. Vitamins and other food supplements should be taken only on the advice of a physician or dentist. If a person decides he is deficient in some dietary element and purchases a patent medicine to treat the problem, he may only make it worse. It is rare to find someone deficient in only one element, and by trying to treat himself, he may delay seeking the advice of a doctor.

BREAKFAST: Many Americans neglect breakfast, an important contribution to good diet. Studies prove that men, women, and children need an adequate breakfast. A good breakfast can provide a start in obtaining the day's vitamin and mineral requirements. It is also a help to dieters and those trying to maintain a stable weight, since those who have eaten a good breakfast are able to avoid mid-morning snacks such as sweet rolls, cakes, and the like, which are usually high in carbohydrates and calories.

Weight and Health

Overweight is one of the biggest deterrents to successful middle age, and is also one of the greatest threats to health and longevity. As one doctor said, "Consider how few really obese persons you see over 60 years of age." Unfortunately, in middle age most of us maintain the eating habits of our youth while we cut down on our exercise. The result: added weight that acts as an anchor to our physical well-being.

The overweight person is more likely to develop arthritis, diabetes, heart disease, high blood pressure, kidney trouble, and many other disabling or fatal disorders. As the American Heart Association said recently: "Pity the fat man; the statisticians number his days."

As reported in *Nation's Business,* "If you are overweight by 10 percent, your chances of surviving the next 20 years are 15 percent less than if you had ideal weight; if you are 20 percent overweight, your chances are 25 percent less; if you are 30 percent overweight, 45 percent less." In other words, the odds are against the overweight.

If you do not know what your ideal weight should be, a doctor can tell you. To check yourself, try the "pinch" test. Take a pinch of skin on your upper arm just below the shoulder. If more than a half-inch separates your fingers, you are too fat. Try the same test on your stomach when you're standing erect. And, of course, your mirror can reval the tell-tale signs of middle-age fat—the double chin, sagging belly, flabby arms and legs.

Good Eating Habits

Is there any magic way to reduce? The only sure way is to *eat less,* and to continue this practice all the time. It will not help if you go on a crash diet and then resume your normal eating habits. And while exercise will help control weight and burn up excess calories, probably the best exercise is to push yourself away from the table before you've overeaten.

Calories do count, and usually the caloric intake of a person in the 40- to 55-year age bracket should be about one-third less than that of a person between ages 25 and 40. Again, your doctor or a good calorie-counter can help you determine what to eat and how much.

Here are some additional tips from nutritionists to help you lose weight:

• *Cut down on quantity.* Eat just enough to satisfy your appetite—not as much as you can. Even low-calorie foods will add weight if you eat enough of them.

• *Eat less more often.* Spread your food intake over several meals or snacks. Some hospitals have been experimenting with five meals a day, spreading the recommended total food intake over two full meals a day (brunch and dinner) and three snacks (continental breakfast, afternoon snack, and night cap). They find that the stomach handles small amounts of food better, that metabolism keeps working at a good pace all day, and that blood sugar levels (your energy reserve) do not drop between meals. Also, the process of digestion burns up calories.

• *Avoid high-calorie foods.* Cut out breads, rolls, jellies, jams, sauces, gravies, dressings, creams, and rich desserts. These are the villains that add calories and are not as rich in nutrients.

• *Look for natural flavors.* Cultivate an interest in the natural flavor of what you eat. Try vegetables without butter, coffee and tea without cream and sugar. You might want to substitute a pinch of salt or a squeeze of lemon on your vegetables or noncaloric sweeteners in your beverages, but chances are you will find the natural flavors new and interesting.

• *Serve only just enough.* Keep portions small and put serving dishes with leftovers out of sight. Taking seconds is often just a habit. Cultivate the idea of just one serving, and you will find it satisfies the appetite. Another idea: serve meals on smaller plates. The portion will look big if only in relationship to the size of the plate.

In order to maintain a healthy body and a youthful appearance while dieting, you must make sure you eat the necessary proteins and nutrients. This can be done by selecting foods from the four basic food groups. See *Basic Nutritional Requirements*, p. 194.

As a panel of experts on middle age said in a recent interview: "Two factors are vital to successful middle age: physical activity and a variety of interests. Move around but don't rush around. Keep an open mind and a closed refrigerator. Remember that variety is more than the spice of life—it's the wellspring of life. The person who pursues a variety of activities will usually stay fit long after middle age."

LIVING LIFE TO THE FULLEST

No wise man ever wished to be younger.   —JONATHAN SWIFT

Staying young is looked on by most of the rest of the world as a peculiarly American obsession. This obsession is certainly fostered and exploited by the advertising industry, but its causes have to be looked for elsewhere.

In many countries, it is the old who are venerated for their wisdom and authority. This point of view is likely to prevail in societies that stay the same or that enjoyed their greatest glories in the past.

America is another matter. Because of its history, it is literally a young country. It is also a nation built on the idea of progress and hope in the future. And to whom does the future belong if not to youth?

Keeping up with change is unfortunately identified by too many people with how they look rather than how they think or feel. To be young in heart and spirit has very little to do with wearing the latest style in clothes—no matter how unbecoming —or learning the latest dances. Maintaining an open mind receptive to new ideas, keeping the capacity for pleasure in the details of daily living, refusing to be overwhelmed by essentially unimportant irritations can make the middle years more joyful for any family.

A Critical Time

Nowadays, the average American can expect to reach the age of 70. Thus, for most people, the middle years begin during the late thirties. Ideally, these are the years of personal fulfillment accompanied by a feeling of pride in accomplishment, a deeper knowledge of one's strengths and limitations, and a growing understanding and tolerance of other people's ideas and behavior.

EMOTIONAL PRESSURES: In many families, however, the pleasures of maturity often go hand in hand with increased pressures. It's no simple matter for the typical husband and wife in their forties to maintain emotional health while handling worries about money, aging parents, anxiety about willful teen-agers, tensions caused by marital friction, and feelings of depression about getting older. To some people, the problems of the middle years are so burdensome that instead of dealing with them realistically—by eliminating some, by compromising in the solution of others—they escape into excessive drinking or into sexual infidelity. It doesn't take much thought to realize that those escapes do nothing except introduce new problems.

PHYSICAL SYMPTOMS OF EMOTIONAL PROBLEMS: For others, deep-seated conflicts that come to a head during the middle years may be expressed in chronic physical symptoms. Many physicians in the past intuitively understood the relationship between emotional and physical health, but it is only in recent years that medical science has proved that feelings of tension, anxiety, suppressed anger, and frustration are often the direct cause of ulcers, sexual impotence, high blood pressure, and heart attacks, not to mention sleeplessness and headaches.

Of course, there are no magic formulas that guarantee the achievement of emotional well-being at any time of life. Nor does any sensible person expect to find a perfect solution to any human problem. However, it is possible to come to grips with specific difficulties and deal with them in ways that can reduce stress and safeguard emotional health.

Sexuality During the Middle Years

In spite of the so-called sexual revolution and all its accompanying publicity, it is still very difficult for most people to sort out their attitudes towards sexual activity. It is a subject that continues to be clouded by feelings of guilt and anxiety, surrounded by taboos, and saddled with misinformation. For each individual, the subject is additionally complicated by personal concepts of love and morality.

Many people were shocked when the Kinsey reports on male and female sexual behavior appeared. More recently, militant efforts have been made in various communities to prevent the schools from including sex education in their courses of study. Yet marriage counselors, family doctors, ministers, and all other specialists in human relations can attest to the amount of human misery caused by ignorance about sex —all the way from the ignorance that results in a 15-year-old's unwanted pregnancy to the ignorance of a 50-year-old man about his wife's sexual needs.

Pioneering Work in Sexual Response

According to the research of Dr. William H. Masters and Mrs. Virginia E. Johnson, directors of the Reproductive Biology Research Foundation in St. Louis and authors of *Human Sexual Response* and *Human Sexual Inadequacy*, 50 percent of all married couples can be considered sexually inadequate. These authorities define sexual inadequacy as the inability to achieve sexual communication in marriage or insecurity about whatever sexual communication does exist.

In the intensive sexual therapy they offer to married couples professionally referred to the Foundation, Dr. Masters and Mrs. Johnson concentrate on the relationship between husband and wife. They stress the concept of sexual activity as communication between two human beings, each with unique needs and desires that must be fulfilled by the other. The basic attitude they hope to instill in those who come to them for help is that pleasure in sex is natural and can be achieved through an understanding of giving and receiving it.

Emotional Causes of Sexual Inadequacy

It is not unusual for a couple whose marriage began with a satisfactory sexual adjustment to find the relationship deteriorating as they approach their forties. From the point of view of how the body itself functions during the middle years, there is rarely a physical reason for a decline in the ability to perform sexually. Almost always, male impotence or lack of female responsiveness is caused by psychological factors, some deeply buried, others superficial.

The Impotent Husband

Because of particular circumstances and differing personalities, many middle-aged men spend their days in a state of impotent anger. They may have suppressed feelings of hostility against an unreasonable boss; they may feel put down by a successful neighbor; they may be unable to deal effectively with a rebellious son. With such men, a chain of cause and effect sometimes develops that cannot be broken without professional help.

The tensions generated by impotent anger may result in impotence during the sex act. Since the underlying causes for sexual impotence are probably unknown to him, a middle-aged husband may develop deep anxieties about his waning sexuality. These anxieties in turn cause the sexual incompetence to continue.

There is also the husband who unconsciously builds up resentments against his wife because he thinks she is paying too much attention to the house and the children or to her career and too little to him. Their surface relationship may not be affected, but his body will express his feelings by withholding itself from her as a form of punishment.

Another typical cause of temporary impotence is a feeling of guilt about an adventure in sexual infidelity. Impotence with the marital partner under these circumstances is usually the husband's way of punishing himself for behavior that he considers sinful.

The Unresponsive Wife

Many men complain about their wives' waning interest in sex during the middle years. It is true that women often give or withhold themselves from their husbands as a reward or a punishment, but more commonly, wives who are unresponsive are likely to be expressing resentment about the fact that the only time they get any attention is in bed, and even there, the attention is apt to be perfunctory rather than personally gratifying and meaningful.

When this is the case, the breach in a marriage is likely to widen unless there is a willingness on the part of both partners to confront the problem openly, if necessary with a marriage counselor, minister, or doctor, so that a satisfactory solution can be found. Otherwise, the wife's resentment of neglect expressed in sexual coldness may lead her husband to look elsewhere for gratification.

Sometimes a woman seems unresponsive only because she feels she is being used as a sex object instead of having her needs satisfied. This unconscious feeling may express itself in the lack of responsiveness that is mistakenly called frigidity. As a result of their experience in helping many couples achieve good sexual relationships, Dr. Masters and Mrs. Johnson assert that the word *frigidity* has little meaning. There are very few women incapable of being physically aroused and satisfied by an understanding sexual partner.

Being Honest

In most cases of sexual inadequacy, insight and honesty about feelings are usually a more effective treatment than hormones, sex manuals, and so-called aphrodisiacs.

Any married couple whose sexual problems have become acute during the middle years should look for the causes in their own emotions about themselves and each other. They should also examine any persistent feelings of tension and anxiety that might be the result of practical matters in their daily lives, such as worry about money or children.

Beyond Motherhood: New Goals

There are many women casting about to find ways of spending their newly found spare time, women who are bored by bridge and gossip, who enjoy being a wife and mother and grandmother but also want an outlet that is their very own, disengaged from their role in the family. Such women might do some thinking about unfulfilled aspirations and the interests of their younger years, abandoned because of practical pressures.

Each one must find a way of spending leisure time in a way that is personally meaningful. Never mind that the children think it's funny for their mother to be going back to school for a college degree; or that the husband doesn't understand why his wife isn't taking it easy instead of taking a part-time job in a department store; or that the neighbors make remarks about the easel and paints that have suddenly appeared on the back porch.

Returning to Work or School

More middle-aged, middle-class women are taking jobs after years of housekeeping than ever before. Many companies are eager to hire them—on a part-time basis if necessary—because they are usually serious, competent, and reliable. Colleges make special provisions for women who want to complete their education after a long absence from studies. Even in small towns, there are many fruitful avenues for earning money or engaging in a productive hobby.

A feeling of pride in accomplishment at a time when household chores and child-raising no longer require much daily attention is usually the best medicine for depressed spirits. Personally meaningful activities outside the home are also an

excellent way to keep in touch with what's happening in the world. Nowadays there is no reason for a woman in her forties or fifties to feel restless, bored, or useless. The opportunities for self-expression and personal fulfillment are sufficiently varied to satisfy anyone's individual needs. All it takes is the genuine desire to find them.

More Than a Breadwinner: Vocation and Avocation

Everybody knows that it takes money to maintain a household and raise a family, and there is no doubt that during the middle years financial pressures reach their highest point, what with sending children through school, helping to support aging parents, and meeting increased medical and dental expenses. At this time, even those men who truly enjoy their work often feel they scarcely have the time or peace of mind to enjoy anything else.

Need for Other Outlets

Just as most women need personal outlets for their individuality away from home and family, so most men can achieve better emotional health if they find avenues of self-expression unrelated to their job or

Many middle-aged women resume their educations after years of absence for child rearing and family responsibilities.

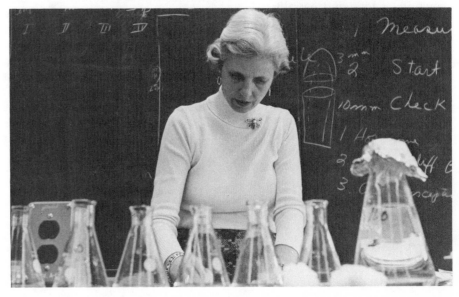

their role as husband and father. This does not mean becoming so passionately involved in playing golf or going fishing that the family is constantly neglected. Nor does it mean spending excessive amounts of money on rare stamps at the expense of the family budget.

On the other hand, if a man chooses a hobby that doesn't include the family, such as singing in a choir or studying a foreign language, rather than choosing one that does—such as going on camping trips, or taking pictures—there is no reason for the rest of the household to be resentful. Togetherness is a good thing to strive for, but it isn't a hard and fast principle to be applied to all activities.

It's healthier for a man to take an occasional fishing trip with his cronies, enjoy every minute of it, and come home relaxed and refreshed, than to take along a wife who will be bored and children who will be restless. In such far-too-frequent cases, no one has a good time. Nor should a father insist on teaching his son how to play chess so that they can share a hobby when his son would rather spend his time otherwise.

A Satisfying Hobby

The choice of a satisfying leisure-time activity is an entirely individual matter. Some men prefer a hobby that is sedentary, such as model-building. Others who have to sit in an office all day find the vigorous play of the handball court physically and emotionally exhilarating.

Some men, oppressed by constant association with other people, enjoy solitary hobbies such as long nature walks; others, whose jobs involve working alone, like to get together with a group for bowling or bridge playing. There are those who like competitive hobbies and those who want to escape the competitiveness of their work by puttering around in the basement or studying the fine points of the Civil War or experimenting in haute cuisine.

Many men as well as women find

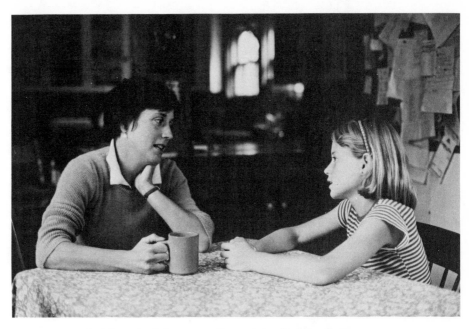

An informal talk between mother and daughter gives both generations an opportunity to express their opinions and exchange ideas.

the idea of community service appealing as a productive way of using free time. The opportunities are endless: going into poorer neighborhoods and training athletic teams; starting a tutoring group as part of a church activity; getting involved in grass-roots politics and pressing for local reforms; organizing a block association for property maintenance and improvement.

Building a collection can be a gratifying hobby, and the collection need not involve much money. The pleasures usually come from finding a rare specimen—whether it's a matchbook cover or an old comic book—from satisfying a need to own something unique, and from learning in the process of looking for items of interest.

Flexing Mental Muscles

Healthy human beings, regardless of age, need a certain amount of intellectual stimulation to keep their spirits refreshed. The arteries of the body may harden slowly with age, but there are people whose minds remain young and limber in spite of their increasing years.

Housewives commonly complain that they do not get enough stimula-

tion from their daily chores. Men talk about getting into a rut on their jobs—going stale. Yet stimulation for the mind is no farther away than the nearest library, if the mind is hungry for food for thought. There's plenty of mental exercise available for those in the middle years who are willing to review their old ideas and to examine some new ones.

FAMILY DISCUSSIONS: Having relaxed discussions with teen-age children can be a fine source of intellectual refreshment if both generations can listen to each other with tolerance and mutual respect. Some parents get huffy and defensive if their views are challenged. This defensiveness—in some cases, downright hostility—results in closing the channels of communication.

This is not to suggest that every idea espoused by the young should be adopted by their elders. But opinions can be exchanged and challenges involving facts and figures can be met in the spirit of civilized discussion. There are areas in which parents can be educated by their children, and the areas can range all the way from trying out new recipes suggested by a venturesome daughter to getting a book on drugs from the library in order to answer a son who cheerfully calls his father a drug addict because he has to have three drinks when he comes home from work.

COMMUNITY RESOURCES: Some families find they need go no farther than their own home for intellectual activity. For those who want broader opportunities to use their heads, there are community resources that can be explored. Church organizations, parent-teacher associations, or social clubs can be used as forums. These might include public discussions, film presentations, and meetings on problems of current interest, such as drug addiction and slum clearance.

For those looking for enlightenment of a specific kind, the facilities of schools in the area should be investigated. Many colleges and universities offer adult education programs that cover a wide range of subjects—from real estate evaluation to philosophy. It's also possible to set up a study group composed of friends and associates who want to find out more about American history or the history of art, to study anthropology or the behavior of social insects, and to hire a lecturer to meet with the group once or twice a week.

Travel

Travel is a wonderful way of broadening interests, even if the trip means going to a nearby city or dairy farm. When children are in their later teens and can safely be left on their own for a few days— with some neighborly supervision —a husband and wife can enjoy going places of special interest to them rather than having to take younger tastes into account

The destination needn't be another continent to provide fascinating new sights and information. People who live in Chicago will find the small seacoast villages of New England a totally new world; Bostonians will find a way of life strange to them if they drive through the Smoky Mountains; people who live in a small town or a farm can

get a big lift out of wandering about in a big city.

In traveling abroad, the more advance planning that is invested in the trip, the greater the rewards. Every effort should be made to learn at least a little of the language of the country to be visited, and instead of settling for a group tour in which each moment is planned, there's much pleasure to be gained from exploring a particular enthusiasm, whether it be food, architecture, history, or a return to the village of one's foreign-born ancestors.

Separation and Divorce

Marriage in this country is based on the highly personal concept of love rather than on such traditional foundations as a property merger between two families or an arrangement determined by the friendship of the young people's parents. It is often assumed, therefore, that if mutual love is the basis for embarking on a marriage, its absence is a valid reason for dissolving it, either by legal separation or divorce.

The idea of divorce is not particularly modern; in practically every time and place where a form of marriage has existed, so has some form of divorce, with reasons ranging from excessive wife-beating to failure to deliver a piece of land mentioned in the marriage contract.

The High Rate of Divorce

What is new is the high rate of divorce. Figures now indicate that in the United States as a whole, approximately one in every four mar-

A divorced parent asks his son for help in the kitchen of his new house, letting the child know that he is always important in his father's life.

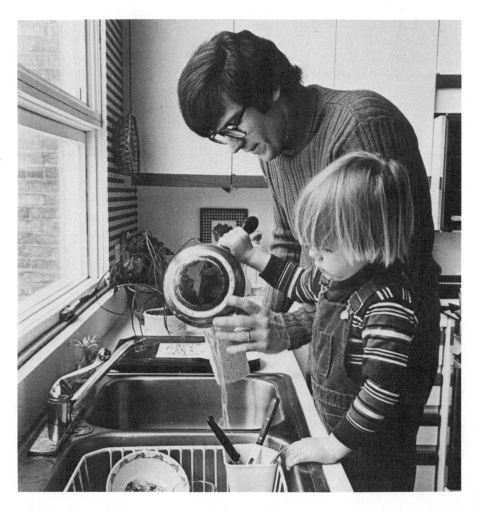

riages is terminated by legal arrangement. However, these figures by no means indicate that the family as an institution is on the way out, since a constantly increasing number of people who get divorced get married again.

There are many reasons for the growing rate of separation and divorce:

• Over the last 50 years, a continually increasing percentage of the population has been getting married.

• Although the trend toward earlier marriages has leveled off in recent years, a significant number of people still marry at earlier ages than was common in the past. (The number of divorces is highest among the poorly educated group who marry under the age of 21.)

• The legal requirements for separation and divorce are less rigid than formerly.

• With increasing independence and earning capacity, women are less frightened of the prospect of heading a family.

• The poorer groups in the population, in which desertion was a common practice, are more often obtaining divorces.

Contrary to popular belief, there are more divorces among the poor than among the rich, and more among the less well-educated than among the educated. Also, most divorces occur before the fifth year of marriage.

Telling the Truth to Children

Most people with children who are contemplating a breakup of their marriage generally make every effort to seek professional guidance that might help them iron out their differences. When these efforts fail and steps are taken to arrange for a separation or divorce, it is far healthier for parents to be honest with each other and with their children than to construct elaborate explanations based on lies.

A teen-ager who is given the real reason for a divorce is less likely to have something to brood about than one who is told lies that he can see through. If the real reason for a divorce is that the parents have tried their best to get along with each other but find it impossible, the child who is in his teens or older can certainly understand this. If the marriage is coming to an end because the husband or wife wants to marry someone else, the explanation to the child should avoid assigning blame. When the rejected parent tries to enlist the child's sympathy by blackening the character of the parent who is supposedly the cause of the divorce, results are almost always unpleasant. Under no circumstances and no matter what his age should a child be called on to take the side of either parent or to act as a judge.

Nor should children be told any more about the circumstances of the breakup of a marriage than they really want to know. Young people have a healthy way of protecting themselves from information they would find hurtful, and if they ask few questions, they need be told only the facts they are prepared to cope with. Of course, as they grow older and live through their own problems, they will form their own view of what really happened between their parents.

After the Separation

Traditionally, in separation and divorce proceedings, the children have remained in the custody of the mother, with financial support arrangements and visiting rights spelled out for the father. Although an increasing number of fathers have been awarded custody of their children in recent years, it is still commonly the mother who must face the problems of single parenthood after divorce. (See below, p. 170.) Although teen-age children may need some extra attention for a while, there is no need for a mother to make a martyr of herself, nor should she feel guilty when she begins to consider remarrying.

The father should be completely reliable in his visiting arrangements, and if he has remarried, should try to establish good relationships between the offspring of his former marriage and his new family.

Stepchildren

People who remarry during the middle years frequently find themselves in the role of stepparent. This is a role with many problems and many rewards; the chief requirements are patience and tact.

The stepchild has to deal with many complicated feelings: his sense of loss, either through death or divorce, of his own parent; his resentment against the parent who has remarried, and his hostility to the stranger who has become his new parent.

A stepparent should proceed affectionately but cautiously, and should not try to be accepted by the child as a replacement for the parent who has gone. If the child and stepparent have achieved a friendly rapport before the remarriage, they should build on the friendship rather than trying to transform it into a parent-child relationship immediately. When the child's trust has been gained, the stepparent can gradually assume some of the authority of a true parent, always waiting for the child to indicate a desire and need for it first.

A Death in the Family

When a husband or wife dies during the middle years, there is a general feeling that the death is unnatural because it is in all ways premature: the normal life expectancy has been cut short, the one who remains is prematurely bereaved, and the children are deprived of a parent too soon.

There are a few consolations in the presence of death: some people are sustained by their religious beliefs, others by the rallying of relatives and friends, and still others by happy memories of the years spent together in a fulfilled relationship.

The bereft parent should share his grief with the children, but they should not be thought unfeeling if they seem to be going about their business almost in the usual way. They may be dealing with a tangle of feelings that will take some time to come to the surface—feelings of guilt about past thoughtlessness, of confusion about wishing that the parent who remains had died instead, and of fear connected with the thought of their own death.

When the time seems right, young people can be encouraged to talk about the parent who died. Remembering funny incidents and times of anger, reliving shared experiences —these can act as a restorative to the living and make family ties closer.

As for remarrying, although the children and the deceased's relatives may consider such a step a disloyalty to the memory of the dead, it is actually a tribute, since it implies that the state of marriage was a happy one.

The Single Parent

When the job of being a single parent has to be faced, either because of death or divorce, the problems may seem overwhelming. Although they differ considerably depending on whether the parent is the father or mother, they are nonetheless difficult to sort out, particularly at a time when morale may be at a low ebb.

The Single Father

The single father with growing children often feels helpless in dealing with household tasks and gains some insight into the number of tasks involved in keeping things running smoothly at home. If he has a teen-age daughter or son, he can depend on him or her to do part of the job, but young people should not be burdened with all the responsibilities of housekeeping if some other arrangement can possibly be made. Perhaps a relative can be called on to help out part-time, or a professional housekeeper can be engaged for a few hours a day. Outside help is particularly important if the care of younger children is involved.

A motherless girl in adolescence may seek out the companionship and occasional guidance of an older woman who was a friend of her mother's, or she may spend more and more time at the home of a friend whose mother she likes and respects. Such a transfer of affection should not be considered as disloyalty.

The Single Mother

The mother who is a single parent usually has to cope with problems of earning and managing money. Fortunately, the job opportunities for middle-aged women are varied, and if the family finances can be worked out on the basis of a part-time job, this is a good transitional solution for making the adjustment of handling a job and running the household. A widow or divorcee may need to call on a friend or relative to help her with such practical matters as income tax, mortgages, loans, or investments. If these matters can be handled by a family lawyer without the fees being prohibitive, so much the better.

A widow or divorced woman should avoid concentrating too much on her children, nor should she give a son in his teens the understanding that he is now the head of the family. He is and must remain her son and nothing more. If an authority figure is needed as partial replacement for the departed husband, he should be sought among neighbors or relatives for whom the children feel respect.

In many communities, single parents have formed groups for discussion and mutual help. Such groups can usually be located through local social work agencies. Parents Without Partners, Inc., 132 Nassau Street, New York, New York 10038, specializes in the problems of single parents and publishes literature of interest to them.

CHAPTER 6

The Later Years

AGING AND WHAT TO DO ABOUT IT

Growing older could mean growing healthier. In many ways you are as old as you think and feel. Consider these points:

• No disease results just from the passage of years.

• We age piecemeal—each organ separately rather than uniformly.

• In retirement you have less daily stress and strain, and you have more time to take better care of yourself.

What, then, makes a person think and feel old?

The Aging Process

Physically, we mature at about age 25 to 30, when the body reaches maximum size and strength. Then, body tissues and cells are constantly being rebuilt and renewed. Nutrition, rest, exercise, and stress influence the length of time that the body can maintain a balance between the wearing down and rebuilding of body tissues. When more cells die than can be reproduced, they are replaced by a fibrous, inert substance called *collagen*. The living process slows down to compensate, and we begin aging; strength and ability start to decline.

But this happens at various intervals. For instance, vision is sharpest at age 25; the eye loses its ability to make rapid adjustments in focus after age 40. Hearing is sharpest at about age 10, then diminishes as you grow older. Sensitivity to taste and smell lessens after age 60.

The decline in strength and muscle ability is long and gradual; there are even gratifying plateaus. At age 50, a man still has about four-fifths of the muscle strength he had when he was 25.

Although physical abilities may decline, mental abilities may actually improve during the middle years, and memory and the ability to learn can remain keen. Dr. Alfred Schwartz, dean of education at Drake University, was asked: "Can a 70-year-old man in reasonably good health learn as rapidly as a 17-year-old boy?" Dr. Schwartz answered:

Indeed he can—provided he's in the habit of learning. The fact that some older people today are not active intellectually is no reflection on their ability to learn. There is ample proof that learning ability does not automatically decline with age.

Regardless of what you may have heard, organic brain damage affects less than one percent of those over age 65.

But in thinking about physical change, remember that this is just one aspect of aging. Age is determined by emotional and intellectual maturity as well as by chronological years.

Can a person do anything to retard aging?

Most *gerontologists* feel that the reason more people don't live longer is that they are not willing to follow a regimen of diet, exercise, rest, recreation—coupled with the exclusion of various excesses. And while there isn't anything you can do to set back the clock, you can keep in good health by making sure to have regular physical examinations, sufficient exercise, adequate rest, nutritious food, and a positive mental attitude.

A Positive Mental Attitude

Mark Twain once said: "Whatever a man's age he can reduce it several years by putting a bright-colored flower in his buttonhole." A lively, fresh outlook is essential for enjoyable living at any age. Most doctors believe there is a direct connection between one's state of mind and physical health. This is especially true when you are faced with the challenges of retirement. Plato said: "He who is of a calm and happy nature will hardly feel the pressure of age, but to him who is of an opposite disposition, youth and

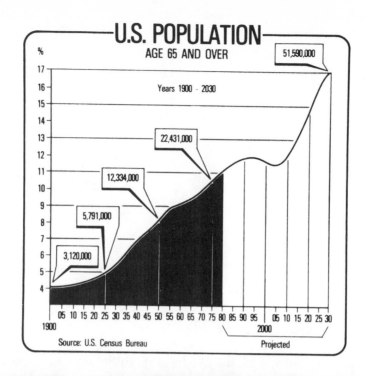

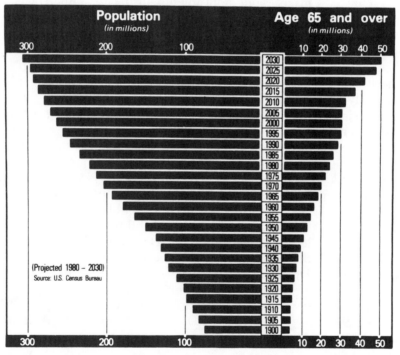

These two graphs show in different ways the number and percentage of Americans of age 65 and over as compared with the total U.S. population. Both graphs indicate actual figures and percentages from 1900–1975 and estimated figures from 1980–2030. *(Top)* This graph shows clearly that the percentage of Americans aged 65 and over has increased from 4 percent of the population in 1900 to about 10.5 percent in 1975, and is expected to climb to 17 percent by the year 2030. *(Bottom)* Look at the vertical column of years as your starting point. Then compare the bar extending to the left of each date—the total population—with the bar extending to the right—the population at age 65 and over at that time. This bar graph provides a good visual comparison between the two groups, and it is worth noting that whereas the total population in 2030 may be over 300 million—more than triple the population of 1900—the 65-and-older population in 2030 is expected to be *ten times* what it was in 1900—more than 50 million people. By 2030, one of every six Americans will be 65 years or older.

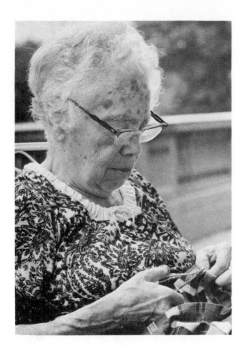

By pursuing new interests or utilizing skills learned through years of experience, a senior citizen can make the years of retirement a fulfilling stage of life.

age are equally a burden."

Experts in the field of aging have found that most older people can relieve transitory depression by a deliberate shift of thought or by physical activity. If you look upon retirement as an opportunity to take better care of yourself and to pursue old and new interests, you'll go a long way toward better health.

The Annual Checkup

For peace of mind and to maintain and improve your health, make it a habit to see your doctor at least once a year. To remind themselves, many people make an appointment on their birthday. An annual checkup is especially important in later years and should not be put off or neglected.

During a routine checkup, the doctor pays special attention to enlarged lymph nodes of the neck, armpits, and groin, and the front of the neck. He also checks the condition of veins and arteries and looks at your knees and arches—which are of particular importance to older people.

He makes tests for arteriosclerosis, high blood pressure, diabetes, brain tumors, and other diseases. He can feel and tap your body to check your lungs, liver, and spleen, and he can take electrocardiographs to detect changes in your heart. Simple tests can note bladder and kidney conditions.

In addition, the doctor usually asks about personal habits—smoking, drinking, eating. He also wants to know about any unusual symptoms you might have. Be completely frank with your doctor, answer his questions as directly as possible, and give all information that might be helpful.

When explaining the nature of your ailment or symptom, tell him what part of the body is involved, what changes are associated with the symptoms, and whether symptoms occurred after a change of diet or medicine. Tell him about any previous experiences with this condition and what treatments you might have had.

It is extremely important to tell your doctor about any pills you are taking—including aspirin, tranquilizers, and sleeping tablets. Even the most common drug can affect the potency of medication he might prescribe.

After he has taken your case history and after he has all the reports from your tests, the doctor will want to talk with you, explain his findings, and perhaps make some recommendations. Take his advice; don't try to be your own doctor.

If you have questions, don't be afraid to ask them. Have him explain the nature of your ailment, how long it may take for relief or cure, how the therapy or medication is expected to work, and the possible impact on your everyday activities.

Hopefully, by following his advice you'll stay healthy and well. However, if you are at home and feel ill, call your doctor if:

• Your symptoms are so severe you can't endure them.

• Apparent minor symptoms persist without explainable cause.

• You are in doubt.

For more information, see *The Physical Examination*, p. 291.

Oral Health

It is especially important in later years to have regular dental checkups. After age 50, over half of the American people have some form of *periodontal disease*, and at age 65 nearly all persons have this disease.

Brushing teeth and gums regularly is a defense against periodontal disease. Use dental floss to remove all food particles and plaque from areas between the teeth, especially after each meal. See *Periodontal Disease*, p. 259, for more information on this subject.

Dentures

If you do lose some teeth, they should be replaced with bridges or partial or full dentures, because the cheeks and lips will otherwise sag and wrinkle and make you look older than you really are. Chewing ability and the clarity of speech are also impaired if missing teeth are not replaced. See *Dentures*, p. 261.

Diet and Health

Just what are your food requirements as you grow older? Basically you need the same essential nutrients that you have always needed, except that you face special problems. You need to:

• Select food more carefully to eat adequate proteins, vitamins, and minerals—while cutting down on calories.

• Get the most nutritious food for the least money and make the most of what you buy.

• Avoid bad eating habits—make mealtime a pleasure rather than a chore.

• Learn new techniques to stretch meals, use leftovers, and substitute lower-priced items with the same nutritional value for higher-price foods. In other words, learn how to shop well.

Basic Requirements

How can you get the essential nutrients every day? A good rule is first to eat recommended servings from the Basic Four Food Groups (see below) established by the National Research Council. Then, eat other foods that you like, as long as they do not go over the recommended daily caloric intake. The average man in the 55-to-75-year age group should consume 2,200 calories a day; the average woman in the same age group, 1,600 calories a day. This is a drop of between 500 and 600 calories a day from what was needed at age 25. As you grow older, your physical activity decreases and your metabolism slows, causing body fats to build up at a much higher rate, and making you more prone to hardening of the arteries and certain heart conditions.

Here are the Basic Four Food Groups:

MEAT GROUP: Two or more servings from this group of foods are recommended daily. A serving is 2 to 3 oz. of cooked meat, fish, or poultry; 2 eggs; occasionally 1 cup of cooked dry beans or peas; 1/2 cup peanut butter; or 1 cup cottage cheese.

DAIRY FOODS: Dairy food requirements may be satisfied by two cups of milk or its equivalent in cheese, ice cream, etc. A 1 1/3 oz. slice of cheddar-type cheese or one scant pint of ice cream is equivalent to 1 cup of milk. Imitation ice cream or ice milk where vegetable fat has been substituted for butterfat has just as much protein.

VEGETABLES AND FRUIT: The daily vegetable and fruit requirement consists of four or more servings. A serving is one-half cup. Include one serving of citrus fruit each day and dark green or deep yellow vegetables every other day.

BREAD AND CEREAL GROUP: Each day have four or more servings of whole grain, enriched, or restored products such as breads, cereals, rice, hominy grits, noodles, or macaroni. One serving is a slice of bread; one-half to three-fourths cup cooked cereal, pasta, or rice; one medium potato.

Use other foods such as sweets, baked goods, desserts to complete meals and treat the sweet tooth. But remember to count calories. Nutritionists have found that skinny animals live longer than fat ones, and this seems to be true of people, too.

Beware of food fads and so-called health foods unless these are recommended by your doctor. Also, do not buy vitamins and mineral tablets unless prescribed. When you obtain vitamins from food, your body uses the amount necessary to maintain proper health, appetite, and resistance to infection. Your body promptly eliminates excesses of vitamin C and the B complex, and stores an excess of vitamins A and D in your liver and other body organs. It may take up to seven years of practically complete deprivation for a previously healthy adult to show signs of a vitamin deficiency.

Some older people may go on low-fat diets because of fear of cholesterol caused by talk and advertisements for unsaturated fats. Get a doctor's recommendation before curtailing your fat intake—too little fat and dairy products can be as harmful as too much.

Also, unless prescribed, do not take iron tonics or pills. Usually, you'll get adequate iron intake if you eat meat, eggs, vegetables, and enriched cereals regularly. Adding more iron to a normal diet may even be harmful.

Eating Habits

If you find that mealtime is a chore rather than a pleasure, try these tips to enhance your meals:

• Try a two-meal-a-day schedule. Have a late breakfast and early dinner when you are really hungry. But be sure to get your Basic Four requirements in these two meals.

• Drink a glass of water as soon as you wake up to promote good digestion, weight control, and bowel movements.

• Try a walk or light exercise to stimulate appetite and to regulate body processes. Moderate exercise also will help regulate weight since it burns up calories.

• You might sip a glass of wine before dinner. Recent research shows wine is very useful to older people in improving appetite and digestion. Port, a light sherry, and vermouth with a dash of soda are good appetite stimulators.

• Make meals interesting by including some food of distinctive flavor to contrast with a mild-flavored food; something crisp for

To maintain good health, an older person should carefully select foods that contain essential nutrients but are low in calories.

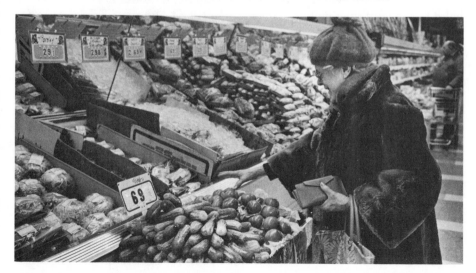

contrast with softer foods, even if it is only a pickle or a lettuce leaf; some brightly colored food for eye appeal.

• Pep up your food with a judicious use of herbs and spices or flavor-enhancers like wine, bottled sauces, fruit juices, and peels.

• If some food causes you distress, eliminate it and substitute something else of equal nutritive value. Green salad may include too much roughage for the intestinal tract; ham or bacon may be supplying your body with too much salt, which increases water retention. Or you may be drinking too much coffee, tea, or soft drinks.

• Be realistic about your chewing ability. Food swallowed whole may be causing digestive problems. If your teeth are not as good as they were or if you are wearing dentures, try cubing, chopping, or grinding foods that are difficult to chew. Let your knife or meat grinder do part of the work.

• Try a different atmosphere or different setting for your meals. Use candlelight, music, and your best linen on occasion. Move outdoors when the weather is good; eat your lunch in the park and dinner on the patio.

• Occasionally invite a friend or relative to dine with you. It's surprising what stimulating conversation and an exchange of ideas can do to boost your mood and appetite.

• Try a new recipe or a new food. Thanks to modern transportation, foods are available in larger cities from many areas and other countries. Eat eggplant or okra, avocado or artichoke, gooseberry jam, or garbanzo beans in a salad. And why not have a papaya with lemon juice for breakfast?

Cooking Hints

Try these ideas for preparing food more easily; they are especially useful if you have only a single gas or electric burner:

• Combine your vegetables and meat—or some other protein food—in a single pot or pan. You can cook many hot, nourishing meals of this kind: Irish stew, braised liver or pot roast with vegetables, ham-and-vegetable chowder or fish chowder, a New England boiled dinner.

• Combine leftovers to make a one-dish meal. Leftover meat combines beautifully with vegetables, macaroni, or rice. Add a cheese or tomato sauce or a simple white sauce and heat in a baking dish. Chopped tomatoes or green onions or chives will give extra flavor and color to the dish.

• Round out one-dish meals with a crisp salad topped with cut strips of leftover cooked meat or poultry or another raw food, bread, a beverage, and perhaps a dessert.

• Mix leftover cooked vegetables with raw fresh ones, such as chopped celery, cucumber slices, tomatoes, green pepper, shredded cabbage, to make an interesting salad.

• Cream vegetables, meat, fish, or chicken. Or serve them with a tasty sauce. Use canned tomato or mushroom soup for a quick and easy sauce. If the dish is a bit skimpy, a hard-boiled egg may stretch it to serving size.

• Add a bit of relish, snappy cheese, or diced cucumber to a cooked dressing for meat or vegetable salad.

• If you cook a potato, an ear of corn, or some other vegetable in the bottom of a double boiler, you can use the top to warm rolls, heat leftover meat in gravy, or heat such foods as creamed eggs or fish.

The Value of Exercise

As you grow older, exercise can help you look, feel, and work better. Various organs and systems of the body, particularly the digestive process, are stimulated through activity, and, as a result, work more effectively.

You can improve your posture through exercise that tones supporting muscles. This not only improves appearance but can decrease the

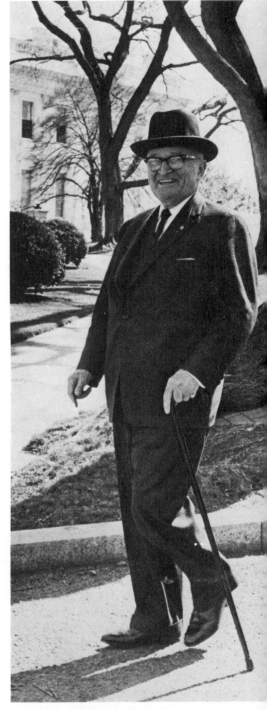

President Harry Truman thrived from the tonic effect of his invigorating 30-minute early morning walks.

frequency of lower-back pain and disability.

Here are some other benefits of exercise: it can increase your ability to relax and tolerate fatigue; it improves muscle tone; reduces fat deposits; increases working capacity of the lungs; improves kidney and liver function; increases volume of blood, hemoglobin, and red blood cells, leading to improved utilization of oxygen and iron.

Also, physically active people are less likely to experience a heart attack or other forms of cardiovascular disease than sedentary people. Moreover, an active person who does suffer a coronary attack will probably have a less severe form. The Public Health Service studied 5,000 adults in Framingham, Mass., for more than a decade. When any member of the group suffered a heart attack, his physical activity was reviewed. It was found that more inactive people suffered more fatal heart attacks than active members.

Walking for Exercise

Exercise need not be something you *must* do but rather something you *enjoy* doing. One of the most practical and enjoyable exercises is walking. Charles Dickens said:

Walk and be happy, walk and be healthy. The best of all ways to lengthen our days is to walk, steadily and with a purpose. The wandering man knows of certain ancients, far gone in years, who have staved off infirmities and dissolution by earnest walking— hale fellows close upon eighty and ninety, but brisk as boys.

The benefits of walking were revealed in a recent Health Insurance Plan study of 110,000 people in New York City. Those who had heart attacks were divided into two groups—walkers and nonwalkers. The first four weeks of illness were reviewed for both groups. At the end of the time 41 percent of the nonwalkers were dead, while only 23 percent of the walkers were. When all physical activity was considered, 57 percent of the inactive had died compared to only 16 percent of those who had some form of exercise.

Walking is as natural to the human body as breathing. It is a muscular symphony; all the foot, leg, and hip muscles and much of the back musculature are involved.

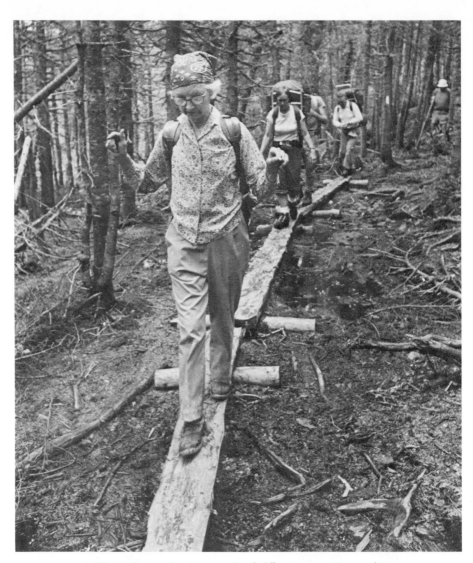

A hike in the woods gives people of different generations a chance to share their interest in nature and get essential exercise.

The abdominal muscles tend to contract and support their share of the weight, and the diaphragm and rib muscles increase their action. There is automatic action of the arm and shoulder muscles; the shoulder and neck muscles get play as the head is held erect; the eye muscles are exercised as you look about you.

Other Types of Exercise

Swimming and bicycling exercise most of the muscles, and gardening is highly recommended. The fresh air is beneficial, the bending, squatting, and countless other movements exercise most parts of the body.

Surprisingly, most games do not provide good exercise. According to a physical fitness research laboratory at the University of Illinois, the trouble with most games is that the action is intermittent—starting and stopping—a burst of energy and then a wait. The bowler swings a ball for 2.5 seconds and gets about one minute of actual muscular work per game. Golf is a succession of pause, swing, walk—or, more often, a ride to the next pause, swing, and so on. Also, you spend a lot of time standing and waiting for the party ahead and for your partners. Tennis gives one more exercise but it too involves a great deal of starting and stopping, as does handball. No game has the essential, tension-releasing pattern of continuous, vigorous, rhythmic motion found in such activities as walking, running, or jogging.

For formal exercises, you could join a gym, but you might find your enthusiasm waning after a few weeks. You could also exercise at home; there are many excellent books on exercise that provide programs for you to follow at home on a daily basis.

But everyone's exercise capacity varies. It is best to discuss any new exercise program with your doctor, especially if you have some illness or are out of practice. Then select an exercise which is pleasant for you and suitable to your condition.

It is most important always to warm up before any strenuous exercise. The U.S. Administration on Aging's booklet, *The Fitness Challenge in the Later Years*, states:

The enthusiast who tackles a keep-fit program too fast and too strenuously soon gives up in discomfort, if not in injury. A warm-up period should be performed by starting lightly with a continuous rhythmical activity such as walking and gradually increasing the intensity until your pulse rate, breathing, and body temperature are elevated. It's also desirable to do some easy stretching, pulling, and rotating exercises during the warm-up period.

The booklet outlines an excellent program—*red* (easiest), *white* (next), and *blue* (the most sustained and difficult). Each program is "designed to give a balanced workout utilizing all major muscle groups." For a copy of this booklet, write to the Superintendent of Documents, U.S. Government Printing Office, Washington, D.C. 20401.

A WORD OF CAUTION: You may be exercising too strenuously if the following happens:

• Your heart does not stop pounding within ten minutes after the exercise.
• You cannot catch your breath ten minutes after the exercise.
• You are shaky for more than thirty minutes afterwards.
• You can't sleep well afterwards.
• Your fatigue (not muscle soreness) continues into the next day.

Sensible, moderate exercise geared to your own physical capacity can help to give you a sense of all-around well-being. As Dr. Ernest Simonson, associate professor of physiological hygiene at the University of Minnesota Medical School, has said:

Those who exercise regularly never fail to mention that it makes them feel better in every way. It's common logic if one feels better, his attitude towards others will be more congenial. When one is in a cordial, happy frame of mind, he will likely make wiser decisions, and his world in general will look better.

Weight Control

Importantly, both diet and exercise affect the individual's ability to control his weight (see "Nutrition and Weight Control," p. 194; and "Weight Problems," p. 269). Healthy habits in both areas provide a complete answer for many older persons. For others, some additional effort is required.

The same diet rules that help the older person feel well and function adequately will make weight control simpler. But persons beyond middle age who have weight problems should make extra efforts to bring their weight down. Extra pounds of fat only make it harder for the vital organs to function; excess poundage also forces the heart to work harder. A variety of diets may be used to bring your weight back to where it should be. But the calorie-counter program may suffice for most persons.

Exercise provides the second key to weight control. Many doctors feel that older persons of both sexes should walk at least a mile daily. Other exercises acclaimed by medical men include golf, gardening, working on or around the house, and similar activities. Some other basic rules regarding exercise and diet should be noted:

• Avoid junk, or high carbohydrate, food where possible
• Make certain you are eating foods that provide enough protein
• Eat to assuage hunger, not to drive away boredom
• Remember that appetite usually decreases with age, and act accordingly
• Avoid vitamins unless they are prescribed by your doctor, and use

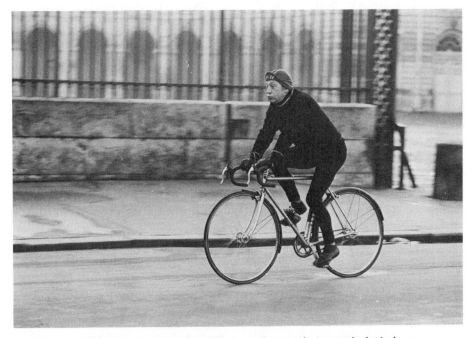

Cycling is an excellent activity for older people in good physical condition, providing fresh air along with needed exercise.

them according to instructions

• Try every day to eat foods in the four basic groups (see "Basic Requirements," p. 174).

• Keep moving; walk daily—to the store, post office, church, around the block

• If you exercise already, do it regularly; a little exercise daily is better than a lot on weekends

• If you don't exercise but are thinking of starting a program of workouts of some kind, start slowly and build up—following your doctor's recommendations

• If stress gives you problems, find ways to relax without eating or drinking; consider light exercises, yoga, meditation, breathing exercises, or some other method

Skin Problems

As a person grows older, his skin begins to wrinkle; oil and sweat glands slow down, causing the skin to become dry. Also, the skin may lack the elasticity and tone of normal skin, and this might cause changes in facial contours.

However, the skin, like other parts of the body, tends to age according to various factors. Among prime agers of the skin are exposure to sunlight and weather; the sailor and chronic sunbather may have older-looking skin than their years. Also, hereditary and racial factors influence skin age.

ITCHING: The skin often itches as one grows older. Itching usually stems from external irritations or internal diseases. External irritations may be more severe in winter because of lack of humidity and because the skin oil does not spread properly. Too many baths or wearing wool garments could also cause itching. You can correct this by cutting down on bathing, maintaining correct temperature and humidity, and applying skin creams.

If itching does not clear up in about two weeks, the trouble may be due to any of a number of internal diseases, some of them serious.

Thus, it is wise to see your doctor if itching persists.

SKIN CANCER: Skin cancer can be easily diagnosed and treated. The two most common types are *basal cell* and *squamous cell.*

The basal cell type begins with a small fleshy *nodule,* usually on the face. It may take several months to reach one-half to one inch in diameter. In about a year it begins to ulcerate and bleed. Then it forms a crust which it sheds at intervals, leaving another ulcer. If you notice anything like this, see your doctor He can usually remove the ulcer by a local operation.

Squamous cell cancer is often aided by smoking and exposure to the sun. The lesions may appear on the lips, mouth, and genitalia, and they tend to spread and increase in size. Horny growths in exposed areas—face, ears, neck, and scalp—may be forerunners of squamous cell cancer. Again, your doctor can treat or operate effectively. See also *Skin Cancer,* p. 438.

VITILIGO: Vitiligo, loss of pigment, is not caused by a disease, but it could be a hereditary problem. The affected area of skin has patches of whiteness throughout, but these can be masked by cosmetics.

SENILE PURPURA: Sometimes the skin develops *senile purpura* as one grows older. The characteristic hemorrhages of this condition usually appear on the extremities, and the purple color gradually fades and leaves mottled areas of yellow-brown. Generally, the skin is thin, fragile, and transparent in appearance.

STASIS DERMATITIS: Sometimes in association with such conditions as varicose veins, the skin may develop *stasis dermatitis,* an acute, chronic condition of the leg, associated with swelling, scaling of the skin, and in some cases, ulcer formation. It may exist for years with or without ulceration.

If any of the above conditions develop, it is wise to consult your doctor rather than try to treat yourself.

OTHER SKIN CONDITIONS: Other skin

conditions that may develop in the later years may include an increase in coarse hairs on exposed places such as the upper lip or chin. The downy hairs in the ears and nose become thicker and more apparent, and the eyebrows may become bushy. Graying hair is popularly associated with aging, but its onset often depends upon genetic factors and varies so much that it cannot be used as a reliable measure of age.

The ear lobes may elongate as you grow older and the nails may become coarse and thickened or thinner and brittle.

RELIEVING SKIN CONDITIONS: As mentioned earlier, you can use some creams to relieve dryness and scaliness in older skin. The best of such creams are the water-in-oil emulsions (cold creams) such as Petrolatum Rose Water Ointment USP XVI, or oil-in-water emulsions such as Hydrophilic Ointment USP XVI. Wrinkle creams will not help much, but some conditions may be masked by regular cosmetic items such as powder, rouge, mascara, hair dyes, etc.

Sunscreens may aid in preventing acute and chronic overexposure to the sun's rays.

Various types of surgery may be performed to correct older skin conditions, but they won't work for everyone. Among some of the more common types of surgery are plastic surgery, dermabrasion (skin planing), chemosurgery (chemical cautery), cryosurgery (freezing of the skin), and electrosurgery (employing electricity). See *Plastic and Cosmetic Surgery,* p. 343.

Hearing Loss

About three out of ten persons over age 65 have some hearing loss; at age 70 to 80 this percentage increases greatly.

Causes

While some hearing loss can be blamed on bad listening habits (tuning out people and conversation a person does not want to hear), the two major causes are conduction loss and nerve defects. A person with conduction loss hears high-pitched sounds best; a person with nerve impairment hears low sounds best. A combination of the two is called mixed deafness.

Conduction loss can be caused by wax, diseases of the ear, disturbances of the eardrum, or abnormalities inside the ear. It can also be caused by *otosclerosis*, a bony growth over the window to the inner ear. Most of these conditions can be treated by an ear doctor (*otologist*). He can remove wax from the ear, repair or replace eardrums, remove bony growths, and loosen or remove fixed ear bones.

Nerve defects may be another story. They are caused by wear and tear on the ear, disease, certain drugs, and blows and skull fractures, and usually cause permanent damage that cannot be helped by surgery or medical treatment.

Some persons complain about ringing in the ears (*tinnitus*) that may start without warning and vary in intensity and quality. What causes tinnitus in one person may not cause it in another, but often it is caused by wax in the ear, middle ear infection, arteriosclerosis, or certain drugs.

Hearing Aids

In some cases, a hearing loss may be helped by a hearing aid, but be sure your doctor refers you to a hearing clinic. A recent survey showed that most persons over 65 bought their aids directly from a hearing aid dealer rather than from a physician or a hearing aid clinic. Many of these older people discontinued using their hearing aids after buying them.

Be sure your doctor thinks a hearing aid will help you and directs you to a nonprofit hearing aid clinic. You can get addresses from your community health organizations or by writing to the National Association of Hearing and Speech Agencies, 814 Mayer Ave., Silver Spring, Md.

20910, or to the American Speech and Hearing Association, 9030 Old Georgetown Rd., Bethesda, Md. 20014.

At a hearing aid clinic, trained *audiologists* will scientifically measure your hearing and will assist you in trying on several kinds of hearing aids. These audiologists do not sell aids, but will give you an idea of what kind is the best for you.

Basically, there are four kinds of aids:

• Body types operate by a cord running to the receiver mold in the ear from a miniature microphone carried in a pocket, pinned to the clothing, or worn in a special carrier. They are about 1 to 1½-inches long and weigh about 2 ounces.

• Behind-the-ear types weigh only about ½ ounce and fit behind the ear. A plastic tube leads from the microphone to the receiver which fits in the ear.

• In-the-ear types are almost invisible. But they are not as powerful as other aids, and they may be affected by dirt, wax, or perspiration.

• Eyeglass models are built into the temple piece of spectacles. The bigger the temple piece the more powerful the aid.

The Veterans Administration, which annually tests aids, points out that there is no best hearing aid for all individuals. "Aids that test well for one person may not test well for someone else."

BUYING A HEARING AID: One good way to test an aid is to have a friend or relative along when you are being fitted. A familiar voice provides a yardstick to help you judge which aid is best.

It takes time to get used to a hearing aid. An aid amplifies all sounds—wanted and unwanted. Voices may sound unnatural or tinny. Normal sounds may be harsh and brutal—mainly because the patient is not used to them and cannot tune them out. However, the maximum power outlet of a hearing aid is below the threshold of pain, and will not amplify sounds over a certain level. Also, special circuiting in some aids limits the sound level reaching the eardrum. Nevertheless, every person who wears an aid must go through some adjustment process.

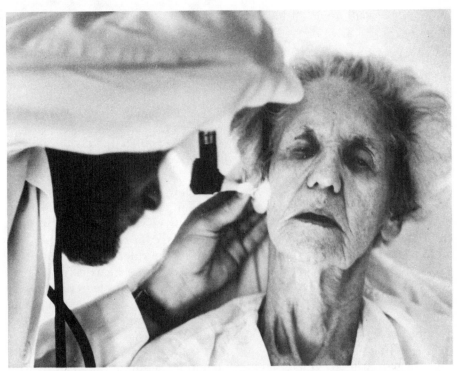

Any earache should be promptly treated by a doctor. Ear infections can be treated simply and safely, but if untreated can cause permanent damage.

If a person does not want to wear an aid or cannot adjust to one, he can try lip reading or speech reading. This involves watching the lips and vocal cords to determine what the person is saying. While you may not catch every word that is spoken, you will be able to understand enough.

TALKING TO THE HARD-OF-HEARING: If you are talking to someone who has some hearing difficulty, he'll understand you better if you speak slowly and distinctly and use the lower range of your voice. Face him when you speak; let him see the movements of your lips. It also helps to point to visible objects.

Above all, don't shout. In fact, raising your voice sometimes pitches it into a higher frequency which a hard-of-hearing person may find difficult to understand.

Other Health Problems

The following health problems might also confront an older person. (Many of these conditions are discussed at greater length elsewhere in the book; in such cases, cross-references are supplied for your convenience at the end of the section.)

Heart Disease

The heart is the strongest, toughest muscle in the body. It is like an engine that could run 70 years or more without an overhaul. The heart has a complete maintenance and repair system, enabling many heart disease victims to continue long and useful lives.

While heart disease is not necessarily a product of aging, some heart and blood vessel problems become more acute as one grows older.

The following symptoms do not necessarily indicate heart disease, but it is wise to see a physician if you notice any of them:

• Shortness of breath
• A feeling of tightness in the chest or pain directly related to exertion or excitement
• Swelling of the feet and ankles

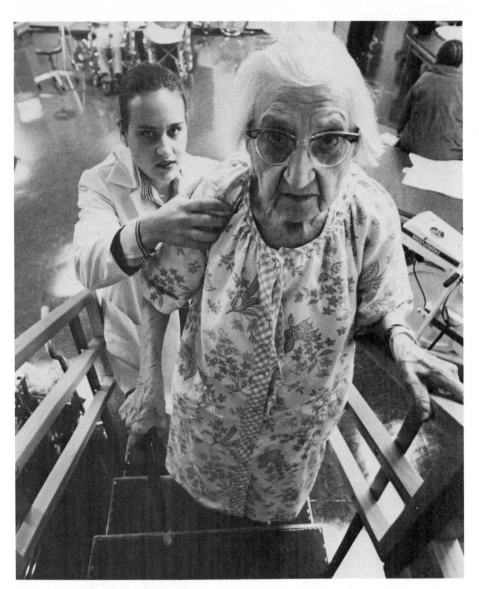

Rehabilitation programs offer stroke victims a good chance for recovery. Even paralyzed patients can make impressive advances in therapy.

• Unusual fatigue

There is much that doctors can do to prevent heart conditions or to relieve them once present. But there is much that you can do to help yourself. You should watch:

WEIGHT: Extra pounds of fat mean more work for the heart.

DIET: The rules of sound nutrition apply to proper heart care.

SMOKING: Heavy cigarette smokers suffer three times as many heart attacks as do pipe or cigar smokers. Nonsmokers are safest.

EXERCISE: Exercise improves the pumping action of the heart as well as circulation, digestion, and general health.

WORRY: Worry increases tension and elevates blood pressure. Try to cultivate a philosophical approach to the daily ups and downs. See *Heart Disease*, p. 360.

Strokes

Strokes are not hopeless; even severely paralyzed patients may make remarkable progress. A *stroke* occurs when the blood supply to a part of the brain tissue is cut off and, as a result, the nerve cells in that part of the brain can't function. When this happens, the part of the body controlled by these nerve cells can't function either.

Whenever the blood supply is cut

off from an area, small neighboring arteries get larger and take over part of the work of the damaged artery. In this way nerve cells that have been temporarily put out of order may recover, and that part of the body affected by the stroke may eventually improve or even return to normal.

Once a stroke has occurred, a sound rehabilitation program can help the patient resume as many normal activities as possible. This program can be worked out in cooperation with the doctor, patient, family, and local organizations. See under *Diseases of the Circulatory System*, p. 349.

Arthritis

There are two main types of arthritis: *rheumatoid arthritis* and *osteoarthritis*.

Rheumatoid arthritis—which can cause pain and swelling in joints, nerves, muscles, tendons, blood vessels, and connective tissue in the whole body—can strike at any age, but it occurs mainly in the 25-to-40-year age group. The exact cause of rheumatoid arthritis is unknown.

Osteoarthritis is a degenerative joint disease that affects almost everyone who lives long enough; it is a product of normal wear and tear on the joints over the years. Poor posture and obesity are contributing causes, as are heredity and trauma.

Osteoarthritis is usually mild, and it seldom cripples. Pain is generally moderate. Unlike rheumatoid arthritis, which is inflammatory, spreads from joint to joint, and affects the whole body, osteoarthritis confines its attack locally to individual joints. Rarely is inflammation a problem.

Osteoarthritis is likely to develop in any joint which has been required to take a lot of punishment or abuse: the knee or hip joints of someone who is overweight; joints injured in an accident; joints injured or overused in sports; joints subjected to unusual stresses and strains in work or play; joints with

hidden defects that were present at birth.

There is no specific cure for arthritis, but the pain and swelling can be controlled. In other than acute cases, common aspirin has proved the safest and most popular medication.

Adequate rest for both the body and the affected joint is a fundamental treatment. Heat, controlled exercise, hydrotherapy, and massage are all effective if done under a doctor's supervision. See *Arthritis and Other Joint Diseases*, p. 450.

Cancer

Cancer strikes at any age, but it does strike more frequently in the later years. Many factors are believed to contribute to cancer: frictional and chemical irritations like cigarette smoking, irritation of the skin and mouth (such as poor dentures), exposure to the sun, X rays, or radioactive elements. Common sites are the lips, mouth, stomach, intestines, rectum, liver, pancreas, lungs, breast, kidney, bladder, skin, uterus, and prostate.

Early detection and prompt treatment are the best protection against cancer. If any of the following seven danger signals lasts longer than two weeks, be sure to get a checkup:

• Unusual bleeding or discharge
• A lump or thickening in the breast or elsewhere
• A sore that does not heal
• Change in bowel or bladder habits
• Hoarseness or cough
• Indigestion or difficulty in swallowing
• Change in wart or mole.

Great strides have been made in treating cancer through surgery, radiotherapy, and chemotherapy. See *Cancer*, p. 434. For cancers affecting women only, see *Cancers of the Reproductive System*, p. 500, and *Cancer of the Breast*, p. 504.

The Eyes

The eye does age. After age 40, failing vision is usually caused by natural hardening of the lens, mak-

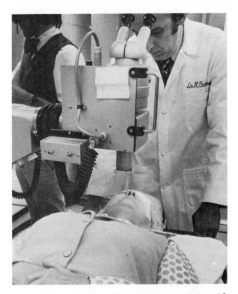

Laser beams are used to treat a patient with advanced glaucoma. Laser surgery is generally quicker and safer than the traditional glaucoma surgery; also, the patient does not have to remain hospitalized.

ing it difficult to see close objects. However, failing vision may also be the first symptom of a serious bodily disorder, or of glaucoma or of a cataract, which requires a physician's immediate attention.

Both glaucoma and cataract can be treated effectively. About 90 percent of glaucoma cases can be checked with eye drops and about 95 percent of cataracts can be removed by a painless operation.

Other diseases that may develop in later years affect the blood vessels of the eye. A common condition is *senile macula degeneration* which causes a blind spot to appear when the victim looks directly at something. The exact cause of senile macula degeneration is not known. See under *Diseases of the Eye and Ear*, p. 417.

Diabetes

Most likely candidates for diabetes are overweight persons past 40, particularly those who have a hereditary history of diabetes, and especially older women.

The exact cause of diabetes is not known, but it is a functional disorder in which the body cannot handle certain foods—mainly sugars and starches. Symptoms include increased thirst, constant hunger, frequent urination, loss of weight, itching, easy tiring, changes in vision, and slow healing of cuts and scratches.

Treatment and control consist of planned diet, exercise, and, in many cases, insulin shots or oral medication. Well-controlled diabetics can lead active lives. See *Diabetes Mellitus*, p. 409.

Constipation

There is no truth in the notion that a daily bowel movement is necessary for good health. A movement every day or twice a day may be all right for one person; for another every three or four days may be enough.

The two most common causes of chronic constipation are physical inactivity and poor food and water habits. Ironically, constipation may be caused by swallowing a cathartic nightly to induce a bowel movement. The habit eventually leads to chronic constipation because normal bowel movement ceases and bowel evacuation depends on using a cathartic.

To maintain proper bowel movement, try the following:

• Drink eight to ten glasses of water a day. Take two glasses of water on an empty stomach as soon as you get up.

• Drink more fruit juices and eat more dried and fresh fruits.

• Get at least one-half hour of moderate exercise daily. Walking, for example, is excellent, particularly if you relax while you walk.

• Give yourself enough time for normal bowel movement and set up a regular time for evacuation.

• If you are constipated, consult your doctor to make sure it is simple and functional. See under *Aches, Pains, Nuisances, Worries*, p. 277.

Back Problems

As we grow older, the back muscles—weakened by inactivity, poor posture, and almost unavoidable wear and tear—start to complain.

Other causes of back problems are muscle and joint strain, changes in the spine, psychological tension, and internal diseases. Here are some tips to help avoid backache:

• Learn to lift correctly. Use your leg muscles, which are stronger than back muscles, by placing your feet closer to the base of the object, bending your knees outward, and pushing up with your legs.

• Avoid subjecting your back to any sudden, erratic motion.

• Try to improve your posture when sitting and walking.

• Sleep on a firm bed; a bed board may be helpful.

• Get regular exercise of a type that stimulates all your muscles rather than just a few.

• If you sit for a long period, get up and stretch occasionally.

• Beware of excess weight. Extra weight on the abdomen pulls on the vertebrae at the small of the back, increasing the spine's normal curve and causing pain.

• Try never to become overfatigued or exhausted, either physically or mentally. Emotional pressure, from work or personal problems, causes muscle tension. See *Backaches*, p. 268.

Since the feet are farthest away from the heart's blood supply, they are often the first areas affected by circulatory diseases. Also, arthritis and diabetes might first show up in the feet.

Warning signs include continued cramping of the calf muscles, pain in the arch and toes, and unusually cold feet—especially if accompanied by a bluish skin. Brittle or thickened toenails or burning, tingling, and numbness may also signal a circulatory disease.

Foot ulcers may be one of the first signs of diabetes. Some *bunions*—swollen, tender, red joints—are caused by arthritis. Swelling around the feet and ankles suggests a possible kidney disorder.

If you have these symptoms, go to a *podiatrist* (a foot doctor) or to your own doctor. They are trained to recognize these symptoms.

Most older people, however, suffer from minor aches and pains in the feet that are caused by poor foot care or abuse. See *The Vulnerable Extremities*, p. 271.

CARE OF THE FEET: To prevent these problems, treat yourself to daily foot care. Dry your feet thoroughly and gently after bathing and inspect the skin for abrasions, rough spots, or cracks. Dry carefully between the toes. If the skin is dry or scaly, lubricate it with lanolin or olive oil. Next, apply a medicated foot powder recommended by your doctor over the entire foot, especially between the toes, as a preventive measure against athlete's foot.

When you cut your nails, do it with a strong light and be careful to cut straight across the nail to prevent ingrown toenails. Avoid the use of strong medications containing salicylate and strong antiseptics like iodine, carbolic acid, lysol, or bleach. Harsh chemicals that attack toughened skin can irritate normal tissue and cause infection. Avoid using hot water bottles, electric pads, or any form of extreme heat or cold. Diabetics should visit a podiatrist regularly.

The Prostate

Men over 50 may have an enlarged *prostate*. (This is not caused by sexual excesses or venereal disease.) The exact cause is not known, but it's estimated that some type of enlarged prostate is present in about 10 percent of 40-year-olds and 80 percent of 80-year-olds.

The prostate is a rubbery mass of glands and muscle tissue about the size and shape of a horse chestnut. It is wrapped around the urethra and base of the bladder at the point where they join. The prostate functions as part of a man's sexual apparatus, providing a fluid that transports and nourishes the spermatozoa.

Symptoms of an enlarged prostate include difficulty in urination. There might be an initial blocking of the urine, or the stream may lack force. You may feel that you can't empty the bladder, and you may have urgent needs to urinate. You may have pain or blood in the urine from straining.

If you have any of these symptoms, your doctor can easily check for enlarged prostate by a simple rectal examination. If he discovers an enlargement, he can usually treat it in early stages with simple massage. But if it has progressed too far, he may have to operate.

An operation is usually performed through the urethra or by an incision in the lower abdomen. The choice depends upon the individual problems of the patient and the judgment of the surgeon. In either case, the patient usually recovers completely in a short time.

A rectal examination can also discover early stages of cancer of the prostate, which is not uncommon in men over 40. Some 20 percent of men over 60 have this condition, and it is most common in men over 70.

Unfortunately, this disease does not manifest itself early, so it is important that men over forty have the diagnostic rectal examination. If the disease is detected early and treated—usually by surgery, hormonal therapy, and possibly radiation—the cure rate is very high. If found late, the cure rate is low.

When treatment is by surgery, the entire prostate and upper urethra may be removed. In some cases, the disease may be retarded or relieved by treatment with female hormones. (The male hormone is known to hasten prostate cancer.)

In both enlargement and cancer of the prostate, early detection is vital to a successful cure. That is why it is important to have a rectal examination. See also *Cancer of the Prostate*, p. 442.

Financing Medical Care

Older people have recourse to many community facilities and programs, all aimed at easing the financial burden of medical care.

There are over 2,000 hospitals, visiting nurse associations, and similar agencies eligible to provide benefits to persons over 65 under Medicare. Those under 65 may also receive aid, although arrangements for payments will differ.

All such agencies provide skilled home-visiting nursing service and one or more additional services, such as physical therapy, occupational therapy, medical-social services, or homemaker-home health aide services.

The Visiting Nurse Service provides a full slate of nursing services: bed baths, injections, physical therapy, diet and nutrition guidance, and related professional nursing services. Cost per visit (as of April, 1977) was $28.75, but fees are adjusted to the patient's ability to pay; fees may be covered by public welfare funds or health insurance benefits.

There are more than 800 agencies in all providing Homemaker-Home Health Aide service in forty-nine states and Puerto Rico. This service offers specially trained women who handle any marketing, cooking, serving, and cleaning requirements of the client.

Many major cities provide a Home Delivered Meals program often sponsored by the women's auxiliaries of county medical associations. This is a catering service for the ill and handicapped confined to their homes. Wholesome, balanced meals are delivered to the homes of the handicapped persons whose finances are slim; those receiving this service pay a minimum fee for the food.

The American Dental Association has entered the home-care program by developing portable equipment for home dental service and dental school programs to train undergraduates in the care of elderly, home-bound patients, and by setting up central-service headquarters and supply departments—usually at a hospital, dental clinic, or state health department.

For those who are able to pay moderate dental costs but can't stand a heavy financial strain, the dental profession has set up prepaid dental care by establishing nonprofit dental service corporations similar to the programs sponsored by Blue Shield and Blue Cross.

Your family doctor should be aware of these community programs. In many cases, your doctor must request the service. He receives regular, periodic reports on your condition.

Also, practically every metropolitan area in the United States and Canada has an Information and Referral Service, usually staffed by the United Crusade or Welfare Department. This service answers many questions, such as how to locate a nursing home or borrow a wheelchair, where to find a doctor or a hospital to meet a specific need, and other inquiries of that nature. To find the number of your Information and Referral Service, consult your local telephone directory.

Medicare and Health Insurance

Medicare offers free hospital benefits to persons 65 and older and optional medical benefits for $7.70 a month (as of July 1, 1977). These benefits are also available to people under 65 who are disabled or who are being treated for chronic kidney disease.

As of July 1, 1977, the hospital insurance program pays the cost of covered services for the following hospital and post-hospital care:
• The first 60 days in a hospital (except for the first $104), and all but $26 per day for an additional 30 days for each spell of illness
• A lifetime reserve of 60 additional hospital days if you need more than 90 days hospital care in the same benefit period and all but $52 a day
• Up to 20 days in an extended-care facility and all but $13 per day for an additional 80 days for each spell of illness—services provided only after a hospital stay of at least 3 days

• Up to 100 home-health visits by nurses or other health workers in the 365 days following your release from a hospital or extended-care facility.

If you sign up for optional medical benefits under Medicare, you agree to pay a premium of $7.70 monthly. The medical insurance will pay 80 percent of the *reasonable* charges for the following services after the first $60 in each calendar year:

• Physicians' and surgeons' services

• Home-health services even if you have not been in a hospital—up to 100 visits a year

• A number of medical and health services, such as diagnostic tests or treatment and certain services by podiatrists.

Benefits have been steadily expanded—some new provisions include coverage for medical equipment needed in your home, provisions for doctors' unpaid but itemized bills to be sent directly to Medicare for payment.

When you reach 65, you are automatically qualified for free hospital benefits. You may sign up for the optional medical benefits during the first three months of any year;

your coverage will begin on July 1 of that year. For each year you delay signing up after your 65th birthday, your monthly medical benefit premium will be increased by approximately 10 percent. To sign up, or for further information, contact your nearest social security office or write for the free booklet, *Your Medicare Handbook,* available from your local social security office.

Private insurance companies offer policies to fill some of the gaps in Medicare coverage and to supplement provisions. Check with your local insurance agent or write to Health Insurance Institute, 277 Park Avenue, New York, N.Y. 10017 for further information.

Nursing Homes

While Medicare pays most of the cost of 100 days in an extended-care facility, you must be referred after a 3-day hospital stay. If your condition—or that of a friend or relative —requires a longer stay in a nursing home, you are faced with different circumstances.

First, there is a confusion of terms. "Nursing home" can mean almost any type of facility that provides some sort of health or custodial care short of that offered by a regular hospital. Thus, convalescent homes, homes for the aged, rest homes, geriatric hospitals, senior care homes all may be loosely classified as nursing homes.

The services they offer vary from skilled nursing and medical attention to strictly personal service. The confusion in terminology has become so great that responsible professionals in the field of health care have recommended that the term "nursing home" be erased from our vocabulary. Others feel that eliminating it might cause even more confusion.

Choosing a Home

Thus, picking the right home for the patient is not easy. The first step would be to have your physician recommend a place suited to the patient's condition. If you are in doubt or if you do not have a family physician, try your local health and welfare or community service agency. Sometimes, these agencies have a referral service that can direct you to a nursing home.

You could also try the Family Service Association or your county medical society. Another source of information is your state affiliate of the American Nursing Home Association, 1025 Connecticut Ave. N.W., Washington, D.C. 20036.

The next step would be to visit the home, if possible. Try to find out as much as you can about the qualifications, staff, and services they offer. The American Nursing Home Association suggests you ask these questions:

• Is the facility licensed by the state or local government? Avoid an unlicensed home.

• What level of nursing care is provided? It should have a Registered Nurse or Licensed Practical Nurse on hand for both day and night shifts.

• Is there a staff physician who spends some time at the nursing home? Can a patient have his own physician? Does the home make a

For older patients who are eligible, Medicare insurance pays a good part of their medical and hospital bills.

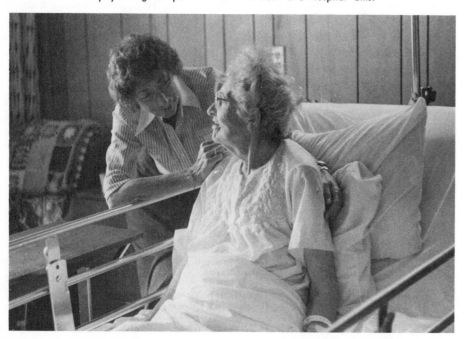

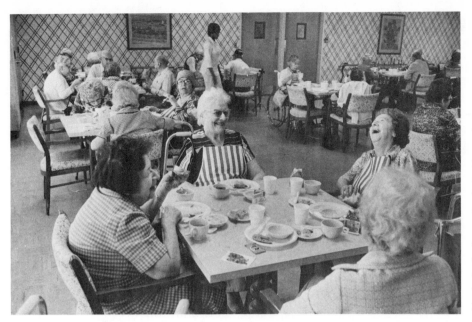

Factors to consider in selecting a nursing home include cost, availability, of medical and nursing care, and licensing by the city or state.

special effort to keep physicians advised of their patients' conditions?

• Does the home have an organized program of diversional activities? What does it include? Are arrangements made for the religious life of the patient?

• What provisions does the home make for visiting patients?

• What facilities are there for rehabilitation and physical therapy?

• Are nursing personnel and other staff members trained in motivation and rehabilitation techniques?

• Does the home have arrangements with a nearby hospital for easy transfer of patients? Is emergency transportation readily available?

• Does the home maintain a planned menu at least a week or two in advance? Are there arrangements for handling patients who require special diets?

• Is the place basically safe? It should have an automatic sprinkler system, be fire resistant, or have an automatic alarm system. It should have escape routes in case of emergencies, and it should have grab bars and rails in hallways and bathrooms.

Also, ask about the food service and dental care. The place should have a general homelike atmosphere rather than a cold, institutional look.

Costs

Most important: *find out about all costs!* Generally, expect to pay about $7,000 to $12,000 a year for a good place ($600 to $1,000 a month) for room, board, and nursing care. You may be charged extra for doctor calls, drugs, special diets, extra nursing care, personal services (shampoos, haircuts, and shaving), etc.

What about tips? Strange as it seems, tipping is a fact of life in many nursing homes. Wages are low, and many staff personnel rely on tips to provide good service. Have a frank talk with the administrator about tipping—it could make a big difference in the service you receive.

In some cases, you might get financial aid to pay part of the cost.

As noted above, Medicare could pay part of the tab if the patient was referred to the home from a hospital. Second, check with your local welfare or public assistance office to determine whether you are eligible for assistance under the Medical Assistance for the Aged program or the Medicaid program. It's *not* always necessary for an individual to be drawing public assistance payments to be eligible for one of these medical assistance programs.

Finally, check with any fraternal organizations you might belong to —they may have their own facilities —and if you are a veteran, check with the Veterans Administration office, or call one of your local veterans organizations for addresses and phone numbers.

Frauds and Quacks

It is estimated that older people spend over $2 billion a year on unnecessary health supplements— worthless electronic devices, skin lotions and cosmetics, and other false products purported to aid health.

Tragically, many claims of quacks and their worthless remedies—particularly in respect to cancer—are death warrants for people who might have been saved had they gone to reliable sources soon enough.

The American Medical Association provides a list to help in spotting quacks. A practitioner may be a quack if he:

• Uses a special or secret machine or formula

• Guarantees a quick cure

• Advertises or uses case histories and testimonials

• Clamors for medical investigation and recognition

• Claims medical men are persecuting him

• Tells you that surgery, X rays, or drugs will do you more harm than good.

MEETING THE CHALLENGE OF LEISURE

Leisure Activities

In ten years of retirement, you will have the leisure time equivalent of working 40 hours a week for 21 years. You cannot fish this time away and you cannot rest it away. Whatever you do for long must have meaning—must satisfy some basic need and want. Certain needs remain constant throughout life:

• Security—good health, income, and a recognized role in society

• Recognition—as an individual with your own abilities and personality

• Belonging—as a member of a family, social group, and community

• Self-expression—by developing abilities and talents in new areas and at new levels

• Adventure—new experiences, new sights, and new knowledge.

There are many activities that can satisfy these basic needs and wants to keep you mentally and physically in top shape.

Travel

Travel satisfies your need for adventure in many ways. If you travel off-season at bargain rates, you'll find that time truly is money. Most travel problems stem from rushing to meet a schedule. Making every minute count on a fast-paced European tour can be expensive and exhausting. For the same transatlantic fare, you can spend a full year in Europe at one-third the daily cost of a three-week vacation.

Wherever you travel, it isn't enough just to sight-see. Try to center your travel around an interest or a hobby. You can take art or music tours—tours that stress education, night life, culture, or special interests. You can travel on your own or with a group. But whatever you do, participate; don't just observe.

Doing things instead of just observing adds new dimensions to the pleasure of going places. For people who participate, travel means the adventure of enjoying exciting new places, people, and experiences. To help plan your trip, write to the government tourist offices of foreign countries (ask your library for addresses); to the National Park Service, Washington, D.C.; to state or local chambers of commerce (no street addresses necessary); to major oil companies that supply free maps and routing services.

Gardening

Gardening satisfies one's need for self-expression in many ways. Being outside in the fresh air and planting living things can bring satisfaction and peace of mind.

Gardening is a many-faceted hobby that offers many challenges. You can go into plant breeding, growing for resale, introducing new plants, collecting the rare and unusual, plant selecting, or simply cultivating what you find personally appealing and satisfying.

Your local library or bookstore has many books on the subject. There are local and national garden clubs that you can join to learn about your hobby and to meet other people who are interested in gardening. Write the Government Printing Office, Washington, D.C. 20401, for help and advice. In addition, state extension directors at state colleges and universities, county agricultural agents, and local plant nurseries can also give expert advice and information.

Reading

Reading offers excitement, adventure, pursuit of knowledge, and an introduction to new people and places. Your local library is the best place to launch a reading program —and you may be surprised to find that it offers more than books. Most libraries have art and music departments, audiovisual services (films and microfilm copies), foreign language departments, periodical rooms (newspapers and magazines), writing classes, genealogy workshops, and special courses of general interest.

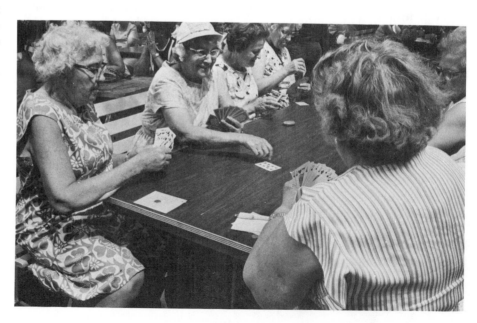

Playing a game of cards with friends in a community group provides rewarding companionship for these senior citizens.

Hobbies

A hobby can be any physical or mental activity that gives you happiness, relaxation, and satisfaction. It should not be just a time killer—it should offer some tangible reward. Also, it should have continuity, not be too expensive, and not make undue demands on time and energy. Perhaps you would prefer a series of hobbies, some serious and some just for fun. They can be related to your work or completely unrelated. In any event, a hobby should be something you've always wanted to do.

Before selecting a hobby, consider these points:

• Do you like to do things alone? Consider arts, crafts, reading, sewing, fishing—activities that are not dependent on others, although you can enjoy them with others.

• Do you like groups? Seek hobbies that include other people—organizational, sport, game, or craft activities.

• Do you like to play to win? Try your luck in competitive or team games that stress winning.

• Do you have to be an expert? Too many of us are afraid to try new activities because we hate to fail or look clumsy. But be fair; judge your efforts in light of your past experience and present progress; do not compare yourself to someone who's been at it longer than you.

• Do you put a price tag on everything? Many people will not engage in an activity if it costs too much. Yet, many hobbies fail because they're tried on a shoestring without adequate equipment. Also, some people do not want to do anything unless it brings in money. If so, perhaps you should look for something that's an offshoot of the work or business you know best.

Creative Crafts

Creative crafts are difficult for most of us because we are conservative, afraid to make mistakes, sensitive because of buried and almost forgotten blunders. Yet creativity is

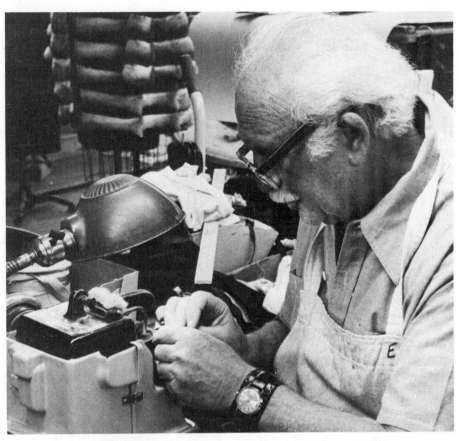

Opportunities for part-time or occasional work are often available for senior citizens who are in good health and wish to work.

essential to life. Without it we don't live fully; through creative skills we refurbish old interests and develop new ones.

Most of us are happiest with creative crafts that do not require intricate work or fine detail and that are not too demanding physically. Some crafts best suited to retirement years include weaving, rug making, sewing, ceramic work, knitting, plastic molding, woodwork, leathercraft, and lapidary.

You can learn these and other

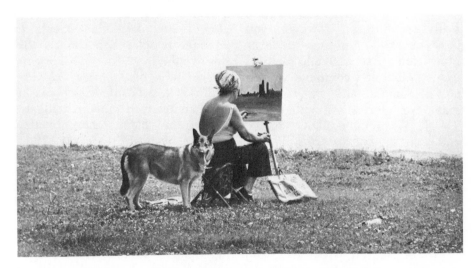

Painting is an outlet for creative expression by this senior citizen; some paint for enjoyment only and others market their work.

crafts and also market your products through senior centers, adult education classes, and senior craft centers.

Volunteer Work

Through community service and volunteer work, thousands are not only helping others but are serving themselves. Such activities keep time from hanging heavy, give purpose to retirement, and in some cases may lead to paying jobs and a second career.

Participating in community activities is not difficult. In some communities a call to the city clerk is enough to get started. In others, a letter to the mayor will bring faster results. In larger cities, call the Volunteer Bureau in your area; this is a United Fund agency that acts as a clearing house for volunteer jobs.

If you wish to have the type of volunteer job that leads to a second career, you might consider doing work for one of the government programs utilizing the skills of older people. All of these programs have been assembled under the umbrella of one organization called ACTION. For additional information about any of the following programs, write to ACTION, Washington, D.C. 20525.

• The Foster Grandparent Program hires low-income men and women over 60 to give love and attention to institutionalized and other needy children.

• The Peace Corps is seeking the skills of retirees. However, you must be skilled in some trade or profession, pass a tough physical examination, and complete a rigorous orientation and training program. For information, write to ACTION, Washington, D.C. 20525, and request a copy of *Older Volunteers in the Peace Corps*. It lists specific skills needed in the Peace Corps.

• Other programs within ACTION include the Retired Senior Volunteer Program, the Service Corps of Retired Executives, and the Active Corps of Executives, and VISTA (Volunteer in Service to

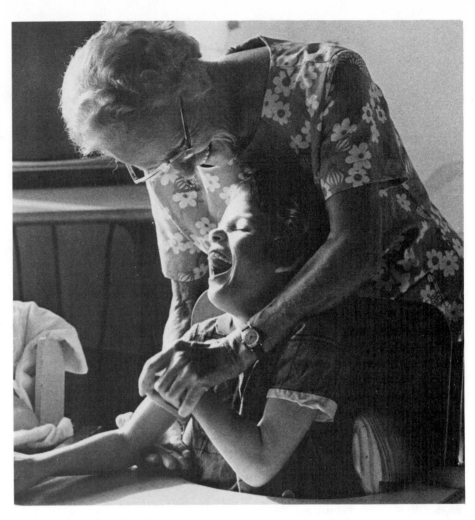

A senior volunteer in a community program provides companionship and affection for a retarded child.

America). Many of the workers in these programs are paid.

There are other volunteer jobs that may not pay a salary, but do fill a basic need by allowing you to pass along your skills and ideals to younger people. You can do this through the Boy Scouts, Girl Scouts, Boys Clubs of America, YMCA's and YWCA's, hospitals, schools for the handicapped and mentally retarded, and many other organizations.

Continuing Social and Intellectual Activities

The one organ we can depend upon in old age is the brain. At 80, a person can learn at approximately the same speed he could when he was

12 years old. But like any organ, the brain must be kept active and alert by constant use.

One of the best ways to exercise the brain is through some process of continuing education. This does not have to mean going back to school or taking formal classes. Continuing education can take the form of participating in discussions in senior centers, "Y's", town meetings, or study courses. You can find out about educational opportunities and possibilities by contacting local, state, or national offices of education; state employment offices; the information service of your Community Council or Health and Welfare Federation; the Adult Education section of the U.S. Office of Education, Washington, D.C. 20202; the National Education Association, 1201 Sixteenth

Street, N.W., Washington, D.C. 20036; the State Commission on Aging (write to your state capital).

Your local library may have some suggestions (and perhaps offers some classes), and your local "Y" is probably offering some programs.

Uncle Sam continues to be a prime source of educational literature. Each year the government prints about 50 million books, pamphlets, brochures, reports, and guidebooks on everything from astrology to zoology. For a free price list of specified subjects, write to the Superintendent of Documents, Government Printing Office, Washington, D.C. 20401.

Formal and informal learning situations can help you keep pace with change and the future. Continuing education prepares you to live contentedly with a free, independent spirit and mind—while providing you with the means for improved social integration, participation, and satisfaction.

Sexual Attitude and Activity in the Aged

We have come far since the Victorian era when talk about sex was taboo. Now science is taking a candid look at sex in the later years and is exploding old myths as well as exploring new truths. Such enlightenment can help reduce any remaining guilt in this area.

After Age 60

In one study to determine the pattern of sexual behavior after 60, researchers at Duke University quizzed 250 people aged 60 to 93 about their sexual activities. Of the 149 who were married, 81 reported they were still sexually active; even in the single group, 7 of the 101 questioned reported "some sexual activity."

Dr. Gustave Newman, who conducted the study, reported 10 percent of the couples over 60 as having sexual relations more than once a week, though couples over 75 unanimously reported less activity.

"No age is an automatic cut-off point for sex," claims the late Dr. Isadore Rubin in his study, *Sexual Life After Sixty*. "But," he continues,

sexuality cannot flourish in a climate where rejection of aging as a worthwhile stage of life leads inevitably to self-rejection by many older persons . . . the men and women who 'act old' in their sexual activity before their bodies have really called a halt become sexually old long before their time.

Sexual Interest After Menopause

Actually, many women take a renewed interest in sex after menopause. Dr. William H. Masters and Mrs. Virginia E. Johnson in their study, *Human Sexual Response*, credit the tendency of many women to experience a second honeymoon in the early fifties to the fact that they no longer have to worry about pregnancy and usually have resolved most of the problems of raising a family.

On the other hand, they tell us:

Deprived of normal sexual outlets, women exhaust themselves physically in conscious or unconscious efforts to dissipate their accumulated and frequently unrecognized sexual tensions. Many demonstrate their basic insecurities by casting themselves unreservedly into their religion, the business world, volunteer social work, or overzealous mothering of their mature children or grandchildren.

Lessened Response of Men

While some women become more responsive as they grow older, Masters and Johnson point out, "There is no question that the human male's responsiveness wanes as he ages." They attribute this to attitudes arising from:

• Boredom—being taken for granted by his wife

• Economic pursuits—occupational competition becomes a demanding, all-consuming activity

• Fatigue from unusual or excessive physical strain, such as that induced by sports; or mental fatigue

induced by such factors as a "bad day at the office"

• Overindulgence in food and drink, usually alcohol

• Physical and mental infirmities

• Fear of failure.

Myths About Sex

One common reason for an older person's termination of sex life is the often mistaken idea that continued sexual activity in middle and old age may adversely affect health. Although the old myths that sex is weakening or speeds the aging process have been largely dismissed by doctors today, some people still cling to them; what sexual activity they do have is troubled by fear.

HEART PATIENTS: Today even cardiac patients are no longer admonished to lead sexless lives except in extreme cases. Even after a heart attack most are able to resume sexual activity within a few months, although patients with angina pectoris may be advised to proceed cautiously.

According to Dr. Philip Reichert, former executive secretary of the American College of Cardiology:

We must get rid of the notion that every heart patient lives under an overhanging sword and that he faces the constant threat of sudden death. The congenial married couple, accustomed to each other and whose technique is habituated through many years of companionship, can achieve sexual satisfaction without too great an expenditure of body energy or too severe a strain upon the heart. . . .

Today, even hypertension sufferers may sometimes indulge in a restricted form of sexual activity with medical supervision. And modern therapy and surgical methods can often prevent or delay impotence caused by prostate disease or diabetes.

OTHER HEALTH PROBLEMS: But where any health problem is involved, it is best to analyze your sex needs and those of your partner; consult with your doctor and partner as to how you can both attain satisfaction without harm to your health; see your doctor regularly and report accurately distress symptoms and the conditions causing them.

Recent research has dispelled other long-held ideas about sex, too—among them the myth that masturbation is childish and harmful to health. Moreover, Rubin points out: "All studies of older persons have shown that autoerotic activity, while not as common as in the younger years, is far more prevalent in later years than most of us have imagined." He quotes a survey by *Sexology Magazine* which showed that of 279 married men studied, 1 out of every 4 masturbated after age 60.

Dr. Lester W. Dearborn, marriage consultant, in pointing out the role masturbation plays in the lives of the single or widowed, comments:

It is to be hoped that those interested in the field of geriatrics will . . . encourage the aging to accept masturbation as a perfectly valid outlet when there is a need and other means of gratification are not available.

The "dirty old man" myth has run its course, too. Although society tends to picture both the child molester and the exhibitionist as older men, experts point out that both typically belong to much younger age groups. Donald Mulcock, child welfare specialist, in studying men who assaulted children sexually in England and Wales, found most offenses against boys were committed by men between the ages of 39 and 50, those against girls by men between 33 to 44. Only six percent of the men he studied were 63, and none was older.

Cellular Therapy and Hormone Treatment

To keep older people vigorous and active, some researchers have experimented with *cellular therapy* as a means of retarding aging. Dr. Paul Niehans, a Swiss physician, introduced the idea of cellular therapy in the 1930s with his theory

that organs begin to deteriorate in old age when the body fails to replace the cells which compose it. He prescribed a treatment whereby a person is injected with cells from healthy embryonic animal organs. (He used sheep, pigs, and calves.) He believed that the animal cells from a particular organ would migrate to the same organ in the aging body and reactivate it. Thus, kidney troubles could be cured with cells from an embryonic animal kidney. Although such notables as Sir Winston Churchill, Pope Pius XII, Somerset Maugham, and Dr. Konrad Adenauer submitted to it, cellular therapy is not widely accepted in the U.S. today as an effective agent against aging.

More to the point, most researchers feel, are the current experiments with hormones. Hormones help women through the tension of menopause and are used to treat impotence and loss of sexual desire. However, some studies have linked estrogen hormone therapy statistically with uterine cancer. For this reason and because of side effects, hormones face many years of testing before they will be used extensively to retard aging.

Mental Outlook

Good health plus a romantic outlook promote sex appeal at any age. Being romantic and showing affection, whether sexually or not, keep you sparkling and lively no matter what your age.

A good wholesome attitude toward life, a hearty sense of humor, a sympathetic interest in other people—all help make up the indefinable something that makes us appealing to the opposite sex. Good grooming plays an important role, too. Cleanliness, neat suitable apparel, and good posture all add to the image we create of ourselves in other people's minds. So do the manners we reflect in the courtesies we show the people around us—the thoughtful little things we do for them, our reactions to the things they do for us.

If you're a woman over 65 who is looking for companionship, you'll probably find a good personality uplift will get you further than a face or bust lift. If you're a man who is hoping to find feminine companionship, you will probably find a good spiritual overhaul more image-enhancing than dyeing your hair. Also, a good night's sleep is the best aphrodisiac.

The Right Housing

Selecting retirement housing is like

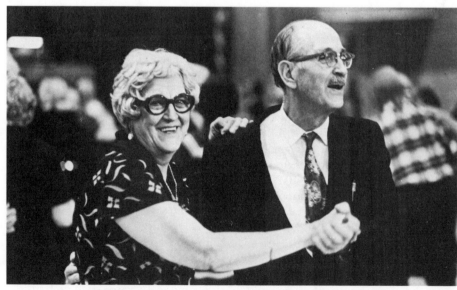

A cheerful mental attitude, combined with a variety of social and intellectual interests, can help keep mind and body youthful.

selecting a spouse; there are many possibilities, but few that are right.

Ideally, the right housing should take care of you rather than requiring you to take care of it. It should give you shelter, security, and privacy; allow you freedom; and keep you near friends, relatives, and a grocer who delivers.

To Move or Not to Move

What is the right housing for you—the one that you are in or some other place? The answer to this question depends upon the state of your pocketbook and the state of your health.

ADVANTAGES OF MOVING: Right now you might be in good health, but this could change. Would stairs become a problem? Could you keep up the house and garden? Would you want more adequate heat? Older people are more comfortable when the temperature is over 75° Fahrenheit. You might also need better lighting in several rooms.

If you are retired, you might find that you cannot keep up expenses on the old house. You might find that your larger, older house does not suit the reduced size of your family or your need for work or recreation. You could probably save money by living in a smaller place that requires less upkeep. You could also arrange to move nearer children and grandchildren, or into an area where you could find new opportunities for work and recreational activities.

ADVANTAGES OF STAYING PUT: But by staying in your home you would remain in familiar surroundings and near old friends. You could maintain your comfortable routine and remain independent as long as possible. If you have unused space, you could move into the first floor and shut off the second floor to save on heat and maintenance. Or you could convert part of the house into apartments.

Where to Live?

Many older persons fulfill ambitions of long standing by moving to warmer climates after retirement. The question whether such a move should be undertaken should be considered with other questions relating to housing.

Moving to a different climate makes sense for many reasons. Many elderly persons feel threatened or restricted by cold winters and their usual accompaniments —snow, sleet, and high winds. Having more leisure time, older persons feel that warmer temperatures will make it possible to take part in more activities for more hours of the day than if they "stay put." Some persons move so that they can live closer to friends who have already moved—or to children or other relatives. Some move to play golf or tennis outdoors the year around.

An individual or couple considering a move to a warmer climate should look at a number of basic considerations. A key one relates to the cost of living in the new area or state. Living on incomes that may have been substantially reduced by retirement, older persons without special preferences may select that state that offers the cheapest living. Studies indicated in 1979 that the "10 best states to retire to" from a personal-financial point of view were, in order:

1. *Utah*, because of lower energy costs, growing job opportunities, moderate living costs. A drawback: Utah may have extremely cold winters.

2. *Louisiana*, because of cheap living costs—about 10 percent lower than other states—and low real estate taxes.

3. *South Carolina*, for the same reasons. A drawback: doctor shortages in some communities.

4. *Nevada*, because of new housing, jobs, no state income or inheritance taxes, and average living costs.

5. *Texas*, with moderate housing costs away from major cities, plenty of service jobs, and normal, if rising, living costs.

6. *New Mexico*, where energy costs are low, jobs are increasing in number, and cheap housing is plentiful.

7. *Alabama*, the cheapest and lowest as regards costs of living. Drawbacks: few new jobs, medical care lacking in some areas.

8. *Arizona*, because of good, relatively inexpensive housing, warm climate, good medical care. Drawbacks: rising living costs, high taxes.

9. *Florida*, with a warm climate, no income tax, good medical services. Drawbacks: living costs high in coastal areas; property taxes rising.

10. *Georgia*, because of mild climate, low living costs. Drawbacks: slow growth in jobs, locally poor medical services.

"Retirement to the sun" entails many other decisions. States like New Mexico offer a wide range of sites, from urban to desert, from high mountains to empty plains. Some of the states with favorable tax laws and cheap living costs have little to offer in the way of cultural attractions. Other states may lack recreational activities.

PSYCHOLOGICAL TRAUMA. Moving 100 or 1,000 or 2,000 miles to live in a warmer climate obviously involves some pain of separation and loss. The psychological trauma occasioned by a departure from old friends and familiar surroundings has caused major problems for some older persons. For that reason, the psychological challenge should be given deep consideration *before* any move is made.

How to alleviate the trauma of leaving the familiar for the unfamiliar? Some persons spend a year in the new locale, return home, and *then* make up their minds to move or not to move. Others, including those who cannot afford such trial living, at least visit the target region to "get a feel" for it and its way of life. Whatever your situation, the wisdom of considering at least five factors cannot be disputed:

• In the new home under the sun, will you be able to entertain family, including children and grandchildren, and in that way to minimize the pain of separation?

• Are friends or relatives already located in the new area—and can you live near them (not *with* them, if possible)?

• Will you be able to swing into enough new activities to eliminate any possibility that you might feel useless, wasted, or frustrated?

• Can you maintain your old, or a decent, standard of living once you have moved?

• Can you stand the first 9 to 12 months in the new home without climbing the walls? Studies have shown that those who can last out a year or more will very likely adjust and continue to enjoy life.

Requirements of Retirement Housing

Whatever you plan to do, your retirement housing should be located near or be easily accessible to shops and recreation centers by public transportation. To make living arrangements more pleasant, individual housing units should contain at least 400 square feet, and there should be two or more rooms.

The new dwelling unit should be equal to or better than the housing you have been used to in the past. It should be suitable for comfortable living in both health and sickness —easily adaptable to convalescent needs with either two bedrooms or a bedroom and sleeping alcove.

In addition, retirement housing should incorporate the following:

• All rooms on one floor, and that floor reached by few, if any, steps

• No thresholds or tripping hazards

• Nonslip surfaces in hallways, bedrooms, and kitchens

• Handrails by all steps and inclines

• Adequate illumination in halls, near steps, and in other potentially hazardous areas

• Fully automatic central heating

• Doors and halls wide enough to accommodate a wheelchair.

Public Housing

If you decide to move and to rent instead of buying, consider public housing projects. These projects are available to single men and women 62 or older, as well as to families whose head is 62 or older or has a spouse at least 62. Local housing authorities build, purchase, or lease the units and set entrance requirements and maximum income limits. Rents are comparatively low.

The Housing and Urban Development Agency also makes loans for nonprofit (and profit) sponsors that will build housing for senior citizens with moderate or higher incomes.

Retirement Hotels and Communities

You might also consider retirement hotels, which are especially numerous in Florida, California, and Texas. These hotels are usually refurbished former resorts that provide room and board at a fixed monthly rent.

Retirement communities offer housing of various types, usually apartments, cooperatives, and individual units. It usually costs about $450 a month or more to cover mortgage payments, living, and maintenance expenses.

Would you like retirement community living? It's usually the life for people who like people and who enjoy being active. For those who don't, it can be a bit tiring. Some couples do not like the closeness and activity found in a retirement community and prefer living in a less social environment.

Lifetime Care Facilities

In contrast to the emphasis on independent living in retirement communities, many projects sponsored by church, union, and fraternal organizations stress lifetime care (room, board, and medical care for life), with fees based on actuarial tables of life expectancy at age of entry. Housing alone costs from $10,000 to $30,000, depending upon age and type of living accommodation, *plus* a monthly charge of

around $250 per person to cover meals, medical care (exclusive of Medicare), maintenance, and other expenses. In many cases, lifetime care for a couple could cost around $90,000.

Cooperatives and Condominiums

In addition to lifetime care facilities, many church, fraternal, and union groups offer other types of housing. In the case of church-sponsored housing, residence usually is not restricted to members of the sponsoring faith.

Some of these units are operated as *cooperatives;* others as *condominiums.* The major difference in the two is that condominium owners have titles to their units, while cooperative residents are stockholders in the cooperative association with occupancy rights to specific units. Condominium owners pay their own taxes; cooperative residents pay taxes in their monthly charges.

Mobile Homes

You might also want to consider a mobile home. A suitable one must be at least 10 feet wide and 50 feet long.

What is it like to live in a mobile-home park? Certainly, there is a closeness in these parks that you would not have in a normal neighborhood. Typically, the mobile home is placed on a lot 25 to 30 feet wide and 75 feet deep. This means that you could have 12 families within a radius of 100 feet.

Residents visit back and forth and hold frequent picnics, barbecues, and other social activities. This would not be the way of life for someone who did not enjoy group activities.

Be Realistic

To find out what type of housing is best for you, look around the area to see where you want to live. Each community is different, shaped by the people who live there. Talk to the residents and do some serious thinking before you move, not forgetting to carefully consider your financial position in regard to the new locale. Try to be realistic; don't expect to find the perfect climate for health and happiness. The nearest thing to it would be a place that encourages outdoor life, is neither too hot nor too cold, has a relative humidity of around 55 percent, and enough variety in weather, with frequent but moderate weather changes, to be interesting and not too monotonous.

If you have any doubts about the location as far as health is concerned, check with your doctor.

When Faced With Ill Health

How can you help yourself or others when faced with a serious or terminal illness?

Alvin I. Goldfarb, M.D., former consultant on Services for the Aged, New York State Department of Mental Hygiene, notes the importance of self-esteem, self-confidence, sense of purpose, and well-being to a person who is seriously ill or dying. Supported by the idea, "I've led a good and full life," older people can face a serious or terminal illness with dignity. Sometimes this acceptance may be almost an unspoken and tacit understanding between the aging and society to help the separation process along.

When a person is terminally ill, the chances are that he is not in severe pain. With the increasing supply of pain-relieving drugs and the possibility of sedation, very few elderly patients suffer greatly with pain. While a fear of death probably exists in most people, when death is actually encountered the fear is seldom overwhelming, even though it may deeply affect others directly involved with the dying patient.

Most patients are at least aware of the possibility of dying soon; those with lingering conditions are particularly adept at self-diagnosis. But more often, they notice a change in social relationships with friends, family, and medical personnel.

Patient-doctor relationships can be vital in helping the seriously ill patient retain peace of mind. It is the doctor's responsibility to give compassion and recognize fear, even when it is hidden. Likewise, he should respond to a patient's hidden wish to discuss his illness. Of course, there is no set formula for communicating with seriously ill patients. Each individual needs a different approach, and most doctors are sensitive to this.

Many doctors report that death, except in unusual cases, is not accompanied by physical pain. Rather, there is often a sense of well-being and spiritual exaltation. Doctors think this feeling is caused by the anesthetic action of carbon dioxide on the central nervous system and by the effect of toxic substances. Ernest Hemingway wrote, "The pang of death, a famous doctor once told me, is often less than that of a toothache."

Stages of Death

According to doctors, man dies in stages—rapidly or slowly, depending on circumstances. First comes *clinical death,* when respiration and heartbeat cease. The brain dies as it is deprived of oxygen and circulating blood, and *biological death* occurs.

Life can be restored in the moments between clinical death and brain death if circulation and respiration are continued through the use of medical devices which stimulate the heart and lungs.

After the brain ceases to function, cellular death begins. Life is not considered to be completely lost until the brain stops functioning. It is possible for doctors to remove viable organs after biological death for transplant or other use.

Many clergymen and doctors insist that we need more honest communication about death, as such communication is probably the single most useful measure to avoid unnecessary suffering. Sound knowledge never made anyone afraid. And although death will probably always remain essentially a mystery to man, scientists will continue to search for a better understanding of its nature. By such means they may learn a great deal more about life.

CHAPTER 7

Nutrition and Weight Control

Food and meals are man's best friends. His health and his social life are tied intimately and everlastingly to what he eats and how he eats it. Of all the physiological functions which maintain his life, eating and all that it entails is the one in which he most expresses his personal preferences and the cultural traditions of his ancestors.

Most people develop eating habits early in life that accord with family patterns and modify them only slightly over the years. Sometimes these habits conform to ideal food recommendations from the viewpoint of maintaining and fostering good health. More often, however, they do not.

Knowledge about food, eating, and their relationship to health is the best way to change inappropriate eating patterns of adults and to introduce youngsters to good eating habits that should last a lifetime.

Basic Nutritional Requirements

In a somewhat oversimplified way, a person can be compared with a working mechanism such as a car. The material of which each is made —tissue cells for the person, metal for the car—has to come from somewhere: the human's, from conception to birth, comes from the food eaten by his mother; after birth, from what he himself eats.

During growth and thereafter, the person's cells must be repaired and replaced just as a car must have new tires, parts, and paint from time to time. And like the car, the human has an engine—his muscular activity—which requires fuel. This fuel is provided by food in the form of calories.

In humans, the process by which food is used by the body is called *metabolism*. It begins with chemical processes in the gastrointestinal tract which change plant and animal food into less complex components so that they can be absorbed to fulfill their various functions in the body.

Protein

Of the several essential components of food, *protein* is in many ways the most important. This is so because much of the body's structure is made up of proteins. For example, the typical 160-pound man is composed of about 100 pounds of water, 29 pounds of protein, 25 pounds of fat, 5 pounds of minerals, 1 pound of carbohydrate, and less than an ounce of vitamins. Since the muscles, heart, brain, lungs, and gastrointestinal organs are made up largely of protein, and since the protein in these organs is in constant need of replacement, its importance is obvious.

Chemically, proteins are mixtures of amino acids which contain various elements, including nitrogen. There are 20 different amino acids that are essential for the body's protein needs. Eight of these must be provided in the diet; the rest can be synthesized by the body itself.

Meat, fish, eggs, and milk or milk products are the primary protein foods and contain all of the necessary amino acids. Grains and vegetables are partly made up of protein, but more often than not, they do not provide the whole range of amino acids required for proper nourishment.

Carbohydrates

Carbohydrates are another essential food component. They are also called *starches* or *sugars* and are present in large quantities in grains, fruits, and vegetables. They serve as the primary source of calories for muscle contraction and must be available in the body constantly for this purpose.

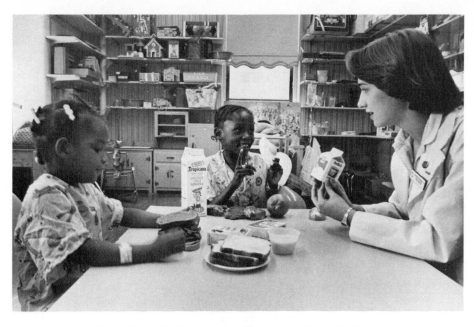

Young hospital patients receive a lesson in basic nutrition from a dietitian who uses props to explain which foods are essential.

It takes one pound of carbohydrates to provide a 160-pound man with fuel for about half a day. Therefore, if he isn't getting new carbohydrate supplies during the day from his food, he will begin to convert his body fat or protein into sugar. This isn't desirable unless he has an excess of body fat, and in any event, could not go on indefinitely.

Fats

Fats are a chemically complex food component composed of *glycerol* (a sweet, oily alcohol) and fatty acids. Fats exist in several forms and come from a variety of sources. One way to think of them is to group them as visible fats, such as butter, salad oil, or the fat seen in meat, and as invisible fats, which are mingled, blended, or absorbed into food, either naturally, as in nuts, meat, or fish, or during cooking. Another way is to think of them as solid at room temperature (fats), or as liquid at room temperature (oils).

SATURATED AND UNSATURATED: Fats are also classified as *saturated* or *unsaturated*. This is a chemical distinction based on the differences in molecular structure of different kinds of fat. If the carbon atoms in a fat molecule are surrounded or boxed in by hydrogen atoms, they are said to be saturated. This type of fat seems to increase the cholesterol content of the blood. *Polyunsaturated* fats, such as those found in fish and vegetable oils, contain the least number of hydrogen atoms and do not add to the blood cholesterol content. In general, fats in foods of plant origin are more unsaturated than in those of animal origin.

Fats play several essential roles in the metabolic process. First of all, they provide more than twice the number of calories on a comparative weight basis than do proteins and carbohydrates. They also can be stored in the body in large quantities and used as a later energy source. They serve as carriers of the fat-soluble vitamins A, D, E, and K, and—of no little importance—they add to the tastiness of food.

Vitamins

Vitamins, which are present in minute quantities in foods in their natural state, are essential for normal metabolism and for the development and maintenance of tissue structure and function. In addition to the fat-soluble vitamins noted above, there are a number of B vitamins, as well as vitamin C, also called *ascorbic acid*. If any particular vitamin is missing from the diet over a sufficiently long time, a specific disease will result.

The understanding of the subtle and complicated role of vitamins in maintaining life and health has come about during this century with the development of highly refined research methods. It is likely that continuing research will shed more light on their importance.

Minerals

Minerals are another component of basic nutritional needs. All living things extract them from the soil, which is their ultimate source. Like vitamins, they are needed for normal metabolism and must be present in the diet in sufficient amounts for the maintenance of good health. The essential minerals are copper, iodine, iron, manganese, zinc, molybdenum, fluorine, and cobalt.

When the normal diet is deficient in certain minerals, these minerals need to be specially added to the diet: iodine for thyroid function, and fluorine for protection against dental cavities. Additional iron for hemoglobin formation may be indicated when the diet is deficient in it, or when there has been an excessive loss of red blood cells, as some women experience with their menstrual periods.

Water

Water is not really a food in the fuel or calorie-producing sense, but it is in many ways a crucial component of nutrition. It makes up from

METRIC EQUIVALENTS OF TRADITIONAL FOOD MEASURES		
1 teaspoon	=	5 milliliters
1 tablespoon	=	15 milliliters
1/4 cup	=	60 milliliters
1/3 cup	=	80 milliliters
1/2 cup	=	120 milliliters
2/3 cup	=	160 milliliters
3/4 cup	=	180 milliliters
1 cup	=	240 milliliters or 0.24 liter

55 to 65 percent of the body's weight, and is constantly being eliminated in the form of urine, perspiration, and expired breath. It must therefore be replaced regularly, for while a person can live for weeks without food, he can live for only a few days without water.

Normally, the best guide to how much water a person needs is his sense of thirst. The regulating mechanism of excretion sees to it that an excessive intake of water will be eliminated as urine. The usual water requirement is on the order of two quarts a day in addition to whatever amount is contained in the solids which make up the daily diet. Information on the protein, fat, and carbohydrate content in specific foods, as well as the number of calories, may be obtained by consulting the table *Nutrients in Common Foods*, pp. 196–202, 207–208. The Metric Equivalents table converts spoon and cup measure into metric measures.

Basic Daily Diets

Everyone should have at least the minimal amount of basic nutrients for resting or basal metabolism. The specific needs of each individual are determined by whether he is still growing, and by how much energy is required for his normal activities. All those who are still growing— and growth continues up to about 20 years of age—have relatively high food needs.

For Infants

That food needs of an infant are especially acute should surprise no one. The newborn baby normally triples his birth weight during his first year and is very active in terms of calorie expenditure.

For his first six months, breast milk or formula, or a combination of both, fills his nutritional needs. The amount of milk he should get each day is about two and a half ounces per pound of his body weight. This provides 50 calories per pound, and in the early months is usually given

NUTRIENTS IN COMMON FOODS

	Food energy	Protein	Fat	Carbohydrate
	Calories	Grams	Grams	Grams
Milk and Milk Products				
Milk; 1 cup:				
Fluid, whole	165	9	10	12
Fluid, nonfat (skim)	90	9	trace	13
Buttermilk, cultured (from skim milk)	90	9	trace	13
Evaporated (undiluted)	345	18	20	24
Dry, nonfat (regular)	435	43	1	63
Yoghurt (from partially skimmed milk); 1 cup	120	8	4	13
Cheese; 1 ounce:				
Cheddar, or American	115	7	9	1
Cottage:				
From skim milk	25	5	trace	1
Creamed	30	4	1	1
Cream cheese	105	2	11	1
Swiss	105	7	8	1
Desserts (largely milk):				
Custard, baked; 1 cup, 8 fluid ounces	305	14	15	29
Ice cream, plain, factory packed:				
1 slice or individual brick, 1/8 quart	130	3	7	14
1 container, 8 fluid ounces	255	6	14	28
Ice milk; 1 cup, 8 fluid ounces	200	6	7	29
Eggs				
Egg, raw, large:				
1 whole	80	6	6	trace
1 white	15	4	trace	trace
1 yolk	60	3	5	trace
Egg, cooked; 1 large:				
Boiled	80	6	6	trace
Scrambled (with milk and fat)	110	7	8	1
Meat, Poultry, Fish, Shellfish				
Bacon, broiled or fried, drained, 2 medium thick slices	85	4	8	trace
Beef, cooked without bone:				
Braised, simmered, or pot-roasted; 3-ounce portion:				
Entire portion, lean and fat	365	19	31	0
Lean only, approx. 2 ounces	140	17	4	0
Hamburger patties, made with				
Regular ground beef; 3-ounce patty	235	21	17	0
Lean ground round; 3-ounce patty	185	23	10	0
Roast; 3-ounce slice from cut having relatively small amount of fat:				
Entire portion, lean and fat	255	22	18	0
Lean only, approx. 2.3 ounces	115	19	4	0
Steak, broiled; 3-ounce portion:				
Entire portion, lean and fat	375	19	32	0
Lean only, approx. 1.8 ounces	105	17	4	0
Beef, canned: corned beef hash: 3 ounces	155	8	10	9
Beef and vegetable stew: 1 cup	220	16	11	15
Chicken, without bone: broiled; 3 ounces	115	20	3	0
Lamb, cooked:				
Chops; 1 thick chop, with bone, 4.8 ounces:				
Lean and fat, approx. 3.4 ounces	340	21	28	0
Lean only, 2.3 ounces	120	18	5	0

NUTRIENTS IN COMMON FOODS *(continued)*

	Food energy	Protein	Fat	Carbohydrate
	Calories	Grams	Grams	Grams
Roast, without bone:				
Leg; 3-ounce slice:				
Entire slice, lean and fat . .	265	20	20	0
Lean only, approx. 2.3 ounces . .	120	19	5	0
Shoulder; 3-ounce portion, without bone:				
Entire portion, lean and fat .	300	18	25	0
Lean only, approx. 2.2 ounces . .	125	16	6	0
Liver, beef, fried; 2 ounces . . .	120	13	4	6
Pork, cured, cooked:				
Ham, smoked; 3-ounce portion, without bone	245	18	19	0
Luncheon meat:				
Boiled ham; 2 ounces	130	11	10	0
Canned, spiced; 2 ounces . .	165	8	14	1
Pork, fresh, cooked:				
Chops; 1 chop, with bone, 3.5 ounces:				
Lean and fat, approx. 2.4 ounces . .	295	15	25	0
Lean only, approx. 1.6 ounces . .	120	14	7	0
Roast; 3-ounce slice, without bone:				
Entire slice, lean and fat . .	340	19	29	0
Lean only, approx. 2.2 ounces . .	160	19	9	0
Sausage:				
Bologna; 8 slices (4.1 by 0.1 inches each), 8 ounces	690	27	62	2
Frankfurter; 1 cooked, 1.8 ounces . .	155	6	14	1
Tongue, beef, boiled; 3 ounces .	205	18	14	trace
Veal, cutlet, broiled; 3-ounce portion, without bone	185	23	9	0
Fish and shellfish:				
Bluefish, baked or broiled; 3 ounces .	135	22	4	0
Clams: raw, meat only; 3 ounces .	70	11	1	3
Crabmeat, canned or cooked; 3 ounces .	90	14	2	1
Fishsticks, breaded, cooked, frozen; 10 sticks (3.8 by 1.0 by 0.5 inches each), 8 ounces	400	38	20	15
Haddock, fried; 3 ounces . . .	135	16	5	6
Mackerel: broiled; 3 ounces . .	200	19	13	0
Oysters, raw, meat only; 1 cup (13–19 medium-size oysters, selects) . .	160	20	4	8
Oyster stew: 1 cup (6–8 oysters) . .	200	11	12	11
Salmon, canned (pink); 3 ounces .	120	17	5	0
Sardines, canned in oil, drained solids; 3 ounces	180	22	9	1
Shrimp, canned, meat only; 3 ounces .	110	23	1	
Tuna, canned in oil, drained solids; 3 ounces	170	25	7	0

Mature Beans and Peas, Nuts

Beans, dry seed:				
Common varieties, as Great Northern, navy, and others, canned; cup:				
Red	230	15	1	42
White, with tomato or molasses:				
With pork	330	16	7	54
Without pork	315	16	1	60

in six feedings a day at four-hour intervals.

If his weight gain is adequate and he appears healthy, and if his stomach is not distended by swallowed air, his appetite is normally a satisfactory guide to how much he needs. The formula-fed baby should get a supplement of 35 milligrams of ascorbic acid each day and 400 international units of vitamin D if the latter has not been added to the milk during its processing.

SOLID FOODS: Between two and six months of age, the baby should begin to eat solid foods such as cooked cereals, strained fruits and vegetables, egg yolk, and homogenized meat. With the introduction of these foods, it is not really necessary to calculate the baby's caloric intake. Satisfaction of appetite, proper weight gain, and a healthy appearance serve as the guides to a proper diet.

By one year of age, a baby should be getting three regular meals a day, and as his teeth appear, his food no longer needs to be strained. By 18 to 24 months, he should no longer need baby foods. For further information on the care and feeding of infants, see under *Birth, Infancy, and Maturation*, p. 50.

Basic Food Groups

The recommended daily amounts of food for people over the age of two have been established with reasonable accuracy. They are called minimal daily amounts, but they always contain a fairly generous safety factor.

THE FOUR GROUP DIVISION: In general, foods are divided into four major groups:
- Meat, fish, eggs
- Dairy products
- Fruits and vegetables
- Breads and cereals.

THE SEVEN GROUP DIVISION: For purposes of planning daily requirements, a more detailed way of considering food groupings is the following:

• Leafy green and yellow vegetables

• Citrus fruits, tomatoes, and raw cabbage

• Potatoes and other vegetables and fruits

• Milk, cheese, and ice cream

• Meat, poultry, fish, eggs, dried peas, and beans

• Bread, flour, and cereals

• Butter and fortified margarine

The Daily Food Guide (see p. 200) is a general guide to planning nutritionally balanced meals for preteens, teens, and adults of any age.

(see p. 200)

The Years of Growth

Even though a child will never again triple his weight in a single year as he did during his first, a proper diet is crucial during the years from 2 to 18, since this is a period of tremendous growth.

Other food goals that should be realized during the childhood and adolescent years are an awareness of what a balanced diet is, a reasonable tolerance for a variety of foods, decent manners at the table, and a sense of timing about when to eat and when not to eat.

These are also the years that a young person should begin to learn something about how to buy and prepare food, how to serve it attractively, and how to clean up after a meal.

CREATING A PLEASANT ATMOSPHERE AT MEALTIME: Although a child's attitudes about food and eating can often be exasperating, it is up to the parent to make mealtime as pleasant as possible, and above all, to avoid any battles of will.

If a young child is too tired, too excited, or too hungry to cope with a meal without ending up in tears or a tantrum, he should not be forced to eat. There are several ways to help children develop a wholesome attitude towards food and eating; here are a few suggestions:

• Children should never be bribed with candy, money, or the promise of special surprises as a way of getting them to eat properly.

• They should not be given the

NUTRIENTS IN COMMON FOODS (continued)

	Food energy	Protein	Fat	Carbohydrate
	Calories	Grams	Grams	Grams
Beans, dry seed:				
Lima, cooked; 1 cup	260	16	1	48
Cowpeas or black-eyed peas,				
dry, cooked; 1 cup	190	13	1	34
Peanuts, roasted, shelled; 1 cup	840	39	71	28
Peanut butter; 1 tablespoon	90	4	8	3
Peas, split, dry, cooked; 1 cup	290	20	1	52
Vegetables				
Asparagus:				
Cooked; 1 cup	35	4	trace	6
Canned; 6 medium-size spears	20	2	trace	3
Beans:				
Lima, immature, cooked; 1 cup	150	8	1	29
Snap, green:				
Cooked; 1 cup	25	2	trace	6
Canned: solids and liquid; 1 cup	45	2	trace	10
Beets, cooked, diced; 1 cup	70	2	trace	16
Broccoli, cooked, flower stalks; 1 cup	45	5	trace	8
Brussels sprouts, cooked; 1 cup	60	6	1	12
Cabbage; 1 cup:				
Raw, coleslaw	100	2	7	9
Cooked	40	2	trace	9
Carrots:				
Raw: 1 carrot (5½ by 1 inch)				
or 25 thin strips	20	1	trace	5
Cooked, diced; 1 cup	45	1	1	9
Canned, strained or chopped; 1 ounce	5	trace	0	2
Cauliflower, cooked, flower buds; 1 cup	30	3	trace	6
Celery, raw: large stalk, 8 inches long	5	1	trace	1
Collards, cooked; 1 cup	75	7	1	14
Corn, sweet:				
Cooked; 1 ear 5 inches long	65	2	1	16
Canned, solids and liquid; 1 cup	170	5	1	41
Cucumbers, raw, pared; 6 slices				
(⅛-inch thick, center section)	5	trace	trace	1
Lettuce, head, raw:				
2 large or 4 small leaves	5	1	trace	1
1 compact head (4¾-inch diameter)	70	5	1	13
Mushrooms, canned, solids and				
liquid; 1 cup	30	3	trace	9
Okra, cooked; 8 pods (3 inches long,				
⅝-inch diameter)	30	2	trace	6
Onions: mature raw; 1 onion (2½-inch				
diameter)	50	2	trace	11
Peas, green; 1 cup:				
Cooked	110	8	1	19
Canned, solids and liquid	170	8	1	32
Peppers, sweet:				
Green, raw; 1 medium	15	1	trace	3
Red, raw; 1 medium	20	1	trace	4
Potatoes:				
Baked or boiled; 1 medium,				
2½-inch diameter (weight raw,				
about 5 ounces):				
Baked in jacket	90	3	trace	21
Boiled; peeled before boiling	90	3	trace	21
Chips; 10 medium (2-inch diameter)	110	1	7	10

NUTRIENTS IN COMMON FOODS (continued)

	Food energy	Protein	Fat	Carbohydrate
	Calories	Grams	Grams	Grams
French fried:				
Frozen, ready to be heated for serving; 10 pieces (2 by ¹/₂ by ¹/₂ inch)	95	2	4	15
Ready-to-eat, deep fat for entire process; 10 pieces (2 by ¹/₂ by ¹/₂ inch)	155	2	7	20
Mashed; 1 cup:				
Milk added	145	4	1	30
Milk and butter added	230	4	12	28
Radishes, raw; 4 small	10	trace	trace	2
Spinach:				
Cooked; 1 cup	45	6	1	6
Spinach:				
Canned, creamed, strained; 1 ounce	10	1	trace	2
Squash:				
Cooked, 1 cup:				
Summer, diced	35	1	trace	8
Winter, baked, mashed	95	4	1	23
Canned, strained or chopped; 1 ounce	10	trace	trace	2
Sweet potatoes:				
Baked or boiled; 1 medium, 5 by 2 inches (weight raw, about 6 ounces):				
Baked in jacket	155	2	1	36
Boiled in jacket	170	2	1	39
Candied; 1 small, 3¹/₂ by 2 inches	295	2	6	60
Canned, vacuum or solid pack; 1 cup	235	4	trace	54
Tomatoes:				
Raw; 1 medium (2 by 2¹/₂ inches), about ¹/₃ pound	30	2	trace	6
Canned or cooked; 1 cup	45	2	trace	9
Tomato juice, canned; 1 cup	50	2	trace	10
Tomato catsup; 1 tablespoon	15	trace	trace	4
Turnips, cooked, diced; 1 cup	40	1	trace	9
Turnip greens, cooked; 1 cup	45	4	1	8

Fruits

Apples, raw; 1 medium (2¹/₂ inch diameter), about ¹/₃ pound	70	trace	trace	18
Apple juice, fresh or canned; 1 cup	125	trace	0	34
Apple sauce, canned:				
Sweetened; 1 cup	185	trace	trace	50
Unsweetened; 1 cup	100	trace	trace	26
Apricots, raw; 3 apricots (about ¹/₄ pound)	55	1	trace	14
Apricots, canned in heavy syrup; 1 cup	200	1	trace	54
Apricots, dried: uncooked; 1 cup (40 halves, small)	390	8	1	100
Avocados, raw, California varieties: ¹/₂ of a 10-ounce avocado (3¹/₂ by 3¹/₄ inches)	185	2	18	6
Avocados, raw, Florida varieties: ¹/₂ of a 13-ounce avocado (4 by 3 inches)	160	2	14	11
Bananas, raw; 1 medium (6 by 1¹/₂ inches), about ¹/₃ pound	85	1	trace	23

idea that dessert is a reward for finishing the earlier part of the meal.

• Relatively small portions should be served and completely finished before anything else is offered.

• Between-meal snacks should be discouraged if they cut down on the appetite at mealtime.

• From time to time, the child should be allowed to choose the foods that he will eat at a meal.

Parents should keep in mind that the atmosphere in which a child eats and the attitudes instilled in him toward food can be altogether as basic as the nourishment for his body.

TEEN-AGE DIET: From the start of a child's growth spurt, which begins at age 10 or 11 for girls and between 13 and 15 for boys, and for several years thereafter, adolescent appetites are likely to be unbelievably large and somewhat outlandish. Parents should try to exercise some control over the youngster who is putting on too much weight as well as over the one who is attracted by a bizarre starvation diet.

Adult Nutrition

Adult nutrition is concerned with more than 50 years of an individual's life span. In typical cases, there is a slow but steady weight gain that may go unnoticed at first; for some, there is an obesity problem that begins at about age 40.

Since it is never easy to lose weight, it is especially important for adults to eat sensibly and avoid excess calories. See under *Weight*, p. 202, for a discussion of weight control and obesity.

FOR OLDER PEOPLE: People over 60 tend to have changes in their digestive system that are related to less efficient and slower absorption. Incomplete chewing of food because of carelessness or impaired teeth can intensify this problem. Avoiding haste at mealtimes ought to be the rule.

In cases where a dental disorder makes proper chewing impossible, food should be chopped or pureed.

Older people occasionally have difficulty swallowing and may choke on a large piece of unchewed meat.

Food for older people should be cooked simply, preferably baked, boiled, or broiled rather than fried, and menus excessively rich in fats should be avoided. A daily multivitamin capsule is strongly recommended for those over 60. A poor appetite can be stimulated by an ounce or two of sherry before a meal unless there are medical reasons for avoiding alcoholic beverages of any kind. See under *Aging and What to Do About It*, p. 171, for a discussion of diet and eating habits in the later years.

DURING PREGNANCY: A pregnant woman needs special foods to maintain her own health as well as to safeguard the health of her baby. She should have additional vitamin D and iron, usually recommended as dietary supplements. More important for most women is the provision of adequate protein in the diet to prevent toxemia of pregnancy or underweight babies. Between 70 and 85 grams of protein a day should be eaten during pregnancy, even if this results in a weight gain of as much as 25 pounds. Adequate nutrition is more important than restricting weight gain to 20 pounds or less.

NURSING MOTHERS: A nursing mother has special dietary needs in addition to those satisfied by the normal adult diet. She should drink an extra quart of milk and eat two more servings of citrus fruit or tomatoes, one more serving of lean meat, fish, poultry, eggs, beans, or cheese, and one more serving of leafy green or yellow vegetables.

Malnutrition

The classic diseases of nutritional deficiency, or malnutrition, such as scurvy and pellagra, are now rare, at least in the United States. The chief reason for their disappearance is the application of scientific knowledge gained in this century of the importance of vitamins and minerals in the diet. Thus most bread is fortified

DAILY FOOD GUIDE				
	Child	Pre-teen and Teen	Adult	Aging Adult
Milk or milk products (*cups*)	2–3	3–4 or more	2 or more	2 or more
Meat, fish, poultry, and eggs (*servings*)	1–2	3 or more	2 or more	2 or more
Green and yellow vegetables (*servings*)	1–2	2	2	at least 1
Citrus fruits and tomatoes (*servings*)	1	1–2	1	1–2
Potatoes, other fruits, vegetables (*servings*)	1	1	1	0–1
Bread, flour, and cereal (*servings*)	3–4	4 or more	3–4	2–3
Butter or margarine (*tablespoons*)	2	2–4	2–3	1–2

1. The need for the nutrients in 1 or 2 cups of milk daily can be satisfied by cheeses or ice cream. (1 cup of milk is approximately equivalent to 1½ cups of cottage cheese or 2–3 large scoops of ice cream.)

2. It is important to drink enough fluid. The equivalent of 3–5 cups daily is recommended.

3. The recommended daily serving of meat, fish, and poultry (3 oz.) may be alternated with eggs or cheese, dried peas, beans, or lentils.

4. Iron-rich foods should be selected as frequently as possible by teen-age and adult females to help meet their high requirement for this mineral (liver, heart, lean meats, shellfish, egg yolks, legumes, green leafy vegetables, and whole grain and enriched cereal products).

From *Your Age and Your Diet* (1971), reprinted with permission from the American Medical Association

NUTRIENTS IN COMMON FOODS (continued)

	Food energy Calories	Protein Grams	Fat Grams	Carbohydrate Grams
Blueberries, raw; 1 cup	85	1	1	21
Cantaloupes, raw, ½ melon (5-inch diameter)	40	1	trace	9
Cherries, sour, sweet, and hybrid, raw; 1 cup	65	1	1	15
Cranberry sauce, sweetened; 1 cup	550	trace	1	142
Dates, "fresh" and dried, pitted and cut; 1 cup	505	4	1	134
Figs:				
Raw; 3 small (1½-inch diameter), about ¼ pound	90	2	trace	22
Dried; 1 large (2 by 1 inch)	60	1	trace	15
Fruit cocktail, canned in heavy syrup, solids and liquid; 1 cup	175	1	trace	47
Grapefruit:				
Raw; ½ medium (4¼-inch diameter, No. 64's)	50	1	trace	14
Canned in syrup; 1 cup	165	1	trace	44
Grapefruit juice:				
Raw; 1 cup	85	1	trace	23
Canned:				
Unsweetened; 1 cup	95	1	trace	24
Sweetened; 1 cup	120	1	trace	32
Frozen concentrate, unsweetened:				
Undiluted; 1 can (6 fluid ounces)	280	4	1	72
Diluted, ready-to-serve; 1 cup	95	1	trace	24
Grapefruit juice:				
Frozen concentrate, sweetened:				
Undiluted; 1 can (6 fluid ounces)	320	3	1	85
Diluted, ready-to-serve; 1 cup	105	1	trace	28
Grapes, raw; 1 cup:				
American type (slip skin)	70	1	1	16
European type (adherent skin)	100	1	trace	26

NUTRIENTS IN COMMON FOODS (continued)

	Food energy	Protein	Fat	Carbohydrate
	Calories	Grams	Grams	Grams
Grape juice, bottled; 1 cup . . .	165	1	1	42
Lemonade concentrate, frozen, sweetened:				
Undiluted; 1 can (6 fluid ounces) . .	305	1	trace	113
Diluted, ready-to-serve; 1 cup . .	75	trace	trace	28
Oranges, raw; 1 large orange				
(3-inch diameter)	70	1	trace	18
Orange juice:				
Raw; 1 cup:				
California (Valencias) . . .	105	2	trace	26
Florida varieties:				
Early and midseason . . .	90	1	trace	23
Late season (Valencias) . .	105	1	trace	26
Canned, unsweetened; 1 cup . .	110	2	trace	28
Frozen concentrate:				
Undiluted; 1 can (6 fluid ounces) .	305	5	trace	80
Diluted, ready-to-serve; 1 cup . .	105	2	trace	27
Peaches:				
Raw:				
1 medium (2½-inch diameter),				
about ¼ pound	35	1	trace	10
1 cup, sliced	65	1	trace	16
Canned (yellow-fleshed) in heavy				
syrup; 1 cup	185	1	trace	49
Dried: uncooked; 1 cup . . .	420	5	1	109
Pears:				
Raw; 1 pear (3 by 2½-inch diameter) .	100	1	1	25
Canned in heavy syrup; 1 cup . .	175	1	trace	47
Pineapple juice; canned; 1 cup . .	120	1	trace	32
Plums:				
Raw; 1 plum (2-inch diameter),				
about 2 ounces	30	trace	trace	7
Canned (Italian prunes), in syrup;				
1 cup	185	1	trace	50
Prunes, dried:				
Uncooked; 4 medium prunes . .	70	1	trace	19
Cooked, unsweetened; 1 cup (17–18				
prunes and ⅓ cup liquid) . .	295	3	1	78
Prune juice, canned; 1 cup . . .	170	1	trace	45
Raisins, dried; 1 cup	460	4	trace	124
Raspberries, red:				
Raw; 1 cup	70	1	trace	17
Frozen; 10-ounce carton . . .	280	2	1	70
Strawberries:				
Raw; 1 cup	55	1	1	12
Frozen; 10-ounce carton . . .	300	2	1	75
Tangerines; 1 medium (2½-inch				
diameter), about ¼ pound . .	40	1	trace	10
Watermelon: 1 wedge (4 by 8 inches),				
about 2 pounds (weighed with rind) .	120	2	1	29

Grain Products

Biscuits, baking powder, enriched flour;				
1 biscuit (2½-inch diameter) . .	130	3	4	20
Bran flakes (40 percent bran) with				
added thiamine; 1 ounce . . .	85	3	1	22
Breads:				
Cracked wheat:				

with vitamins and minerals, and in addition, commercial food processing has made it possible for balanced diets of an appealing variety to be eaten all year round.

Many people do not get an adequate diet, either through ignorance or because they simply cannot afford it. A number of food programs have been created to assist them, but unfortunately, the programs don't reach everyone who needs help.

Causes of Malnutrition

Some people, either because of ignorance or food faddism, do not eat a balanced diet even though they can afford to. There are also large numbers of people with nutritional deficiency diseases who can be described as abnormal, at least in regard to eating. Some are alcoholics; others live alone and are so depressed that they lack sufficient drive to feed themselves properly. Combination of any of these factors increase the likelihood of poor nutrition and often lead to health-damaging consequences.

DISEASE: People can also develop nutritional deficiencies because they have some disease that interferes with food absorption, storage, and utilization, or that causes an increased excretion, usually in the urine, of substances needed for nutrition. These are generally chronic diseases of the gastrointestinal tract including the liver, or of the kidneys or the endocrine glands.

MEDICATIONS: Nutritional deficiencies can also result from loss of appetite caused by medications, especially when a number of different medications are taken simultaneously. This adverse affect on the appetite is a strong reason for not taking medicines unless told to do so by a doctor for a specific purpose.

Most people are not aware of inadequacies in their diet until there are some dramatic consequences. Nor is it easy to recognize the presence of a disorder that might be causing malnutrition. A doctor should

NUTRIENTS IN COMMON FOODS *(continued)*

	Food energy	Protein	Fat	Carbohydrate
	Calories	Grams	Grams	Grams
1 pound (20 slices)	1,190	39	10	236
1 slice (1/2 inch thick)	60	2	1	12
Italian; 1 pound	1,250	41	4	256
Rye:				
American (light):				
1 pound (20 slices)	1,100	41	5	236
1 slice (1/2 inch thick)	55	2	trace	12
Pumpernickel; 1 pound	1,115	41	5	241
White:				
1–2 percent nonfat dry milk:				
1 pound (20 slices)	1,225	39	15	229
1 slice (1/2 inch thick)	60	2	1	12
3–4 percent nonfat dry milk:				
1 pound (20 slices)	1,225	39	15	229
1 slice (1/2 inch thick)	60	2	1	12
5–6 percent nonfat dry milk:				
1 pound (20 slices)	1,245	41	17	228
1 slice (1/2 inch thick)	65	2	1	12
Whole wheat, graham, or entire wheat:				
1 pound (20 slices)	1,105	48	14	216
1 slice (1/2 inch thick)	55	2	1	11
Cakes:				
Angelfood: 2-inch sector (1/12 of cake, 8-inch diameter)	160	4	trace	36
Butter cakes:				
Plain cake and cupcakes without icing:				
1 square (3 by 3 by 2 inches)	315	4	12	48
1 cupcake (2 3/4-inch diameter)	120	2	5	18
Butter cakes:				
Plain cake with icing:				
2-inch sector of iced layer cake (1/16 of cake, 10-inch diameter)	320	5	6	62
Rich cake:				
2-inch sector layer cake, iced (1/16 of cake, 10-inch diameter)	490	6	19	76
Fruit cake, dark; 1 piece (2 by 1 1/2 by 1/4 inches)	60	1	2	9
Sponge; 2-inch sector (1/12 of cake, 8-inch diameter)	115	3	2	22
Cookies, plain and assorted; 1 cookie (3-inch diameter)	110	2	3	19
Cornbread or muffins made with enriched, degermed cornmeal; 1 muffin (2 3/4-inch diameter)	105	3	2	18
Cornflakes: 1 ounce	110	2	trace	24
Corn grits, degermed, cooked: 1 cup	120	3	trace	27
Crackers:				
Graham; 4 small or 2 medium	55	1	1	10
Saltines; 2 crackers (2-inch square)	35	1	1	6
Soda, plain: 2 crackers (2 1/2-inch square)	45	1	1	8
Doughnuts, cake type; 1 doughnut	135	2	7	17
Farina, cooked; 1 cup	105	3	trace	22
Macaroni, cooked; 1 cup:				
Cooked 8–10 minutes	190	6	1	39
Cooked until tender	155	5	1	32

be consulted promptly when there is a persistent weight loss, especially when the diet is normal. He should also be informed of any changes in the skin, mucous membranes of the mouth or tongue, or nervous system function, since such symptoms can be a warning of dietary deficiency.

The family or friends of a person with a nutritional deficiency can often detect his condition because they become aware of changes in his eating patterns. They can also note early signs of a deficiency of some of the B vitamins, such as cracks in the mucous membranes at the corners of the mouth, or some slowing of intellectual function.

Correction of Nutritional Deficiencies

Nutritional deficiencies are among the most easily preventable causes of disease. It is important to realize that even mild deficiencies can cause irreparable damage, particularly protein deprivation in young children, which can result in some degree of mental retardation. Periodic medical checkups for everyone in the family are the best way to make sure that such deficiencies are corrected before they snowball into a chronic disease. In most cases, all that is required is a change in eating habits.

Weight

Probably the most important dietary problem in the United States today is obesity. It is certainly the problem most talked about and written about, not only in terms of good looks, but more important, in terms of good health.

All studies indicate that people who are obese have a higher rate of disease and a shorter life expectancy than those of average weight. From a medical point of view, people who are too fat may actually suffer from a form of malnutrition, even though they look overnourished.

BEEF CHART

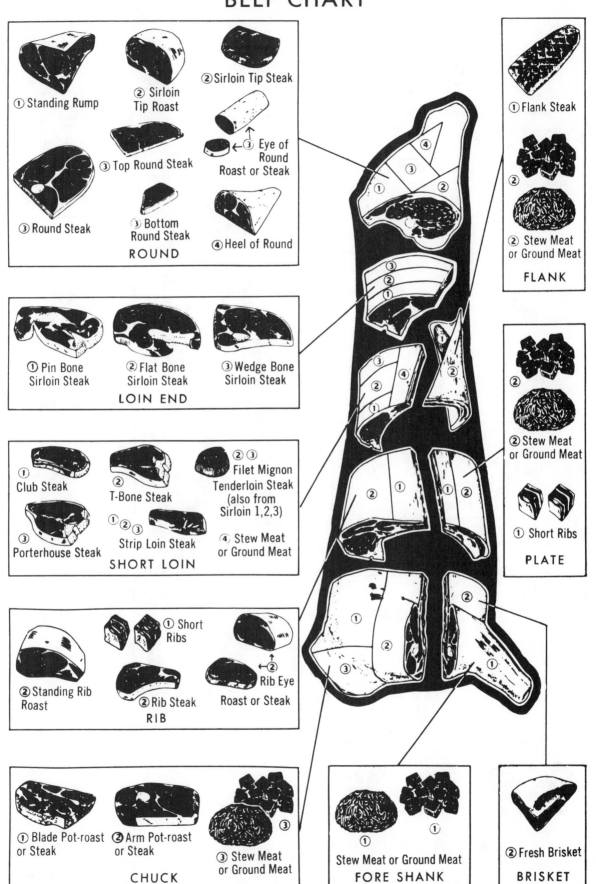

ROUND
① Standing Rump
② Sirloin Tip Roast
② Sirloin Tip Steak
③ Top Round Steak
③ Eye of Round Roast or Steak
③ Round Steak
③ Bottom Round Steak
④ Heel of Round

LOIN END
① Pin Bone Sirloin Steak
② Flat Bone Sirloin Steak
③ Wedge Bone Sirloin Steak

SHORT LOIN
① Club Steak
② T-Bone Steak
②③ Filet Mignon Tenderloin Steak (also from Sirloin 1,2,3)
③ Porterhouse Steak
①②③ Strip Loin Steak
④ Stew Meat or Ground Meat

RIB
② Standing Rib Roast
① Short Ribs
② Rib Steak
② Rib Eye Roast or Steak

CHUCK
① Blade Pot-roast or Steak
② Arm Pot-roast or Steak
③ Stew Meat or Ground Meat

FLANK
① Flank Steak
② Stew Meat or Ground Meat

PLATE
② Stew Meat or Ground Meat
① Short Ribs

FORE SHANK
① Stew Meat or Ground Meat

BRISKET
② Fresh Brisket

LAMB CHART

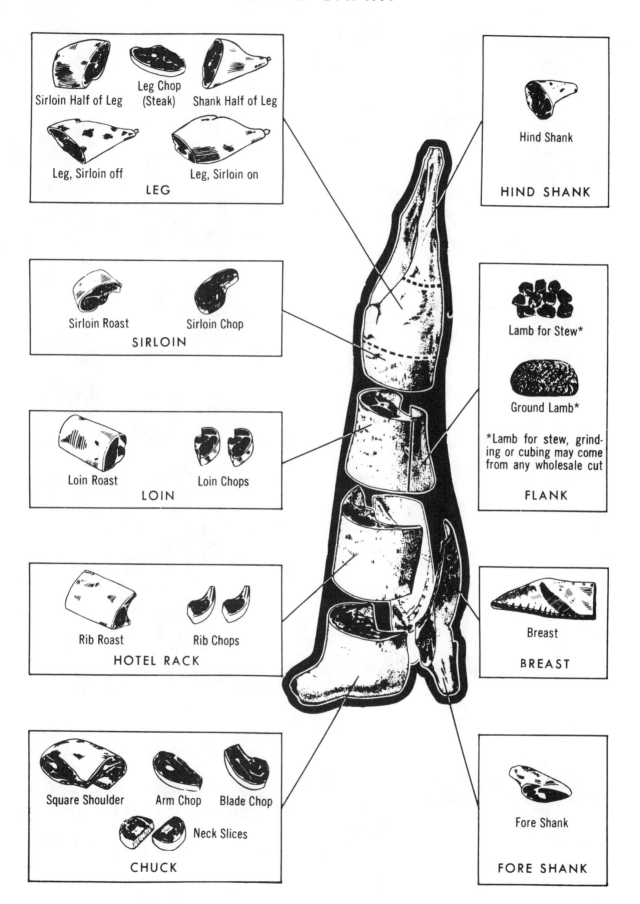

LEG

Sirloin Half of Leg   Leg Chop (Steak)   Shank Half of Leg

Leg, Sirloin off   Leg, Sirloin on

SIRLOIN

Sirloin Roast   Sirloin Chop

LOIN

Loin Roast   Loin Chops

HOTEL RACK

Rib Roast   Rib Chops

CHUCK

Square Shoulder   Arm Chop   Blade Chop

Neck Slices

HIND SHANK

Hind Shank

FLANK

Lamb for Stew*

Ground Lamb*

*Lamb for stew, grinding or cubing may come from any wholesale cut

BREAST

Breast

FORE SHANK

Fore Shank

PORK CHART

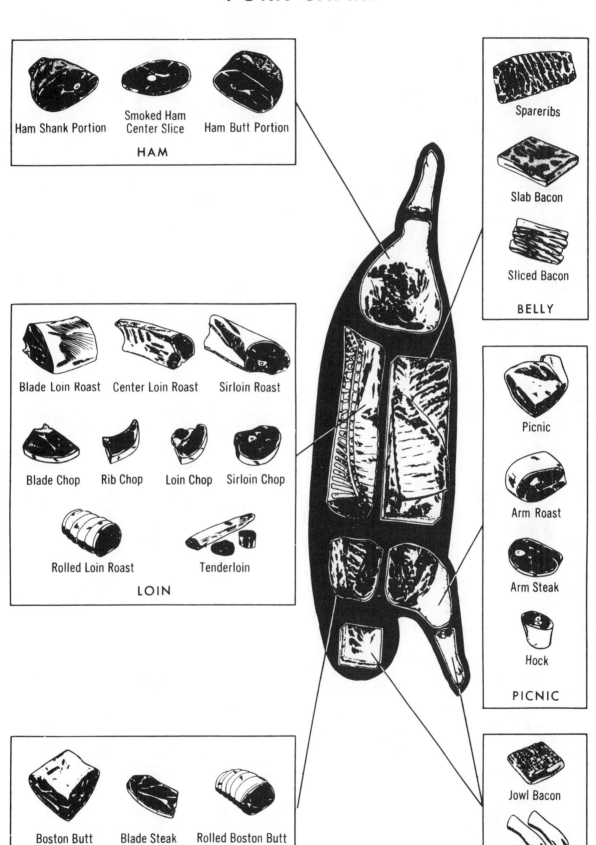

HAM
Ham Shank Portion — Smoked Ham Center Slice — Ham Butt Portion

BELLY
Spareribs — Slab Bacon — Sliced Bacon

LOIN
Blade Loin Roast — Center Loin Roast — Sirloin Roast — Blade Chop — Rib Chop — Loin Chop — Sirloin Chop — Rolled Loin Roast — Tenderloin

PICNIC
Picnic — Arm Roast — Arm Steak — Hock

BOSTON BUTT
Boston Butt — Blade Steak — Rolled Boston Butt

Jowl Bacon — Pig's Feet

Being too fat and being over-weight are not necessarily the same. Heavy bones and muscles can make a person overweight in terms of the charts, but only an excess amount of fat tissue can make someone obese. However, height and weight tables are generally used to determine obesity.

Table 1 lists standard desirable weights for people of various heights, calculated with indoor clothing and shoes on. Frame sizes are estimated in a general way. This table applies to anyone over the age of 25, indicating that weight gain for the rest of the life span is unnecessary for biological normalcy.

Table 2 gives average weights of American men and women, according to height and age. These measurements are made without clothing or shoes. Note that the weights are considerably higher than the corresponding ones of Table 1. There is a modest weight gain until the middle years and then a gradual loss.

To determine whether a person is obese according to the tables, the percent that he is overweight has to be calculated. An individual is usually considered obese in the clinical sense if he weighs 20 percent more than the standard tables indicate for his size and age.

THE PINCH TEST: Another method of determining obesity is to use the "pinch" test. In most adults under 50 years of age, about half of the body fat is located directly under the skin. There are various parts of the body, such as the side of the lower torso, the back of the upper arm, or directly under the shoulder blade, where the thumb and forefinger can pinch a fold of skin and fat away from the underlying bone structure.

If the fold between the fingers—which is, of course, double thickness when it is pinched—is thicker than one inch in any of these areas, the likelihood is that the person is obese.

TABLE 1

Desirable Weights for Men and Women Aged 25 and Over[1]
(in pounds by height and frame, in indoor clothing)

MEN (in shoes, 1-inch heels)				WOMEN (in shoes, 2-inch heels)			
Height	Small Frame	Medium Frame	Large Frame	Height	Small Frame	Medium Frame	Large Frame
5' 2"	112–120	118–129	126–141	4' 10"	92– 98	96–107	104–119
5' 3"	115–123	121–133	129–144	4' 11"	94–101	98–110	106–122
5' 4"	118–126	124–136	132–148	5' 0"	96–104	101–113	109–125
5' 5"	121–129	127–139	135–152	5' 1"	99–107	104–116	112–128
5' 6"	124–133	130–143	138–156	5' 2"	102–110	107–119	115–131
5' 7"	128–137	134–147	142–161	5' 3"	105–113	110–122	118–134
5' 8"	132–141	138–152	147–166	5' 4"	108–116	113–126	121–138
5' 9"	136–145	142–156	151–170	5' 5"	111–119	116–130	125–142
5' 10"	140–150	146–160	155–174	5' 6"	114–123	120–135	129–146
5' 11"	144–154	150–165	159–179	5' 7"	118–127	124–139	133–150
6' 0"	148–158	154–170	164–184	5' 8"	122–131	128–143	137–154
6' 1"	152–162	158–175	168–189	5' 9"	126–135	132–147	141–158
6' 2"	156–167	162–180	173–194	5' 10"	130–140	136–151	145–163
6' 3"	160–171	167–185	178–199	5' 11"	134–144	140–155	149–168
6' 4"	164–175	172–190	182–204	6' 0"	138–148	144–159	153–173

[1]Adapted from Metropolitan Life Insurance Co., New York. New weight standards for men and women. *Statistical Bulletin* 40:3.

TABLE 2

Average Weights for Men and Women[1]
(in pounds by age and height, in paper gown and slippers)

MEN						
Height	18–24 Years	25–34 Years	35–44 Years	45–54 Years	55–64 Years	65–74 Years	75–79 Years
5' 2"	137	141	149	148	148	144	133
5' 3"	140	145	152	152	151	148	138
5' 4"	144	150	156	156	155	151	143
5' 5"	147	154	160	160	158	154	148
5' 6"	151	159	164	164	162	158	154
5' 7"	154	163	168	168	166	161	159
5' 8"	158	168	171	173	169	165	164
5' 9"	161	172	175	177	173	168	169
5' 10"	165	177	179	181	176	171	174
5' 11"	168	181	182	185	180	175	179
6' 0"	172	186	186	189	184	178	184
6' 1"	175	190	190	193	187	182	189
6' 2"	179	194	194	197	191	185	194
WOMEN							
4' 9"	116	112	131	129	138	132	125
4' 10"	118	116	134	132	141	135	129
4' 11"	120	120	136	136	144	138	132
5' 0"	122	124	138	140	149	142	136
5' 1"	125	128	140	143	150	145	139
5' 2"	127	132	143	147	152	149	143
5' 3"	129	136	145	150	155	152	146
5' 4"	131	140	147	154	158	156	150
5' 5"	134	144	149	158	161	159	153
5' 6"	136	148	152	161	164	163	157
5' 7"	138	152	154	165	167	166	160
5' 8"	140	156	156	168	170	170	164

[1]Adapted from National Center for Health Statistics: Weight by Height and Age of Adults, United States. *Vital Health Statistics.* PHS Publication No. 1000–Series 11, No. 14.

NUTRIENTS IN COMMON FOODS (continued)

	Food energy Calories	Protein Grams	Fat Grams	Carbohydrate Grams
Noodles (egg noodles), cooked: 1 cup .	200	7	2	37
Oat cereal (mixture, mainly oat flour), ready-to-eat; 1 ounce	115	4	2	21
Oatmeal or rolled oats, regular or quick cooking, cooked; 1 cup	150	5	3	26
Pancakes, baked; 1 cake (4-inch diameter):				
Wheat (home recipe) . . .	60	2	2	7
Buckwheat (with buckwheat pancake mix)	45	2	2	6
Pies; 3½-inch sector (⅛ of 9-inch diameter pie):				
Apple	300	3	13	45
Cherry	310	3	13	45
Custard	250	7	13	27
Lemon meringue	270	4	11	40
Mince	320	3	14	49
Pumpkin	240	5	13	28
Pretzels; 5 small sticks	20	trace	trace	4
Rice, cooked; 1 cup:				
Converted	205	4	trace	45
White	200	4	trace	44
Rice, puffed or flakes; 1 ounce . . .	110	2	trace	25
Rolls:				
Plain, pan (16 ounces per dozen); 1 roll .	115	3	2	20
Hard, round (22 ounces per dozen); 1 roll	160	5	2	31
Sweet, pan (18 ounces per dozen); 1 roll	135	4	4	21
Spaghetti, cooked until tender; 1 cup .	155	5	1	32
Waffles, baked, with enriched flour:				
1 waffle (4½ by 5½ by ½ inches) .	215	7	8	28
Wheat, puffed: 1 ounce	100	4	trace	22
Wheat, rolled, cooked; 1 cup . . .	175	5	1	40
Wheat flakes; 1 ounce	100	3	trace	23
Wheat flours:				
Whole wheat; 1 cup, sifted . .	400	16	2	85
All purpose or family flour: 1 cup, sifted	400	12	1	84
Wheat germ; 1 cup, stirred . .	245	17	7	34

Fats, Oils, Related Products

	Food energy Calories	Protein Grams	Fat Grams	Carbohydrate Grams
Butter; 1 tablespoon	100	trace	11	trace
Fats, cooking:				
Vegetable fats:				
1 cup	1,770	0	200	0
1 tablespoon	110	0	12	0
Lard:				
1 cup	1,985	0	220	0
1 tablespoon	125	0	14	0
Margarine; 1 tablespoon . . .	100	trace	11	trace
Oils, salad or cooking; 1 tablespoon .	125	0	14	0
Salad dressings; 1 tablespoon:				
Blue cheese	90	1	10	1
Commercial, plain (mayonnaise type) .	60	trace	6	2
French	60	trace	6	2

The Problem of Overweight

The percentage of overweight people in this country has been increasing steadily, chiefly because people eat more and use less physical energy than they used to. Americans do very little walking because of the availability of cars; they do very little manual labor because of the increasing use of machines. They may eat good wholesome meals, but they have the time for nibbling at all hours, especially when sitting in front of the television screen.

These patterns usually begin in childhood. Youngsters rarely walk to school any more; they get there by bus or car. They often have extra money for snacks and soft drinks, and frequently parents encourage them to overeat without realizing that such habits do them more harm than good.

Most overweight children remain overweight as adults. They also have greater difficulty losing fat, and if they do lose it, tend to regain it more easily than overweight adults who were thin as children. Many adults become overweight between the ages of 20 and 30. Thus, by age 30, about 12 percent of American men and women are 20 percent or more overweight, and by age 60, about 30 percent of the male population and 50 percent of the female are at least 20 percent overweight. As indicated above, the phenomenon of weight gain while aging does not represent biological normalcy.

		Calories
	Sedentary	2,500
	Moderately active	3,000
	Active	3,500
	Very active	4,250
	Sedentary	2,100
	Moderately active	2,500
	Active	3,000
	Very active	3,750

Guidelines for average daily calorie consumption by men and women. With increasing use of labor-saving devices, most Americans fall into the sedentary category.

Why People Put On Weight

Why does weight gain happen? Excess weight is the result of the imbalance between caloric intake as food and caloric expenditure as energy, either in maintaining the basic metabolic processes necessary to sustain life or in performing physical activity. Calories not spent in either of these ways become converted to fat and accumulate in the body as fat, or *adipose* tissue.

A *calorie* is the unit of measurement that describes the amount of energy potentially available in a given food. It is also used to describe the amount of energy the body must use up to perform a given function.

An ounce of protein contains 130 calories, as does an ounce of carbohydrate. An ounce of fat, by contrast, contains 270 calories. This biochemical information isn't too helpful in calculating the calories in a particular piece of meat, slice of bread, or pat of butter. For such practical figures, there are useful pocket guides, such as *Calories and Weight*, a U.S. Government publication that can be obtained by sending $1.00 to the Superintendent of Documents, U.S. Government Printing Office, Washington, D. C. 20401, and asking for the Agriculture Information Bulletin No. 364.

Counting Calories

If an adult gets the average 3,000 calories a day in his food from the age of 20 to 70, he will have consumed about 55 million calories. About 60 percent of these calories will have been used for his basic metabolic processes. The rest—22 million calories—might have resulted in a gain of about 6,000 pounds of fat, since each group of 3,500 extra calories could have produced one pound of fat.

In some ways, it's a miracle that people don't become more obese than they do. The reason, of course, is that most or all of these extra calories are normally used to provide energy for physical activity. On this page are some examples of

NUTRIENTS IN COMMON FOODS (continued)

	Food energy	Protein	Fat	Carbohydrate
	Calories	Grams	Grams	Grams
Mayonnaise	110	trace	12	trace
Thousand Island	75	trace	8	1
Sugars, Sweets				
Candy; 1 ounce:				
Caramels	120	1	3	22
Chocolate, sweetened, milk . .	145	2	9	16
Fudge, plain	115	trace	3	23
Hard	110	0	0	28
Marshmallow	90	1	0	23
Jams, marmalades, preserves; 1 tablespoon	55	trace	trace	14
Jellies; 1 tablespoon	50	0	0	13
Sugar; 1 tablespoon	50	0	0	12
Syrup, table blends; 1 tablespoon . .	55	0	0	15
Miscellaneous				
Beverages, carbonated, cola types; 1 cup .	105	—	—	28
Bouillon cubes; 1 cube	2	trace	trace	0
Chocolate, unsweetened; 1 ounce . .	145	2	15	8
Gelatin dessert, plain, ready-to-serve; 1 cup	155	4	0	36
Sherbet, factory packed; 1 cup (8-fluid-ounce container)	235	3	trace	58
Soups, canned, prepared with equal amount of water; 1 cup:				
Bean with pork	168	8	6	22
Beef noodle	140	8	5	14
Bouillon, broth, and consomme . .	30	5	0	3
Chicken consomme	44	7	trace	4
Clam chowder, Manhattan style . .	80	2	3	12
Tomato	90	2	3	16
Vegetable beef	80	5	2	10
Vinegar; 1 tablespoon	2	0	—	1

Adapted from *Nutritive Value of American Foods* by Catherine F. Adams, Agriculture Handbook No. 456, U.S. Department of Agriculture, issued November 1975. The cup measure used in the following table refers to the standard 8-ounce measuring cup of 8 fluid ounces or one-half liquid pint. When a measure is indicated by ounce, it is understood to be by weight—1/16 of a pound avoirdupois—unless a fluid ounce is indicated. All weights and measures in the table are in U.S. System units. To find the metric equivalents, see the table on this page.

calorie expenditure during various activities.

A reasonably good way for an adult to figure his daily caloric needs for moderate activities is to multiply his desirable weight (as noted in Table 1) by 18 for men and by 16 for women. If the typical day includes vigorous or strenuous activities, extra calories will, of course, be required.

Parental Influences and Hereditary Factors

Although there are exceptions, almost all obese people consume more calories than they expend. The reasons for this imbalance are complex. One has to do with parental weight. If the weight of both parents is normal, there is only a 10

TYPE OF ACTIVITY	CALORIES PER HOUR
Sedentary: reading, sewing, typing, etc.	30–100
Light: cooking, slow walking, dressing, etc.	100–170
Moderate: sweeping, light gardening, making beds, etc.	170–250
Vigorous: fast walking, hanging out clothes, golfing, etc.	250–350
Strenuous: swimming, bicycling, dancing, etc.	350 and more

percent likelihood that the children will be obese. If one parent is obese, there is a 50 percent probability that the children will be too, and if both are, the probability of obese offspring is 80 percent.

No one knows for certain why this is so. It is probably a combination of diet habits acquired in youth, conditioning during early years to react to emotional stress by eating, the absence of appropriate exercise patterns, and genetic inheritance.

Some obese people seem to have an impairment in the regulatory mechanism of the area of the central nervous system that governs food intake. Simply put, they do not know when to stop eating. Others, particularly girls, may eat less than their nonobese counterparts, but they are considerably less active. Some researchers think that obese people have an inherent muscle rhythm deficiency. A few people appear to have an abnormality in the metabolic process which results in the accumulation of fat even when the balance between calories taken in and expended is negative and should lead to weight loss.

Obesity and Health

There are many reasons why obesity is a health hazard. The annual death rate for obese people between the ages of 20 and 64 is half again as high as that for people whose weight is close to normal. This statistical difference is due primarily to the increased likelihood that the obese person will suffer from diabetes mellitus and from diseases of the digestive and circulatory systems, especially of the heart.

One possible reason for the increased possibility of heart disease is that there are about two-thirds of a mile of blood vessels in each pound of adipose tissue. Thus 20 or more pounds of excess weight are likely to impose a great additional work load on the heart.

Obese people are also poorer surgical risks than the nonobese, and it is often more difficult to diagnose and therefore to treat their illnesses correctly.

Permanent loss of excess weight makes the formerly obese person come closer to matching the life expectancy of the nonobese. However, losing and regaining weight as a repeated pattern is even more hazardous in terms of health than consistent obesity.

Psychological Consequences of Obesity

In ways that are both obvious and subtle, obesity often has damaging psychological consequences. This is particularly true for obese children, who tend to feel isolated and rejected by their peers. They may consider themselves victims of prejudice and blame their obesity for everything that goes wrong in their lives. In many cases, the destructive relationship between obesity and self-pity keeps perpetuating itself.

Obese adults are likely to experience the same feelings, but to a somewhat lesser degree. For some, obesity is an escape which consciously or unconsciously helps them to avoid situations in which they feel uncomfortable—those that involve active competition or relationships with the opposite sex.

Avoiding Excess Weight

Clearly, obesity is a condition that most people would like to avoid. Not putting on extra pounds does seem to be easier, in theory at least, then taking them off. One possible explanation for this is that additional adipose tissue consists of a proliferation of fat cells. Shrinking these cells is one thing, eliminating them is another. Our present lack of fundamental knowledge about the regulatory and metabolic mechanisms relating to obesity limits the technique of preventing overweight to recommending a balance between caloric intake and expenditure.

The real responsibility for preventing the onset of obesity in childhood rests with parents. All of the fundamentals of good nutrition and healthy eating habits are of the utmost importance in this connection. Caloric expenditure in the form of regular exercise is equally important.

EXERCISING BY HABIT: This does not necessarily mean that exercise

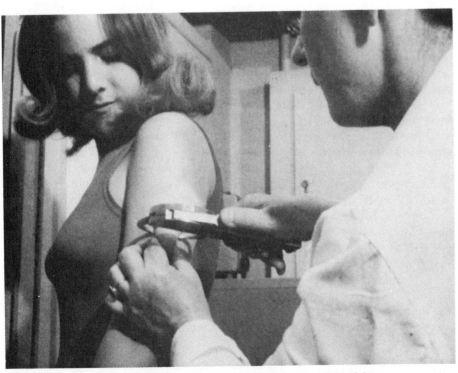

A doctor demonstrates the pinch test for obesity. A fold of skin and fat of the upper arm should be no thicker than one inch.

should be encouraged for its own sake. What it does mean is making a habit of choosing an active way of approaching a situation rather than a lazy way: walking upstairs rather than taking the elevator; walking to school rather than riding; walking while playing golf rather than riding in a cart; running to get the ball that has rolled away rather than ambling toward it. These choices should be made consistently and not just occasionally if obesity is to be avoided. Those people who naturally enjoy the more active way of doing things are lucky. Those who don't should make an effort to develop new patterns, especially if obesity is a family problem.

Anyone with the type of physical handicap that makes a normal amount of exercise impossible should be especially careful about caloric intake.

Weight Reduction

The treatment of obesity is a complicated problem. In the first place, there is the question of who wants or needs to be treated and how much weight should be lost. Except in unusual situations, anyone who wants to lose weight should be encouraged to do so. Possible exceptions are teen-agers who are not overweight but who want to be as thin as they can possibly be—the boy who is involved in an athletic event such as wrestling, or the girl who has decided she wants to look like a fashion model.

Crash dieting is usually unwise if the goal is to lose too much weight too rapidly and should be undertaken only after consulting a doctor about its advisability. As for adolescents who have become slightly overweight during puberty, they may be ill-advised to try to take off the extra pounds that probably relate to a temporary growth pattern.

Losing Weight Must Be Self-Motivated

Unless there are compelling medical reasons for not doing so, anyone

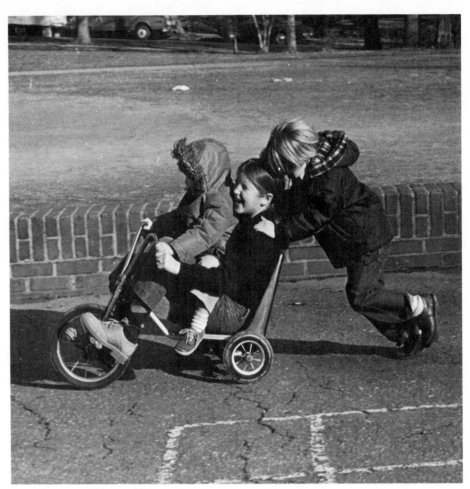

Most children naturally love to exercise regularly in play. Maintaining the habit of exerting oneself is the secret of avoiding obesity.

weighing 20 percent or more over the normal limit for his age and body build should be helped to slim down. It is extremely important, however, for the motivation to come from the person himself rather than from outside pressure.

Unless an overweight person really wants to reduce, he will not succeed in doing so, certainly not permanently, even though he appears to be trying. He must have convinced himself—intellectually and emotionally—that the goal of weight loss is truly worth the effort.

It is very difficult not only for his friends and family but for the person himself to be absolutely sure about the depth of his motivation. A doctor treating an overweight patient has to assume that the desire to reduce is genuine and will try to reinforce it whenever he can. However, if a patient has made a number of attempts

to lose weight over a period of years and has either been unable to reduce to any significant degree, or has become overweight again after reducing, it is probably safe to assume that the emotional desire is absent, or that there are emotional conflicts that stand in the way.

It is very possible that such a person could be harmed psychologically by losing weight, since he might need to be overweight for some deep-seated reason. This can be true for both children and adults. Occasionally it is possible for a psychiatrist or psychologist to help the patient remove a psychological block, and then weight reduction can occur if the caloric balance is straightened out.

Effective Planning for Weight Loss

The ultimate key to successful weight reduction is proper eating combined with proper physical activity. This balance is extremely difficult for many people to achieve because it involves a marked change in attitudes and behavior patterns that are generally solidly established and of long duration. Furthermore, once the changes are made, they will have to endure for a lifetime if the weight that has been lost is not to be regained.

It is therefore important that the reducing diet should be somewhat similar to the person's usual eating pattern in terms of style and quality. Ideally, only the caloric content should be changed, and probably the word "dieting" should not be used to describe the process, since most people don't find the idea of permanent dieting congenial.

Similarly, the increased physical activity that must accompany the new eating style should be of a type that the person enjoys. It is virtually impossible for an overweight person to reduce merely by restricting his

Patent remedies that promise quick and effortless release from obesity have long been on the market; this 1878 ad sells one such product.

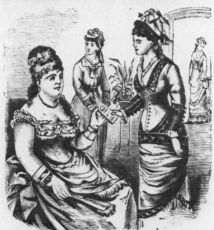

ANTI-FAT

The Great Remedy for Corpulence

ALLAN'S ANTI-FAT

is composed of purely vegetable ingredients, and is perfectly harmless. It acts upon the food in the stomach, preventing its being converted into fat. Taken in accordance with directions, **it will reduce a fat person from two to five pounds per week.**

LOW CALORIE DIET					
Sample Menus					
800 calories		1,200 calories		1,600 calories	
Weight grams	Household measure	Weight grams	Household measure	Weight grams	Household measure
Breakfast					
Orange, sliced	125	1 medium	125	1 medium	125	1 medium
Soft cooked egg	50	One	50	One	50	One
Toast	25	1 slice	25	1 slice	25	1 slice
Butter	5	1 teaspoon	5	1 teaspoon	5	1 teaspoon
Coffee or tea	—	As desired	—	As desired	—	As desired
Milk	240	1 cup skim	240	1 cup skim	240	1 cup whole
Luncheon					
Clear broth	—	As desired	—	As desired	—	As desired
Salad (cottage cheese, tomato, plain lettuce leaf)	90	½ cup	90	½ cup	90	½ cup
Egg			50	One	50	One
Green peas					100	½ cup
Baked apple, unsweetened	80	1 small	80	1 small	80	1 small
Bread			25	1 slice	25	1 slice
Butter			5	1 teaspoon	5	1 teaspoon
Milk	240	1 cup skim	240	1 cup skim	240	1 cup whole
Coffee or tea	—	As desired	—	As desired	—	As desired
Dinner					
Roast beef, lean	60	2 ounces	90	3 ounces	120	4 ounces
Carrots, plain	100	½ cup	100	½ cup	100	½ cup
Tossed vegetable salad with vinegar	50	¾ cup	50	¾ cup	50	¾ cup
Pineapple, unsweetened	80	½ cup	80	½ cup	80	½ cup
Bread			25	1 slice	25	1 slice
Butter			5	1 teaspoon	10	2 teaspoons
Coffee or tea	—	As desired	—	As desired	—	As desired
Nourishment					
Peach					100	1 medium

These diets contain approximately 800, 1,200, and 1,600 calories. The 800 calorie diet, even with variations in selections of food, will not meet the recommended daily allowances in iron and thaimine. The approximate composition is as follows:

	800 calories	1,200 calories	1,600 calories
Protein	60 gm.	75 gm.	85 gm.
Fat	30 gm.	50 gm.	80 gm.
Carbohydrate	75 gm.	110 gm.	130 gm.

From the *Clinical Center Diet Manual*, revised edition, prepared by the Nutrition Department, The Clinical Center, National Institutes of Health, Public Health Service, U.S. Department of Health, Education, and Welfare (Public Health Service Publication No. 989), pp. 67–68.

caloric intake, or merely by increasing his caloric expenditure. The two must go together.

Cutting Down Step by Step

The first thing to determine when planning to lose weight is the number of pounds that have to go. A realistic goal to set is the loss of about one pound a week. This may seem too slow, but remember that at this rate, fifty pounds can be lost in a year.

GETTING STARTED: Start by weighing yourself on arising, and then for two weeks try to eat in your customary manner, but keep a careful record of everything that you eat, the time it is eaten, and the number of calories it contains. During this period, continue to do your usual amount of physical activity.

When the two weeks are over, weigh yourself again at the same time of day as before. If you haven't gained any weight, you are in a basal caloric state. Then check over your food list to see what might be eliminated each day without causing discomfort.

Try to think in terms of eliminating fats and carbohydrates first, because it is essential that you continue to get sufficient vitamins and minerals which are largely found in proteins. The foods described in the chart on page 202 should all continue to be included in your daily food consumption. If you are in the habit of having an occasional drink, remember that there are calories in alcohol but no nutrients, and that most alcoholic beverages stimulate the appetite. See *Low Calorie Diet* sample menus on page 211, and *Nutrients in Common Foods*, pp. 196–202 and 207–208, for estimating calories in particular foods.

PLANNING MEALS: When you replan your meals, keep in mind that the items you cut down on must add up to between 300 and 400 calories a day if you are going to lose one pound a week.

Your total daily food intake should be divided among at least three meals a day, more if you wish. If you need to eat more food or to eat more often, try snacking on low calorie foods such as cabbage, carrots, celery, cucumber, and cauliflower. All of these can be eaten raw between meals.

There is definitely something to be said in favor of having breakfast every morning, or at least most mornings. This may be psychologically difficult, but try to do it, because it will be easier to control your urge to eat too much later in the day.

INCREASING EXERCISE: At the same time that you begin to cut down on your food intake, start to increase your daily exercise in whatever way you find congenial so that the number of calories expended in increased exercise plus the number of calories eliminated from your diet comes to 500 or more. This is your daily caloric loss compared with your so-called basal caloric state.

ACHIEVING YOUR GOAL: You may wish to double your daily caloric loss so that you lose two pounds a week. Do not try to lose any more than that unless you are under close medical supervision.

If you gained weight during your two-week experimental period, you will have to increase your daily caloric loss by 500 for every pound gained per week. Thus, if you gained one pound during the two weeks, you will have to step up your daily caloric loss to 750 to lose a pound a week.

You'll have to keep plugging away to achieve your goal. It will be trying and difficult in many ways. You may get moody and discouraged and be tempted to quit. Don't. You'll probably go on periodic food binges. All this is natural and understandable, so try not to brood about it. Just do the best you can each day. Don't worry about yesterday, and let tomorrow take care of itself.

In many ways it can help, and in some cases it's essential, to have the support and encouragement of family and friends, particularly of those with whom you share meals. You may find it helpful to join a group that has been formed to help its members lose weight and maintain their weight loss. This is good psychological support.

MAINTAINING YOUR WEIGHT LOSS: Once you have achieved your desired weight, you can test yourself to see what happens if you increase your caloric intake. Clearly, anyone who can lose weight in the manner described can't stay in a state of negative caloric imbalance indefinitely. But you will have to be careful, or you'll become overweight again. It's a challenge, but people who stick to a disciplined program can be rewarded by success.

Special Problems

If you do not succeed in losing weight in spite of carrying out the program described above, you may need professional help because of some special problem. A qualified physician may try some special diets, or he may even suggest putting you into a hospital so that he can see to it that you have no caloric food at all for as long as three weeks.

Perhaps the situation is complicated by a metabolic abnormality that can be corrected or helped by medication. Although such conditions are rare, they are not unheard of.

Obesity is almost never caused by a "glandular" problem—which usually means an underactive thyroid. Do not take thyroid pills to reduce unless your thyroid has been found to be underactive on the basis of a specific laboratory test.

The indiscriminate use of pills to reduce, even when prescribed, is never helpful in the long run, although it may appear to be at first. The unsupervised use of amphetamines, for example, can be extremely dangerous. See *Stimulant Drugs*, p. 553, for further information about the dangers of amphetamine abuse.

Because so many people are eager to reduce, and because losing weight isn't easy, there are many unethical professionals who specialize in the problem. Avoid them. All they are likely to do for you is take your money and make your situation no better—and often worse—than it was to begin with.

Underweight

Weighing too little is a problem which is considerably less common than weighing too much. In fact, in many cases, it isn't accurate to call it a problem at all, at least not a medical one.

There are some times, however, when underweight may indicate the presence of a disease, especially when a person rather suddenly begins and continues to lose weight, even though there has been no change in his eating habits. This is a situation that calls for prompt medical evaluation. Such a person may already be under a doctor's care at the time the weight loss is first noticed.

More often, however, underweight is a chronic condition that is of concern to the person who feels his looks would improve if he could only add some extra pounds. This is especially true in the case of adolescent girls and young women.

What To Do About Weighing Too Little

Chronic underweight is rarely a reflection of underlying disease. It is rather an expression of individual heredity or eating patterns, or a combination of both. Treatment for the condition is the opposite of the treatment for overweight. The achievement of a positive caloric balance comes first; more calories have to be consumed each day than are expended. An underweight person should record his food history over a two-week period in the manner described for an overweight one. Once this has been done, various adjustments can be made.

First of all, he should see that he eats at least three meals a day and that they are eaten in a leisurely way and in a relaxed frame of mind. All of the basic foods should be represented in the daily food intake, with special emphasis on protein. The daily caloric intake should then be gradually increased at each meal and snacks added, so long as the snacks don't reduce the appetite at mealtimes.

Carbohydrate foods are the best ones to emphasize in adding calories. Since the extra food intake may cause a certain amount of discomfort, encouragement and support from family and friends can be extremely helpful. Just as there may be psychological blocks against losing weight, there may well be a compli-

SOFT AND BLAND SOFT DIETS

SOFT DIET

Foods allowed on this diet are left whole. The fiber content is modified by using only cooked or canned fruits and vegetables (with skins and seeds removed); refined or finely ground cereals and breads are included. Some restrictions have been placed on highly seasoned and rich foods because of the specific needs for which the soft diet is usually ordered.

BLAND SOFT DIET

If further restrictions on seasonings and food items are necessary, a bland soft diet may be ordered. This diet follows the same pattern as the soft diet outlined below but is modified to eliminate all stimulants, such as meat extractives, spices, condiments (except salt), strongly flavored foods, and beverages that contain caffeine, such as coffee, tea, or cola drinks. The following foods are also omitted: all whole grain breads, rolls, muffins, and cereals; all gravies and salad dressings; pork; broth and soups with a meat base (use only strained cream soups); lettuce. Limit quantities of jelly, sugar, and hard candies. Extremely hot or cold foods are avoided. The foods allowed may be divided into five or six small meals with each feeding containing a good source of protein.

SOFT DIET

Type of food	Foods included	Foods excluded
Beverages	Coffee, decaffeinated coffee, tea, carbonated beverages, cereal beverages, cocoa, milk.	None
Breads	White; whole wheat, finely ground; rye (without seeds), finely ground; white or whole wheat rolls or muffins, finely ground; plain crackers.	Coarse whole wheat breads; breads, rolls, and muffins with seeds, nuts, raisins, etc.
Cereals	Cooked or prepared cereals, such as corn flakes, strained oatmeal, cream of rice or wheat, farina, hominy grits, cornmeal, puffed rice, other rice cereals.	Cooked or prepared coarse cereals, such as bran, shredded wheat.
Desserts	Plain cake and cookies, sponge cake; custards, plain puddings, rennet desserts; gelatin desserts with allowed fruits; plain ice cream, sherbets (except pineapple), fruit ices.	Pies; pastries; desserts made with coconut, nuts, pineapple, raisins, etc.
Fats	Butter, cream, fortified fats, plain gravies, mayonnaise, cream sauces.	Fried foods; rich highly seasoned sauces and gravies with mushrooms, pimento, etc.
Fruits	Raw ripe bananas; canned or cooked fruits without skins or small seeds, such as applesauce, baked apple without skin, apricots, sweet cherries, peaches, pears; fruit juices as desired.	Raw fruits except bananas; canned or cooked fruits with skins, coarse fibers, or seeds, such as figs, raisins, berries, pineapple, etc.
Meat, poultry, fish	Bacon, beef, ham, lamb, pork, veal, poultry, and fish that has been baked, boiled, braised, broiled, or roasted.	Fried meat, poultry, or fish; highly seasoned meats; stews containing celery, onions, etc.; cold cuts, sausages.
Cheese	All except strongly flavored cheeses.	Cheeses with pimento, caraway seeds, etc.; strongly flavored cheeses.

SOFT DIET (continued)		
Type of food	Foods included	Foods excluded
Eggs	Any raw, soft cooked, hard cooked, soft scrambled, poached; omelets made with allowed foods.	Fried eggs, omelets containing mushrooms, etc.
Potato or substitute	Hominy, macaroni, noodles, rice, spaghetti; white or sweet potatoes without skins.	Fried potatoes; potato chips; highly seasoned sauces for spaghetti, macaroni, etc.
Soups	Broth, strained soups; cream soups made with allowed vegetables.	All others
Sweets	Hard candies, simple chocolate candies without nuts or fruit; strained honey, jelly, sugar, syrup.	Candies with whole fruit, coconut, or nuts; jam, marmalade.
Vegetables	Cooked or canned asparagus tips, string beans, wax beans, beets, carrots, chopped spinach, winter squash; tomato puree, tomato juice; raw lettuce leaf as garnish.	Cooked broccoli, brussels sprouts, cabbage, cauliflower, celery, corn, mustard greens, turnip greens, mushrooms, onions, fresh and dried peas, summer squash, whole tomatoes; dried beans, lima beans, lentils. All raw vegetables except lettuce as a garnish.
Miscellaneous	Salt; small amounts of white or black pepper used in cooking; creamy peanut butter.	Hot seasonings, such as chili sauce, red pepper, etc.; coconut, nuts, olives, pickles; spiced fruit.

From the *Clinical Center Diet Manual*, revised edition, prepared by the Nutrition Department, The Clinical Center, National Institutes of Health, Public Health Service, U.S. Department of Health, Education, and Welfare (Public Health Service Publication No. 989), pp. 45–52.

cated underlying resistance to adding it.

Anyone trying to gain weight should remain or become reasonably active physically. Adding a pound or two a month for an adult—and a little more than that for a growing youngster—is an achievable goal until the desired weight is reached. When this happens, there will probably have to be some adjustments in eating and exercise patterns so that a state of caloric balance is achieved.

How Food Relates to Disease

Just as proper food is essential in the prevention of some diseases, it is helpful in the treatment of others. It also plays an important role in protecting and fortifying the general health of a patient while a specific illness is being treated.

The components of therapeutic diets are usually prescribed by the physician in charge, but some general principles will be presented here. Remember that diets designed to treat a given disease must supply the patient's basic nutritional requirements.

Ulcers

Special diet is a major treatment consideration in the case of peptic ulcer, whether located in the stomach (gastric) or in the small intestine (duodenal). A major aim of such a diet is the neutralizing of the acidity of gastric juices by the frequent intake of high protein foods such as milk and eggs. Foods which irritate an ulcer chemically, such as excessive sweets, spices, or salt, or mechanically, such as foods with sharp seeds or tough skins, and foods that are too hot or too cold, should be avoided. It is also advisable to eliminate gravies, coffee, strong tea, carbonated beverages, and alcohol, since all of these stimulate gastric secretion. Such a diet is called a *bland* diet. See *Soft and Bland Soft Diets*, pp. 213–215. A soft diet is recommended for some forms of gastrointestinal distress and for those people who have difficulty chewing. It is often combined with the bland diet recommended for peptic ulcer patients to reduce the likelihood of irritation. See under *Diseases of the Digestive System*, p. 373, for further information about ulcers.

Diabetes

As the section on diabetes mellitus indicates (see Ch. 21, p. 409), the major objectives of the special diet are weight control, control of the abnormal carbohydrate metabolism, and as far as possible, psychological adjustment by the patient to his individual circumstances. To some extent, he must calculate his diet mathematically. First, his daily caloric needs have to be determined in terms of his activities:

TYPE OF ACTIVITY	CALORIES PER POUND OF BODY WEIGHT
Sedentary	13.5
Moderate	16
Marked	18

If he is overweight or underweight, the total calories per pound of body weight will have to be adjusted downward or upward by about five calories per pound.

After his total daily caloric needs have been figured out, he can calculate the number of grams of carbohydrate he should have each day by dividing his total calories by 10. The number of grams of protein per day as well as the number of grams of fat should be **half the number of grams of carbohydrate**.

This will mean that 40 percent of his daily calories will come from carbohydrate, 40 percent from fat, and 20 percent from protein. One-fifth of the total should be obtained at breakfast and the rest split between lunch and dinner. Snacks that are taken during the day should be subtracted equally from lunch and dinner.

It is important that meals and planned snacks be eaten regularly and that no food servings be added or omitted. Growing children from 1 to 20 years of age who have diabetes will require considerably more daily calories. A rough estimate is 1,000 calories for a one-year-old child and 100 additional calories for each year of age.

Salt-Free Diets

There are a number of chronic diseases which are treated in part by restricting the amount of sodium in the diet. These diseases, which are associated with fluid retention in the body, include congestive heart failure, certain types of kidney and liver diseases, and hypertension or high blood pressure.

The restriction of sodium intake helps to reduce or avoid the problem of fluid retention. The normal daily diet contains about seven or more grams of sodium, most of it in the form of sodium chloride or table salt. This amount is either inherent in the food or added during processing, cooking, or at mealtime. Half the weight of salt is sodium.

For people whose physical condition requires only a small restriction of the normal sodium intake, simply not salting food at the table is a sufficient reduction. They may decide to use a salt substitute, but before doing so should discuss the question with their physician.

A greater sodium restriction, for example, to no more than 5 grams a day, requires the avoidance of such high salt content foods as ham, bacon, crackers, catsup, and potato chips, as well as almost entirely eliminating salt in the preparation and serving of meals. Severe restriction—1 gram or less a day—involves special food selection and cooking procedures, as well as the use of distilled water if the local water has more than 20 milligrams of sodium per quart. In restricting sodium to this extent, it is important to make sure that protein and vitamins are not reduced below the minimum daily requirements. See *Sodium Restricted Diets*, pp. 216–218.

SOFT DIET
Sample Menu
Breakfast
Orange juice . . . . ½ cup
Corn flakes . . . . ½ cup
Poached egg . . . . One
Whole wheat toast . . 1 slice
Butter or fortified fat . 1 teaspoon
Milk, whole . . . . 1 cup
Coffee or tea . . . . As desired
Cream . . . . As desired
Sugar . . . . As desired
Luncheon
Creamed chicken on toast ½ to ¾ cup
Mashed potato . . . ½ cup
Buttered carrots . . ½ cup
Bread, enriched . . 1 slice
Butter or fortified fat . 1 teaspoon
Canned pear halves . . 2 halves
Milk, whole . . . . 1 cup
Coffee or tea . . . . As desired
Cream . . . . As desired
Sugar . . . . . As desired
Dinner
Roast beef, gravy . . . 2 to 3 ounces
Baked potato . . . . 1 medium
Buttered asparagus spears 1 serving
Bread, enriched . . . 1 slice
Butter or fortified fat . 1 teaspoon
Vanilla ice cream . . . ½ cup
Coffee or tea . . . . As desired
Cream . . . . As desired
Sugar . . . . . As desired

BLAND SOFT DIET
Sample Menu (six small meals)
Breakfast
Egg, poached . . . . One
White toast, enriched . . 1 slice
Butter or fortified fat . 1 teaspoon
Hot cocoa . . . . . 1 cup
10:00 a.m.
Orange juice . . . . ½ cup
Corn flakes . . . . ½ cup
Cream . . . . ¼ cup
Sugar . . . . . . 2 teaspoons
Luncheon
Creamed chicken on toast ½ cup
Mashed potato . . . ½ cup
Buttered carrots . . . ½ cup
Milk . . . . . 1 cup
Canned pears . . . . 1 half
2:30 p.m.
Milkshake . . . 1 cup
Soda crackers . . . . Three
Dinner
Roast beef . . . . 2 ounces
Baked potato . . . . 1 medium
Buttered asparagus . . 1 serving
Butter or fortified fat . 1 teaspoon
Milk . . . . . 1 cup
Vanilla ice cream . . . ½ cup
8:30 p.m.
Baked custard . . . ½ cup
Vanilla wafers . . . Two

Other Diseases
Requiring Special Diets

There are several other disorders in which diet is an important consideration: all chronic gastrointestinal disorders, such as ulcerative colitis, enteritis, gall bladder stones, and diverticulitis; a variety of hereditary disorders such as phenylketonuria and galactosemia; atherosclerosis, especially when it is associated with elevated blood levels of cholesterol or triglycerides or both; liver disease such as cirrhosis; many of the endocrine diseases; kidney stones; and sometimes certain neurological diseases such as epilepsy. Diet also plays a special role in convalescence from most illnesses and in post-surgical care. The *Modified Fat Diet* (pp. 219–220) and *Low Fat Diet* (pp. 221–222) are recommended for some diseases of the liver and gall bladder. The *Minimal Residue Diet* (pp. 223) is recommended for some digestive troubles and before and after gastrointestinal surgery.

Diet and Individual Differences

Most discussions about food and eating tend to suggest that all normal people have identical gastrointestinal and metabolic systems. This is simply not true. There are many individual differences that explain why one man's meat is another man's poison. A person's intolerance for a given food may be caused by a disorder, such as an allergy or an ulcer, and it is possible that many of these intolerances will ultimately be related to enzyme deficiencies or some other biochemical factor.

More subtle are the negative physical reactions to particular foods as a result of psychological conditioning. In most such cases, the choice is between avoiding the food that causes the discomfort or eating it and suffering the consequences. Of course, compulsive overeating can also cause or contribute to discomfort. Practically no one can eat unlimited quantities of anything without having gastrointestinal discomfort or *dyspepsia*.

The establishment of so-called daily minimum food requirements suggests that every day's intake should be carefully balanced. Although this is beneficial, it is by no means necessary. Freedom from such regimentation can certainly be enjoyed during a holiday, or a trip to another country, or on a prolonged visit to relatives with casual food habits.

Sometimes a change in diet is dictated by a cold or an upset stomach or diarrhea. Liquids containing carbohydrates, such as tea with sugar and light soups, should be emphasized

---

SODIUM RESTRICTED DIETS
DIETS MODERATELY RESTRICTED IN SODIUM

If only a moderate sodium restriction is necessary, a normal diet *without added salt* may be ordered. Such an order is interpreted to mean that the patient will be offered the regular salted food on the general selective menu with the following exceptions:

1. No salt will be served on the tray.
2. Soups that are salted will be omitted.
3. Cured meats (ham, bacon, sausage, corned beef) and all salted cheeses will be omitted.
4. Catsup, chili sauce, mustard, and other salted sauces will be omitted.
5. Salt-free gravies, sauces, and salad dressings will be substituted for the regular salted items.
6. Salted crackers, potato chips, nuts, pickles, olives, popcorn, and pretzels will be omitted.

This diet contains approximately 3 grams of sodium or 7.5 grams of sodium chloride, depending on the type and quantity of the food chosen.

LOW SODIUM DIETS[1]		
(1,000 mg. Sodium and 800 mg. Sodium Diets)		
Type of food	Foods included	Foods excluded
Beverages	Coffee, tea, carbonated beverages, cereal beverages; milk, cream, or cocoa within stated milk limitations.	All others.
Breads	Any unsalted yeast bread or rolls; quick breads made with "sodium-free" baking powder; unsalted matzoth.	All bread and rolls containing salt, baking powder or baking soda; salted or soda crackers; pretzels.
Cereals	Any cereal that is cooked without salt; puffed rice, puffed wheat; shredded wheat; specially prepared "sodium-free" corn flakes and rice flakes; unsalted popcorn.	All prepared cereals containing salt; hominy grits.

[1]Approximate composition is indicated in the following table. 1,000 milligrams (abbreviated *mg.*) equals 1 gram. The 500, 800, and 1,000 milligram sodium diets meet the recommended nutrient levels of the normal diet.

Nutrient	Unit	500 mg. sodium	800 mg. sodium	1,000 mg. sodium
Sodium	Milligrams	485	775	970
Protein	Grams	70	95	95
Fat	Grams	90	90	90
Carbohydrate	Grams	185	250	250
Calories°		1,830	2,190	2,190

°Calories can be augmented by using additional salt-free fats and oils, white sugar, and pure jellies.

From the *Clinical Center Diet Manual*, revised edition, prepared by the Nutrition Department, The Clinical Center, National Institutes of Health, Public Health Service, U.S. Department of Health, Education, and Welfare (Public Health Service Publication No. 989), pp. 77–86.

LOW SODIUM DIETS (continued)		
Type of food	Foods included	Foods excluded
Desserts	Any unsalted dessert; custards and puddings made with allowed milk; puddings made without milk; unflavored gelatin desserts; fruit ices; unsalted fruit pie and fruit whips.	Desserts made with salt, baking powder, or baking soda; flavored gelatin desserts.
Fats	Any unsalted fat or oil, vegetable or animal; unsalted salad dressings.	Salted butter, salted margarine; commercial salad dressings; bacon drippings.
Fruits	Any fresh, canned, or frozen fruit or juice.	Dried fruits prepared with sodium preservatives.
Meat, poultry, fish	Prepared without salt: beef, lamb, fresh pork, veal; poultry; fresh-water fish;[2] liver (limit to one serving per week).	Salted meats; bacon; smoked or canned meats or fish; shellfish; all glandular meats except liver as allowed.
Cheese	Unsalted cottage cheese; specially prepared "sodium-free" yellow cheese.	All other.
Eggs	Limit to one daily, prepared without salt.	Any prepared with salt.
Potato or substitute	Dried beans (navy, pea), macaroni, noodles, potato, rice, spaghetti, sweet potato, all prepared without salt.	Salted potato chips, hominy.
Soups	Unsalted meat broth; cream soups prepared with allowed milk and allowed vegetables.	Bouillon; all soups prepared with salt.
Sweets	Hard candies, honey, jam, jelly, white sugar, syrup.	Commercial candy prepared with sodium salts; brown sugar.
Vegetables, cooked and raw	Two servings (½ cup) of vegetables listed below, fresh, frozen, or canned without salt: asparagus, lima beans,[3] navy beans, snap beans (green or yellow wax), broccoli, brussels sprouts, cabbage, carrots, cauliflower, corn, cucumbers, eggplant, dried lentils, lettuce, mushrooms, okra, onions, parsley, parsnips, black eyed peas, green peas,[3] green peppers, radishes, rutabaga, squash, tomatoes, turnips, turnip greens.	Beets, beet greens, celery, dandelion greens, kale, frozen lima beans, mustard greens, frozen peas, sauerkraut, spinach, frozen succotash, swiss chard.
Miscellaneous	Herbs and spices, except salt. Unsalted peanut butter.	Salt, celery salt, garlic salt; celery seed, parsley flakes; sauces containing salt, such as catsup, chili sauce, mustard, steak sauces; salted nuts and popcorn; olives, pickles; monosodium glutamate.

[2]Unsalted salt-water fish is usually avoided because of the difficulty of obtaining a consistently unsalted supply.
[3]Use only fresh or canned without salt.

children with diarrhea can become dehydrated in a day or so, professional advice is indicated when cutting down liquid intake.

Diet and Disease Prevention

Whether or not diet can be helpful in preventing various diseases other than those caused by nutritional deficiency is an unsettled question. Some specialists think that a diet low

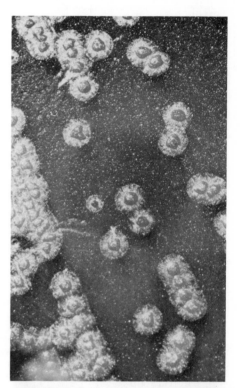

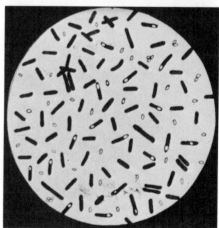

Scientists have isolated the bacterium *Clostridium botulinum (above)*, which causes botulism food poisoning. If a seriously ill patient is suspected of having botulism, cultures of his blood and stool are made. The lab technician sees colonies of *C. botulinum (left)* under the microscope, confirming botulism.

in treating a cold, while at the same time solid food intake should be somewhat reduced. In the case of an upset stomach or diarrhea, the discomfort may be eased by not eating or drinking anything at all for a whole day. This form of treatment may be helpful for an adult, but since

LOW SODIUM DIETS *(continued)*				
Sample Menus				
	500 mg. Sodium		800 mg. Sodium	
	Weight grams	Household measure	Weight grams	Household measure
Breakfast				
Orange, sliced	125	1 medium	125	1 medium
Soft cooked egg	50	One	50	One
Unsalted oatmeal	100	½ cup	100	½ cup
Unsalted toast	25	1 slice	25	1 slice
Unsalted butter	10	2 teaspoons	10	2 teaspoons
Jelly	—	As desired	—	As desired
Milk, low sodium	None		None	
Milk (or cream)	240	1 cup	240	1 cup
Coffee or tea	—	As desired	—	As desired
Sugar	—	As desired	—	As desired
Luncheon				
Unsalted beef patty	60	2 ounces	60	2 ounces
Unsalted fried potatoes	100	½ cup	100	½ cup
Unsalted asparagus	100	½ cup	100	½ cup
Lettuce and tomato salad	100	1 small	100	1 small
Unsalted French dressing	15	1 tablespoon	15	1 tablespoon
Unsalted chocolate cookies	None			1 serving
Canned peaches	100	1 serving	—	As desired
Unsalted bread	25	1 slice	25	1 slice
Unsalted butter	10	2 teaspoons	10	2 teaspoons
Jelly	—	As desired	—	As desired
Milk, low sodium	None		None	
Milk	240	1 cup	240	1 cup
Coffee or tea	—	As desired	—	As desired
Sugar	—	As desired	—	As desired
Dinner				
Unsalted roast chicken	60	2 ounces	90	3 ounces
Unsalted gravy	30	2 tablespoons	30	2 tablespoons
Unsalted mashed potatoes	100	½ cup	100	½ cup
Unsalted green beans	100	½ cup	100	½ cup
Banana salad	100	One	100	One
Unsalted mayonnaise	15	1 tablespoon	15	1 tablespoon
Fresh fruit cup	100	½ cup	100	½ cup
Unsalted bread	25	1 slice	25	1 slice
Unsalted butter	10	2 teaspoons	10	2 teaspoons
Jelly	—	As desired	—	As desired
Milk, low sodium	—	As desired	None	
Milk	None		240	1 cup
Coffee or tea	—	As desired	—	As desired
Sugar	—	As desired	—	As desired
Nourishment				
Orange juice	240	1 cup	—	As desired
Milk	None		240	1 cup

in cholesterol and saturated fats can help prevent cardiovascular disease caused by atherosclerosis, but the evidence for this point of view is not yet definitive. It has been said for years that vitamin C is helpful in preventing the common cold, and this point of view has recently re-ceived a great deal of publicity, but the evidence is not conclusive.

FOOD-BORNE DISEASES: There are several ways in which food can be the *cause* of disease, most commonly when it becomes contaminated with a sufficient amount of harmful bac-teria, bacterial toxin, viruses, or other poisonous substances. The gastrointestinal diseases typically accompanied by nausea, vomiting, diarrhea, or stomach cramps that are produced in this way are not, strictly speaking, caused by the foods them-selves, and are therefore called food-borne diseases.

Most food-borne illnesses are caused by a toxin in food contami-nated by staphylococcal or sal-monella bacteria. In general, milk, milk products, raw shellfish, and meats are the foods most apt to be contaminated. This is most likely to happen when such foods are left standing at room temperature for too long between the time they are pre-pared and the time they are eaten. However, food can also become con-taminated at many different points in time and at various stages of process-ing. Standards enforced by federal and local government agencies pro-vide protection for the consumer for foods bought for the home as well as for use in restaurants, although whether the protection is adequate is a matter of dispute.

Food Storage

Food is best protected from con-tamination when it is stored below 40 degrees Fahrenheit or heated to 145 degrees or more. Cold slows bacterial growth; cooking kills it. Bacteria present in food can double in number every 15 minutes at room temperature.

All food stored in the refrigerator should be covered except ripe fruits and vegetables. Leftover foods can-not be kept indefinitely, nor can fro-zen foods be stored beyond a certain length of time. Specific information about these time periods for indi-vidual items is available from the Agricultural Extension Service in each state.

Commercially processed foods sold in the United States are under government control and generally are safe. However, any food can spoil or become contaminated at any point in time, and the consumer should not buy or serve food whose container

MODIFIED FAT DIET		
Type of food	Foods included	Foods excluded
Beverages	Coffee, tea, carbonated beverages, cereal beverages; skimmed milk, nonfat dried milk and buttermilk (made from skimmed milk).	Cream, evaporated milk, whole milk, whole milk beverages.
Breads	Whole wheat, rye, or enriched white bread; plain yeast rolls.	All others, including biscuits, cornbread, French toast, muffins, sweet rolls.
Cereals	Any; whole grain or enriched preferred.	None.
Desserts	Angel food cake; plain puddings made with skimmed milk; gelatin desserts; fruit ices, sherbets; fruit whips; meringues.	Cakes except angel food; cookies; ice cream; pastries; rich desserts.
Fats	Oils: corn, cottonseed, olive, peanut, safflower, soy bean. (If calories permit, 1½ to 3 ounces will be included daily.) Specially prepared margarines.	Bacon drippings, butter, coconut oil, regular fortified fats, salt pork, vegetable shortenings, commerical salad dressings.
Fruits	Any fresh (except avocado), canned, frozen, or dried fruit or juice (one citrus fruit to be included daily).	Avocado.
Meat, fish, poultry, cheese	Limit to 4 ounces daily from Group I or the equivalent from Groups II or III (below). Lean meat trimmed of all visible fat.	Fried meats; fat meats, such as bacon, cold cuts, duck, goose, pork, sausage; fish canned in oil; all other fish except those allowed. All cheese except dry cottage cheese.
Eggs	Egg whites as desired; whole eggs (a maximum of one per day or about 3 per week) poached, soft or hard cooked, fried in allowed oil.	Eggs or egg whites cooked with fat, except those fats allowed.
Group I	7 gms. fat per 30 gms. (1 ounce).	Lean beef, ham, lamb, and pork; tongue; veal; trout.
Group II	3 gms. fat per 30 gms. (1 ounce).	Beef liver, heart, kidney, dried or chipped beef; chicken, turkey; lean fish, such as codfish, haddock, halibut, mackerel, shad, salmon, tuna, whitefish.
Group III	Less than 1 gm. fat per 90 gms. (3 ounces).	Crab, clams, flounder, lobster, oysters, perch, scallops, shrimp.
Potato or substitute	Hominy, macaroni, noodles, popcorn (prepared with allowed oil), potato, rice, spaghetti.	Potato chips; any of these items fried or creamed unless prepared with allowed fats.
Soups	Bouillon, clear broth, vegetable soup; cream soups made with skimmed milk.	All others.
Sweets	Hard candies, jam, jelly, sugar, syrup; chocolate syrup made only with cocoa, sugar, and water.	All other candies; chocolate.
Vegetables	Any fresh, frozen, or cooked without added fat (one green or yellow vegetable should be included daily).	Buttered, creamed, or fried vegetables unless prepared with allowed fats.

(package or can) has been broken, cracked, or appears unusual.

Food Additives

From time to time, concern is expressed about one or another food additive as a hazard to health. Most of these additives are put into foods during processing in order to increase their nutritional value, or to improve their chemical or physical characteristics, such as taste and color. Perhaps as many as 2,000 different substances are used in this way in the United States. Some are natural products such as vanilla, others are chemicals derived from other foods, and a few, like artificial sweeteners, are synthetic. Other additives are referred to as indirect, since they are residues in the food from some stage of growing, processing, or packaging. Although additives are controlled and approved by agencies such as the federal Food and Drug Administration, they continue to be a cause of concern to many people. See under *Food Hazards*, p. 231, for further discussion of food additives.

Organic Foods

Some people feel that industrial methods of food farming and processing introduced during the past century, and more particularly in the last four or five decades, have resulted in foods that are deficient in nutritional value. They have recommended a return to the techniques of food production of an earlier era, in which only organic fertilizers were used. Foods so produced are called *organic foods*. Standard, commercially prepared foods, they feel, lack the health benefits and better tastes of organic foods and may even be damaging to health.

The damage, they believe, is caused because chemical fertilizers, pesticides, and food additives make foods toxic in some way or other. These toxins include female hor-

MODIFIED FAT DIET (continued)		
Type of food	Foods included	Foods excluded
Miscellaneous	Condiments, pickles, salt, spices, vinegar.	Gravies, nuts, olives, peanut butter.

This diet is planned to reduce the intake of fats containing a high degree of either saturated or short-chain fatty acids and to avoid the excessive carbohydrate intake associated with a very low fat diet. This is done through replacement of saturated fat sources with those containing higher quantities of polyunsaturated fatty acids. The fats ordinarily used are corn oil, cottonseed oil, safflower oil, olive oil, peanut oil, and soybean oil. Fats containing large amounts of saturated fatty acids are restricted to approximately 30 grams daily. Carbohydrate and protein are planned to conform to normal levels, with approximately 300–350 grams carbohydrate and approximately 70–80 grams protein. The modified fat diet is planned to meet normal dietary allowances. Calories can be adjusted to fit the needs of the individual. If normal or higher than normal calories are required, fats containing a high percentage of unsaturated fatty acids, such as corn oil, cottonseed oil, etc., may be added.

From the *Clinical Center Diet Manual*, revised edition, prepared by the Nutrition Department, The Clinical Center, National Institutes of Health, Public Health Service, U.S. Department of Health, Education, and Welfare (Public Health Service Publication No. 989), pp. 69–72.

MODIFIED FAT DIET (continued)	
Sample Menu	
	Household measure[1]
Breakfast	
Orange juice	½ cup
Oatmeal	½ cup
Nonfat milk[2]	1 cup
Sugar	2 teaspoons
Poached egg	One
Toast, enriched or whole grain	2 slices
Jelly	1 tablespoon
Coffee or tea	As desired
Luncheon	
Clear broth, fat free	As desired
Lean roast beef	2 ounces
Baked potato	1 medium
Green beans	½ cup
Lettuce and tomato salad, oil dressing	1 serving
Bread, enriched or whole grain	1 slice
Jelly	1 tablespoon
Canned peach halves	2 halves
Nonfat milk[2]	1 cup
Coffee or tea	As desired
Sugar	1 teaspoon
Dinner	
Roast chicken (no skin)	4 ounces
Diced potato	½ cup
Green peas	½ cup
Head lettuce salad, oil dressing	1 serving
Bread, enriched or whole grain	1 slice
Jelly	1 tablespoon
Nonfat milk[2]	1 cup
Fruited gelatin	½ cup
Coffee or tea	As desired
Sugar	1 teaspoon

[1]Household measure is given to indicate the quantity of food necessary to supply 2,200 calories.

[2]As an example of the manner in which oil can be incorporated into the modified fat diet, a recipe for nonfat milk with oil follows:

For one quart of nonfat milk including one and one-half ounces of oil:

Dried powdered skim milk°	3¼ ounces (1⅓ cup)
Corn oil	1½ ounces
Water	to make 1 quart

Blend water with powdered skimmed milk in food blender until thoroughly mixed. Add corn oil and blend at a high speed until fully blended. Fresh skimmed milk may be substituted in the recipe for the powdered skimmed milk and water. The skimmed milk should be served cold, and the addition of flavoring is not recommended.

°Dried skimmed milk powders vary in weight. They may be reliquefied according to the directions on each package.

mones, antibiotics, and an inordinate number of organic and inorganic chemicals. They are thought to cause or contribute to the development of some cancers, arteriosclerosis, and other degenerative diseases, the causes of which really are unknown.

Organic foods are also said to make people less susceptible to viral infections such as common colds, and to tooth decay. All of these claimed health benefits could also be the result of having preserved in organically prepared foods various substances that are eliminated in normal commercial processing.

The organic food philosophy calls for growing your own foods, using only organic fertilizers such as compost or animal (not human) manure, and without using pesticides or herbicides. For those unable to grow their own foods, commercial sources of organic foods are becoming more and more readily available.

Typical Organic Foods

Whole grain cereals such as brown rice, and wheat, beans, vegetables, and fruits are the major sources of organic foods. Unsulfured molasses and natural honey are the primary sweeteners. Sea salt and herbs are used for flavoring. Organic meat is available, but many organic food people are vegetarians. Fertile eggs, cheeses, especially those from raw goat or cow milk, and yogurt also are basic parts of an organic diet. Cold pressed vegetable oils, filtered in a special way, and made from sesame, corn germ, or soy are used regularly; they are not only unsaturated fats and therefore have low cholesterol contents but also contain many natural vitamins. Herb teas, fruit juices, and raw milk are among the preferred liquids. Ideally, all organic foods should be eaten when fresh or in season, since canning or freezing requires the addition of chemicals.

Natural Foods

Several other food styles are associated with organic foods. *Natural*

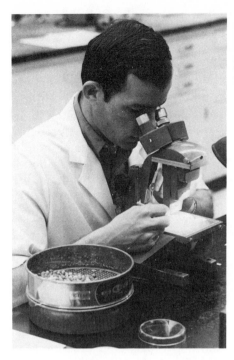
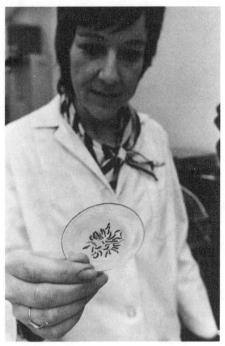

Acting on a consumer complaint, a Food and Drug Administration chemist *(left)* examines popcorn kernels under a microscope for the presence of moth larvae. The picture at right shows the larvae found in the sample.

LOW FAT DIET		
Type of food	Foods included	Foods excluded
Beverages	Coffee, tea, carbonated beverages, cereal beverages, skimmed milk or nonfat buttermilk.	Cream, whole milk, whole milk beverages.
Breads	Whole wheat, rye, or enriched white bread; plain yeast rolls.	Muffins, biscuits, sweet rolls, cornbread, pancakes, waffles, french toast.
Cereals	Any: whole grain or enriched preferred.	None.
Desserts	Plain angel food cake; custards and puddings made with skimmed milk and egg allowances; fruit puddings; gelatin desserts; ices; fruit whips made with egg white.	Rich desserts, pastries; sherbets, ice cream; cakes, except angel food.
Fats	None	All fats and oils; salad dressings.
Fruits	Any fresh (except avocado), canned, frozen, or dried fruit or juice (one citrus fruit to be included daily).	Avocado.
Meat, poultry, fish, cheese	Limit to 5 ounces daily: lean meat, such as lean beef, lamb, liver, veal; chicken, turkey, canned salmon or tuna (canned without oil); shellfish, lean whitefish; dry cottage cheese.	Fried meats; fat meats, such as bacon, cold cuts, duck, goose, pork, sausage; fish canned in oil. All cheese except dry cottage cheese.
Eggs	Any poached, soft or hard cooked; limit to one egg daily.	Fried eggs; eggs scrambled with fat.

foods are not necessarily grown organically, but are not processed very much. *Macrobiotics* is a special natural food concept, oriental in origin, and based upon the idea of maintaining an equilibrium between foods that make one active *(Yang)* and foods that make one relax *(Yin)*. A proper mixture of grain and vegetables contains an excellent balance of Yin and Yang. Yoga diets center around such natural foods as fruits and nuts.

Psychological Aspects of Food and Meals

Food and meals play an important role in emotional well-being and interpersonal relationships as well as in physical health and appearance.

During Infancy

The infant whose needs are attended to by a loving family develops a general sense of trust and security. The major contribution to his emotional contentment is probably made at mealtimes, and perhaps in a special way if he is breast-fed.

For most infants, food comes to be identified with love, pleasure, protection, and the satisfaction of basic needs. If there is an atmosphere of tension accompanying his feeding times, his digestion can be impaired in such a way as to cause vomiting, fretting, or signs of colic. If the tension and the baby's reaction to it—and inevitably the mother's increasing tension as a consequence—become a chronic condition, the result may be a failure to gain weight normally, and in extreme cases, some degree of mental retardation. Throughout life, good nutrition depends not only on eating properly balanced meals that satisfy the body's physiological requirements, but also on a reasonable degree of contentment and relaxation while eating.

Everybody develops individual emotional reactions and attitudes about food and its role as a result of conditioning during the years of in-

	LOW FAT DIET (continued)	
Type of food	Foods included	Foods excluded
Potato or substitute	Hominy, macaroni, noodles, potatoes, rice, spaghetti.	Any of these items fried or creamed; potato chips.
Soups	Bouillon, clear broth, vegetable soup; cream soups made with milk.	All others.
Sweets	Hard candies, jam, jelly, sugar, syrup; chocolate syrup made only with cocoa, sugar, and water.	All other candies or chocolate.
Vegetables	Any fresh, frozen or cooked without added fat (one green or yellow vegetable should be included daily).	Buttered, creamed or fried vegetables.
Miscellaneous	Condiments, pickles, salt, spices, vinegar.	Gravies, nuts, olives, peanut butter.

The low fat diet contains approximately 40 grams of fat. To maintain normal calorie intake with fat restricted, it has a high carbohydrate content. The low fat diet is adequate in all nutrients. Calories can be adjusted to fit the needs of the individual patient. Approximate composition is as follows:

Protein	85 gm.
Fat	40 gm.
Carbohydrate	325 gm.
Calories	2,000

From the *Clinical Center Diet Manual*, revised edition, prepared by the Nutrition Department, The Clinical Center, National Institutes of Health, Public Health Service, U.S. Department of Health, Education, and Welfare (Public Health Service Publication No. 989), pp. 73–75.

LOW FAT DIET (continued)

Sample Menu

	Household measure[1]
Breakfast	
Orange juice	½ cup
Oatmeal	½ cup
Skimmed milk	1 cup
Sugar	1 tablespoon
Poached egg	One (limit to one daily)
Toast, enriched or whole grain	2 slices
Jelly	1 tablespoon
Coffee or tea	As desired
Luncheon	
Beef broth, fat free	As desired
Sliced chicken	2 ounces
Baked potato	1 small
Peas	½ cup
Lettuce and tomato salad	1 serving
Lemon ice	½ cup
Bread, enriched or whole grain	1 slice
Jelly	1 tablespoon
Skimmed milk	1 cup
Coffee or tea	As desired
Sugar	1 tablespoon
Nourishment	
Pineapple juice	1 cup
Dinner	
Lean roast beef	3 ounces
Steamed potato	1 small
Carrots	½ cup
Mixed fruit salad	1 serving
Angel food cake	1 serving
Bread, enriched or whole grain	1 slice
Jelly	1 tablespoon
Coffee or tea	As desired
Sugar	1 tablespoon
Nourishment	
Tomato juice	1 cup
Crackers	Five

[1]Household measures are given to indicate the quantity of food necessary to supply 2,000 calories.

fancy and childhood. These attitudes relate not only to food itself and to mealtimes in general, but also to other aspects of eating, including the muscle activities of sucking, chewing, and swallowing.

If food symbolized contentment during the early years, it probably will have the same role later on. If it was associated with conflict, then it may be associated throughout life with strife and neurotic eating patterns.

During Childhood

For the preschool child, mealtimes should provide the occasion for the development of interpersonal relationships, since they are a daily opportunity for both verbal and nonverbal self-expression. The child who eats with enthusiasm and obvious enjoyment is conveying one message; the one who dawdles, picks at food, and challenges his mother with every mouthful is conveying quite a different one.

Meals can become either positive or negative experiences depending in large part on how the adults in the family set the stage. Communication can be encouraged by relaxed conversation and a reasonably leisurely schedule. It can be discouraged by watching television or reading while eating, by not eating together, or by eating and running.

Reasonably firm attitudes about eating a variety of foods in proper quantities at proper times and avoiding excessive catering to individual whims can also help in the development of wholesome eating patterns.

Those who select and prepare the food can transmit special messages of love and affection by serving favorite dishes, by setting the table attractively, and by creating an atmosphere of grace and good humor. Or they can show displeasure and generate hostility by complaining about all the work involved in feeding everyone, or by constant criticism of table manners, or by bringing up touchy subjects likely to cause arguments at the table.

MINIMAL RESIDUE DIET

Type of food	Foods included	Foods excluded
Beverages	Black coffee, tea, carbonated beverages, cereal beverages.	Milk, milk drinks.
Breads	Salted and soda crackers.	All breads.
Cereals	Cooked rice cereals or refined wheat cereals, made with water.	Whole grain cereals.
Desserts	White angel food cake, arrowroot cookies; ices; clear gelatin dessert.	Custards, puddings; desserts made with milk; ice cream.
Fats	Bacon, butter, fortified fats.	Cream.
Fruits	Strained fruit juices only.	All fruits.
Meat, eggs, poultry, fish, cheese	Beef, lamb, veal; chicken, turkey; white fish; eggs.	Fried meats, poultry, or fish; all cheese.
Potato or substitute	Macaroni, noodles, rice, spaghetti.	Potatoes, hominy.
Soups	Bouillon, broth.	Cream soups.
Sweets	Hard candies without nuts or fruit; honey, jelly, sugar, syrup.	Candies with fruit or nuts; jam, marmalade.
Vegetables	Tomato juice only.	All other vegetables.
Miscellaneous	Salt, small amounts of pepper used in cooking.	All other spices; condiments; nuts, olives, pickles, etc.

Minimal residue diet. The foods included on the minimal residue diet are selected on the basis of the small amount of residue left in the intestines after digestion. Since milk, milk products, fruits, and vegetables are thought to leave a large residue, these foods (except fruit and vegetable juices) have been omitted from the diet. The minimal residue diet is adequate in protein and calories. All other nutrients are below the recommended allowances.

From the *Clinical Center Diet Manual*, revised edition, prepared by the Nutrition Department, The Clinical Center, National Institutes of Health, Public Health Service, U.S. Department of Health, Education, and Welfare (Public Health Service Publication No. 989), pp. 45, 56–57.

MINIMAL RESIDUE DIET (continued)

Sample Menu

Breakfast

Orange juice	½ cup
Cream of wheat (cooked in water with butter)	½ cup; 1 teaspoon butter
Poached egg	One
Salted crackers	4 to 5
Butter	2 teaspoons
Jelly	1 tablespoon
Coffee or tea	As desired
Sugar	As desired

Luncheon

Roast beef	3 ounces
Buttered noodles	½ cup
Tomato juice	½ cup
Salted crackers	4 to 5
Butter	2 teaspoons
Jelly	1 tablespoon
Plain gelatin dessert	½ cup
Coffee or tea	As desired
Sugar	As desired

Dinner

Grapefruit juice	½ cup
Clear broth	As desired
Baked chicken	4 ounces
Buttered rice	½ cup
Salted crackers	4 to 5
Butter	2 teaspoons
Fruit ice	½ cup
Coffee or tea	As desired
Sugar	As desired

Nourishment

Strained fruit juices	As desired
Plain gelatin desserts	As desired
Fruit ices	As desired

How Food Can Relieve Tension

Food can be instrumental in relieving individual tension as well as in smoothing over minor family conflicts. Most people are familiar with the type of individual who is grumpy before a meal and who visibly brightens when he begins to eat. Sometimes this is due to the condition of *hypoglycemia* in which the blood sugar is too low for comfort. More often, the good spirits come from the psychological uplift brought about by the comradeship of eating.

People often turn to food as a way of relieving tension, thus reverting to a pattern established in childhood. Milk, for example, is often sought in times of stress. The relationship between food and anxiety is a complex one, and if it becomes so distorted that neurosis results, the physical consequences can be extremely unpleasant. Gastrointestinal disorders such as ulcers, bloating, belching, passing gas, diarrhea, and constipation are more often than not emotional rather than purely physical in origin.

The Symbol of Food

Food has many symbolic aspects: it can transmit and reinforce ethnic traditions either regularly or on special holidays. It can be used at lavish dinner parties as an expression of economic success; it can denote worldliness and sophistication in the form of complicated gourmet dishes of obscure origin.

A great deal can be learned about a person by knowing something about his attitudes toward food—not only what, how, when, and where he eats, but also how the groceries are bought, how the refrigerator and pantry shelves are stocked, how the cooking is organized, and how the dishes are cleaned up. In many significant ways, all of us are not only *what* we eat; we truly express who we are by *how* we eat.

CHAPTER 8

The Environment and Health

"Ecology . . . pollution . . . deterioration of the environment . . . the quality of life. . . ."

These words are with us constantly, in the news, political speeches, informed conversation. Heated controversy flairs over just how contaminated the globe is, the extent of the danger, the cost of cleaning up the mess, and whether any solution is realistically possible.

One thing is clear and incontestable: the quality of the environment is crucial to health, perhaps more important than any individual personal health measures you can employ. According to the federal Task Force on Research Planning in Environmental Health Science: ". . . the environment plays a predominant role in man's health; . . . rapid technologic change, increased population, and greater concentration of people into urban centers are compounding the problems of maintaining the environment at a healthful level."

Kinds of Pollution

Harmful ingredients in the environment are often the result of pollution; however, natural components—ultraviolet radiation in sunlight, for example—can also be contributing factors. These pollutants and the occasional natural counter-

parts can damage health in a variety of ways; even though there is as yet no scientific proof linking some of these pollutants with a specific malady, the statistical or circumstantial evidence is impressive. Most health experts believe, for example, that there is a direct connection between air pollution and various forms of respiratory illness.

Excessive noise, sometimes referred to as the "third pollution," after air and water pollution, is known to cause temporary and permanent hearing loss, anxiety, tension, and insomnia; it is strongly suspected of contributing to cardiovascular disease.

Many of the products of the technological age are toxic. Quantities of them find their way into the air, water, and food. Apart from outright poisoning, some of these contaminants are implicated in the development of cancer. Others are thought to cause mutations in the consumer, resulting in abnormal and sometimes nonviable offspring.

OCCUPATIONAL DISEASE: Because of our jobs, some of us are vastly more exposed to these dangerous contaminants than others. Occupational disease linked to specific pollutants has a long and unpleasant history. Chimney sweeps in 18th-century London developed cancer of the scrotum from long exposure to coal

soot, which contained potent cancer-producing agents (carcinogens). The malady was called "soot-wart." The Mad Hatter in Lewis Carroll's Alice in Wonderland represents a well-known type, a victim of "hatter's disease"—chronic mercury poisoning. (Mercury was used in the preparation of felt for hats.) During the latter part of the 19th century, skin cancer was a frequent hazard of work in the coal tar, paraffin, oil, and lignite tar industries. Bladder cancer began to appear among workers in the new aniline dye industry; it wasn't until 1938 that the carcinogen responsible was identified.

Today, miners contract black lung disease and silicosis from inhaling coal and other dusts. Cotton workers suffer chest-tightening byssinosis ("white lung disease") from inhaling cotton dust. Asbestos workers have seven times more lung cancer than the general population, and risk several other lung diseases, among them silicosis. Recently, some clothing workers were exposed to similar risks when they unknowingly manufactured 100,000 women's coats from a cloth containing eight percent asbestos fiber. One authority advised any woman in possession of such a coat to "bury it." Merely rubbing or brushing the coat would produce asbestos levels in the air 10,000 times higher than normal. See also *Lung Disease*, p. 396.

Added to all these and other traditional occupational hazards are those from a bewildering new profusion of synthetic chemicals whose dangerous properties may become known only long after they are in production.

RADIATION: Finally, there is a category of contaminants about which so little is known that they are provoking raging debate: ionizing radiation (such as that from nuclear reactors and other radioactive sources), microwave radiation (such as that from microwave ovens), and laser radiation. The Task Force quoted earlier points out with some asperity that the United States allows a level of microwave radiation for occupational exposure that is 1,000 times higher than the maximum set by Soviet Russia and other Eastern European countries. Microwaves, similar to radio waves and used in communications as well as ovens, are measurable in the environment of one-half the U.S. population.

Air Pollution

Most air pollution results from the incomplete burning of fuels and other materials, such as garbage. There are hundreds of different pollutants; some are visible as the yellowish brown haze that hangs over most large cities, but most are invisible. There is some debate over the precise relation between these various contaminants and the level of respiratory disease among the general population, although many experts think that the evidence now linking them with asthma, emphysema, and bronchitis is very strong.

Inversions

No one can doubt that high concentrations of air pollution are dead-ly. Modern history has seen some appalling examples. They usually occur in a region that is subject to a freak weather condition called an *inversion*, during which a mass of warm air sits like a lid on top of cool air, trapping it and preventing the pollutants that are produced daily from being ventilated. The pollutants accumulate in this stagnant air until they sometimes reach high concentrations, with lethal results.

The Meuse valley in Belgium, a center of heavy industry with many coal-burning factories, experienced an inversion in 1930 that trapped the smoke for five days. Some 60 people died as a result and 6,000 were sickened.

A killer smog brought a new menace to London's notorious pea-soupers in December, 1952. For five days an impenetrable, smoky fog paralyzed the city. Hospitals were jammed with people gasping for breath. When the smog finally lifted, medical statisticians calculated that 4,000 deaths during and immediately after the siege could be attributed to the smog.

The United States has known its share of such tragedies. Perhaps the worst and most famous was the inversion that hit Donora, Pennsylvania, in October, 1948, in a valley similar in topography and in pollution-creating industry to the Meuse. The inversion lasted six days—six days of ever more unhealthy air. At its peak, more than half of the valley's 14,000 persons had been stricken; at least 20 deaths were blamed on the pollution. Many more persons suffered irreversible damage to their health, according to a U.S. Public Health Service study.

Sulfur Dioxide

Today, numbers of cities still report unsatisfactory or unhealthy air conditions with some frequency, but at least local and national officials are aware of the seriousness of the problem. New York City officials have stated that between 1,000 and 2,000 deaths a year there

Smog produced by copper mines east of Phoenix, Arizona. Should an inversion trap such concentrated pollution, the health hazards can be enormous.

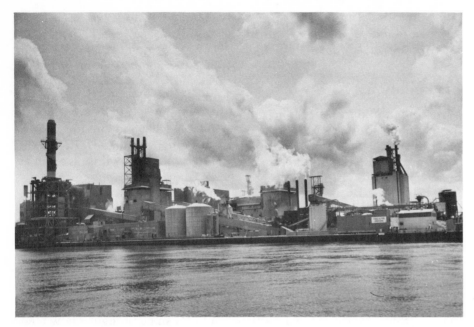

Sulfur dioxide in factory emissions becomes air-borne quickly and is a major source of air pollution over large areas of the U.S.

probably result from sulfur dioxide—the main toxic component of killer smogs—and other particles suspended in the air. Sulfur dioxide is spewed into the air—more than 23 million tons in the country, and 380,000 tons in New York City alone—when heavy fuel oil and coal are burned to provide heat, generate electricity, and provide industrial power. These fuels are generally rich in sulfur. Recently, some localities have passed legislation requiring the use of low-sulfur coal and oil for certain uses.

No one knows exactly how sulfur dioxide affects the respiratory tract. The likelihood is that it irritates the lungs and contributes to a reduction of the lungs' oxygen-handling capacity. Persons especially vulnerable to smogs are those suffering from bronchial asthma, chronic bronchitis (some studies show 13 percent of U.S. men have the disease) and emphysema, because their respiratory capacity is already defective. In emphysema, for example, the elasticity of the air sacs in the lungs has progressively broken down, usually after prolonged infection or repeated bronchial irritation (such as is produced by cigarette smoking). Deaths from emphysema are twice as high in cities as in rural areas.

Other Contaminants

Other major contaminants that have been identified as dangerous are nitrogen oxides, lead, carbon monoxide, hydrocarbons, and soot—the visible particles of carbon suspended in the air.

Dust may be harmful by transporting corrosive chemicals or other irritants to the lungs. Ordinarily, particles in the air are trapped in the nasal passages, but very small ones can slip past into the lungs. These tiny motes are called submicron particles—less than one twenty-five-thousandth of an inch in size.

Auto Exhausts

The major contributor of these harmful agents is the automobile. Auto exhausts contribute more than one-half the total of all atmospheric contaminants; in large cities, the figure is much higher. For example, in New York City cars, buses, and trucks contribute an estimated 77% by weight of all air pollution.

How can these substances affect your health? Nitrogen oxides irritate the eyes and the respiratory tract. Moreover, when nitrogen oxide and hydrocarbons mix in the presence of sunlight, they form other noxious substances in what is called a photochemical smog that has a typical yellowish cast. The new ingredients produced include ozone—a poisonous form of oxygen—and peroxyacetyl nitrate (PAN), which is intensely irritating to the eyes. Los Angeles was the first city to experience these smogs; they now occur in many other cities as well.

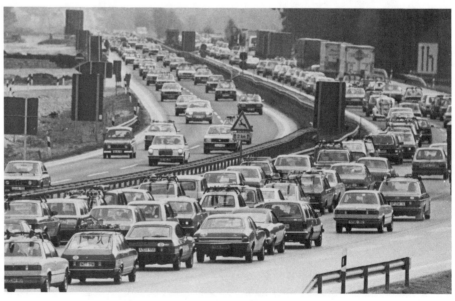

Auto emissions, particularly hydrocarbons and lead, are a major source of air pollution in industrialized countries.

Auto exhaust hydrocarbons include varieties that are suspected of being carcinogens, that is, of contributing to the development of cancer in susceptible individuals. This link so far has been proven only in animals. Dr. Ernest Wynder of the Sloan-Kettering Institute for Cancer Research, however, got some provocative results by painting the skin of laboratory mice with the residues collected from filters exposed to New York air. The mice developed cancer.

Carbon monoxide is an odorless, colorless gas that is lethal even in very small concentrations because it combines with hemoglobin readily and thus replaces oxygen in the blood. In concentrations that have been measured in heavy city traffic, it can make you tired, headachy, drowsy, and careless.

LEAD POISONING: Lead is an extremely poisonous substance. Acute cases of lead poisoning produce headache, nausea, cramps, anemia, numbness, loss of control of wrist and ankle, and finally, coma and death. The symptoms of chronic lead poisoning are much more subtle and harder to pinpoint. Test animals that have consumed lead in amounts comparable to those ingested by men over long periods have had their life spans reduced by 20 percent, experienced increased infant mortality rates, sterility, and birth defects. Testifying before the Senate Subcommittee on Energy, Natural Resources and the Environment, Carl L. Klein, an assistant Secretary of the Interior, said that "there can be little doubt that exposure of mothers to lead has a damaging effect upon fertility, the course of pregnancy, and the development of the fetus."

One expert estimated that auto exhausts were releasing 300,000 tons of lead annually into the air, some of which winds up in the water supply. Industrial users also vent large quantities of lead into lakes and rivers.

Experts are now debating exactly how much airborne lead can be tol-

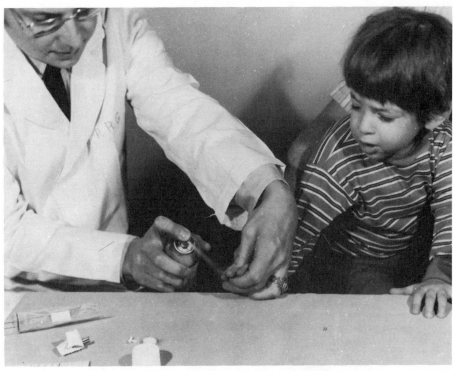

After taking a few drops of blood to test for lead poisoning, a technician sprays the finger with collodion, a coating agent for wounds.

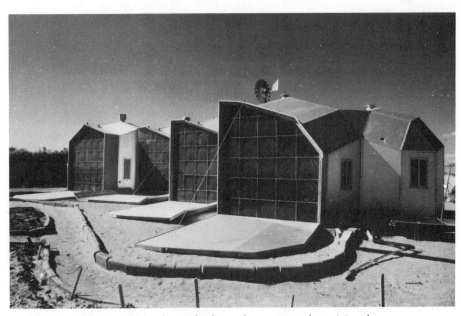

Solar energy can be used to heat a home, as seen here. It is a clean source of energy, but it is not yet practicable on a large scale.

erated. But a strange phenomenon is occurring in big cities such as New York. The tragedy of slum children developing lead poisoning has been explained readily because it is known that they nibble lead-bearing paint peeling from their walls. Yet a number of instances of high lead levels in the blood of middle-class children have been discovered. Those children live in dwellings painted with modern house paints containing no lead. Some doctors have concluded that the children have been poisoned by auto exhausts. Lead levels in high

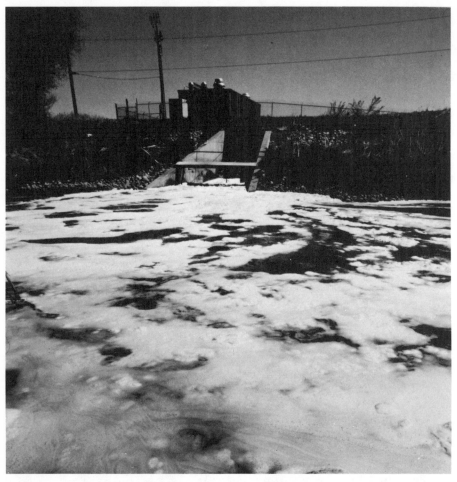

Foamy discharge from a water treatment plant in Colorado is the end product of a water supply that has been infiltrated with detergents.

Water Pollution

The quality of water is intimately tied to our physical well-being, and we have, therefore, come to expect high standards of cleanliness and purity in the water we drink and bathe in. Public health authorities are increasingly concerned, however, at the progressive deterioration of this country's water supply. This deterioration results from years of abuse in which natural waterways were inundated with quantities of raw sewage, waste products of industrial and chemical plants and slaughterhouses, petroleum residues, poisonous herbicides and insecticides—the list is almost endless, but our water supply is not. In 1970, the Division of Water Hygiene, part of the federal Environmental Protection Agency, concluded that some 969 of the nation's individual water supplies were substandard.

Many householders do not need to be told that their water is less than sparkling and delicious. Bad tastes and odors, off colors and cloudiness plague many regions and make water drinking distasteful, even if it is not yet dangerous. In Suffolk County on New York's Long Island, for example, water in the region's wells had become so

traffic areas of New York are sometimes 25 times higher than the legal limit in California.

The outlook for any drastic improvements in the air pollution scene is not good. The federal government has extended the deadline for auto manufacturers to reduce exhaust emissions until 1979. In any event, the pollution contribution of older cars will continue into the '80s.

Energy production, the other major air polluter, also offers little hope for immediate improvement, because it will be many years before we can rely heavily on other than fossil fuels such as coal and oil. Supplies of nonpolluting natural gas are in too short supply to do us much good. There is still a good deal of controversy over the safety of nuclear power plants, and it will be some time before solar energy can make a dent in the energy crisis.

See under *Lung Disease,* p. 396, for additional information about the effects of air pollution on health.

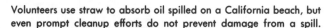

Volunteers use straw to absorb oil spilled on a California beach, but even prompt cleanup efforts do not prevent damage from a spill.

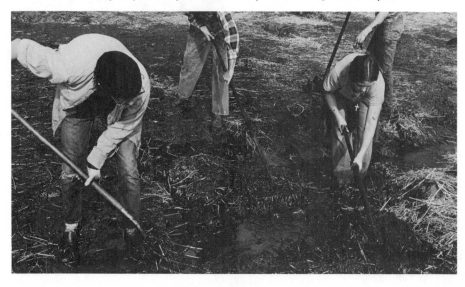

infiltrated with detergents that a glass of water was likely to have a head of detergent foam. After much controversy, the County banned the sale of all laundry products containing detergents.

The problem is that some synthetic detergents are not *biodegradable*—they are not broken down by microorganisms in the soil and water, and thus become water pollutants. Even biodegradable synthetic detergents may add another pollutant—phosphates—to water. Phosphates overstimulate the growth of the primitive water plants called algae, which overrun lakes and streams; the algae consume vast quantities of oxygen, thereby choking out other life, such as game and food fish.

Oil Spills

With the increasing reliance on supertankers to carry industrial and heating oil from abroad, the danger of major oil spills occurring near a coastal area is becoming ever greater. Several of these huge ships have been grounded and broken apart by the seas, their vast cargoes spilling out heavy oil into the ocean, where currents can carry it many miles before it disperses and gradually sinks to the ocean floor. Sometimes, of course, the currents carry the oil toward land, where it fouls beaches and kills water birds. Other accidents have involved smaller tankers plying the inland waterways; their oil cargoes have polluted rivers and lakes, killing fishes and despoiling recreational areas.

Microbes in Sewage

The risk to health from drinking contaminated water depends on the contaminant. It is fairly rare in this country for cases of typhoid, for example, caused by a pathogenic bacillus, to be contracted through an impure water supply. But you may risk gastrointestinal upsets caused by other organisms if you swim at a beach that is posted "Polluted Waters," as so many beaches now are. The cause is generally the dumping

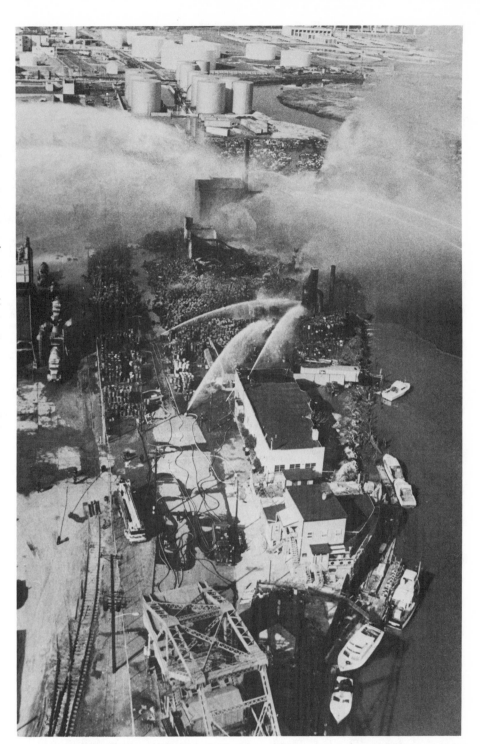

An explosion and fire in a chemicals' warehouse sent toxic fumes into the atmosphere rapidly—a common type of industrial accident.

of raw sewage nearby, or of sludge, the solid mass that is left after some kinds of sewage treatment. In New York Harbor there is a dead sea 21 miles square where nothing can live.

Chemical Contamination

In addition to the danger of infection from viral and microbial agents in polluted water, there is mounting danger from chemical contamination. Literally hundreds of chemical compounds find their way into the water supply, some of them in potentially dangerous quantities. Attention has focused most recently on the heavy metals and especially mercury. In a recent study, the U.S. Geological Survey reported that small amounts of seven toxic metals were present in many of the country's lakes and streams, with dangerous concentrations seemingly rare. The metals are mercury, arsenic, cadmium, chromium, cobalt, lead, and zinc. Aside from being generally poisonous, some of these metals are implicated in specific health problems. Cadmium, for example, has been linked to hypertension due to kidney malfunction. In Taiwan, skin cancer has been proved to rise with the quantity of arsenic in well water.

The Dangers of Mercury

Mercury represents a special case. For years, experts thought that since mercury was heavier than water and couldn't dissolve in it, it was therefore safe to dump large quantities of the metal into the waterways on the assumption that it would lie harmlessly on the bottom. They were, however, wrong. Bacteria can convert some of the metallic form of the element into a water-soluble form, which enters the food chain and eventually winds up, concentrated, in fish. When dangerous levels of this form of mercury were found in some waters and in food fish, the boom was lowered. There was a scare over canned tuna (the government later said that 97 percent of the canned tuna on the market was safe to eat) and swordfish. Lakes and rivers across the country were closed to commercial and sport fishing, and some remain closed.

The reason is not hard to understand. Mercury is an exceedingly toxic substance. The U.S. Food and Drug Administration has established the safe limit of mercury in food at half a part per million, comparable to a thimbleful in an Olympic-sized swimming pool. Even infinitesimal amounts absorbed by the body over a period of time can produce blindness, paralysis, and brain damage.

SWORDFISH: In an extremely unusual action, the Food and Drug

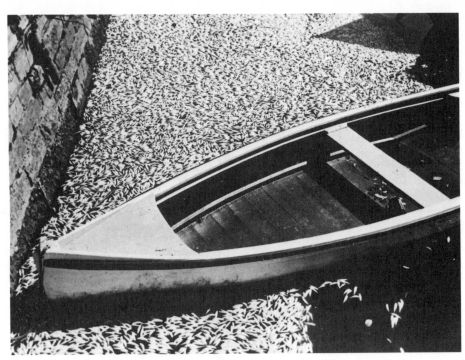

Thousands of dead shad float in the Anacostia River, Washington, D.C. The oxygen content of the water was decreased by industrial pollution.

Administration in 1971 advised the public to stop eating swordfish. The FDA had no power to ban the fish legally, but the move curtailed the consumption of swordfish in this country for some time. FDA investigators had discovered that only 42 of 853 samples of the fish contained acceptable levels of mercury. The average level of the remaining samples was twice the permissible amount. Soon after the announcement, doctors disclosed the first death in this country attributable to eating mercury-contaminated swordfish—that of a woman who had been eating large quantities of the fish on a weight-reducing diet.

The population of Minimata, a Japanese coastal town, was afflicted in 1953 by a strange malady that killed 40, crippled 70. The Minimatans had eaten the local fish and shellfish, which had absorbed mercury discharged into the water in a water soluble form by a nearby plastics factory. Similar cases of mass mercury poisoning have occurred in Italy, Guatemala, and Pakistan.

Pollution experts are particularly worried about mercury because even if we stopped producing mer-

cury compounds and discharging mercury wastes into the country's waters today, the problem would continue to worsen. The enormous store of metallic mercury already discharged and sitting on river and lake bottoms continues to be converted slowly into soluble forms. One chemist has estimated that in the St. Clair River system alone (between Detroit and southwestern Ontario), about 200,000 pounds of metallic mercury have been discharged in the last 20 years.

Recently, high amounts of selenium, an element considered more toxic than mercury, have been found in microscopic animal life in Lake Michigan downwind from Chicago and Milwaukee.

PCBs: Among the chief water pollutants today are the *polychlorinated biphenyls* (PCBs), highly toxic chemicals used industrially in carbonless copying paper and as an additive in lubricants, paints, and other products. PCBs, which require many years for the process of being altered chemically (biodegraded) to take place, have been found in unusually large quantities in waterways downstream from manufacturing plants. In January, 1977, the federal Environmental Protection Agency banned the direct discharge of PCBs into any U.S. waterway. Tests had shown that fish in some rivers, such as the Hudson River, had levels of PCB far higher than the permissible level. PCBs, which are related chemically to DDT—banned in 1972—are found in major bodies of water throughout the world because of their many industrial uses. No one knows what the long-term effects of ingesting small quantities of PCBs will be.

Food Hazards

Contaminants found in water often make their way into food products in the cooking and packaging processes, so that many of the comments on water apply here. Some dilute water pollutants become highly concentrated as they pass up the food chain and end in fish or other foods for man. Mercury was cited earlier as one example. Contamination of food with harmful microorganisms is an everpresent concern wherever standards of cleanliness and sanitation are low.

Additives

Food entails a whole new set of problems because of the thousands of new ingredients that have been added to it, directly and indirectly, in recent years. These substances include many that have been deemed necessary because of the revolution in food technology—the rise of packaged convenience foods of all kinds. Labels on today's convenience foods list preservatives, thickeners, mold inhibitors, fillers, emulsifiers, and artificial colors and flavors. The trouble with food additives is that we have had little time to learn about their effect on the body, especially over a long period of time. The Food and Drug Administration does set standards in this area; but in the opinion of many experts, these safeguards are inadequate. According to Bess Myerson, then Commissioner of New York

City's Department of Consumer Affairs, "The food that we eat is becoming as polluted as the air we breathe. Inadequate federal regulations allow manufacturers of prepared foods to ignore potential health hazards. No reasonable person would knowingly drink a glass full of the chemicals he unwittingly consumes in his daily diet."

What are some of these chemicals, and how could they be dangerous? One that was imbibed freely by large numbers of Americans and in great quantities was sodium cyclamate, the artificial sweetener used in diet drinks and foods. It was eventually withdrawn after it was linked to cancer and chromosome damage in experimental animals. The controversy continues, however, and some accused the government of acting precipitately in this case. Cyclamates are still recommended for diabetics and dieters.

Nitrates and nitrites are used in enormous quantities as preservatives in food. Recently, Food and Drug Administration chemists found that these chemicals had apparently given rise to substances called nitrosamines in samples of fish. Ni-

trosamines are powerful carcinogenic agents, even in small amounts. The amounts found in the fish were minuscule, up to 26 parts per billion. These chemicals are also thought to be capable of producing genetic and birth defects.

Recently, a red dye used to color maraschino cherries and other food substances was ordered withdrawn from the market because it was implicated in certain studies as having potentially carcinogenic properties.

In Sweden, a geneticist and microbiologist named Dr. Bjorn Gillsberg has warned that unless we start to screen potentially mutagenic (causing changes in the genes) substances from our food we face an epidemic of birth defects, loss of fertility, and other genetic damage. He cited sodium bisulphate, a chemical used to prevent peeled potatoes from darkening, as a potentially dangerous additive.

The federal Task Force on Research Planning in Environmental Health Science estimates there are some 10,000 of these chemicals—additives and residues—to be found in our foods, and it holds that "only a portion . . . have been studied thoroughly enough to meet

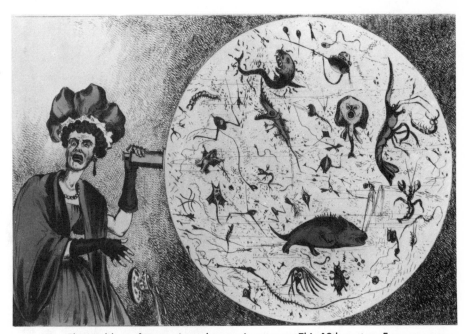

The problem of contaminated water is not new. This 19th-century English etching shows a horrified citizen with a cup of drinking water enormously magnified according to the artist's imaginative conception.

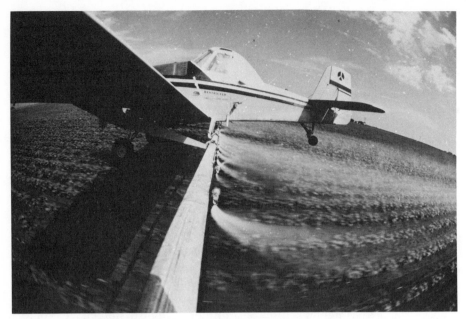

Pesticides are sprayed on crops to combat insect pests, but residues of chemical pesticides contaminate the crops and the soil, too.

exacting, present-day standards."

Pesticide Residues

Every year until recently, synthetic organic pesticides have drenched the territory of the United States in an amount equivalent to 220 pounds for every square mile. American mother's milk now contains four times the level of DDT that is permitted in cow's milk. We know that DDT and similar compounds have had devastating effects on many forms of wildlife, especially fish and birds. Some scientists fear the genetic and other effects of these compounds on human beings. As the result of widespread clamor, the use of DDT and related pesticides is on the wane in many parts of the world.

Noise Pollution

Most people are aware that their health may be threatened by the contamination of the air they breathe or the water they drink or swim in. Some know that dangerous substances may pollute the food they eat. But few realize that we are all adversely affected by a pollutant so common it tends to be overlooked—noise.

Noise is generally defined as any unwanted sound. It is the most widespread form of pollution in the United States. Who has not been driven to distraction by the wail of

sirens, the din of construction noise, cars, trucks, and buses? The old joke about city-dwellers being so used to noise that they were kept awake by the silence of a vacation retreat in the country is an expression of just how much noise most of us have accepted as inevitable.

The joke has a new twist now, because rural and suburban areas are plagued by their own varieties of noise. Farms have become increasingly more mechanized, and agricultural machinery contributes its ear-splitting toll. The once-inviolate stillness of snow-blanketed wilderness is now ruptured by the buzz of snowmobiles. Suburban homes are filled with the sound of electric dishwashers, garbage disposals, air conditioners, vacuum cleaners, and power tools—all potent noise makers—while from their backyards comes the insistent roar of power lawn mowers.

Worst of all is the situation of some workers, who, in addition to all this domestic noise, must suffer

Noise pollution is on the rise. These jackhammer operators will suffer a hearing loss from their continual exposure to loud noise.

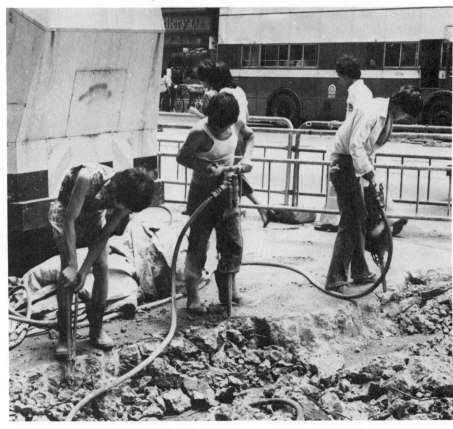

high noise levels on the job. Boilermakers and jackhammer operators are obvious examples, but cab drivers, bookkeeping machine operators, and parents of young children are all subject to special, if less conspicuous, hazards.

For noise is not just annoying, it is potentially dangerous, both physically and mentally. Dr. Vern Knudsen, a specialist in sound and chancellor emeritus at UCLA, has said, "Noise, like smog, is a slow agent of death. If it continues to increase for the next 30 years as it has for the last 30, it could become lethal."

Effect of Sound on the Eardrum

How can mere sound have such dire effects? Sound is a form of energy, and energy can be destructive as well as constructive. Sound is caused by anything that moves back and forth—vibrates. For us to hear sound over a distance, the energy of this vibrating motion must be transmitted to our ears over a distance, via sound waves. A sound wave in air is a succession of regions of compressed air and partial vacuums, or areas of high and low air pressure. (Sound waves can also travel through liquids and solids.) We hear sound because our eardrums are moved back and forth by these changes in air pressure. The eardrum, or *tympanic membrane*, can be incredibly delicate, perceiving a sound that moves it only one billionth of a centimeter—the threshold of hearing—equivalent, perhaps, to the rustle of one blade of grass against another. If the intensity of sound pressure becomes too great, at something like a billion billion times the energy at the threshold of hearing, we experience pain, and the eardrum or the delicate structures inside the ear may be damaged.

The intensity of sounds is often measured in units called *decibels*, or *db*. These units are logarithmic—that is, 10 db is ten times as powerful as 1 db, 20 db is 100 times as powerful, 30 db is 1,000 times as powerful, and so on. On this scale,

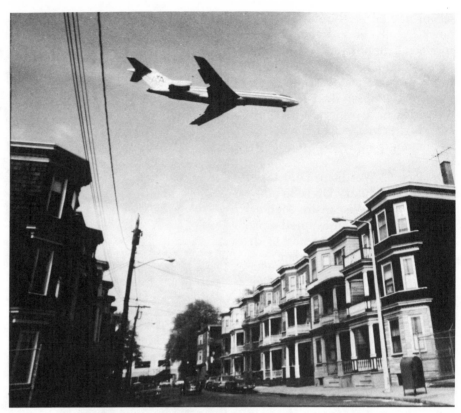

It is easy to understand the protests lodged against jet aircraft by people who endure the hearing hazards posed by living near a major airport.

0 db is at the threshold of hearing; rustling leaves, 20 db; a quiet office, about 50 db; conversation,· 60 db; heavy traffic, 90 db; a pneumatic jackhammer six feet away, 100 db; a jet aircraft 500 feet overhead, 115 db; a Saturn rocket's takeoff, 180 db.

For most people, the pain threshold is about 120 db; deafening ear damage will result at 150 db. But damage of various kinds can come from much lower exposures. Temporary hearing impairment can result from sounds over 85 db now found in modern kitchens with all appliances going. If the ears don't get a chance to recover, the impairment will become permanent.

Damage to the Inner Ear

Although very loud noise can damage the eardrum, most physiological damage from noise occurs in the snail-shaped, liquid-filled cochlea, or inner ear. Sound transmitted to the cochlea produces waves in the liquid, which in turn move delicate and minute structures called hair cells or *cilia* in that part of the coch-

lea known as the organ of Corti. The motion of the cilia is transformed into electrical impulses that conduct the sensation of sound to the brain.

The cilia can easily be fatigued by noise, causing a temporary loss of hearing, or a shift in the threshold of hearing. If they are not given a chance to recuperate, they will be permanently damaged, and irreversible hearing loss will result. There are some 23,000 cilia in the average cochlea; different sets of cilia respond to different frequency bands. The cilia responding to sound frequencies of 4,000 to 6,000 cps (cyles per second) are especially vulnerable to damage. The region of 85–95 db is generally regarded as the beginning of dangerous sound intensities. In general, the louder the noise, the longer it lasts, the higher it is, and the purer in frequency, the more dangerous it is. Thus, jet engines and powerful sirens are particularly hazardous.

Noise and Mental Illness

Moreover, noise has a definite effect on mental well-being. No one knows exactly how, but noise can produce irritability, tension, and nervous strain. Extreme noise conditions can cause, or at least contribute to, mental illness. British medical authorities have reported a significantly higher incidence of mental illness among people exposed to aircraft noise.

Dr. Jack C. Westman, Director of the Child Psychiatry Division of the University of Wisconsin Medical School, thinks that unwanted noise in the home is contributing to divorce and the generation gap:

> We scapegoat, take out our tensions in other ways. Mothers yell at the youngsters, and parents bicker and fight between themselves. The average kitchen is like a boiler room, and what we thought was our friendly dishwasher is adding to the unhealthy surroundings by contributing to the noise.

A Growing Problem

Unfortunately, the noise problem seems to be getting worse. The U. S. Surgeon General states that as many as 16 million citizens are now losing their hearing from on-job noise. The U. S. Department of Commerce's Panel on Noise Abatement recently observed that noise pollution in the United States is reaching a serious level—a conclusion that most authorities had reached some time ago. Noise experts generally agree that the overall sound level in this country is rising at the rate of 1 db per year—or doubling every decade. There is every reason to believe that the rate of increase will rise in the coming years. Some scientists predict that even at the current rate, everyone in America will be deaf by the year 2000. Measurements conducted in average American towns show that noise levels have boomed four times higher than 1956 values and 32 times those in 1938. A New York City task force on noise control found that noise had reached a level "intense, continuous and persistent enough to threaten basic community life." The Federal Council for Science and Technol-

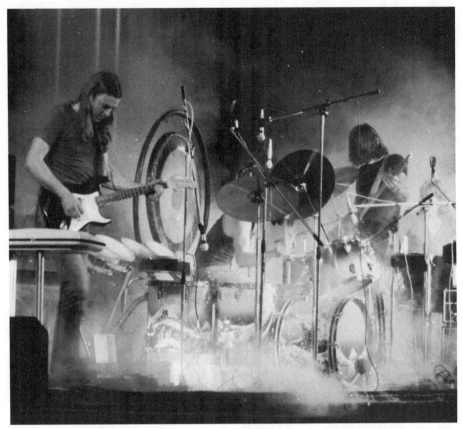

Listening to rock music at levels typical of those at which it is played or reproduced may blow not only one's mind but one's hearing as well.

ogy reckons that this major health hazard costs the nation $4 billion a year in decreased efficiency and lost compensation.

Some experts have linked the rise in diseases of the cardiovascular system to this steady increase in noise pollution. Noise elevates blood pressure and raises the amount of cholesterol in the blood. A group of Africans living in the hushed environment of the Southeast Sudan retain acute hearing and youthful arteries into advanced old age. But when they move to their noisy capital, their hearing deteriorates, and their rate of heart disease goes up.

Protection Against Noise

What can you do to protect yourself and your family from the effects of noise pollution? You can't do much to control some forms of noise—such as traffic noise—directly. But you can support local, state, and federal legislation that

seeks to control or eliminate some forms of noise. For example, many communities have laws that forbid blowing car horns except in emergencies; regrettably, such laws are poorly enforced, and the noise contribution from impatient drivers in our metropolitan areas is staggering.

You have at your constant command two effective noise-control instruments—your hands. Cupping your ears with them during noise of extraordinary pitch and intensity may help preserve your hearing. If you regularly encounter loud or irritating noise on your job or travels, buy a pair of ear protectors and wear them. This solution is no more farfetched than wearing sunglasses on dazzling days at the beach.

If you're responsible for the running of an office or plant, seek professional sound engineers' advice to make sure that you've taken advantage of the latest techniques and materials to cut noise to a minimum.

One of the most important things you can do is to stay clear of avoidable dangerous noise. A prevalent source of this kind of sound is rock music played or reproduced at damaging levels. If you or your children pooh-pooh this threat, here are the facts: listening to this music at levels typical of those now current may blow not only your mind, but your hearing, too.

Dr. Ralph R. Rupp, head of the audiology division of the speech clinic of the University of Michigan, together with his assistant, Larry J. Koch, measured sound levels produced by a rock combo. In the rehearsal room, these averaged 120–130 db during loud passages. All members of the combo reported ringing in their ears or other uncomfortable symptoms for from eight hours to several days after their get-togethers—signs of temporary or permanent hearing damage. Dr. Rupp says that people who either play or listen to music at such high levels may pay an enormous price in terms of eventual hearing loss. He suggests that rock musicians wear ear protectors that could reduce the sound levels at the ear by 20 or 30 db. He also proposes that local governments set safe maximum allowable noise limits for electronic amplification in clubs and discothèques.

In another test, Dr. Kenneth Pollock of the University of Florida found that the sound levels at a swinging teen club dropped to a safe 90 db only when he moved his equipment 40 feet outside the club. Ten teen-agers suffered hearing losses after dancing for three hours near the bandstand, where the din averaged 120 db. Listening to music via earphones offers a particularly effective means of going deaf—all it takes is a twist of the dial and you are instantly assaulted with sound levels that are practically unbearable. Dr. David M. Lipscomb of the University of Tennessee says, "We are apparently reaching the point where young people are losing sufficient hearing to jeopardize their occupational potential."

Yet another form of noise introduced to our novelty-hungry society is that from snowmobiles—those off-road vehicles that have enjoyed an amazing boom in recent years. Some ranch hands, foresters, and Arctic Indians and Eskimos have found the snowmobile literally a lifesaver in their harsh, snowbound winters, but most snowmobiles are used for recreational purposes. If you ride a snowmobile for any reason, you should know that its snarl is a definite hazard to your hearing, and wear special ear protectors. John G. Bollinger, a professor of mechanical engineering at the University of Wisconsin, measured snowmobile noise in a project to determine how they might be quietened. He recorded levels of about 110 db at a point six inches in front of the driver's head. Noise of this intensity can cause temporary hearing loss for an occasional rider, and permanent hearing loss for someone who spends several hours a day on the snowmobile.

CHAPTER 9

Skin and Hair

Not many people have perfectly proportioned faces and bodies, but practically anyone, at any age, can present an attractive appearance if skin is healthy-looking and glowing and hair is clean and shining. Healthy skin and hair can be achieved through good health habits, cleanliness, and personal grooming. Expensive skin-and-hair products may boost self-confidence, but they are a poor substitute for proper diet, exercise, enough sleep, and soap and water or cleansing creams.

The condition of skin and hair reflects a person's physical and emotional health. Of course, general appearance is determined not only by what is going on inside the body, but by outward circumstances, such as extremes of temperature or the use of harsh soaps. Appearance can also be altered temporarily by cosmetics and permanently by surgery.

THE SKIN

The skin is one of the most important organs of the body. It serves as protection against infection by germs and shields delicate underlying tissue against injury. Approximately one-third of the bloodstream flows through the skin, and as the blood vessels contract or relax in response to heat and cold, the skin acts as a thermostat that helps control body temperature. The two million sweat glands in the skin also regulate body temperature through the evaporation of perspiration. The many delicate nerve endings in the skin make it a sense organ responsive not only to heat and cold, but to pleasure, pain, and pressure.

Certain cells in the skin produce a protective pigmentation that determines its color and guards against overexposure to the ultraviolet rays of the sun. By absorption and elimination, the skin helps regulate the body's chemical and fluid balance. One of the miracles of the skin is that it constantly renews itself.

Structure of the Skin

The skin is made up of two layers. The outer layer or *epidermis* has a surface of horny, nonliving cells that form the body's protective envelope. These cells are constantly being shed and replaced by new ones which are made in the lower or inner layer of the epidermis.

Underneath the epidermis is the *dermis,* the thicker part of the skin. It contains blood vessels, nerves, and connective tissue. The sweat glands are located in the dermis, and they collect fluid containing water, salt, and waste products from the blood. This fluid is sent through tiny canals that end in pores on the skin's surface.

The oil or *sebaceous* glands that secrete the oil which lubricates the surface of the skin and hair are also located in the dermis. They are most often associated with hair *follicles.* Hair follicles and oil glands are found over most of the body, with the exception of the palms of the hands and the soles of the feet.

The layer of fatty tissue below the dermis, called *subcutaneous* tissue, acts as an insulator against heat and cold and as a shock absorber against injury.

Skin Color

The basic skin color of each person

ANATOMY OF THE SKIN

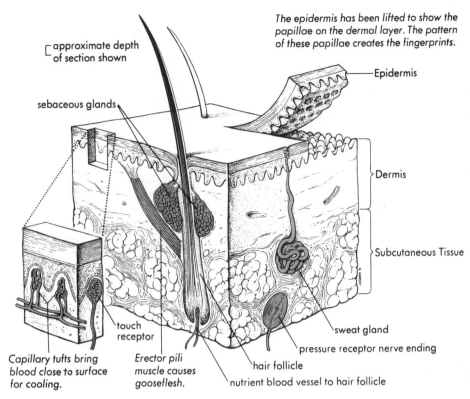

The epidermis has been lifted to show the papillae on the dermal layer. The pattern of these papillae creates the fingerprints.

approximate depth of section shown

sebaceous glands

Epidermis

Dermis

Subcutaneous Tissue

touch receptor

Capillary tufts bring blood close to surface for cooling.

Erector pili muscle causes gooseflesh.

sweat gland

pressure receptor nerve ending

hair follicle

nutrient blood vessel to hair follicle

is determined at birth, and is a part of his heritage that cannot be changed.

MELANIN: There are four pigments in the normal skin that affect its color: melanin, oxygenated hemoglobin, reduced hemoglobin, and various carotenes. Of these, *melanin* is the most powerful. The cells that produce it are the same in all races, but there is wide variation in the amount produced, and wide variation in its color, which ranges from black to light tan. Every adult has about 60,000 melanin-producing cells in each square inch of skin.

Melanin cells also affect eye color. When the cells are deep in the eye, the color produced is blue or green. When they are close to the surface, the eye is brown. An *albino*, a person with no melanin, has eyes that appear pink because the stronger pigment that ordinarily masks the blood vessels is lacking.

HEMOGLOBIN: The pigment that gives blood its color, called hemoglobin, has the next greatest effect on skin color. When it is combined with oxygen, a bright red is the result, and this in turn produces the rosy complexion associated with good health in light-skinned people. When such people suffer from reduced hemoglobin due to anemia, they appear to be excessively pale. A concentration of reduced hemoglobin gives the skin a bluish appearance. Since hemoglobin has a weaker coloring effect than the melanin that determines basic skin color, these variations are more visible in lighter-skinned individuals.

CAROTENES: The weakest pigments in the skin are the *carotenes*. These produce a yellowish tone that is increased by eating excessive amounts of carrots and oranges. In people with black or brown skin, excess carotene is usually masked by the melanin pigment.

Aging Skin

Skin appearance is affected by both internal and external factors. The silken quality of a baby's skin is due mainly to the fact that it has not yet begun to show the effects of continued exposure to sun and wind. The skin problems associated with adolescence reflect the many glandular changes that occur during the transition to adulthood. As the years pass, the skin becomes the most obvious indicator of aging.

Heredity, general health, and exposure to the elements are some of the factors that contribute to aging skin. Because people with darker skin have built-in protection against the ravages of the sun, their skin usually has a younger appearance than that of lighter-skinned people of comparable age.

In general, the skin of an older person is characterized by wrinkles and shininess. It feels thinner when pinched because it has lost its elasticity and part of the underlying fat that gives firmness to a younger skin.

Constant exposure to sunlight is now thought to play a more important role in the visible aging of skin than the aging process itself. Such exposure also appears to be directly related to the greater frequency of skin cancer among farmers, sailors, and others who spend most of their working hours out-of-doors.

Care of the Skin

Healthy, normal skin should be washed regularly with mild soap and warm water to remove grease, perspiration, and accumulated dirt. For those with a limited water supply or inadequate bath and shower facilities, sponge baths are a good substitute if the sponge or washcloth is thoroughly rinsed as various parts of the body are washed. Many people feel that a shower is a much more efficient way of getting clean than a bath, since the bath water becomes the receptacle for the dirt washed from the body, instead of its being rinsed away.

No matter what method is used, all soap should be thoroughly rinsed off the skin after washing. Unless specifically prescribed by a doctor, medicated or germicidal soaps

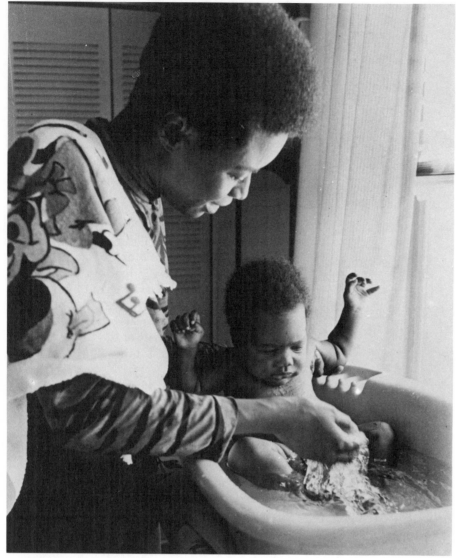

When bathing a baby, care must be taken to see that soap is thoroughly rinsed off after washing, since it can act as a skin irritant.

To correct the condition, the use of soap and water should be kept to a minimum for those parts of the body where the skin is dry. Cleansing creams or lotions containing lanolin should be used on the face, hands, elbows, and wherever else necessary. If tub baths are taken, a bath oil can be used in the water or applied to the skin after drying. Baby oil is just as effective and much cheaper than glamorously packaged and overadvertised products. Baby oil or a protective lotion should also be used on any parts of the body exposed to direct sunlight for any extended length of time. Applying oil to the skin will not, however, prevent wrinkles.

OILY SKIN: The amount of oil that comes to the surface of the skin through the sebaceous glands is the result not only of heredity, but also of temperature and emotional state. In warm weather, when the skin perspires more freely, the oil spreads like a film on the surface moisture. Non-oily foundation lotions can be helpful in keeping the oil spread to a minimum, and so can frequent washing with soap and water. When washing is inconvenient during the day, cleansing pads packaged to fit in pocket or purse are a quick and efficient solution for both men and women.

Too much friction from complexion brushes, rough washcloths, or harsh soaps may irritate rather than improve an oily skin condition.

Deodorants and Antiperspirants

Sweat glands are present almost everywhere in the skin except for the lips and a few other areas. Most of them give off the extremely dilute salt water known as sweat, or perspiration. Their purpose is to cool the body by evaporation of water. Body odors are not produced by perspiration itself, but by the bacterial activity that takes place in the perspiration. The activity is most intense in warm, moist parts of the body from which perspiration cannot evaporate quickly, such as the underarm area.

should not be used, since they may be an irritant. Skin should be dried with a fluffy towel, and bath towels should never be shared. Hands should be washed several times a day, and fingernails kept clean.

Facial skin requires special care because of its constant exposure. The face should be cleaned in the morning and before bedtime. Some women may prefer to use a cleansing cream rather than soap and water. Everyone should avoid massaging soap into the skin, since this may cause drying.

Dry and Oily Skin

Both heredity and environment account for the wide variation in the amount of oil and perspiration secreted by the glands of different people. Also, the same person's skin may be oily in one part of the body and dry in another.

DRY SKIN: This condition is the result of loss of water from the outer surface of the epidermis and its insufficient replacement from the tissues below. Some causes of the moisture loss are too frequent use of soap and detergents, and constant exposure to dry air. Anyone spending a great deal of time in air-conditioned surroundings in which the humidity has been greatly lowered is likely to suffer from dry skin.

DEODORANTS: The basic means of keeping this type of bacterial growth under control is through personal cleanliness of both skin and clothing. Deodorant soaps containing antiseptic chemicals are now available. Though they do not kill bacteria, they do reduce the speed with which they multiply.

Underarm deodorants also help to eliminate the odor. They are not meant to stop the flow of perspiration, but rather to slow down bacterial growth and mask body odors with their own scent. Such deodorants should be applied immediately after bathing. They are usually more effective if the underarm area is shaved, since the hair in this unexposed area collects perspiration and encourages bacterial growth.

ANTIPERSPIRANTS: Antiperspirants differ from deodorants in that they not only affect the rate of bacterial growth, but also reduce the amount of perspiration that reaches the skin surface. Since the action of the chemical salts they contain is cumulative, they seem to be more effective with repeated use. Antiperspirants come under the category of drugs, and their contents must be printed on the container. Deodorants are considered cosmetics, and may or may not name their contents on the package.

No matter what the nature of the advertising claim, neither type of product completely stops the flow of perspiration, nor would it be desirable to do so. Effectiveness of the various brands differs from one person to another. Some may produce a mild allergic reaction; others might be too weak to do a good job. It is practical to experiment with a few different brands, using them under similar conditions, to find the type that works best for you.

Creams and Cosmetics

The bewildering number of creams and cosmetics on the market and the exaggerated claims of some of their advertising can be reduced to a few simple facts. In most cases, the higher price of such products is an indication of the amount of money spent on advertising and packaging rather than on the ingredients themselves. Beauty preparations should be judged by the user on their merits rather than on their claims.

COLD CREAMS AND CLEANSING CREAMS: These two products are essentially the same. They are designed to remove accumulated skin secretions, dirt, and grime, and should be promptly removed from the skin with a soft towel or tissue.

LUBRICATING CREAMS AND LOTIONS: Also called night creams, moisturizing creams, and conditioning creams, these products are supposed to prevent the loss of moisture from the skin and promote its smoothness. They are usually left on overnight or for an extended length of time. Anyone with dry skin will find it helpful to apply a moisturizer under foundation cream. This will help keep the skin from drying out even further, and protect it against the effects of air

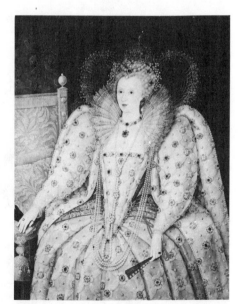

England's Queen Elizabeth I, who reigned in the 1500s, is usually portrayed as very pale. An amateur cosmetician, she almost always wore white-lead powder.

conditioning.

VANISHING CREAMS AND FOUNDATION CREAMS: These products also serve the purpose of providing the skin with moisture, but are meant to be applied immediately before putting on makeup.

REJUVENATING CREAMS: There is no scientific proof that any of the "royal jelly," "secret formula," or "hormone" creams produce a marked improvement on aging skin. They cannot eliminate wrinkles, nor can they regenerate skin tissue.

MEDICATED CREAMS AND LOTIONS: These products should not be used except on the advice of a doctor since they may cause or aggravate skin disorders of various kinds.

LIPSTICKS: Lipsticks contain lanolin, a mixture of oil and wax, a coloring dye, and pigment, as well as perfume. Any of these substances can cause an allergic reaction in individual cases, but such reactions are uncommon. Sometimes the reaction is caused by the staining dye, in which case a "nonpermanent" lipstick should be used.

COSMETICS AND THE SENSITIVE SKIN: Anyone with a cosmetic problem due to sensitive skin should consult a *dermatologist*, a physician specializing in the skin and its diseases. Cosmetic companies will inform a physician of the ingredients in their products, and he can then recommend a brand that will agree with the patient's specific skin problems. He may also recommend a special nonallergenic preparation.

EYE MAKEUP: Eye-liner and mascara brushes and pencils—and lipsticks for that matter—can carry infection and should never be borrowed or lent. *Hypoallergenic* makeup, which is specially made for those who get allergic reactions to regular eye makeup, is available and should be used by anyone so affected.

SUNTANNING LOTIONS: See under *Aches, Pains, Nuisances, Worries,* p. 265, for a discussion of sunburn.

HAIR

Hair originates in tiny sacs or follicles deep in the dermis layer of skin tissue. The part of the hair below the skin surface is the root; the part above is the shaft. Hair follicles are closely connected to the sebaceous glands which secrete oil to the scalp and give hair its natural sheen.

Hair grows from the root outward, pushing the shaft farther from the scalp. Depending on its color, there may be as many as 125,000 hairs on an adult's head. The palms of the hands, the soles of the feet, and the lips are the only completely hairless parts of the surface of the body.

Texture

Each individual hair is made up of nonliving cells that contain a tough protein called *keratin*. Hair texture differs from one part of the body to another. In some areas, it may be soft and downy; in others, tough and bristly. Hair texture also differs between the sexes, among individuals, and among the different races.

If an individual hair is oval in cross-section, it is curly along its length. If the cross-section is round, the hair is straight. Thick, wiry hair is usually triangular or kidney-shaped. The fineness or coarseness of hair texture is related to its natural color.

CURLING: Anyone using a home permanent preparation should read and follow instructions with great care. If a new brand is tried, the instructions should be read all over again, since they may be quite different from the accustomed ones.

Electric curling irons are not safe because they may cause pinpoint burns in the scalp which are hardly noticeable at the time but may lead to permanent small areas of baldness. The danger can be minimized, however, if instructions for use are followed exactly and the recommended moisturizing lotions are used. It is especially important that the iron not be hot enough to singe the hair. The results, even if there is no damage, are not long lasting and

are adversely affected by dampness. Setting lotions used with rollers or clips have a tendency to dull the hair unless they are completely brushed out.

STRAIGHTENING: The least harmful as well as the least effective way of straightening the hair temporarily is the use of pomades. They are usually considered unsatisfactory by women because they are too greasy, but are often used by men with short unruly hair. Heat-pressing the hair with a metal comb is longer-lasting but can cause substantial damage by burning the scalp. When this method is used, humidity or scalp perspiration will cause the hair to revert to its natural curl. The practice of ironing the hair should be discouraged since it causes dryness and brittleness, with resultant breakage. Chemical straighteners should be used with great care since they may cause serious burns. Special efforts must be made to protect the eyes from contact with these products.

Hair Color

In the same way that melanin colors the skin, it also determines hair color. The less melanin, the lighter the hair. As each hair loses its melanin pigment, it gradually turns gray, then white. It is assumed that the age at which hair begins to gray is an inherited characteristic and therefore can't be postponed or prevented by eating special foods, by taking vitamins, or by the external application of creams. The only way to recolor gray hair is by the use of a chemical dye.

DYES AND TINTS: Anyone wishing to make a radical change in hair color should consult a trained and reliable hairdresser. Trying to turn black hair

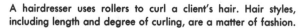

A hairdresser uses rollers to curl a client's hair. Hair styles, including length and degree of curling, are a matter of fashion.

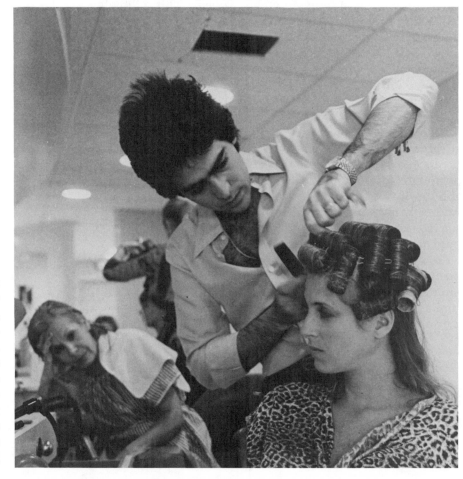

bright red or dark red hair to blonde with a home preparation can sometimes end up with unwanted purplish or greenish results. When tints or dyes are used at home to lighten or darken the hair color by one or two shades, instructions accompanying the product must be followed carefully. Anyone with a tendency to contract contact dermatitis (see page 245) should make a patch test on the skin to check on possible allergic reactions. Hair should be tinted or dyed no more often than once a month.

DYE STRIPPING: The only safe way to get rid of an unwanted dye color that has been used on the hair is to let it grow out. The technique known as stripping takes all color from the hair and reduces it to a dangerously weak mass. It is then redyed its natural color. Such a procedure should never be undertaken by anyone except a trained beautician, if at all.

BLEACHING: Hydrogen peroxide is mixed with a hair-lightener to pre-bleach hair before applying blond tints. Bleaching with peroxide alone can cause more damage to the hair than dyeing or tinting it with a reliable commercial preparation, because it causes dryness, brittlenesss, and breakage.

General Hair Care

Properly cared for hair usually looks clean, shiny, and alive. Unfortunately, too many people mask the natural good looks of their hair with unnecessary sprays and "beauty" preparations.

WASHING THE HAIR: Hair should be washed about once a week—more often if it tends to be oily. The claims made by shampoo manufacturers need not always be taken too seriously, since most shampoos contain nothing more than soap or detergent and a perfuming agent. No shampoo can restore the natural oils to the hair at the same time that it washes it. A castile shampoo is good for dry hair, and one containing tincture of green soap is good for oily hair.

Thorough rinsing is essential to

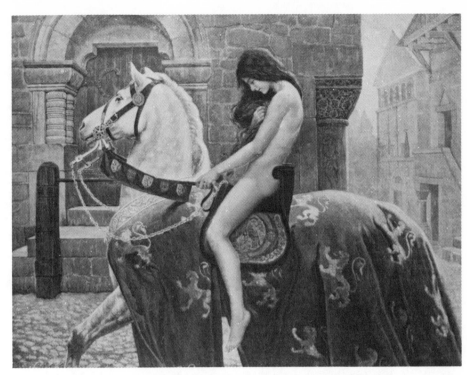

An old etching portrays Lady Godiva's infamous ride through the streets of Coventry, England, clad only in her long, beautiful hair.

eliminate any soap deposit. If the local water is hard, a detergent shampoo can be rinsed off more easily than one containing soap.

DRYING THE HAIR: Drying the hair in sunlight or under a heat-controlled dryer is more satisfactory than trying to rub it dry with a towel. Gentle brushing during drying reactivates the natural oils that give hair its shine. Brushing in general is excellent for the appearance of the hair. Be sure to wash both brush and comb as often as the hair is washed.

Hair pomades should be avoided or used sparingly, since they are sometimes so heavy that they clog the pores of the scalp. A little bit of olive oil or baby oil can be rubbed into dry hair after shampooing. This is also good for babies' hair.

There is no scientific evidence that creme rinses, protein rinses, or beer rinses accomplish anything for the hair other than making it somewhat more manageable if it is naturally fine and flyaway.

Dandruff

Simple dandruff is a condition in which the scalp begins to itch and

flake a few days after the hair has been washed. There is no evidence that the problem is related to germ infection.

Oiliness and persistent dandruff may appear not only on the scalp, but also on the sides of the nose or the chest. In such cases, a dermatologist should be consulted. Both light and serious cases often respond well to prescription medicines containing tars. These preparations control the dandruff, but there is no known cure for it.

Nits

Head lice sometimes infect adults as well as children. These tiny parasites usually live on the part of the scalp near the nape of the neck, and when they bite, they cause itching. They attach their eggs, which are called *nits*, to the shaft of the hair, and when they are plentiful, they can be seen by a trained eye as tiny, silvery-white ovals. This condition is highly contagious and can be passed from one head to another by way of combs, brushes, hats, head scarfs, and towels. A doctor can be consulted for information on effective ways of eliminating nits—usually by the application of chemicals and the use of a fine-toothed comb.

Baldness

Under the normal circumstances of combing, brushing, and shampooing, a person loses anywhere from 25 to 100 hairs a day. Because new hairs start growing each day, the loss and replacement usually balance each other. When the loss rate is greater than the replacement rate, thinning and baldness are the result.

ALOPECIA: The medical name for baldness is *alopecia,* the most common form of which is *male pattern baldness.* Dr. Eugene Van Scott, Professor of Dermatology of Temple University's Health Sciences Center, sums up the opinion of medical authorities on the three factors responsible for this type of baldness: sex, age, and heredity. Unfortunately, these are three factors over which medical science has no control.

OTHER CAUSES OF BALDNESS: Other forms of baldness may be the result of bacterial or fungus infections, allergic reactions to particular medicines, radiation, or continual friction. It has also been suggested that constant stress from hair curlers or tightly pulled ponytails can cause loss of hair. These forms of baldness usually disappear when the cause is eliminated.

Although diet has very little to do with baldness, poor nutrition can result in hair that is dry, dull, and brittle enough to break easily. Any serious illness can lead to hair loss as well. It is thought that vitamin A taken in grossly excessive amounts can contribute to hair loss.

Women ordinarily lose some of their hair at the end of pregnancy, after delivery, and during the menopause, but regrowth can be expected in a few months.

It is now possible for anyone suffering from temporary baldness or from male pattern baldness to choose from a wide variety of attractively styled wigs and hairpieces.

A surgical procedure for treating

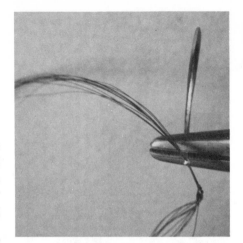
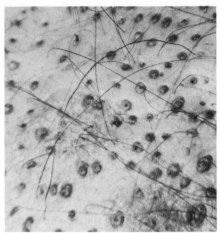

Synthetic fibers, (*above, left*) are sometimes used as hair implants, but scalp tissue can be badly infected (*above, right*) by the operation.

male pattern baldness and baldness in women is called hair transplantation; it is discussed under *Surgery,* p. 346.

Hair Removal

Over the centuries and around the world, fashions in whiskers and beards come and go, but the average American male still subjects at least part of his face to daily shaving. Although feminine shaving practices are a more recent phenomenon, most American women now consider it part of good grooming to remove underarm and leg hair with a razor as often as twice a week. Shaving removes not only the dead skin cells that make up the protective layer of the body's surface, but also some of the living skin underneath. Instead of being harmful, this appears to stimulate rather than damage new skin growth.

Male Shaving

The average beard grows about two-tenths of an inch a day. However, the density of male face hair

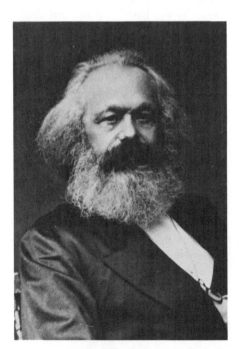
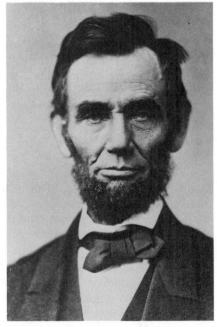

Beards were fashionable in the 1800s, and we are accustomed to seeing portraits of Karl Marx (*above, left*) and Abraham Lincoln with beards.

varies a great deal depending on skin and hair color. In all races, the concentration is usually greatest on the chin and in the area between the nose and upper lip.

There is no proof that an electric razor is safer or better for all types of skin than a safety razor. Both types result in nicks and cuts of the living skin tissue, depending on the closeness of the shave.

Twice as many men prefer wet shaving to dry because the use of soap and hot water softens the hair stubble and makes it easier to remove. Shaving authorities point out that thorough soaking is one of the essentials of easy and safe shaving. Leaving the shaving lather on the face for at least two minutes will also soften whiskers a good deal.

The razor should be moistened with hot water throughout the process, and the chin and upper lip left for last so that the heavier hair concentration in these areas has the longest contact with moisture and lather.

OILY SKIN: Men with oily skin should use an aerosol shaving preparation or a lather type applied with a brush. These are really soaps and are more effective in eliminating the oils that coat the face hair, thus making it easier to shave.

DRY SKIN: A brushless cream is advisable for dry skin since it lubricates the skin rather than further depriving it of oil.

INGROWN HAIRS: One of the chief problems connected with shaving is that it often causes ingrown hairs, which can lead to pore-clogging and infection. Hair is more likely to turn back into the skin if it is shaved against the grain, or if the cutting edge of the blade is dull and rough rather than smooth. Men with coarse, wiry, curly hair may find that whisker ends are more likely to become ingrown than men with fine hair. The problem is best handled by shaving with the grain, using a sharp blade, and avoiding too close a shave, particularly in the area around the neck.

SHAVING AND SKIN PROBLEMS: For men with acne or a tendency to skin problems, the following advice is offered by Dr. Howard T. Behrman, Director of Dermatological Research, New York Medical College:

• Shave as seldom as possible, perhaps only once or twice a week, and always with the grain.

• If wet shaving is preferred, use a new blade each time, and shave as lightly as possible to avoid nicking pimples.

• Wash face carefully with plenty of soap and hot water to make the beard easy to manage, and after shaving, rinse with hot water followed by cold.

• Use an antiseptic astringent face lotion.

• Instead of plucking out ingrown hairs, loosen them gently so that the ends do not grow back into the skin.

• Although some people with skin problems find an electric shaver less irritating, in most cases, a wet shave seems best.

Female Shaving

Millions of American women regularly shave underarm and leg hair, and most of them do so with a blade razor. In recent years, various types of shavers have been designed with blade exposure more suited to women's needs than the standard type used by men. To make shaving easier and safer, the following procedures are recommended:

• Since wet hair is much easier to cut, the most effective time to shave is during or immediately following a bath or shower.

• Shaving cream or soap lather keeps the water from evaporating, and is preferred to dry shaving.

• Underarm shaving is easier with a contoured razor designed for this purpose. If a deodorant or antiperspirant causes stinging or irritation after shaving, allow a short time to elapse before applying it.

• Light bleeding from nicks or scrapes can be stopped by applying pressure to a sterile pad placed on the injured area.

Unwanted Hair

The technical word for excess or unwanted hair on the face, chest, arms, and legs is *hirsutism*. The condition varies greatly among different ethnic strains, and so does the attitude toward it. Women of southern European ancestry are generally hairier than those with Nordic or Anglo-Saxon ancestors. Caucasoid peoples are hairier than Negroid peoples. The sparsest amount of body hair is found among the Mongolian races and American Indians.

Although heredity is the chief factor in hirsutism, hormones also influence hair growth. If there is a sudden appearance of coarse hair on the body of a young boy or girl or a woman with no such former tendency, a glandular disturbance should be suspected and investigated by a doctor.

A normal amount of unwanted hair on the legs and under the arms is usually removed by shaving. When the problem involves the arms, face, chest, and abdomen, other methods of removal are available.

Temporary Methods of Hair Removal

BLEACHING: Unwanted dark fuzz on the upper lip and arms can be lightened almost to invisibility with a commercially prepared bleach or with a homemade paste consisting of baking soda, hydrogen peroxide (bleaching strength), and a few drops of ammonia. Soap chips can be used instead of baking soda. The paste should be left on the skin for a few minutes and then washed off. It is harmless to the skin, and if applied repeatedly, the hair will tend to break off as a result of constant bleaching.

CHEMICAL DEPILATORIES: These products contain alkaline agents that cause hair to detach easily at the skin surface. They can be used on and under the arms, and on the legs and chest. However, they should not be used on the face unless the label says it is safe to do so. Timing instructions should be followed carefully. If skin irritation results, this type of depilatory should be discontinued in favor of some other method.

ABRASIVES: Devices which remove hair from the skin surface by rubbing are cheap but time-consuming. However, if an abrasive such as pumice is used regularly, the offending hairs will be shorter with each application. A cream or lotion should be applied to the skin after using an abrasive.

WAXING: The technique of applying melted wax to the skin for removal of excess facial hair is best handled by an experienced cosmetician. The process involves pouring hot wax onto the skin and allowing it to cool. The hairs become embedded in the wax, and are plucked out from below the skin surface when the wax is stripped off. Since this method is painful and often causes irritation, it is not very popular, although the results are comparatively long-lasting.

PLUCKING: The use of tweezers for removing scattered hairs from the eyebrows, face, and chest is slightly painful but otherwise harmless. It is not a practical method for getting rid of dense hair growth, however, since it takes too much time.

Permanent Hair Removal by Electrolysis

The only permanent and safe method of removing unwanted hair is by *electrolysis*. This technique destroys each individual hair root by transmitting electric current through fine wire needles into the opening of the hair follicle. The hair thus loosened is then plucked out with a tweezer. The older type of electrolysis machine uses galvanic current. The newer type, sometimes called an electrocoagulation machine, uses modified high frequency current. In either case, the efficiency and safety of the technique depends less on the machine than on the care and skill of the operator.

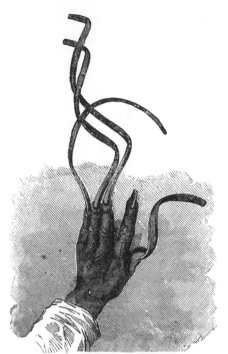

An old engraving portrays the long fingernails supposedly in vogue among the upper classes in ancient China.

Since the process of treating each hair root is expensive, time-consuming, and uncomfortable, it is not recommended for areas of dense hair growth such as the arms or legs. Before undertaking electrolysis either at a beauty salon or at home, it would be wise to consult a dermatologist about individual skin reaction.

Nails

Fingernails and toenails are an extension of the epidermis or outer layer of the skin. They are made of elastic tissue formed from keratin, the substance that gives hair its strength and flexibility.

Some of the problems associated with fingernails are the result of too much manicuring. White spots, for example, are often caused by too much pressure at the base of the nail when trying to expose the "moon" —the white portion which contains

tissue not yet as tough as the rest of the nail.

To ensure the health of toenails, feet should be bathed once a day and the nails cleaned with a brush dipped in soapy water. Shoes should fit properly so that the toenails are not subjected to pressure and distortion. In order to avoid ingrown toenails, trimming should be done straight across rather than by rounding or tapering the corners.

SPLITTING: Infection or injury of the tissue at the base of a fingernail may cause its surface to be rigid or split. Inflammation of the finger joints connected with arthritis will also cause nail deformity. For ordinary problems of splitting and peeling, the nails should be kept short enough so that they don't catch and tear easily. For practical purposes, the top of the nail should not be visible when the palm is held about six inches from the eye. As the nails grow stronger, they can be grown longer without splitting.

BRITTLENESS: This condition seems to be caused by external factors such as the chemicals in polish removers, soaps, and detergents. It is also a natural consequence of aging. Commercial nail-hardening preparations that contain formaldehyde are not recommended, since they are known to cause discoloration, loosening, or even loss of nails in some cases.

Nail damage can be reduced by wearing rubber gloves while doing household chores. Hand cream massaged into the skin around the nails will counteract dryness and lessen the possibility of hangnails. Although nail polish provides a shield against damage, it should not be worn all the time, particularly if the nail is polished right down to the base, since this prevents live tissue from "breathing."

DISORDERS OF THE SKIN

The skin is subject to a large number of disorders, most of which are not serious even though they may be temporarily uncomfortable. A disorder may be caused by one or another type of allergy; by excessive heat or cold; or by infection from fungi, bacteria, viruses, or parasites. There are also many skin ailments that are caused or aggravated by emotional disturbances.

The symptoms and treatment of the more common disorders are discussed in the following pages. Any persistent change in skin condition should be brought to the attention of a doctor.

Allergies and Itching

Itching and inflammation of the skin may be caused by an allergic reaction, by exposure to poisonous plants, or by a generalized infection.

Dermatitis

Dermatitis is the term used for an inflammation of the skin. The term for allergic reactions of the skin resulting from surface contact with outside agents is *contact dermatitis*. This condition is characterized by a rash and may be brought on by sensitivity to cosmetics, plants, cleaning materials, metal, wool, and so on. Other forms of dermatitis can be caused by excesses of heat or cold, by friction, or by sensitivity to various medicines. Dermatitis is usually accompanied by itching at the site of the rash.

Poison Ivy

This common plant, unknown in Europe, but widespread everywhere in the United States except in California and Nevada, produces an allergic reaction on the skin accompanied by a painful rash and blisters. Some people are so sensitive to it that they are affected by contact not only with the plant itself, but with animal fur or clothing that might have picked up the sap weeks before.

A mild attack of poison ivy produces a rash and small watery blisters that get progressively larger. The affected area of the skin becomes crusty and dry, and after a few weeks, all symptoms vanish. If the exposed area is thoroughly washed with laundry soap immediately after contact, the poison may not penetrate the skin.

If the symptoms do develop, they can be relieved with Burow's solution—one part solution to fifteen parts of cool water—or with the application of calamine lotion. If the symptoms are severe, and especially if the area around the eyes is involved, a doctor should be consulted. He may prescribe an application or an injection of cortisone.

The best way to avoid the unpleasantness of a poison ivy attack is to learn to recognize the plant and stay away from it. Children especially should be warned against putting the leaves and berries in their mouths.

Poison oak and poison sumac produce somewhat the same symptoms and should also be avoided.

Under no circumstances should these plants be burned in order to eliminate them, since the inhaling of the contaminated smoke even from a distance can cause a serious case of poisoning. The application

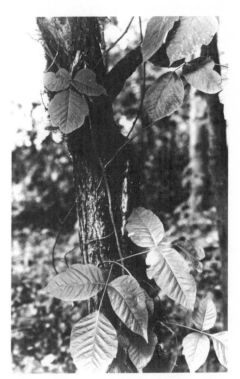

The glossy leaves of the poison ivy plant are arranged in clusters of three, and often have irregularly-shaped notches.

of special sprays, if the instructions are followed carefully, will get rid of the plants without affecting people or the neighborhood greenery.

Hives

These are large, irregularly shaped swellings on the skin that burn and itch. The cause is unknown, but allergic reactions to certain foods and medicine or to insect bites have been suggested as possible causes. The swellings of hives usually disappear within a day or so, but they can be very uncomfortable while they last. The itching and burning can often be relieved by applying cold water and a calamine solution. However, some people are sensitive to cold and develop wheals when subjected to intense cold. Commercial preparations containing surface anesthetics are seldom effective and may cause allergic reactions.

If the outbreak of hives can be traced to a specific food such as shellfish or strawberries, the food

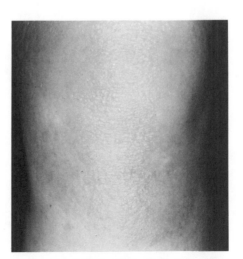

A close-up of contact dermatitis of the knee, an allergic skin reaction caused by surface contact with a substance such as wool.

should be eliminated from the diet. If a medicine such as penicillin or a sulfa drug is the cause, the doctor should be told about the reaction.

Eczema

This condition is an allergic reaction that produces itching, swelling, blistering, oozing, and scaling of the skin. It is more common among children than among adults and may sometimes cover the entire body, although the rash is usually limited to the face, neck, and the folds of the knees and elbows. Unlike contact dermatitis, it is likely to be caused by an allergy to a food or a pollen or dust. Advertised cures for eczema cannot control the cause and sometimes make the condition worse. A doctor should be consulted if the symptoms are severe, particularly if the patient is an infant or very young child.

Itching

The technical name for the localized or general sensation on the skin which can be relieved by scratching is *pruritus*. Itching may be caused by many skin disorders, by infections, by serious diseases such as nephritis or leukemia, by medicines, or by psychological factors such as tension. A doctor should always be consulted to find the cause of persistent itching, since it may be the symptom of a basic disorder. Repeated scratching may provide some relief, but it can also lead to infection.

Anal Pruritus

If itching in the anal area is so severe that only painful scratching will relieve it, the condition is probably *anal pruritus*. It is often accompanied by excessive rectal mucus that keeps the skin irritated and moist. This disorder is most commonly associated with hemorrhoids, but many other conditions, such as reactions to drugs, can cause it. Anxiety or tension can also contribute to it. Sitz baths with warm water are usually recommended. Every effort should be made to reduce scratching and to keep the anal skin clean and dry. Cortisone cream may be prescribed in persistent cases.

Skin Irritations and Weather

Extremes of weather produce local inflammations and other skin problems for many people.

Chapping

In cold weather, the sebaceous glands slow down the secretions that lubricate the skin, causing it to become dry. When dry skin is exposed to wintry weather, it becomes irritated and is likely to crack, particularly around the lips. Chapped skin is especially sensitive to harsh soaps. During such periods of exposure, the skin can be protected with a mild cream or lotion. A lubricating ointment should be used on the lips to prevent them from cracking. Children who lick their lips constantly no matter what the weather can benefit from this extra protection. Chapped hands caused by daily use of strong soaps and detergents can be helped by the use of a lubricating cream and rubber gloves during housework.

Frostbite

Exposure to extreme cold for a prolonged period may cause freezing of the nose, fingers, toes, or ears, thus cutting off the circulation to the

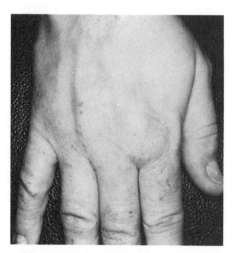

Unlike contact dermatitis, eczema (or *atopic dermatitis*) is caused by an allergic reaction to a food or an airborne substance such as pollen.

affected areas. Frostbitten areas are of a paler color than normal and are numb. They should not be rubbed with snow or exposed to intense heat. Areas should be thawed gradually, and a doctor should be consulted for aftercare in extreme cases.

Chilblain

A localized inflammation of the skin, called *chilblain*, is common among people who are particularly sensitive to cold because of poor circulation. Chilblains may occur in the ears, hands, feet, and face, causing itching, swelling, and discoloration of the skin. Anyone prone to chilblain should dress protectively during the cold weather and use an electric pad or blanket at night. Affected parts should not be rubbed or massaged, nor should ice or extreme heat be applied directly, since these measures may cause additional damage. Persistent or extreme attacks of chilblain should be discussed with a doctor.

Chafing

This condition is an inflammation of two opposing skin surfaces caused by the warmth, moisture, and friction of their rubbing together. Diabetics, overweight people, and those who perspire heavily are particularly prone to chafing. Chafing is accompanied by itching and burning, and sometimes infection can set in if the superficial skin is broken. Parts of the body subject to chafing are the inner surfaces of the thighs, the anal region, the area under the breasts, and the inner surfaces between fingers and toes.

To reduce the possibility of chafing, cool clothing should be worn and strenuous exercise avoided during hot weather. Vaseline or a Vitamin A and D ointment may be applied to reduce friction. In general, the treatment is the same as that for diaper rash in infants. If the condition becomes acute, a doctor can prescribe more effective remedies.

Prickly Heat

This skin rash is usually accompanied by itching and burning. It is caused by an obstruction of the sweat ducts so that perspiration does not reach the surface of the skin, but backs up and causes pimples the size of a pinhead. If the obstruction is superficial, the pimples are white; if it is deeper, they are red. The condition can be brought on by other minor skin irritations, by continued exposure to moist heat such as a compress, or by exercise in humid weather. Infants and people who are overweight are especially prone to prickly heat.

The discomfort can be eased by wearing lightweight, loose-fitting clothing, especially at night, and keeping room temperature low. Alcoholic beverages, which tend to dehydrate the body, should be avoided. Tepid baths and the application of cornstarch to the affected skin areas will usually relieve itching. If the rash remains for several days, a doctor should be consulted to make sure it does not arise from some other cause.

Calluses and Corns

As a result of continued friction or pressure in a particular area, the skin forms a tough, hard, self-protecting layer known as a *callus*. Calluses are common on the soles of the feet, the palms of the hands, and, among guitarists and string players, on the tips of the fingers. A heavy callus which presses against a bone in the foot because of poorly fitted shoes can be very painful. The hard surface can be reduced somewhat by the use of pumice, or by gently paring it with a razor blade that has been washed in alcohol.

Corns are a form of callus that appear on or between the toes. They usually have a hard inner core that causes pain when pressed against underlying tissue by badly fitted shoes. A hard corn that appears on the surface of the little toe can be removed by soaking for about ten minutes and applying a few drops of ten percent salicylic acid in collodion. The surface should be covered with a corn pad to reduce pressure, and the corn lifted off when it is loose enough to be released from the skin. Anyone suffering from a circulatory disease and particularly from diabetes should avoid home treatment of foot disturbances. Those with a tendency to callus and corn formations should be especially careful about the proper fit of shoes and hose. A *chiropodist* or *podiatrist* is a trained specialist in foot care who can be visited on a regular basis to provide greater foot comfort.

Fungus Infections

Fungi are plantlike parasitic growths found in the air, in water, and in the soil. They comprise a large family that includes mushrooms, and are responsible for mildew and mold. Only a small number cause disease.

Ringworm

This condition is not caused by a worm, but by a group of fungi that live on the body's dead skin cells in those areas that are warm and damp because of accumulated perspiration. One form of ringworm attacks the scalp, arms, and legs, especially of children, and is often spread by similarly affected pets. It appears as reddish patches that scale and blister and frequently feel sore and itchy. Ringworm is highly contagious and can be passed from person to person by contaminated objects such as combs and towels. It should therefore be treated promptly by a doctor. Ringworm can best be prevented by strict attention to personal cleanliness.

Athlete's Foot

Another form of ringworm, *athlete's foot*, usually attacks the skin between the toes and under the toenails. If not treated promptly, it can cause an itching rash on other parts of the body. Athlete's foot causes the skin to itch, blister, and crack, and as a result, leaves it vulnerable to more serious infection

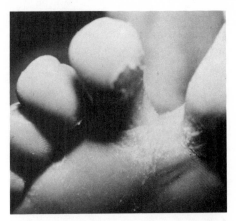

Athlete's foot, a form of ringworm, is marked by a cracking of the skin between the toes or under the toenails. Itching and soreness are usual symptoms.

from other organisms. The disorder can be treated at home by gently removing the damaged skin, and, after soaking the feet, thoroughly drying and dusting between the toes with a medicated foot powder. Some of the powder should be sprinkled into shoes. If the condition continues, a fungicidal ointment can be applied in the morning and at night. Persistent cases require the attention of a doctor.

Scabies

An insectlike parasite causes the skin irritation called *scabies*, otherwise known as "the itch." The female itch mite burrows a hole in the skin, usually in the groin or between the fingers or toes, and stays hidden long enough to build a tunnel in which to deposit her eggs. The newly hatched mites then work their way to the skin surface and begin the cycle all over again. There is little discomfort in the early period of infestation, but in about a week, a rash appears accompanied by extreme itching, which is usually most severe at night. Constant scratching during sleep can lead to skin lesions that invite bacterial infection.

Scabies is very contagious and can spread rapidly through a family or through a community, such as a summer camp or army barracks. It can also be communicated by venereal contact.

Treatment by a doctor involves the identification of the characteristic tunnels from which sample mites can be removed for examination. Hot baths and thorough scrubbing will expose the burrows, and medical applications as directed by the doctor usually clear up the condition in about a week.

Bacterial Infections

The skin is susceptible to infection from a variety of bacteria. Poor diet and careless hygiene can lower the body's resistance to these infectious agents.

Boils

These abscesses of the skin are caused by bacterial infection of a hair follicle or a sebaceous gland. The pus that accumulates in a boil is the result of the encounter between the bacteria and the white blood cells that fight them. Sometimes a boil subsides by itself and disappears. Sometimes the pressure of pus against the skin surface may bring the boil to a head; it will then break, drain, and heal if washed with an antiseptic and covered with a sterile pad. Warm water compresses can be applied for ten minutes every hour to relieve the pain and to encourage the boil to break and drain. A fresh dry pad should be applied after each period of soaking.

Anyone with a serious or chronic illness who develops a boil should consult a doctor. Since the bacteria can enter the bloodstream and cause a general infection with fever, a doctor should also be consulted for a boil on the nose, scalp, upper lip, or in the ear, groin, or armpit.

Carbuncles

This infection is a group of connected boils and is likely to be more painful and less responsive to home treatment. Carbuncles may occur as the result of poor skin care. They tend to occur in the back of the neck where the skin is thick, and the abscess tends to burrow into deeper tissues. A doctor usually lances and drains a deep-seated carbuncle, or he may prescribe an antibiotic remedy.

Impetigo

This skin infection is caused by staphylococcal or streptococcal bacteria, and is characterized by blisters that break and form yellow crusted areas. It is spread from one person to another and from one part of the body to another by the discharge from the sores. Impetigo occurs most frequently on the scalp, face, and arms and legs. The infection often is picked up in barber shops, swimming pools, or from body contact with other infected people or household pets.

Special care must be taken, especially with children, to control the spread of the infection by keeping the fingers away from infected parts. Bed linens should be changed daily, and disposable paper towels as well as paper plates and cups should be used during treatment. A doctor should be consulted for proper medication and procedures to deal with the infection.

Barber's Itch

Sycosis, commonly called *barber's itch*, is a bacterial infection of the hair follicles of the beard, accompanied by inflammation, itching, and the formation of pus-filled pimples. People with stiff, curly hair are prone to this type of chronic infection, since their hair is more likely to curve back and reenter the skin. The infection should be treated promptly to prevent scarring and the destruction of the hair root. In some cases, doctors recommend antibiotics. If these are not effective, it may be necessary to drain the abscesses and remove the hairs from the inflamed follicles. During treatment, it is best to avoid shaving, if possible. If one must shave, the sterilization of all shaving equipment and the use of a brushless shaving cream are recommended.

Erysipelas

An acute streptococcal infection of the skin, *erysipelas* can be fatal, particularly to the very young or very old, if not treated promptly. One of its symptoms is the bright redness of the affected areas of the skin. These red patches enlarge and spread, making the skin tender and painful. Blisters may appear nearby. The patient usually has a headache, fever, chills, and nausea. Erysipelas responds well to promptly administered antibiotics, particularly penicillin. The patient is usually advised to drink large amounts of fluid and to eat a nourishing, easily digested diet.

Viral Infections

The most common skin conditions caused by viruses are cold sores, shingles, and warts, discussed below.

Cold Sores

Also called fever blisters, *cold sores* are technically known as *herpes simplex*. They are small blisters that appear most frequently in the corners of the mouth, and sometimes around the eyes and on the genitals. The presumed cause is a virus that lies dormant in the skin until it is activated by infection or by excessive exposure to sun or wind. There is no specific cure for cold sores, but the irritation can be eased by applying drying or cooling agents such as camphor ice or cold water compresses. Recurrent cold sores, especially in infants, should be called to a doctor's attention.

Recent studies have shown that a variety of the herpes simplex virus called HSV-2 (for Herpes simplex virus-Type 2) can be a serious danger to the fetus of a pregnant woman. For a discussion of this condition, see Ch. 27, p. 488. The variety that causes cold sores is called Type I.

Shingles

The virus infection of a sensory

nerve, accompanied by small, painful blisters that appear on the skin along the path of the nerve—usually on one side of the chest or abdomen—is called *shingles*. The medical name for the disorder, which is caused by the chicken pox virus, is *herpes zoster,* Latin for "girdle of blisters." When a cranial nerve is involved, the blisters appear on the face near the eye. The preliminary symptom is neuritis with severe pain and, sometimes, fever. The blisters may take from two to four weeks to dry up and disappear. Although there is no specific cure, the pain can be alleviated by aspirin. In severe cases, or if the area near the eye is involved, a doctor should be seen.

Warts

These growths are caused by a virus infection of the epidermis. They never become cancerous, but can be painful when found on the soles of the feet. In this location, they are known as *plantar warts,* and they cause discomfort because constant pressure makes them grow inward. Plantar warts are most likely to be picked up by children because they are barefooted so much of the time, and by adults when their feet are moist and they are walking around in showers, near swimming pools, and in locker rooms. Warts can be spread by scratching, by shaving, and by brushing the hair. They are often transmitted from one member of the family to another. Since warts can spread to painful areas, such as the area around or under the fingernails, and since they may become disfiguring, it is best to consult a doctor whenever they appear.

In many ways, warts behave rather mysteriously. About half of them go away without any treatment at all. Sometimes, when warts on one part of the body are being treated, those in another area will disappear. The folklore about "witching" and "charming" warts away has its foundation in fact, since apparently having faith in the cure,

no matter how ridiculous it sounds, sometimes brings success. This form of suggestion therapy is especially successful with children.

There are several more conventional ways of treating warts. Depending on their size and the area involved, electric current, dry ice, or various chemicals may be employed. A doctor should be consulted promptly when warts develop in the area of the beard or on the scalp, since they spread quickly in these parts of the body and thus become more difficult to eliminate.

Sebaceous Cysts

When a sebaceous gland duct is blocked, the oil which the gland secretes cannot get to the surface of the skin. Instead, it accumulates into a hard, round, movable mass contained in a sac. This mass is known as a *sebaceous cyst.* Such cysts may appear on the face, back, ears, or in the genital area. A sebaceous cyst that forms on the scalp is called a *wen,* and may become as large as a billiard ball. The skin in this area will become bald, because the cyst interferes with the blood supply to the hair roots.

Some sebaceous cysts just disappear without treatment. However, those that do not are a likely focus for secondary infection by bacteria, and they may become abscessed and inflamed. It is therefore advisable to have cysts examined by a doctor for possible removal. If such a cyst is superficial, it can be punctured and drained. One that is deeper is usually removed by simple surgical procedure in the doctor's office.

Acne

About 80 percent of all teen-agers suffer from the skin disturbance called *acne.* It is also fairly common among women in their twenties. Acne is a condition in which the skin of the face, and often of the neck, shoulders, chest, and back, is covered to a greater or lesser extent with pimples, blackheads, whiteheads, and boils.

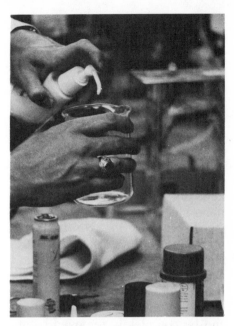

An FDA inspector analyzing commercial cosmetics. The use of such products should be discontinued if they cause irritation.

The typical onset of acne in adolescence is related to the increased activity of the glands, including the sebaceous glands. Most of the oil that they secrete gets to the surface of the skin through ducts that lead into the pores. When the surface pores are clogged with sebaceous gland secretions and keratin, or when so much extra oil is being secreted that it backs up into the ducts, the result is the formation of the skin blemishes characteristic of acne. Dirt or make-up does not cause acne.

The blackheads are dark not because they are dirty, but because the fatty material in the clogged pore is oxidized and discolored by the air that reaches it. When this substance is infected by bacteria, it turns into a pimple. Under no circumstances should such pimples be picked at or squeezed, since the pressure can rupture the surrounding membrane and spread the infection further.

Although a mild case of acne usually clears up by itself, it is often helpful to get the advice of a doctor so that it does not get any worse.

CLEANLINESS: Although surface dirt does not cause acne, it can contribute to its spread. Therefore, the affected areas should be cleansed with a medicated soap and hot water twice a day. Hair should be shampooed frequently and brushed away from the face. Boys who are shaving should soften the beard with soap and hot water. The blade should be sharp and should skim the skin as lightly as possible to avoid nicking pimples.

CREAMS AND COSMETICS: Nonprescription medicated creams and lotions may be effective in reducing some blemishes, but if used too often, they make the skin dry. They should be applied according to the manufacturer's instructions and should be discontinued if they cause additional irritation. If makeup is used, it should have a non-oily base and be completely removed before going to bed.

FORBIDDEN FOODS: Although acne is not caused by any particular food, it can be made worse by a diet overloaded with candy, rich pastries, and fats. Chocolate and cola drinks must be eliminated entirely in some cases.

PROFESSIONAL TREATMENT: A serious case of acne, or even a mild one that is causing serious emotional problems, should receive the attention of a doctor. He may prescribe antibiotics, usually considered the most effective treatment, or recommend sunlamp treatments. He can also be helpful in dealing with the psychological aspects of acne that are so disturbing to teen-agers.

Psoriasis

Psoriasis is a noncontagious chronic condition in which the skin on various parts of the body is marked by bright red patches covered with silvery scales. The areas most often affected are the knees, elbows, scalp, and trunk, and less frequently, the areas under the arms and around the genitals.

The specific cause of psoriasis has not yet been discovered, but it is thought to be an inherited abnormality in which the formation of new skin cells is too rapid and disorderly. In its mild form, psoriasis responds

well to a variety of long-term treatments. When it is acute, the entire skin surface may be painfully red, and large sections of it may scale off. In such cases, prompt hospitalization and intensive care are recommended.

CONDITIONS THAT CAN BRING ON AN OUTBREAK: It has been observed that the onset or aggravation of psoriasis can be triggered by some of the following factors:

• Bruises, burns, scratches, and overexposure to the sun
• Sudden drops in temperature—a mild, stable climate is most beneficial
• Sudden illness from another source, or unusual physical or emotional stress
• Infections of the upper respiratory tract, especially bacterial throat infections and the medicines used to cure them.

TREATMENT: Although there is no specific cure for psoriasis, these are some of the recommended treatments:

• Controlled exposure to sunlight or an ultraviolet lamp
• Creams or lotions of crude coal tar or tar distillates, used alone or in combination with ultraviolet light
• Psoralen and ultraviolet light (PUVA), a combined systemic-external therapy in which a psoralen drug is taken orally before exposure to ultraviolet light
• Systemic drugs, such as methotrexate, which can be taken orally
• Steroid hormone medications applied to the skin surface under dressings.

Pigment Disorders and Birthmarks

The mechanism which controls skin coloration is described above under *Skin Color*. Abnormalities in the creation and distribution of melanin result in the following disorders, some of which are negligible.

Freckles

These are small spots of brown pigment which frequently occur

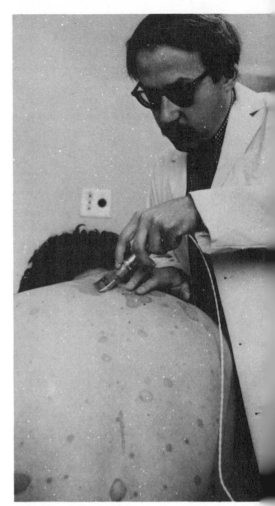

Research techniques involving the removal of tissue from a psoriatic back for study hold out hope for a cure.

when fair-skinned people are exposed to the sun or to ultraviolet light. For those whose skin gets red rather than tan during such exposure, freckles are a protective device. In most cases, they recede in cold weather. A heavy freckle formation that is permanent can be covered somewhat by cosmetic preparations. No attempt should be made to remove freckles with commercial creams or solutions unless supervised by a doctor.

Liver Spots

Flat, smooth, irregularly placed markings on the skin, called *liver spots*, often appear among older people, and result from an increase in pigmentation. They have nothing to do with the liver and are completely harmless. Brownish markings of similar appearance sometimes show up during pregnancy or as a result of irritation or infection. They usually disappear when the underlying cause is eliminated.

Liver spots are permanent, and the principal cause is not aging, but the accumulated years of exposure to sun and wind. They can be disguised and treated in the same way as freckles. A liver spot that becomes hard and thick should be called to the doctor's attention.

Moles

Clusters of melanin cells, called *moles*, may appear singly or in groups at any place on the body. They range in color from light tan to dark brown; they may be raised and hairy or flat and smooth. Many moles are present at birth, and most make their appearance before the age of twenty. They rarely turn into malignancies, and require medical attention only if they become painful, if they itch, or if they suddenly change in size, shape, or color.

There are several ways of removing moles if they are annoying or particularly unattractive. They can be destroyed by the application of an electric needle, by cauterizing, and by surgery. A mole that has been removed is not likely to reappear. The hairs sometimes found in moles can be clipped close to the surface of the skin, or they can be permanently removed. Hair removal often causes the mole to get smaller.

Vitiligo

The condition called *vitiligo* stems from a loss of pigment in sharply defined areas of the skin. There is no known cause for this abnormality of melanin distribution. It may affect any part of the body and may appear any time up to middle age. It is particularly conspicuous when it occurs among blacks, or when a lighter skinned person becomes tanned except around the paler patches. There is no cure for vitiligo, but cosmetic treatment with pastes and lotions can diminish the contrast between affected areas and the rest of the skin.

Birthmarks

About one-third of all infants are born with the type of birthmark called a *hemangioma*, also known as a vascular birthmark. These are caused by a clustering of small blood vessels near the surface of the skin. The mark, which is flat, irregularly shaped, and either pink, red, or purplish, is usually referred to as "port wine stain." There is no known way to remove it, but with cosmetic covering creams, it can usually be successfully masked.

The type of hemangioma which is raised and bright red—called a strawberry mark—spontaneously disappears with no treatment in most cases during early childhood. If a strawberry mark begins to grow rather than fade, or if it begins to ulcerate, a physician should be promptly consulted.

See under *Cancer*, p. 438, for a discussion of skin cancer; see under *Puberty and Growth*, p. 112, for a discussion of adolescent skin problems; see under *Aches, Pains, Nuisances, Worries*, p. 273, for further discussion of minor skin problems.

CHAPTER 10

The Teeth and Gums

Although a human baby is born without teeth, a complete set of 20 *deciduous*, or baby teeth (also called *primary teeth*) already has formed within the gums of the offspring while it still is within the mother's womb. The buds of the permanent or secondary teeth are developing even before the first baby tooth appears at around the age of six months. The baby teeth obviously are formed from foods eaten by the mother. Generally, if the mother follows a good diet during pregnancy, no special food items are required to insure an adequate set of deciduous teeth in the baby.

It takes about two years for the full set of deciduous teeth to appear in the baby's mouth. The first, usually a central incisor at the front of the lower jaw, may erupt any time between the ages of three and nine months. The last probably will be a second molar at the back of the upper jaw. Like walking, talking, and other characteristics of infants, there is no set timetable for the eruption of baby teeth. One child may get his first tooth at three months while another must wait until nine months, but both would be considered within a normal range of tooth development.

The permanent teeth are never far behind the deciduous set. The first permanent tooth usually appears around the age of six years, about four years after the last of the baby teeth has erupted. But the last of the permanent molars, the third molars or *wisdom teeth*, may not break through the gum line until the offspring is an adult.

Types of Teeth

The permanent teeth number thirty-two. In advancing from deciduous to permanent teeth, the human gains six teeth in the lower jaw, or *mandible*, and six in the upper jaw, or *maxilla*, of the mouth. The primary set of teeth includes the following:

UPPER JAW	LOWER JAW
2 central incisors	2 central incisors
2 lateral incisors	2 lateral incisors
2 cuspids	2 cuspids
2 first molars	2 first molars
2 second molars	2 second molars

The permanent set of teeth has an equivalent combination of incisors, cuspids, and first and second molars. But it also includes:

2 first bicuspids	2 first bicuspids
2 second bicuspids	2 second bicuspids
2 third molars	2 third molars

An *incisor* is designed to cut off particles of food, which is then pushed by muscles of the tongue and cheeks to teeth farther back in the mouth for grinding. The front teeth, one on each side, upper and lower, are central incisors. Next to each central incisor is a lateral incisor.

A *cuspid* is so named because it has a spear-shaped crown, or *cusp*. It is designed for tearing as well as cutting. Cuspids sometimes are called *canine teeth* or *eye teeth; canine teeth* owe their name to the use of these teeth by carnivorous animals such as dogs for tearing pieces of meat. There are four cuspids in the mouth, one on the outer side of each lateral incisor in the upper and lower jaws.

Bicuspids sometimes are identified as *premolars*. The term bicuspid suggests two cusps, but a bicuspid may in fact have three cusps. The function of the bicuspids is to crush food passed back from the incisors and cuspids. The permanent set of teeth includes a total of eight bicuspids.

The *molars*, which also number eight and are the last teeth at the

THE STRUCTURE OF A TOOTH

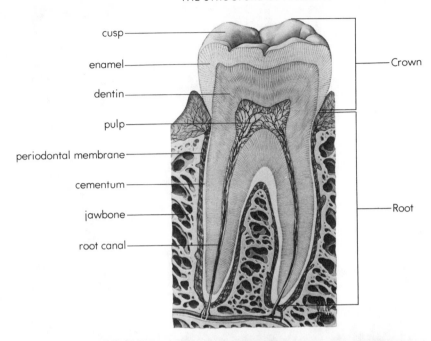

cusp
enamel
dentin
pulp
periodontal membrane
cementum
jawbone
root canal

Crown

Root

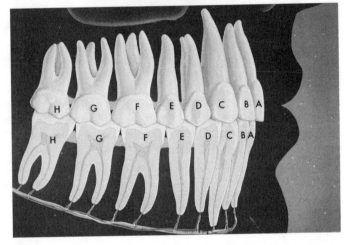

THE ADULT TEETH

A. central incisors
B. lateral incisors
C. cuspids
D. first bicuspids
E. second bicuspids
F. first molars
G. second molars
H. third molars
X. artery, vein, and nerve

back of the mouth, are the largest and strongest teeth, with the job of grinding food. The third molars, or wisdom teeth, are smaller, weaker, and less functional than the first and second molars.

Structure of the Tooth

The variety of shapes of teeth make them specialized for the various functions in preparing food for digestion—biting, chewing, and grinding. All varieties, however, have the same basic structure.

Enamel

The outer covering of the part of the tooth that is exposed above the gum line is *enamel,* the hardest substance in the human body. Enamel is about 97 percent mineral and is as tough as some gemstones. It varies in thickness, with the greatest thickness on the surfaces that are likely to get the most wear and tear.

Enamel begins to form on the first tooth buds of an embryo at the age of about 15 weeks, depending upon substances in the food eaten by the mother for proper development. Once the tooth has formed and erupted through the gum line, there is nothing further that can be done by natural means to improve the condition of the enamel. The enamel

has no blood supply, and any changes in the tooth surface will be the result of wearing, decay, or injury.

While the health and diet of the mother can affect the development of tooth enamel in the deciduous teeth, certain health factors in the early life of a child can result in defective enamel formation of teeth that have not yet erupted. Some infectious or metabolic disorders, for example, may result in enamel pitting.

Dentin

Beneath the enamel surface of a tooth is a layer of hard material—though not as hard as enamel—called *dentin,* which forms the bulk of a tooth. The dentin forms at the same time that enamel is laid down on the surface of a developing tooth, and the portion beneath the crown of the tooth probably is completed at the same time as the enamel. However, the dentin, which is composed of calcified material, is not as dense as the enamel; it is formed as myriad tubules that extend downward into the pulp at the center of the tooth. There is some evidence that dentin formation may continue slowly during the life of the tooth.

Cementum

The *cementum* is a bonelike substance that covers the root of the tooth. Though harder than regular bone, it is softer than dentin. It contains attachments for fibers of a periodontal ligament that holds the tooth in its socket. The periodontal ligament serves as a kind of hammock of fibers that surround and support the tooth at the cementum surface, radiating outward to the jawbone. This arrangement allows the tooth to move a little while still attached to the jaw. For example, when the teeth of the upper and lower jaws are brought together in chewing, the periodontal ligament allows the teeth to sink into their sockets. When the teeth of the two jaws are separated, the hammocklike ligament permits the teeth to float outward again.

Pulp

The cavity within the dentin contains the *pulp*. There is a wide pulp chamber under the crown of the tooth and a pulp canal that extends from the chamber down through the root or roots. Some teeth, such as the molars, may contain as many as three roots, and each of the roots contains a pulp canal.

The pulp of a tooth contains the blood vessels supplying the tooth and the lymphatic system. Although the blood supply arrangement is not the same for every tooth, a typical pattern includes a dental artery entering through each passageway, or *foramen*, leading into the root of a tooth. The artery branches into numerous capillaries within the root canal. A similar system of veins drains the blood from the tooth through each foramen. A lymphatic network and nerve system also enter the tooth through a foramen and spreads through the pulp, as branches from a central distribution link within the jawbone. The nerve fibers have free endings in the tooth, making them sensitive to pain stimuli.

Supporting Structures

The soft, pink gum tissue that surrounds the tooth is called the *gingiva*, and the bone of the jaw that forms the tooth socket is known as *alveolar bone*. The gingiva, alveolar bone, and periodontal ligaments sometimes are grouped into a structural category identified as the *periodontium*. Thus, when a dentist speaks of periodontal disease he is referring to a disorder of these supporting tissues of the teeth. The ailment known as *gingivitis* is an inflammation of the gingiva or gum tissue around the teeth.

Care of the Teeth and Gums

Years ago, loss of teeth really was unavoidable. Today, thanks to modern practices of preventive dentistry,

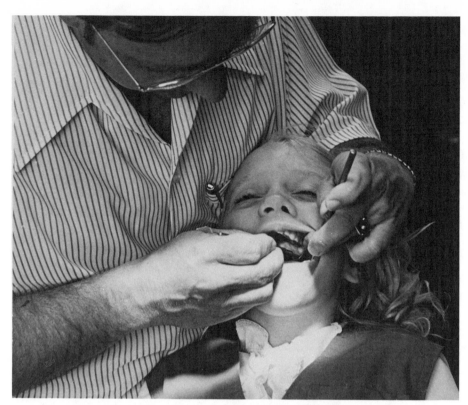

Preventive medicine is the best medicine involving teeth. Dentists recommend regular checkups for everyone, but especially for children.

it is possible for nearly everyone to enjoy the benefits of natural teeth for a lifetime. But natural teeth can be preserved only by daily oral-hygiene habits and regular dental checkups.

The Dental Examination

During the teen years, careful supervision by the dentist and cooperation from the teen-ager are especially necessary. The poor eating habits of many youngsters are reflected in high cavity rates, which may be greater during adolescence than in later life. Neglect of proper dental care also occurs in the middle years when an often-used excuse is that eventual loss of teeth is inevitable. After the permanent teeth are established, the dentist should be visited every six months, or at whatever intervals he recommends for an individual patient who may need more or less care than the typical patient.

The dentist, like the family doctor, usually maintains a general health history of each patient, in addition to a dental health history. He examines each tooth, the gums and other oral tissues, and the *occlusion*, or bite. A complete set of X-ray pictures may be taken on the first visit and again at intervals of perhaps five to seven years. During routine visits, the dentist may take only a couple of X-ray pictures of teeth on either side of the mouth; a complete set of X rays may result in a file of 18 or 20 pictures covering every tooth in the mouth.

X rays constitute a vital part of the dental examination. Without them the dentist cannot examine the surfaces between the teeth or the portion of the tooth beneath the gum, a part that represents about 60 percent of the total length of the tooth. The X rays will reveal the condition of the enamel, dentin, and pulp, as well as any impacted wisdom teeth and the alveolar bone, or tooth sockets. Caps, fillings, abscessed roots, and bone loss due to gum disease also are clearly visible on a set of X rays.

Other diagnostic tests may be made, such as a test of nerve response. Sometimes the dentist will make an impression of the teeth, an accurate and detailed reverse reproduction, in plaster of Paris, plastic impression compound, or other material. Models made from these impressions are used to study the way the teeth meet. Such knowledge is often crucial in deciding the selection of treatment and materials.

After the examination, the dentist will present and explain any proposed treatment. After oral restoration is completed, he will ask the patient to return at regular intervals for a checkup and *prophylaxis*, which includes cleaning and polishing the teeth. Regular checkups and prophylaxis help prevent periodontal diseases affecting the gum tissue and underlying bone. Professional cleaning removes hard deposits that trap bacteria, especially at the gum

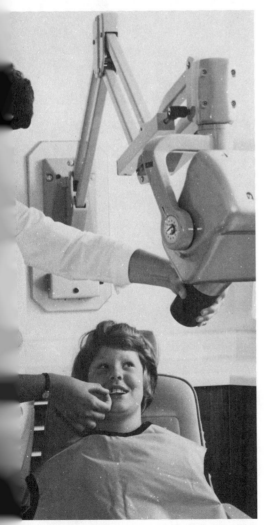

A complete set of X rays helps a dentist determine whether a child's teeth are growing in correct alignment.

line, and polishing removes stains and soft deposits.

Dental Care in Middle Age

Although periodontal (gum) disease and cavities—called *dental caries* by dentists—continue to threaten oral health, two other problems may assume prominence for people of middle age: replacing worn-out restorations, or fillings, and replacing missing teeth. No filling material will last forever. The whitish restorations in front teeth eventually wear away. Silver restorations tend to crack and chip with age because they contract and expand slightly when cold or hot food and drinks come in contact with them. Even gold restorations, the most permanent kind, are subject to decay around the edges, and the decay may spread underneath.

If a needed restoration is not made or a worn-out restoration is not replaced, a deep cavity may result. When the decay reaches the inner layer of the tooth—the dentin—temporary warning twinges of pain may occur. If the tooth still is not restored, the decay will spread into the pulp that fills the inner chamber of the tooth. A toothache can result from inflammation of the pulp, and although the pain may eventually subside, the pulp tissue dies and an abscess can form at the root of the tooth.

Dental Care During Pregnancy

It may be advisable for a pregnant woman to arrange for extra dental checkups. Many changes take place during pregnancy, among them increased hormone production. Some pregnant women develop gingivitis (inflammation of the gums) as an indirect consequence of hormonal changes. A checkup by the dentist during the first three months of pregnancy is needed to assess the oral effects of such changes, and to make sure all dental problems are examined and corrected. Pregnant women should take special care to brush and floss their teeth to minimize these problems.

INFECTION: To avoid the problem of toxic substances or poisons circulating in the mother's bloodstream, all sources of infection must be removed. Some of these sources can be in the mouth. An abscessed tooth, for example, may not be severe enough to signal its presence with pain, but because it is directly connected to the bloodstream it can send toxic substances and bacteria through the mother's body with possible harmful effects to the embryo.

It is during pregnancy that tooth buds for both the deciduous and permanent teeth begin to form in the unborn child. If the mother neglects her diet or general health care during this period, the effects may be seen in the teeth of her child.

What You Can Do: Observing Good Oral Hygiene

FLUORIDATION: Among general rules to follow between dental checkups are using fluorides, maintaining a proper diet, and removing debris from the teeth by brushing and by the use of dental floss. Fluorides are particularly important for strengthening the enamel of teeth in persons under the age of 15. Many communities add fluorides to the water supply, but if the substance is not available in the drinking water, the dentist can advise the patient about other ways of adding fluoride to water or other fluids consumed each day. Studies show that children who drink fluoridated water from birth have up to 65 percent fewer cavities than those who do not drink fluoridated water. However, using excessive amounts of fluoride in the drinking water can result in mottled enamel.

DIET: Although a good diet for total health should provide all of the elements needed for dental health, several precautions on sugars and starches should be added. Hard or sticky sweets should be avoided. Such highly refined sweets as soft drinks, candies, cakes, cookies, pies, syrups, jams, jellies, and pastries should be limited, especially between meals. One's intake of starchy foods, such as bread, potatoes, and pastas, should also be controlled. Natural sugars contained in fresh fruits can provide sweet flavors with less risk of contributing to decay if the teeth are brushed regularly after eating such foods. Regular chewing gum may help remove food particles after eating, but it deposits sugar; if you chew gum, use sugarless gum.

Since decay is promoted each time sugars and other refined carbohydrates are eaten, between-meals snacks of sweets should be curtailed in order to lessen the chances of new or additional caries. Snack foods can be raw vegetables, such as carrots or celery, apples, cheese, peanuts, or other items that are not likely to introduce refined carbohydrates into the mouth between meals.

BRUSHING: Brushing the teeth is an essential of personal oral hygiene. Such brushing rids the mouth of most of the food debris that encourages bacterial growth, which is most intense twenty minutes after eating. Therefore, the teeth should be

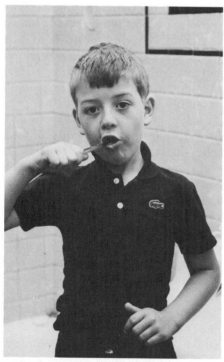

A good tooth-brushing should hit the top, front, and inside of each and every tooth and should also include the area where the gums meet the teeth.

cleaned as soon as possible after a meal.

There is no one kind of toothbrush that is best for every person. Most dentists, however, recommend a soft toothbrush with a straight handle and flat brushing surface that can clean the gums without irritating them. As for claims about whether toothbrushes should have bristles with square corners or rounded shapes, a dentist may point out that there are both curved and straight surfaces in the mouth so what one design offers in advantages may be offset by equivalent disadvantages. There also are special brushes for reaching surfaces of crooked teeth or cleaning missing-tooth areas of the mouth.

Although several different methods may be used effectively, the following is the technique most often recommended. Brush the biting surfaces, or tops, of the back upper and lower teeth. The lines and grooves on these surfaces make them prone to decay. They should be brushed first, before moisture has softened the brush. The cheek and tongue surfaces of the lower teeth are brushed next. Hold the brush parallel to the teeth with the bristle edges angled against and touching the gums. Using short strokes, move the brush back and forth several times before proceeding to the next one or two teeth. Use the same technique on all the inner surfaces of your teeth as well. For the hard-to-brush inner surfaces of the front teeth, hold the handle of the brush out in front of the mouth and apply the tip in an up-and-down motion. For all brushing, a scrubbing motion —but without too much pressure— should be used.

Some people prefer electric toothbrushes, which require less effort to use than ordinary toothbrushes. These are available with two basic motions—up-and-down and back-and-forth. Your dentist may advise which kind best serves an individual needs and proper use of equipment. Some dentists point out that back-

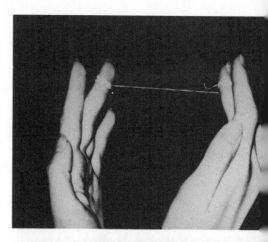

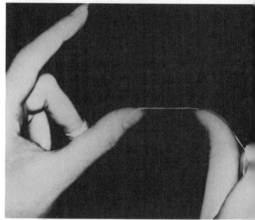

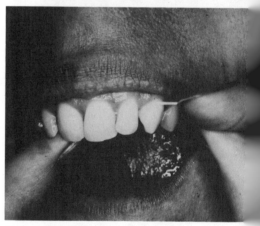

How to use dental floss: (top) wrap ends of floss several times around middle fingers; (middle) hold center part of floss between thumbs; (bottom) insert floss between teeth and work back and forth gently.

and-forth brushing applied with too much pressure can have an abrasive effect on tooth enamel because it works against the grain of the mineral deposits. The American Dental Association also evaluates electric toothbrushes and issues reports on the safety and effectiveness of various types.

REMOVING DEBRIS WITH DENTAL FLOSS: Brushing often does not clean debris from between the teeth. But plaque and food particles that stick between the teeth usually can be removed with dental floss. A generous length of floss, about 18 inches, is needed to do an effective job. The ends can be wrapped several times around the first joint of the middle finger of each hand. Using the thumbs or index fingers, the floss is inserted between the teeth with a gentle, sawing, back-and-forth motion. Then it is slid gently around part of a tooth in the space at the gum line and gently pulled out; snapping the floss in and out may irritate the gums. After brushing and flossing, the mouth should be rinsed with water. A mouthwash is unnecessary, but it may be used for the good taste it leaves in the mouth.

The dentist may recommend the use of an oral irrigating device as part of dental home care. These units produce a pulsating stream of water that flushes food debris from between teeth. They are particularly useful for patients wearing orthodontic braces or for those who have had recession of the gums, creating larger spaces between the teeth.

The person who wants to see the areas of plaque on his teeth can chew a *disclosing tablet*, available at most pharmacies, which leaves a harmless temporary stain on plaque surfaces. Some dentists recommend the use of disclosing tablets about once a week so that patients can check on the effectiveness of their tooth cleaning techniques.

TOOTH DECAY

In addition to wear, tear, and injury, the major threat to the health of a tooth is bacteria. Bacteria can cause tooth decay, and the human mouth is a tremendous reservoir of bacteria because the mouth is warm, dark, moist, and usually contains tiny particles of food which help nourish the organisms. The bacteria found in the mouth are of two kinds, *aerobic* and *anaerobic*. Aerobic bacteria need oxygen to survive; anaerobic bacteria do not. Anaerobic bacteria can find their way through cracks and crevices into areas of the mouth or teeth where there is little or no oxygen and continue their *cariogenic*, or decay, activity.

Saliva

Saliva offers some protection against the decay germs, for reasons not well understood, but there are crevices and deep pockets around the teeth and gums where saliva does not penetrate. Paradoxically, saliva itself contains millions of different bacterial organisms. Dental scientists have calculated that one ounce of saliva may contain as many as 22 billion bacteria. Even a presumably healthy mouth may contain more than ten varieties of bacteria, plus protozoa and yeast cells. The yeast cells and at least three of the different kinds of bacteria are capable of producing acids that erode the tough enamel surface of a tooth.

Bacterial Acids and Plaque

The acids produced by decay bacteria actually are waste products of the organisms' digestive processes; bacteria, like other living creatures, eventually excrete waste products after a meal. As unpleasant as the thought may be, tooth decay can be the result of feeding a colony of germs in the mouth. Bacterial growth—hence the production of harmful acids—is encouraged by the consumption of too many foods composed of refined sugars. The sugars of candies, cakes, soft drinks, and the like are easier for the bacteria to eat and digest than those of fruits, vegetables, and other less thoroughly processed foods. Even a tiny bit of food remaining in the mouth after a meal may be enough to support many millions of bacteria for 24 hours or more.

An additional contributing factor to tooth decay is *plaque* formation. Plaque is a sticky, transparent substance that forms a film over the surface of the teeth. Plaque forms every day, which is the reason that the teeth must be brushed every day. Plaque frequently begins with deposits of soft food debris along the gum line after a meal; it consists mainly of bacteria and its products. When mixed with mucus, molds, tissue cells from the membranes lining the mouth, and mineral salts, it takes the form of a white, cheesy substance called *materia alba*. If not removed regularly by brushing and the use of dental floss, this substance becomes a thick, sticky mass which has been compared to epoxy cement. Then it becomes a rough-surfaced hard substance with the texture of stone, otherwise known as *dental calculus*, or *tartar*.

Other Causes of Decay

Bacterial acid is not the only way in which the tooth enamel may be damaged to permit the entry of decay bacteria. Certain high acid foods and improper dental care can erode the molecules of enamel. Temperature extremes also can produce cracks and other damage to the enamel; some dental scientists have suggested that repeated exposure to rapid temperature fluctuations of 50°F., as in eating alternately hot and cold foods or beverages, can cause the enamel to develop cracks.

Complications of Tooth Decay

Once decay activity breaks through the hard enamel surface, the bacteria can attack the dentin. Since the dentin is about 30 percent organic material, compared to 5 percent in the enamel layer, the decay process can advance more rapidly there. If the tooth decay is not stopped at the dentin layer, the disease organisms can enter the pulp chamber where they will multiply quickly, producing an acute inflammation and, if unchecked, spread through the blood vessels to other parts of the body. Osteomyelitis, an infection of the membrane covering the skeletal bones, and endocarditis, an extremely dangerous heart ailment, are among diseases in other parts of the body that can begin with untreated tooth decay.

Periodontal disease, described below, is another possible complication of tooth decay.

Treatment of Tooth Decay

The portion of a tooth invaded by decay is called a *cavity;* it may be compared to an ulcer that develops because of disease in soft tissues. In treating the decay process, the dentist tries to prevent further destruction of the tooth tissue. The dentist also tries to restore as much as possible the original shape and function of the diseased tooth. The procedure used depends on many factors, including the surfaces affected (enamel, dentin, etc.) and the tooth face and angle involved as well as whether the cavity is on a smooth area or in a pit or fissure of the tooth surface.

The decayed portions of the tooth are removed with various kinds of carbide burrs and other drill tips as well as with hand instruments. The dentist may also use a caries removal system that reduces or eliminates drilling. In this system two solutions are combined in one liquid and squirted in a pulsating stream onto the decayed area. The stream does not harm gums or healthy teeth;

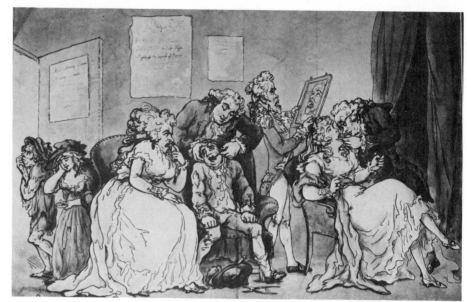

"The Transplanting of Teeth," an early painting, portrays the shambles of a dentist's office before licensing requirements were introduced.

rather, it softens the caries so that it can easily be scraped away. Used, generally, in conjunction with rotary or hand instruments, the "squirt" system may make anesthesia unnecessary.

In other cases an anesthetic may be injected for the comfort of the patient. The dentist usually asks whether the patient prefers to have an anesthetic before work commences. In the cleaning process, an effort is made to remove all traces of diseased enamel or dentin, but no more of the tooth material than is necessary.

The cleaned cavity is generally filled in a layering procedure. The layers of liners and bases used before insertion of the filling are determined by the depth of the cavity and other factors. If pulp is exposed, special materials may be applied to help the pulp recover from the irritation of the procedure and to form a firm base for the amalgam, inlay, or other restorative substance that becomes the filling.

In the 1980s, new ceramic materials came into use for fillings. Many dentists believed that ceramics could provide more natural-looking restorations. With ceramics, also, teeth would be less sensitive to changes of temperature—a problem with some more traditional materials.

Tooth Extraction

When it becomes necessary to remove a diseased, damaged, or malpositioned tooth, the procedure is handled as a form of minor surgery, usually with administration of a local anesthetic to the nerves supplying the tooth area. However, there is no standard routine for extraction of a tooth because of the numerous individual variations associated with each case. The dentist usually has a medical history of the patient available, showing such information as allergies to drugs, and medications used by the patient which might react with those employed in oral surgery. Because the mouth contains many millions of bacteria, all possible precautions are taken to prevent entry of the germs into the tooth socket.

The condition of the patient is checked during and immediately after tooth extraction, in the event that some complication develops. The patient is provided with analgesic (pain-killing) and other needed medications along with instructions regarding control of any postoperative pain or bleeding. The dentist also may offer special diet information with suggested meals for the recovery period, which usually is quite brief.

DRY SOCKET: Severe pain may develop several days after a tooth has been extracted if a blood clot that forms in the socket becomes dislodged. The condition, commonly called *dry socket*, can involve infection of the alveolar bone that normally surrounds the roots of the tooth; loss of the clot can expose the bone tissue to the environment and organisms that produce *osteitis*, or inflammation of the bone tissue. Dry socket may be treated by irrigating the socket with warm salt water and packing it with strips of medicated gauze. The patient also is given analgesics, sedatives, and other medications as needed to control the pain and infection.

General anesthetics are sometimes necessary for complicated oral surgery. In such cases, there are available dental offices or clinics that are as well equipped and staffed as hospital operating rooms.

Endodontic Therapy

Tooth extraction because of caries is less common today than in previous years, although an estimated 25 million Americans have had all of their teeth removed. Modern preventive dentistry techniques of *endodontics* now make it possible to save many teeth that would have been extracted in past decades after the spread of decay into the pulp canal. The procedures include *root canal therapy*, *pulp capping*, and *pulpotomy*.

ROOT CANAL THERAPY: Once the tooth has fully developed in the jaw, the nerve is not needed, so if the pulp is infected the nerve as well as the pulp can be removed. Only minor effects are noticeable in the tooth structure after the pulp is removed, and the dentist compensates for these in filling the tooth after root canal therapy.

Briefly, the procedure of root canal work begins by examination and testing of the pulp viability. The pulp may be tested by heat, cold, or by an electrical device called a *vitalometer*, which measure the degree of sensation the patient feels in a tooth. If the pulp is dead, the patient will feel no sensation, even at the highest output of current.

After the degree of vitality in the pulp has been determined, a local anesthetic is injected and the dentist begins removing the pulp, using rotary drills and hand instruments. By means of X-ray pictures, the dentist measures the length of the root, which may be about one and a half times the length of the crown. Stops or other markers are placed on the root excavation tools to show the dentist when the instrument has reached the end of the root. The canal is then sterilized and filled with gutta-percha—a tough plastic substance—silver, or a combination of the two, and a cap is added.

PULP CAPPING: Pulp capping consists of building a cap over the exposed pulp with layers of calcium hydroxide paste, which is covered by zinc oxide and topped with a firm cement.

PULPOTOMY: A pulpotomy procedure involves removal of the pulp in the pulp chamber within the crown of the tooth, while leaving the root-canal pulp in place. The amputated pulp ends are treated and a pulp capping procedure is used to restore the crown of the tooth.

PERIODONTAL DISEASE

It is important in the middle years of life and later to continue good oral-hygiene habits and the practice of having regular dental checkups. Studies have found that after the age of 50 more than half the people in America have periodontal disease. At the age of 65, nearly everybody has this disease.

The Course of the Disease

The combination of bacterial action described above and the roughness of the resulting calculus injures the surrounding gum tissue and makes it susceptible to infection and recession. The irritation causes swelling, inflammation, and bleeding into the crevices between the teeth and gums, which is one of the early signs of impaired tissue health.

The inflammation of the gums, known as *gingivitis*, can spread to the roots of the teeth if not treated. The gums separate from the teeth, forming pockets that fill up with more food particles and colonies of bacteria. As the disease progresses, the bone support for the teeth is weakened and the affected teeth begin to loosen and drift from their normal position. Finally, unless the disease is treated in time, the teeth may be lost.

Periodontal disease is sometimes called *pyorrhea*, a Greek word meaning a discharge of pus. But pyorrhea is a somewhat misleading term because it identifies only one manifestation of the disease, an abscess that usually forms along the side of an affected tooth. In some cases, a membrane forms around the abscess, creating a pus-filled cyst in the tooth socket.

Other Signs and Complications

Another manifestation of periodontal disease is periodontal atrophy, or recession of the gingiva, or gum tissue, and the underlying bone away from the outer layer of the tooth that joins it to its socket. Recession tends to expose the dentin below the gum line, which is not pro-

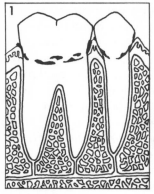
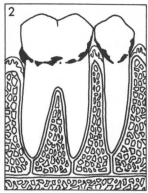
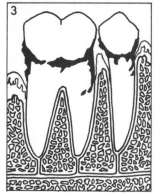
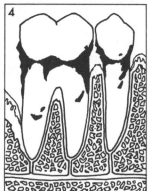
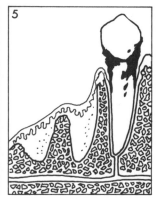

Periodontal diseases are often caused by neglect. *(1 and 2)* Plaque and calculus deposits accumulate. *(3)* The irritated, swollen gums bleed easily and have begun to retract. *(4)* Most of the bony support for the teeth has been destroyed. *(5)* One tooth is lost; another weakened.

tected by a layer of enamel. The exposed dentin may be hypersensitive to hot or cold foods or beverages, air, and sweet or sour food flavors.

Inflammation of the gingival tissue in periodontal disease may be increased in intensity by toxic chemicals from tobacco smoke, bacterial infections, vitamin deficiencies, and defective dental restorations. The normal pink color of the gingival tissue may be altered by periodontal disease to a bright red or a darker coloration ranging to bluish purple.

The inflamed gingival tissue may lead to a complication called *periodontitis* in which the bone under the gum tissue is gradually destroyed, widening the crevice between the tooth and surrounding tissues. Pregnant women seem particularly vulnerable to periodontitis and gingivitis if they have been experiencing periodontal disorders, because the temporary hormonal imbalance of the pregnancy tends to exaggerate the effects of this condition.

One kind of gingivitis that involves projections of gum tissue between the teeth is sometimes referred to as *trench mouth*, because it was not an uncommon form of periodontal disease affecting soldiers during World War I. The infection is associated with poor oral hygiene along with nutritional deficiencies and general depressed condition of health.

Causes

At one time it was assumed that periodontal diseases were associated with the life styles of persons living in more technologically advanced societies, where soft, rich foods are eaten regularly, providing materials toward the formation of plaque and support of bacteria in the plaque. But recent investigations show that people living in the less developed nations, who are relatively free of tooth decay, eventually develop periodontal disease. However, this does not alter the fact that the accumulation of plaque and harmful bacteria are the chief cause of periodontal disease as well as of tooth decay.

Although periodontal disease generally becomes troublesome in middle age, there is some evidence that early symptoms of gingival disorders occur during childhood or adolescence. Also, because more people live longer today, periodontal disease has become more common than in the past.

BRUXISM: *Bruxism*—the nervous habit, often unconsciously done, of clenching and grinding the teeth—can contribute to the development of periodontal disease. Bruxism frequently occurs during sleep.

MALOCCLUSION: Another contributing cause to periodontal disease is repeated shock or undue pressure on a tooth because of *malocclusion,* or an improper bite. This effect accelerates damage to the tooth and gum structure during such simple activities as biting and chewing.

Treatment

Periodontal treatment may include a variety of techniques ranging from plaque removal to oral surgery

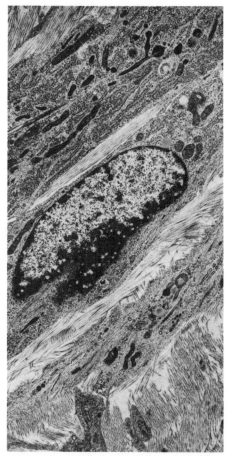

The periodontal ligaments, shown here in an electron micrograph, anchor the teeth in the sockets, allowing a slight amount of movement.

to form new contours on the alveolar bone surrounding the tooth. If treatment is not begun until periodontal disease is well advanced, it may be difficult to fit replacement teeth, or *dentures*, as substitutes for lost teeth. Dentures fit over the ridges of the jaws, and if the top edge of the ridge has been destroyed by periodontal disease, the procedure for holding the denture firmly in place will be complicated.

DENTURES

If it becomes necessary to have some teeth removed, they should be replaced as soon as possible with a *bridge*—a mounting for false teeth anchored to natural teeth on either side—or a partial or full denture.

Why Missing Teeth Must Be Replaced

Chewing ability and clarity of speech may be impaired if missing teeth are not replaced. Also, each tooth functions to hold the teeth on either side and opposite it in place. If a tooth is lost, the tooth opposite may erupt further and the teeth on either side shift in their positions because there is no counterforce to keep them in place. Food particles lodge in the spaces created by the shifting teeth, plaque forms, and periodontal disease develops, causing the loss of additional teeth. This loss may take years if the movement of intact teeth is slow, but if they tilt and shift rapidly into the empty spaces, the remaining teeth may be lost in a much shorter time.

The loss of a few teeth can also alter a person's appearance. The cheeks may become puckered and the lips drawn together, making the individual look older than he is.

Fitting of Dentures

Modern techniques and materials of construction and the skill of modern dentists should assure well-fitting, natural-looking dentures. The dentist selects the tooth shade and shape that are best for an individual's face size, contours, and coloring. No one, however, has perfectly arranged, perfectly white natural teeth. Tooth coloring depends upon genetic factors and changes as one grows older. These factors must be considered in designing dentures.

Bridges and Partial Dentures

Several different types of dental appliances may be constructed to fill empty spaces. Some, such as dental bridges, may be attached to the remaining natural teeth by cementing them. Others, such as complete sets of dentures, are removable.

A bridge may be made entirely of gold, a combination of gold and porcelain, or combinations of gold and porcelain and other materials. If there is a sound natural tooth on either side of the space, a *pontic*, or suitable substitute for the missing tooth, may be fused to the metal bridge. The crown retainer on either side of the pontic may then be cemented to the crowns of the neighboring natural teeth.

If there are no natural teeth near the space created by an extracted tooth, a partial denture may be constructed to replace the missing teeth. This appliance usually fastens by a clasp onto the last tooth on each side of the space. A bar on the inside of the front teeth provides stability for the partial denture.

A "Maryland bridge," a fixed partial denture developed by the University of Maryland's Baltimore College of Dental Surgery, eliminates the need for crowns to anchor false teeth. With the Maryland bridge, hidden metal "wings" are used to anchor the partial denture. The wings are bonded to the backs of neighboring teeth. Because it eliminates the need for drilling, the Maryland bridge saves healthy teeth, makes anesthesia unnecessary, and reduces costs considerably.

New materials have brought bonding into more common use as an alternative to crowning and for cosmetically restoring chipped, malformed, stained, or widely spaced teeth. In the bonding process the dentist isolates a tooth with a rubber dam, cleans and dries the tooth, and applies a phosphoric acid solution that produces microscopic pores in the enamel. The etched area is then filled in with a liquid plastic. To that base the dentist applies thin layers of tooth-colored plastics known as composite resins. The layers can be sculpted, hardened with a beam of light or by some other method, contoured, and polished.

A removable partial denture should be taken out and cleaned whenever the natural teeth are brushed. A special brush, usually cone-shaped to fit into the clasp, is available as a cleaning tool. The pontic, or tooth substitute of a bridge, remains in place permanently and is brushed like a natural tooth.

A bridge or partial denture helps prevent further deterioration of the mouth if it is kept clean and in good condition. But a dentist should check bridges and partial dentures periodically to make sure they have not become loosened. A loose clasp of a partial denture can rock the teeth to which the device is attached, causing damage and possible loss.

Complete Dentures

Although dentures do not change with age, the mouth does. Therefore, it is necessary for the denture-wearer to have occasional dental checkups. At denture checkup appointments, the dentist examines oral tissues for irritation and determines how the dentures fit with respect to possible changing conditions of the mouth. If the dentures no longer fit properly, a replacement may be recommended. The dentist also seeks to correct any irritations of the oral tissues of the mouth and polishes the dentures, making them smooth and easier to keep clean between checkups. If any of the teeth in the dentures has become damaged, the dentist can repair or replace the denture tooth.

Care of Dentures

Dentures should be cleaned daily with a denture brush and toothpaste; once a week they should be soaked for seven or eight hours in a denture cleaner. To avoid breaking them during the brushing process, fill a wash basin with water and place it under the dentures while they are being cleaned; if they are dropped, the dentures will be cushioned by the water. A harsh abrasive that could scratch the denture surface should not be used. Scratches allow stains to penetrate the surface of the dentures, creating permanent discoloration.

The use of adhesives and powders is only a temporary solution to ill-fitting dentures. In time, the dentist may rebuild the gum side of the denture to conform with the shape of the patient's gum ridge. The patient should never try to make his own changes in the fit of dentures. Rebuilding the gum side of the dentures, or *relining*, as it is called, usually begins with a soft temporary material if the patient's gums are in poor condition, and requires several appointments over a period of two or three weeks while the gum tissues are being restored to good health.

Most patients show some concern over the replacement of natural teeth with dentures, even when a set of complete dentures is needed to replace an earlier set. Some people associate the loss of teeth with old age in the same way that others resist the advice that they should wear eyeglasses or a hearing aid. The fact is that many millions of persons of all ages have found they can improve their eating, speaking, and physical appearance by obtaining attractive and well-fitted dentures.

Before a full set of removable dentures is constructed, the dentist will take Xrays to determine whether there are any abnormalities in the gum ridges, such as cysts or tooth

root tips that may have to be removed. If the gums are in poor condition, treatments may be needed to improve the surfaces of the ridges on which the dentures will be fitted. The dentist may also have to reconstruct the bone underlying the gums —the alveolar ridge. Human bone "harvested" from another part of the patient's body has for decades been used in such reconstruction, but is today giving way to ceramic materials.

Two ceramic materials used in such surgery are hydroxylapatite and beta tricalcium phosphate. Oral surgeons have reported good results with both. The new materials are said to be safer and simpler to use and less expensive than human bone. They also eliminate the need for preliminary surgery to obtain transplants of the patient's bone.

With preliminary work done, the dentist makes an impression of the patient's mouth. Tooth and shade choices are discussed. Several other appointments may be arranged before the new dentures are delivered to the patient. Appointments may be needed for "try-ins" of dentures as they are being constructed and for adjustments after completion of the set.

ORTHODONTICS

Orthodontics is a term derived from the Greek words for straight, or normal, teeth. Straight teeth are easier to keep clean and they make chewing food more efficient. There also is a cosmetic benefit in being able to display a smile with a set of straight teeth, although many dentists consider the cosmetic aspect of orthodontics as secondary to achieving proper occlusion, or bite.

Causes of Improper Bite

The causes of orthodontic problems can be hereditary or due to an infectious or other kind of disease, to the premature loss of primary teeth, to the medications used in treatment, or to individual factors such as injury or loss of permanent teeth. A person may have congenitally missing teeth resulting in spaces that permit drifting of neighboring teeth or collapse of the dental arch. Or he

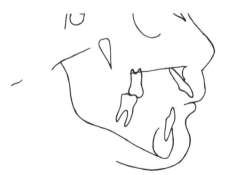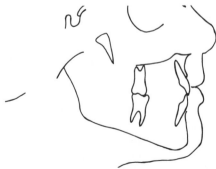

These drawings illustrate a malocclusion *(left)* in which the upper arch is too far forward and the front incisors do not meet. *(Right)* After orthodontic treatment, the molars and incisors have been brought into proper alignment. Note the improved physical appearance.

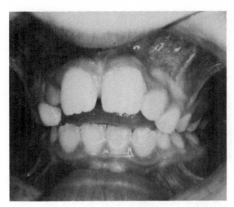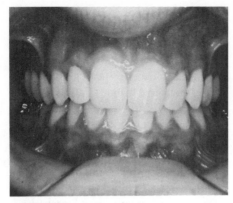

(Left) An open bite, in which the upper and lower incisors do not meet. *(Right)* The same patient after orthodontic correction.

may develop extra (supernumerary) teeth due to an inherited factor. The supernumerary teeth may develop during the early years of life while the deciduous teeth are in use. A supernumerary tooth may force permanent teeth into unnatural positions.

Nutritional disorders can also affect the development of jaws and teeth, while certain medications can cause abnormal growth of gingival, or gum, tissues, resulting in increased spaces between the teeth.

Teeth that erupt too early or too late, primary teeth that are too late in falling out when permanent teeth have developed, and habits such as grinding of the teeth, thumb-sucking, or pushing the tongue against the teeth are among other factors that can result in *malocclusion,* or improper bite, and the need for orthodontic treatment.

Diagnosis of Orthodontic Problems

Each child should visit a dentist before the eruption of his permanent teeth for an examination that may determine the need for orthodontic treatment. Since there are many genetic and other influences that help shape the facial contours and occlusion of each individual, there are no standard orthodontic procedures that apply to any or all children. The dentist may recommend what treatment, if any, would be needed to produce normal occlusion and when it should begin; some dentists advise only that necessary pro-

cedures for correcting malocclusion be started before the permanent set of teeth (excluding wisdom teeth) has become established, or around the age of 12 or 13. However, there are few age limits for orthodontic care, and an increasing number of adults are receiving treatment today for malocclusion problems that were neglected during childhood.

In the normal or ideal occlusion

positions of the teeth, the first and second permanent upper molars fit just slightly behind the same molars of the lower jaw; all of the teeth of the upper jaw are in contact with their counterparts of the lower jaw. In this pattern of occlusion, all of the biting surfaces are aligned for optimum use of their intended functions of cutting, tearing, or grinding.

There are numerous variations of malocclusion but generally, in simple deformities, the teeth of the upper jaw are in contact with lower jaw teeth once removed from normal positions. Other variations include an *open bite,* in which the upper and lower incisors do not contact each other, or *closed bite,* in which there is an abnormal degree of overlapping *(overbite)* of the front teeth.

Diagnosis is made with the help of X-ray pictures, photographs of the face and mouth, medical histories, and plaster models of the patient's teeth and jaws. The plaster models are particularly important because

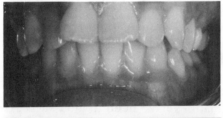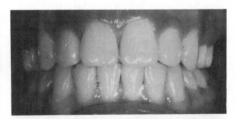

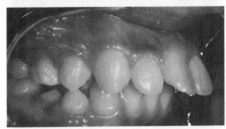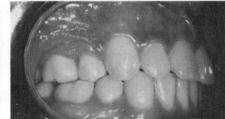

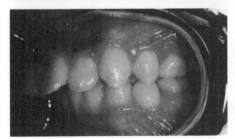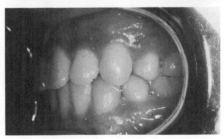

The photographs demonstrate the orthodontic correction of one patient's closed bite, in which the front teeth overlap the bottom abnormally. Each pair of pictures shows the teeth from a particular angle before and after correction. The pictures at the right were taken about 28 months after those on the left.

the dentist can use them to make experimental reconstructions without touching an actual tooth of a patient. For example, the dentist can remove one or more teeth from the plaster model and reorganize neighboring teeth in the jaw bones to get an accurate representation of the effects of extracting teeth or forcing teeth into different developmental situations.

Orthodontic Appliances

Once a plan of orthodontic treatment has been determined by the dentist, he may choose from a dozen or more types of bands, braces, or other orthodontic appliances, some removable and some nonremovable, for shaping the teeth and jaws of the patient. A typical orthodontic appliance may include small curved strips or loops of metal cemented to the surfaces of the teeth as anchors for arch wires which pass around the dental arch. Springs and specially designed rubber bands, called elastics, are sometimes used to bring about alignment of the two jaws, or to align teeth within a dental arch.

In addition to the appliances that are attached to and between the upper and lower dental arches, the dentist may prescribe the use of an elastic tape device with a strap that fits around the back of the patient's neck and is attached also to the arch wire inside the mouth, thus providing a force from outside the mouth to bring teeth into alignment.

Orthodontic appliances are custom-designed and built for the individual patient. This requires several rather long sessions or one all-day session in the dental chair while the appliance is being organized and properly anchored. Thereafter, the patient must return at regular intervals spaced a few weeks to a month apart so the dentist can make adjustments in the appliance, determine if any of the bands have pulled away from tooth surfaces, and prevent plaque from building up in places that the braces may make impervious to brushing.

The patient, meanwhile, must follow a diet that prohibits sticky foods or items that may damage the appliance or any of its parts. A conscientious program of oral hygiene including regular cleaning by the dentist or hygienist, also is necessary because, as indicated above, it is more difficult to do a thorough job of cleaning the teeth when orthodontic appliances are in the mouth.

Orthodontics for Adults

Although orthodontic treatment originally was applied only to children, the technique has been requested with increasing frequency for the correction of a variety of facial and dental disorders. Receding chins, buck teeth, sunken cheeks, sunken mouths, and other abnormalities have been treated successfully in adults beyond the age of 40. Orthodontists have observed that adult patients usually are more patient and cooperative during the long periods of treatment than youngsters.

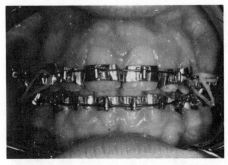

In this orthodontic appliance, arch wires are held in place by metal bands cemented to the surface of the teeth.

The upper age limit for orthodontic work has not really been established, but doctors at the National Institute of Dental Research believe it is possible to treat adult patients with protrusion of the upper jaw and related disfigurements until the age of 70. This is possible because the upper jaw does not completely unite with the frontal bone of the skull, according to the experts, until after the age of 70 in most people.

Orthodontic treatments can be relatively expensive and involve many visits to a dentist's office over a long period of time. Any parent of a prospective patient or a responsible older patient seeking orthodontic work for himself should have a frank discussion with the dentist regarding the time and money to be invested in the corrective procedures before making an agreement to begin the work. In nearly every case some arrangement can be made for covering the costs of dental work that is vital to the health and welfare of a patient.

CHAPTER 11

Aches, Pains, Nuisances, Worries

And Other Things You Can Live With But Could Get Along Very Well Without

None of the variety of discomforts discussed in this chapter is a laughing matter. The best thing about most of them is that they will pass, given your common-sense attention, or will disappear if you follow your doctor's advice. This includes taking the medications prescribed by your doctor exactly as directed. In a few cases, such as allergies or gout, long-term drug therapy may be necessary on a self-supervised basis, once treatment has been established by a doctor. Of course, when symptoms of any kind persist or get worse, you should waste no time in seeking a professional diagnosis.

There may be somebody, somewhere, who has never felt rotten a day in his life. But most of us are not so fortunate. Among the most common nuisance ailments are:

- Upper respiratory infections
- Allergies
- Occasional headaches
- Backaches
- Weight problems
- Weather discomforts
- Disturbances of normal sleep patterns
- Aching feet
- Indigestion.

The unpleasant feeling associated with any of these common disorders can almost always be banished with a modicum of care and thought. For example, allergic reactions to particular foods can be avoided by identifying the offending food and avoiding it. Self-diagnosis and self-discipline can often cope with weight problems. A backache may be cured by attention to posture, or adjusting your office chair. A sensible approach to clothing and exposure can often do away with weather discomforts.

But when symptoms do not respond to self-help—as when sporadic difficulty in sleeping burgeons into a string of near-sleepless nights, or when abdominal pain you interpret as indigestion is intense or frequent in spite of avoiding rich or heavy foods, it's time to see a doctor.

The Common Cold and Upper Respiratory Infections

Common cold is the label attached to a group of symptoms that can be caused by one or more of some 20 different viruses. Colds are considered highly contagious, but some doctors think that people don't entirely catch others' colds—in a sense they catch their own. While the viruses that carry the infection are airborne and practically omnipresent, somebody in good health is usually less susceptible to a cold than someone who is run down. Both environmental factors (such as air pollution) and emotional ones (such as anxiety or depression) seem to increase susceptibility.

SYMPTOMS: Symptoms differ from person to person and from cold to cold with the same person. Generally, a cold starts with sneezes, a running nose, teary eyes, and a stuffed head. Sometimes the nasal membranes become so swollen that a person can breathe only through the mouth; sometimes the senses of smell and taste simply disappear. The throat may be sore; a postnasal drip may cause a constant cough when the person is lying down at night.

When these symptoms are acute and are accompanied by fever and aching joints, the illness is usually referred to as influenza or "the flu." There are many different viruses that cause influenza, and new ones are always turning up. Unfortunately, there is as yet no medicine that can cure either a cold or a flu attack, although many people do get relief from symptoms by taking various cold remedies. Antibiotics are sometimes prescribed by doctors to prevent more serious bacterial diseases, such as pneumonia, from developing, but antibiotics are not effective against the cold viruses.

TREATMENT: Some people can get

265

away with treating a cold with contempt and an occasional aspirin, and go about their business. Others are laid low for a few days. If you are the type who is really hit hard by a cold, it isn't coddling yourself to stay home for a couple of days. In any event, a simple cold usually runs its course, lasting anywhere from a few days to two weeks.

Discomfort can be minimized and recovery speeded by a few simple steps: extra rest and sleep, drinking more liquids than usual, and taking one or two aspirin tablets every four hours. Antihistamine preparations or nose drops should be avoided unless specifically prescribed by a physician.

A painful sore throat accompanied by fever, earache, a dry hacking cough, or pains in the chest are symptoms that should be brought to the attention of a physician.

PREVENTION: Although taking massive doses of vitamin C at the first sign of a cold is said by some authorities to prevent the infection from developing, there is not yet general agreement on the effectiveness of this treatment.

Actually, there are several common-sense ways of reducing the risk of infection, particularly for those people who are especially susceptible to catching a cold. For most people, getting a proper amount of sleep, eating sensibly, avoiding exposure to sudden chill, trying to stay out of crowds, and trying to keep emotional tensions under control can increase resistance to colds and other minor respiratory infections.

Inoculation against particular types of viruses is recommended by many physicians in special cases: for pregnant women, for the elderly, and for those people who have certain chronic heart and lung diseases. Flu shots are effective against a particular virus or viruses for a limited period.

Allergies

Discomforts of various kinds are considered allergies when they are brought on by substances or conditions that ordinarily are harmless. Not too long ago, perturbed allergy sufferers would say things like:

"I can't use that soap because it gives me hives."

"Smelling roses makes me sneeze."

"Eating almonds gives me diarrhea."

Nowadays, such complaints are commonly recognized as allergies.

SYMPTOMS: Allergic symptoms can range from itching eyes, running nose, coughing, difficulty in breathing, welts on the skin, nausea, cramps, and even going into a state of shock, depending upon the severity of the allergic individual's response. Almost any part or system of the body may be affected, and almost anything can pose an allergic threat to somebody.

ALLERGENS: Substances that trigger an allergic reaction are called *allergens*. The system of an allergic individual reacts to such substances as if they were germs, producing *antibodies* whose job it is to neutralize the allergens. But the body's defense mechanism overreacts: in the process of fighting off the effects of the allergens, various chemicals, particularly *histamines*, are dumped

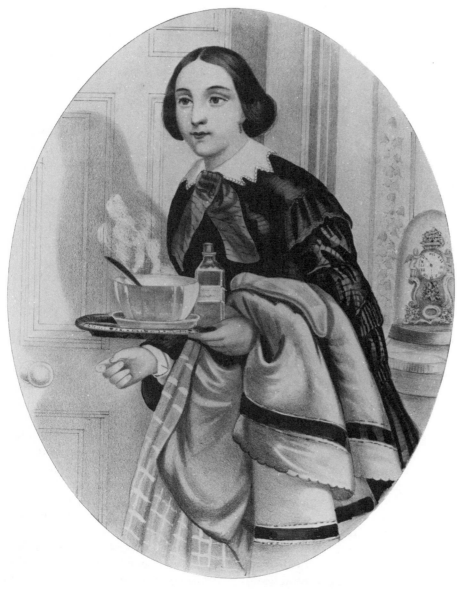

A Currier and Ives lithograph shows a woman bringing hot soup and an extra blanket for the patient with a cold—a treatment still in use.

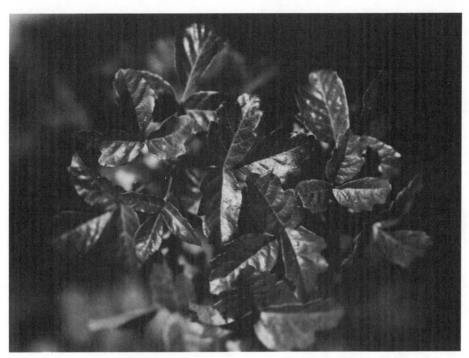

Western poison oak (shown here) is one of the common poisonous plants that cause allergic reactions in many people.

As soon as the source of the allergen is identified, the best thing for the allergic person to do is avoid it—if possible. But a person may find it more convenient to be relieved of the allergy by desensitization treatments administered by a doctor. Sometimes allergies that resist these treatments are kept under control by medicines such as adrenaline, ephedrine, cortisone, or the antihistamines.

Any person subject to severe, disabling allergy attacks by a known allergen should carry a card describing both the allergic reactions and the allergen. Detailed information on the latest developments in the treatment of allergies is available from the Allergy Foundation of America, 801 Second Avenue, New York, New York 10017. See also *Allergies and Hypersensitivities*, p. 283.

indiscriminately into the bloodstream. It is the overabundance of these "good" chemicals that causes the discomforts associated with allergies.

Allergens are usually placed in the following categories:

• Those that affect the respiratory tract, or *inhalants*, such as pollens, dust, smoke, perfumes, and various airborne, malodorous chemicals. These bring on sneezing, coughing, and breathing impairment.

• Food substances that affect the digestive system, typically eggs, seafood, nuts, berries, chocolate, and pork. These may not only cause nausea and diarrhea, but hives and other skin rashes.

• Medicines and drugs, such as penicillin, or a particular serum used in inoculations.

• Agents that act on the skin and mucous membranes, such as insecticides, poison oak, and poison ivy, particular chemical dyes, cosmetics, soaps, metals, leathers, and furs.

• Environmental agents such as sunlight or excessive cold.

• Microbes, such as particular bacteria, viruses, and parasites.

TREATMENT: Some allergic reactions are outgrown; some don't develop until adulthood. In many cases, the irritating substance is easy to identify and then avoid; in others, it may take a long series of tests before the allergen is finally tracked down.

Headaches

The common headache is probably as ancient as primitive man. The headache, a pain or ache across the forehead or within the head, may be severe or mild in character, and can last anywhere from under half an

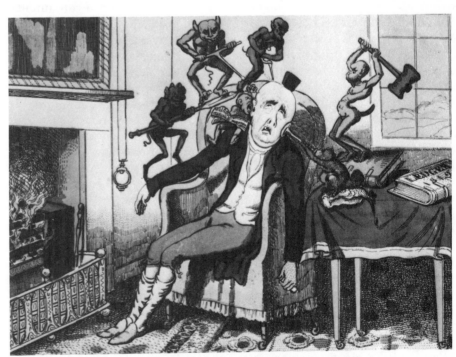

This 19th-century etching by George Cruikshank (1792–1878) vividly illustrates the diabolical misery of a headache.

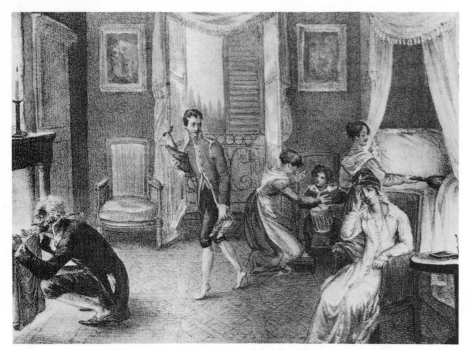

Family and servants tiptoe around trying to alleviate the suffering of a migraine patient (foreground) in a lithograph from the 1800s.

hour to three or four days. It may be accompanied by dizziness, nausea, nasal stuffiness, or difficulty in seeing or hearing. It is not a disease or illness, but a symptom.

Causes

Headaches in today's modern world can arise from any of a number of underlying causes. These include excessive drinking or smoking, lack of sleep, hunger, drug abuse, and eyestrain. Eyestrain commonly results from overuse of the eyes, particularly under glaring light, or from failure to correct defective vision.

Headaches can also be caused by exposure to toxic gases such as carbon monoxide and sulfur dioxide, which are common components in polluted air. Some headaches are symptoms of illness or disease, including pneumonia, constipation, allergy, high blood pressure, and brain tumor. Finally, emotional strain or tension can cause headache by unconsciously constricting the head and neck muscles. Many of these causes give rise to the common physiological cause of headache— dilation of the blood vessels in the head.

Headaches may be suffered on an occasional basis, or they may be chronic. Chronic headaches are usually *tension headaches* or *migraine*.

Migraine

Migraine, also called *sick headache,* is a particularly severe intense kind of headache. An attack may last several days and necessitate bed rest. Dizziness, sensitivity to light, and chills may accompany a migraine headache.

The exact cause of migraine is unknown, but researchers suspect a hereditary link, since the majority of migraine patients have one or more close relatives with migraine.

Migraine headaches can be precipitated by changes in body hormone balance (as from oral contraceptives), sudden changes in temperature, exposure to bright light or noise, shifts in barometric pressure, or by the intake of alcoholic beverages or the abuse of drugs. An attack can also be triggered by allergic responses to certain foods or beverages, such as chocolate or milk, and by emotional stress. Women, who outnumber

men by a 2 to 1 ratio in the incidence of migraine, may have an attack brought on by premenstrual tension. Many migraine sufferers have been found to conform to a personality type characterized as compulsive; their standards of achievement are exacting, their manner of work meticulous, and they tend to avoid expression of their anxieties.

Anyone suffering from very severe or chronic headaches should see a doctor and get a complete physical checkup.

Tension Headaches

Tension headaches can be avoided by getting adequate amounts of sleep and exercise and by learning to cope with frustrations and anxieties. Find time to relax each day, and resist the temptation to be a perfectionist or overachiever in all things. Tension headaches can be helped by neck massage, use of a heating pad, or a long, hot bath.

Headache Relief

Aspirin is often effective against headaches, but should be taken according to directions. A double dose is dangerous, and is not doubly effective. A cup of coffee or other caffeine beverage may prove helpful, since caffeine helps constrict blood vessels. In some cases headaches can be helped by nothing more than a few deep breaths of fresh air. Excess use of alcohol and tobacco should be avoided. If you must skip a meal, have a candy bar, piece of fruit, or some soup to prevent or relieve a hunger headache.

Take care of your eyes. Do not read in dim or glaring light. Have your eyes checked regularly, and if you have glasses, wear them when you need them.

Backaches

"Oh, my aching back" is probably the most common complaint among people past the age of 40. Most of the time, the discomfort—wherever it occurs, up or down the backbone—can be traced to some simple cause. However, there are continuous backaches which have their origin in some internal disorder that needs the attention of a physician. Among the more serious causes are kidney or pancreas disease, spinal arthritis, and peptic ulcer.

SOME COMMON CAUSES: Generally a backache is the result of strain on the muscles, nerves, or ligaments of the spine. It can occur because of poor posture, carelessness in lifting or carrying heavy packages, sitting in one position for a long time in the wrong kind of chair, or sleeping on a mattress that is too soft. Backache often accompanies menstruation, and is common in the later stages of pregnancy. Emotional tension can also bring on back pain.

PREVENTION: In general, maintaining good posture during the waking hours and sleeping on a hard mattress at night—if necessary, inserting a bedboard between the mattress and bedsprings—are the first line of defense against backaches. Anyone habitually carrying heavy loads of books or groceries, or even an overloaded attaché case, should make a habit of shifting the weight from arm to arm so that the spine doesn't always get pulled in one direction. Workers who are sedentary for most of the day at a desk or factory table should be sure that the chair they sit in provides firm support for back muscles and is the right height for the working surface.

TREATMENT: Most cases of simple backache respond to rest, aspirin, and the application of heat, applied by a hot water bottle or heating pad. In cases where the pain persists or becomes more acute, a doctor should be consulted. He may find that the trouble is caused by the malfunctioning of an internal organ, or by pressure on the sciatic nerve (*sciatica*). With X rays he may also locate a slipped disk or other abnormality in the alignment of the vertebrae of the spine. See *Back Pain and Its Causes*, p. 460.

Weight Problems

A few people can maintain the weight that is right for their body build without ever having to think about it. However, most experts believe that just about half the people in the United States may be risking shorter lives because they are too heavy. By one estimate, approximately one out of five American men and one out of four American women are ten percent or more overweight, a group that may be called the borderline obese.

There is no longer any reasonable doubt that, if you are overweight, you have statistically a greater chance of high blood pressure, diabetes, and *atherosclerosis* (lumpy deposits in the arteries). And since atherosclerotic heart disease alone accounts for 20 percent of deaths among adults in the United States, it is understandable why doctors consider weight truly a national problem.

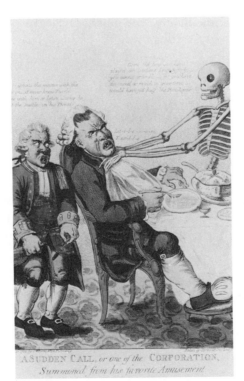

Death claims a man guilty of gluttony in a caricature published in 1799. Death says, "You have devoured as much in your time as would have fed half the . . . poor."

CAUSES: In practically all cases, weighing too much is the result of eating too much and exercising too little. In many cases, the food eaten is of the wrong kind and leisure time is used for riding around in a car rather than walking, or for watching television rather than playing tennis.

Many people like to think that they weigh too much only because they happen to like good food; but the real explanations may be considerably more complicated. In some cases, overeating has been found to have emotional sources: feelings of inadequacy; the need to compensate for a lack of affection or approval, or an unconscious desire to ward off the attention of the opposite sex. Psychological weight problems of this kind can be helped by consulting a psychiatrist or psychologist.

TREATMENT: There are many overweight people who merely need the support and encouragement that comes from participating in a group effort, and for them, joining one of the various weight-control organizations can be extremely beneficial in taking off extra pounds and keeping them off.

Permanent results are rarely achieved by crash diets, faddish food combinations, or reducing pills. Not only are such solutions usually temporary, they may actually be harmful. See *Weight*, p. 202 for further information about weight problems.

Weather Discomforts

Using good sense about clothing, exercise, and proper diet is probably our best protection against the discomforts caused by extremes of temperature. Sometimes circumstances make this exercise of good sense impossible, with unpleasant but rarely serious results, if treatment is promptly administered. Following are some of the more common disorders resulting from prolonged exposure to excessive heat or cold, and what you can do to alleviate them.

Heat Cramps

In a very hot environment, a person may drink great quantities of water while "sweating buckets" of salty perspiration. Thus, the body's water is replaced, but its salt is not. This salt-water imbalance results in a feeling of faintness and dizziness accompanied by acute stomach cramps and muscle pains in the legs. When the symptoms are comparatively mild, they can be relieved by taking coated salt tablets in five-to-ten-grain doses with a full glass of tepid or cool—not iced—water. Salt tablets along with plenty of fluids should be taken regularly as a preventive measure by people who sweat a great deal during hot weather.

Sunburn

If you have not yet been exposed to much sun, as at the beginning of summer, limit your exposure at first to a period of 15 or 20 minutes, and avoid the sun at the hours around mid-day even if the sky is overcast. Remember, too, that the reflection of the sun's rays from water and beach sand intensifies their effect. Some suntan lotions give effective protection against burning, and some creams even prevent tanning; but remember to cover all areas of exposed skin and to reapply the lotion when it's been washed away after a swim.

TREATMENT: A sunburn is treated like any other burn, depending upon its severity. See *Burns*, p. 590. If there is blistering, take care to avoid infection. Extensive blistering requires a physician's attention.

Heat Exhaustion

This condition is different from heatstroke or sunstroke, discussed below. Heat exhaustion sets in when large quantities of blood accumulate in the skin as the body's way of increasing its cooling mechanism during exposure to high temperatures. This in turn lowers the amount of blood circulating through the heart and decreases the blood supply to the brain. If severe enough, fainting may result. Other symptoms of heat exhaustion include unusual pallor and profuse cold perspiration. The pulse may be weak and breathing shallow.

TREATMENT: A person suspected of having heat exhaustion should be placed in a reclining position, his clothing loosened or removed, and his body cooled with moist cloths applied to his forehead and wrists. If he doesn't recover promptly from a fainting spell, smelling salts can be held under his nose to revive him. As soon as he is conscious, he can be given salt tablets and a cool sugary drink—either tea or coffee—to act as a stimulant. Don't give the patient any alcoholic beverages.

Sunstroke or Heatstroke

Sunstroke is much more of an emergency than heat exhaustion and requires immediate attention. The characteristic symptom is extremely high body temperature brought on by cessation of perspiration. If hot, dry, flushed skin turns ashen gray, a doctor must be called immediately. Too much physical activity during periods of high temperature and high humidity is a direct contributing cause.

TREATMENT: See *Heatstroke*, p. 598, for a description of the emergency treatment recommended for this condition.

Chapped Skin

One of the most widespread discomforts of cold weather is chapped skin. In low temperatures, the skin's sebaceous glands produce less of the oils that lubricate and protect the skin, causing it to become dry. Continued exposure results in reddening and cracking. In this condition, the skin is especially sensitive to strong soaps.

TREATMENT: During cold, dry weather, less soap should be used when washing, a bath oil should be used when bathing, and a mild lotion or cream should be applied to protect the skin from the damaging effects of wind and cold. A night

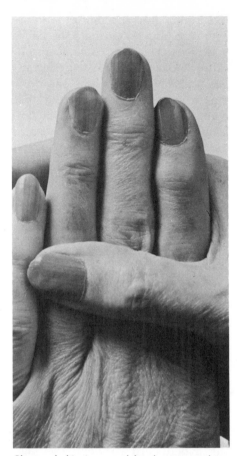

Chapped skin is caused by dryness resulting from the effect of cold weather on the sebaceous glands. The secretions of the glands are reduced at low temperatures.

cream or lotion containing lanolin is also helpful, and the use of cleansing cream or oil instead of soap can reduce additional discomfort when cleansing chapped areas. The use of a colorless lip pomade is especially recommended for children when they play out of doors in cold dry weather for any length of time.

Chilblain

A *chilblain* is a local inflammation of the skin brought on by exposure to cold. The condition commonly affects people overly sensitive to cold because of poor circulation. When the hands, feet, face, and ears are affected, the skin in these areas itches and burns, and may swell and turn reddish blue.

TREATMENT: The best way to avoid chilblains is to wear appropriate clothing during cold weather, especially warm socks, gloves, and ear coverings. The use of bed socks and a heating pad at night is also advisable. Cold wet feet should be dried promptly, gently, and thoroughly, once indoors. Rubbing or massaging should be avoided, since these can cause further irritation. People who suffer from repeated attacks of chilblains should consult a doctor for diagnosis of circulatory problems.

Frostbite

Frostbite is a considerably more serious condition than chilblains, since it means that a part or parts of the body have actually been frozen. The fingers or toes, the nose, and the ears are most vulnerable. If frostbitten, these areas turn numb and pale, and feel cold when touched. The dangerous thing about frostbite is that pain may not be a warning. If the condition is not treated promptly, the temperature inside the tissues keeps going down and eventually cuts off blood circulation to the overexposed parts of the body. In such extreme cases, there is a possible danger of gangrene.

TREATMENT: In mild cases, prompt treatment can slowly restore blood circulation. The frozen parts should be rewarmed *slowly* by covering them with warm clothing or by soaking them in lukewarm water. Nothing hot should be applied—neither hot water nor a heating pad. Nor should the patient be placed too close to a fireplace or radiator. Since the affected tissues can be easily bruised, they should not be massaged or rubbed. If you are in doubt about restoring circulation, a doctor should be called promptly or the patient taken to a hospital for emergency treatment.

Sleep and the Lack of It

Until rather recently, it was assumed that sleep was the time when the body rested and recovered from the activities of wakefulness. Although there is still a great deal to learn about why we sleep and what

happens when we are sleeping, medical researchers have now identified several different phases of sleep, all of them necessary over the long run, but some more crucial than others.

How much sleep a person needs varies a great deal from individual to individual; and the same individual may need more or less at different times. Children need long periods of unbroken sleep; the elderly seem to get along on very little. No matter what a person's age, too little sleep over too long a time leads to irritability, exhaustion, and giddiness.

Insomnia

Almost everybody has gone through periods when it is difficult or impossible to fall asleep. Excitement before bedtime, temporary worries about a pressing problem, spending a night in an unfamiliar place, changing to a different bed, illness, physical discomfort because of extremes of temperature—any of these circumstances can interfere with normal sleep patterns.

But this is quite different from *chronic insomnia*, when a person consistently has trouble falling

asleep for no apparent reason. If despite all your common-sense approaches insomnia persists, a doctor should be consulted about the advisability of taking a tranquilizer or a sleeping pill. Barbiturates should not be taken unless prescribed by a physician.

The Vulnerable Extremities

Aches and pains in the legs and feet occur for a wide variety of reasons, some trivial and easily corrected, others serious enough to require medical attention. Those that originate in such conditions as arthritis and rheumatism can often be alleviated by aspirin or some of the newer prescription medications.

Gout

Gout, which is actually a metabolic disorder, is a condition that especially affects the joint of the big toe, and sometimes the ankle joint, causing the area to become swollen, hot, and acutely painful. Although the specific cause of gout is not yet clearly understood, the symptoms can be alleviated by special medication prescribed by a physician. An attack of gout can be triggered by a

Do your feet hurt? Then you can readily sympathize with the gout patient shown in this 1799 lithograph. Gout was once very common.

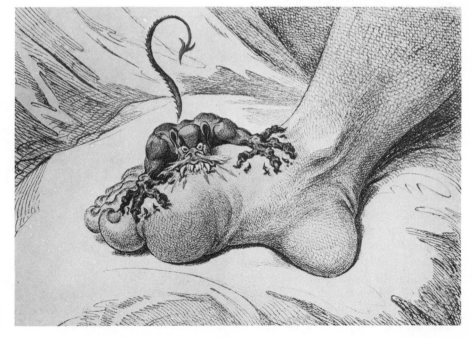

wide variety of causes: wearing the wrong shoes, eating a diet too rich in fats, getting a bad chill, surgery in some other part of the body, or chronic emotional anxiety, as well as the use of certain medicines such as diuretics ("water pills"). See also p. 456.

Fallen Arches

Fallen arches can cause considerable discomfort because the body's weight is carried on the ligaments of the inside of the foot rather than on the sole. When the abnormality is corrected by orthopedic shoes with built-in arches for proper support, the pressure on the ligaments is relieved. A doctor rather than a shoe salesman should be consulted for a reliable diagnosis. In some cases, the doctor may also recommend special exercises to strengthen the arch.

Flat Feet

Flat feet can usually be revealed by a simple test—making a footprint on level earth or hard-packed sand. If the print is solid rather than indented by a curve along the big-toe side of the foot, the foot is flat. Aching ligaments in the area of the instep are often a result, but can be relieved by proper arch supports inside the shoes. Corrective arch supports are particularly important for young children, for anyone who is overweight, and for anyone who has to stand a great deal of the time.

Blisters

Although blisters are sometimes a sign of allergy, fungus infection, or sunburn, they most commonly appear on the feet because of the friction of a shoe or of hosiery that does not fit properly. A *water blister* is a collection of lymph that forms inside the upper level of the skin; a *blood blister* goes down deeper and contains some blood released from broken capillaries. A normal amount of walking in shoes and hosiery that fit comfortably—neither too loose nor too tight—rarely results in blisters. When blisters do appear, it is best to protect them from further friction by the use of a sterile bandage strip.

TREATMENT: A blister that causes acute pain when walking can be treated as follows: after cleaning the area with soap and water, pat it dry and swab it with rubbing alcohol. Sterilize the tip of a needle in a flame, let it cool a little, and then puncture the edge of the blister, absorbing the liquid with a sterile gauze. The loose skin can be removed with manicure scissors that have been sterilized by boiling for ten minutes. The surface of raw skin should then be covered with an adhesive bandage. This procedure is best done before bedtime so that healing can begin before shoes are worn again.

If redness appears around the area of any blister and inflammation appears to be spreading, a doctor should be consulted promptly.

Bunions

A *bunion* is a deformation in the part of the foot that is joined by the big toe. The swelling and pain at the joint is caused by inflammation of the *bursa* (a fluid-filled sac) that lubricates the joint. Although bunions often develop because of wearing shoes that don't fit correctly, they most frequently accompany flat feet.

Pain that is not too severe can be relieved by the application of heat; the condition may eventually be cured by doing foot exercises recommended by a physician, who will also help in the choice of correct footwear. A bunion that causes acute pain and difficulty in walking can be treated by a simple surgical procedure.

Calluses

A *callus* is an area of the skin that has become hard and thick as a result of constant friction or pressure against it. Pain results when the callus is pressed against a nerve by poorly-fitting shoes. A painful callus can be partially removed by rubbing it—very cautiously—with a sandpaper file or a pumice stone sold for that purpose. The offending shoes should then be discarded for correctly fitted ones. Foot care by a podiatrist is recommended for anyone with recurring calluses and corns (see below), and especially for those people who have diabetes or any disorder of the arteries.

Corns

A *corn* is a form of callus that occurs on or between the toes. When the thickening occurs on the outside of the toe, it is called a *hard corn*; when it is located between the toes,

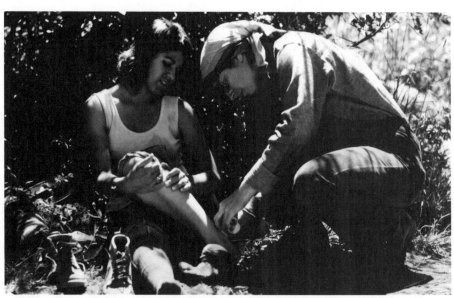

First aid being administered to a hiker. Painful blisters should be opened under sterile conditions and protected with a sterile bandage strip.

it is called a *soft corn*. The pain in the affected area is caused by pressure of the hard inside core of the corn against the tissue beneath it. The most effective treatment for corns is to wear shoes that are the right size and fit. Corns can be removed by a podiatrist or chiropodist, but unless footwear fits properly, they are likely to return.

TREATMENT: To remove a corn at home, the toes should be soaked in warm water for about ten minutes and dried. The corn can be rubbed away with an emery file, or it can be treated with a few drops of ten percent salicylic acid in collodion, available from any druggist. Care should be exercised in applying the solution so that it doesn't reach surrounding tissue, since it is highly irritating to normal skin. The area can then be covered with a corn pad to relieve pressure. This treatment may have to be repeated several times before the corn becomes soft enough to lift out. Diabetics or those suffering from any circulatory disorder should never treat their own corns.

Housemaid's Knee

Housemaid's knee is actually a form of *bursitis*, in which the fluid-filled bursa in front of the kneecap becomes inflamed by injury or excessive pressure, as because of constant kneeling. When the inflammation is mild, it can usually be corrected by rest. In the acute stage, the knee becomes swollen and painful, particularly when bent. It is especially prone to infection if scratched, bruised, or cut. Acute housemaid's knee is usually treated by anti-inflammatory type drugs, injections of cortisone, or by surgery under local anesthesia in the doctor's office. Anyone whose daily activities involve a great deal of kneeling should make a habit of using a thick rubber mat.

Tennis Elbow

This disorder can affect not only tennis players but also people who have injured their elbow joint or

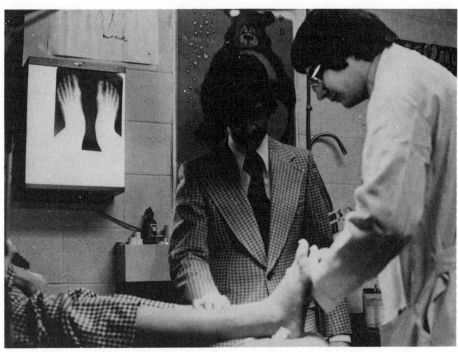

Corns can sometimes be removed by over-the-counter preparations, but diabetics should never treat their own corns.

subjected it to various stresses and strains. It may be a form of bursitis similar in nature to housemaid's knee, but it is more correctly called *tendinitis,* that is, an inflammation of the tendons which can affect any joint in the arms and legs. Rest and the application of heat usually relieve the painful symptoms. If the pain becomes acute, a doctor should be consulted.

Tenosynovitis

Tenosynovitis is an inflammation of a tendon sheath. One of the commoner sites of trouble is that of the wrist muscles. It can be caused by injury, infection, or constant use of the wrist muscles in piano-playing, typing, or some form of labor involving the wrist. The condition is usually treated by splinting the wrist and resting it for a while. Pain can be relieved with aspirin.

Writer's Cramp

Writer's cramp is a muscular pain caused by constant use of a set of muscles for a particular activity. The same set of muscles will function with no difficulty when the activity is changed. The best way to treat the

discomfort is to give the muscles a rest from the habitual activity and to relieve the pain with heat and aspirin.

Other Muscle Cramps

A sharp cramp or pain in the leg muscles, and sometimes in the arm, can occur because blood circulation has been impaired, either by hardening of the arteries, or because of undue pressure, such as habitually sitting with one leg tucked under the upper thigh. The cramp is usually relieved by either changing the activity involved or by shifting the position of the affected limb. Constant or acute muscle cramps should be brought to the attention of a doctor.

The Exposed Integument

Common skin and scalp annoyances such as rashes, itches, dandruff, excessive perspiration, and infections of various kinds (such as athlete's foot and ringworm), as well as acne, wrinkles, and baldness, are discussed under *Skin and Hair*, p. 236.

Splinters

If lodged superficially in the hand,

a splinter will usually work its own way out, but a splinter of no matter what size in the sole of the foot must be removed promptly to avoid its becoming further embedded by pressure and causing infection. The simplest method of removal is to pass a needle through a flame; let the needle cool; then after the skin surface has been washed with soap and water or swabbed with alcohol, press the point of the needle against the skin, scraping slightly until the tail of the splinter is visible and loosened. It can then be pulled out with tweezers that have been sterilized in boiling water or alcohol.

Hangnails

Hangnails are pieces of partly living skin torn from the base or side of the fingernail, thus opening a portion of the underskin to infection. A hangnail can cause considerable discomfort. It should not be pulled or bitten off; but the major part of it can be cut away with manicuring scissors. The painful and exposed area should then be washed with soap and water and covered with a sterile adhesive bandage. Hangnails are likely to occur when the skin is dry. They can therefore be prevented by the regular use of a hand cream or lotion containing lanolin.

"Normal" Disorders of the Blood and Circulation

Almost everybody is bothered occasionally by minor disturbances of the circulatory system. Most of the time these disturbances are temporary, and in many cases where they are chronic they may be so mild as not to interfere with good health. Among the more common disturbances of this type are the following.

Anemia

Anemia is a condition in which there is a decrease in the number of red blood cells or in the hemoglobin content of the red blood cells. *Hemoglobin* is the compound that carries oxygen to the body tissues

from the lungs. Anemia in itself is not a disease but rather a symptom of some other disorder, such as a deficiency of iron in the diet; excessive loss of blood due to injury or heavy menstrual flow; infection by industrial poisons; or kidney or bone marrow disease. A person may also develop anemia as a result of hypersensitivity (allergy) to various medicines.

In the simple form of anemia, caused by a deficiency of iron in the diet, the symptoms are rarely severe. There may be feelings of fatigue, a loss of energy, and a general lack of vitality. Deficiency anemia is especially common among children and pregnant women, and can be corrected by adding foods high in iron to the diet, such as liver, lean meat, leafy green vegetables, whole wheat bread, and dried peas and beans.

If the symptoms persist, a doctor should be consulted for diagnosis and treatment. For more information on anemia; see under *Diseases of the Blood*, p. 349.

Varicose Veins

Varicose veins are veins that have become ropy and swollen, and are therefore visible in the leg, sometimes bulging on the surface of the skin. They are the result of a sluggish blood flow (poor circulation), often combined with weakened walls of the veins themselves. The condition is common in pregnancy and occurs frequently among people who find it necessary to sit or stand in the same position for extended periods of time. A tendency to develop varicose veins may be inherited.

Even before the veins begin to be visible, there may be such warning symptoms as leg cramps, feelings of fatigue, or a general achiness. Unless the symptoms are treated promptly, the condition may worsen, and if the blood flow becomes increasingly impeded, ulcers may develop on the lower area of the leg.

TREATMENT: Mild cases of varicose veins can be kept under control, or

even corrected, by giving some help to circulation, as follows:
• Several times during the day, lie flat on your back for a few minutes, with the legs slightly raised.
• Soak the legs in warm water.
• Exercise.
• Wear lightly reinforced stockings or elastic stockings to support veins in the legs.

If varicose veins have become severe, a physician should be consulted. He may advise you to have injection treatment or surgery. See also p. 356.

Chronic Hypertension

Hypertension, commonly known as *high blood pressure*, is a condition that may be a warning of some other disease. In many cases, it is not in itself a serious problem and has no one underlying specific cause: this is called *functional, essential,* or *chronic hypertension*. The symptoms of breathing difficulty, headache, weakness, or dizziness that accompany high blood pressure can often be controlled by medicines that bring the pressure down, by sedatives or tranquilizers, and in cases where overweight is a contributing factor, by a change in diet, or by a combination of these.

More serious types of high blood pressure can be the result of kidney disease, glandular disturbances, or diseases of the circulatory system. Acute symptoms include chronic dizziness or blurred vision. Any symptoms of high blood pressure call for professional advice and treatment. See *Hypertensive Heart Disease*, p. 366.

Tachycardia

Tachycardia is the medical name for a condition that most of us have felt at one time or another—abnormally rapid heartbeat, or a feeling that the heart is fluttering, or pounding too quickly. The condition can be brought on by strong feelings of fear, excitement, or anxiety, or by overtaxing the heart with sudden exertion or too much exercise. It may also be a sign of heart disease, but in such cases, it is usually accompanied by other symptoms.

The most typical form of occasional rapid heartbeat is called *paroxysmal tachycardia*, during which the beat suddenly becomes twice or three times as fast as it is normally, and then just as suddenly returns to its usual tempo. When the paroxysms are frequent enough to be disturbing and can be traced to no specific source, they can be prevented by medicines prescribed by your physician.

Nosebleed

Nosebleeds are usually the result of a ruptured blood vessel. They are especially common among children, and among adults with high blood pressure. If the nosebleed doesn't taper off by itself, the following measures should be taken: the patient should be seated—he should not lie down—his clothing loosened, and a cold compress placed on the back of his neck and his nose. The soft portion of the nostril may be pressed gently against the bony cartilage of the nose for at least six minutes, or rolled wads of absorbent cotton may be placed inside each nostril, with part of the cotton sticking out to make its removal easier. The inserted cotton should be left in place for several hours and then gently withdrawn.

Fainting

Fainting is a sudden loss of consciousness, usually caused by an insufficient supply of blood and oxygen to the brain. Among the most common causes of fainting are fear, acute hunger, the sight of blood, and prolonged standing in a room with too little fresh air. Fainting should not be confused with a loss of consciousness resulting from excessive alcohol intake or insulin shock. A person about to faint usually feels dizzy, turns pale, and feels weak in the knees.

TREATMENT: If possible, the person should be made to lie down, or to sit with his head between his knees for several minutes. Should he lose consciousness, place him so that his legs are slightly higher than his head, loosen his clothing, and see that he gets plenty of fresh air. If smelling salts or aromatic spirits of ammonia are available, they can be held under his nose. With these procedures, he should revive in a few minutes. If he doesn't, a doctor should be called.

Troubles Along the Digestive Tract

From childhood on, most people are occasionally bothered by minor and temporary disturbances connected with digestion. Most of the disturbances listed below can be treated successfully with common sense and, if need be, a change in habits.

The Mouth

The digestive processes begin in the mouth, where the saliva begins chemically to break down some foods into simpler components, and the teeth and the tongue start the mechanical breakdown. Disorders of the teeth such as a malocclusion or poorly fitted dentures that interfere with proper chewing should be brought to the prompt attention of a dentist.

INFLAMMATION OF THE GUMS: Also known as *gingivitis*, inflammation of the gums is caused by the bacteria that breed in food trapped in the spaces between the gums and the teeth. The gums become increasingly swollen, may bleed easily, and be sore enough to interfere with proper chewing. The condition can be prevented by cleaning the teeth thoroughly and frequently, which includes the use of dental floss or the rubber tip on the toothbrush to remove any food particles lodged in

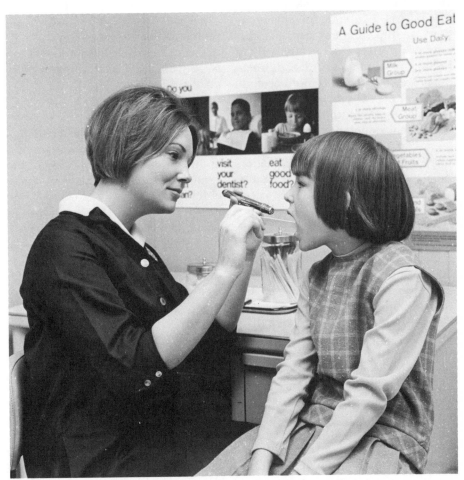

A school nurse examines a student's throat and mouth for signs of inflammation or other symptoms of illness. Contrary to popular impression, a coated tongue is not necessarily an indication of illness.

the teeth after eating. Since gingivitis can develop into the more serious condition of *pyorrhea*, persistent gum bleeding or soreness should receive prompt professional treatment. See *The Teeth and Gums*, p. 252.

CANKER SORES: Canker sores are small ulcers inside the lips, mouth, and cheeks. Their specific cause is unknown, but they seem to accompany or follow a virus infection, vitamin deficiency, or emotional stress. They may be additionally irritated by citrus fruit, chocolate, or nuts. A canker sore usually clears up in about a week without special treatment. A bland mouth rinse will relieve pain and, in some cases, speed the healing process.

COATED TONGUE: Although a coated tongue is commonly supposed to be a sure sign of illness, this is not the case. The condition may occur because of a temporary lack of saliva.

GLOSSITIS: Glossitis, an inflammation of the tongue causing the tongue's surface to become bright red or, in some cases, glazed in appearance, may be a symptom of an infection elsewhere in the body. It may also be a symptom of anemia or a nutritional deficiency, or it may be an adverse reaction to certain forms of medication. If the inflammation persists and is accompanied by acute soreness, it should be called to a doctor's attention.

HALITOSIS OR BAD BREATH: Contrary to the millions of commercial messages on television and in print, bad breath cannot be cured by any mouthwash, lozenge, spray, or antiseptic gargle now on the market. These products can do no more than mask the odor until the basic cause is diagnosed and cured. Among the many conditions that may result in bad breath (leaving out such fleeting causes as garlic and onions) are the following: an infection of the throat, nose, or mouth; a stomach or kidney disorder; pyorrhea; respiratory infection; tooth decay; improper mouth hygiene; and excessive drinking and smoking. Anyone who has been made self-conscious about the

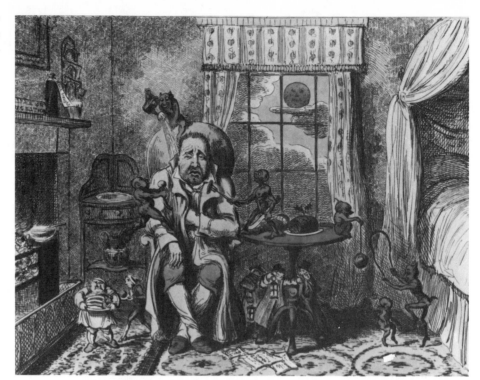

Morning-after remorse does little to counter the effects of overindulgence, as this 1825 etching by George Cruikshank so graphically illustrates.

problem of bad breath should ask his doctor or dentist whether his breath is truly offensive and if it is, what to do about it.

Gastritis

Gastritis, one of the most common disorders of the digestive system, is an inflammation of the lining of the stomach which may occur in acute, chronic, or toxic form. Among the causes of *acute gastritis* are various bacterial or viral infections; overeating, especially heavy or rich foods; excessive drinking of alcoholic beverages; or food poisoning. An attack of acute gastritis may be severely painful, but the discomfort usually subsides with proper treatment. The first symptom is typically sharp stomach cramps, followed by a bloated feeling, loss of appetite, headache, and nausea. When vomiting occurs, it rids the stomach of the substance causing the attack but usually leaves the patient temporarily weak. If painful cramps persist and are accompanied by fever, a doctor should be consulted about the possibility of medication for bacterial infection. For a few days

after an attack of acute gastritis, the patient should stay on a bland diet of easily digested foods, taken in small quantities.

TOXIC GASTRITIS: Toxic gastritis is usually the result of swallowing a poisonous substance, causing vomiting and possible collapse. It is an emergency condition requiring prompt first aid treatment and the attention of a doctor. See *Poisoning*, p. 578.

CHRONIC GASTRITIS: Chronic gastritis is a recurrent or persisting inflammation of the stomach lining over a lengthy period. The condition has the symptoms associated with indigestion, especially pain after eating. It can be caused by excessive drinking of alcoholic beverages, constant tension or anxiety, or deficiencies in the diet. The most effective treatment for chronic gastritis is a bland diet from which caffeine and alcohol have been eliminated. Heavy meals should be avoided in favor of eating small amounts at frequent intervals. A tranquilizer or a mild sedative prescribed by a doctor may reduce the tensions that contribute to the condition. If the discomfort continues, a physician should be consulted about the possibility of ulcers. See under *Diseases of the Digestive System*, p. 380.

Gastroenteritis

Gastroenteritis is an inflammation of the lining of both the stomach and the intestines. Like gastritis, it can occur in acute or toxic forms as a result of food poisoning, excessive alcohol intake, viral or bacterial infections, or food allergies. Vomiting, diarrhea, and fever may be more pronounced and of longer duration. As long as nausea and vomiting persist, no food or fluid should be taken; when these symptoms cease, a bland, mainly fluid diet consisting of strained broth, thin cereals, boiled eggs, and tea is best. If fever continues and diarrhea doesn't taper off, a doctor should be called.

Diarrhea

Diarrhea is a condition in which bowel movements are abnormally frequent and liquid. It may be accompanied by cramps, vomiting, thirst, and a feeling of tenderness in the abdominal region. Diarrhea is always a symptom of some irritant in the intestinal tract; among possible causes are allergy, infection by virus or bacteria, accidentally swallowed poisonous substances, or excessive alcohol. Brief attacks are sometimes caused by emotions, such as overexcitement or anxiety.

Diarrhea that lasts for more than two days should be diagnosed by a physician to rule out a more serious infection, a glandular disturbance, or a tumor. Mild attacks can be treated at home by giving the patient a light bland diet, plenty of fluids, and the prescribed dosage of a kaolin-pectin compound available at any drugstore.

Constipation

Many people have the mistaken notion that if they don't have a bowel movement every day, they must be constipated. This is not necessarily so. From a doctor's viewpoint, constipation is not determined by an arbitrary schedule of when the bowel should be evacuated, but by the individual's discomfort and other unpleasant symptoms. In too many instances, overconcern and anxiety about bowel movements may be the chief cause of constipation.

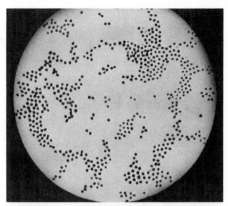

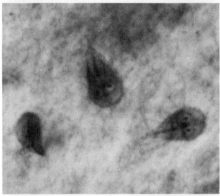

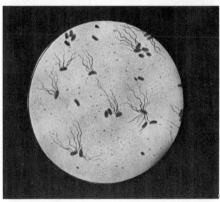

Diarrhea results from a variety of causes. In severe cases, a physician may do extensive testing and find one of these culprits responsible: *Staphylococcus aureus* bacteria (*top*), *Giardia lamblia* protozoans (*center*), or *Salmonella* bacteria (*bottom*).

The watery waste that results from the digestion of food in the stomach and small intestine passes into the large intestine, or colon, where water is absorbed from the waste. If the waste stays in the large intestine for too long a time, so much water is removed that it becomes too solid and compressed to evacuate easily. The efficient removal of waste material from the large intestine depends on wavelike

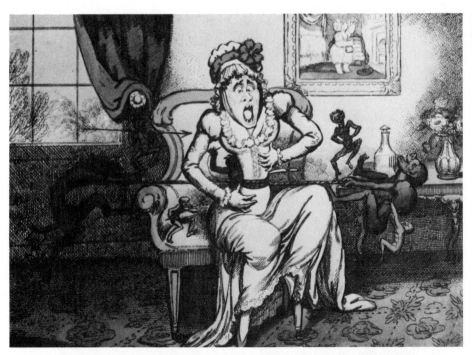

It must have been something she ate! Digestive demons attack an overindulgent lady of fashion in this 19th-century caricature by George Cruikshank.

muscular contractions. When these waves are too weak to do their job properly, as often happens in the elderly or the excessively sedentary, a doctor may recommend a mild laxative or mineral oil.

TREATMENT: Constipation is rarely the result of an organic disorder. In most cases, it is caused by poor health habits; when these are corrected, the disorder corrects itself. Often, faulty diet is a major factor. Make sure that meals contain plenty of roughage in the form of whole-grain cereals, fruit, and leafy green vegetables. Figs, prunes, and dates should be included from time to time. Plenty of liquid intake is important, whether in the form of juices, soups, or large quantities of water. Scheduling a certain amount of exercise each day strengthens the abdominal muscles and stimulates muscle activity in the large intestine. Confronting the sources of worries and anxieties, if necessary with a trained therapist, may also be helpful.

An enema or a laxative should be considered only once in a while rather than as regular treatment. The colon should be given a chance to function properly without relying on artificial stimulation. If constipation resists these common-sense approaches, the problem should be talked over with a physician.

Hemorrhoids

Hemorrhoids, commonly called *piles,* are swollen veins in the mucous membrane inside or just outside the rectum. When the enlargement is slight, the only discomfort may be an itching sensation in the area. Acute cases are accompanied by pain and bleeding. Hemorrhoids are a very common complaint and occur in people of all ages. They are usually the result of straining to eliminate hard, dry stools. The extra pressure causes a fold of the membranous rectal lining to slip down, thus pinching the veins and irritating them.

Since hemorrhoids may be a symptom of a disorder other than constipation, they should be treated by a physician. If neglected, they may bleed frequently and profusely enough to cause anemia. Should a blood clot develop in an irritated vein, surgery may be necessary.

TREATMENT: Advertised cures should be avoided since they are not only ineffective but can cause additional irritation. Laxatives and cathartics, which may temporarily solve the problem of constipation, are likely to aggravate hemorrhoids.

If pain or bleeding becomes acute, a doctor should be consulted promptly. Treatment can be begun at home. Sitting for several minutes in a hot bath in the morning and again in the evening (more frequently if necessary) will provide temporary relief. Preventing constipation is of the utmost importance.

Anal Fissure

This is a condition in which a crack or split or ulcerated place develops in the area of the two anal sphincters, or muscle rings, that control the release of feces. Such breaks in the skin are generally caused by something sharp in the stool, or by the passage of an unusually hard and large stool. Although discomfort often accompanies a bowel movement when there is a fissure, the acute pain typically comes afterward. Healing is difficult because the injured tissue is constantly open to irritation. If the condition persists, it usually has to be treated by a minor surgical procedure. Intense itching in this area is called *anal pruritis.*

Minor Ailments in the Air Pipes

In addition to all the respiratory discomforts that go along with the common cold (see p. 265), there are various other ailments that affect breathing and normal voice production.

Bronchitis

Usually referred to as a chest cold, *bronchitis* is an inflammation of the bronchial tubes that connect the windpipe and the lungs. If bronchitis progresses down into the lungs, it can develop into pneumonia. Old people and children are especially susceptible to acute bronchitis. The symptoms include pain in the chest, a feeling of fatigue, and a nagging cough. If the infection is bacterial, it will respond to antibiotics. If it is viral, there are no specific medicines. The attack usually lasts for about ten days, although recovery may be speeded up with bed rest and large fluid intake.

CHRONIC BRONCHITIS: Chronic bronchitis is a condition that may recur each winter, or may be present throughout the year in the form of a constant cough. The condition is aggravated by smoking and by irritants, such as airborne dust and smog. The swollen tissues and abnormally heavy discharge of mucus interfere with the flow of air from the lungs and cause shortness of breath. Medicines are available which lessen the bronchial phlegm and make breathing easier. People with chronic bronchitis often sleep better if they use more than one pillow and have a vaporizer going at night.

Coughing

Coughing is usually a reflex reaction to an obstruction or irritation in the trachea (windpipe), pharynx (back of mouth and throat), or the bronchial tubes. It can also be the symptom of a disease or a nervous habit. For a simple cough brought on by smoking too much or breathing bad air, medicines can be taken that act as sedatives to inhibit the reflex reaction. Inhaling steam can loosen the congestion (a combination of swollen membranes and thickened mucus) that causes some types of coughs, and hot drinks such as tea or lemonade help to soothe and relax the irritated area. Constant coughing, especially when accompanied by chest pains, should be brought to a doctor's attention. For a discussion of whooping cough and croup, see the respective articles under the *Alphabetical Guide to Child Care* beginning on p. 60.

Laryngitis

Laryngitis is an inflammation of the mucous membrane of the larynx (voice box) that interferes with breathing and causes the voice to become hoarse or disappear altogether. This condition may accompany a sore throat, measles, or whooping cough, or it may result from an allergy. Prolonged overuse of the voice, a common occupational hazard of singers and teachers, is also a cause. The best treatment for laryngitis is to go to bed, keep the room cool, and put moisture into the air from a vaporizer, humidifier, or boiling kettle. Don't attempt to talk, even in a whisper. Keep a writing pad within arm's reach and use it to spare your voice. Drinking warm liquids may help to relieve some of the discomfort. If you must go out, keep the throat warmly protected.

Chronic laryngitis may result from too many acute laryngitis attacks, which can cause the mucous membrane to become so thick and tough that the voice remains permanently hoarse. The sudden onset of hoarseness that lasts for more than two weeks calls for a doctor's diagnosis.

Hiccups

Hiccups (also spelled *hiccoughs*) are contractions of the diaphragm, the great muscle responsible for forcing air in and out of our lungs. They may be brought on by an irritation of the diaphragm itself, of the respiratory or digestive system, or by eating or drinking too rapidly. Common remedies for hiccups include sipping water slowly, holding the breath, and putting something cold on the back of the neck. Breathing into a paper bag is usually effective because after a few breaths, the high carbon dioxide content in the bag will serve to make the diaphragm contractions more regular, rather than spasmodic. If none of

these measures helps, it may be necessary to have a doctor prescribe a sedative or tranquilizer.

The Sensitive Eyes and Ears

Air pollution affects not only the lungs but the eyes as well. In addition to all the other hazards to which the eyes are exposed, airborne smoke, chemicals, and dust cause the eyes to burn, itch, and shed tears. Other common eye troubles are discussed below.

Sty

This pimplelike inflammation of the eyelid is caused by infection, which may be linked to the blocking of an eyelash root or an oil gland, or to general poor health. A sty can be treated at home by applying clean compresses of hot water to the area for about 15 minutes at a time every two hours. This procedure should cause the sty to open, drain, and heal. If sties are recurrent, a health checkup may be indicated.

Pinkeye

Pinkeye, an acute form of *conjunctivitis*, is an inflammation of the membrane that lines the eyelid and covers the eyeball, causing the eyes to become red and the lids to swell and stick together while sleeping. The condition may result from bacterial or viral infection—in which case it is extremely contagious—or from allergy or chemical irritation. A doctor should be consulted.

Conjunctivitis can be treated by washing the eyes with warm water, drying them with a disposable tissue to prevent the spread of infection, and applying a medicated yellow oxide of mercury ophthalmic ointment (as recommended by your physician) on the inner edges of the lids. This should be done upon rising in the morning and upon retiring at night. The eyes should then be closed until the ointment has spread. Apply compresses of hot water three or four times a day for five-minute periods.

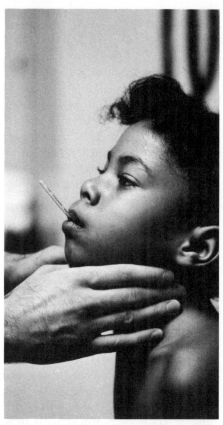

The presence of a respiratory infection calls for a check of the lymph nodes in the neck. Swollen glands are characteristic of a number of diseases, including scarlet fever.

Eyestrain

Eyestrain—with symptoms of fatigue, tearing, redness, and a scratchy feeling in the eyelids—can be caused by a need for corrective glasses, by a disorder of the eye, or by overuse of the eyes that brings about fatigue. One of the most common causes of eyestrain, however, is improper lighting. Anyone engaged in close work, such as sewing or minature model building, and at all times when reading, should have light come from behind and from the side so that no shadow falls on the book or object being scrutinized. The light should be strong enough for comfort—not dazzling. Efforts should be made to avoid a shiny or highly polished work surface that produces a glare. To avoid eyestrain when watching television, the picture must be in sharp focus; the viewer should sit at least six feet from the screen; and the room should not be in total darkness.

Ear Infections

Ear infections related to colds, sore throats, or tonsillitis can now be kept from spreading and entering the mastoid bone by the use of sulfa drugs and antibiotics. Any acute earache should therefore be called to a doctor's attention promptly. Aspirin can be taken for temporary relief from pain; holding a heating pad or a hot water bottle to the affected side of the face may also be helpful until proper medication can be prescribed.

Earwax

An excessive accumulation of earwax can sometimes cause pain as well as interfere with hearing. When the ear canal is blocked in this way, gently rotating a small wad of cotton may clean it. The ears should never be cleaned with sharp objects such as hairpins or matchsticks. If earwax has hardened too much to be removed with cotton, it can be softened by a few drops of hydrogen peroxide. When the wax is so deeply and firmly imbedded that it can't be removed at home, a physician may have to flush it out with a syringe.

Ear Blockage

A stopped-up feeling in the ear can be caused by a cold, and also by the change in air pressure experienced when a plane makes a rapid descent. The obstruction of the Eustachian tube can usually be opened by swallowing hard or yawning.

Ringing in the Ear

The general word for a large variety of noises in the ear is *tinnitus*. People who experience such noises describe the sounds in many ways: hissing, ringing, buzzing, roaring, whistling. When they are heard only occasionally for brief periods, without any other symptoms, they can be ignored. However, when they are constant, they should be considered a symptom of some disorder such as

an infection, high blood pressure, allergy, or an improper bite (malocclusion). Sounds in the ears may also be caused by excessive smoking or drinking, or by large doses of aspirin or other medicines. In cases where the source of the ear disturbance can't be diagnosed and the noises become an unsettling nuisance, the doctor may recommend a sedative or tranquilizer.

The Path From the Kidneys

Cystitis

Cystitis is the general term for inflammation of the bladder caused by various types of infection. It is more common in women than in men. Infecting microbes may come from outside the body by way of the urethra, or from some other infected organ such as the kidney. When the bladder becomes inflamed, frequent and painful urination results.

Cystitis may also occur as a consequence of other disorders, such as enlargement of the prostate gland, a structural defect of the male urethra, or stones or a tumor in the bladder. Although there is no completely reliable way to prevent cystitis, some types of infection can be prevented by cleansing the genital region regularly so that the entrance of the urethra is protected against bacterial invasion. Cystitis is usually cured by medicines prescribed by a physician. For a detailed discussion of cystitis and related conditions affecting women, see *Disorders of the Urinary System*, p. 494.

Prostatitis

Prostatitis is an inflammation of the prostate gland (present in males only), caused by an infection of the urinary tract or some other part of the body. It may occur as a result of venereal infection. The symptoms of painful and excessive urination generally respond favorably to antibiotics. *Acute prostatitis* is less common: the patient is likely to have a high fever as well as a dis-

charge of pus from the penis. These symptoms should be brought to a doctor's attention without delay.

Excessive Urination

A need to empty the bladder with excessive frequency can be merely a nuisance caused by overexcitement or tension, or it can be the sign of a disorder of the urinogenital system. A doctor should be consulted if the problem persists.

The All-Important Feet

The *podiatrist* is the specialist who treats foot problems. Causes of foot ailments range from lack of cleanliness to ill-fitting shoes and over-indulgence in athletic activities (see "Care of the Feet," p. 156, "The Vulnerable Extremities," p. 271, and other sections on foot problems and foot care).

An ache, pain, or other disorder of the foot can be particularly annoying because it usually hampers mobility. A severe problem can keep a person bedridden, sometimes in the hospital, for substantial periods of time. As humans, we move about on our feet. They deserve the best of care from us, as their owners, and from the podiatrist in case a serious problem arises.

PODIATRICS, the science of foot care, has become more and more important as Americans have taken to athletics and exercises of various kinds. Most of these activities require the use of the feet. Increasing numbers of persons in the adult years are also taking up walking, jogging, or running as diversions or exercises.

Podiatrists believe that some persons "walk old"—they give the appearance, by the way they walk, of greater age than their chronological years. Others "walk young," or walk normally. Those who walk old may be inviting foot problems, and a fact of podiatric science is that every foot problem has its reflection in another part, or other parts, of the body.

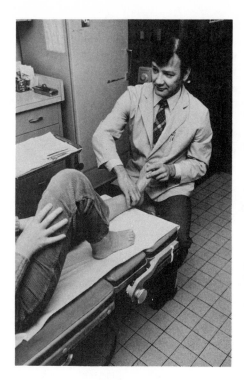
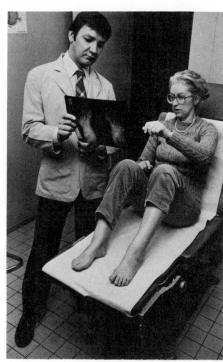

A podiatrist examines a patient with chronic foot problems and then uses X rays to explain the course of treatment he thinks is needed.

By contrast, good foot and body posture often suggests that the owner of the feet enjoys good health in other parts of the body. Foot care may in effect help other body parts to function better. Because many problems with parts of the body remote from the feet make good foot posture and normal walking difficult or impossible, individuals with diverse problems, such as back pains, sometimes go to a podiatrist for treatment. The back pain may disappear when the feet have been brought into good working order.

Diabetes and the Feet

"Care" for the feet of diabetics means prevention. The diabetic tries to keep his feet so healthy that he avoids major problems. He knows that diabetes affects blood circulation, and that the leg and foot are extremely vulnerable to circulatory problems. Where blood cannot reach a limb or member, gangrene becomes a possibility.

FOOT CARE: What kind of care serves the diabetic best? Effective care means that the diabetic takes steps quickly to treat such problems

as abrasions or ulcers that refuse to heal. Other conditions that warn of possible future problems are dry skin, numbness, and dried or brittle nails. Ulcers that appear in the skin of the foot and that appear to have roots in deeper layers of tissue serve as danger signals. Such ulcers may appear on the site of an injury, cut, or scratch. A physician will usually prescribe medication, dietary adjustments, or other measures.

Ulcers may result from neglect of a corn or callus. But such neglect itself indicates the risks that diabetics incur: they may neglect to have a foot problem such as a corn treated because their disease has, over time, reduced the sensitivity of their feet. They may lose much of their ability to feel pain, heat or cold, or stress in the foot. Because of such problems, diabetics generally follow certain rules of foot care, including the following:

• Give the feet a daily examination for cuts, bruises, or other abnormalities

• Use only prescribed medications in caring for the feet—and avoid over-the-counter preparations

• Visit a podiatrist regularly, as often as once a month, and avoid medical "treatment" of one's own feet or even cutting one's own toenails

• Wash the feet daily in warm, not hot, water, and dry them carefully, including the area between the toes

• Use a gentle lubricant on the feet after washing and drying—and never go barefoot

• Avoid the use of items of clothing that may interfere with circulation, including wrap-around garters and support hosiery

• Avoid "holey" socks, darned socks, or anything else that may irritate the soles of the feet

• Avoid constrictive boots or shoes

JOGGING AND RUNNING: The podiatrist usually tries to learn about a patient's work, his hobbies and sports, and other facts before undertaking treatment. In particular, the foot-doctor asks whether the patient runs or jogs or takes part in other strenuous exercises. With such background information, the podiatrist can suggest appropriate treatment.

A podiatrist will advise runners or joggers on the kind of footwear that would be best—especially if problems have been encountered or may be expected. Shoe inserts may be custom-designed if needed. The podiatrist may also advise runners and joggers to run on softer surfaces rather than cement. Jogging or running "in place," without forward movement, is to be avoided if possible; even when jogging inside the home or apartment, the jogger should move from room to room.

Podiatrists point out that even the more serious knee and ankle problems incurred in running and jogging can be treated. "Jogger's ankle," pain resulting from too much jogging and the attendant strain, can be controlled if the jogger will use moderation. Beginning joggers in particular should start slowly and gradually increase their level of participation. Runners' knee problems may be cured in many cases by treatment that enables the feet to carry the weight of the body properly. In part, the treatment requires practice in throwing the body weight onto the balls of the feet, not on the inner sides of the feet. The remainder of the body, including the knees, can be kept in proper alignment with the feet if the weight falls where it should.

Podiatrists also advise runners, joggers, and others taking part in sports to make certain *all* their clothing and equipment are appropriate. That applies especially in skiing, ice skating, and other sports requiring extensive foot use. Proper equipment helps runners and joggers avoid colds and similar respiratory problems.

With proper equipment, including good shoes, and a moderate approach, runners and joggers can avoid many other potentially troublesome physical difficulties that could require podiatric care. These others include fallen arches; corns, calluses, and bunions; and "aging feet" that grow weaker from lack of proper foot attention.

CHAPTER 12

Allergies and Hypersensitivities

Allergy is a broad term used to describe an unusual reaction of the body's tissues to a substance which has no noticeable effect on other persons. About 17 out of every 100 persons in America are allergic, or hypersensitive, to one or more substances that are known to precipitate an unusual reaction. Such substances, known as *allergens*, include a variety of irritants, among them mold spores, pollens, animal dander, insect venoms, and house dust. Some individuals are allergic to substances in soap, which produce a skin irritation. Others react to the smell of a rose by sneezing. Still others react with an outbreak of hives, diarrhea, or other symptoms to allergens in foods.

How Allergens Affect the Body

Allergic symptoms can range from itching eyes, running nose, coughing, difficulty in breathing, and welts on the skin to nausea, cramps, and even going into a state of shock, depending upon the severity of the particular individual's sensitivity and response. Almost any part or system of the body can be affected, and almost anything can pose an allergic threat to somebody.

The Role of Antibodies

The system of an allergic individual reacts to such substances in the way it would react to an invading disease organism: by producing *antibodies* whose job it is to neutralize the allergen. In the process of fighting off the effects of the allergen, the body's defense mechanism may overreact by dumping a chemical mediator, *histamine*, indiscriminately into the individual's bloodstream. It is the overabundance of this protective chemical that causes the discomforts associated with allergies.

At the same time, the antibodies can sensitize the individual to the allergen. Then, with each new exposure to the allergen, more antibodies are produced. Eventually the symptoms of allergy are produced whenever the allergen is encountered. Most allergic reactions, including hay fever, asthma, gastrointestinal upsets, and skin rashes, are of the type just described; their

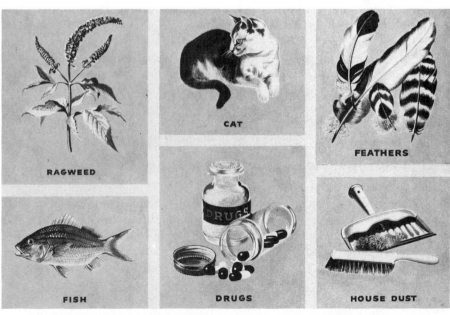

RAGWEED   CAT   FEATHERS

FISH   DRUGS   HOUSE DUST

The illustrations above provide a sampling of the enormous number of creatures and substances that can cause allergic reactions.

effect is more or less immediate. A second type, known as the delayed type, seems to function without the production of antibodies; contact dermatitis is an example of the delayed type.

Eosinophils

Some individuals seem to be sensitive to only one known allergen, but others are sensitive to a variety of substances. Persons who suffer acute allergic reactions have abnormally high levels of a type of white blood cell called *eosinophil*. The eosinophil contains an enzyme that may have some control over the allergic reaction, and varying degrees of the enzyme's efficiency appear to account for individual differences in the severity of allergic reactions.

Allergic Symptoms in Children

Many of the common allergies appear during the early years of life. It has been estimated that nearly 80 percent of the major allergic problems begin to appear between the ages of 4 and 9 years of age. Allergic youngsters may have nasal speech habits, breathe through the mouth, have coughing and wheezing spells, or rub their eyes, nose, and ears because of itching. A not uncommon sign of allergic reaction in a child may be dark circles under the eyes caused by swelling of the mucous membranes to such an extent that blood does not drain properly from the veins under the lower eyelids. Nose twitching and mouth wrinkling also are signs that a youngster has allergic symptoms.

Common Allergens

The allergens responsible for so many unpleasant and uncomfortable symptoms take a variety of forms too numerous and sometimes too obscure for any book to enumerate. Discussed below are some of the more common types of allergens.

Foods

Foods are among the most com-

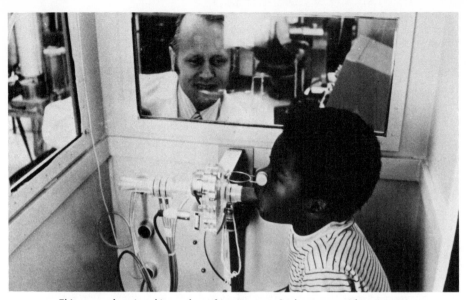

This young boy is taking a lung function test. Such tests provide accurate measurements which are of great value in asthma and allergy evaluations.

mon causes of allergic reactions. While nearly any food substance is a potential allergen to certain sensitive individuals, those most frequently implicated are cow's milk, orange juice, and eggs, all considered essential in a child's diet. However, substitute foods are almost always available. Many natural foods contain vitamin C, or ascorbic acid, found in orange juice. Ascorbic acid also is available in vitamin tablets. All of the essential amino acids and other nutrients in cow's milk and eggs also can be obtained from other food sources, although perhaps not as conveniently packaged for immediate use. Other common food offenders are chocolate, pork, seafoods, nuts, and berries. An individual may be allergic to the gluten in wheat, rye, and oats, and products made from those grains.

Inhaled Allergens

Allergens also may affect the respiratory tract, bringing on sneezing, coughing, and breathing impairment. The substances involved can be pollens, dust, smoke, perfumes, and various airborne chemicals.

MOLD SPORES: A person also can become allergic to a certain mold by inhaling the spores, or reproductive particles, of fungus. In the nose, the mold spores trigger a reaction in cells of the tissues beneath the mucous membranes which line the nasal passages. This in turn leads to the symptoms of allergy. Because they are small, mold spores can evade the natural protective mechanisms of the nose and upper respiratory tract to reach the lungs and bring on an allergic reaction in that site. Usually, this leads to the buildup of mucus, wheezing, and difficulty in breathing associated with asthma.

Less frequently, inhaling mold spores can result in skin lesions similar to those of eczema or chronic hives. In all but the very warmest areas of the United States, molds are seasonal allergens, occurring from spring into late fall. But unlike pollens, molds do not disappear with the killing frosts of autumn. Actually, frost may help increase the activity of molds, which thrive on dying vegetation produced by cold temperatures.

DUST AND ANIMAL HAIR: House dust and animal hair (especially cat and dog hair) are also responsible for respiratory allergies in many people. Asthma attacks are often triggered by contact with these substances. Symptoms of dust allergy are usually most severe in the spring and fall, and tend to subside in the summer.

MAN-MADE ALLERGENS: An example of respiratory allergy caused by man-made allergens is the complaint known as "meatwrappers' asthma," which results from fumes of the price-label adhesive on the polyvinyl chloride film used to package foods. The fumes are produced when the price label is cut on a hot wire. When the fumes are inhaled, the result is burning eyes, sore throat, wheezing and shortness of breath, upset stomach, and other complaints. Studies show that exposure to the fumes from the heat-activated label adhesive for as little as five minutes could produce airway obstruction in food packagers.

Another source of respiratory allergy is the photochemical smog produced by motor vehicle exhaust in large city areas. The smog is composed of hydrocarbons, oxides of nitrogen, and other chemicals activated by the energy of sunlight.

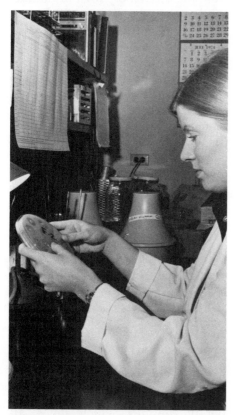

A laboratory technician conducting an experiment designed to test the allergic reaction of patients to various antibiotics.

When inhaled in the amounts present along the nation's expressways, the smog has been found to impair the normal function of membranes in the lungs.

Drugs

Medicines and drugs, such as penicillin, or serums used in inoculations, can cause allergic reactions. Estimates of the incidence of allergy among those receiving penicillin range from one to ten percent. The National Institutes of Health has calculated that just three common drugs—penicillin, sulfonamides, and aspirin—account for as much as 90 percent of all allergic drug reactions. The allergic reactions include asthmatic symptoms, skin rash, shock, and other symptoms similar to tissue reactions to other allergens. Medical scientists theorize that chemicals in certain drugs probably combine with protein molecules in the patient's body to form a new substance which is the true allergen. However, it also has been noted that some persons show allergic reactions to placebo drugs, which may contain sugar or inert substances rather than real drugs.

Insect Venom

Insect stings cause serious allergic reactions in about four of every 1,000 persons stung by bees, fire ants, yellow jackets, wasps, or hornets. A single sting to a sensitive person may lead to a serious drop in blood pressure, shock, and possibly death. There are more than 50 reported fatalities a year, and experts suspect that other deaths occur as a result of insect stings but are listed as heart attacks, stroke, or convulsions.

Sensitivity tests of persons who might be acutely allergic to insect stings have been difficult to develop because allergic individuals reacted in the same way as nonallergic persons to skin tests performed with extracts from insect bodies. More recently, doctors have found that using pure insect venom produces a reaction that determines

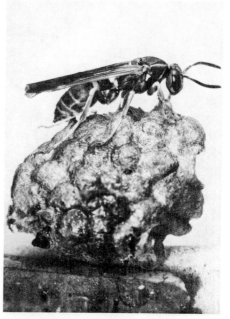

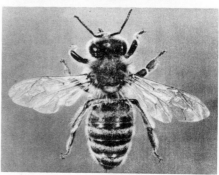

Stings of the wasp (top) and bee (bottom) can cause serious allergic reactions in susceptible individuals, who should take extra precautions to avoid them.

whether a person is allergic to the sting. Medical scientists also have isolated the major allergen in an insect venom for use in diagnosing and treating patients who are particularly sensitive to stings.

Skin Allergies

Allergies affecting the skin take many forms, the most common being eczema, urticaria (hives), angioedema (swelling of the subcutaneous tissues), and contact dermatitis. Among the most common causes are foods, cosmetics, fabrics, metals, plants and flowers, plastics, insecticides, furs and leather, jewelry, and many industrial chemicals. Studies of patients who seem to be especially sensitive

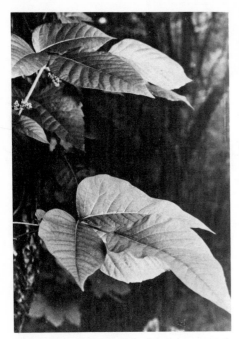

The shiny-surfaced leaves of the common poison ivy plant grow in clusters of three.

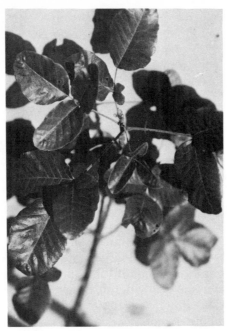

The leaves of this western poison oak plant have a thick, leathery appearance.

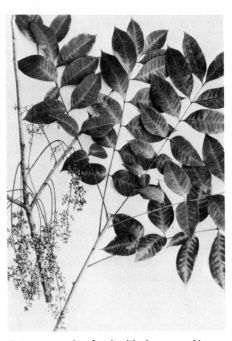

Poison sumac has featherlike leaves and hanging clusters of small, grayish fruit.

to skin allergies show that they have higher than average amounts of a body protein called *immunoglobulin E* in their systems.

In certain instances, a person who is sensitive to an allergen in a plant food also may be allergic to the pollen of the plant. The fava bean, for example, produces severe reactions when eaten by individuals who are allergic to the food; inhaling the pollen of the growing plant can cause similar reactions.

Poisonous Plants

Poison ivy, poison oak, and poison sumac contain an extremely irritating oily resin which sensitizes the body; repeated contact seems to increase the severity of the allergic reactions. About 50 percent of the population that comes in contact with the resin will experience a severe form of dermatitis and up to ten percent will be temporarily disabled by the effects. Exposure to the resin may come from direct contact with the plant, by contact with other objects or animals that have touched the plant, or by inhaling smoke from the burning plant.

Cosmetics and Jewelry

A wide variety of cosmetics and jewelry can cause allergic reactions through skin contact. Even jewelry that is presumably pure gold can contain a certain amount of nickel which will produce a mild reaction that causes a skin discoloration, sometimes aided by chemical activity resulting from perspiration in the area of jewelry contact. Among cosmetics that may be involved in allergic reactions are certain permanent-wave lotions, eyelash dyes, face powders, permanent hair dyes, hair spray lacquers, and skin tanning agents. Of course, not all persons are equally sensitive to the ingredients known to be allergens, and in most cases a similar product with different ingredients can be substituted for the cosmetic causing allergic reactions. For more information on skin allergies, see *Disorders of the Skin*, p. 245.

Environmental Allergies

Environmental agents such as sunlight, excessive cold, light, and pressure are known to produce allergic reactions in certain individuals. Cold allergy, for example, can result in hives and may even lead to a drop in blood pressure, fainting, severe shock, and sometimes death.

Research into the causes of cold allergy has shown that cold urticaria, or hives, results from a histamine released from body tissues as they begin to warm up after a cold stimulus. Extremely high histamine levels coincide with episodes of very low blood pressure, the cause of fainting.

Although reaction of the body tissues to the invasion of microbes, such as bacteria, viruses, and other microorganisms, generally is not thought of as an allergic situation, the manner in which the body musters its defenses against the foreign materials is essentially the same as the way the antibodies are mobilized to neutralize other allergens. Thus, there is a similarity between infectious diseases and allergies.

Temporary Allergies

Occasionally, a change in the body's hormonal balance may trigger a hypersensitivity to a substance that previously had no effect on the individual. Pregnant women are especially susceptible to these temporary allergies, which almost always disappear after childbirth. Some women, on the other hand, experience complete relief during pregnancy from allergies that have plagued them since childhood.

People who suffer from seasonal allergies, such as hay fever, often have heightened allergic reactions to dust, animal dander, and even certain foods, such as chocolate and pineapple, during the season when ragweed pollen or other airborne allergens are plentiful.

Diagnosis of Allergies

Some allergic reactions are outgrown; some don't develop until adulthood; some become increasingly severe over the years because each repeated exposure makes the body more sensitive to the allergen. In many instances, the irritating substance is easily identified, after which it can be avoided. In other cases, it may take a long series of tests before the offending allergen is tracked down.

Medical History

If a person suspects he may have an allergy, the first thing he should do is consult a doctor to see if the help of an allergy specialist should be sought. The doctor or allergist

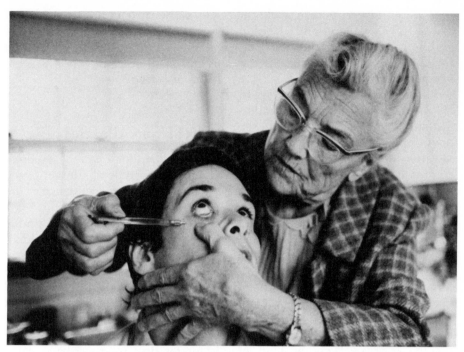

A physician puts drops of pollen extract in a patient's eye to find the pollen strength he reacts to—which in turn determines treatment.

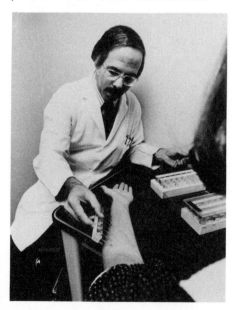

An allergy specialist applies seven substances to a patient's arm for skin testing. He will then perform a scratch test for each substance.

will first take a complete medical history and check the patient's general health. Not infrequently the source of an allergy can be found by general questioning about the patient's life style. For example, the reaction may occur only on or immediately after the patient eats seafood. Or a patient may have an apparently chronic allergy, but is not aware that it may be related to daily meals that include milk and eggs. A patient who keeps several cats or sleeps every night with a dog in the bedroom may not realize that an asthmatic condition actually is an allergic reaction to dander from the fur of a pet animal.

The history taken by the doctor will include questions about other known allergies, allergies suffered by other members of the family, variations in symptoms according to the weather, time of day, and season of the year. The symptoms may be related to a change in working conditions or the fact that the symptoms, if perhaps due to house dust, diminish during periods of outdoor exercise. A person sensitive to cold may unwittingly exacerbate the symptoms with cold drinks

while another person who is sensitive to heat may not realize that symptoms can be triggered by hot drinks but relieved by cold drinks, and so on.

Skin Testing

If the patient is referred to an allergy specialist, the allergist will continue the detective story by conducting skin tests.

SCRATCH TEST: Based on information in the medical history of the patient and the allergist's knowledge of molds, pollens, and other airborne allergens in the geographical area, he will conduct what is called a *scratch test*.

A diluted amount of a suspected allergen is applied to a small scratch on the patient's arm or back. If the results of the scratch test are inconclusive, a more sensitive test may be tried.

INTRACUTANEOUS TEST: In the *intracutaneous* test, a solution of the suspected allergen is injected into the underlayer of skin called the dermis. The intracutaneous test also may be used to verify the results of a positive scratch test. With either test, a positive reaction usually consists of a raised reddish welt, or *wheal*. The welt should develop within 15 or 20 minutes if that particular allergen is the cause of the symptoms.

CULTURE PLATES: If the allergen has been identified, or if the allergist still suspects a substance in the environment of the patient despite negative or inconclusive tests, the patient may be given a set of culture plates to place around his home and office or work area. If the allergen has been identified, the culture plates can help the doctor and patient learn where his exposure to the substance takes place. If the allergen is not known, the cultures may pick up samples of less common allergens which the specialist can test.

MUCOSAL TEST: Another kind of approach sometimes is used by allergists when skin tests fail to show positive results despite good evidence that a particular allergen is the cause of symptoms. It is called the mucosal test. The allergist using the mucosal test applies a diluted solution of the suspected allergen directly to the mucous membranes of the patient, usually on the inner surface of a nostril or by aerosol spray into the bronchial passages. In some cases, the allergic reaction occurs immediately and medication is administered quickly to counter the effects. Because of the possibility of a severe reaction in a hypersensitive patient, the mucosal test is not employed if other techniques seem to be effective.

Relief From Allergies

AVOIDANCE: For a patient sensitive to a particular type of allergen, such as molds, complete avoidance of the substance can be difficult, but some steps can be taken to avoid undue exposure. For example, the mold allergy sufferer should avoid areas of his home, business, or recreational areas that are likely spots for mold spores to be produced. These would include areas of deep shade or heavy vegetation, basements, refrigerator drip trays, garbage pails, air conditioners, bathrooms, humidifiers, dead leaves or wood logs, barns or silos, breweries, dairies, any place where food is stored, and old foam rubber pillows and mattresses.

MEDICATION: To supplement avoidance measures, the allergist may prescribe medications that will significantly reduce or relieve the irritating symptoms of the allergic reaction. Antihistamines, corticosteroids, and a drug called cromolyn sodium are among medications that may be prescribed, depending upon the nature and severity of the patient's reactions to the allergen.

IMMUNOTHERAPY: If avoidance measures and medications do not control the symptoms effectively, the allergist may suggest *immunotherapy*. Immunotherapy consists of injections of a diluted amount of the allergen, a technique similar to that used in the skin tests. A small amount of a very weak extract is injected once or twice a week at first. The strength of the extract is gradually increased, and the injections are given less frequently as relief from the symptoms is realized. The injections are continued until the patient has experienced complete relief of the symptoms for a period of two or three years. However, some people may have to continue the injections for longer time spans. Even though the treatments may relieve the symptoms, they may not cure the allergy.

IDENTIFICATION CARDS: Any person subject to severe disabling allergy attacks by a known allergen should carry a card describing both the allergic reaction and the allergen. Detailed information can be obtained from the Allergy Foundation of America, 801 Second Avenue, New York, New York 10017. See also *Allergic Respiratory Diseases*, p. 394 and *Asthma Attack*, p. 587.

CHAPTER 13

Physicians and Surgeons and Their Diagnostic Procedures

Perhaps a few words are called for in explanation of the title of this chapter. *Medicine* is the umbrella term for the entire profession dealing with the maintenance of health and treatment of disease. In a narrower sense, however, it is often used in distinction to *surgery*, which deals with the correction of disorders or other physical change by operation or by manual manipulation. Thus the term *medical* is often used in distinction to *surgical*, and a *physician*, who treats his patients by medical means, may likewise be distinguished from a *surgeon*. The term *physician*, however, is also used broadly to apply to any authorized practitioner of medicine, including surgeons.

The two kinds of physicians most likely to be encountered when we have an undefined symptom or ailment that requires professional diagnosis and treatment are general or family practitioners and internists. These are the generalists of the medical profession, physicians who treat a wide variety of disorders and illnesses. Unlike other specialists, they usually do not require a referral from another doctor and are the first to interview a person about his condition and any complaints he may have.

The General Practitioner

The *general practitioner* or GP is about the closest thing we have to the old country doctor who hung out his shingle in front of his small-town house and made midnight carriage rides to deliver babies. The GP not only delivers babies, but also listens to our problems, treats skin rashes, sets broken bones, sees children through difficult diseases, dispenses antibiotics and pain-killers, and does all the other things we expect a doctor to do. He may also perform appendectomies.

Internal Medicine

The *internist* is really a specialist in the branch of medicine called internal medicine. He usually refers surgery, and may also refer special problems affecting specific body systems, to physicians specializing in such areas. The internist's training is longer and more intensified than that of the GP. In addition, most internists spend one or two years of study in a subspecialty, such as cardiology (heart), hematology (blood), etc. An internist is usually associated with at least one major hospital, its specialists, and its operating and laboratory facilities.

The field of an internist has been defined as "medical diagnosis and treatment"—obviously a very broad definition, to which must be added the observation that one of the responsibilities of the internist is to know when his knowledge is insufficient and when he should refer a patient to another specialist.

An internist should not be confused with an *intern* (or *interne*), who is a medical school graduate serving a year in residence at a hospital. The intern is, in a sense, an apprentice doctor, putting the finishing practical touches on the knowledge he has accumulated in medical school by first-hand diagnosis and treatment of patients under the supervision of an experienced doctor.

The medical profession officially recognizes and licenses physicians and surgeons to become specialists in 19 fields (listed below). Before becoming a certified specialist in any of these fields, a doctor must qualify in training and pass examinations supervised by a board made up of physicians already practicing that specialty. This training is known as *residency* training.

Subspecialties of Internal Medicine

There are also a number of subspecialties in which an internist may develop a special interest, such as *cardiology*, the study of the diseases of the heart, or *gastroenterology*, dealing with disorders of the digestive tract. Both cardiology and gastroenterology are unusual subspecialties in that passing of examinations is required for certification as a *cardiologist* or a *gastroenterologist*.

There are a number of other subspecialties of internal medicine, some having a quite familiar ring. *Allergology*, the treatment and diagnosis of allergies, is the interest of the *allergist*. The circulatory system (heart and blood vessels) is the special concern of the *cardiovascular specialist*. *Endocrinology* is the study of the endocrine system and its glands; the specialist is an *endocrinologist*. The study of blood chemistries and treatment of blood diseases, such as anemia and leukemia, are called *hematology*, the province of the *hematologist*. The study of the connecting and supporting tissues of the body is called *rheumatology*, and the specialist is a *rheumatologist*.

Apart from these subspecialties, a number of internists have satisfied the requirements of boards for both internal medicine and one of the other special branches of medicine.

Specialties Approved by the American Medical Association

The following major specialties are recognized by the American Medical Association:

ANESTHESIOLOGY: The *anesthesiologist*, especially during major surgery, administers a patient's state of anesthesia (loss of the sensation of pain) either in parts of or all of the body.

COLON AND RECTAL SURGERY: *Proctology* is the field dealing with diseases of the rectum and colon.

DERMATOLOGY: The *dermatologist* is a specialist in the diagnosis and treatment of skin diseases.

INTERNAL MEDICINE: The role of the *internist*, a kind of general specialist, is discussed above.

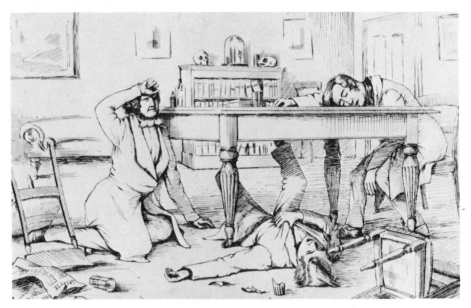

Doctors at one time tested new remedies by trying them personally. This nineteenth century drawing shows scientists taking chloroform.

NEUROLOGICAL SURGERY: The neurological surgeon deals with the diagnosis, treatment, and surgical management of disorders and diseases of the brain, spinal cord, and nervous systems.

OBSTETRICS AND GYNECOLOGY: A physician can be an *obstetrician*, a *gynecologist*, or both. The obstetrician's specialty is pregnancy and childbirth; the gynecologist specializes in the care and treatment of women and their diseases, especially of the reproductive system. In practice, he usually treats women who are not pregnant.

OPHTHALMOLOGY: The *ophthalmologist* is a specialist in medical and surgical treatment of the eye.

ORTHOPEDIC SURGERY: The *orthopedist* or "*orthopod*" specializes in diagnosing, treating, and surgically correcting, where possible, disorders and injuries associated with the bones, joints, muscles, cartilage, and ligaments.

A pediatrician examines a patient with a sore throat. Pediatrics as a specialty deals with all types of disease experienced by children.

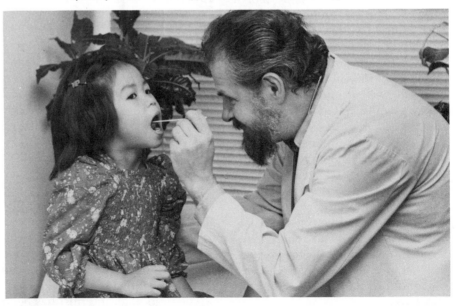

OTOLARYNGOLOGY: The *otolaryngologist* is a specialist, with surgical competence, in practically all the cavities of the head except those holding the eyes and the brain. He is the doctor of the ear, nose, and throat, often abbreviated to ENT.

PATHOLOGY: The pathologist investigates the course and causes of diseases with a mastery of the laboratory devices and techniques at his disposal.

PEDIATRICS: The pediatrician specializes in all medical aspects of child care.

PHYSICAL MEDICINE AND REHABILITATION: This specialist deals with the full or partial restoration of use and function to body parts that have been affected by disease or injury, or have been defective at birth.

PLASTIC SURGERY: The plastic surgeon specializes in operations designed to give a more normal appearance to parts of the body that are disfigured or that the owner feels are unsightly.

PREVENTIVE MEDICINE: This specialist is concerned with predicting and preventing disease, usually in one specific institution or sector, such as an industry or an urban community.

PSYCHIATRY AND NEUROLOGY: Broadly speaking, the psychiatrist deals with the subjective feelings of his patients; the neurologist deals with the objective facts of the nervous system.

RADIOLOGY: The radiologist is an expert in using electromagnetic radiations (*e.g.*, X rays) for the diagnosis and treatment of diseases.

SURGERY: The general surgeon has been trained to perform surgery anywhere on the body, but he usually specializes in a particular area.

THORACIC SURGERY: A thoracic surgeon specializes in operations involving the organs of the chest, or thoracic cavity.

UROLOGY: The urologist specializes in the diagnosis, treatment, and surgical management of diseases affecting the male urinogenital tract and the female urinary tract.

THE PHYSICAL EXAMINATION

The use of physical examinations to determine the health of people is not new. Medical literature reveals that periodic health examinations were required of the Spartans of ancient Greece. American doctors have encouraged periodic examinations of children and adults as a preventive health measure since the beginning of the Civil War. But only in the last few decades has the general public accepted the idea that many physical disorders can be detected in the earliest stages by an examining physician and corrective measures prescribed to insure the maximum number of productive years for the patient. Heart disease, cancer, diabetes, hypertension, and glaucoma are just a few examples of diseases that a doctor can detect during a routine physical examination long before disabling symptoms begin to be noticeable to the patient. The Pap test for women is a specific example of an examination technique that can predict the development of cervical cancer several years before the woman might notice signs and symptoms of the insidious disease.

On the other hand, physical examinations may determine that bothersome symptoms do not herald a dangerous disease. A man who suffers from abdominal pains and fears he has stomach cancer would be relieved to learn after an examination that the problem is only nervous tension, which can be corrected by other means. Heart palpitations and breathlessness similarly might be found through a doctor's examination to be due to anxiety rather than heart disease.

The Importance of Periodic Physicals

Health examinations for most Americans unfortunately tend to be sporadic. During infancy and upon entering school, there may be detailed physical examinations, followed by possibly additional checkups during later childhood when required by the local educational system, and finally, a thorough examination for persons entering the military service or applying for a job or insurance policy. But there may follow a period of 30 to 40 "lost years" for many persons before they feel the need for a checkup because of the symptoms of one of the degenerative diseases that may appear when they have reached their 50s or 60s. Unfortunately, statistics show that nearly 30 percent of chronic and disabling diseases begin before the age of 35 and about 40 percent appear between the ages of 35 and 55, with evidence that many chronic disabilities actually developed more or less unnoticed by the patients during the "lost years" when periodic physical examinations were considered unnecessary.

Periodic physical examinations are now encouraged for persons of all age groups with four objectives:

• to detect abnormalities so that early diagnosis and treatment can prevent disability and premature death, especially from chronic diseases

• to improve the individual's understanding of health and disease

• to establish good relations between patient and doctor as a basis for continuing health maintenance

• to provide specific preventive

health measures such as immunizations and advice about such life style matters as cigarette smoking and weight control.

General Diagnostic Procedures

A typical physical examination will include a careful health appraisal by an examining physician, including a detailed health history of the patient and study of the patient's body appearance and functions, an X ray of the chest area, and electrocardiogram of the heart in some cases, and laboratory analysis of blood and urine samples. Other appropriate procedures, such as a Pap test smear, may be added to the routine. Since no two persons are exactly alike and the differences between patients are likely to increase with advancing years, the examining doctor's interest in a set of signs and symptoms may vary with different patients as he pieces evidence together to come up with a complete evaluation of a particular patient.

Medical History

The examination almost invariably begins with the *medical history* and includes details which may seem trivial or unimportant to the patient. But the information sometimes can provide important clues to a physician compiling data about a patient. This information usually includes the age, sex, race, marital status, occupation, and birthplace of the patient. The examiner also may want to know about any previous contacts with the doctor's medical group, clinic, hospital, or other medical facility, in the event that previous medical records of the individual are on file.

SYMPTOMS: The doctor may ask a simple, obvious question, like "What is bothering you?" or "Why did you want to see a doctor?" The answer given may become for examining purposes the chief complaint and usually will involve any current or recent illness. If there is a current or recent illness to discuss, the doctor will want to know more about it: when did it begin, how did it begin, and how has it affected you? If the doctor asks about *symptoms*, he usually is probing for information about what the patient feels, and where. A symptom may be a pain, ache, bloated feeling, and so on. A *sign* is, in medical terminology, what somebody else, such as the doctor, observes; signs and symptoms usually go together in solving a medical problem.

The doctor's view of the importance of some symptoms may not be the same as the patient's. The doctor may try to pursue complaints that may not seem important to the patient but actually can be more significant than the chief complaint. The doctor's training and experience give him some advantages in concluding, for example, that a 45-year-old woman who has had a chronic cough for several years probably does not have lung cancer, even though that may be her chief concern.

PAST ILLNESSES: Other questions included in the medical history would be a list of childhood diseases, adult diseases such as pneumonia or tuberculosis, broken bones suffered, burns or gunshot wounds, unconsciousness as a result of an injury, a description of past operations, information about immunizations, medicines taken and side effects experienced from medications, and, for women, information about pregnancies, if any. Family history questions would cover information about the parents and blood relatives, including a variety of diseases they may have suffered.

LIFE STYLE AND ATTITUDE: Next, the doctor may review the body systems, asking questions about any difficulties experienced with the head, eyes, ears, mouth, nose, lungs, heart, etc. Changes in body weight, hair texture, appetite, and other factors will be recorded, along with information about occupation, military service, and travel in foreign countries. Life style questions could cover sleeping habits, sex life, use of coffee, tea, alcoholic beverages, vitamin tablets, sleeping pills, tobacco, exercise, and social activities. In addition to the answers given, the doctor may record how the answers to questions are presented by a patient, since the patient's attitude can offer additional insight into the person's mental and physical health. For example, a patient who tries to dominate the examination interview or who answers the doctor's questions with a response like "What do you mean by that?" may reveal more by the quality than the content of the answers.

Observation

After the medical history has been recorded or updated, the doctor may begin a general inspection of the patient's body, beginning with the head and neck and working down to the feet. The doctor looks for possible deformities, scars or wounds including insect bites, or pulsations or throbbing areas. Bruises, areas of skin peeling or flaking, areas of heavy skin pigmentation or loss of pigmentation, hair distribution, perspiration or goose bumps, firmness or slackness of the skin, warts, calluses, and other features are noted.

Palpation

The doctor usually checks the exterior of the body by a method known as *palpation,* which means feeling with the fingers and hands. Because some parts of the hand are more sensitive to warmth and others are more sensitive to vibrations, the doctor may shift from finger tips to palms at various times in his search for health clues. Rough vibrations from a disorder in the respiratory system, the trembling sensation of blood encountering an obstruction, or the grating feeling of a bone deformity can be detected during palpation. The doctor also can tell from palpation where areas are tender or abnormally warm to the touch. If he finds a raised area of the skin, he can tell by palpation whether there is a growth within or beneath the skin.

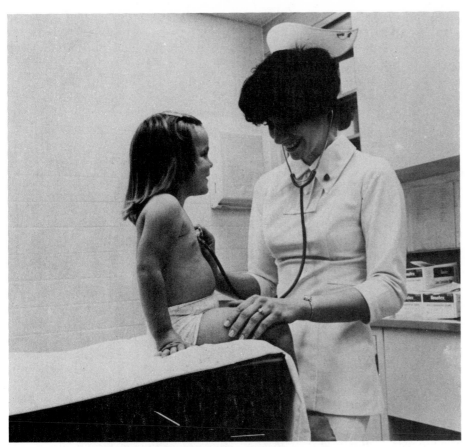

The familiar stethoscope utilizes auscultation, the listening to sounds within the body, to check the condition of the lungs.

Percussion and Auscultation

In addition to palpation, the examining physician may apply *percussion*, or tapping, of certain body areas. Tapping the chest, for example, gives the doctor some information from the sounds produced about the condition of the lungs. He also uses a related technique of *auscultation*, or listening to sounds within the body, either with his ear against the body or through a stethoscope, the familiar Y-shaped instrument used to amplify internal sounds.

In percussion, the doctor usually places one hand on the surface of the patient's body with the fingers slightly spread apart and taps on one of the fingers with the middle finger of the other hand. By moving the lower hand around on various areas of the chest surface while tapping one finger on the other, the doctor can get a fairly accurate "sound pic-

ture" of the condition of organs within the chest. He can outline the heart and the distance moved by the diaphragm in filling and emptying the lungs by listening for changes in percussion sounds that range from resonance over hollow spaces to dullness over solid or muscular areas. Lack of resonance over a normally resonant area of the lung might indicate fluid, pneumonia, or perhaps an abnormal mass. Percussion may also give the first sign of enlargement of organs such as the liver, heart, or spleen.

During auscultation, the doctor listens for normal or abnormal breathing sounds. He can usually detect specific aberrations in lung function by noises made as the air rushes in and out of the lungs through the bronchi. A sound of frictional rubbing can suggest a rough surface on the lining of the pleura, a membrane surrounding the lung tissue; a splashing or slapping sound

would indicate the presence of fluid in the lungs. In auscultation of the heart, the doctor listens for extra heartbeats, rubbing sounds, the rumbling noises of a heart murmur, or the sounds of normally functioning heart valves opening and closing.

An experienced physician may use his stethoscope for listening to sounds beyond the chest area. He may listen to the sounds of blood flowing through vessels of the neck, bowel sounds through the wall of the abdomen, and the subtle noises made by joints, muscles, and tendons as various limbs are moved.

During examination of the chest, the doctor usually asks the patient to perform certain breathing functions: take a deep breath, hold your breath, inhale, exhale, etc. On one or more of the exhalation commands, the doctor may make a quick check of the air exhaled from the lungs to determine if there is any odor suggesting a disease that might be unnoticed by the patient. Just as the doctor learns to recognize the meaning of percussion and auscultation sounds, he learns the meaning of certain odors of bacterial activity or other disorders.

Body Structure and Gait

Weight and height are checked as part of any routine examination. These factors are important in a health examination for children to determine the rate of growth, even though youngsters of the same age can vary considerably in height and weight and still be within the so-called normal range. Sudden changes in the rate of growth or abnormal growth may be signs that special attention should be given to possible problems. Adults also can vary greatly in weight and height, but special concern may be indicated by the doctor if the individual is exceptionally tall, short, fat, or skinny. In addition to a possible disease associated with unusual stature, the facts and figures obtained about body build can be important because certain disorders tend to

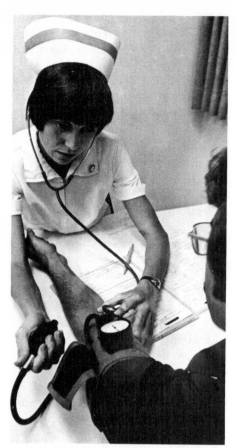

In taking blood pressure with a sphygmomanometer, a stethoscope is used to listen for the heartbeat as pressure is released.

alongside it. Either kind of device also has attached to it an inflatable cuff, which is wrapped around the upper arm; a rubber bulb is used to inflate the cuff and increase pressure in it so that it can control the blood flow in the arm. The doctor places the bell-shaped end of the stethoscope on a point on the inside of the elbow where the pulse can be felt. The bulb is squeezed to increase the cuff pressure until the heartbeat, in the form of the pulse, can no longer be heard through the stethoscope. The reading on the sphygmomanometer at that stage may be well over 200. Then the doctor slowly deflates the cuff and lets the reading on the gauge fall gradually until he hears the first beat of the heart. The reading on the gauge at that point is recorded as the *systolic pressure*. The doctor continues to relax the pressure in the cuff and watches for the reading at the point where the thumping of the heart disappears. That number is recorded as the *diastolic pressure*.

If the systolic pressure is, for example, 130 and the diastolic pressure is 72, the doctor may make a notation of "BP 130/72," which is the patient's blood pressure at the time of the examination. The records also may indicate whether the patient was sitting or lying down at the time and whether the pressure was taken on the right arm or the left arm. Sometimes the pressure is checked on both arms. If the patient appears tense or anxious, which could produce a higher than normal blood pressure reading, the doctor may encourage the patient to relax for a few minutes and try again for a more meaningful reading.

Pulse Rate

The pulse itself usually is studied for rate and quality, or character, which means the force of the pulse beat and the tension between beats. The pulse beat for small children may be well over 100 per minute and still be considered normal. But in an adult who is relaxed and resting any pulse rate over 100 suggests that something is wrong. An adult pulse rate of less than 60 also might indicate an abnormal condition.

develop in individuals of a particular body structure. Posture also provides clues to the true condition of a patient; a person who has a slouch or who holds one shoulder higher than the other may have an abnormal spinal curvature. The doctor may watch the patient's manner of walking because a person's gait can suggest muscle, bone, or nervous-system disorders; a person who seems to lean forward and take short steps, for example, may have muscles that do not relax normally during movement of the legs.

Blood Pressure

Blood pressure is measured with the help of a device called a *sphygmomanometer* and the stethoscope. The sphygmomanometer has either a dial with a face that shows the blood pressure reading in millimeters of mercury, or a column of mercury in a glass tube with numbers

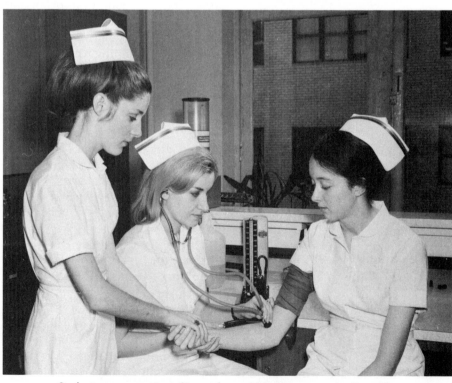

Student nurses practice taking pulse and blood pressure readings. The sphygmomanometer here utilizes a column of mercury rather than a dial.

Eyes

Inspection of the eyes, is usually done with the aid of an *ophthalmoscope*, by means of which the doctor can visualize the retina on the back inner surface of each eye, and its associated arteries, veins, and nerve fibers. Distended retinal veins may be a sign of a variety of disorders, including diabetes or heart disease; signs of hardening of the arteries also may be observed in the eyes before other indications are found elsewhere in the body. The condition of retinal blood vessels may, in addition, signal the development of hypertension.

Mouth, Nose, and Ears

The mouth, nose, and ears are inspected for signs of abnormalities. A device called an *otoscope* is inserted in the outer ear to examine the external auditory canal and eardrum. If the patient wears dentures, the doctor may ask that they be removed during examination of the mouth so that the health of the gums can be checked. The condition of the tongue, teeth, and gums can reveal much about the health habits of the individual. An inadequate set of teeth, for example, can indicate that certain important food items that require chewing are being avoided. Tobacco stains obviously are a sign of tobacco use.

X Rays

A chest X ray is usually a routine part of the examination; the X ray usually covers the chest area, showing the condition of the heart and lungs. The finished X-ray picture looks something like a large photographic negative but the film is designed so that areas filled with gas, such as the lungs or fatty tissues, appear almost transparent, and bone or solid metal objects appear sharply opaque. Muscle, blood, and other objects, including gall bladder stones, can be identified through a hazy kind of contrast between opaque and translucent. A number of special kinds of X rays may be

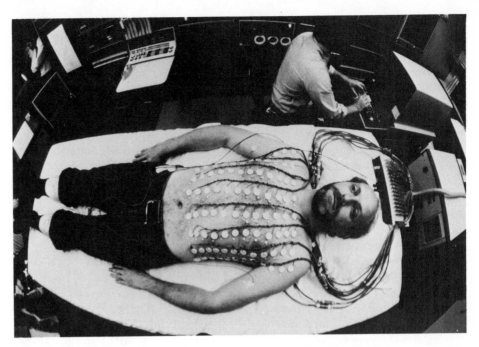

An experimental electrocardiogram uses 190 electrodes to give a clearer picture of the heart's movements than the traditional EKG.

ordered if the doctor wants to make a more detailed check of some possible disorder involving a specific body cavity, such as a peptic ulcer in the stomach wall.

Electrocardiogram

An increasing number of health examinations today include an electrocardiographic study of the heart. An *electrocardiogram,* or *EKG,* is made as a kind of "picture" traced by a pen on a moving sheet of paper, with the movements of the pen controlled by electrical impulses produced by the heart. All muscle activity produces tiny electrical discharges, and the rhythmic contractions of heart muscle result in a distinctive pattern of electrical pulsations which form the electrocardiogram picture. The tracing appears to the patient as simply a long wavy line, but the doctor can identify each of the wave crests and dips in terms of different parts of the heart muscle contracting or relaxing in proper sequence, or—if the heart is not functioning normally—not in proper sequence.

The electrocardiogram is recorded by attaching electrodes, or leads, to the chest, arms, and legs, in a series

of differing arrangements depending upon the kind of heart picture the doctor wants to record. The wires from the electrodes are connected to the machine that translates the heartbeat rhythms into the electrocardiogram. There is no danger of electrical shock because the only electricity flowing through the wires is the current produced continuously by the human body as part of its natural functions.

It is always an advantage for the patient to have an electrocardiogram taken early in adult life and when in a good state of health, because that record can serve as a benchmark for comparing electrocardiograms made later in life when the condition of the heart may have changed. This rule applies to all other health examination records as well.

Urinalysis

No patient health evaluation is complete without the findings of laboratory tests of blood and urine. The doctor or his assistant may give special instructions about food and water intake well in advance of the time for delivering a urine specimen because those factors can influence the chemical makeup of the sample. The time of day of the collection also can affect the composition of the urine sample; urine voided early in the morning is likely to be more acid in content, while urine collected after a meal may be more alkaline. Thus, for a routine physical, the doctor may advise that a urine sample be taken at his office at 9 a.m. but that nothing be eaten since the previous evening meal. The doctor also may want not the first, but the second specimen of the day. In some cases, depending upon the patient's complaint, the doctor may request a collection of all the urine voided during a period of 12 or 24 hours.

CHEMICAL CONTENT OF THE URINE: A typical urine sample is, of course, mostly water. But it also may contain about two dozen identifiable minerals and other chemicals, including sodium, potassium, calcium, sulfur, ammonia, urea, and several different acids. A urine sample can range in color from pale straw to dark amber, depending upon the concentration. It also can be other colors, including orange or blue, or even colorless, depending upon foods eaten, medi-

cations taken, diseases, or exposure to toxic substances.

APPEARANCE AND ACIDITY: The urine sample's general appearance, including color, is noted by the laboratory technician. The sample also is tested for acidity or alkalinity, normal urine being just slightly on the acid side of neutral. Urine that is definitely acidic can be a sign of a variety of disorders, including certain metabolic problems. Urine that is markedly on the alkaline side of neutral also can suggest a number of possible disorders, including an infection of the urinary tract. Alkalinity could also be caused by certain medications, or even by the patient's use of large doses of bicarbonate of soda. Foods rich in protein can make the urine more acidic, while citrus fruits and some vegetables may tend to make a patient's urine more alkaline.

WHAT THE URINE SHOWS: A thorough analysis of a person's urine can turn up some clues to the condition of almost every part of the body and verify or rule out the presence of myriad physical disorders. The specific gravity of the urine, for example, can indicate the general health of the urinary tract; protein (albu-

min) tests may tell something about the condition of the kidneys and prostate and, in a pregnant women, indicate toxemia; glucose (sugar) in the urine could suggest diabetes; the presence of ketone bodies could be a sign of metabolic disorders; bilirubin (bile) in the urine could be a sign of liver disease, and so on. Various urine tests check for the presence of red blood cells or white blood cells, tissue cells from the lining of organs, various hormones, traces of drugs taken. fat bodies, parasites, indications of renal calculi (kidney stones), and a variety of bits of tissue, often microscopic, called *casts*. One kind of cast might be a sign of heart failure or shock, another might be a warning of heavy-metal poisoning, a third might indicate a kidney infection.

Blood Tests

Laboratory blood studies also can reveal bits of information about organ systems throughout the body. For a simple blood test, a few drops may be drawn from a capillary through a finger prick; more detailed blood tests can require the equivalent of a couple of teaspoonfuls of blood drawn from a vein in the arm. The amount of blood taken for a laboratory test is not harmful; a normal body manufactures a couple of ounces of new blood every day, several times the amount used for a laboratory test.

RED CELLS: For a count of red blood cells (RBC), or *erythrocytes,* a small part of the original blood sample may be diluted and a bit of the solution placed on a special microscope slide that enables the technician to estimate the average number of red blood cells per cubic millimeter of blood. The normal RBC range for a man is in the neighborhood of 4.8 to 5.8 million red blood cells per cubic millimeter of blood; for a woman, the RBC count is about 4.4 to 5.4 million. For a child, the normal figure is slightly less than that of a woman.

The blood sample also may be checked for the level of hemoglo-

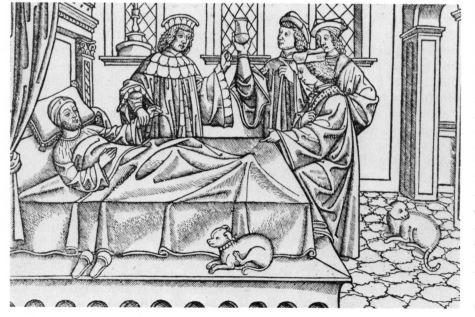

Examining a patient's urine is a time-honored method of diagnosing disease, as is evident in this sixteenth century woodcut from Italy.

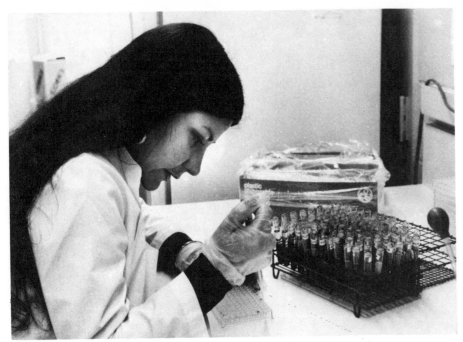

A lab technician conducting a test of blood samples.

bin, an iron-protein substance that gives the blood its red color and makes it possible for blood to carry oxygen to all parts of the body. A below-normal level of hemoglobin could be a sign of anemia due to a number of possible causes, including actual loss of blood from hemorrhage, vitamin deficiencies, lack of iron in the diet, or a disease.

WHITE CELLS: White blood cell (WBC), or *leukocyte*, counts are made the same way as RBC counts. The total normal WBC count for both men and women ranges from 5,000 to 10,000 per cubic millimeter. A higher count would indicate the presence of an infection or other disease problem.

OTHER FACTORS: Other blood studies may be performed for information about the coagulation characteristics of a patient's blood sample, levels of calcium, sodium, potassium, and other chemicals present, presence of certain enzymes, acidity of the blood, levels of sugar, bilirubin, urea nitrogen, cholesterol and other fatty substances, alcohol and other drugs, and proteins, including albumin.

Not all of these tests are performed during a routine physical examination, but they could be used if needed to track down the cause of an otherwise elusive set of symptoms. By comparing the results of two blood enzyme tests, for example, it would be possible to sort out symptoms of six different kinds of liver disease as well as a heart attack and infectious mononucleosis. The results might not be the final answer to a medical problem, but the laboratory test data could be important pieces of the jigsaw puzzle that the doctor needs to complete the health picture that begins to take form when the patient enters the doctor's office for a physical examination.

Specialties and Their Diagnostic Procedures

If a definite diagnosis cannot be made on the basis of the medical history and preliminary physical examination, more specialized tests are employed. These are usually made under the direction of a specialist. These specialists and some of the most important of their diagnostic procedures—there are literally hundreds of them—are described below, arranged according to the major body systems.

The Skeleton and the Muscles

The *orthopedic surgeon*, or *orthopedist*, is the major specialist in the diagnosis, treatment, and surgical correction of diseases and injuries of the bones, joints, and musculature. Because the healthy functioning of muscles is closely involved with the nervous system, the *neurologist* is frequently consulted. The branch of internal medicine called *rheumatology* is specially concerned with the joints.

The teeth and their supporting structures are, of course, the concern of *dentistry* and the *dentist*. The *orthodontist* is a dentist specializing in the alignment of teeth and their proper positioning in the mouth. A *pediatric dentist* specializes in teeth problems of young people up to the time that the second set of teeth erupt. An *oral surgeon* (dental surgeon) performs surgery within the oral cavity, including tooth extraction. He and the orthodontist have had additional training after receiving the dental degree, and the oral surgeon may have a medical degree (M.D.) as well. The *periodontist* treats gum disorders.

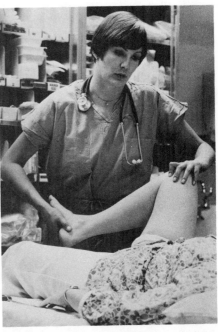

Orthopedic surgery, which deals with bone defects and diseases, was long considered a specialty for men only; recently women have entered the field.

DIAGNOSTIC PROCEDURES: *X rays* are probably relied upon more than any other technique for special investigations of the bones, joints, and teeth. They can reveal a tiny tooth cavity, a hairline fracture of a major bone, a bony deposit, or an eroded surface around a joint. *Serum analysis*—laboratory investigation of the clear portion separated from a person's blood sample—can also reveal underlying chemical irregularities that accompany or precede bone and joint diseases.

Synovial aspiration (also called *synovial fluid exam*) involves the withdrawal of a tiny amount of fluid (synovial fluid) with a needle inserted into a joint. The laboratory analysis of the fluid can diagnose gout and some forms of arthritis.

Electromyography can give an electrical tracing of muscle nerve function and reveal the presence of disorders.

Muscle biopsy is the surgical excision of a small piece of muscle tissue for laboratory examination and tests.

Skin, Hair, and Nails

The *dermatologist* is the principal specialist. *Skin biopsy*, the removal of a piece of skin tissue for laboratory testing and microscopic study, is used for difficult diagnoses.

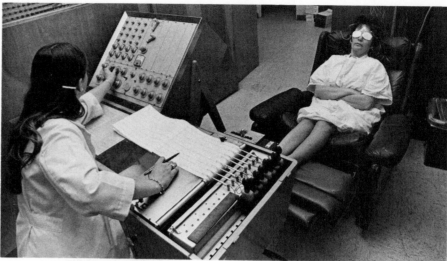

The electroencephalogram gives a detailed picture of brain activity. Electrodes placed on the patient's head record brain waves in detail.

The Nervous System and the Brain

The *neurosurgeon*, sometimes popularly referred to as a brain surgeon, is qualified for diagnosis, treatment, and surgery of the brain and nervous system. The term *neurologist* is generally restricted to a physician who does not perform surgery. The neurologist may be an internist having neurology as a subspecialty.

DIAGNOSTIC PROCEDURES: A *spinal fluid exam* or spinal tap involves the withdrawal by special needle under sterile conditions, and subsequent laboratory examination, of a small amount of cerebrospinal fluid for the diagnosis of polio, meningitis, brain tumors, and other conditions. The *electroencephalogram* (EEG) gives a picture of, and shows irregularities in, a person's "brain waves." The *echoencephalogram* uses ultrasonic waves, rather than the electric currents of the EEG, to investigate the functioning of the brain. A *brain scan* calls for the injection of a radioactive element into the brain tissue or fluid and records its movements on a photographic plate.

Recently, an X-ray technique utilizing a computer and known as *CAT scanning* (for *computerized axial tomography*) has proved to be most effective for visualizing "slices" of the brain that would otherwise be inaccessible, and no injection is necessary. Sometimes called a *brain scanner*, the device takes a series of pictures as it is rotated around the patient. From data fed into a computer, the computer generates composite pictures of the brain.

The *cerebral arteriogram* is a method of visualizing and assaying brain damage by injecting a dye into the blood vessels serving the brain and then X-raying them. It is especially useful in judging the severity and location of hemorrhages and strokes. A *pneumoencephalogram* is an X-ray picture of the brain taken

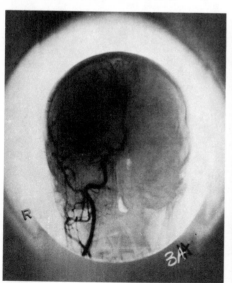
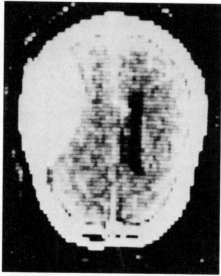

A cerebral arteriogram *(left)* shows evidence of a blood clot on the surface of a patient's brain. A CAT scan *(right)* of the same individual clearly shows the clot as a white area in the upper left section of the scan.

after air or gas has been injected into the ventricles of the brain.

The Circulatory System, the Heart, and Blood

The *cardiologist* is an internist who has special knowledge in the diagnosis and medical treatment of heart disease. The *hematologist* is an internist who has special training in the techniques of diagnosing and treating diseases of the blood (including lymph) and bone marrow.

The *thoracic surgeon* is a surgeon who has satisfied the requirements of licensing boards for both general surgery and thoracic (chest cavity) surgery. He has special training in the surgical treatment of defects and diseases of the heart and large blood vessels. The *vascular surgeon* is a general surgeon specializing in the surgical treatment of diseases of blood vessels.

DIAGNOSTIC PROCEDURES: The *electrocardiogram* graphically records the electrical activity of the heart associated with contraction of the cardiac muscle. It can provide valuable information regarding disorders of or damage to the heart muscle (i.e. heart attack), disturbances in rhythm, or enlargement of any of the four chambers of the heart. A *vectorcardiogram* is similar to the electrocardiogram, but more specifically attuned to the magnitude and direction of the electrical currents of the heart. Abnormalities not apparent on the electrocardiogram may often be revealed by a vectorcardiogram.

The *phonocardiogram* is a recording on paper of the heart sounds, which enables the physician to evaluate murmurs and abnormal heart sounds with more accuracy than by listening with the stethoscope. The timing of the murmur with relation to the specific events of heart muscle contraction may also be precisely evaluated. The *echocardiogram* provides a paper tracing of sound waves which are directed towards, and subsequently bounced back from, various internal heart structures. The technique is useful in diagnosing abnormalities of the heart valves,

as well as abnormal collections of fluid in the sac (pericardium) enveloping the heart.

The *fluoroscope* visualizes the heart in action by use of X rays. It is useful in the evaluation of heart and vessel pulsation as well as valve or vessel calcification. Plain *chest X rays* may reveal enlargement of the heart, abnormal calcification of vessels or heart valves, and signs of a congestive heart valve. These are only three examples of the great number of abnormalities that can be revealed by a routine chest X ray.

The *cardiac X-ray series* are a number of X rays of the chest taken in several positions as the patient swallows a liquid, for example, barium sulfate, which makes the esophagus stand out on the X ray. This is usually called a barium swallow. Indentation of the esophagus by abnormally enlarged heart chambers may be revealed by this technique. "Barium meals" are also important in the radiologic diagnosis of disorders of the esophagus, stomach, and small intestine.

Cardiac catheterization is the insertion of a small tubular surgical instrument, via a vein in the arm or artery of the leg, through the blood vessels, directly into the right or left side of the heart. This procedure is employed to confirm suspected intracardiac (within the heart) anomalies, determine intracardiac pressures, and take blood samples. Catheterization enables the physician to confirm suspected defects in the walls dividing the heart chambers or to estimate the severity of a lesion and the need for corrective surgery.

Angiocardiography (or simply *angiography*), if warranted, is performed at the same time as cardiac catheterization. Its principle involves the injection of a contrast material (e.g., a substance visible on a fluoroscopy screen or X-ray film) by means of the catheter, with consequent visualization of the heart and major blood vessels. Angiography is not limited to investigation of the heart chambers but can reveal abnormalities of large vessels such as the aorta, coronary arteries, and renal arteries.

CAT scanning, mentioned above on p. 298, is becoming an increasingly important diagnostic tool and may in many cases make angiocardiography unnecessary. Sometimes called a *body scanner,* the CAT scanner takes a series of computer-assisted X-ray pictures as it slowly rotates around the patient, thus pro-

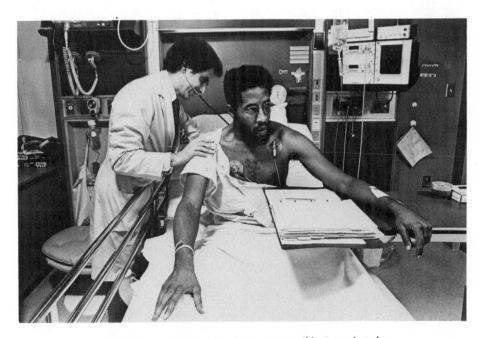

A physician examines a heart patient to see if he is ready to be transferred out of the hospital's cardiac intensive care unit.

viding cross-sectional pictures of the target organ. It is a painless and safe procedure, and is capable of providing pictures of areas of the body that would be very difficult to visualize by any other means.

HEMATOLOGICAL (BLOOD SAMPLING) DIAGNOSTIC TECHNIQUES: Routine laboratory tests performed in all hospital admissions are the *peripheral smear* and *complete blood count*. Approximately 5 milliliters (ml) of blood are *aspirated* (withdrawn by suction) from a vein, typically in the crease of the elbow. From this sample, a determination of the patient's hemoglobin and percentage of red corpuscles per milliliter of plasma may be calculated. Microscopic analysis of the number and character of the red cells, white cells, and platelets provides additional essential information. See also p. 296.

If an abnormality such as decreased hemoglobin or overpopulation of white cells is noted on complete blood count and peripheral smear, the physician might request that a sample of the patient's bone marrow be obtained for evaluation —a procedure called *bone marrow biopsy*. Following local anesthesia of the operative site, typically the hip bone, a biopsy needle is inserted into the marrow of the bone and a small sample of marrow is withdrawn. If performed by an experienced physician, the patient feels only some pressure and very slight pain as the marrow sample is aspirated.

In suspected cases of *neoplastic diseases*—diseases involving abnormal growths that may be or may become malignant—a *lymph node biopsy* (surgical excision and microscopic examination of lymph node tissue) is performed. A *lymphangiogram* is used when tumors of the lymphatic system are suspected. A dye or contrast material visible on an X ray is injected into a lymphatic vessel, usually one on the top of the foot. X rays of the abdomen taken over the next several days are studied for abnormalities in the size and structure of internal lymph nodes.

There are numerous other hematological tests, including radioactive (radio-isotope) tests, which are used in special situations when diagnosis by other means is inadequate.

The Digestive System and the Liver

The internist is generally able to treat most gastrointestinal disorders. The *gastroenterologist* is an internist who has special knowledge of disorders of the digestive tract. *Colon and rectal surgeons* operate on the large intestine, rectum, and anus; *proctology* deals with the diagnosis and treatment of disorders in this area. Surgeons and internists specializing in this region are called *proctologists*.

DIAGNOSTIC PROCEDURES: Examination can be made of the esophagus, stomach, and duodenum, and sometimes of the entire length of the small intestine, by using a sequence of many fluoroscope, motion-picture, and X-ray pictures. This is called the *gastrointestinal series*, or simply the *GI series*. So that the internal walls of the digestive organs will stand out clearly in the pictures, the patient eats nothing for eight hours before, and when the examination begins, he is asked to swallow a glassful of chalky, sticky barium sulfate. The GI series is one of the first tests administered when an ulcer or cancer is suspected in the stomach or duodenum.

Gastric analysis is the extraction and study of stomach juices for clues to intestinal disorders.

A *barium enema* is the injection via the anus of a barium solution; it usually precedes X-ray examination of the large intestine for signs of cancer or other diseases. *Stool exams*, laboratory studies of the feces, may also reveal cancer as well as the presence of parasitic worms and amebas.

There are a wide variety of slender, hollow, tubular instruments, equipped with a light and a lens to enable the physician to see into the GI tract: the *esophagoscope* for insertion by way of the mouth into the esophagus; the *gastroscope* for inspection of the stomach; the *gastroduodenal fiberscope* for inspection of the stomach and duodenum. "Scopes" inserted via the anus include the *proctosigmoidoscope* for visual examination of the rectum and lower colon, and the *colonoscope* for investigating farther up the large intestine. These are called *fiberoptic* instruments because they transmit light by means of a bundle of fibers of glass or plastic which permit observation of curved interior spaces of the body that would otherwise be inaccessible.

Special tests for the liver's health and function include the removal of a tiny piece of liver tissue, by means of a long needle inserted through the skin, and the tissues' subsequent laboratory examination; this procedure is called *needle biopsy of liver* and often is used to confirm diagnosis of cirrhosis. An injection of a chemical called *BSP*, followed later by analysis of a blood specimen, is used to investigate liver function. A *liver scan*, like a brain scan, employs a radioactive substance to visualize the function of the organ.

X-ray examination of the gall bladder, resulting in a *cholecystogram*—*cholecyst* is a medical name for gall bladder—is used to diagnose gall bladder disease and to locate gallstones. A dye is swallowed before the test.

The Respiratory System and the Lungs

The internist handles most nonsurgical disorders, and the thoracic surgeon specializes in surgical procedures involving the respiratory organs.

DIAGNOSTIC PROCEDURES: In the *sputum exam* a number of bacteriological, chemical, and microscopic tests are performed on the sputum (saliva, often mixed with mucus or other substances); these tests can detect a hidden abscess in the respiratory tract, pneumonia,

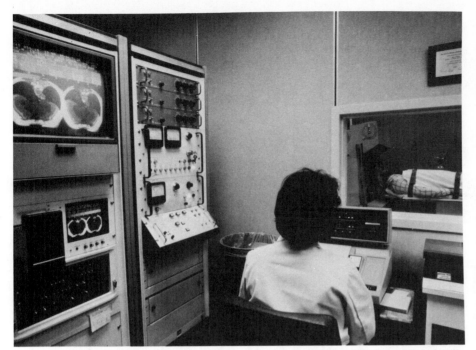

CAT scanning, an important diagnostic tool, provides detailed black-and-white or full-color TV images of a cross-section or "slice" of the body.

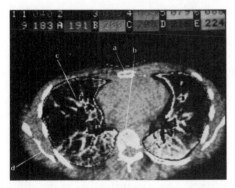

A CAT scan of a normal chest shows (a) sternum, (b) spine, (c) lung, (d) shoulder blade. Panel above indicates tissue densities.

tuberculosis, and other lung diseases.

Practically everybody is aware of the value of *chest X rays* in the diagnosis of diseases and disorders of the lungs, heart, and ribs. Many diseases of the lungs and respiratory system are also revealed by tests administered on the skin. For example, the skin's reaction to a substance called PPD (*p*urified *p*rotein *d*erivative) is used in diagnosing tuberculosis. *Bronchoscopy* is inspection of the bronchial tubes with the tube and scope instrument called the *bronchoscope*.

Special tests that measure lung volume, capacity, and function have become more common as doctors have become conscious of the adverse effects of air pollution and the growing incidence of irreversible diseases such as emphysema.

The Endocrine Glands

There is no AMA-licensed specialty, but the internist-endocrinologist is the expert.

DIAGNOSTIC PROCEDURES: There are a great many tests, using both blood and urine samples, that suggest or confirm the excess or insufficiency of a specific hormone in the body. In turn, these tests point to the overactivity or underactivity of one of the hormone-secreting endocrine glands.

The Sense Organs—Eye, Ear, Nose

The two specialists in this area are both licensed to perform surgery in their special areas of competence. The *ophthalmologist* is the eye doctor. The *otolaryngologist* is the ear, nose, and throat specialist.

DIAGNOSTIC PROCEDURES: We are all familiar with the lettered test charts that determine whether we are nearsighted or farsighted or have some other defect in our eye's focusing apparatus, such as an astigmatism. Color charts to test for color blindness are also commonly used.

With the *ophthalmoscope* and the *slit-lamp microscope*, which magnifies a beam of concentrated light, the ophthalmologist can examine the structures within the eye in great detail. The *retinoscope* reveals the actual structural abnormalities that account for nearsightedness or farsightedness. The *gonioscope* enables the ophthalmologist to inspect the angle between the cornea and the iris, which is of importance in diagnosing glaucoma. The fluid pressure itself within the anterior chamber can be measured by an extremely delicate spring-balance gauge called a *tonometer*. Finally, *perimeter* can be used to map boundaries of the visual field; the narrowing of these boundaries ("tunnel vision" is the extreme example) is a symptom of glaucoma and other eye disorders.

Hearing and hearing loss are measured by a device called the *audiometer*, with which a physician can measure accurately the whole range of vibrations heard as sound by the human ear. The *otoscope* is an instrument for examining the external auditory canal and eardrum.

The Urinogenital System and the Kidneys

The *urologist* is the acknowledged specialist. He does not deal, however, with the female reproductive organs, which are the specialty of the obstetrician and gynecologist.

DIAGNOSTIC PROCEDURES: The collective name for a number of tests that analyze the contents or urine is *urinalysis*. These include tests of the urine's physical properties, as well as chemical and microscopic analysis. Telltale signs of diseases of the kidneys and bladder often show up in urine, and sugar in the urine may be an indication of diabetes. *Urine culture* is a test for microbial infec-

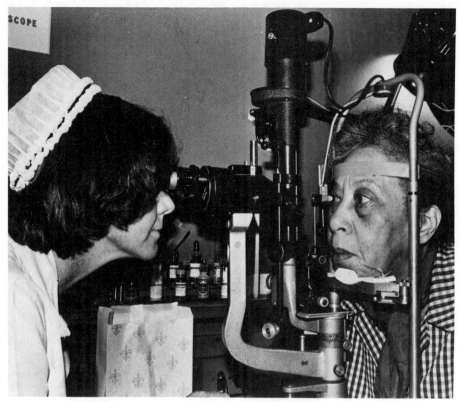

This patient is undergoing a test for glaucoma with a device known as a tonometer, which measures fluid pressure within the eye.

tions of the urinary tract.

Pyelograms are X-ray examinations of the interior of the kidney (kidney pelvis) and of the tube (ureter) carrying urine away from the kidney to the bladder. Pyelograms may involve the injection of a substance into the patient's bloodstream to facilitate viewing of the kidney area.

The special hollow tube, lens, and light instrument called a *cystoscope* is used to view the inside of the bladder after being inserted up the urethra. *Voiding cystometrics* test the condition and capacity of the bladder by pumping water into it, measuring the resulting pressures, and timing the onset of the desire to void.

The technique of *needle biopsy,* discussed in respect to the liver under *The Digestive System and the Liver,* p. 300, is also used to examine kidney and prostate tissue.

For a discussion of diagnostic procedures for the female reproductive system, see *The Gynecological Examination,* p. 483. Diagnostic procedures are also discussed under *Surgery,* p. 304.

Patients' Rights

Diagnostic procedures have raised many questions centering on patients' rights. The questions concern both physicians and hospitals, and relate to the general right of a patient to know what is happening to him or her and why.

Efforts to develop lists of specific rights that the patient enjoys have gone far beyond the specific area of diagnosis and treatment. The lists touch on such matters as the patient's need to maintain privacy, his or her right to be informed of any surgical or other procedures to be performed, and the right to refuse treatment to the extent permitted by law. One such "Bill of Rights" was issued by the American Hospital Association in 1973. It noted in part:

Equitable and humane treatment at all times and under all circumstances is a right. This principle entails an

obligation on the part of all those involved in the care of the patient to recognize and to respect his individuality and his dignity. This means creating and fostering relationships founded on mutual acceptance and trust.

Like other statements on patients' rights, the AHA list stressed *informed consent.* That meant the need on the part of the patient to be able to agree to medical and surgical treatment on the basis of complete, accurate information. Informed consent as a principle provided the foundation for many other specific or general rights. These include:

• The right to considerate and respectful care
• The right to take part in planning for one's own care
• The right to have records kept confidential
• The right to full explanation of the hospital bill

Questions to Ask the Doctor

The various rights suggest some of the questions the patient may want to ask the doctor—either at the time of the first visit or later. For example, most patients want to know the results of diagnostic tests and procedures. Patients may also ask about planned treatments, the risks and chances of success or failure with particular types of treatment, and the period of time for which the patient may be hospitalized.

Many other factors become important. Where one patient may want to know about alternative forms of care or treatment, another may ask about the surgeons who may perform an operation, the specialists who may be called in, and so on. Typically, most questions relate to the patient's situation: how far it has progressed, whether danger to life or health is involved, the doctor's estimate of the chances of recovery, and other points. Doctors themselves suggest that patients ask questions to find out . .

1. whether hospitalization, if it has been recommended, is really necessary;

2. whether consultation with another doctor or other doctors may be called for;

3. whether—if necessary—medical terms or wordings can be clarified; and

4. whether, in case the patient is in doubt, the doctor understood what the patient reported about symptoms, history, prescriptions already taken, and similar data.

Common sense usually indicates what other questions the patient should ask the doctor. The patient may have to make allowances for medical procedures. For instance, a thorough physical examination always requires that the patient undress—but no invasion of privacy is intended. Most important, the patient's right to free communication should be respected, and the patient should understand that it is.

Diagnostic Tests and Patients' Rights

Many diagnostic tests and procedures have been discussed. Many others could be listed.

One reason is that as medical costs have risen in recent years, some persons have questioned the necessity of various diagnostic tests. Consumer advocates have insisted that patients in some hospitals have been charged for tests that only increased their hospital bills. In some cases the tests were given in *batteries*, or sets. The question that has come up: Did the patients actually understand all those tests and what they involved?

Cost, as both outsiders and members of the medical profession admit, has definitely become a factor in medical care. An electrocardiogram may cost only $20 or $30; but a computerized axial tomography (CAT) scan can cost $500 to $600.

Another reason why questions about patients' rights have been raised centers on the nature of test batteries and the time available to doctors. The batteries can be complex, and the physician may often be short of time. He may find it difficult or impossible to explain every test he has ordered—and to do so in enough detail so that the patient knows what each test requires and what it means in terms of discomfort, risk, and cost.

Hospital admission tests may be simple or complex. They may involve only "vital signs" tests of temperature, pulse rate, respiratory rate, and blood pressure. But they can include the *admission labs*—screening tests done by automated machines. These tests may include a urinalysis (UA), a complete blood count (CBC), and serum chemistries—Simultaneous Multiple Analyzer tests of 12 (SMA-12) or 24 (SMA-24) factors. The SMA-12 would typically call for chemical analyses for calcium, inorganic phosphorus, glucose, and nine other body elements.

Admission labs usually also include a test for syphilis, a chest X-ray, and an EKG. The latter is often considered essential for patients over 40. Together, the admission labs tell the physician a number of important facts about the state of the patient's health.

Literally dozens of other tests could be noted. All involve some degree of risk and discomfort for the patient. But for most admission tests, both risk and discomfort are minimal. When the patient agrees to undergo them in batteries, is his or her right of informed consent being violated?

The Doctor's Challenge

That question cannot be answered in a single word. The doctor faces a dilemma in nearly all cases. He or she has to ask how much information can and should be transmitted—and how much the patient can absorb without becoming confused. He or she has also to ask what degree of risk is involved in any test or series of tests. Then the doctor has to weigh the advantages of having test readings against the disadvantages involved in not having those test results. For a woman under 35, a test for cancer such as the mammogram may entail some risk if administered regularly (annually). For an older woman the risk is considered minimal.

With some tests, the risk for the patient is slight to virtually nonexistent. But all tests given in batteries involve some risk, however minor. Does that mean that administration of tests in batteries increases the risk element significantly? It may, say those who argue against administration of tests by sets or groups.

The protocols or understandings on patients' rights establish fairly loose standards. That applies particularly in the area of information to be given to the patient. Thus the physician has to make a judgment decision in many cases. He or she tries to find out what the patient wants to know and whether all the needed information is readily available. The doctor may even have to do some "homework" to answer the patient's questions.

Authorities agree that doctors should spend time with patients and their families to the extent necessary to clarify procedures, risks, and prognoses. Doctors are also advised to talk to patients in a direct and honest manner, and in layman's terms. By such means the patient's rights are protected. The doctor also finds out what he or she needs to know to make an accurate diagnosis.

CHAPTER 14

Surgery

WHAT YOU SHOULD KNOW BEFORE UNDERGOING SURGERY

Almost everyone can expect to be wheeled into an operating room at some point in his lifetime. Surveys of hospitals during the 1970s indicated that about 12,000,000 people in the United States were surgery patients in a typical year. The range of surgical procedures performed every year is vast—correction of broken bones, organ transplants, facial uplifts, hernia repairs, hysterectomies, Caesarian sections, vasectomies, appendectomies, and so on. It is obviously impossible for a work of this sort to describe more than a fraction of the thousands of surgical procedures and their variations that are widely performed. For a representative sampling of some specific surgical procedures, see *Common Surgical Procedures*, beginning on p. 317.

The seriousness of surgical procedures within the same category can vary widely. For example, one case of inguinal hernia may be repaired quickly and simply in a young man physically able to leave the hospital on the same day he arrived. Another inguinal hernia case could be a real emergency if a portion of the small intestine were to become trapped in the hernia sac protruding into the abdominal wall, resulting in the death of the bowel-tissue cells. Easy generalizations about the seriousness of a given procedure are simply not warranted.

Types of Surgery

Surgery is sometimes categorized according to whether it is vital to life, necessary for continued health, or desirable for medical or personal reasons. Although there are many ways in which surgical procedures are classified, the following breakdown is one that is widely accepted among surgeons.

Emergency Surgery

Most disorders requiring surgery do not improve by delaying the trip to the hospital. Some can be planned and scheduled so as to coincide with periods in which a few days in the hospital will be unlikely to interfere with job or family responsibilities. But unfortunately there are also unpredictable events that precipitate an immediate need for surgery. An automobile accident, a fire, a violent crime, or even a sudden change in a chronic medical problem like a perforated ulcer or a strangulated hernia, can create situations in which the life of the patient depends upon the time it takes to get the victim into the hands of a trained surgeon. Emergency surgery cases typically involve the treatment of gunshot and stab wounds, fractures of the skull and other major bones, severe eye injuries, or life-threatening situations such as obstruction of the windpipe caused by choking on a piece of food.

Emergency surgery may be one of the most common routes for patients entering the operating room. Accident patients, according to one estimate, require four times as many hospital beds as cancer patients and more hospital beds than all heart patients. They account for more than a half-million deaths and disabilities in America each year. They present tremendous challenges to surgeons because emergency room patients frequently have multiple injuries involving several organ systems.

Such victims are often unconscious or otherwise unable to communicate coherently about their injuries, and there may be little or no time to obtain medical histories or information about their blood types, allergies to medicines, etc.

When possible, vital information about the patient and the circumstances surrounding the injury or sudden need for surgery is obtained by medical personnel who question anybody who might provide one or more clues. Efforts to maintain life are begun even while blood samples are taken for laboratory analysis and X-ray photographs made of the chest, abdomen, and other body areas that may be involved. Many *heroic* measures—extreme measures taken when a life is in immediate peril—may be used in critical cases; for example, resuscitation, induction of anesthesia, and surgery might proceed simultaneously as soon as a diagnosis is made. When several teams are working on the patient at the same time, a general surgeon may be called upon to coordinate the multiple operating room procedures.

The Emergency Room

As the first part of the hospital to which patients with emergency problems are admitted, the emergency room (ER) plays a key role in making total medical care available. Not all patients admitted to the emergency room will require surgery; in fact, estimates place the number of *nonemergency cases* encountered in the typical emergency room at 50 to 75 percent. That means one-half to two-thirds of all ER patients cannot be classified as true emergency cases. But the ER staff has to be prepared to deal with cuts and bruises as well as with major emergencies that can, at worst, result in death.

The emergency room may or may not be part of the hospital's outpatient department. In either case, the ER remains what has been called a "stepchild" of the hospital system: it has its own record-keeping and admission procedures, and in general operates fairly independently of the rest of the hospital. But the ER physician makes the initial decisions regarding the seriousness of an emergency. He or she also provides initial treatment, and may ask for immediate tests of various kinds to make possible rapid diagnoses.

The patient reporting to the emergency room becomes an "emergency outpatient." He is thus distinguished from the "general outpatient" who receives various hospital services on an outpatient basis and is the responsibility of the hospital for further care and treatment. The emergency outpatient is different also from the "referred outpatient" who is referred by a doctor and who remains the doctor's responsibility while utilizing hospital services.

The inpatient, by contrast, is formally admitted to the hospital and assigned to a ward and bed. Special types of records are kept. Where the outpatient typically occupies a bed for a few hours, if at all, an inpatient may remain for weeks or even months. Once the emergency outpatient moves on to utilize the hospital's regular clinical or medical service – including surgery—he or she ceases to be the responsibility of the outpatient department and becomes an inpatient.

Like all medical costs, the fees for emergency outpatient care have been rising steadily. In the early 1980s the basic per-visit fee reached $25 to $35. Other charges were regularly made for tests according to schedules that varied from hospital to hospital. For example, of the chemical analyses that could be ordered, a bilirubin test might cost $7.50 to $10. A complete blood count (CBC) might cost $12 to $15. Depending on the area of the body examined, an X-ray could cost from $50 to $90.

Urgent Surgery

Next in priority for the surgeon are cases in which an operation is vital but can be postponed for a few days. A person injured in an automobile accident, but conscious and suffering a minor bone fracture may be classed as an urgent rather than emergency surgery case, and the delay would give surgeons and other medical personnel time to study X rays carefully, evaluate blood tests and other diagnostic data, and otherwise plan corrective therapy while under less pressure. A penetrating ulcer of the stomach likely would be classed as urgent surgery, but the ulcer case would become emergency surgery if it were to rupture through the stomach wall. An acute, inflamed gall bladder, kidney stones, or cancer of a vital organ would be examples of urgent surgery cases.

Elective Surgery

Elective surgery is usually subdivided into three categories: required, selective, and optional.

REQUIRED SURGERY: Physical ailments that are serious enough to need corrective surgery, but which can be scheduled a matter of weeks or months in advance, generally are designated as required surgery cases. Conditions such as a chronically inflamed gall bladder, cataracts, bone deformities, or diseased tonsils and adenoids would be examples of conditions that require surgery. Also in this classification might be cases of uncomplicated inguinal hernia, hiatal hernia, and surgery of the reproductive organs that do not need immediate attention.

SELECTIVE SURGERY: Selective surgery covers a broad range of conditions which are of no real threat to the health of the patient but nevertheless should be corrected by surgery in order to improve his comfort and well-being. Certain congenital defects such as cleft lip (harelip) and cleft palate would be included in this classification, as well as removal of certain cysts and non-malignant fatty or fibrous tumors. Selective surgery also might include operations to correct crossed eyes in children so that normal binocular vision can develop properly.

OPTIONAL SURGERY: Of the lowest priority are operations that are primarily of cosmetic benefit, such as removal of warts and other non-malignant growths on the skin, blemishes of the skin, and certain cases of varicose veins. Optional surgery also includes various kinds of plastic surgery undertaken for cosmetic effect. Among popular types of plastic surgery are operations to change the shape of female breasts; this would include the correction of unusually large or pendulous breasts as well as the enlargement of unusually small breasts. Other common plastic surgery procedures are *rhinoplasty*, or nose shaping; *otoplasty*, the correction of protuding ears; *blepharoplasty*, the removal of bags under the eyes; and *rhytidoplasty*, known popularly as a facelift. Rhytidoplasty is relatively simple, virtually painless, and effective; because the benefits usually are temporary, it is an operation which many patients volunteer to undergo more than once. For fuller information on these procedures, see *Plastic and Cosmetic Surgery*, p. 343.

Since the end of World War II, there has been a proliferation of surgical specialties. The general surgeon of past eras who handled all kinds of operations is gradually being replaced by a battery of highly specialized experts who may work only on the nervous system, the eye, the ear, the bones and muscles, and so on. When warranted, a patient's case may be handled by several different surgical specialists. The result has been safer, more effective surgical treatment for the average patient.

Pre-operative Procedures

Preparation of a patient for surgery involves a variety of procedures determined by the urgency of the operation, the anatomical area involved, the nature of the disease or injury requiring surgery, the general condition of the patient, and other factors. Emergency surgery of an accident victim in critical condition obviously requires a greatly accelerated pace of preparing the patient for the operating room; medical personnel may cut away the clothing of the victim in order to save precious minutes. An operation on the intestine, on the other hand, may require a full week of preparation, including the five or so days needed to sterilize the bowel with drugs and evaluate laboratory tests. However, most pre-op procedures, as they are commonly called, generally follow a similar pattern designed to insure a safe and sound operation. Even in a case of emergency surgery, certain information must be compiled to help guide the surgeon and other hospital staff personnel in making the right decisions affecting proper care of the patient during and after the operation.

Medical History

This pattern begins with a medical history of the patient. The medical history should reveal the general health of the patient and any factors that might increase the risk of surgery. Perhaps one of his parents or another close relative suffered from heart disease or diabetes; such facts might suggest a predisposition of the patient to problems associated with those disorders. The data should also show whether the patient has a tendency to bleed easily, and whether he has been following a special diet such as a sodium-restricted diet.

It is important that the patient reveal quite frankly to his own doctor, the surgeon, and the anesthetist the names of any drugs or other medications used. It also is vital that the medical personnel have a complete record of any patient experiences, including allergic reactions to certain drugs, that might help predict drug sensitivities that could complicate the surgery. The simple fact that a patient suffers from asthma or hay fever might indicate that he may be more sensitive than other individuals to drugs that might be administered.

ALLERGIC REACTIONS: Some patients are allergic to penicillin or other antibiotics. Others may be sensitive to aspirin or serums. Still others could be allergic to iodine, Merthiolate, or even adhesive tape. All of these factors should be brought to the attention of the medical staff, if they are known and if they apply to the patient about to undergo surgery.

MEDICATIONS CURRENTLY BEING USED: Among medications routinely used by the patient that should be brought to the attention of the surgeon and anesthetist are insulin for diabetes, digitalis drugs for heart diseases, and cortisone for arthritis. Depending upon various factors relating to the individual case, the patient may be directed to continue using the medication as usual, change the size of the dose before or after surgery, or discontinue the drug entirely for a while.

A patient who has been taking certain sedatives or drinking alcoholic beverages regularly for a prolonged period before surgery may have developed a tolerance for the anesthetic used, which means that he would require a larger than usual dose to get the desired effect. A patient who has been using epinephrine-type eye drops for glaucoma may be asked to increase the dosage before surgery as an adjustment to one of the drugs used in conjunction with a general anesthetic.

Diuretics, tranquilizers, and anti-coagulant drugs are among other medications commonly used by patients that could affect the manner in which a surgical procedure is carried out. When possible, the patient should take a sample of the medication, a copy of the prescription, or the pharmacist's label from a container of the medication to the hospital so the medical staff can verify the type of drug used.

PSYCHOLOGICAL EVALUATION: Of increasing importance in recent years has been a psychological evaluation of the patient. Individuals with a past history of mental disease or patients whose complaints may be based on psychoneurotic factors may react differently to surgery than persons who could be described as psychologically well-balanced. The pre-operative interviews also may seek to obtain information about the patient's use of drugs of abuse or alcohol; a patient who has developed a physical dependence upon alcohol could develop withdrawal symptoms after suddenly being separated from alcoholic beverages during his hospital stay.

Physical Examination

In addition to the medical history evaluation, the surgeon will need vital information about the physical condition of the patient. This requires a complete physical examination, including a chest X ray, an electrocardiogram of the heart activity, a neurological examination, and a check of the condition of the blood vessels in various areas of the body. Other body areas may be checked as warranted by complaints of the patient or by the type of surgery to be performed. An examination of the rectum and colon may be suggested, for example, if the medical history includes problems related to the digestive tract. Adult women patients usually receive a Pap test and possibly a pelvic examination. Samples of blood and urine are taken for laboratory analysis, including blood typing in the event a transfusion is needed. The laboratory tests for older patients frequently are more detailed and may include an examination of a stool sample.

Many hospitals and surgeons will accept information obtained from a pre-op examination conducted several days or more before admission to the hospital for surgery, especially for elective surgery. By completing the blood and urine tests, physical examination, X rays, elec-

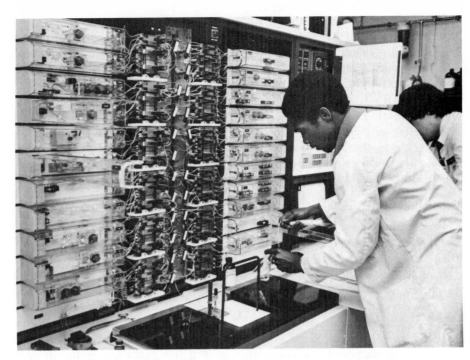

A wealth of tests precedes surgery. A high-speed computerized machine can analyze 150 blood samples an hour, making up to 20 tests on each.

trocardiograms, and medical history interview in advance of the trip to the hospital, the patient can reduce the length of the hospital stay. In some instances, the patient may be able to report to the hospital the night before the surgery is scheduled or even a few hours ahead of actual surgery. However, additional blood and urine samples may be taken immediately after admission to recheck the body chemistry, and a brief physical examination may be made to make sure the patient does not have any open wounds or infections that might complicate the chances of recovery or introduce a dangerous strain of bacteria into the sterile environment of the operating room.

Preparation for Anesthesia

After the patient is settled in his assigned bed, he is visited by the anesthetist who will be working with the surgeon. The anesthetist usually has an advance copy of all the information obtained by the surgeon and other doctors who have examined the patient, along with laboratory reports of blood chemis-

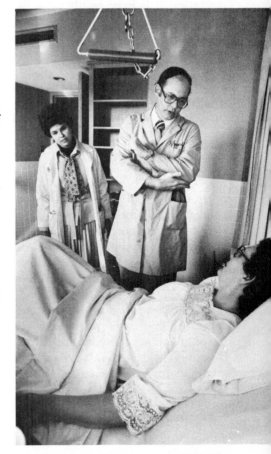

A surgeon explains what he will do and why to a patient the night before her surgery. The patient can also expect visits from the anesthesiologist and any specialists consulting her doctor.

try, etc. He may want to review the information with the patient and examine him briefly to learn more about his particular problem. If the patient uses a medication that might interfere with the intended effects of the anesthetic to be used, the anesthetist will make a decision regarding the best way to avoid a possible chemical conflict during surgery.

Other Preparations

In a typical case of elective surgery, the patient can expect to experience the actual pre-operative preparations on the afternoon or evening before surgery is scheduled. If blood transfusions may be required, there will be a final check by the hospital staff to make sure enough units of the correct cross-matched type are available.

If the surgery involves the lower digestive tract, or is an abdominal operation that may result in a disturbance of normal bowel function, the patient can expect to be given an enema. However, enemas are not administered routinely to surgery patients who are being prepared for other kinds of operations. An exception to the rule would be patients who complain of constipation.

Legal Authorization

Before the pre-operative preparations are completed, chances are good that a member of the hospital staff will make sure that the patient has signed a permit authorizing the operation. The permit is a legal form describing the operation to be performed, or a special diagnostic or therapeutic procedure other than surgery if that is the purpose of the hospitalization. The statement may be signed by a close relative or legal guardian if for some reason the patient is unable to take responsibility for this action. For example, a parent will be asked to sign a permit authorizing an operation on his or her child.

Exceptions may be made in cases of emergency surgery where the patient is unable to sign a permit and a relative or guardian cannot be located in time. But there are in-house procedures of consultation among staff members who accept the responsibility. Laws regarding permission to perform surgery may vary locally; and in some communities, for example, a married patient cannot authorize surgery that may affect his or her reproductive organs without consent of the spouse. Abortion, likewise, may be illegal in some areas without the husband's consent.

Pre-op Meals

A light but adequate evening meal is served if the surgery is scheduled for the following morning, but no solid food is permitted for 12 hours before surgery. No fluids are allowed during the eight hours before surgery. Children and patients with certain diseases, such as diabetes, may be given special orders regarding nutrients. An infant, for example, may be allowed sweetened orange juice up to four hours before surgery in order to prevent the child from developing restless anxiety because of hunger.

Preparation of the Skin Area

The area of the skin around the surgery site is carefully prepared beginning the evening before the operation. A member of the hospital staff may assist or direct the cleaning of the area with soap and warm water. The cleansing may be done in a shower or tub, or simply with a pan of water and soap brought to the patient's bedside. The cleaned skin area is usually scrubbed again in the operating room as further protection against possible infection.

SHAVING: Whether or not the skin area is to be shaved depends upon the amount of hair present. If there is no hair, the tiny nicks or cuts made by a razor would constitute an unnecessary hazard of infection. Where hair is present, however, shaving is essential in order to make available a very clean skin surface. Also, it is important that no hair or hair fragments be close enough to the surgical incision to fall beneath the skin; the bit of hair beneath the skin could cause a serious infection after surgery. Thus, to clean an area for an inguinal hernia the patient's abdomen may be shaved and scrubbed from a point above the navel down to the mid-thigh level.

Sedation

After all these pre-op steps have been completed, the patient usually is given a bedtime sedative or other medication and additional sedatives plus special medications in the morning, about 30 minutes to an hour before surgery is scheduled to begin.

The Surgical Team

Most surgical operations are performed not by the surgeon alone, but by a surgical team. Depending upon the complexity of the surgical procedure involved, the surgeon may have one or more assistants working with him. The assistants may be interns or hospital residents who participate in the operation as a part of their advanced training in surgical techniques, or they may be other surgeons who are specialists in a particular field. An abdominal surgeon or orthopedic surgeon, for example, may be assisted by a neurosurgeon if the operation is likely to require a special knowledge of the nervous system as it affects another organ system.

The Anesthetist

The anesthetist, who is also likely to be a physician, specializes in maintaining the proper degree of anesthesia in the patient, while also helping to maintain the body's life systems. The job of the anesthetist is more complicated than one might suppose, because in addition to making the patient unaware of pain during the operation—sometimes by making him unconscious, sometimes without affecting consciousness—the muscles and nervous reflexes must be kept in proper state for the type of surgery to be performed.

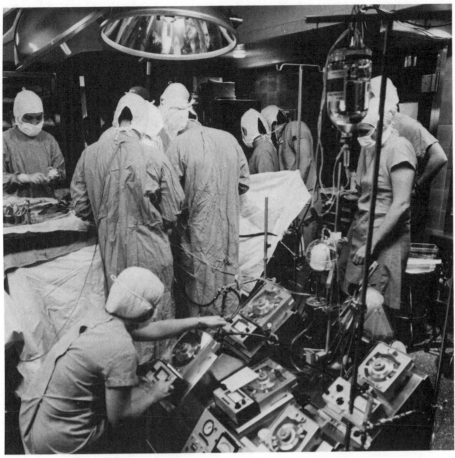

Most operations are performed not by a surgeon alone but by a surgical team, as seen here, with the anesthesiology unit in the foreground.

room also may be headed by a Chief Operating Room Nurse, whose responsibility is to supervise and coordinate the activities of the scrub nurses who assist the surgeon in the actual operation and the supply and circulating nurses who aid the rest of the surgical team by making available as needed the various towels, drapes, sponges, sutures, instruments, and other equipment.

One or more of the nurses wear gowns and gloves that have been sterilized so they can work directly with the surgeon and hand him equipment or supplies that he requests. Such a nurse is called a *scrub nurse* because she scrubs her hands and arms for ten minutes before the operation—just as the surgeon does. Other nurses in the operating room, who do not wear sterilized gowns and gloves, are not permitted to handle equipment directly but may be permitted to pick up sterilized materials with an instrument that has been sterilized. One or more orderlies, who are responsible for lifting the patient and keeping the operating room in tidy condition, complete a typical surgical team.

Each of the various functions—muscle relaxation, reflex paralysis, etc.—requires a different anesthetic drug. Their performance must be perfectly coordinated to prevent complications during the operation. In some cases, it may be necessary for the patient to remain awake during the procedure so that he can follow instructions of the surgeon in moving certain muscle groups. At the same time, the patient must have an anesthetic that eliminates pain. Obviously, the anesthetist must prepare a different combination of drugs for a child, an elderly person, a pregnant woman in labor, or a man with a heart disease.

Other Members of the Surgical Team

As noted earlier, there are occasions when several surgeons are working more or less simultaneously on an accident victim with injuries to multiple organ systems. In such cases of emergency surgery, a general surgeon may supervise and coordinate the work of the other surgeons. The nursing staff in the operating

Operating Room Equipment

When the operating room is in use by the surgical team, an impressive array of equipment is mobilized.

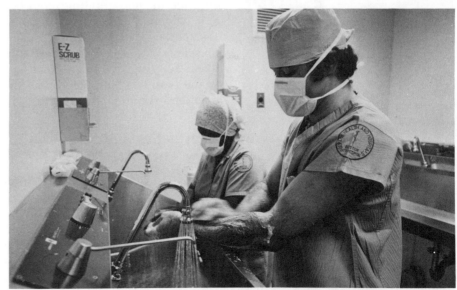

Members of a surgical team scrub before operating to ensure that their hands are sterile—free of germs that could infect the patient.

The center of activity, of course, is the operating table, a massive metal device equipped with numerous levers and gears to permit the surface of the table to be raised, lowered, tilted to various angles, or to raise or lower the head, feet, or other parts of the patient's body. The table is equipped with straps to hold the patient firmly in place during the surgical procedure.

Above the operating table is a very large and powerful lamp with lenses designed to focus a bright, shadowless light on the area in which the surgical team is working. Additional lights also are available to provide illumination at various sides or angles not adequately lighted by the overhead lamp.

Near the head of the operating table is a cart containing tanks of gases used as general anesthetics, plus oxygen tanks and equipment

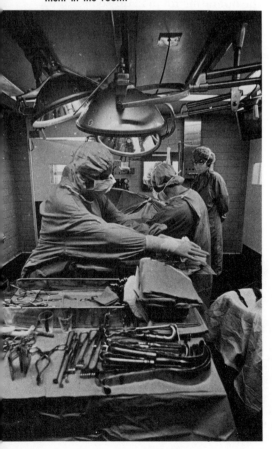

A table holding surgical instruments is placed conveniently near the operating table in the operating room. Of course, the instruments have all been sterilized, along with the other equipment in the room.

for administering anesthetics and monitoring the life processes of the patient.

Also in the operating room are a variety of other wheeled carts, small tables, and stands containing myriad instruments, suction machines to clear mucus from the patient's throat and blood and other fluids from the incision area. Several stands in the area hold basins which, during an operation, can be filled with sterile solutions for rinsing hands, cleaning instruments, or moistening towels and sponges used by the surgeon and his assistants. One tall metal stand near the operating table is designed to hold bottles of intravenous fluids or containers of blood for transfusions. Another special stand is used to collect sponges used in the operation. One cart contains jars or bottles of alcohol and other solutions, soap, and gauze pads, all of which are available for careful cleansing and sterilizing of the skin around the area of the incision just before the surgeon begins the actual operation.

A large clock on the wall of the operating room is intended for timing various functions and procedures involved in an operation, such as the number of minutes that have elapsed since sterilization of certain instruments was started. For many patients the clock is the last thing they see in the operating room before they begin the deep sleep of anesthesia; patients who remain conscious under a local anesthetic like to keep one eye on the clock face so they can tell how much time the operation requires.

Anesthetics and How They Are Used

Anesthesia is a word derived from ancient Greek, meaning "without perception," or a loss of sensation. During a major or minor operation, as in having a tooth extracted by a dentist, it is helpful to both the patient and the doctor if there is a lack of sensation during the procedure. But eliminating pain isn't the only

consideration in the choice of anesthetic and other drugs used in conjunction with it. The age of the patient, chronic ailments, the site of the operation, and the emotional status of the patient are among factors considered. If a patient has undergone surgery previously and had an adverse effect from a particular kind of anesthesia, this information would have an important influence on the choice of an alternative type of anesthetic.

For many types of surgery, the kind of anesthetic chosen may be the result of an agreement among the surgeon, the patient, and the anesthetist. Some patients, given a choice, would prefer to remain conscious during an appendectomy or hernia repair; others would rather not. The surgeon frequently recommends the use of a general anesthetic because the procedure may require more time than the patient can be comfortable with in an operating room situation. Therefore, patients should realize that when a surgeon recommends a general anesthetic for an operation in which a local or spinal anesthetic might be adequate, it is for their own welfare.

General Anesthetics

General anesthetics are those that produce "sleep," or unconsciousness, along with *analgesia*, or absence of pain. They also cause a kind of amnesia in that the patient remembers nothing that occurs during the period in which the anesthetic is effective. At the same time, general anesthetics produce a certain loss of muscle tone and reflex action. A general anesthetic, however, should not interfere significantly with such normal bodily functions as respiration and circulation, nor should it produce permanent damage to body tissues.

HOW THEY WORK: General anesthetics cause the patient to fall into a kind of sleep state by depressing the central nervous system, an effect that is reversible and lasts only until the drug has been eliminated by the body tissues. The general anesthet-

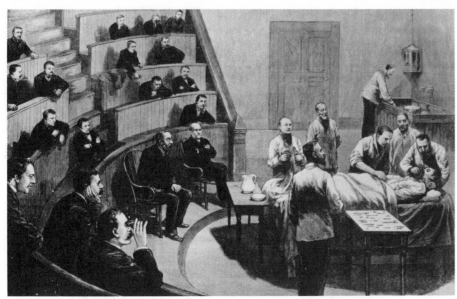

A doctor administers ether to a patient before surgery in an old print depicting instruction for surgeons at a Boston hospital.

ic reaches the central nervous system rather quickly because it is introduced directly or indirectly into the bloodstream. The use of a gas to produce anesthesia is an indirect method of producing unconsciousness.

A gas-type anesthetic, such as nitrous oxide or cyclopropane, can be delivered under compression from tanks or cylinders, or it may be stored in the operating room as a liquid that is converted to a vapor, like ether or halothane. The compressed gas anesthetics are administered with the help of an anesthetic machine. The liquid forms of gases may be dripped through a mask over the patient's face; or the liquid may be vaporized and directed to the patient by anesthetic equipment. Whether the source of the anesthetic is compressed gas or a volatile liquid, the purpose is the same: to get the anesthetic into the patient's lungs. There the gas enters the bloodstream through the walls of the blood vessels of the tiny sacs that make up the lungs.

KINDS OF GENERAL ANESTHETICS: Nearly a dozen different kinds of gases are available as general anesthetics. Each has certain advantages and disadvantages and interacts differently with other drugs used by the patient. The effects of each on chronic diseases of the patient must be weighed. Some gases induce anesthesia more rapidly than others; some are tolerated better by patients. These are among the many factors that can determine which gas or mixture of gases might be selected by the anesthetist for a particular surgical procedure.

INTRAVENOUS ANESTHETICS: Not all general anesthetics come in the form of compressed gases or volatile liquids. Several commonly used general anesthetics are administered intravenously, by injection into the bloodstream. The group includes barbiturates, such as thiopental, and narcotics, such as morphine. Ketamine is a general anesthetic drug that can be injected into the muscles as well as into the bloodstream. The intravenous anesthetics may be used instead of the gaseous general anesthetics or in combination with them. Thiopental is often administered to a patient first, to bring on sleep quickly, after which an inhaled general anesthetic is applied. Like the gaseous general anesthetics, each of the injected general anesthetics has its own peculiarities and may have different effects on different individuals. The rate of recovery from thiopental anesthesia varies according to the ability of a patient's body tissues to eliminate the drug; narcotics can affect the patient's respiration; ketamine may produce hallucinations in some patients.

Regional Anesthetics

Regional anesthetics include *local anesthetics* and *spinal anesthetics*. They are more likely to be used than general anesthetics when the patient is ambulatory and the surgery involves removal of moles or cysts, plastic surgery, certain eye, ear, nose, and throat procedures, and certain operations such as hernia repair that generally are uncomplicated. Regional anesthetics also may be recommended by the surgeon for operations to correct disorders in the arms or legs.

The surgical procedure may require that the patient remain conscious so he can follow instructions of the surgeon in manipulating muscles or bones to test the function of a body part being repaired. In such cases, a regional anesthetic would be preferred; a regional also would be advised for a patient with

A gas-type anesthetic, such as nitrous oxide or cyclopropane, can be delivered under compression from tanks or cylinders.

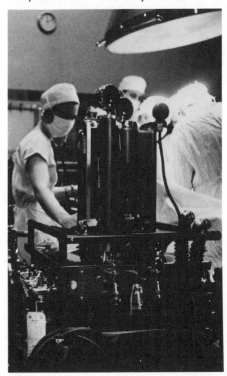

severe heart or lung disease that might be complicated by the effects of a general anesthetic. A restless child, on the other hand, might be given a general anesthetic for a relatively minor operation because the youngster would not be likely to remain motionless for the duration of the operation.

TOPICAL ANESTHETICS: Regional anesthetics generally are administered by infiltration of a drug into the tissues involved or into the nerve trunks leading into the area of incision. A simple kind of regional anesthesia is the topical application of a substance to a sensitive membrane of a body organ. For example, the eye drops applied by an opthalmologist may anesthetize a patient's eyes to make it easier for him to examine them. Topical anesthetics are not very effective when applied to the skin, which forms a tough barrier against most invasive substances, but they can effectively anesthetize the inner surfaces of the mouth, nose, throat, and other inner body surfaces. The anesthetic might be administered by sprays, gargles, or by direct application. Topical anesthetics commonly are used to prepare the throat and upper lung passages for examination with medical instruments.

LOCAL ANESTHETICS: Local anesthetics, which are similar to those used by the dentist, are usually injected by a hypodermic needle into the tissues surrounding the area to be operated on. The injection of an anesthetic into the tissue area sometimes is referred to as a *field block*. A variation of this technique is the *nerve* or *plexus block*, in which a hypodermic needle is used to inject the drug into the region of one or more key nerve trunks leading to the site of the incision. Local anesthetics are not recommended by most surgeons if there is an inflammation or infection of the tissues around the surgery site. The drugs used for local anesthetics can lower the patient's resistance to the infection while at the same time the inflammation may reduce the effec-

tiveness of the drug as a pain-killer.

INTRAVENOUS ADMINISTRATION: Sometimes a regional anesthetic is administered intravenously by injecting it into a vein that runs through the site of the surgery. The drug is confined to the area, such as an arm or leg, by applying a tourniquet about the limb. Because of the possible dangers in suddenly releasing a potent anesthetic drug into the general bloodstream after the operation is ended, the tourniquet is intermittently tightened and released to slow the flow to a mere trickle. A sudden release also would quickly end the pain-killing effect in the area of the incision.

SPINAL ANESTHETICS: Spinal anesthesia is similar to a nerve trunk or plexus block method of eliminating pain sensation in a region of the body, except that the nerves receive the drug at the point where they leave the spinal cord. The drugs may be the same as those used as local anesthetics. They are injected either by hypodermic needle or catheter into tissues surrounding the spinal cord. Although there are several variations of spinal anesthesia—each involving the precise layer of tissue or space around the spinal cord that is the immediate target area of the injection—for all practical purposes the objective is the same. They are all intended to produce a lack of sensation in the spinal nerves along with a loss of motor function so there will be no movement of the body area to be operated on during surgery.

The spinal anesthetic may affect not only the targeted nerve system but neighboring spinal nerves as well, generally all the spinal nerves below the point of drug injection. For its purposes, spinal anesthesia can be a highly effective alternative to a general anesthetic. However, side effects are not uncommon. Severe headache is one of the most frequent complaints of patients. Temporary adverse effects can occur after use of other regional anesthetics as well and may be due in part to individual allergic reac-

tions to the drug used.

Care After Surgery

The last thing you may remember as a patient, before receiving a general anesthetic, is being wheeled into the operating room and lifted by hospital orderlies onto the operating table. You may not see the surgeon, who could be scrubbing for the operation or reviewing the information compiled on your case. The anesthetist and a few nurses may be in the operating room. You are feeling relaxed and drowsy because of the pre-anesthetic medications. A tube may be attached to your arm to drip an intravenous solution into a vein. The anesthetist may administer a dose of a drug such as sodium pentothal, a not unpleasant medication that brings on a deep sleep within a matter of seconds.

The Recovery Room

You will probably remember nothing after that point until you gradually become aware of the strange sounds and sights of a recovery room. The recovery room may contain a number of patients who have undergone surgery at about the same time, especially in a large hospital. Each is reclining in a bed equipped with high railings to prevent a groggy, confused patient just recovering from a general anesthetic from falling onto the floor.

Nurses move briskly about the room, checking the conditions of the various patients. As each patient gains some awareness of the situation, a nurse puts an oxygen mask over his face and explains the purpose: to help restore the tiny air sacs of the lungs to their normal condition. During administration of the anesthetic, the air sacs can become dry and partially collapsed. The humidified oxygen mixture helps restore moisture to the inner surfaces of the lungs; by breathing deeply of the oxygen the patient expands the air sacs to their normal capacity. Before the use of oxygen masks in the recovery room and

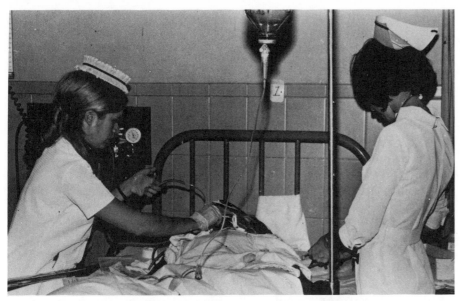

As patients in recovery rooms begin to regain consciousness, nurses apply oxygen masks to their faces to assist respiration.

enced; the incision may cause no more discomfort than the problem that required surgical therapy. Obviously, a minor operation will result in less painful discomfort than a major operation. Generally, the pain or discomfort associated with a surgical incision may last for one or two days, then subside over a period of perhaps three or four days. After that an occasional twinge may be felt in the area of the incision when shifting the body puts extra stress on the muscles or other tissues involved in the operation. During the hospital stay medications will be available to help relieve any serious pain resulting from the operation.

Signs of Recovery or Complication

While the patient may be concerned about pain following surgery, the physicians and nurses are more likely to direct their attention toward other signs and symptoms that

deep breathing techniques for patients recovering from the effects of an anesthetic gas, there was a much greater danger of pneumonia developing as a post-operative complication.

Nurses assigned to the recovery room are given a report on each patient arriving from the operating room and instructions about such matters as the position of the patient in the bed. One patient may have to lie flat on his back, another on his side, a third in a sitting position, and still another with the head lower than the feet. If the patient has received a general anesthetic, the nurses may be instructed to turn him from one side to the other at regular intervals until he is able to turn himself.

The patient's blood pressure, pulse, and respiration are checked at regular intervals by the recovery room nurses, who also watch for any signs of bleeding or drainage from the area of incision. The surgeon is notified immediately of any signs of complications. Since the recovery room usually is located next to the operating room, the surgeon can quickly verify any threatened complication and attend to the problem without delay. Most surgical patients will remain in the recovery

room for a few hours at the most, and when they appear to be able to manage somewhat on their own they are returned to their beds in the regular nursing area of the hospital.

The Intensive Care Unit

Critically ill patients or those with heart, lung, kidney, or other serious disorders usually are assigned to an intensive care unit where each bed may be isolated from the others in a glass booth designed to provide privacy and quiet during the recovery period. Patients can still be clearly observed from the central nursing station.

Patients in an intensive care unit are given continuous care by nurses. Electronic equipment is used to monitor pulse, blood pressure, heartbeat, and, when needed, brain function and body temperature. Other devices are available for making bedside measurements of bodily function and to obtain laboratory data such as blood chemistry without moving the patient from his bed.

Pain

Most surgical patients will be concerned about how much pain they will feel after leaving the operating room. It is not unusual to expect greater pain than is actually experi-

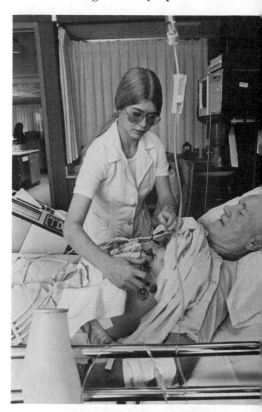

A patient who has undergone surgery for a coronary bypass needs careful and thorough monitoring afterwards, usually in a cardiac intensive care unit.

will help them to gauge the rate of recovery, such as the patient's body temperature, skin coloring, urine output, and his ability to cough. The health professionals are well aware that surgery, and drugs or anesthetics administered in conjunction with surgery, can be disruptive to normal bodily activities. The major operation is more likely to cause changes in the patient's physiology than a minor operation.

Vital Signs

Nurses can be expected to make regular checks of temperature, pulse, and respiration because these common measures of body functions (sometimes called *vital signs*) can provide early-warning signals of possible post-operative complications. A patient may have a temperature of 100°F. even after a major operation, but because of increased metabolic activity of the body following surgery a slightly elevated thermometer reading is considered normal. The pulse and respiration also may be slightly above the patient's rate before surgery, but the mild change again is due to a normal stress reaction of the body. However, a temperature rising above 100°F. and/or a significantly faster pulse or respiration rate suggests that a complication may have developed.

If a nurse seems interested in the patient's ability to cough, it is because the cough reflex helps the patient get rid of mucus accumulation in his lungs, especially after the use of a general anesthetic. If coughing is difficult, a plastic tube may be inserted into the patient's throat to help clear the breathing passages. Normal breathing can also be restored by steam inhalation, aerosol sprays of water or special medications, or positive pressure breathing equipment that forces air into the lungs. Failure to expand the air passages of the lungs leads to serious respiratory complications.

Urine output is also checked. This is just one more way of watching the rate of recovery of a patient and alerting the staff to any signs of complications. If for some reason the patient is unable to pass urine, a *catheter*, or plastic tube, is inserted into the bladder to drain it. The volume of urine drained is collected and measured.

The Incision Area

Some blood may accumulate under the skin in the area of the incision or in nearby tissues, causing a discoloration of the skin. But this effect is seldom a serious matter, and the discoloration gradually vanishes. In some cases of excess blood accumulation, the surgeon may simply remove one or two sutures and drain away the blood. Any continued bleeding about the incision would, of course, be a complication.

A more common complication is infection of the incision area by bacteria that enter the wound. An infection may develop any time from one day to one week after an operation. However, most post-operative infections of incision wounds are easily controlled by antibiotics, drainage, or natural defenses against disease. The surgeon or other physicians will make regular inspections of the incision during the first few days after surgery to make sure it is healing properly.

Post-operative Nourishment

A light meal may be offered the patient a few hours after surgery. The patient may or may not feel like eating, especially if he still feels a bit nauseated from the effects of a general anesthetic. At this stage fluid intake is probably more important, especially if the patient has not been allowed to have even a sip of water since the previous evening. If the surgery was not performed on the stomach or intestinal tract, a small amount of water or tea may be permitted within a few hours after the operation. It is unlikely in any case that the patient will feel a great desire for fluid because intravenous solutions may have been dripping slowly into a vein since he entered the operating room. Intravenous solutions can satisfy hunger as well as thirst, since they may contain proteins, carbohydrates, and essential vitamins and minerals dissolved in a finely formulated broth. Perhaps unnoticed by the patient, the amount of fluid intake will be routinely measured by members of the hospital staff.

Ambulation

Ambulation—getting the patient out of bed and moving about—is an important part of post-operative care. Experience has shown that recovery from surgery is more effective if the patient spends increasing amounts of time each day in simple physical activity. The degree of ambulation depends upon the magnitude of the surgery and the general physical health of the patient. But in a typical case of hernia surgery or an appendectomy, the patient may be asked, on the first or second day after the operation, to sit on the edge of his bed and dangle his legs for a while. On the second or third day, he may be allowed to walk about the room, and may in fact prefer to walk to the bathroom rather than use a bedpan or urinal. On the following day, he may walk up and down the halls with the help of a nurse or other hospital staff member.

Each patient is encouraged to handle the ambulation phase of recovery at his own pace, and there are few hard and fast rules. Of two persons entering the operating room on the same day for the same kind of elective surgery, one may feel like walking to the bathroom a few hours after surgery while the second may prefer to remain in bed and use a bedpan a week after surgery. The surgeon and attending physicians may encourage and in some cases even insist upon early ambulation, however, because it reduces the rate of complications.

Back at Home

Dressings used to cover the incision are changed regularly, as the incision is inspected once each day, more frequently if warranted. If the patient is anxious to be discharged from the hospital as early as possible, the surgeon may give him instructions for changing his own dressings. The surgeon will also outline a plan for recovery procedures to be followed after he leaves the hospital. The plan will include a schedule of visits to the surgeon's office for removal of stitches that may remain and a final inspection of the incision. The surgeon will also offer his advice on how the patient should plan a return to normal activities, including a return to his job and resumption of sports or recreational programs.

Special Diets

Proper foods are as important as proper medicines in helping a patient recover from surgery. Despite the common complaints about hospital meals, the nutrients that are provided in certain special diets for surgical patients are as carefully prescribed and prepared as are some medications that are served in pill or capsule form.

Surgical nutrition has become increasingly important in recent years because of an awareness by physicians that an operation, minor or major, is not unlike an organic disease that creates physiological stresses and a nutritional imbalance in the patient's body. To help compensate for alterations in the patient's physiology as it recovers from the effects of surgery, special diets may be ordered.

Bland Soft Diet

A bland soft diet frequently is ordered for patients who are unable to handle a regular diet but whose condition is not serious enough to require a liquid diet. The foods are selected because they are low in cellulose and connective tissue; they are bland, smooth, and easily digested. The choice of food, nevertheless, represents as great a variety as one might be served in a restaurant or at home, except for an absence of spices and other substances that would be stimulating to the gastrointestinal tract. Included in the surgical soft diet might be lean meat, fish, poultry, eggs, milk, mild cheese, cooked tender or pureed fruits and vegetables, refined cereals and breads with butter or margarine, plus gelatin deserts, puddings, custards, and ice cream. See pp. 213–215.

Liquid Diet

Liquid diets for surgical patients may be prepared with or without milk. They are usually ordered for patients with impaired function of the gastrointestinal tract. A liquid diet without milk may include a cereal gruel made with water, clear bouillon or broth, gelatin, strained fruit juice, and coffee or tea. Liquid diets with milk are similar but may also include creamed soups, sherbets, ice cream, cereal gruel made with milk instead of water, cocoa and beverages of milk or cream. Beverage options permitted are tomato juice and some carbonated beverages such as ginger ale.

Diets Following Particular Kinds of Surgery

PEPTIC ULCERS: A special diet for peptic ulcer patients may include a half-and-half mixture of milk and cream, plus mashed potatoes, eggs, toast and butter, pureed vegetables, cottage cheese, rice, plain puddings and gelatin desserts. But meat soups, tea, coffee, raw vegetables, and fried foods are prohibited.

RECTAL SURGERY: Following rectal surgery, and other procedures in which it is necessary to prevent bowel movements for a period of several days, a low residue diet is ordered. A low residue diet (or *minimal residue diet*, as it is also called) might offer eggs, poached or boiled, rice, soda crackers, cereals made with water, butter, bouillon or clear broths, carbonated beverages, tea, coffee and certain meats including oysters, sweetbreads, and tender bits of beef or veal. See p. 223. An attractive low residue diet is the bland soft diet with all milk-containing items eliminated.

GALL BLADDER SURGERY: Gall bladder surgical patients may expect a modified fat diet that eliminates as much as possible fats and gas-producing food items. It includes foods that provide protein and carbohydrate sources of energy to replace fats and includes primarily fish, poultry, lean cuts of beef, cottage cheese, cereal products and bread, and certain fruits and vegetables. However, foods prohibited are mainly pork products and fatty cuts of other meats, cream, chocolate, melons, apples, fried foods of any kind, onions, cabbage, turnips, cucumbers, radishes, green peppers, and dried beans and peas. See pp. 219–220.

RESTRICTED SALT INTAKE: Chronic heart failure patients and those with liver ailments or edema are placed on a low-sodium diet before and after surgery. The low-sodium diet is fairly simple in that it is prepared mainly with foods from which sodium or salt either is naturally absent or has been removed. Many salt-free or low-sodium foods are available commercially from manufacturers that also supply special dietetic foods for persons suffering from diabetes. See pp. 216–218.

FRACTURES OR BURNS: Special consideration is given the diets of patients who are recovering from accidents that result in fractures or burns. Because of complex body responses to such injuries, there may be an abnormal loss of nitrogen from the tissues and a breakdown of muscle tissue, which is a rich source of nitrogen, an important component of protein. As a result, adequate amounts of protein need to be provided to surgical patients with burn injuries and broken bones.

Potassium Loss

Normal body stores of potassium also may be diminished during and immediately after surgery, but potassium can be replaced in the tissues by including in the meals adequate amounts of meats, fish, poultry, bananas, raisins, figs, dates, and prunes, as well as dried peaches and dried apricots. Prune, tomato, orange, and pineapple juices also are a rich source of potassium for post-operative patients.

Replacement of Water Losses

While water is not always thought of as a food, it is an important part of the gastronomic intake of the surgical patient; adequate amounts of water need to be provided the person recovering from an operation. The post-operative patient usually requires larger than normal amounts of water even though he may not feel inclined to help himself to as much fluid intake as he would at home or on the job. In addition to normal water losses through perspiration, urine, and breathing, there may be additional water losses through vomiting. Water replacement may be provided through sufficient amounts of fruit juices and other beverages offered during meals and between meals.

Apprehensions About Surgery

Most people feel anxious when faced with the need for surgery. This is to be expected. After all, a certain amount of anxiety normally accompanies any prolonged or incapacitating illness or infirmity. When surgery is the recommended therapy, it's natural for the patient to feel some anxiety about the surgery even if he's optimistic about a favorable result.

Factors That Reduce the Risk of Modern Surgery

Much of the risk of surgery these days is eliminated through the careful pre-operative screening examinations reviewed earlier. A patient with a chronic disease who might have been a surgical risk a generation ago may have one or more options not available in past years, such as regional anesthetics that allow surgeons alternatives to general anesthetics that would be less than

satisfactory. Antibiotics and other backup medications are available to control possible complications after surgery. Recovery room techniques and intensive care units with electronic monitoring of vital life systems provide added insurance of safe recovery. And, of course, surgeons today have the added experience of many millions of successful operations involving a range of procedures such as kidney and heart transplants, open heart surgery, and replacement of important organ parts with plastic substitutes. These and other procedures, including the implanting of electronic heart pacemakers, were beyond the dreams of surgeons of past years.

Surgery for the Older Patient

With the rapid increase in the proportion of older people in the population, the surgical patient is more likely to be an older person with problems associated with aging. An older man who underwent surgery to remove his prostate gland before World War II had a life expectancy of a few years after the operation. Today, such procedures in older men are considered routine cases with little or no effect on longevity. It is not unusual nowadays to find men and women in their

70s and 80s who have undergone five or six major operations since reaching the traditional retirement age and without any significant restrictions on their physical activities.

Part of the reason for the greatly improved outlook for surgery on older patients may be that older persons today are simply in better health because of the improved medical care available. Thus they are better surgical risks than their parents would have been at the same age. Advanced pre-operative and post-operative care has also improved the outlook for the older patient. He may be admitted to the hospital a few days earlier than the younger patient for more intensive examinations, and he may remain a few days longer for post-operative care. Convalescence for the older patient may take longer, and in some instances the recovery may not be as complete as that of a younger person. But in general, modern surgical techniques are likely to offer a safe and effective therapy for people of advanced age with complaints that can be corrected by an operation.

In addition to the physical benefits, surgery may improve the mental capacity, personality, and sensitivity of older persons who had

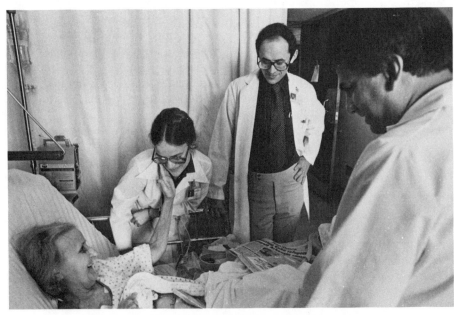

Many surgery patients are senior citizens; special preoperative and postoperative techniques for the aging have been developed.

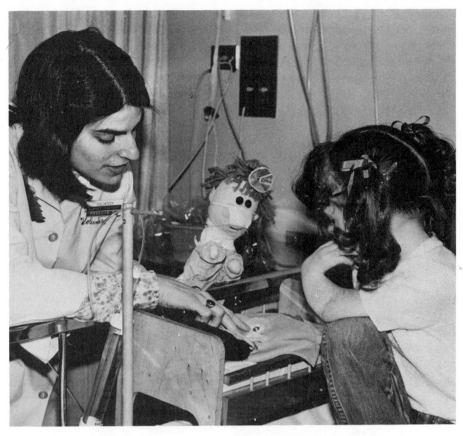

A volunteer at Children's Memorial Hospital in Chicago uses puppets to explain to a young patient what will happen to her in surgery.

prehensive about the trip to a hospital for surgery. Most children seem to worry that the operation will hurt or that other procedures, such as taking a blood sample for testing, will be painful.

TELLING THE TRUTH: Many surgeons recommend that the child be told as realistically as possible, in terms he can understand, what can be expected. The youngster should not be given a sugar-coated story about the operation which might give the impression that he is embarking upon a happy adventure. At the same time, the child should not be frightened by suggestions that he may be given drugs to make him unconscious while he is strapped to a table so that strangely masked and gowned strangers can cut him open with sharp knives.

Children are more likely to appreciate surgery if they are told that a friendly person will help them go to sleep; that the operation will hurt a little but the pain will go away after a while; and that the operation will make them feel better or help correct a problem so they can be more active like other children. A small child should always understand that he may have to remain overnight at the hospital without his parents, but that he will have other adults to take care of him and there probably will be other children at the hospital to keep him company.

been depressed about a disorder before surgery. The patient who complained that he is "no longer the person he used to be" physically may have assumed that his medical problem was simply a result of growing old and overlooked the possibility that the complaint was due to a disease that might respond to treatment.

Surgery for the Child

A child, on the other hand, may have his own reasons to be ap-

COMMON SURGICAL PROCEDURES

In this section some of the more common surgical procedures are described. The operations discussed are organized by the system or region of the body with which they are concerned. The following areas are covered in this order:

• Male Reproductive System (For surgical procedures involving the female reproductive system, see under *Women's Health*, p. 483.

• Urinary Tract
• Abdominal Region
• Oral Cavity and Throat
• Ear Surgery
• Eye surgery
• Chest Region
• Vascular Surgery
• Orthopedic Surgery
• Neurosurgery

For *Plastic and Cosmetic Surgery*, see p. 343. *Uncommon Surgical Procedures*, including transplants, are discussed beginning on p. 346.

Many of the conditions treated in this chapter from a surgical point of view are also treated elsewhere, in the chapter devoted to diseases of the appropriate body system or organ; the reader is invited to turn to those chapters for additional information. For example, although heart surgery is discussed in this chapter, heart disease is treated in greater detail in Ch. 16, p. 360. Likewise, many of the tumors described in this chapter are also discussed in Ch. 28, p. 502.

Male Reproductive System

Surgical procedures of the prostate, testis, scrotum, and penis are considered in this section. Undescended testicles and vasectomy are also among the subjects discussed.

Prostate Surgery

The prostate gland is a small cone-shaped object that surrounds the male urethra, the tube that carries urine from the urinary bladder to the penis. It is normally about one-half inch long and weighs less than an ounce. Ejaculatory ducts empty through the prostate into the urethra and other ducts drain glandular secretions of the prostate into the urethra. Because of the intimate association of the prostate gland and the urinary tract, a disorder in one system can easily affect the other. A urinary infection can spread to the prostate and an abnormality of prostate can interfere with the normal excretion of urine.

ENLARGEMENT OF THE PROSTATE: A relatively common problem is the tendency of the prostate to grow larger in middle-aged men. The gradual enlargement continues from the 40s on but the symptoms usually go unnoticed until the man is in his 60s. At that point in life, the prostate may have become so enlarged that it presses on the urethra and obstructs the flow of urine from the neighboring bladder. The older man may experience various difficulties in emptying his bladder. He may have to urinate more frequently, and suddenly find himself getting out of bed at night to go to the bathroom. He may not be able to develop a urine stream of the size and force he had in earlier years. He may have trouble getting the stream of urine started and it may end in a dribble.

In addition to the somewhat embarrassing inconveniences caused by prostate enlargement, the urinary bladder may not drain properly and can eventually lose its own muscle tone needed for emptying. Residual urine in the bladder can become a source of infection, and backflow into the ureters can gradually affect those tissues and the kidneys. It has been estimated that 20 percent of all older men may need treatment of some kind, including surgery, for correcting this problem of the prostate gland.

FACTORS INDICATING THE NEED FOR SURGERY: Factors that may decide in favor of surgical removal of the prostate include residual urine in the patient's bladder; blood in the urine, with evidence that the blood comes from the prostate; the severity of the inconveniences associated with irregular urination; and complications such as the presence or threat of failure of the wall of the urinary bladder, the formation of stones, and symptoms and signs of infection.

SURGICAL METHODS: There are several methods of performing a *prostatectomy* (excision of all or part of the prostate) for relief of the symptoms of an enlarged prostate, a condition that may appear on the patient's medical records as *benign prostatic hyperplasia*. All of the methods are relatively safe and in none of the techniques is the entire prostate removed. One method, called *transurethral resection*, requires insertion of an instrument into the urethra through the penis. The instrument, a *resectoscope*, uses a high-frequency electric current to cut away the tissue inside the gland. This technique avoids open surgery and requires a postoperative hospital stay of only a few days.

OPEN SURGERY: The other techniques involve *open surgery*, that is, surgery in which an incision is made in the pelvic or rectal area to make the prostate gland accessible so that its inner tissues can be removed. The differences in the various open surgery techniques depend upon such factors as where the incision should be made and the risks associated with the approaches. The incision is made either in the *perineum*, the region between the rectum and the testicles, or through the abdomen. Only a small percentage of patients experience complications or regrowth of the prostate tissues to produce a second enlargement problem. Impotence is usually not an aftereffect of the surgery, and libido is normal.

INFECTIONS OF THE PROSTATE: Infections of the prostate gland can involve obstruction of the urethra,

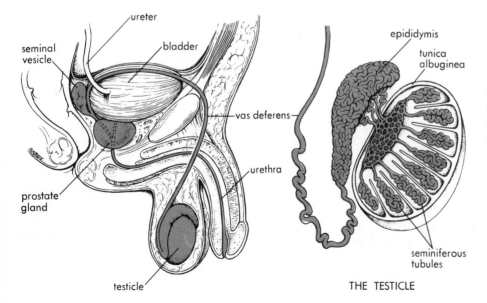

THE MALE REPRODUCTIVE SYSTEM

ureter
seminal vesicle
bladder
epididymis
tunica albuginea
vas deferens
prostate gland
urethra
seminiferous tubules
testicle

THE TESTICLE

but the problem usually can be resolved by the use of medications and techniques other than surgery. An abscess, however, may require an incision to drain the prostate. Surgery also may be recommended for the treatment of stones, or calculi, that develop in the prostate and cause obstruction or contribute to infections.

CANCER OF THE PROSTATE: Cancer of the prostate also may occur in older men, causing obstruction of the urinary flow or contributing to infection of the urinary tract. If examination including biopsy studies confirms the presence of cancer, the surgeon may recommend radical prostatectomy. In this procedure an incision is made either through the lower abdomen or through the perineum to remove the entire prostate gland and surrounding tissues such as the seminal vesicles. Hormonal therapy, chemotherapy, and radiation treatments also may be administered. See also p. 442.

Tumors of the Testis

Tumors of the testis occur most frequently in younger men between the ages of 18 and 35. Such a tumor appears as a firm and enlarged testis and usually without pain unless bleeding is involved as a symptom. Testicular tumors generally are malignant and spread rapidly to other parts of the body, including the lungs. The onset of the disorder can be so insidious that the patient may seek medical advice for a more obvious secondary problem such as the apparent development of mammary glands on his chest, the result of disruption of his normal male hormonal balance.

Special laboratory tests and other examination techniques usually are required to determine which of several possible kinds of testicular tumors may be involved and the extent of metastasis of the cancer cells to other body areas. If cancer of a testicle is confirmed it is removed by an incision through the groin area, and neighboring lymph nodes also will be taken out. The surgical procedure usually is supplemented with chemotherapy and radiation. The prognosis, or chances for recovery, following surgical removal of a testicular tumor depends upon the particular kind of cancer involved and how far the disease had progressed before medical treatment was begun.

Tumors of the Scrotum and Penis

Tumors of the scrotum and penis are relatively uncommon but do occur. Cancer of the scrotum is usually associated with exposure to cancer-causing chemicals. Boys who worked as chimney sweeps a century ago tended to develop cancer of the scrotum from body contact with soot in coal-burning fireplaces. Cancer of the penis occurs usually in men who have not been circumcised. In either type of cancer, the treatment usually requires removal of the affected tissues. This can mean castration in the case of scrotal cancer or amputation of a part or all of the penis, depending upon the extent of the cancerous growth. Surgery that requires removal of a part of the reproductive system can have a devastating psychological effect on a man, but the alternative is likely to be early death from the spread of cancer.

Undescended Testicles

About ten percent of cases of tumors of the testis occur in men with an undescended testicle. Since the chances of a tumor developing in an undescended testicle are as much as 50 times greater than the incidence for the normal male population, the existence of an undescended testicle can warrant corrective surgery.

Ordinarily, the testicles descend from their fetal location in the abdomen into the scrotum about two months before birth. But in one case in 200 male births, a child is found with a failure of one or, less commonly, both testicles to descend properly into the scrotum. In addition to the risk of cancer, undescended testicles are associated with lack of fertility and other problems such as hernias.

CRYPTORCHIDISM: In male babies and small children, an undescended testicle sometimes can be encouraged to enter the scrotum by manipulation or administration of hormones. Many surgeons recommend that the developmental problem of undescended testicles, or *cryptorchidism*, be corrected before a child enters school, although the surgical procedure for correcting the situation can be postponed until adolescence or adulthood. The operation for correcting an undescended testicle is called *orchidopexy* and involves an incision in the groin to release the testicle and its attached cord from fibrous tissue holding it in the abdomen. The testicle may be brought directly down into the scrotum where it may be anchored temporarily with a suture. Or it may be brought down in stages in a series of operations to permit the growth and extension of blood supply to the testis. The original location of the undescended testicle determines which procedure is used.

Vasectomy

Vasectomy is a birth control technique that is intended to make a man permanently sterile. It does not involve the removal of any of the male reproductive system and does not result in a loss of potency or libido. A vasectomy is a relatively simple operation that can be performed in a doctor's office in less than 30 minutes and requires only a local anesthetic. The operation is similar to, but much less complicated, than the procedure in which a woman may be sterilized by cutting or tying her Fallopian tubes. A vasectomy requires no hospitalization, and the man is able to return to work or other normal activities after a day or two.

HOW THE PROCEDURE IS DONE: The vasectomy procedure requires a small incision, about one-half inch in length, on either side of the scrotum. The surgeon removes through the incision a short length of the *vas deferens*, the tube that carries spermatozoa from the testicles, and ties a piece of surgical thread at two points about an inch apart. Then a small piece of the vas deferens between the tied off points is snipped out of the tube. The procedure is done on each side. With the ducts of the vas deferens cut and tied, sperm from the testicles can no longer move through their normal paths to the prostate where they would become mixed with semen from the prostate and seminal vesicles and be ejaculated during sexual intercourse.

STERILITY IS USUALLY PERMANENT: A vasectomy does not immediately render a man sterile. Sperm already stored in the seminal "pipeline" can still be active for a period of a month to six weeks, and a woman who has intercourse with a vasectomized man during that period can become pregnant. On the other hand, a man who undergoes vasectomy should not expect that the severed ducts can be connected again should he want to become a father in the future. Sperm banks have been offered as a possible alternative for the man who might want to store some of his spermatozoa for future use, but there is little evidence that the sperm will remain fertile in a sperm bank for more than a year or 18 months. In rare cases, men who have undergone vasectomies have unintentionally become fertile again because of *canalization*, or creation of a new channel connecting the severed ends of the vas deferens; in one case the canalization occurred eight years after the vasectomy was performed.

The vasectomy is regarded as an extremely safe operation, and complications are infrequent. Some swelling and discomfort are reported by a small percentage of men undergoing the operation. Steroid hormone drugs are sometimes administered to control these aftereffects.

Urinary Tract

Surgical procedures involving uri-

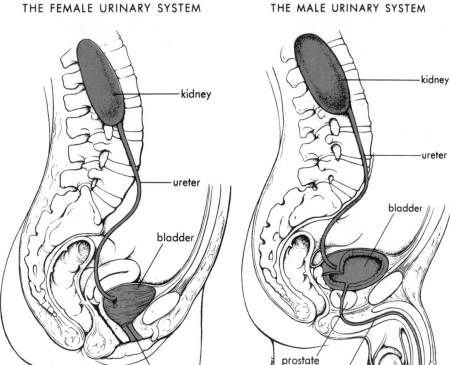

THE FEMALE URINARY SYSTEM — kidney, ureter, bladder, urethra

THE MALE URINARY SYSTEM — kidney, ureter, bladder, prostate gland, urethra

nary stones and tumors of the bladder, ureter, urethra, and kidney are considered in this section. Also discussed are kidney cysts and conditions affecting the adrenal glands that might require surgery.

Urinary Stones

Most stones that occur in the urinary tract are formed in the kidneys, but kidney stones can travel to other areas such as the ureters and cause problems there. Various types of stones can develop in the kidneys from several different causes. A common cause is a metabolic disorder involving calcium, proteins, or uric acid. Other causes are infections or obstructions of the urinary tract, the use of certain drugs, such as diuretics, or vitamin deficiency.

SYMPTOMS: Kidney stones seldom cause problems while they are forming, but movement of the stones irritates the urinary tract and can cause severe pain; the irritation of the tissues may cause bleeding that will result in blood appearing in the urine. Other symptoms may indicate obstruction of the flow of urine

and infection. In some cases obstruction of a ureter can lead to failure of the kidney. X-ray techniques can usually verify the cause of the patient's symptoms and locate the urinary stone. Most stones cast a shadow on X-ray film, and by injecting special dyes into the urinary system the degree of obstruction by a stone can be determined.

URETER STONES: Most stones released by the kidney are small enough to pass through a ureter to the bladder and be excreted while urinating. But if a stone is large enough it can become lodged in a ureter, causing excruciating pain that may be felt both in the back and the abdomen along the path of the ureter. Ureter stones often can be removed by manipulation, using catheter tubes that are inserted through the bladder. If the stuck stone cannot be manipulated from the ureter, an operation in a hospital is required. However, the surgical procedure is relatively simple and direct. An incision is made over the site of the stuck stone, the ureter is exposed and opened just far enough to permit removal of the stone. The operation is safe and requires perhaps a week in the hospital.

KIDNEY STONES: If the urinary stone is lodged in the kidney, the surgical procedure also is a relatively safe one although more complicated and requiring a longer hospital stay. The surgeon must work through skin and muscle layers to reach the kidney, then cut into the kidney if necessary to remove the stone. If the obstruction has been serious enough to impair normal kidney function or if infection has damaged the kidney tissue, the surgeon may elect to remove the affected kidney. Fortunately, the human body can get along fairly well with one good functioning kidney, so a *nephrectomy*, as the procedure is called, may not be as drastic a maneuver as the patient might imagine. If, on the other hand, the affected kidney has not been seriously damaged, the stone or stones can be removed with instruments or by the surgeon's fingers and the incision in the kidney sewed up so that it can resume its normal functions.

VESICAL STONES: Occasionally, urinary stones are found in the neck of the bladder or in the bladder itself. They are called *vesical stones* and, depending upon their size and other factors, may be removed by several techniques including use of a cystoscope inserted through the urethra. In some cases the stone can be broken into smaller pieces for removal. If it appears unlikely that the stone can be removed directly or by crushing it, the surgeon can make an incision directly to the bladder in a manner similar to the approach used in removing a stone from the ureter.

Bladder Tumors

About three-fourths of the tumors of the bladder occur in men past the age of 45. Although the specific cause of bladder tumors is unknown, doctors suspect that a cancer-producing chemical is involved. Several studies have found an association between the disease and cigarette smoking or occupations that require contact with organic chemicals used in making dyes. Tumors that appear in the female bladder are less likely to be cancerous than those that occur in the male bladder.

SYMPTOMS AND DIAGNOSIS: The first symptom of bladder tumor is blood in the urine. The tumor itself may cause no pain but an early complication could be an infection producing inflammation and discomfort in the region of the bladder. If the tumor blocks the normal flow of urine, the patient may feel pain or discomfort in the area of the kidneys; this condition is most likely to happen if the tumor is located at the opening of a ureter leading from a kidney to the bladder. An early examination of the bladder may fail to locate a small tumor, although X rays might show the growth as a bit of shadow on the film, and obstruction of a ureter could be seen. Nonetheless, examination of the interior of the bladder by a cystoscope is necessary to confirm the presence of the tumor. A biopsy can be made by removing a few tissue cells from the area in a manner quite like the procedure for making a Pap smear test for possible cancer of the cervix in a female patient.

TREATMENT: Most early and simple cases of bladder tumor can be corrected by a procedure called *saucerization* by an instrument that removes the abnormal tissue, leaving a shallow wound that normally will grow over with healthy tissue cells. But a tumor that invades deeply into the wall of the bladder requires more radical therapy, such as surgery to cut away the part of the bladder that is affected by the growth. Radiation also may be employed to control the spread of tumor cells, particularly if laboratory tests indicate that the type of tumor cells involved are sensitive to radiation.

SURGICAL PROCEDURE: If it is necessary to cut away a part of the bladder, the surgeon simply shapes

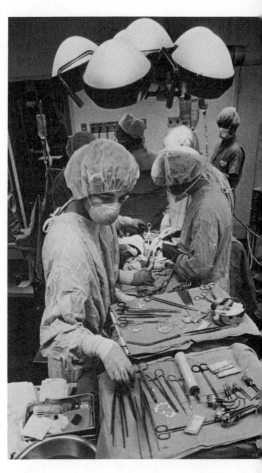

During a lengthy, complicated tumor operation, a scrub nurse must remain alert to the doctor's requests for forceps, clamps, and other instruments.

a new but smaller organ from the remaining tissues. If a total *cystectomy* is required to save the life of the patient, the entire bladder is removed, along with the prostate if the patient is a man. When the bladder is removed, a new path for the flow of urine is devised by the surgeons, usually to divert the urine into the lower end of the intestinal tract.

Tumors of the Ureter or Urethra

Tumors of the ureter, above the bladder, or of the urethra, below the bladder, may begin with symptoms resembling those of a bladder tumor, although X rays might show the growth as a bit of shadow on the normal flow of urine. Treatment also usually requires removal of the affected tissues with reconstructive surgery as needed to provide for a normal flow of urine from the kidneys.

Kidney Tumors

WILMS' TUMOR: Tumors of the kidney generally occur either in children before the age of eight years or in adults over the age of 25. The type of tumor that affects children usually is the Wilms' tumor, one of the most common kinds of cancer that can afflict a youngster. The tumor grows rapidly and may be painful even though there may be no obvious signs of urinary tract disorder in the child's urine. The tumor frequently becomes so large that it appears as an abdominal swelling. A Wilms' tumor usually occurs only on one side of the body, but in a small percentage of the cases the disorder can develop in both right and left kidneys. Kidney function may continue normally during growth of the tumor, but cancerous cells from the tumor may be carried by the bloodstream to other parts of the body, by metastasis, causing the problem to spread to the lungs and other vital organs.

Treatment usually requires surgical removal of the affected kidney and radiation therapy; the tumor cells responsible for the growth are sensitive to radiation. The younger the child and the earlier treatment is started, the better are the child's chances for recovery from a Wilms' tumor.

ADULT KIDNEY TUMOR: The adult type of kidney tumor, which is more likely to afflict men than women, may also appear as an enlarged abdominal mass. But unlike the Wilms' tumor, the adult kidney tumor presents as an early symptom blood in the urine. Bleeding from the kidney may be painless. X-ray studies may show an enlarged and sometimes distorted kidney. The patient may have symptoms indicating metastasis of the tumor cells to the lungs, bones, or other body systems. Adult kidney tumors are almost always malignant.

Treatment usually requires nephrectomy, or surgical removal of the diseased kidney. Radiation therapy may be provided in addition to the surgery, although the kind of tumor cells involved in the adult type of kidney tumor usually are resistant to radiation. Chemotherapy also may be offered. The chances for complete recovery from a kidney tumor depend upon several factors such as the location of the tumor in the kidney and the extent of metastasis of the cancerous cells to other organ systems.

Kidney Cysts

A *cyst* is a small pouch enclosed by a membrane; technically, the urinary bladder and gall bladder are cysts. But the cysts of medical disorders are small pouches or sacs filled with a fluid or viscous substance; they may appear on the skin, in the lungs, or in other body systems such as the kidneys.

SYMPTOMS: Kidney cysts produce symptoms that resemble the symptoms of cancer of the kidney; in a few cases kidney cysts are associated with tumors that cause bleeding into the cysts. In addition to the troublesome symptoms of flank pain and blood in the urine, untreated cysts can grow until they damage normal kidney tissue and impair the function of the organ's functions. Simple or solitary kidney cysts usually do not occur before the age of 40.

DIAGNOSIS: X-ray techniques are made to determine the exact nature of kidney cyst symptoms, but in some cases exploratory surgery is recommended to differentiate a cyst from a tumor. The cyst is excised, frequently by cutting away the exposed wall of the growth. The chances of the cyst re-forming are very slight.

POLYCYSTIC KIDNEY DISEASE: A different kind of kidney cyst disease, consisting of many small cysts, may be found in younger persons, including small children. The symptoms again may be flank pain and blood in the urine; examination may show some enlargement of the kidney. This form of the disease, sometimes called *polycystic kidney disease*, can be complicated by uremia and hypertension as the patient grows older. Treatment usually is medical unless the cysts interfere with urine flow by obstructing the upper end of the ureter. If the outlook for recovery through conservative treatment is poor, the surgeon may consider a kidney transplant operation. See p. 347.

Adrenal Glands

The adrenal glands are small hormone-producing organs that are located just above the kidneys. Although the combined weight of the two glands may be only one-fourth of an ounce, the adrenals affect a number of important body functions, including carbohydrate and protein metabolism and fluid balance. Surgery of the adrenal glands may be needed for the correction of various bodily disorders associated with oversecretion of the adrenal hormones; it may also be indicated to help control of cancer of the breast in women and cancer of the prostate in men.

TUMORS OF THE ADRENAL GLANDS: Tumors of the adrenal glands produce a disorder known as *primary hyperaldosteronism*, which is marked by symptoms of muscle weakness, hypertension, abnormally large outputs of urine, and excessive thirst. Another kind of tumor invasion of the adrenal glands can

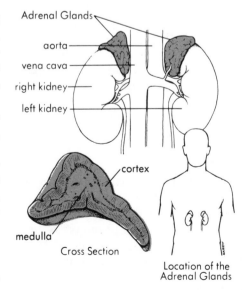

THE ADRENAL GLANDS

Adrenal Glands
aorta
vena cava
right kidney
left kidney
cortex
medulla
Cross Section

Location of the Adrenal Glands

produce symptoms of hypertension with headaches, visual blurring, and severe sweating. Still another adrenal related disorder, called *Cushing's syndrome*, tends to affect women under the age of 40. The symptoms may range from hypertension and obesity to acne, easy bruising, and *amenorrhea* (cessation of menstruation). Adrenal tumors may also alter secondary sex characteristics of men and women; they may result in body hair and baldness in women and increased sex drive in men.

Despite the tiny size of the adrenal glands, they are complex organs and the varied disorders caused by tumors of the glands may depend upon the precise kind of tumor cells involved and the precise area of the glands affected by the tumor, as well as the interactions of the adrenal hormones with hormones from other glands such as the pituitary, or master gland of the body, located at the base of the brain.

PRE-OPERATIVE TESTS: Before adrenal surgery for correction of a disorder is begun, the surgeon may ask for detailed laboratory tests and other diagnostic information. A radioactive scan to help locate and identify the kind of tumor more precisely may be ordered. Women patients who have been using oral contraceptives usually have to discontinue use of "the pill" for two months or more because the medication can interfere with laboratory studies of hormones in the bloodstream.

LONG-RANGE EFFECTS: Doctors handling the case also must evaluate the long-range effects of an adrenal gland operation because normal metabolism is likely to be disrupted by removal of the glands, if that should be necessary. Hormone medications usually are needed in such cases to replace the hormones normally secreted. An *adrenalectomy* (removal of an adrenal gland) sometimes is explained as the substitution of a controllable disease for a life-threatening disease that can-

not be controlled by medical therapy. If only one of the adrenal glands must be removed, however, the patient may be able to recover and resume a normal life without the need for hormone medications.

SURGICAL PROCEDURE: The surgical approach to the adrenal glands is similar to that used in kidney operations. The incision may be made through the abdomen or through the flank. The surgery may be primarily exploratory, or the surgeon may excise a part of a gland, an entire gland, or both glands, depending upon the extent of the disease, or upon other factors such as the need to control cancers in other parts of the body.

Abdominal Region

This section discusses the following procedures or conditions: appendicitis, peptic ulcers, hiatus hernia, adhesions, cancer of the stomach and of the intestines, gall bladder surgery, inguinal hernia, and hemorrhoids.

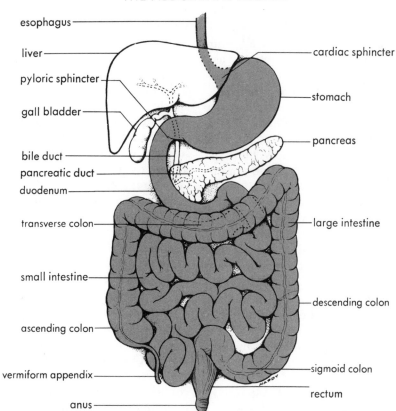

THE ABDOMINAL REGION

esophagus
liver
pyloric sphincter
gall bladder
bile duct
pancreatic duct
duodenum
transverse colon
small intestine
ascending colon
vermiform appendix
anus
cardiac sphincter
stomach
pancreas
large intestine
descending colon
sigmoid colon
rectum

Appendicitis

Inflammation of the appendix is one of the most common causes of abdominal surgery today, particularly among children. But appendicitis was not recognized as a disease until 1886, leading some doctors to believe that this digestive tract infection may be related to a change in eating habits that occurred within the past century. The vermiform appendix, the site of the inflammation, is a short, wormlike (or *vermiform*) appendage at the junction of the small and large intestines. Its function in humans is unknown; plant-eating animals have an appendix but carnivorous animals, like cats, do not. Humans live quite well without an appendix, so it seems reasonable to have a diseased appendix removed.

SYMPTOMS: The appendix can cause trouble if it becomes obstructed by a foreign body, a tumor, an infection, or other cause of inflammation. Pain is a common symptom; there may be two kinds of pain at the same time: one, localized on the lower right side of the abdomen, near the site of the appendix; the other, more generalized and colicky, of the kind sometimes associated with gas in the intestine. Some patients experience diarrhea or a constant urge to defecate, an effect attributed to irritation of the bowel by the abnormal activity of the appendix. Frequently there is loss of appetite, nausea and vomiting, and a fever.

The symptoms of appendicitis may begin suddenly but frequently take from six to 18 hours to develop into a pattern typical of the disease, so most cases permit ample time for a doctor to examine the patient and make a diagnosis before the problem becomes critical. During the period that any symptoms suggest a possibility of appendicitis, the patient should avoid the use of any laxatives.

RUPTURED APPENDIX: A potentially serious complication of untreated appendicitis is rupture of the appendix, which can produce a slightly different set of symptoms because of the onset of *peritonitis*, a dangerous inflammation of tissues outside the intestinal tract. The contents of the ruptured appendix leak into the body cavity, spreading the bacterial infection and irritating the lining (peritoneum) of the abdominal cavity. Diarrhea and a fever of more than 101°F. are frequently associated with a perforated or ruptured appendix. The colicky pain may disappear suddenly because the internal pressure ends with perforation of the wall of the appendix, but it is quickly replaced by the pain of peritonitis. The severe pain of peritonitis usually is made worse by any body movement, including the abdominal muscle movement required for coughing or sneezing.

Appendicitis with perforation is much more common in older persons, perhaps because the early symptoms of colicky pain that younger people notice are not felt by older people, so the disease is not detected until it has reached an advanced stage. Appendicitis also requires special attention in pregnant women because the enlarged uterus crowds and repositions segments of the intestinal tract and the potential threat grows more serious during the last trimester of pregnancy.

SURGICAL PROCEDURE: Laboratory tests usually are checked before surgery proceeds if there is no evidence of perforation. The usual symptoms of appendicitis can be produced by a number of other ailments, and the symptoms may diminish with bed rest, time, and medications. However, appendicitis must be considered in any case of acute abdominal complaints, and many doctors follow the rule of "When in doubt, operate." Surgery for appendicitis is fairly simple and safe if the appendix has not perforated. An incision is made in the lower right side of the abdomen, the connection between the end of the large intestine and appendix is tied off with surgical thread, and the appendix cut away from the stump. The actual operation, if uncomplicated by peritonitis or other factors, may require only a few minutes. A hospital stay of a few days is usually required while the diet is readjusted from nothing by mouth at first, to a liquid diet, then a soft diet, etc. Normal work activities usually can be resumed within two or three weeks following surgery. Complications other than those related to peritonitis are rare. In untreated cases involving peritonitis, however, the risk is very high.

Peptic Ulcers

The cause of peptic ulcers is still unknown, although the disease affects about ten percent of the population at some time in life. Men are four times as likely as women to develop ulcers; the incidence is highest in young and middle-aged men. Peptic ulcers may occur in the stomach, where they are called *gastric ulcers*, or in the duodenum, where they are called *duodenal ulcers*. Ninety percent of the ulcer cases that reach the doctor's office for treatment are in the duodenum, a short length of the small intestine just beyond the stomach. Autopsy studies indicate that gastric ulcers may be as common as duodenal ulcers, but are frequently not detected during the life of the individual.

CAUSES: The development of ulcers is associated with the possible action of gastric acid on the lining of the stomach and duodenum in people who may have inherited a sensitivity to the substances. Ulcers are also related to the use of certain drugs and exposure to severe burns, injury, emotional stress, and disease.

SYMPTOMS: A common symptom is a gnawing pain in the area of the stomach from 30 minutes to several hours after eating; the pain is relieved by food or antacid medications. The pain sometimes is described as heartburn and may be described as radiating from the abdomen to the back. Some patients report the discomfort is more like a feeling of hunger or cramps; they may be awakened from sleep by the feeling which is relieved by a midnight snack of milk or other foods. Attacks of ulcers may be seasonal, occurring in certain patients only in the spring and autumn. In severe cases there may be bleeding without any sensation of abdominal pain; bleeding occurs from erosion of the lining of the stomach or duodenum and penetration of blood vessels in those membranes.

Complications other than bleeding can include perforation of the wall of the stomach or duodenum by continued erosion, or inflammatory swelling and scarring by an ulcer at a narrow part of the digestive tract, causing an obstruction. A duodenal ulcer can erode into the head of the pancreas, which secretes its digestive juices into the small intestine in that area. The pain may then become more or less continuous regardless of efforts to palliate it with food or antacids.

Symptoms vary only slightly between duodenal and gastric ulcers.

Gastric ulcer pain usually begins earlier after a meal, attacks generally last longer, and symptoms, including vomiting and loss of appetite, may be more severe than in duodenal ulcer. But because of the similarities, doctors usually rely on laboratory tests and X-ray studies to determine the precise location in the digestive tract of the peptic ulcer.

DUODENAL ULCERS: Duodenal ulcers nearly always occur within an inch of the pyloric valve separating the stomach from the small intestine. The pain or discomfort follows a cycle. The patient may experience no pain until after breakfast. The pain is relieved by the noon meal but returns in the afternoon and occurs again in the evening. Milk or other bland food or medications relieve the pain that may appear at various times in the cycle. The symptoms of duodenal ulcers also go through periods of remission and recurrence over periods of months or years. Most duodenal ulcers are treated with diet, drugs, and measures that encourage rest and relaxation.

SURGICAL PROCEDURES: Surgery for either duodenal or gastric ulcer is designed to reduce gastric acid secretion rather than simply to excise the ulcer from the normal digestive tract tissue. One surgical approach, called *subtotal gastrectomy*, involves cutting away a portion of the stomach in the area where it joins the duodenum. There are several variations of this technique, including one in which the remaining portion of the stomach is attached to the jejunum, a segment of the small intestine. The ulcerated portion of the duodenum may be removed during the reconstructive surgery of the digestive tract, or it may be left in the duodenal segment which is closed during the gastrectomy procedure. An interesting effect is that a duodenal ulcer usually heals, when left in place, after the gastric juices are routed into the intestine through the jejunum. The reconstructed stomach and stomach-to-intestine connection cause no serious problems in eating after the patient has recovered.

A second surgical approach, called a *vagotomy*, involves cutting a part of the vagus nerve trunk that controls the secretion of stomach acid. There are several variations of vagotomy, each technique affecting a different portion of the vagus nerve distribution to the stomach.

GASTRIC ULCERS: Stomach or gastric ulcers tend to develop in older persons more often than duodenal ulcers, and the problem seems to be less importantly related to the overproduction of gastric acid. The real hazard of stomach ulcers is that a significant percentage are found to be a kind of cancer and do not respond to the usual therapies for controlling peptic ulcer symptoms. If it is determined that a stomach ulcer is a malignant growth, a partial gastrectomy is performed in the same manner as an operation of that type for duodenal ulcers. The vagotomy approach is not used for treatment of a stomach ulcer unless the ulcer is excised at the same time.

Hiatus Hernia

The term *hiatus hernia* actually describes a diaphragmatic hernia or weakness in the diaphragm, the horizontal muscular wall separating the organs of the chest from the organs of the abdomen. A *hernia* is an abnormal protrusion of an organ or tissue through an opening. A *hiatus*, or opening, occurs naturally to permit the esophagus to carry food from the mouth to the stomach. Blood vessels and nerves also pass through the diaphragm. The diaphragm is an important group of muscles for contracting and expanding the lungs, forcing air in and out of the lung tissues.

Hiatus hernias are rare in children, but as people grow older there may be a weakening of the diaphragm muscles and associated tissues. Aided by a tendency toward obesity and the use of girdles and other tight garments, a portion of the stomach may be pushed through the opening designed by nature for use of the esophagus. Aside from the discomfort of having a part of the stomach in the chest, there are potential dangers of incarceration of the stomach, with obstruction, strangulation, and hemorrhage with erosion of the stomach lining. In severe complications, the entire stomach along with intestines and other abdominal organs may be forced through the hiatus hernia into the chest area.

The most common kind of hiatus hernia is sometimes called sliding hiatus hernia from the tendency of the stomach to slide in and out of the thorax, or chest cavity, when the patient changes body positions or as a result of the pressure of a big meal in the gastrointestinal tract. Sometimes the herniated stomach does not move at all but remains fixed, with a significant portion of the stomach above the diaphragm. Hiatus hernia causes heartburn symptoms, including regurgitation of digested food and gastric acid from the stomach, while lying down or when straining or stooping. The effect also may be noticeable in a woman during pregnancy.

NONSURGICAL TREATMENT: Many cases of hiatal hernia can be treated without surgery through a change of eating habits and the use of antacid medications. The patient may be advised to eat small amounts more frequently during the day with dietary emphasis on high-protein, low-fat foods. Some doctors recommend that patients use liquid antacid medications rather than antacid tablets or lozenges.

SURGICAL TREATMENT: When surgery is recommended to correct hiatus hernia, the repair may be performed either through the abdominal wall or through the chest. About three-fourths of the procedures are handled through abdominal incisions because doctors often find other abdominal problems that need to be corrected at the same time, such as peptic ulcers or gall bladder disease. The opening through the diaphragm is firmly closed with sutures to prevent upward movement of the stomach. The stomach and lower end of the esophagus may be anchored in place in the abdomen. The chances of recurrence are about one in ten, although some patients may continue to have a few of the symptoms of the disorder for a while after the hernia repair.

Adhesions

Adhesions may develop between various abdominal organs and the peritoneum, the membrane lining the abdominal cavity. The bowel may acquire adhesions that result in obstruction of the intestinal tract. Adhesions may form between the liver and the peritoneum or between the liver and the diaphragm. The symptoms may be pain or cramps in the area where tissues are literally stuck together; in more serious cases that involve bowel obstruction, symptoms may include constipation, vomiting, and distension of the abdomen. Adhesions do not show on X-ray film and can be difficult to diagnose unless the patient's medical history suggests a cause for the bands or filaments of tissues responsible for the adhesions.

CAUSES: The causes may be peritonitis, injury, infection, internal bleeding, or foreign objects. Adhesions occur after an operation, perhaps because of a bit of blood resulting from surgery or as a result of a speck of talc from the surgeon's glove or a fiber from a surgical drape that produces a foreign body reaction, much like an allergic reaction, when it comes in contact with the abdominal tissues. Disease organisms may enter the female abdominal cavity through the Fallopian tubes to produce adhesions, especially in the case of gonorrhea, which can escape early detection in women because of the lack of obvious symptoms.

COMPLICATIONS: Adhesions can cause complications such as changing the position of the intestinal tract through twisting or otherwise distorting its path so that bowel movements are obstructed. If the involved portion of the intestine becomes seriously damaged so that it no longer functions properly, the surgeon may have to remove that section. Generally, when the surgeon is correcting the problem of adhesions, a relatively simple procedure of cutting away the tissue bands or filaments holding organs in abnormal ways, he inspects the organs to determine if they appear to be in good working order. That part of the operation may add 15 or 20 minutes to the time spent on an operating table but it helps insure that the patient will not have to be returned soon for further surgery.

Cancer of the Stomach

There are several possible types of stomach tumors but one kind, called *adenocarcinoma*, is one of the greatest killers of men over the age of 45. Although the incidence of stomach cancer in the United States has declined considerably since the end of World War II, the death rate from this problem in the U.S. alone is about 15,000 per year. In central and eastern Europe the incidence of stomach cancer is about four times, and in Japan seven times, that of the United States. Almost two-thirds of the stomach cancers develop near the pylorus, the opening from the stomach into the small intestine; only five percent involve the entire stomach area.

SYMPTOMS: Symptoms include a feeling of heaviness rather than pain following a meal. The patient in many cases mysteriously loses his appetite for meat and begins to lose weight. There may be vague symptoms of an upset stomach, with some vomiting, especially if the tumor begins to obstruct the pylorus so that stomach contents cannot be emptied into the intestine. The vomitus usually is the color of coffee grounds, suggesting a loss of blood from the stomach lining because of the tumor, and the patient's stools also may be dark in coloration because of internal bleeding. The doctor frequently can confirm his suspicions about the cause of the symptoms by laboratory analysis of a specimen of cells from the stomach, by X-ray studies of the stomach, or by an examination with a gastroscope that permits a direct view of the interior of the stomach. In some cases the doctor will be able to feel an abnormal mass in the stomach by palpating the stomach area of the abdomen with his hands.

TREATMENT: Treatment is by cutting away the tumor and surrounding tissues that may be involved, including parts of neighboring organs. The lymph nodes in the region of the stomach are also removed. The remaining part of the stomach is used to build a new digestive organ, as in a case of partial gastrectomy for correcting a peptic ulcer problem. However, before beginning reconstructive surgery the doctor usually orders biopsy tests of the remaining tissues to make sure the new stomach will not be made of tissues in which tumor cells have spread. If the edges of the remaining stomach wall are found to contain tumor cells, the surgeon simply extends the area to be removed. As in subtotal gastrectomy for peptic ulcers, the remaining portion of the stomach may be connected directly to the upper portion of the small intestine, at the duodenum or the jejunum.

Meals are provided in the form of intravenous feedings for the first few days following surgery. Sips of water may be permitted on the second or third day after the operation with the amounts gradually increased to one or two ounces of water per hour as the new digestive system adjusts to fluid intake. Then soft or bland foods can gradually be taken orally in a half-dozen small feedings each day. It may take three or four months for the new stomach to distend and adjust to normal eating habits of the patient.

POST-OPERATIVE EFFECTS: Some patients may experience a variety of symptoms ranging from nausea to cramps and diarrhea while recovering from stomach surgery. The symptoms form what is known as the dumping syndrome which occurs within a half hour after a meal, presumably by rapid distention of the upper portion of the small intestine as fluid rushes, or is dumped, into that part of the digestive tract from the new stomach. The effects can be controlled by a change of diet to eliminate starches and sugars, by delaying the intake of fluids until after the meal, by medications, and by training the patient to lie in a recumbent or semirecumbent position to lessen discomfort following a meal. The symptoms occur in only a small proportion of stomach surgery patients, and they usually diminish gradually during the period of recovery.

Cancer of the Intestines

SMALL INTESTINE: Tumors of the small intestine are not common but they also are not rare. It has been estimated that less than five percent of all tumors of the gastrointestinal tract occur in the small intestine. Of tumors that do develop in this portion of the gastrointestinal tract, about 90 percent are benign, or noncancerous, growths. The symptoms of small intestine tumors may include bleeding, obstruction, and perforation of the intestinal wall. However, most tumors of the small intestine produce no symptoms at all. When tumors are found in the small intestine they usually are found at the same time in other parts of the body, and usually in a patient over 40 years of age, although the more malignant growths can occur in younger persons. Treatment of a cancer of the small bowel is by removing the affected section and administration of radiation therapy for certain kinds of cancerous tumors.

LARGE INTESTINE: Tumors of the large intestine, unlike those of the small bowel, account for a large proportion of cancers of the human body and for most of the malignant growths of the entire gastrointestinal tract. Over 40,000 deaths each year in the United States are due to cancers of the colon and rectum portions of the large bowel. And about three-fourths of all large-intestine tumors develop near the rectal portion of the bowel where, ironically, they should be easily available for detection during physical examination.

Tumors of the large intestine can be found in persons of any age, but they occur most frequently in patients who are of middle age or older, reaching a peak of incidence around the age of 65. Men are more likely to develop cancer of the rectum, but women are more frequently affected by cancer of the colon. While cancer of the large intestine tends to occur among members of the same families at a rate that is two or three times the normal incidence, it is believed that family environment factors, such as life style and diet, are the causative influences rather than hereditary factors. People who develop cancer of the large intestine usually eat foods that are low in cellulose and high in animal fats and refined carbohydrates.

Bowel cancers appear to grow in size at a very slow rate, doubling about once every 20 months, so a number of years may elapse between the start of a bowel tumor and the appearance of signs or symptoms of cancer.

SYMPTOMS: The location of the growth can influence the type of symptoms experienced. Cancer in the right colon may be found as an abnormal mass during a physical examination by a physician after complaints of fatigue and weakness and signs of anemia. The tumor can develop to a rather large size without producing signs of blood in the stools. Cancer in the left colon, by contrast, may be found after complaints of alternate periods of constipation and frequent urge to defecate, pain in the abdomen, and stools marked by dark or bright red blood. When the cancer is in the rectum, the patient may find blood mixed with the bowel movements but experience no pain in the early stages. Other symptoms of cancer of the large intestine may mimic those of appendicitis, hemorrhoids, peptic ulcer, or gall bladder disease.

As noted above, most cancers of the large bowel are close enough to the end of the intestinal tract to be observed directly by palpation or the use of fiberoptic instruments such as a sigmoidoscope or colonoscope that can be inserted into the rectum or colon. Biopsy samples can be removed for study and X-ray pictures taken after a barium enema has coated the bowel membrane so that abnormal surfaces are marked in black-and-white contrast.

SURGICAL PROCEDURES: Surgical procedures for treatment of cancer of the large intestine vary somewhat according to the location of the growth, but the objective is the same: to remove the affected portion and reconstruct the bowel so that normal digestive functions can resume. Radiation therapy and chemotherapy may be used in the treatment of certain advanced cases. When surgical treatment is begun soon after the first symptoms are diagnosed, the chances of curing cancer of the large bowel are very good.

If there are complications, such as obstruction of the portion of the large intestine, the surgery may be conducted in a series of stages over a period of several weeks. The several stages involve a colostomy procedure in which an opening is made in the wall of the abdomen to permit a portion of the intestinal tract to be brought to the surface of the body. After the complicating problem is treated and resection of the cancerous segment is completed, the colostomy is closed by sewing the open end of the bowel to the remaining portion and closing the opening in the abdomen.

PRE-OPERATIVE STEPS: Some special pre-operative measures are ordered for patients awaiting surgery for treatment of bowel cancer. They consist primarily of several days of liquid diets, laxatives, and enemas to make the interior of the intestinal tract as clean as possible. Other measures will be directed toward correction of anemia and compensation for possible loss of blood resulting from the cancer's invasion of bowel tissues.

Gall Bladder Surgery

Gall bladder disease is one of the most common medical disorders in the United States. It has been estimated that more than 15 million Americans are affected by the disease and about 6,000 deaths a year are associated with it. The incidence increases at middle age; one of every five women over the age of 50 and one of every 20 men can expect to be treated for gall bladder symptoms. Approximately 1,000 people in the United States enter operating rooms each day for removal of gallstones, a primary cause of the symptoms of the disorder.

GALLSTONES: Gallstones generally are formed from crystals of cholesterol that gradually increase in size in the gall bladder; some, however, are formed from other substances such as bile salts and breakdown products of old red blood cells. Because they are very small in size, the stones may produce no symptoms at first. But as they grow in size they become more threatening and eventually can block the normal flow of bile from one of the bile ducts emptying into the intestine. Bile contains substances needed by the body to digest fats in the diet.

SYMPTOMS: A common symptom of *chronic cholecystitis*, or gallstone disease, is a pain that appears suddenly in the upper abdomen and subsides slowly over a period of several minutes to several hours. The pain may occur after a meal or with no apparent relationship to meals. There can be tenderness in the upper right side of the body, with pain extending to the shoulder. The pain also can appear on the left side or near the center of the upper abdomen, producing misleading symptoms suggesting a heart attack. Nausea, heartburn, gas, indigestion, and intolerance of fatty foods are among other possible symptoms. The gall bladder attacks may occur frequently or there may be remissions (periods without symptoms) lasting for several months or years.

A careful and extensive physical examination, including X-ray studies of the gall bladder area, may be needed to confirm the presence of gallstones. Until recently, the most commonly used test was the oral cholecystogram (OCG), in which the patient swallowed an iodine-based "dye," or contrast agent. X rays taken about 12 hours after administration of the dye might or might not provide useful "pictures" of the gallstones. As a result, ultrasound has largely replaced X rays as a primary test for suspected gallstones.

ACUTE CHOLECYSTITIS: About three-fourths of the cases of acute cholecystitis are patients who have had previous attacks of gallstone disease. In the acute phase there is persistent pain and abdominal tenderness, along with nausea and vomiting in many cases and a mild fever. Complications may include perforation, or rupture, of the gall bladder, leading to peritonitis, or development of adhesions to neighboring organs such as the stomach or intestine.

TREATMENT: Surgical treatment of chronic or acute cholecystitis is basically an elective procedure that can be scheduled at a time convenient to the patient. But acute cases with complications may require emergency operations. The patient can usually be maintained after surgery on intravenous fluids and pain-killing medications.

A number of alternatives to surgery have been developed. A gastroenterologist may use an endoscope on older patients or those in poor health. The endoscope, a tube inserted through the chest wall, enables the physician to view the gall bladder's duct area and to widen its opening so that small gallstones can slip through the small intestine. Using a small basket on the endoscope, the physician can sometimes catch and withdraw or crush the stones.

In gallstone surgery, the abdomen is opened so that the surgeon can examine the gall bladder and the ducts leading from it for stones. The gall bladder may be freed of stones and a temporary drainage tube inserted, with an opening to the outside of the upper abdomen. But usually the surgeon removes the entire gall bladder in an operation called a *cholecystectomy*. The bile duct, which remains as a link between the liver and the small intestine, gradually replaces the gall bladder in function. Most patients require no more than ten days to two weeks of hospitalization, and can resume normal work activities in a month to six weeks.

Other nonsurgical treatments include chemical preparations. Chenodeoxycholic acid or chenodiol has been given orally to dissolve smaller, floating cholesterol stones. But the drug has little effect against pigment stones or stones with a high calcium content, and can cause diarrhea as a side effect. Researchers have worked experimentally with ursodeoxycholic acid and other drugs that have been found to dissolve gallstones in both animals and humans.

Among the most advanced techniques is *choledocholithotripsy*, a nonsurgical method using shock waves to destroy gallstones. Already in use as a method of shattering kidney stones, lithotripsy requires only a local anesthetic and the recovery period lasts only a few days. The physician uses a hollow tool—the lithotripter—that is inserted through the patient's chest until it approaches the stones. With a foot switch, the physician then triggers a jolt of high-voltage, low-current electricity that shatters the stones.

Inguinal Hernia

An inguinal hernia (hernia of the groin) can develop in either men or women at almost any age from infancy to late adult years. But the incidence of inguinal hernia is much more common in males. An inguinal hernia is one in which the intestinal tract protrudes through the opening

INGUINAL HERNIA

muscular wall of abdomen

intestine

bladder

inguinal canal

vas deferens

loop of intestine in scrotum

In this type of indirect hernia, a loop of small intestine has pushed through the weakened inguinal canal in the abdominal wall and descended into the scrotal sac.

of one of the inguinal rings on either side of the groin. In males, the inguinal rings are temporary openings through which the testicles descend into the scrotum before birth; in females, the openings permit the passage of a ligament supporting the ovary.

CAUSES: Normally, the inguinal rings are closed after the birth of the child. However, they may fail to close completely or the muscles and connective tissues may become stretched or weakened in later years to permit a portion of the abdominal contents, usually part of the intestine, to protrude. A number of factors can contribute to the development of a hernia, including physical strain from exercise or lifting, straining over a bowel movement, coughing spells, pregnancy, pressure of abdominal organs, or obesity.

REDUCIBLE AND IRREDUCIBLE HERNIAS: The hernia may be *reducible*, that is, the bulge in the abdominal wall may disappear when the body position is changed, as in lying down, only to reappear upon standing. An *irreducible* hernia does not allow the hernia sac contents to return to the abdominal cavity; an irreducible hernia also may be called *incarcerated*, a term aptly describing the hernia as being trapped. A serious complication is strangulation of the hernia contents, which usually involves obstruction of normal blood flow and resulting damage or destruction of the incarcerated intestines. A strangulated hernia may be life-threatening because of the possibility of gangrene in body tissues damaged by incarceration.

SURGICAL PROCEDURE: Some hernias are called direct, some indirect, for purposes of medical records. These terms indicate to the surgeon specific layers of muscle and connective tissue that have been breached and are of no real significance to the patient because the surgical repair procedures are essentially the same for either type. In the absence of complications, the operation is fairly simple and usually can be performed with either a general or local anesthetic. An incision is made in the lower abdomen in the area of the hernia, the protruding organ is returned to its normal position, and the weakened or ruptured layers of muscle and connective tissue are repaired and reinforced to provide a strong internal wall that will hold the abdominal contents in place. In some cases the surgeon will use available tissues from the patient's own body in building a new wall against future hernias. The surgeon also may use a variety of materials including silk, catgut, stainless steel, tantalum mesh gauze, or mesh screens made of plastics in building a new barrier.

RECOVERY: The hospital stay for hernia repair is relatively brief, usually from three days to a week; some healthy children undergo surgery early in the morning and return home in the evening of the same day. The patient usually is instructed to avoid exercise or exertion for a couple of weeks and can return to work in a month to six weeks, depending upon the work load expected. Hernias tend to recur in only a small percentage of cases among adults and very rarely in children.

Femoral Hernia

About five percent of all hernias of the groin area are femoral hernias, with the hernia bulge appearing along the thigh. Femoral hernias occur about four times as frequently among women and usually appear in middle age. While a femoral hernia is not necessarily limited to obese patients, it is more likely to be associated with being overweight and the movement of a bowel segment or the urinary bladder into the hernia frequently is preceded by a fat pad—a mass of fatty tissue. Femoral hernias are more prone to incarceration and strangulation than inguinal hernias. The surgical treatment of femoral hernias is similar to that used in the repair of inguinal hernias, although the incision may be made through the thigh in a few cases.

Hemorrhoids

Hemorrhoid, a term derived from Greek words meaning "blood flowing," refers to a system of arteries and veins that serve the rectal area. The medical problem known as *hemorrhoids,* or *piles,* is a tortuous enlargement of the hemorrhoidal veins, a problem similar to the varicose veins of the legs. Causes of the varicosities of the hemorrhoidal veins include the human peculiarity of standing and walking in an erect posture—animals that walk on all fours do not get hemorrhoids.

Women during pregnancies are particularly subject to hemorrhoidal problems because of the pressure on the veins of the lower body area. Other causes are constipation and straining at stool; diseases of the digestive tract resulting in anal infection; and cirrhosis of the liver, which obstructs blood flow and puts increased pressure on the hemorrhoidal veins.

SYMPTOMS: Symptoms usually include bleeding, which may stain the patient's clothing; irritation and discomfort, including itching, in the anal region; and occasionally pain with inflammation. Because rectal bleeding also can be a sign of a number of other diseases, the doctor usually makes a thorough examination to rule out other possible causes, such as cancer or ulcerative colitis.

TREATMENT: If the hemorrhoids do not warrant surgery, medical treatments may be prescribed. *Prolapsed hemorrhoids* (veins that protrude from the anus) can be reduced by gentle pressure. Bed rest, warm baths, and medications are also a part of medical treatments. A type of injection chemotherapy sometimes is used to control bleeding and eliminate the varicosed veins.

Surgery can be used to excise all the affected tissues, and the disorder also can be treated by cryosurgery in which the hemorrhoids are destroyed by a probe containing supercold liquid nitrogen or carbon dioxide. The patient usually is able to recover and return to work within one or two weeks after surgical removal of the hemorrhoidal tissues.

Oral Cavity and Throat

This section discusses oral cancers, tonsils and adenoids, and surgery of the thyroid. For a discussion of cosmetic surgery of the face area, see pp. 343–345.

Oral Cancers

There are many potential problems of the mouth, or oral cavity, besides an occasional toothache. Surgical treatment frequently is needed to correct a disorder or to prevent a life-threatening situation from developing. Cancers of the lips, tongue, hard and soft palate, and other areas of the mouth, for example, affect about 25,000 people in the United States each year. Elsewhere in the world, the incidence varies considerably according to sex and location; the rate in Hong Kong for men is three times the figure for women, and the incidence of oral cancer for women in Hong Kong is nearly 10 times as high as that of women in Japan. Environmental factors such as tobacco and contact with chemical and physical agents have been suggested as causes, although

one form of oral cancer, known as *Burkitt's lymphoma,* is believed to be transmitted by a mosquito-borne virus.

CANCER OF THE LIP: Oral cancers tend to occur after the age of 45. Some types of oral cancer, particularly when the lips are affected, are found most frequently in persons exposed to a great deal of sunlight. Farmers, sailors, and other outdoor workers develop such tumors around the age of 60, with the lesion appearing on the lower lip. Like other cancers, cancer of the lip may begin as a tiny growth but if untreated can spread through neighboring tissues and eventually destroy part of the chin. Treatment may include both radiation therapy and surgical excision of the growth; if surgery is performed when the tumor is small the scar is likewise small. Obviously, the larger the tumor is allowed to grow, the more difficult the treatment.

CANCER OF THE CHEEK: Similarly, cancers that develop on the inner surface of the cheek usually can be excised and the wound closed with simple surgery if treatment is started early. If the cancer is allowed to grow before treatment, the surgery becomes more complicated with removal of tissues extending to the outer skin layers and repair of the wound with skin grafts. Radiation therapy also may be used to augment the surgical repair.

CANCER OF THE MOUTH: Cancer of the floor of the mouth may be second only to lip cancer in rate of occurrence of oral cavity tumors; together they may account for half of the oral cavity cancers in the United States. A tumor of the floor of the mouth may involve the under surface of the tongue, the lower jawbone, and other tissues of the area. A small lesion detected early can be controlled in most cases by excision of the growth and radiation therapy.

CANCER OF THE TONGUE: The tongue may be the site of cancerous growths beginning in the 30s of the patient's life, particularly if the individual is a heavy user of tobacco and alcohol and has been neglectful

of proper oral hygiene, such as brushing the teeth regularly. If the growth is at the tip of the tongue rather than underneath or along the sides, the operation is easier and there is less chance that the normal function of the tongue will be impaired by removing the growth and surrounding tissue cells. Radiation therapy for cancer of the tongue sometimes involves the implantation of needles containing radium into the tongue. The procedure is done while the patient is under a general anesthetic. Tumors at the base of the tongue, as well as some growths on the floor of the mouth, sometimes are approached through an incision in the neck.

OTHER SURGERY: Apart from cancers, surgery of the oral cavity may be needed to treat genetic defects, such as cleft lip and cleft palate, damage to tissues from injuries, and noncancerous tumors of the soft tissues, such as cysts. For information on cleft lip and cleft palate, see pp. 343, 344. For a discussion of cosmetic surgery, see pp. 343–345.

Tonsils and Adenoids

Tonsils and adenoids are glands of lymphoid tissue lying along the walls near the top of the throat. The tonsils are located on the sides of the pharynx, or throat, near the base of the tongue. Unless an adult's tonsils are inflamed, they may not be easily visible to a doctor or other person looking into the throat, but when inflamed and swollen they can be seen without difficulty. The adenoids are located higher in the pharynx and cannot be seen by look-

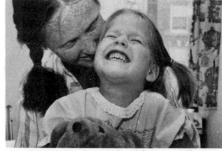

A young patient hospitalized for a tonsillectomy gets some loving comfort from her mother before the operation. Tonsillectomies are no longer routinely performed on young sore-throat victims.

ing into the back of the mouth without special instruments because the palate, or roof of the mouth, blocks the view.

TONSILLITIS: The function of the tonsils and adenoids apparently is that of trapping infectious organisms that enter the body through the nose and mouth. But sometimes the glands do such a good job of collecting infections that they lose their effectiveness, becoming enlarged and inflamed, a condition known as *tonsillitis*. The patient develops fever and sore throat and the breathing passages become obstructed. The infections can spread through the nearby Eustachian tubes to the ears, causing *otitis media* (inflammation of the middle ear), resulting in deafness. Disease organisms also can spread from the tonsils and adenoids to the kidneys, joints, heart, eyes, and other body areas. Many youngsters survive occasional bouts of tonsillitis and the infections can be treated with antibiotics and medications to relieve pain and fever symptoms. But many surgeons recommend that the tonsils and adenoids be removed if tonsillitis occurs repeatedly.

TONSILLECTOMY: A *tonsillectomy* (removal of the tonsils) is not a complicated operation but it usually is performed under a general anesthetic if the patient is a child. A local anesthetic may be used for an adult. The adenoids usually are removed at the same time; they consist of the same type of lymphoid tissue in the same general area, and adenoids develop similar problems from the same kind of infectious agents. An overnight stay in the hospital may be required or it may be possible for the patient to have the tonsils and adenoids removed in the morning and be released from the hospital in the evening of the same day, after a few hours of post-operative rest under medical observation.

PRE-OPERATIVE AND POST-OPERATIVE CARE: The patient may receive antibiotic medications two or three days prior to surgery and is instructed to avoid eating foods or drinking fluids

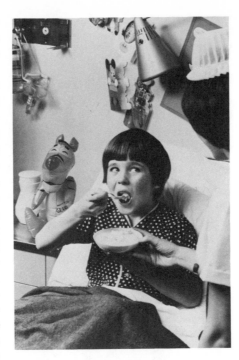

Following a tonsillectomy, the young patient is fed bland liquid or semi-liquid foods such as ice cream, pudding, and milk. This staves off irritation of sensitive throat tissue.

for at least 12 hours before the operation. If the patient has a cold or other viral infection, the surgery may be delayed or postponed. Some surgeons also prefer to avoid tonsillectomy operations during the hay fever season. If there is any evidence of bleeding after the patient is released, such as spitting blood, he is returned to the hospital and the surgeon is notified; the bleeding usually can be controlled without difficulty. The patient also returns for checkups a couple of weeks after the operation and again about six months later.

ADENOIDECTOMY: In some cases, a doctor may recommend an *adenoidectomy* (removal of the adenoids) without a tonsillectomy. This is particularly true when the patient suffers from recurrent ear infections and hearing loss. An adenoidectomy is a relatively simple operation performed under a local anesthetic when the patient is an adult or older teen-ager; a general anesthetic is preferred for younger patients.

The surgeon can reach the adenoid mass through the open mouth of the patient. The tissue grows on a

palate ledge near the point where the nasal passage enters the back of the mouth cavity. Using a special instrument, the surgeon cuts away the adenoid tissue within a few minutes. A medicated pack is inserted into the postnasal area to help control bleeding and the patient is moved to a recovery room. The only aftereffects in most cases are a soreness in the postnasal area for a few days and, occasionally, a temporary voice change that is marked by a nasal tone while the wound heals.

Thyroid Surgery

The thyroid gland lies along the trachea, or windpipe, at a point just below the Adam's apple. Secretions of the thyroid gland are vital for metabolic activities of the body, and the gland's functions are closely orchestrated with those of other endocrine glands of the body. When the thyroid is less active than normal, mental and physical functions are slow and the patient gains weight. When the gland is overly active, body functions operate at an abnormally fast pace, with symptoms of weight loss, irritability, heart palpitations, and bulging eyes. Occasionally, lumps develop on the thyroid, requiring medical or surgical treatment. A lump on the thyroid gland may be a nodular, or nontoxic, goiter. Or it could be a tumor. A nodular goiter poses several threats: it can make the thyroid gland become overactive, it can press on the windpipe and cause hoarseness, or it can develop into a cancer. Some growths of the thyroid gland can be treated effectively with medica-

THE THYROID GLAND

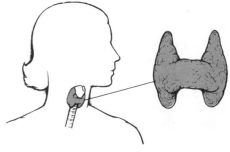

tions, radiation, or a combination such as radioactive iodine. However, when conservative forms of therapy no longer appear to control the condition, or when it is suspected that a thyroid growth may be a malignant cancer, surgical removal of the affected area is advised promptly.

SURGICAL PROCEDURE: The operation itself is fairly simple. An incision is made through the skin folds of the neck, neck muscles beneath the skin are separated, and the affected portion of the gland is cut away. The neck and throat area may be sore and painful for a few days after the operation; within a few weeks the patient can resume normal activities. A thin scar remains at the line of incision but it is usually partly concealed by skin folds of the neck.

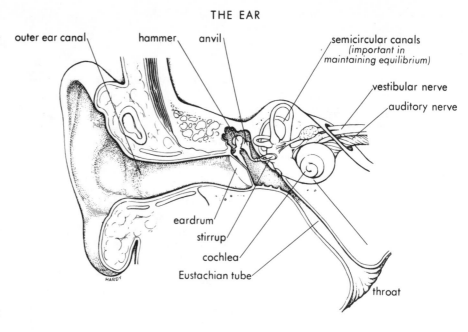

THE EAR

outer ear canal — hammer — anvil — semicircular canals *(important in maintaining equilibrium)* — vestibular nerve — auditory nerve — eardrum — stirrup — cochlea — Eustachian tube — throat

HARDY

Ear Surgery

Surgical treatment of the ear usually is directed toward restoring the function of normal hearing which may have been lost or impaired by disease or injury. The eardrum, or tympanic membrane, can be perforated or ruptured by direct injury, by the shock waves of an explosion, or by an infection of the middle ear. Infection or injury also can disrupt hearing function by damaging the ossicles, a chain of tiny bones that transmit sound waves from the eardrum to the inner ear. Disease, aging effects, and exposure to loud noises can cause hearing loss or impairment.

Surgery of the ear usually involves working with the middle ear, the compartment between the eardrum and the inner ear, which contains the nerve endings that carry impulses to the auditory centers of the brain. The middle ear contains three ossicles, known by their common names of *hammer, anvil,* and *stirrup*—terms that suggest their functions in translating movements of air molecules into the vibrations the brain understands as sounds.

Otitis Media

One common disease of the middle ear is otitis media, which can occur by infection from a number of different kinds of organisms. Otitis media also can develop from secretions or fluids such as milk being forced into the ear through the Eustachian tube, particularly in infants that are fed while they are in a reclining position. The symptoms of otitis media are pain in the ear, fever, and loss of hearing; a small child may indicate the symptoms by crying and tugging at the ear.

SURGICAL PROCEDURE: Many cases of otitis media respond to medical treatment, such as the use of antibiotics, but for patients who suffer severe pain or who have middle ears filled with pus a surgical procedure called *myringotomy* is performed. Myringotomy means simply perforating the eardrum. But the operation usually is performed in a hospital, under a local anesthetic, and with great care to avoid disturbing the ossicles or other ear structures beyond the eardrum. The middle ear is drained and the eardrum either heals spontaneously or can be subsequently repaired with a graft from the patient's own tissues.

Surgery to Correct Hearing Loss

Occasionally surgery is required to correct a conductive hearing loss involving the structures of the middle ear. Such problems happen more frequently among older persons due to abnormal tissue growths that in effect "freeze" the ossicles so they no longer work with their normal flexibility. Ossicular disorders also can occur in younger persons, including children, because of congenital defects, injury, or repeated infections, as of otitis media. The exact procedure for restoration of hearing depends upon the type of disorder. If one of the ossicles has slipped out of position or has become rigidly attached to another structure like the tympanic membrane, the tiny bones can be repositioned or freed from the tissues that may have immobilized them. It is not unusual for the surgeon, working in a space about the size of a pea and viewing his progress through a microscope, to literally take the middle ear structures apart, rebuild the organ with bits of plastic or metal shaped like the ossicles, and reconstruct the eardrum with tissue grafts. This kind of surgery is called *microsurgery.*

THE EYE

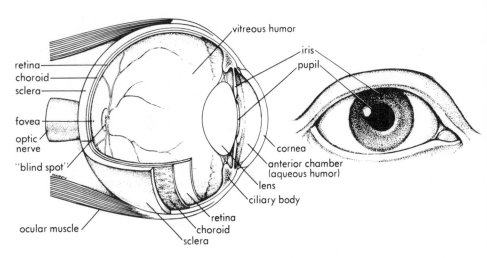

retina
choroid
sclera

fovea

optic
nerve

"blind spot"

ocular muscle

vitreous humor

iris
pupil

cornea
anterior chamber
(aqueous humor)
lens
ciliary body

retina
choroid
sclera

Inner Ear Disturbances

Disorders of the inner ear usually are treated with medications. Surgery in that area is seldom performed unless there is a great risk to the life of the patient. Little can be done to restore hearing loss due to nerve deafness except with hearing aids; these are designed to pick up sounds on the affected side of the head and route the sounds by electronic circuitry to an area where they can be picked up by remaining functional auditory nerves. See p. 346 for a discussion of plastic surgery on the ears.

Eye Surgery

Among common types of eye surgery are procedures for correcting eye muscles, glaucoma, cataracts, cornea, and retina disorders. Operations on the eye muscles are in-tended to correct crossed eyes or similar problems in which the two eyes fail to work together.

Crossed Eyes

The condition technically known as *strabismus*, in which one eye drifts so that its position is not parallel with the other, is caused by a congenitally weak muscle. Infants often appear to have crossed eyes, but in most cases the drifting corrects itself by the time the baby is six months old. If the condition persists beyond that time, a doctor should be consulted. He may recommend the use of an eye patch over the stronger eye so that the weaker one will be exercised. If this does not achieve the desired result, he may prescribe special glasses and eye exercises as the child gets older so that there is no impairment of vision.

CORRECTIVE SURGERY: If corrective surgery proves necessary after these measures, it is usually done before the child enters school. The operation is a simple one involving the muscle and not the inside of the eye itself. Each eye has six *extraocular* muscles—muscles originating outside the eyeball—to move the eye up, down, left, right, etc.; the surgeon lengthens or shortens these muscles, as may be required, to coordinate the eye movements. The operation is safe and requires only a brief hospital stay.

AMBLYOPIA: If the lack of eye coordination is not corrected a kind of blindness called *amblyopia* can result in one of the eyes. This condition occurs particularly in young children who depend upon the vision of one good eye; the function of

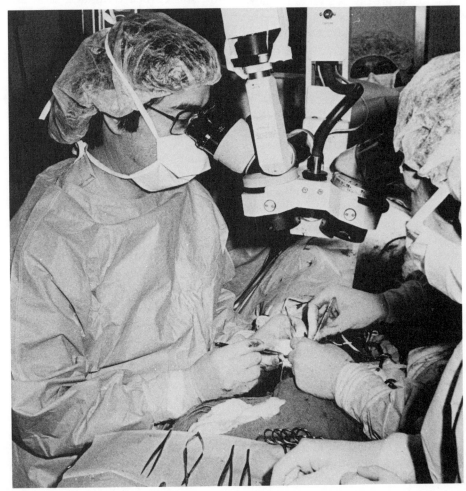

Microsurgery, which makes use of a microscope and often of tiny and delicate instruments, is particularly helpful in treating eyes and ears.

the other eye is allowed to deteriorate. It has been estimated that about two million Americans have lost a part of their vision in this manner. Crossed eyes should receive professional attention early enough to prevent a permanent visual handicap.

Cataract

Cataract is a condition in which there is a loss of transparency of the lenses of the eyes. Each lens is made up of layers of cells naturally formed to focus a visual image on the retina at the rear of the eyeball. As a result of aging, or because of an injury to the eye, the lens may develop cloudy or opaque areas, or *cataracts*, that result in a blurring of vision. About five percent of the population of the United States has cataracts. Some doctors claim that anyone who lives long enough can expect to have cataracts, although age is not the only determining factor.

SURGICAL CORRECTION: The condition can be corrected rather easily by several different kinds of surgical procedures. Among these, a relatively simple, advanced technique involves a microsurgery procedure called extracapsular extraction followed by implantation of a new lens. Using this method, the surgeon first makes a tiny incision in the cornea. Reaching through that incision, the surgeon then makes a circle of tiny cuts in the lens. The lens and its cataract are then drawn through the opening in the cornea. The back part of the lens remains in place to support the implant lens.

Extracapsular extraction has begun to replace older techniques. These include dissolving the tissues holding the lens in place with a liquid enzyme, freezing the lens with a supercold probe, and grinding the lens tissue with a high-speed instrument. Extracapsular extraction requires only a local anesthetic injected into the facial muscles. Because the sutures are tiny, healing time can be as short as a few weeks.

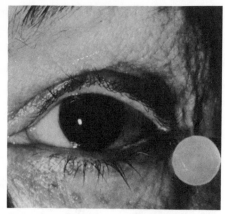

Cataract is a condition in which there is a loss of transparency of the lenses of the eyes. The picture above shows a normal eye and a cataract (opaque lens) outside the eye.

The timing of cataract surgery presents the patient with a difficult decision. To help you make up your mind, the doctor may use a potential acuity meter (PAM) to show what kind of vision you should have after a cataract is removed. The PAM projects a light beam that flashes a standard eye chart through tiny clear areas in the cataract. Because the beam hits your retina directly, you can read the chart without interference.

Lens implants normally effect greatly improved vision. But for optimum results most patients need to wear eyeglasses or contact lenses after the operation. Because implanted lenses cannot focus as your eye's natural lens does, you will probably need reading glasses. The artificial lenses may require some adjustments to compensate for visual illusions as to distances and shapes, but the blurring of progressive blindness will have been eliminated.

Sometimes after cataract operations, patients notice that the rear part of the lens left in to support the implant has begun to cloud. In such a case a surgeon may use a laser beam to punch a tiny hole in the clouded area. The hole lets light rays reach the retina unimpeded.

Cornea Transplant

The cornea of the eye is a clear window of several cells in thickness at the very front of the eye. While it is protected by the constant sweeping of the corneal surface by the eyelid and the washing of the surface by tears, it is vulnerable to injury and infection, allergies, and metabolic disorders. The simple habit of rubbing the eyes can distort the shape of the cornea, changing the normal round shape to a cone shape. Eventually, a cornea may degenerate from wear and tear and become clouded so that the patient can no longer see clearly, if at all. It is possible, however—and has been since the 1930s—to replace a clouded cornea with an undamaged cornea from a deceased person. Corneas are contributed by donors and stored in eye banks.

SURGICAL PROCEDURE: When only a portion of the cornea needs to be replaced, as is often the case, a disk encompassing the damaged cornea is carefully cut out and a piece of new cornea of precisely the same size and shape is sewn into the remaining tissue of the old cornea. The reconstructed cornea is treated with antibiotics and bandaged for several weeks. More than three-fourths of the cornea transplants are successful; the chances of success depend upon many factors, including the health of the remaining tissues of the original cornea.

Glaucoma

Glaucoma, a leading cause of blindness, is a disease caused by a failure of the fluid produced inside the eye to drain properly. The fluid, or *aqueous humor,* is produced in the anterior chamber of the eye, between the cornea and the lens. In a normal eye it drains through a duct at the base of the cornea at the same rate at which it is produced. But if the drainage system is obstructed, fluid buildup creates pressure backwards through the eye. If untreated, such pressure can cause gradual blindness by crushing the nerves at the back of the eye.

TREATMENT: Some cases of glaucoma can be treated with medications that control the rates of fluid production and drainage. But when medications are no longer effective

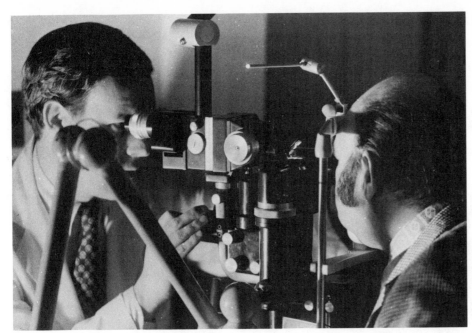

A patient being treated by laser beam. This form of therapy is used in some cases of retinal bleeding associated with diabetic retinopathy.

or when an acute attack occurs, with symptoms of severe eye pain sometimes accompanied by abdominal pain, nausea, and vomiting, surgery within a matter of hours is recommended. Several surgical procedures for the treatment of glaucoma are available; all are designed to release the fluid pressure in the eye. One common procedure involves cutting a small opening in the iris. Another technique is to insert a fine wire into the duct that normally drains the fluid and literally ream it open.

An estimated ten million people in the world are afflicted by glaucoma, and the chances of it developing increase with age. Women are twice as likely to develop the disease as men, and there is some evidence that the risk is hereditary. However, it also is easily preventable and controllable, since glaucoma usually develops slowly and can be detected during routine eye examinations in its early stages.

Retinal Detachment or Disease

Retinal detachment can occur from bleeding in the retinal area, an injury, a change in the shape of the eyeball, or other causes. The surgi-cal treatment to correct the problem usually is related to the specific cause. For example, if fluid or blood has accumulated behind the retina, it is drained away. Alternatively, pressure may be directed within the eyeball to push the retina back into its proper position. For some cases, such as those associated with *diabetic retinopathy*, a kind of retinal bleeding in diabetes patients, a laser beam is used to seal the blood vessels responsible for the tiny hemorrhages in the eye.

Chest Region

This section deals with surgery of the lungs and heart. For a discussion of cosmetic surgery of the chest area, as of the breast, see p. 344.

The Lungs

Before the era of modern drugs such as antibiotics, lung disorders were the leading cause of death in the United States. Lung diseases are still common enough. With every breath taken in, the lungs are vulnerable to damage from disease organisms, chemicals, and air pollutants, many of which did not exist 50 years ago when pneumonia and tuberculosis were among the greatest threats to human life. Because the lungs are not as sensitive to pain as some other organs, a respiratory disorder may develop insidiously with few or no symptoms. When pain is felt in the chest area, the source of the pain may be the chest wall, the esophagus, or the bronchial tubes that branch from the trachea into smaller units that distribute air through the lung tissues. Other symptoms of respiratory disease may be coughing, shortness of breath, or sputum that contains blood.

TUBERCULOSIS: Any of the above signs or symptoms could be associated with tuberculosis, which also can cause loss of appetite, weight loss, lethargy, and heavy perspiration, especially during the night. Tuberculosis is still one of the most common causes of death in the world, and new cases are found in the United States each year at a rate of 18 per 100,000 population. In addition, an estimated 35 million Americans are tuberculin-positive, indicating they have been in contact with the infectious organism but have developed an immune response to it. For an explanation of how tuberculosis is spread and of tests devised to check its spread, see pp. 391–392.

SURGICAL TREATMENT OF TUBERCULOSIS: A dozen different drugs are available for medical treatment of tuberculosis and several types may be taken in combination by a patient. Intensive treatment may require a hospital stay of several months and use of the drugs for at least 18 months. However, because of adverse side effects of drugs, resistance of the bacterium to the drugs, and other reasons, surgery may be required. If one of the five lobes of lung tissue—the right lung has three lobes, the left lung two—has been severely damaged by tuberculosis, it may be removed by surgeons. In some instances, doctors may recommend that surgery be undertaken to allow one of the lungs to rest while it recovers from the infection.

THE RESPIRATORY SYSTEM

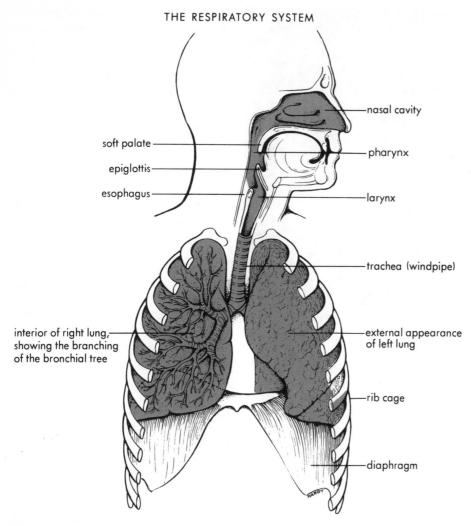

soft palate

epiglottis

esophagus

nasal cavity

pharynx

larynx

trachea (windpipe)

interior of right lung, showing the branching of the bronchial tree

external appearance of left lung

rib cage

diaphragm

This is accomplished by crushing the phrenic nerve, under a local anesthetic, creating a partial paralysis of the diaphragm. Partial lung collapse also can be accomplished by removing parts of the ribs over the affected lung.

LUNG CANCER: Cancer of the lung may appear with early symptoms of coughing, wheezing, or the appearance of blood in sputum; in about ten percent of cases there is chest pain or shortness of breath. However, it is not unusual for the lung-cancer patient to have no complaints of illness. Chest X-rays during a routine physical examination may reveal the disease. In many cases, the cancer develops from metasases of cancers that have spread from other body systems. Medical therapy for lung cancer patients, including the use of radiation, is primarily for the

purpose of relieving pain or other symptoms. The only effective cure is surgical excision of the affected lung tissue along with the nearby lymph nodes. Surgical treatment is most effective in young adults when the tumor has not invaded neighboring tissues, although the five-year survival rate for lung cancer is still poor.

Heart Surgery

Heart surgery procedures that are routine in many hospitals today were unheard of a generation ago. Since World War II techniques have been devised to permit attachment of a heart-lung machine to the human body so that the patient's blood can be circulated and refreshed with oxygen while the heart itself is stopped temporarily for surgery.

HEART VALVE REPAIR: While the blood flow is shunted away from the heart, surgeons can replace a diseased heart valve which may have become calcified with deposits that keep it from closing normally. An artificial valve made of metal and plastic may be used to replace the patient's diseased mitral valve that no longer effectively controls the flow of blood from the left atrium to the left ventricle of the heart. Artificial valves also can be installed between the right chambers of the heart. In some cases, a diseased valve leaf may be repaired with a graft of tissue from the patient's body.

Installation of artificial heart valves has had a remarkably good record of success; some surgeons recommend the procedure over other techniques for treatment of heart valve diseases and report the operation has been well tolerated by patients more than 70 years of age. Life expectancy is increased for most patients, and while some activities may be restricted, they are able to have comfortable and more normal lives after such operations.

SEPTAL DEFECT: Another kind of heart surgery is used to correct a septal defect. The right and left atria of the heart are separated by a septum, a wall of muscular tissue. A similar but much thicker septum separates the left and right ventricles. Occasionally, usually because of a birth defect, the septum does not close completely and blood flows from one side to the other through the opening in the heart wall. The problem is solved by putting the patient on a heart-lung machine while the heart is opened and the septum closed either by sewing the opening or by stitching into the septum a patch of plastic material. See the illustrations on p. 337.

COARCTATION OF THE AORTA: An equally dramatic bit of heart surgery is used to correct a defect called *coarctation,* or narrowing, of the aorta, the main artery leading from the heart. This short, pinched section interferes with normal blood flow. If untreated, the patient may

THE HEART

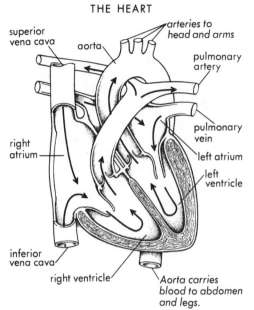

superior vena cava

aorta

arteries to head and arms

pulmonary artery

pulmonary vein

left atrium

left ventricle

right atrium

inferior vena cava

right ventricle

Aorta carries blood to abdomen and legs.

die of a ruptured aorta or heart failure. Treatment requires an operation in which the narrowed section of the aorta is cut away and the two normal-sized ends sewed together. In some cases, a piece of plastic material is sewed into the reconstructed aorta to replace the coarctated section.

AORTAL-PULMONARY ARTERY SHUNT: A comparatively simple bit of heart surgery is employed to correct a defect that occurs in some newborn children. Before birth, when the lungs are not needed because fresh blood is supplied from the placenta via the umbilical cord, the aorta is connected by a shunt to the pulmonary artery. After birth the shunt closes in most cases so the pulmonary artery can carry the blood from the heart to the lungs for oxygenation. In some children this shunt fails to close. To correct the defect and prevent heart failure, the surgeon opens the child's chest, ties off the open shunt, and cuts the ligated connection.

Vascular Surgery

This section consists of discussions of aneurysms, varicose veins, phlebitis, and intermittent claudication.

Aneurysm

When a blood vessel develops a balloonlike malformation the defect is called an aneurysm. A common

complication of the aneurysm is that it may rupture if not treated. A ruptured aneurysm of a large blood vessel, or of a small blood vessel in a critical area such as the brain, can be fatal or severely disabling.

SURGICAL PROCEDURES: If the aneurysm develops at a vital site such as the aorta, heroic surgical measures may be required to correct the problem. Before the important artery can be clamped off, the patient may have to be attached to a heart-lung machine and the body temperature lowered so as to reduce normal body functions to a minimum. After the aneurysm is removed, that section of the aorta may have to be replaced with a piece of plastic artery. Not all aneurysms require such complicated methods of repair; if the ballooning section of artery develops as a saclike appendage, it frequently can be tied off and removed while the relatively small opening between the blood vessel and the sac is sewed closed.

Surgical removal of an aneurysm is the only available treatment for the disorder. The surgery is much less complicated if the abnormal section of the blood vessel is replaced before it ruptures than after. When the patient has recovered from correction of the aneurysm he can resume a rather active, normal life style.

Varicose Veins

Varicose veins can develop in many parts of the body. But they are most obvious and commonly a problem when they appear in the legs, especially in the *saphenous veins*, large veins that lie close to the surface of the skin.

CAUSES: The cause of varicose veins is a failure of tiny valves in the blood vessels to function properly so that venous blood destined for the heart flows backwards and forms pools which can make the veins distended, tortuous, and painful. Varicose veins are related to the erect posture of humans; the heart pumps blood through arteries to the extremities but the return flow must fight the pull of gravity. Ordinarily,

SEPTAL DEFECTS

Interventricular defect

Interatrial defect

A normal heart in cross section *(top)*, showing the circulation of the blood. An interventricular defect *(bottom left)* allows blood to pass directly between the left and right ventricles. An interatrial defect *(bottom right)*, with the aorta seen in cross section over the left atrium, allows blood to pass freely between the two atria. Any septal defect interferes with the effectiveness of the pumping action of the heart.

THE SAPHENOUS VEINS

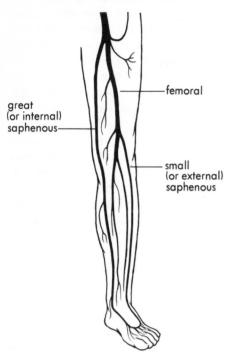

great
(or internal)
saphenous

femoral

small
(or external)
saphenous

The saphenous veins of the leg, which lie close to the surface of the skin, are those most likely to become varicosed. Although the external saphenous is sometimes called "small" to distinguish it from the internal saphenous, both are large veins.

venous blood gets a boost up the legs by a pumping action of leg muscle contractions. Valves in the legs are designed to let the blood move upward but are supposed to block any backward flow. People whose jobs require them to stand all day are among those likely to suffer from a breakdown of the normal functioning of the valves. Women who have had multiple pregnancies and obese individuals are also apt to develop varicose veins.

ULCERATION: Varicose veins can cause ulcers in the lower leg near the ankle that bleed through the skin after an injury to the area.

TREATMENT: One kind of surgical treatment of the varicosed vein is *ligation,* which means tying or binding. An incision is made in the leg, usually in the area of the groin. The diseased saphenous vein is severed from its connection with the larger femoral vein and is tied off. The function of a ligated vein is taken over by other veins in the leg. An al-

ternate kind of surgery for varicose veins, sometimes called *stripping,* requires either a series of small incisions along the path of the vein, from the groin to the ankle, or an internal stripping by use of a special, long, threadlike instrument. The diseased vein is then removed and any connections with other veins ligated.

Varicose vein surgery is used for treatment of the *superficial* veins— those that are close to the skin. The operation is simple and can be performed under a local anesthetic in many cases. When multiple varicose veins are on both legs, all of the problem veins can be stripped and ligated at the same time. A hospital stay of several days may be required, and dressings are needed on the treated legs for two or three weeks after the operation.

Phlebitis

A problem related to varicose veins is *phlebitis,* a disease that usually involves the larger, deep veins of the legs with inflammation, pain, and swelling. Phlebitis is much more serious than varicose veins because a large vein is involved and a clot usually forms, obstructing return blood flow of the limb. The danger is that the clot will break loose— that is, become an *embolus*—and travel to the lungs where it can obstruct a vital blood vessel, with serious or even fatal results. The obstructing clot is called an *embolism.*

CAUSES AND TREATMENT: Causes of phlebitis can be injury, infection, poor circulation, or simply sitting for long periods of time. Medical therapy may include wet dressings and medications, especially anticoagulant drugs to thin the blood and reduce the chances of clot formations. Supportive bandages, leg exercises, and elevation of the legs may also be recommended.

SURGICAL PROCEDURE: Surgery is reserved usually for cases in which medical therapy fails to control the risk of emboli forming. The surgical procedure is directed toward treatment of the deep vein that is the source of the phlebitis symptoms.

The surgeon may open the vein to remove the clot, or a device can be inserted in the vein to strain out any clots that may form in the vein and travel toward the lungs. In some cases the surgeon may block the upward flow of blood from the affected vein, allowing other veins in the leg to assume that function. However, if other veins already have been stripped or ligated in the treatment of varicose veins it is unlikely that a surgeon would occlude or block the flow of blood in a deep leg vein.

Intermittent Claudication

Intermittent claudication is a disorder of blood circulation of the legs involving the arteries. It is primarily a disease of aging, with gradual, progressive narrowing of the lumen (interior space) of the arteries by atherosclerosis. Atherosclerosis of the arteries occurs in other parts of the body, including the arms. Intermittent claudication is marked by muscle fatigue and pain when the leg muscles are used, as in walking. The symptoms are relieved by rest. The condition can be relieved by drugs, particularly medications that help dilate the arteries, but in severe cases surgery to reconstruct the leg arteries is the solution.

SURGICAL PROCEDURE: The surgeon may build a bypass artery by grafting a length of plastic tubing into the affected blood vessel and around the area blocked by atherosclerotic narrowing. Sometimes surgeons will use a piece of a vein from the patient's body to make a bypass artery; for example, a vein from the arm may be transformed into an artery for the leg. Another procedure involves simply removing the portion of the artery blocking the normal flow of blood.

Orthopedic Surgery

Orthopedics originally was the name given the subject of treating deformities of children; the original Greek term could be translated as "normal child." But the medical world now uses the word to describe treatment of the bones, muscles, joints, and associated tissues of the body's locomotion apparatus. Orthopedic surgery, therefore, might involve repair of a broken big toe as well as treatment of a whiplash injury to the neck.

This section discusses disorders of the spine, including herniated (or "slipped") disk, fractures, and torn ligaments.

Slipped Disk

The spinal column of 33 stacked vertebrae is a common source of painful problems that require orthopedic treatment. In addition to helping support the weight of the body above the hips, the vertebrae are subjected to a variety of twists, turns, and strains during a typical day. Much of the nearly continuous shock exerted on the spinal column is absorbed by the gel-like disks between the vertebrae.

SYMPTOMS: Eventually, one of the disks may *herniate,* or slip out of place, causing pressure on a spinal nerve. The result can be severe pain that radiates along the pathway of the nerve as far as the lower leg. The pain may be accompanied by muscular weakness and loss of reflexes, even perhaps by a loss of feeling in part of the leg affected by a pinched or squeezed nerve. This condition, known popularly as a slipped disk, has symptoms of low back pain or leg pain that are similar to those of other disorders such as intermittent claudication, arthritis, strained muscles, and prostatitis. Also, a herniated disk can occur near the top of the spinal column with symptoms of head and neck-area pains. But more than 90 percent of herniated disk cases involve the lumbar region of the spinal column, in the lower back.

DIAGNOSIS: Doctors usually can confirm a herniated disk problem by a technique called *myelography,* in which a dye is injected into the spinal canal and X-ray pictures taken. Another procedure, called *electromyography,* can help determine which nerve root is involved.

TREATMENT: Conservative measures generally are used at first to re-

duce the pain and other symptoms. They include bed rest on a hard mattress, medications, and sometimes the use of traction and back braces. If conservative therapy fails to correct the problem and the diagnosis has been well established by a myelogram, surgery may be advised to remove the herniated disk.

SPINAL FUSION: The surgeon may recommend a procedure called spinal fusion, in which the edges of several of the vertebrae are roughened and a piece of bone from the pelvis grafted onto the roughened edges. The bone graft will fuse with the vertebrae and in effect make the several vertebrae a single bone. However, the fused vertebrae will not interfere noticeably with body movements after the fusion is completed, which takes about six months. The operation requires a hospital stay of from one to two weeks and the patient must wear a body cast for the first few weeks and then use a back brace for a period of possibly several months. The patient usually can return to work and resume some normal activities within a couple of months after the operation. Strenuous activity, however, is usually restricted after an operation on the spinal column.

Other Spinal Disorders

SPONDYLOLISTHESIS: Spinal fusion surgery also may be used to correct two other kinds of spinal disorders. One disorder is known as *spondylolisthesis,* a condition in which one of the vertebrae slips out of alignment. Spondylolisthesis usually occurs at the bottom of the group of lumbar vertebrae, where that section of the spinal column rests on the sacrum.

SCOLIOSIS: The other disorder is *scoliosis,* or abnormal curvature of the spinal column. If the case of scoliosis is mild and causes no severe symptoms, it may be treated with conservative measures such as braces and special exercises. Surgical treatment of scoliosis may involve not only spinal fusion but reinforcement of the spinal column with

metal rods attached to the vertebrae to hold them in proper alignment.

Disorders of the cervical portion of the spinal column, in the area of the neck, may cause symptoms similar to those of a herniated disk in the lower back. But there is pain in the neck and shoulders and weakness in the arms. Surgical treatment also is similar, with removal of a herniated disk portion or fusion of cervical vertebrae when conservative therapy, with bed rest, neck braces, and medications, does not prove helpful.

Fractures

Many fractures of the spinal column also are treated by fusion operations, use of casts or braces, bed rest, or traction, in addition to therapy directed toward the specific problem. Spinal fractures frequently are compression fractures of vertebrae caused by falling in a sitting or standing position or mishaps in which a bony process of a vertebra is broken. Spinal fractures that result in permanent damage to the spinal cord, with resulting paralysis, are relatively uncommon.

REDUCTION OF FRACTURES: Fractures of the long bones of the arms and legs are treated by a method called *reduction,* the technique of aligning the broken ends of the bones properly so the healing process will not result in a deformity. Reduction also requires that the muscles and surrounding tissues be aligned and held in place by immobilizing them as the break heals.

If the break is simple enough, the limb can be immobilized by putting a plaster cast around the part of the limb involved after the fractured ends of the bone and associated tissues have been realigned. In complicated cases with a number of bone fragments resulting from the fracture and surrounding tissues in some disarray, the patient usually is given a general anesthetic while the surgeon reorganizes the shattered limb like a player assembling pieces of a jigsaw puzzle. If some of the needed pieces are missing, the surgeon may fill in the gaps with bone from a bone bank, although bone bank materials usually are not as effective in the healing process as pieces of the patient's own bones.

USE OF INTERNAL APPLIANCES: A common technique of modern fracture surgery is the application of wires, screws, pins, metal plates, and other devices to provide internal fixation of a broken long bone during the healing process. Nails and pins may be used to fasten the fractured neck of a femur, the long bone of the upper leg, to the shaft of that bone. A steel rod may be driven through the shaft of a long bone to align the broken sections. Screws may be used to hold together bone ends of a fracture in which the break runs diagonally across the shaft. Screws also may be employed to hold a metal plate or strip of bone from the patient's own body across the break. The screws, nails, and other devices generally are well tolerated by the body and may be left in the bones indefinitely if they do not cause adverse reactions after the healing process is completed. See the illustration to the right.

TRACTION: Traction frequently is employed to hold a limb in alignment while a fracture is healing. A clamp sometimes is placed at one end of the fractured limb and a weight attached by wires over a pulley is connected to the clamp. Depending upon the kind of fracture and type of traction prescribed, a system of several weights and pulleys may be rigged around the bed of a patient to fix the bone and related tissues in correct positions.

Torn Cartilage

Joints of the body can be vulnerable to damage from sudden twisting and turning actions, particularly when the force of the individual's body weight is added to the pressure on the joint. The effect of such forces on the knee joint can result in tearing of the half-moon-shaped cartilages that cushion friction of the upper and lower leg bones where they are joined. Sports fans are particularly aware of the vulnerability of the

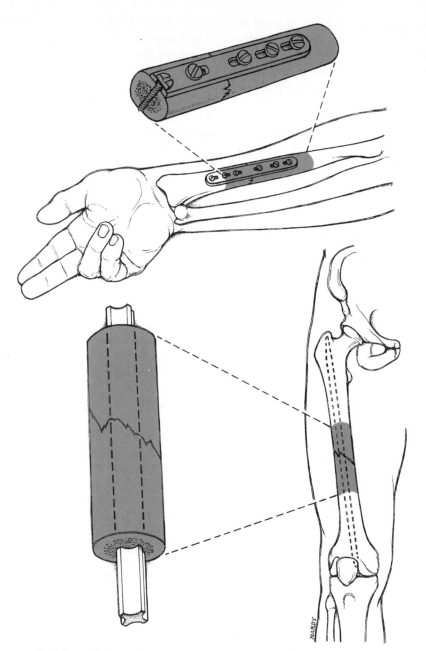

(Top) A metal plate is fastened with screws to secure a fractured bone in the arm (the radius). The enlarged portion shown in cross section in color is also shown as it appears in the patient's arm. (Bottom) A steel rod has been driven through the center of the femur of the leg to hold the jagged ends of the fractured bone in proper alignment. Such appliances are sometimes left in place indefinitely when there are no adverse reactions.

knee joint because of the high incidence of knee injuries to athletes, especially in football and basketball. Obese individuals are also particularly liable to develop cartilage problems in the knee.

SYMPTOMS: When a cartilage of the knee joint is torn, the patient may feel pain and weakness in the area of the injury. Swelling usually occurs

and in more than half the cases the knee cannot be straightened because it has become "locked" by the cartilage. There may be a remission of symptoms, but surgery frequently is required sooner or later.

SURGICAL PROCEDURE: The surgeon makes an incision in the area of the kneecap and cuts away the torn cartilage. Full recovery takes several weeks after the first few post-operative days, during which the patient remains in bed with the affected leg elevated. Special exercises are required to overcome muscle weakness in the leg and to help the patient learn to use the leg with part of the cartilage cushion missing.

Neurosurgery

Neurosurgery may be employed to treat a wide assortment of disorders involving the nervous system, from the brain to nerve endings in the fingers and toes. Neurosurgery may involve treatment of epilepsy, Parkinson's disease and psychiatric disorders, as well as herniated disks of the spinal column and aneurysms that affect the nervous system. Causes of neurosurgical problems can be injury, tumors, infectious diseases, or congenital disorders.

This section includes discussions of trigeminal neuralgia, brain tumors, and head injuries.

Trigeminal Neuralgia

Trigeminal neuralgia is one of many types of pain that sometimes can be treated by surgery. The disorder, also known as *tic douloureux* or *facial neuralgia,* tends to develop in persons between 40 and 60 years of age, causing attacks of acute pain and muscular twitching in the area of the face containing branches of the trigeminal nerve. The painful attacks occur with no apparent reason but seem to be associated with certain stimuli such as touch or temperature changes at points around the face and mouth. During periods of attacks, the patient may avoid eating, shaving, or any other activity that might trigger a spasm of severe pain. But the pain attacks also may cease, with or without treatment, for three or four months, only to resume for weeks or months.

TREATMENT: Alcohol injections and medications may offer relief of symptoms, but when symptoms continue surgery frequently is recommended. The operation consists of an incision to reach the root of the nerve and cut the divisions that appear to be involved with the painful symptoms. However, cutting the nerve can result in loss of feeling for the entire side of the face, including the cornea of the eye, so that the patient must wear special glasses to protect the cornea. An alternative procedure that is not always effective involves exposing the nerve root and rubbing it, a technique that seems to produce a temporary loss of sensation in the nerve fibers.

Brain Tumor

Brain tumors are popularly associated with neurosurgery skills. And while brain surgery requires great skill and knowledge of brain anatomy, which in itself is quite complicated, most brain tumor operations are conducted safely and successfully. Diagnosing, locating, and identifying a brain tumor are challenges faced by the doctor before surgery begins. There are a dozen major types of brain tumors plus some minor types. The types of tumors tend to vary according to the age of the patient; the patient's age and the type of tumor may suggest where it develops.

SYMPTOMS: Because brain tumors can cause organic mental changes in the patient, the symptoms of changed behavior can be mistaken for neurotic or psychotic disorders with the result that a patient may spend valuable time receiving psychiatric treatment rather than surgical treatment; autopsies of a significant number of patients who die in mental hospitals reveal the presence of brain tumors. In addition to mental changes, the person suffering from a brain tumor may complain of headaches, experience convulsions, or display signs of neurological function loss such as abnormal vision.

DIAGNOSIS: The specific signs and symptoms along with X-ray studies, electroencephalograms, and other tests help the doctors determine the site and extent of growth of a brain tumor. A recently developed technique called *CAT scanning* (for *computerized axial tomography*) aids the neurosurgeon by producing a series of X-ray pictures of the interior of the skull as if they were "slices" of the brain taken in thicknesses of about two-thirds of an inch. The detailed anatomical por-

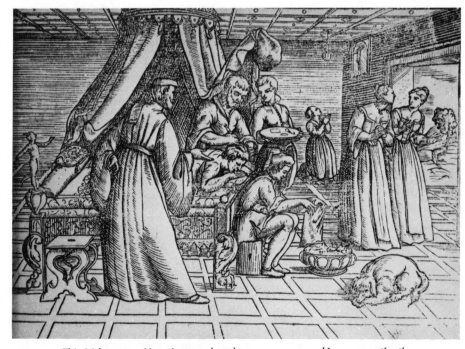

This 16th-century Venetian woodcut shows a surgeon working on a patient's skull with a trephine, a drill specially designed for such an operation.

trait of the patient's brain helps pinpoint the disorder and indicate whether it is a tumor or another kind of abnormality.

SURGICAL PROCEDURE: The usual method of removing a brain tumor after it has been diagnosed and located is a procedure called a *craniotomy*. The entire head is shaved and cleaned to eliminate the possibility that a stray bit of hair might fall into the incision that is made in the scalp. After the scalp has been opened, a series of holes are drilled in a pattern outlining the working area for the surgeon; a wire saw is used to cut the skull between the drilled holes.

Removing the tumor is a delicate operation, not only because of the need to avoid damage to healthy brain tissue but because accidental severing of a blood vessel in the brain could produce a critical hemorrhage. The surgeon tries to remove the entire tumor, or as much of the tumor as appears possible without damaging vital brain tissues or blood vessels. All of the various types of brain tumors are considered dangerous, whether malignant or benign, because within the rigid confines of the skull there is no opportunity for outward release of pressure. Therefore any growth may compress or destroy vital brain tissues if left untreated.

After the tumor is removed, the piece of skull removed at the start of the operation is replaced and the scalp flap is sewed in place. Radiation therapy may be administered for a month to six weeks after surgery to destroy any tumor tissue left behind or tumor cells that may have drifted into the spinal canal. Some tumors near the base of the brain may be treated effectively with radiation alone if the tumor cells are radiosensitive. Tumors of the pineal gland and the pituitary gland also may be treated with radiation.

Head Injuries

BRAIN HEMORRHAGE: Head injuries, such as a blow to the head, can pro-
duce massive hemorrhages within the skull. As in the case of brain tumors, the expanding pool of blood within the skull gradually compresses the brain tissue and can result in death unless the problem is corrected. The damage of a brain hemorrhage can be insidious, with no immediate signs or symptoms of the problem until irreversible changes have occurred in the brain tissue. The patient may receive what may appear to be a minor head injury, for example, and not lose consciousness. Or he may be unconscious for a brief period, then recover and appear very alert. But gradually, over a period of hours or even days, neurological signs of disintegrating brain function appear.

TREATMENT: The treatment requires a procedure similar to that used for removing brain tumors. An opening is made in the skull to remove the blood or blood clot and relieve pressure on the brain tissues.

The chances for full recovery depend somewhat on the extent of brain damage caused by the hemorrhage before treatment.

SKULL FRACTURE: Surgical treatment for a skull fracture may combine techniques of various other methods for fractures and brain injuries. The scalp is shaved and cleaned carefully so the surgeon can determine the extent of the injury and its location with respect to vital tissues under the skull. With the help of X rays and signs of neurological damage, the surgeon frequently can tell how severe the fracture may be and whether there is bleeding beneath the skull.

TREATMENT: If the skull appears to be intact but there are signs of a brain hemorrhage, the skull is opened to remove the blood or blood clot and relieve pressure on the brain. If the skull fracture is compound and depressed, or with skull fragments in the brain tissue, efforts also must be

The location and size of a brain aneurysm can be identified by X-ray pictures after an opaque dye has been injected into the bloodstream.

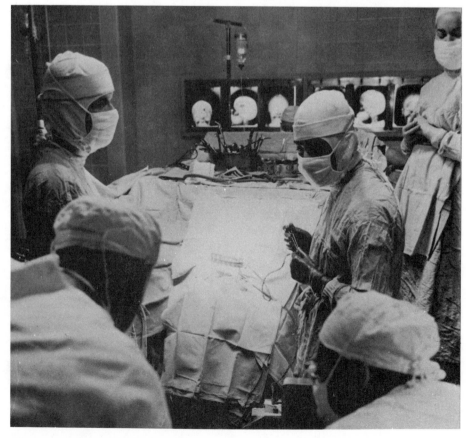

made to elevate the depressed bone section so it does not press on vital brain areas and to remove bits of bone or other foreign materials that may have entered the brain.

Surgeons frequently can rebuild a fractured skull by replacing missing bits of bone or adding appropriate synthetic materials such as a piece of metal plate. Full recovery depends upon such factors as the age of the patient and the severity of damage before treatment was started. Younger patients generally respond better to the repair procedures, but full recovery from a severe skull fracture may take as long as a year.

ANEURYSM IN THE BRAIN: Aneurysms can develop in blood vessels of the brain, and like aneurysms in other parts of the body they can be corrected surgically. A ruptured aneurysm produces a brain hemorrhage. The condition is most likely to develop in people over the age of 30; in patients over 40, women are more likely than men to be victims of the disorder. The approach to repair of an intracranial aneurysm depends upon the condition of the patient and the location and size of the aneurysm, which frequently can be identified by X-ray pictures after an opaque dye has been injected into the bloodstream. The diseased blood vessel may be ligated, reinforced, or repaired, depending upon the conditions found by the surgeon after the aneurysm has been exposed and examined.

PLASTIC AND COSMETIC SURGERY

The use of surgical techniques for the correction of physical deformities is by no means a modern development. The practice goes back to ancient India, where as early as the sixth century B.C. Hindu specialists were reconstructing noses, reshaping ears, and grafting skin for reducing scar tissue.

Through the centuries, improvements in procedure and new types of operations became part of the common fund of information. During World War I, great technical advances were made when the Medical Corps of the United States Army created a special division of *plastic surgery* to treat the deformities caused by battle injuries. Today's plastic surgery is based on many of the procedures perfected then and during World War II.

In recent years, attention has been focused not only on birth and injury deformities, but on lesser irregularities as well. Surgeons in the field of *cosmetic surgery* perform such procedures as nose reconstruction, face lifting, reshaping of breasts, removal of fatty tissue from upper arms and legs, and the transplanting of hair to correct baldness.

There is no longer any reason for someone to suffer from the emotional and professional problems caused by abnormalities in appearance. No child should be expected to live with the disability of a cleft lip or crossed eyes. A young woman tormented by what she considers to be a grotesque nose can have it recontoured to her liking. An older woman who finds wrinkles a social liability can have them removed. Anyone interested in undergoing any form of cosmetic surgery should stay away from so-called beauty experts, and deal only with a reputable surgeon or physician.

Some surgical specialists, called *plastic surgeons,* perform cosmetic or plastic surgery exclusively. Other surgeons and physicians, including general surgeons, dermatologists, ophthalmologists, and others are qualified to do some kinds of plastic surgery, usually the techniques related to their particular specialties. The kind of surgery desired should first be discussed with the family doctor, who can then evaluate the problem and recommend a qualified surgeon to deal with it.

Before undergoing any kind of plastic surgery, the prospective patient should realize that it is neither inexpensive nor totally painless. Most cosmetic surgery is performed in hospitals, which means that in addition to the surgeon's fees there can be a bill for the anesthetist, use of the operating and recovery rooms, and for the hospital stay itself. Also, because cosmetic surgery is often optional surgery, surgery not needed to ensure the patient's physical health, it may not be covered by a health-insurance policy. Getting one's nose fixed, for example, may cost between $500 and $1,500.

Reshaping the Nose

Known technically as a *rhinoplasty,* the operation for the reconstruction of the nose is not only one of the oldest, but also one of the most common forms of cosmetic surgery. Depending on the demands of facial symmetry and individual taste, the nose can be shortened, straightened, narrowed, or even lengthened. If a nose deformity has caused breathing problems, the surgeon will take the correction of this into account in planning the reconstruction.

Barring accidents, most children's noses are perfectly adequate until they enter their teens, when the facial bones begin to take on the contours determined by inheritance. Teen-agers are especially sensitive about their looks. If nose surgery seems advisable, therefore, it is usually undertaken when the child is between 14 and 16 years of age, though the operation is also performed on adults.

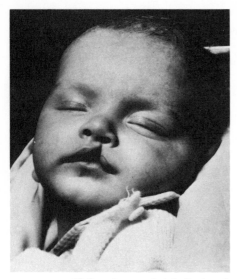
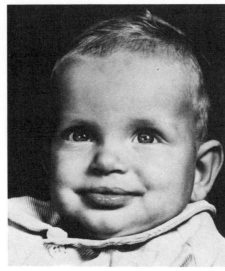

Cleft palate and cleft lip interfere with the infant's ability to suck and, if uncorrected, would later cause speech impairment. These pictures show how surgery can correct the disfigurement.

In many cases, parents agree with the youngster about the need for surgery. In some families, however, the parent who has lived with a nose very similar to the one which the child finds so objectionable may take a negative view of the need for correction. If a serious disagreement results, it may be necessary to seek family counseling from a professional source to resolve it.

SURGICAL PROCEDURES: When a nose reconstruction is being planned, the surgeon requires photographs of both the left and right profiles as well as front and under views of the nose. Transparent paper is placed on top of the photos, and the recommended changes are drawn over the original nose structure. The patient's preferences are always taken into account, but the surgeon has a final say in determining the suitability of the new shape in terms of appearance and function. In some cases, facial surgery to build up an underdeveloped chin, called a *mentoplasty,* is recommended so that better balance of the features is achieved.

The surgery itself is performed under local anesthesia in a hospital. It is done through the nostrils so that there is no scarring of facial tissue. The skin is loosened from the bone and cartilage, and these are reshaped to the desired specifications. The skin then resettles on its new frame, and the new shape is retained by packing the nostrils and splinting the nose.

THE HEALING PROCESS: The packing is left in place for about three to five days or until it can be removed without sticking. The total dressing stays on for about a week. During the healing period, the nose is cleaned with cotton swabs. All swelling in the area vanishes in about a month, and within a year the reconstructed nose is as strong if not stronger than its original counterpart.

Cosmetic Breast Surgery

INVERTED NIPPLES: The condition in which the nipples are turned back into the breasts rather than projecting from them can be corrected by a simple operation. The breast tissue is cut to release the nipple so that it can be pulled outward to the normal position. This surgical procedure is sometimes recommended to facilitate the nursing of a newborn baby.

BREAST LIFTING: Breasts that sag even though they are not too large can be lifted to a more attractive contour by an operation that consolidates the tissue. The surgical procedure consists of removing strips of skin from the base of the breasts and bringing the rest of the skin together under tension so that it is tight enough to support the tissue in an upward position.

BREAST REDUCTION: In spite of all the publicity given to breast augmentation, most cosmetic surgery

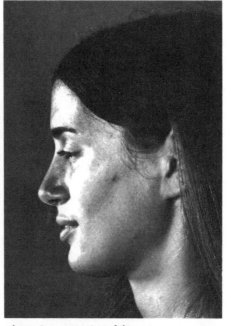

Pictures taken before and after rhinoplasty. Reconstruction of the nose is done through the nostrils so that there is no scarring of facial tissue. The surgery is performed under local anesthesia in a hospital.

involving the breasts is concerned with reducing rather than enlarging them. Breast reduction is frequently undertaken not only to improve appearance, but also for purposes of health and comfort.

The operation, called a *mastoplasty,* is performed under general anesthesia and consists in cutting out fatty tissue and skin. Although the incision may be large, the resulting scars are no thicker than a hairline and are hidden in the fold below the breasts.

The most remarkable thing about this type of surgery—and the reason for its being considerably more complicated than breast enlargement—is the repositioning of the nipples so that they are properly placed relative to the newly proportioned breast contours.

BREAST ENLARGEMENT: The techniques used in this operation, called a *mammoplasty,* have changed over the years. Early operations to augment the size of the breasts involved the injection of paraffin, but this was soon abandoned as unsatisfactory. Considerable experimentation with the use of various synthetics as well as with the use of fatty tissue taken from the buttocks didn't provide good results either.

Silicone—a form of man-made plastic material of great versatility—was first used in this connection in the form of sponges, and later was injected in liquid form directly into the tissue. However, the federal Food and Drug Administration has ruled that the use of liquid silicone is unsafe and illegal, since its presence would mask signs of malignancy. Another problem with liquid silicone is that it has a tendency to drift to other parts of the body.

In the latest techniques of breast augmentation, a silicone gel or saline solution is placed in a flexible silicone bag shaped to resemble the breast. The bags are inserted through incisions under the breast tissue, and to date appear to be the safest and most satisfactory solution to the problem of breast enlargement.

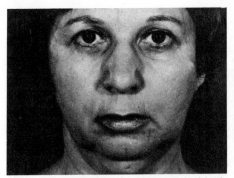 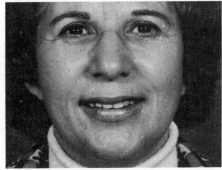

This patient underwent rhytidoplasty (face lift) and mentoplasty (chin buildup). Face lift removes wrinkles by tightening facial skin and removing the excess. Scars are hidden under hair and behind the ears.

Face Lift

Face lifting, or *rhytidoplasty,* is a form of cosmetic surgery designed to eliminate as far as possible signs of aging such as wrinkles, pouches under the chin and eyes, and sagging tissue generally. About 7,000 such operations are performed each year with satisfactory results.

In deciding on the advisability of a face lift, a reputable surgeon will take into account the person's age, emotional stability, and physical condition. The main procedure involves tightening the skin after the surplus has been removed. The resulting scars are usually hidden in the hair and behind the ears. Those directly in front of the ears are visible only under very close scrutiny. Even after a face lift, however, the same wrinkles will eventually reappear because of the characteristic use of the individual's facial muscles.

Recently, interest has grown in the application of cosmetic surgery to the problem of removing surplus fat from various parts of the body. Once considered controversial, the operation is being performed by many plastic surgeons. But these specialists emphasize that each person with a problem of surplus fat requires individual consultation and treatment.

Traditionally, to reduce the size of the upper arms or legs, the abdomen, or the buttocks, an incision was made in a natural fold of the body area in question. The surrounding skin was loosened, the surplus fat and the excess skin re-

moved, and the remaining skin was stretched tight and sutured. The procedure usually left a long scar.

In *suction lipectomy,* a new, alternative procedure, the surgeon does not make a long incision. Instead, the specialist makes a series of tiny, half-inch-long incisions. A suction device called a blunt cannula (which looks like a long straw) is inserted into the incisions. The cannula suctions out, or "vacuums" out, the excess fat. The operation can be performed on the stomach, buttocks, chin, calf, and ankle areas.

Suction lipectomy, also called *lipolysis,* involves normal surgical risks. The skin in the area of the operation may acquire a rippling effect. Some damage could be done to nerves and blood vessels. Bruising could last for several weeks. The patient may have to wear supportive clothing for four to six weeks. Plastic surgeons stress that the procedure is not a weight-reduction technique for the obese, but a contouring operation.

Eyelids

The shape and size of the eyelids can be changed by an operation called a *blepharoplasty.* In this procedure, an incision is made in the fold of the upper eyelid, and excess skin and fat are removed. The technique can be used to correct congenital deformities such as hanging upper eyelids that do not fully open. When a comparable incision is made below the lash line on the lower lid, the surgeon can remove the fat which causes bags under the eyes.

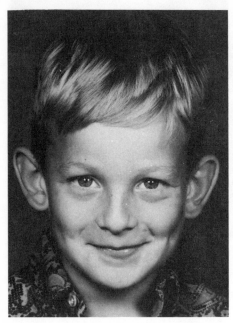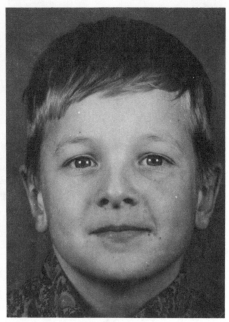

Surgery to correct protruding or overlarge ears is called otoplasty. It is usually performed on children before they enter school to prevent the psychological problems that often result from teasing.

Ears

Surgery to correct protruding or overlarge ears is called *otoplasty*. Though it can be performed on adults, it is usually performed on children before they enter school to prevent the psychological problems that often result from teasing. In the procedure, an incision is made behind the ear, cartilage is cut, and the ear is repositioned closer to the skull. Otoplasty can also build up or replace an ear missing because of a birth defect or accident.

Scar Reduction

Unsightly scars that are the result of a birth defect or an injury can usually be reduced by plastic surgery to thin hairlines. The procedure is effective only if there has been no extensive damage to surrounding areas of underlying tissue, as sometimes occurs in severe burns. The operation involves the removal of the old scar tissue, undermining the surrounding skin, and pulling it together with very fine stitches.

Hair Transplant

A comparatively new solution to the problem of baldness is the technique called hair transplantation. This involves the surgical grafting of hair-bearing skin taken from the back part and sides of the scalp onto the bald areas of the head. The transplanting is usually done in the surgeon's office with the patient receiving a local anesthetic. The surgeon can make anywhere from 10 to 60 transplants in an hour's session.

Within about a month, the hairs in the grafted skin fall out, but the roots remain, and most of these eventually produce new hair. The areas from which the grafts are taken remain hairless, but since each transplant is very small, about 150 or 200 graftings can be done without creating any conspicuous bald spots. Transplanted hair has the same thickness and appearance that it had in its former location.

UNCOMMON SURGICAL PROCEDURES

Organ Transplants

The notion of man's ability to rebuild human bodies from parts of other humans or from artificial organs probably is as old as the dreams that men might some day fly like birds or travel to the moon. Some of the oldest documents, thousands of years old, tell of medical efforts to transplant organs, limbs, and other tissues to save lives or enable disabled persons to pursue normal activities. In recent decades, medical scientists have discovered how to overcome some of the obstacles to organ transplanting, just as other scientists have learned to fly higher and faster than birds and travel beyond the moon.

Tissue Compatibility

A major obstacle to organ transplants has been one of *histoincompatibility* (*histo* means "tissue"): the tissues of the person receiving the transplant tend to reject the tissues of the transplanted organ. The problem is quite similar to that of allergies or the body's reaction to foreign bodies, including infectious organisms. Each individual has a set of antigens that are peculiar to that person, because of genetic variations among different persons. The histoincompatible antigens are on the surfaces of the tissue cells. But in most cases the antigens on the cells of the transplanted organ do not match those of the person receiving the transplant, so the recipient's body in effect refuses to accept the transplant.

The major exception to this rule is found in identical twins, who are born with the same sets of antigens. The organs of one twin can be transplanted to the body of the other twin with a minimum risk of rejection. Antigens on the tissue cells of brothers and sisters and of the parents will be similar, because of the biological relationship, but they will not be as compatible as those of identical twins. Even less compatible are antigens of people who are not related.

TYPES OF GRAFTS: There is virtually no problem in transferring tissues from one area to another of the same patient. Skin grafts, bone grafts, and blood-vessel transplants are commonly made with a patient's own tissues, which have the same antigens, as in spinal fusions, repair of diseased leg arteries, and so on. Tissue transplants within an individual's body are called *autografts*. Transplants of tissues or organs from one human to another are called *homografts*. *Heterografts* are tissues from one species that are transplanted to another; they offer the greatest risk of histoincompatibility and are used mainly as a temporary measure, such as covering a severely burned area of a person with specially treated pieces of pigskin. The heterograft will be rejected but it will provide some protection during the recovery period.

Much of the experience of surgeons in handling tissue transplants between humans came from early experiments in skin grafting. It was found that histoincompatibility in transplants of skin appeared to sensitize the recipient tissues in the same way that allergy sensitivity rises. Thus, when a second skin graft from the same donor is attempted, the graft is rejected more rapidly than the first graft because of the buildup of antibodies from the first rejection. The same sort of rejection reaction can occur in transplants of kidneys, hearts, and other organs unless the problem of histoincompatibility is overcome.

IMMUNOSUPPRESSIVE CHEMICALS: In order to make the host body more receptive to an organ transplant, *im-munosuppressive* chemicals are injected into the recipient's tissues to suppress their natural tendency to reject the foreign tissue. However, the technique of suppressing the immune response of the host tissues is not without hazards. By suppressing the natural rejection phenomenon, the transplant recipient is made vulnerable to other diseases. It has been found, for example, that persons who receive the immune response suppression chemicals as part of transplant surgery develop cancers at a rate that is 15 times that of the general population. Transplant patients also can become extremely vulnerable to infections, such as pneumonia.

ANTIGEN MATCHING: The breakthrough in human organ transplantation was helped by the development of a system of matching antigens related to lymphocytes—a type of white blood cell—of the donor and recipient. At least a dozen lymphocyte antigens have been identified, and it is possible to match them by a process similar to matching blood factors of patients before making a blood transfusion. If all or most of the antigens of the donor tissue and the recipient match, the chances for a successful transplanting procedure are greatly enhanced.

Antigen matching is less important in some kinds of homografts, such as replacing the cornea of the eye. The cornea is a unique kind of tissue with no blood vessels, and therefore is unlikely to be invaded by antibodies of the recipient. Pieces of human bone also may be used in homografts with a minimum risk of rejection, although surgeons usually prefer to use bone from the patient's own body in repairing fractures and other orthopedic procedures.

Types of Transplants

CORNEA TRANSPLANT: Cornea transplants helped to pioneer the art of homografts. The first successful cornea transplants were made during the 1930s. In addition to the absence of rejection problems because of incompatible antigens, cornea transplants probably succeeded in the early days of homografts because only small pieces of the tissue were used. See p. 334.

KIDNEY TRANSPLANT: Kidney transplants began in the 1950s. Antigen typing was unknown at that time, but doctors had learned of the genetic factors of blood groups and found from experience that although kidney transplants from siblings and parents could eventually be rejected, the rejection phenomenon was delayed. The first truly successful kidney transplant operation was performed in Boston in 1954 between twin brothers; doctors had tested the tissue compatibility of the twins first by making a small skin transplant to see if it would be rejected. Knowledge acquired later of immunosuppressive drugs enabled surgeons to make kidney transplants between persons who were not twins.

More than 5,000 kidney-transplant operations have been performed with an 82 percent survival rate of two years or more when the donor was related to the recipient. When a cadaver kidney was transplanted, the two-year survival rate was 65 percent. It has been estimated that as many as 10,000 kidney-disease patients each year could benefit from a transplanted organ, but a lack of available kidneys in satisfactory condition restricts the number of transplants. An alternative for some kidney patients awaiting an organ transplant is hemodialysis, a process which performs as an artificial kidney. See p. 425 for further information on dialysis.

HEART TRANSPLANT: The first successful human heart transplant was performed by Dr. Christiaan Barnard in Cape Town, South Africa, in 1968. The patient survived more than 18 months and led a relatively active life until the second heart failed because of a rejection reaction. Many heart transplant operations have been performed since 1968, with varying success, sometimes leading to complete recovery and sometimes to recovery for long periods of time. Heart transplants were found to be more difficult than some other organ transplants, such as of the kidney, because the heart must be taken from the donor at virtually the moment of death and immediately placed in the body of the recipient. Because of concern about determining the moment of death, the medical profession has offered guidelines for answering this complex ethical and legal question.

Success of a heart transplant operation may depend on the health of other organ systems in the patient's body; persons in need of heart transplants usually have medical problems involving the lungs and kidneys as a result of the diseased heart. And heart transplant patients frequently seem less able to tolerate the use of immunosuppressive drugs that must be administered after surgery. The introduction of cyclosporine as an immunosuppressant in the early 1980s changed the picture substantially, however. Medical evidence indicated that cyclosporine would lead to a five-year survival rate among heart transplant patients of 50 percent or more. Because cyclosporine speeds rehabilitation after an operation, average hospital stays for patients receiving the immunosuppressant have been reduced from 72 to 42 days.

Conducted before cyclosporine came into common use, one study of a group of transplant patients showed that fewer than 40 percent survived beyond the first year. Several lived more than two years after the operation.

BONE-MARROW TRANSPLANT: Limited success has been reported in efforts to perform bone-marrow transplants. Bone-marrow transplants are performed to supply patients with active leukocytes to fight cancer and other diseases. The successful early cases have involved transplants between sisters and brothers who had been typed for tissue compatibility.

OTHER KINDS OF TRANSPLANTS: Surgeons also have experimented with varying success with human transplants of livers, lungs, and pancreas tissue. Lung transplant efforts have been hampered by infection, rejection, and hemorrhage. Because the lungs are exposed to pathogenic organisms in the environment they are especially vulnerable to infections when the host tissues have been treated with immunosuppressive chemicals. Liver transplants are difficult to perform because of a lack of satisfactory donor organs and the complex circuitry of arteries, veins, and bile duct that must be connected to the recipient before the liver can begin to function.

Most major organ transplants are considered only in terms of a "last ditch" effort to prolong the life of a patient who is critically ill. While homografts are not always a perfect success and may lengthen a patient's life by only a few years, remarkable strides in these surgical techniques have been made over a relatively short period of time. Surgeons who specialize in organ transplants state that even greater progress could be made if a greater supply of donor organs were available.

Reattachment of Severed Members

Because an individual's tissues present no histocompatibility problem with other parts of his own body, severed fingers and other members can be rejoined to the rest of the body if vital parts are not damaged beyond repair. Children sometimes suffer amputation of a part of a finger during play or in accidents at home. For example, a finger tip can be severed when caught in a closed door of an automobile. If the severed part of the finger is saved and the patient is given immediate medical care, the finger usually can be rejoined and sutured in place with a very good chance of survival of the graft.

Rejoining a Severed Limb

One of the most dramatic cases of a rejoined limb in American medical annals involved a 12-year-old whose right arm was severed at the shoulder when he was crushed between a train and a tunnel wall in 1962. Railroad workers called an ambulance, and the boy, his severed arm still encased in his sleeve, was rushed to a hospital. The boy was given plasma by doctors who packed the severed arm in ice and flushed out the blood vessels of the arm with anticoagulant drugs and antibiotics. During three hours of surgery, the major veins and artery of the arm were carefully stitched to the vessels at the shoulder. For the next five hours, doctors joined the bones, located the main nerve trunks and connected them to the nerve ends in the shoulder, and repaired the muscles. The boy was released from the hospital three weeks after the accident but returned for additional operations to connect various nerve fibers. That operation was a success, but similar attempts to rejoin severed arms of middle-aged men have failed despite heroic attempts by surgeons to restore the limbs as functioning parts of the body.

A Chinese factory worker suffered accidental amputation of his right hand when it was caught in a metal-punching machine, and was rushed to a hospital in Shanghai. Chinese medical reports of the case indicate that a procedure similar to the one used on the American boy was followed. Blood vessels were rejoined first to permit the flow of blood to tissues. This was followed by surgery to connect the tendons and main nerve trunks. The bones of the forearm, where the amputation occurred, were joined and held in place with metal plates and screws. Doctors reported that the graft was successful, and the patient, a 27-year-old man, was able to move his fingers again within three weeks after the accident.

Medical records indicate that major reattachments of severed limbs are still rare, although rejoined finger tips, ears, and other parts not involving main arteries, veins, or nerve trunks are not as uncommon.

CHAPTER 15

Diseases of
the Circulatory System

It's called the river of life, the five or six quarts of blood that stream through the 60,000 tortuous miles of arteries, veins, and capillaries.

Blood contains many elements with specific functions—red cells to transport oxygen from the lungs to body tissues, white cells to fight off disease, and tiny elements called *platelets* to help form clots and repair tears in the blood vessel wall. All float freely in an intricate complex of liquid proteins and metals known as *plasma*.

Because of the blood's extreme importance to life, any injury to it—or to the grand network of channels through which it flows—may have the most serious consequences. The troubles that beset the circulation may be grouped conveniently into two categories: diseases of the blood and diseases of the blood vessels.

DISEASES OF THE BLOOD

Diseases of the blood include disorders that affect the blood elements directly (as in the case of *hemophilia,* where a deficiency in clotting proteins is at fault) as well as abnormalities in the various organs involved in maintaining proper blood balance (i.e., spleen, liver and bone marrow). The various ills designated and described below are arranged according to the blood component most affected (i.e., clotting proteins, red blood cells, and white blood cells).

Hemorrhagic or
Clotting-Deficiency Diseases

The blood has the ability to change from a fluid to a solid and back to a fluid again. The change to a solid is called *clotting*. There are mecha-nisms not only for sealing off breaks in the circulatory system when serious blood loss is threatened, but also for breaking down the seals, or clots, once the damage has been repaired and the danger of blood loss is eliminated. Both mechanisms are in continuous, dynamic equilibrium, a delicate balance between tissue repair and clot dissolution to keep us from bleeding or literally clogging to death.

Clotting involves a very complex chain of chemical events. The key is the conversion of an inactive blood protein, *fibrinogen*, into a threadlike sealant known as *fibrin*. Stimulus for this conversion is an enzyme called *thrombin*, which normally also circulates in an inactive state as *prothrombin* (formed from vitamin K in the daily diet).

For a clot to form, however, inactive prothrombin must undergo a chemical transformation into thrombin, a step requiring still another chemical—*thromboplastin*. This agent comes into play only when a tissue or vessel has been injured so as to require clot protection. There are two ways for thromboplastin to enter the bloodstream to spark the chain of events. One involves the release by the injured tissue of a substance that reacts with plasma proteins to produce thromboplastin. The other requires the presence of blood platelets (small particles that travel in the blood) and several plasma proteins, including the so-called antihemophilic factor. Platelets tend to clump at the site of vessel injury, where they disintegrate and ultimately release thromboplastin, which, in the presence of blood calcium, triggers the pro-

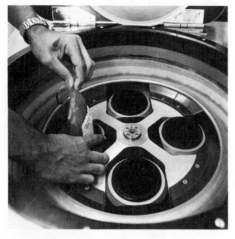
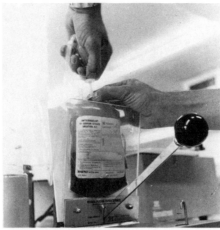
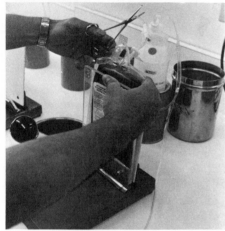
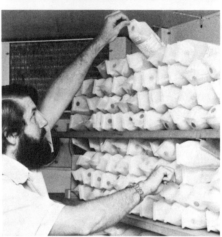

Modern blood bank techniques can make large quantities of whole blood and blood components available to hemophiliacs and others in need of transfusions. *(Top left)* Blood taken from a donor is placed in a centrifuge, which spins around to separate the red cells from the plasma. *(Top right)* Centrifuging has caused the plasma to rise to the top of the bag and the red cells to settle to the bottom. The bag is placed in an extracting device to draw off the plasma. *(Bottom left)* The plasma has been withdrawn and the bag of red blood cells is being detached. *(Bottom right)* Plasma is stored in a freezer to await use in the manufacture of medicines and in diagnostic products.

thrombin-thrombin conversion.

The clot-destroying sequence is very similar to that involved in clot formation, with the key enzyme, *fibrinolysin*, existing normally in an inactive state *(profibrinolysin)*. There are also other agents (e.g., *heparin*) in the blood ready to retard or prevent the clotting sequence, so that it doesn't spread to other parts of the body.

Naturally, grave dangers arise should these complex mechanisms fail. For the moment, we shall concern ourselves with hemorrhagic disorders arising from a failure of the blood to clot properly. Disorders stemming from excessive clotting are discussed below under *Diseases of the Blood Vessels*, since they are likely to happen as a consequence of pre-existing problems in the vessel walls.

Hemophilia

Hemophilia is probably the best known (although relatively rare) of the hemorrhagic disorders, because of its prevalence among the royal families of Europe. In hemophilia the blood does not clot properly and bleeding persists. Those who have this condition are called *hemophiliacs* or bleeders. The disease is inherited, and is transmitted by the mother, but except in very rare cases only the male offspring are affected. Hemophilia stems from a lack of one of the plasma proteins associated with clotting, *antihemophilic factor (AHF)*.

The presence of hemophilia is generally discovered during early childhood. It is readily recognized by the fact that even small wounds bleed profusely and can trigger an emergency. Laboratory tests for clotting speed are used to confirm the diagnosis. Further investigation may occasionally turn up the condition in other members of the family.

In advanced stages, hemophilia may lead to anemia as a result of excessive and continuous blood loss. Bleeding in the joints causes painful swelling, which over a long period of time can lead to permanent deformity and hemophilic arthritis. Hemophiliacs must be under constant medical care in order to receive quick treatment in case of emergencies.

Treating bleeding episodes may involve the administration of AHF alone so as to speed up the clotting sequence. If too much blood is lost a complete transfusion may be necessary. Thanks to modern blood bank techniques, large quantities of whole blood can be made readily available. Bed rest and hospitalization may also be required. For bleeding in the joints, an ice pack is usually applied.

Proper dental hygiene is a must for all hemophiliacs. Every effort should be made to prevent tooth decay. Parents of children with the disease should inform the dentist so that all necessary precautions can be taken. Even the most common procedures, such as an extraction, can pose a serious hazard. Only absolutely essential surgery should be performed on hemophiliacs, with the assurance that large amounts of plasma are on hand.

Purpura

Purpura refers to spontaneous hemorrhaging over large areas of the skin and in mucous membranes. It results from a deficiency in blood platelets, elements essential to clotting. Purpura is usually triggered by other conditions: certain anemias, leukemia, sensitivity to drugs, or exposure to ionizing radiation. In newborns it may be linked to the prenatal transfer from the maternal circulation of substances that depress platelet levels. Symptoms of purpura include the presence of blood in the urine, bleeding from the mucous membranes of the mouth, nose, intestines and uterus. Some forms of the disease cause arthritic changes in joints, abdominal pains, diarrhea and vomiting—and even gangrene of the skin, when certain infectious organisms become involved.

To treat purpura in newborns, physicians may exchange the infant's blood with platelet-packed blood. Sometimes drug therapy with *steroids* (i.e., cortisone) is prescribed. In adults with chronic purpura it may be necessary to remove the spleen, which plays an important role in eliminating worn-out blood components, including platelets, from the circulation. Most physicians prescribe large doses of steroids coupled with blood transfusions. Purpura associated with infection and gangrene also requires appropriate antibiotic therapy.

Red Cell Diseases

Half the blood is plasma; the other half is made up of many tiny blood cells. The biggest group in number is the red blood cells. These cells contain a complicated chemical called *hemoglobin*, which brings oxygen from the lungs to body cells and picks up waste carbon dioxide for expiration. Hemoglobin is rich in iron, which is what imparts the characteristic red color to blood.

Red blood cells are manufactured by bones all over the body—in the sternum, ribs, skull, arms, spine and pelvis. The actual factory is the red bone marrow, located at bone ends. As red cells mature and are ready to enter the bloodstream, they lose their nuclei to become what are called *red corpuscles* or *erythrocytes*. With no nucleus, a red corpuscle is relatively short-lived (120 days). Thus, the red cell supply must be constantly replenished by bone marrow. And a busy factory it is, since 20 to 25 trillion red corpuscles normally travel in the circulation. The spleen is responsible for ridding the body of the aged corpuscles, but it is not an indiscriminate sanitizer; it salvages the hemoglobin for reuse by the body.

To measure levels of red cells, physicians make a blood count by taking a smidgen of blood from a patient's fingertip. The average number of red cells in healthy blood is about five million per cubic millimeter for men, and four and one-half million for women.

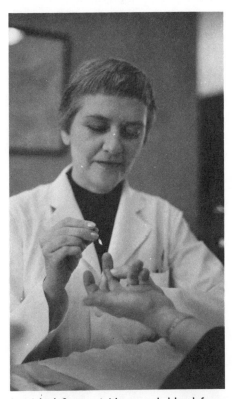

A pricked finger yields enough blood for a test sample that can determine the proportion of red blood cells in a blood count.

Anemia

Anemia exists when the red cell count stays persistently below four million. Abnormalities in the size, shape, or hemoglobin content of the erythrocytes may also account for anemic states. Any such irregularity interferes with the red cell's ability to carry its full share of oxygen to body tissues. It also tends to weaken the red cells so that they are more likely to be destroyed under the stresses of the circulation.

Anemia may result from:

• Nutritional deficiencies which deprive the body of elements vital to the production of healthy cells

• Diseases or injuries to organs associated with either blood cell formation (bone marrow) or blood cell destruction (spleen and liver)

• Excessive loss of blood, the consequences of surgery, hemorrhage, or a bleeding ulcer

• Heredity, as in the case of *sickle cell anemia* (where the red cells are misshapen).

HEMOLYTIC ANEMIA: There are also several kinds of disorders known as *hemolytic anemias* that are linked to the direct destruction of red cells. Poisons such as snake venom, arsenic, and lead can cause hemolytic anemia. So can toxins produced by certain bacteria as well as by other organisms, such as the parasites that cause malaria, hookworm, and tapeworm. Destruction of red cells may also stem from allergic reactions to certain drugs or transfusions with incompatible blood.

The various anemias range from ailments mild enough to go undetected to disorders which prove inevitably fatal. Many are rare; among the more common are:

PERNICIOUS ANEMIA: Pernicious anemia, or *Addison's anemia,* is associated with a lack of hydrochloric acid in the gastric juices, a defect which interferes with the body's ability to absorb vitamin B_{12} from the intestine. Since the vitamin acts as an essential stimulus to the production of mature red blood cells by the bone marrow, its lack leads to a reduced output. Moreover, the cells tend to be larger than normal, with only half the life-span of the normal erythrocyte.

The symptoms are characteristic of most anemias: pale complexion, numbness or a feeling of "pins and needles" in the arms and legs, shortness of breath (from a lack of oxygen), loss of appetite, nausea, and diarrhea (often accompanied by significant weight loss). One specific feature is a sore mouth with a smooth, glazed tongue. Advanced stages of the disease may be marked by an unsteady gait and other nervous disorders, owing to degeneration of the spinal cord. Red cell count may drop to as low as 1,000,000. Several kinds of tests may be necessary to differentiate pernicious anemia from other blood diseases—a test for hydrochloric acid levels, for example.

Pernicious anemia, however, is no longer so pernicious, or deadly, as it once was—not since its cause was identified. Large, injected doses of vitamin B_{12} usually restore normal blood cell production.

SICKLE-CELL ANEMIA: Sickle-cell anemia, an inherited abnormality, occurs almost exclusively among black people. Widespread in tropical Africa and Asia, sickle-cell anemia is also found in this country, affecting perhaps 1 in 500 American blacks. The blood cells are sickle-shaped rather than round, a structural aberration arising from a defect in the manufacture of hemoglobin, the oxygen-carrying component. Such misshapen cells have a tendency to clog very small capillaries and cause the complications discussed below.

A differentiation should be made between sickle-cell anemia, the full-blown disease, and sickle cell trait. Anemia occurs when the offspring inherits the sickle-cell gene from both parents. For these people life stretches out in endless bouts of fatigue punctuated by a series of crises of excruciating pain lasting days or even weeks. In some cases there is permanent paralysis. The crises often require long-term hospitalization. The misshapen cells increase the patient's susceptibility to blood clots, pneumonia, kidney and

heart failure, strokes, general systemic poisoning due to bacterial invasions, and, in the case of pregnant women, spontaneous abortion. Ninety percent of the patients die before age 40, with most dead by age 30. Half are dead by age 20, with a number also suffering from poor

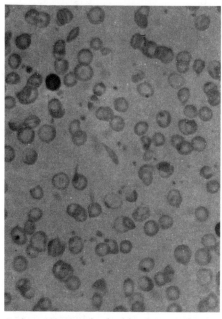

A photomicrograph of a blood smear showing sickle cells amidst the normal red cells. The solid dark circles are lymphocytes, a type of white blood cell. The very small dark spots are platelets, which are abnormally numerous.

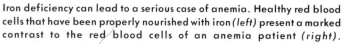

Iron deficiency can lead to a serious case of anemia. Healthy red blood cells that have been properly nourished with iron *(left)* present a marked contrast to the red blood cells of an anemia patient *(right)*.

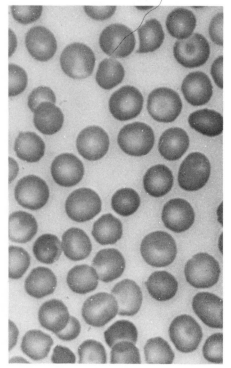

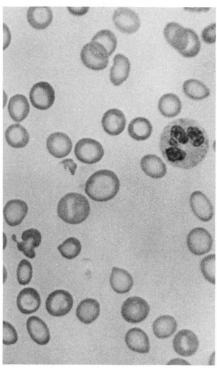

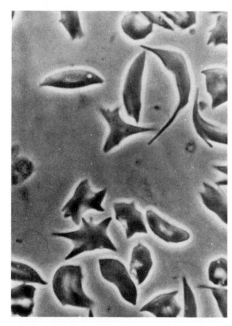

A photomicrograph of sickle cells. Sickle-cell anemia is an inherited disease affecting about one black American in 500.

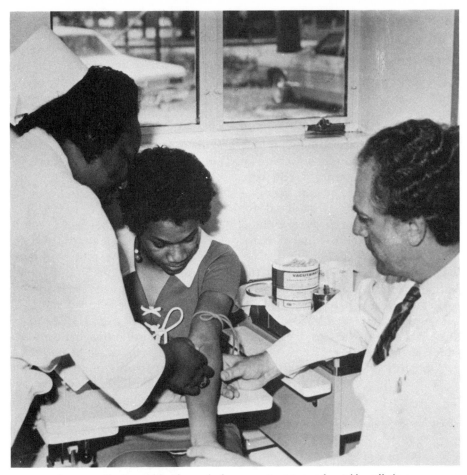

A nurse collecting a blood sample from a patient to test for sickle-cell characteristics. Two out of every 25 black Americans carry the sickle-cell trait.

digestive disturbances (e.g., a lack of hydrochloric acid) which may hinder the absorption of dietary iron from the intestines. Some women may not observe proper dietary habits, thereby aggravating the anemic state. Successful treatment involves increasing iron intake, with iron supplements and an emphasis on iron-rich foods, including eggs, cereals, green vegetables, and meat, especially liver.

Polycythemia

Polycythemia is the opposite of anemia; the blood has too many red corpuscles. The most common form of the disease is *polycythemia vera* (or *erythremia*). In addition to the rise in corpuscle count, there is a corresponding rise—as much as three-fold—in blood volume to accommodate the high cell count, and increased blood viscosity. Symptoms include an enlarged spleen, bloodshot eyes, red mouth and red mucous membranes—all due to excess red cells. Other common characteristics are weakness, fatigue, irritability, dizziness, swelling in the ankles, choking sensations, vise-

physical and mental development.

Those with only one gene for the disease have *sickle cell trait*. They are not likely to have too much trouble except in circumstances where they are exposed to low oxygen levels (the result, say, of poor oxygenation in a high-altitude plane). Administration of anesthesia or too much physical activity may also bring on some feverish attacks. Those with the trait are also carriers of the disease, since they can pass it on to the next generation. Two out of every 25 black Americans are said to be carrying the trait.

IRON-DEFICIENCY ANEMIA: Iron-deficiency anemia is a common complication of pregnancy, during which time the fetus may rob the maternal blood of much of its iron content. Iron is essential to the formation of hemoglobin. The deficiency can be further aggravated by

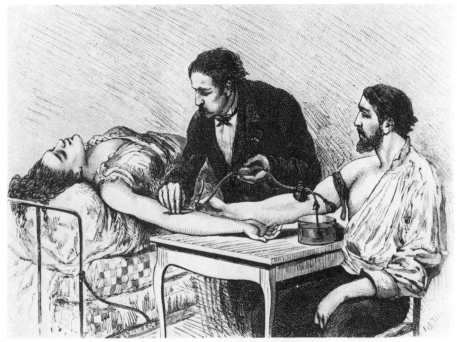

The illustration above was taken from a medical book of the 19th century. It shows an early blood transfusion employing the direct method, in which the blood of the donor flowed directly into the bloodstream of the patient.

like chest pains (angina pectoris), rapid heartbeat, and sometimes severe headaches. There is also an increased tendency toward both clotting and hemorrhaging.

The disease occurs primarily in the middle and late years and is twice as prevalent in males as in females. The cause is unknown, but polycythemia is characterized by stepped-up bone marrow production activity.

Radioactive phosphorus therapy is one method for controlling this hyperactivity. Low iron diets and several forms of drug therapy have been tried with varying degrees of effectiveness. A one-time panacea, bloodletting—to drain off excess blood—appears to be of considerable value. Many patients survive for years with the disease. Premature death is usually the result of vascular thrombosis (clotting), massive hemorrhage, or leukemia.

The Rh Factor

Rh disease might also be considered a form of anemia—in newborns. The disorder involves destruction of the red blood cells of an as-yet unborn or newborn infant. It is brought about by an incompatibility between the maternal blood and fetal blood of one specific factor—the so called *Rh* factor. (*Rh* stands for *rhesus* monkey, the species in which it was first identified.) Most of us are *Rh* positive, which is to say that we have the *Rh* protein substance on the surface of our red cells. The *Rh* factor is, in fact, present in 83 percent of the white population and 93 percent of the black. Those lacking it are classified as *Rh* negative.

A potentially dangerous situation exists when an *Rh* negative mother is carrying an *Rh* positive baby in her uterus. Although the mother and unborn baby have separate circulatory systems, some leakage does occur. When *Rh* positive cells from the fetus leak across the placenta into the mother's blood, her system recognizes them as foreign and makes antibodies against them. If these antibodies then slip across into the fetal circulation, damage is inevitable.

The first baby, however, is rarely affected because it takes time for the mother's body to become sensitized to the *Rh* positive cells. But should she become pregnant with another child, the now-sensitized mother's blood produces a large quantity of destructive antibodies that could result in stillbirth, death of the infant shortly after birth or, if the child survives, jaundice and anemia.

Modern medicine has reduced the fatality rate and considerably improved the prognosis. Severely affected newborns are being treated by complete blood transfusion—even while still in the womb—to draw off all the *Rh* positive cells. After birth and as it grows older, the child will once again produce *Rh* positive cells in its bone marrow—but by that time the danger from the mother's antibodies is past. Recently an *Rh* vaccine to prevent the problem from ever occurring was developed. After *Rh* negative women give birth to their first *Rh* positive baby, they are immunized with the anti-*Rh* serum to prevent them from manufacturing these dangerous antibodies.

White Blood Cell Diseases

For every 600–700 or more red corpuscles, there is one white blood cell, or *leukocyte*. White cells, unlike red corpuscles, have nuclei; they are also larger and rounder. About 70 percent of the white cell population have irregularly-shaped centers, and these are called *polymorphonuclear leukocytes* or *neu-*

A blood donor watches intently as her contribution is taken. Many hospitals keep a record of donors with rare blood types for future reference.

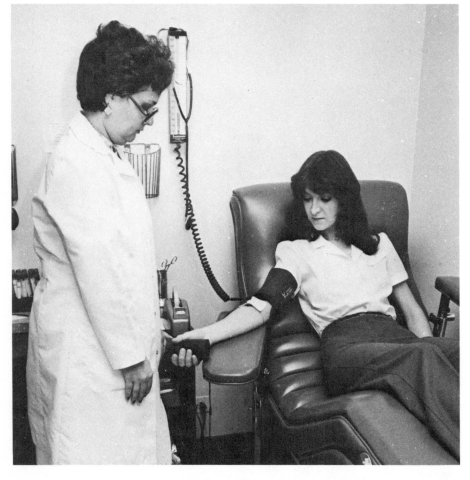

trophils. The other 30 percent are made up of a variety of cells with round nuclei called *lymphocytes.* A cubic millimeter of blood normally contains anywhere from 5,000 to 9,000 white cells (as compared with the 4–5 million red cells).

White cells defend against disease, which explains why their number increases in the bloodstream when the body is under infectious assault. There are some diseases of the blood and blood-forming organs themselves that can increase the white count. Disorders of the spleen, for example, can produce white cell abnormalities, because this organ is a major source of lymphocytes (cells responsible for making protective antibodies). Diseases of the bone marrow are likely to affect neutrophil production.

Leukemia

Leukemia, characterized by an abnormal increase in the number of white cells, is one of the most dangerous of blood disorders. The cancerlike disease results from a severe disturbance in the functioning of the bone marrow. Chronic leukemia, which strikes mainly in middle age, produces an enormous increase in neutrophils, which tend to rush into the bloodstream at every stage of their development, whether mature or not. Patients with the chronic disease may survive for several years, with appropriate treatment.

In acute leukemia, more common among children than adults, the marrow produces monster-sized, cancerous-looking white cells. These cells not only crowd out other blood components from the circulation, they also leave little space for the marrow to produce the other elements, especially the red cells and platelets. Acute leukemias run their fatal course in a matter of weeks or months—although there have been dramatic instances of sudden remission. The cause is unknown, but recent evidence strongly suggests that a virus may be responsible for at least some forms of the disease.

Modern treatment—radiation and drugs—is aimed at wiping out all of the malignant cells. A critical stage follows treatment, however. For with the disappearance of these abnormal cells and the temporary disruption of marrow function, the patient is left with his defenses against infection down. He also runs a great risk of hemorrhage. Therefore, he is usually kept in isolation to ward off infections. In addition he may be given white cell and platelet transfusions along with antibiotic therapy. Eventually—and hopefully—the marrow will revert to normal function, freed of leukemic cell production. For additional information on leukemia, see p. 447.

Other White Cell Diseases

AGRANULOCYTOSIS: Agranulocytosis is a disease brought on by the direct destruction of neutrophils (also called *granulocytes*). Taken over a long period of time, certain types of drugs may bring about large-scale destruction of the neutrophil supply. Symptoms include general debilitation, fatigue, sleeplessness, restlessness, headache, chills, high fever (often up to 105°F.), sore mouth and throat, along with psychologically aberrant behavior and mental confusion. White cell count may fall as low as 500 to 2,000. Sometimes agranulocytosis is confused with leukemia.

Treatment involves antibiotic therapy to ward off bacterial invasion, a likelihood that is increased owing to the lowered body resistance. In advanced cases, hospitalization and transfusions with fresh blood are necessary. Injections of fresh bone marrow may also be prescribed.

LEUKOPENIA: Leukopenia is less severe than agranulocytosis. It too involves a reduction of circulating white cells to counts of less than 5,000. It is usually the result of allergic reactions to some chemical or drug.

INFECTIOUS MONONUCLEOSIS: Infectious mononucleosis, also known as *glandular fever* or *kissing disease,* is characterized by the presence in the bloodstream of a large number of lymphocytes, many of which are abnormally formed. The disease is mildly contagious—kissing is thought to be one popular source of transmission—and occurs chiefly among children and adolescents. The transmitting agent, however, has yet to be discovered, though some as yet unidentified organism is strongly suspected.

The disease is not always easy to diagnose. It can incubate anywhere from four days to four weeks, at which point the patient may experience fever, headache, sore throat, swollen lymph nodes, loss of appetite, and a general feeling of weakness.

The disease runs its course in a matter of a week or two, although complete recovery may take a while longer. Bed rest and conservative medical management is often enough for complete patient recovery. A few severe cases may require hospitalization because of occasional complications, such as rupture of the spleen, skin lesions, some minor liver malfunctions, and occasionally hemolytic anemia or purpura.

DISEASES OF THE BLOOD VESSELS

Diseases of the blood vessels are the result primarily of adverse changes in the vessel walls, such as hardening of the arteries, stroke, and varicose veins.

A healthy circulation depends to a large extent not only on the condition of the blood-forming organs but on the pipelines through which this life-sustaining fluid flows. The arteries, which carry blood away from the heart, and the veins, which bring it back, are subject to a wide range of maladies. They may become inflamed, as in the case of arteritis, phlebitis, and varicose veins; or they may become clogged—especially the arteries—as a result of atherosclerosis (hardening of the arteries) or blood clots (thrombosis and embolism), which can prevent the blood from reaching a vital organ.

The Inflammatory Disorders

Arteritis

Arteritis, or inflammation of the arterial wall, usually results from infections (e.g., syphilis) or allergic

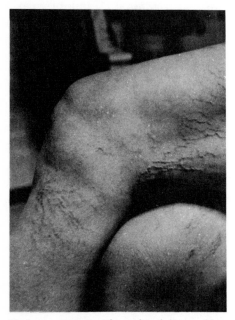

Varicose veins are enlarged and distorted because the walls or valves of veins have become weakened. In most cases veins close to the surface of the skin are affected.

reactions in which the body's protective agents against invading organisms, the antibodies, attack the vessel walls themselves. In these instances, the prime source of inflammation must be treated before the arterial condition can heal.

Phlebitis

Phlebitis is an inflammation of the veins, a condition that may stem from an injury or may be associated with such conditions as varicose veins, malignancies, and infection. The extremities, especially the legs, are vulnerable to the disorder. The symptoms are stiffness and hot and painful swelling of the involved region. Phlebitis brings with it the tendency of blood to form blood clots (*thrombophlebitis*) at the site of inflammation. The danger is that one of these clots may break away and enter the bloodstream. Such a clot, on the move, called an *embolus*, may catch and become lodged in a smaller vessel serving a vital organ, causing a serious blockage in the blood supply.

Physicians are likely to prescribe various drugs for phlebitis—agents to deal with the suspected cause of the disorder as well as *anticoagulants* (anti-clotting compounds) to ward off possible thromboembolic complications.

Varicose Veins

Varicose veins, which are veins that are enlarged and distorted, primarily affect the leg vessels, and are often troublesome to people who are on their feet for hours at a time. Varicose veins develop because either the walls or the valves of veins are weakened. Some people may be born with weakened veins or valves. In others, the damage may develop from injury or disease, such as phlebitis. More women than men seem to have this condition, but it is common among both sexes. In women, the enlarged veins sometimes occur during pregnancy, but these

may well diminish and disappear after delivery. Some elderly people are prone to this condition because the blood vessels lose their elasticity with aging, with the muscles that support the vein growing less sturdy.

In most instances, the surface veins lying just beneath the skin are involved. If there are no other complications, these cases are seldom serious, although they may be disturbing because of unsightliness. Doctors have remedies, including surgery, for making varicose veins less prominent.

When varicose veins become severe, it is usually because the vessels deeper in the leg are weak. Unchecked, this situation can lead to serious complications, including swelling (*edema*) around the ankles and lower legs. The skin in the lower leg may become thin and fragile and easily irritated. Tiny hemorrhages may discolor the skin. In advanced stages, hard-to-treat leg ulcers and sores may erupt.

Most of the complicating problems can be averted with early care and treatment. Doctors generally prescribe elastic stockings even in the mildest of cases and sometimes elastic bandages to lend support to the veins. They may recommend some newer techniques for injecting certain solutions that close off the affected portion of the vein. On the other hand, surgery may be indicated, especially for the surface veins, in which the varicose section is either tied off or stripped, with the blood being rerouted to the deeper vein channels. See under *Vascular Surgery*, p. 337, for more information about surgical treatment of varicose veins.

While long periods of standing may be hard on varicose veins, so are uninterrupted stretches of sitting, which may cause blood to collect in the lower leg and further distend the veins. Patients are advised to get up and walk about every half hour or so during any extended period of sit-

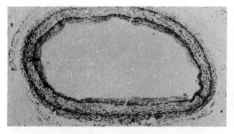
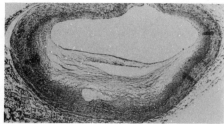
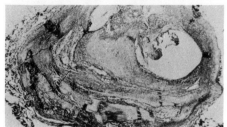
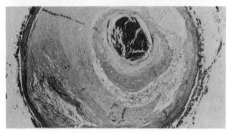

These extraordinary photographs show a coronary artery being progressively narrowed by artherosclerosis. *(Top left)* The artery is normal. *(Top right)* Deposits are beginning to form on the inner lining. *(Bottom left)* The deposits harden. *(Bottom right)* The channel through which blood normally flows has been dangerously narrowed and is blocked by a blood clot.

ting. A good idea, too, is to sit with the feet raised, whenever possible, to keep blood from collecting in the lower legs.

The Vessel-Clogging Disorders

Atherosclerosis

Atherosclerosis (hardening of the arteries) is the nation's most serious health problem, the underlying cause of a million or more deaths each year from heart attack and stroke. It is the process whereby fats carried in the bloodstream gradually pile up on the walls of arteries, like rust in a pipe. The vessels become brittle and roughened; the channel through which blood flows grows narrower. Eventually the organs and tissues supplied by the diseased arteries may be sufficiently deprived of their normal oxygen delivery so as to interfere with proper function. Such a cutback in the pipeline supply is called *ischemia*. This fat deposit poses its greatest hazard when it occurs in the vessels serving the heart, brain and, sometimes, the lower extremities.

A reduced supply of blood to the lower extremities may cause irre-

versible damage and ultimately lead to death of the leg tissues unless proper circulation is restored. Bacterial invasion may follow; the area may swell, blacken, and emit the distinctly offensive smell of the deadly infection. Such a condition is known as *gangrene*, a severe disorder that may require amputation above the site of blockage if other measures, including antibiotic therapy, fail. Diabetics more commonly than others may develop atherosclerotic obstructions in leg arteries. Such persons must take care to avoid leg injuries, since even minimal damage in an already poorly served tissue area can bring on what is termed *diabetic gangrene.*

When the coronary arteries nourishing the heart are involved, even a moderate reduction in blood delivery to the heart muscle may be enough to cause angina pectoris, with its intense, suffocating chest pains.

Thrombosis

Thrombosis, a blood clot that forms within the vessels, is a great ever-present threat that accompanies atherosclerosis. The narrowed arteries seem to make it easier for normal blood substances to adhere

to the roughened wall surfaces, forming clots. If the clot blocks the coronary arteries, it may produce a heart attack—damage to that part of the heart deprived by vessel obstruction. For a detailed account of atherosclerosis and heart attack, see under *Heart Disease,* p. 360.

Stroke

Stroke, like heart attack, is a disorder usually due to blockage brought on by the atheroslerotic process in vessels supplying the brain. This sets the stage for a *thrombus,* or blood clot fixed within a vessel, which would not be likely to occur in arteries clear of these fatty deposits. A stroke may be a result of an interruption of blood flow through arteries in the brain or in neck vessels leading to the brain.

Sometimes the shutoff of blood flow, or *embolism,* may be triggered by a wandering blood clot that has become wedged in cerebral vessels. This kind of clot, known as an *embolus,* is a thrombus that has broken free into the circulation.

A stroke may also stem from hemorrhaging, where a diseased artery in the brain bursts. A cerebral

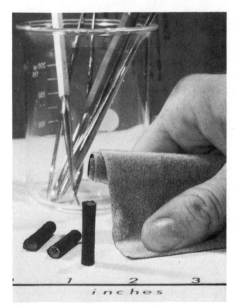

Man-made blood vessels fashioned from polyester velour fabric *(right)* simulate functions of veins and arteries. Still in the experimental stage, they may soon aid people suffering from vascular diseases.

hemorrhage is most likely to occur when a patient has atherosclerosis in combination with hypertension (high blood pressure). (For a discussion of hypertension, see *Hypertensive Heart Disease*, p. 366.) Hemorrhage is also a danger when an aneurysm forms in a blood vessel. An *aneurysm* is a blood-filled pouch that balloons out from a weak spot in the artery wall. Sometimes, too, pressure from a mass of tissue—a tumor, for example—can produce a stroke by squeezing a nearby brain vessel shut.

When the blood supply is cut off, injury to certain brain cells follows. Cells thus damaged cannot function; neither, then, can the parts of the body controlled by these nerve centers. The damage to the brain cells may produce paralysis of a leg or arm; it may interfere with the ability

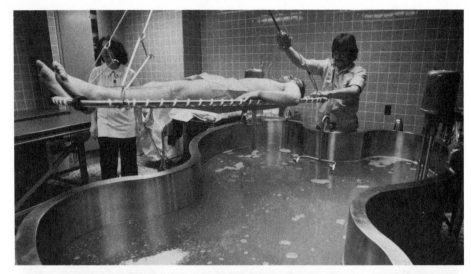

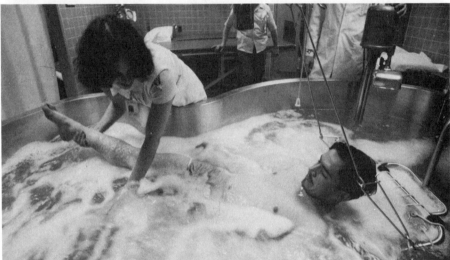

Rehabilitation for stroke victims, most of whom generally suffer some paralysis, may involve the use of hydrotherapy. Water makes movement easier by reducing body weight as well as by relaxing the muscles.

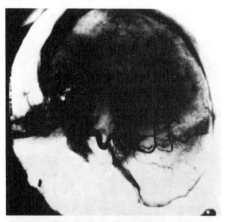

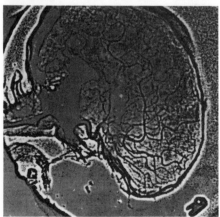

Digital computer techniques can be used effectively to clarify X rays. The computer-enhanced X ray of a human skull *(below)* shows the frontal blood vessels much more clearly than an ordinary X ray *(above)*.

to speak or with a person's memory. The affected function and the extent of disability depend on which brain region has been struck, how widespread the damage is, how effectively the body can repair its supply system to this damaged area, and how rapidly other areas of brain tissue can take over the work of the out-of-commission nerve cells.

SYMPTOMS: Frequently there are symptoms of impending stroke: headaches, numbness in the limbs, faintness, momentary lapses in memory, slurring of speech, or sudden clumsiness. The presence of these symptoms does not always mean a stroke is brewing; sometimes they are quite harmless. But should

they be stroke warning signals, the physician can take some preventive action. He may recommend anticoagulant therapy as well as drugs to bring down elevated blood pressure. In some cases, he might decide to call for surgical replacement of diseased or weakened sections of arteries leading to the brain.

TREATMENT: Once a stroke has occurred, the most important step is intensive rehabilitation. Not everyone needs such a program, inasmuch as some people are only slightly affected by a stroke. Others may recover quickly from what seems like a severe stroke. But still others may suffer such serious damage that it may take a long time to regain even partial use of the faculty involved. A great deal, however, can be done to help, especially for patients who are partially paralyzed and those with *aphasia*—the inability to deal with language properly because of damage to the brain's speech center. For rehabilitation to be most effective, it should be started as soon as possible after the stroke.

Embolism

An embolus, or thrombus that has broken away into the bloodstream, is, as we have seen, sometimes the direct cause of a stroke. A heart attack may also cause a stroke. Bacterial action may soften a thrombus so that it separates into fragments and breaks free from its wall anchorage.

Thrombi are not the only source of emboli; any free-floating mass in the bloodstream, be it an air bubble, clumps of fat, knots of cancer cells, or bacteria, can prove dangerous.

Usually, however, emboli originate as thrombi in the veins, especially the leg veins. Breaking free, the clump of clot material wanders into the bloodstream to be carried towards the right chamber of the heart and then onward into the lungs, unless dissolved before that. Once in the pulmonary arteries there is a growing threat that the moving mass will catch in one of the smaller branches of the lung circulation. This life-threatening blockage is called a *pulmonary embolism*.

This disorder takes at least 50,000 lives a year; most occur during or following prolonged periods of hospitalization and bed rest. The lack of activity slows the blood flow and increases the danger of thrombi—and ultimately emboli. Prevention requires getting the patient out of bed as soon and as often as possible to stimulate leg circulation. The non-ambulatory patient, meanwhile, is encouraged to move his legs by raising them, or changing position so as to step up blood flow.

The detection of a large embolus—symptoms include shortness of breath and chest pains—may require emergency surgery for removal. In most instances, however, treatment means administering anticoagulants to prevent new clots from emerging while allowing the body to rid itself of the embolus.

CHAPTER 16

Heart Disease

Heart disease is the commonly used, catch-all phrase for a number of disorders affecting both the heart and blood vessels. A more apt term is cardiovascular disease, which represents America's worst health scourge. More than 27,000,000 Americans of all ages are afflicted with some kind of cardiovascular ailment. When considered together, heart and circulatory system diseases, including stroke, account for more than one-half of all deaths each year in the United States, a total of over 1,000,000 people.

The most frequent cause of death from cardiovascular disease is *coronary artery disease,* brought on by obstructions that develop in the coronary vessels nourishing the heart muscle. These fatty blockages impair adequate delivery of oxygen-laden blood to the heart muscle cells. The result may be *angina pectoris*: short episodes of viselike chest pains that strike when the heart fails to get enough blood; or it may be a full-blown heart attack, where blood-starved heart tissue dies.

One out of every five American males will have a heart attack before the age of 60. Heart attacks strike about 1.6 million annually, killing over 600,000. Overall, more than 6 million adults either definitely have or are suspected of having some de-

gree of coronary disease; for this reason it has been labeled the "20th-century epidemic," or the "black plague of affluence."

Hypertensive heart disease is an impairment of heart-pumping function stemming from persistent *hypertension* (high blood pressure). Untreated, elevated pressure makes the heart work harder, causing it to enlarge and sometimes to fail. It can also lead to serious damage to the kidneys and acceleration of the vessel-clogging process responsible for most heart attacks and strokes. Hypertension is the most common of the cardiovascular diseases, affecting about 22 million Americans, with more than half having some degree of heart involvement. A little more than 60,000 deaths are directly attributable to hypertension and hypertensive heart disease.

Rheumatic heart disease, the left-over scars of a rheumatic fever attack, claims the lives of 13,000 annually. It generally strikes children between the ages of 5 and 15. All told, 1,600,000 persons are suffering from rheumatic heart disease, with about 100,000 new cases reported each year.

Congenital heart disease includes that collection of heart and major blood vessel deformities that exist at birth in 8 out of every 1,000 live

births, or 25,000 cases yearly. Nine thousand deaths annually are attributed to these inborn heart abnormalities.

This grim portrait of death and disability is improving rapidly, however, because of research uncovering new knowledge for protecting the heart and its pipelines. For example:

• Rheumatic fever, once a major menace of childhood, has been subdued effectively through the use of antibiotics, which can eradicate streptococcal infections, the precursor of rheumatic disease; theoretically, the disease has been made wholly preventable. In the last two decades the death rate from rheumatic heart disease has dropped more than 85 percent within the 5- to 24-year-old age group.

• Bold new surgery makes it possible to cure or alleviate most congenital heart defects, to replace defective heart valves with plastic substitutes, and to open new sources of blood to a heart with diseased coronary arteries.

• A broad arsenal of drugs that makes almost all cases of hypertension—whether mild or severe—controllable, helps explain the 63 percent drop in the death rate as compared with that recorded in 1950.

• Advances in coronary care are

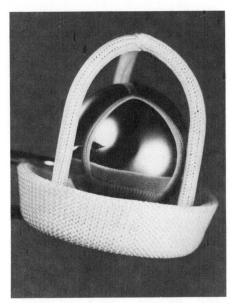

This aortic valve prosthesis consists of a metal frame and seating ring covered with a synthetic fabric, and a hollow ball of stellite.

lowering the heart attack death rate. Physicians, having learned to recognize the coronary-prone individual, are able to prescribe life styles to forestall heart attack.

• Out-of-kilter heart rhythms are being restored to normal with permanently implanted pacemakers.

Coronary Artery Disease

To keep itself going, the heart relies on two pencil-thick main arteries. Branching from the aorta, these vessels deliver freshly oxygenated blood to the right and left sides of the heart. The left artery is usually somewhat larger and divides into two sizable vessels, the circumflex and anterior branches. The latter is sometimes called the artery of sudden death, since a clot near its mouth is common and leads to a serious and often fatal heart attack. These arteries wind around the heart and send out still smaller branches into the heart muscle to supply the needs of all cells. The network of vessels arches down over the heart like a crown—in Latin, *corona*—hence the word *coronary*.

Atherosclerosis

Coronary artery disease exists when flow of blood is impaired because of narrowed and obstructed coronary arteries. In virtually all cases, this blockade is the result of atherosclerosis, a form of *arteriosclerosis*, the thickening and hardening of the arteries. *Atherosclerosis*, from the Greek for porridge or mush, refers to the process by which fat carried in the bloodstream piles up on the inner wall of the arteries like rust in a pipe. As more and more fatty substances, including cholesterol, accumulate, the once smooth wall gets thicker, rougher, and harder, and the blood passageway becomes narrower.

This fatty clogging goes on imperceptibly, a process that often begins early in life. Eventually, blood flow may be obstructed sufficiently to cause the heart muscle cells to send out distress signals. The brief, episodic chest pains of angina pectoris announce that these cells are starving and suffering for lack of blood and oxygen. Flow may be so severely diminished or totally plugged up that a region of the heart muscle dies. The heart has been damaged; the person has had a heart attack.

Angina

Angina pectoris means chest pain. Usually the pain is distinctive and feels like a vest being drawn too tightly across the chest. Sometimes it eludes easy identification. As a rule, however, the discomfort is felt behind the breastbone, occasionally spreading to the arms, shoulders, neck, and jaw. Not all chest pain indicates angina; in most cases it may simply be gas in the stomach.

Symptoms

Angina attacks are likely to appear when sudden strenuous demands are placed on the heart. They may come from physical exertion—walking uphill, running, sexual activity, or the effort involved in eating and digesting a heavy meal. Watching an exciting movie or sporting event can trigger it; so might cold weather. An attack can occur even when the individual is lying still or asleep—perhaps the result of tension or dreams.

Whatever the trigger, the heart is called upon to pump more blood to meet the body's stepped-up needs. To do so means working harder and faster. If one or more of the heart's supply lines is narrowed by disease, the extra blood and oxygen required to fuel the pump cannot get through to a region of the heart muscle. Anginal pain is a signal that muscle cells are being strained by an insufficiency of oxygen; they are, as it were, gasping for air.

The attacks usually are brief, lasting only a matter of minutes. Attacks stop when the person rests. Some people, apparently, can walk through an attack, as if the heart has gotten a second wind, and the pain subsides.

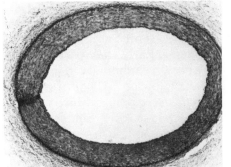 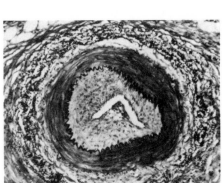

At left, a cross section of a normal coronary artery. At right, an artery almost completely blocked by fatty deposits; the narrow inverted V opening is the only channel through which blood can flow. If this opening should become blocked by a clot, a heart attack would result.

Treatment

Treatment may involve merely rearranging activity to avoid overly taxing physical labors or emotional situations likely to induce discomfort. A major medication used for angina is *nitroglycerine*. It dilates small coronary blood vessels, allowing more blood to get through. Nitroglycerine pellets are not swallowed but are placed under the tongue, where they are quickly absorbed by blood vessels there and sped to the heart; discomfort passes in minutes. Often anginal attacks can be headed off by taking the tablets before activities likely to bring on an attack.

Still other drugs have been found to relieve angina pains. One group, called the beta-blockers, slows down the heart's action and thus its need for oxygen. Widely used to treat high blood pressure as well as heart disease, the beta-blockers may cause shortness of breath. For that reason, physicians usually prescribe other medications for persons with asthma.

The first of the beta-blockers to come into use was *propranolol*. But at least five chemically related drugs may be prescribed: atenolol, timolol, metoprolol, nadolol, and pindalol. Doctors generally try to fit one of these drugs to the problems of the individual patient. There is some evidence that propranolol and nitroglycerin taken together may increase the effectiveness of therapy.

A second group of drugs for angina is known as the calcium slow channel blockers, or simply calcium channel blockers. These drugs prevent coronary spasms, one cause of angina chest pains, by blocking the flow of calcium ions to the heart. Unblocked, the calcium ions enter the muscle cells of coronary arteries, in some cases causing the muscles to contract suddenly. Three chemically different calcium channel blockers in use are verapamil, nifedipine, and diltiazem.

Angina does not mean a heart attack is inevitable. Many angina patients never have one, probably because their hearts have developed collateral circulation. Fortunately, an auxiliary system of very tiny pipelines lacing the heart exists in a dormant state as a potential escape hatch for the diseased heart. As the coronary arteries narrow, the collateral vessels gradually grow larger and wider, switched on, presumably, by the oxygen shortage. Thus, they may provide an alternate route for blood to the afflicted area of the heart muscle. As the collateral system continues to develop, it may cause anginal symptoms to lessen. Although this may not prevent a heart attack, these newly activated pathways might make the attack less severe.

Coronary Artery Surgery

In general, surgery for angina is reserved for the severely restricted, incapacitated patient for whom medical treatment has been a failure. A procedure devised in Canada for bringing new sources of blood to the heart with clogged arteries may be of value in some cases. It involves implanting into the wall of the left ventricle an artery that normally supplies blood to the chest. One drawback is the time it takes—often a matter of months—for the implanted artery to develop the necessary collateral linkages to be of help to the heart.

Ideally, surgeons would like to operate directly on the coronary arteries, especially when the obstructing atherosclerotic deposits are confined to short, accessible vessel segments. Early attempts to do this, however, have brought high mortality and a low percentage of cures.

Endarterectomy, which means reaming out the trouble-making blockage, is still in the experimental stage. Carbon dioxide, forced in under high pressure to blow the deposits loose, has been used as a reaming tool in experiments. The diseased core is then cut free and pulled out through an incision in the coronary artery. Still another direct technique involves bypassing the diseased portion of the artery with a synthetic blood vessel graft taken from the patient's leg artery.

Heart Surgery

Direct surgery on the heart is possible because of the development of the heart-lung machine, which takes over the job of oxygenating and pumping blood into circulation, thus giving surgeons time to work directly on a relatively bloodless heart.

To choose patients appropriate for surgery, physicians use a reviewing system called *arteriography*, which allows them to watch blood flowing through the coronary artery system and to evaluate with accuracy the degree and location of obstruction. A substance opaque to X rays is injected into the coronary arteries and then followed by X ray as it runs its course through the vessels supplying the heart muscle.

Later diagnostic methods dispense with injections of the opaque fluid and with X-ray technology. Nuclear magnetic resonance (NMR), for example, uses magnetic forces to scan the interior of the body for abnormalities. In heart disease diagnoses, a NMR can identify specific problems in specific areas of the heart and its arteries.

Despite the newspaper headlines and dramatic history-making operations of recent years, heart transplants must still be considered experimental. One reason is the logistics problem: getting and storing enough donor hearts to meet the demand. More important, however, is the immunological barrier. The body's defense against disease regards the new heart as foreign and attacks it, just as it would bacteria and viruses. Until scientists have learned how to thwart rejection consistently, heart transplants will have to be performed only on a limited, highly selective basis. For more information on heart surgery, see p. 336. See also *Organ Transplants*, p. 346.

Heart Attack

Physicians have other names for heart attack: coronary occlusion, coronary thrombosis, myocardial infarction. *Coronary occlusion* means total closure of the coronary artery. This may be caused by fatty deposits that have piled up high enough to dam the flow channel.

Or it may be that a blood clot, or *thrombus*, forming in the coronary artery, has suddenly caught on the roughened, fat-clogged area and plugged up the vessel. In this case the occlusion is called a *coronary thrombosis. Myocardial infarction* refers to the actual damage or death of heart muscle (*myocardium*) resulting from the occlusion.

Heart attacks hit males hardest. The frequency of heart attacks begins to build rapidly among men between the ages of 30 and 40 but is almost unknown in women of the same age group. The odds begin evening out as women approach and pass menopause. Despite this, during the same 40- to 44-age period, the ratio of male to female heart attacks may be as high as 24 to one.

The incidence of heart attacks increases with age. The peak years for male heart attacks are in the 55- to 59-age bracket. The percentage of deaths from first heart attacks, however, is higher among men in their forties than those in their sixties, presumably because the younger men do not have as well-developed collateral circulation to protect them.

Symptoms

Sometimes heart attacks are so vague or indistinct that the victim may not know he has had one. Often a routine electrocardiogram—the squiggly-lined record of the heart's activity—turns up an abnormality indicative of an *infarct,* or injured area. This is another instance of the importance of periodic check-ups. Special blood tests can also detect substances which may leak out into the circulation when heart muscle cells are injured.

Most heart attacks, however, do not sneak by. There are well-recognized symptoms. The most common are:

- A feeling of strangulation
- A prolonged, oppressive pain or unusual discomfort in the center of the chest that may radiate to the left shoulder and down the left arm
- Abnormal perspiring
- Sudden, intense shortness of breath
- Nausea or vomiting (Because of these symptoms, an attack is sometimes taken for indigestion; usually, coronary pains are more severe.)
- Occasionally, loss of consciousness.

Treatment

Knowing these warning signals and taking proper steps may make the difference between life and death. Call a physician or get to a hospital as soon as possible. Time is crucial. Most deaths occur in the initial hours after attack. About 25 percent, for example, die within three hours after onset of their first heart attack.

ALTERNATIVES TO SURGERY: Medical researchers have sought for years to find ways to stop heart attacks before they damage heart tissue permanently. The hope has been that such methods may provide fast relief and even serve as alternatives to surgery. Artificial clot destroying agents like the enzymes *streptokinase* and *urokinase* have been administered through a thin tube, or catheter. The catheter is inserted through the arterial system until it reaches the coronary vessels. Then the enzyme is released.

Often, death is not due to any widespread damage to the heart muscle, but rather to a disruption in the electric spark initiating heart muscle contraction—the same spark measured by the electrocardiogram. These out-of-kilter rhythms, including complete heart stoppage or cardiac arrest, are often reversible with prompt treatment.

Nonsurgical methods of treating coronary occlusions in particular have multiplied in recent years. Among the techniques, balloon angioplasty has proved most effective. In this procedure, a catheter is pushed through blood channels into a coronary artery that has been narrowed by atherosclerosis, or fatty deposits in the artery that gradually cut off the flow of blood. Inflated inside the artery, the balloon com-

A close-up of an open-heart operation. Metal retractors hold back layers of skin and fat to enable surgeons to work directly on the heart.

presses the fatty deposits against the artery wall. The catheter and balloon are then removed. The blood can resume its normal flow.

Like all methods of treating heart diseases, balloon angioplasty has both advantages and disadvantages. Among persons with severe heart defects, for example, only one in 10 is eligible for angioplasty. Others must undergo bypass surgery.

CORONARY CARE UNITS: Special hospital centers called coronary care units have been created to provide for heart attack victims. Here, around-the-clock electronic sentries keep watch over the patient's vital functions, particularly the heart's electrical activity. The critical period is the first 72 hours, during which time as many as 90 percent of heart attack patients experience some type of electrical disturbance or *arrhythmia* (rhythmic irregularity). Not all are dangerous in themselves, but they may be the forerunner of chaotic rhythms that are dangerous indeed. The onset of any irregular beat alerts a member of the 24-hour-a-day, specially-trained nursing staff to initiate the appropriate countermeasures while a physician is being summoned.

In planning the coronary care unit, or CCU, each hospital considers its own situation. It assesses the number of heart attack victims reaching the hospital annually. It tries to find out how many patients would have to be kept in the CCU at any given time, and for approximately what periods. The question whether the pattern of patient referrals to the hospital will be changed nearly always arises. The CCU must also, of course, be integrated into the entire hospital system so that it can work with other departments and facilities. If possible, it should be remote from the emergency room so that the highest degree of peace and quiet can be maintained.

In some hospitals the CCU is located close to, or virtually as part of, the intensive care unit, or ICU. but hospital planners and hospital staff members generally feel that the CCU should be kept separate where possible. The reason is that many patients receiving care in the ICU need an environment that may not encourage the quiet recovery of the heart attack victim.

Patient rooms in the CCU are designed to ensure privacy and a tranquil, cheerful environment. Rooms may be separated from one another by curtains or partial or full walls. Beds are comfortable, and usually stand in a space adequate for movement of heavy equipment such as the portable X-ray apparatus. CCU's commonly have acousticaal ceiling and floors; good lighting, including bright lights for emergency use; and adequate electrical, suction, and other outlets.

Very importantly, the CCU provides for electrocardiographic or heart monitoring at each bed. A "slave" monitor that duplicates the bedside oscilloscope readings makes it possible for nurses to check the patient's condition without leaving the nurses' station. The station has one slave for every bedside monitor. Like the bedside unit, the slave unit has a pulse rate meter and a readout trigger that enables a nurse or doctor to take a recorded electrocardiogram (EKG) simply by pressing a button. The slave unit also has an audio and visual alarm system that is connected to the pulse rate meter. The alarm notifies the nurse that a major change is taking place in the patient's condition.

Provision has to be made in the CCU for various types of emergencies. A defibrillator, for example, makes it possible to treat the condition called ventricular fibrillation. Where possible, CCUs have two defibrillators one for standby use. An adequate supply of intravenous pacemakers is usually kept on hand. A crash cart is stocked with all the various drugs needed for emergency cardiac care (ECC), as well as endotracheal tubes, laryngoscopes, and other equipment.

The staff of the CCU is always chosen with care. Staff members are generally selected on the basis of their experience with acute coronary care. Even with such experience, additional training is normally provided to make certain they can deal with all possible problems. In the course of such training the potential CCU nurse or aide learns that the period of greatest danger for the cardiac patient is the first 24 hours. Some 40 percent of all patients who die while under acute coronary care are stricken during the first day.

Fibrillation

The most dangerous rhythmic disorder is ventricular *fibrillation,* in which the lower chambers of the heart contract in an uncoordinated manner, causing blood-pumping to cease completely. Treated within one minute, the patient has a 90 percent or better chance of surviving. A delay of three minutes means a survival rate of less than 10 percent because of extensive and irreversible brain and heart damage.

Treatment involves use of an instrument called a *defibrillator.* Through plates applied to the chest, the device sends a massive jolt of electricity into the heart muscle to get the heart back on the right tempo.

More significantly, it is now also possible to head off ventricular fibrillation, so that the already compromised heart will not have to tolerate even brief episodes of the arrhythmia. Ventricular fibrillation is invariably heralded by an earlier, identifiable disturbance in the heartbeat. Most frequently, the warning signal is a skipped or premature ventricular beat. Picked up by the coronary care monitoring equipment, the signal alerts the unit staff to administer heart-calming medicaments that can ward off the danger. One such drug is *lidocaine,* a long-used dental anesthetic found to have the power to restore an irritated heart to electrical tranquillity.

The advent of coronary care has produced striking results. Where in use, these units have reduced heart attack deaths among hospitalized patients up to 30 percent. If all heart victims surviving at least a few hours received such care, more than 50,000 lives could be saved annually.

Failure of Heart Muscle

Most deaths in coronary care units, however, result not from electrical failure but power failure—the result of massive injury to the heart muscle. So large an area of the muscle is put out of commission, at least temporarily, that the still healthy portion is unable to cope with the body's ceaseless blood needs.

Success in treating failures of the heart muscle has not been great. Various devices for assisting the weakened heart with its pumping burden are still in the experimental stage. The problem is to create a device that will do most, if not all, of the work for the struggling left ventricle over a period of days or weeks to give the heart muscle a chance to rest and recover.

Emergency Care

Most heart attack victims never reach the hospital. About 400,000 die before getting there, as many as 60 percent in the first hour. Evidence suggests that many of these sudden deaths result from ventricular fibrillation or cardiac arrest—reversible disturbances when treated immediately.

These considerations led to the concept of mobile coronary care units—of bringing the advanced techniques of heart resuscitation to the victims. Originated in 1966 in Belfast, Northern Ireland, the practice of having a flying squad of specially equipped ambulances ready to race with on-the-spot aid to heart attack patients has been spreading to more U.S. communities, successfully reducing mortality.

An emergency technique called *external cardiopulmonary resuscitation* (ECPR), more popularly known as *cardiac massage* or *closed-chest massage,* has also reduced out-of-hospital heart attack mortality figures. Used in conjunction with mouth-to-mouth breathing, ECPR is an emergency procedure for treating cardiac arrest. The lower part of the breastbone is compressed rhythmically to keep oxygenated blood flowing to the brain until appropriate medical treatment can be applied to restore normal heart action; often ECPR alone is enough to restart the heart. The technique should be performed only by trained personnel, however, because it involves risks, such as the danger of fracturing a rib or rupturing a weakened heart muscle if too much pressure is applied.

Recuperation

Beyond the 72-hour crisis period, the patient will still require hospitalization for three to six weeks to give the heart time to heal. During the first two weeks or so, the patient is made to remain completely at rest. In this period, the dead muscle cells are being cleared away and gradually replaced by scar tissue. Until this happens, the damaged area represents a dangerous weak spot. By the end of the second week, the patient may be allowed to sit in a chair and then to walk about the room. Recently, some physicians have been experimenting with getting patients up and about earlier, sometimes within a few days after their attack. Although most patients are well enough to be discharged after three or four weeks, not everyone mends at the same rate, which is why doctors hesitate to predict exactly when the patient will be released or when he will be well enough to resume normal activity.

About 15 percent of in-hospital heart attack deaths come in the post-acute phase owing to an *aneurysm,* or ballooning-out, of the area where the left ventricle is healing. This is most likely to develop before the scar has toughened enough to withstand blood pressures generated by the heart's contractions. The aneurysm may kill either by rupturing or by so impairing pumping efficiency that the heart fails and the circulation deteriorates.

Most heart attack patients are able to return to their precoronary jobs eventually. Some, left with anginal pain, may have to make adjustments in their jobs and living habits. What kind of activity the patient can ultimately resume is an individual matter to be worked out by the patient with his physician. The prescription usually involves keeping weight down and avoiding undue emotional stress or physical exertion; moderate exercise along with plenty of rest is encouraged.

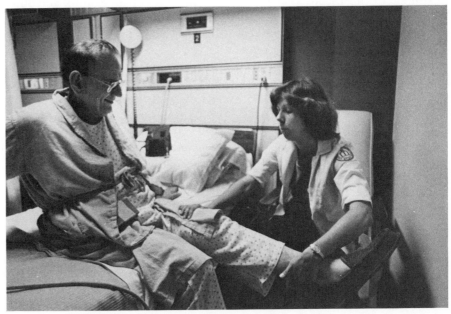

A physical therapist helps a heart attack patient with appropriate exercises that will aid his recovery but not endanger his weakened heart.

The Holter Monitor

Before or after a heart attack victim returns to work and more normal life habits, physicians may want to know how he or she will react to stresses, medicines, and other factors and conditions. A "Holter monitor," named after the physicist Dr. Norman J. Holter, makes such measurements possible. The portable monitor delivers electrocardiographic readings for 6 to 24 hours or longer while the patient goes about his normal activities.

Called "ambulatory electrocardiographic monitoring," the process of recording heart signals is relatively simple. Electrodes are attached to the patient's chest over the heart. The electrodes connect with a tape recorder that makes electrocardiograms. Completely portable because of its weight—less than two pounds—the tape recorder/monitor is carried on a strap hung over the patient's shoulder or is attached to the wearer's belt.

The monitor's recordings tell physicians a number of things that may be crucial to the patient's survival. Where a patient has experienced heart palpitations or irregularities, the doctor can adjust treatment to the recorded findings. Medication designed to prevent rhythm disorders may be adjusted as regards dosage and timing. These readings would typically be taken before the patient returns to work, either in the hospital or at home.

Where a patient has dizzy spells, the monitor can often detect the specific problems affecting heart functioning. Those problems, mainly slow or rapid nonrhythmic beats or heart blockage, may be found to be causing the dizziness. The possibility of pacemaker failure may also be indicated. The pacemaker provides a regular electrical impulse to keep heart action regular.

Patients using the ambulatory monitor are generally asked to supplement the cardiographic record by keeping notes on their activities. These notes show the doctor the activities in which the patient was engaged from hour to hour during the day. The notes may be matched up with the EKG to show what stresses accompanied particular activities. Some monitors have a special band on which the patient can record oral reports of his activities. With the monitor's tape record and the patient's written or dictated notes, the physician can often

• give the patient specific instructions on when and to what extent he or she can resume normal home activities;

• provide an accurate schedule for resuming work tasks;

• guide the patient on the need for future evaluations and therapy.

Prevention

Scientists do not have all the answers to atherosclerosis as yet. What is apparent, though, is that not one but a mosaic of factors is involved.

Long-term population studies have helped to point up individual characteristics and living habits that raise heart attack risk. These include such factors as sex, heredity, overweight, high blood pressure, lack of exercise, cigarette smoking, high blood levels of cholesterol and other fatty substances, and the presence of diabetes.

The identification of these risk factors has given the physician an important new weapon: a way to spot coronary-prone individuals years before any overt symptoms appear and—because so many of the risk factors are controllable—a promising program for reducing this risk.

These are some of the recommendations:

• Eat less saturated fat and cholesterol. Egg yolks are rich in cholesterol. Saturated animal fats—as in butter, cheese, cream and whole milk—help to raise cholesterol levels. Use skimmed (fat-free) milk. Substitute polyunsaturated vegetable fats for saturated fats as often as possible. This means, for example, cooking with vegetable oils and eating poultry and fish. Polyunsaturates tend to lower blood cholesterol. The more cholesterol in the circulation, presumably, the more material is available to build up the blood-blocking atherosclerotic deposits.

• Control high blood pressure. Hypertension sharply increases the chances of heart attack. A man whose blood pressure at *systole* (the moment the heart contracts) is higher than 160 runs four times the risk of an individual with a systolic blood pressure under 120. In almost all cases, elevated blood pressure can be brought under control.

• Don't smoke. The heart attack death rate is 50 to 200 percent higher, depending on age and number of cigarettes consumed, among men who smoke as compared with nonsmokers. Giving up the habit can decrease the coronary risk to that of the nonsmoker; the danger from smoking appears to be reversible. A combination of two or more risk factors not only increases the risk, it compounds it. A male cigarette smoker with high cholesterol and high blood pressure may be ten times as likely to have a heart attack as a nonsmoker with normal blood pressure.

• Count calories. Get down to your proper weight and stay there. Excess weight taxes the heart, makes it work harder. Middle-aged men who are 20 percent overweight run as much as two to three times the risk of a fatal heart attack than their trimmer counterparts.

• Exercise regularly. Your physician can tell you what the best exercise program is for your age and physical condition. Studies show active men to be better able to survive a heart attack than sedentary individuals. The belief is that exercise promotes the development of collateral circulation.

Children can benefit most of all, perhaps, if they are trained from the start in this life-long prescription.

Hypertensive Heart Disease

Hypertension, or elevated blood

pressure, results from a persistent tightening or constriction of the body's very small arterial branches, the *arterioles*. This clenching increases the resistance to blood flow and sends the blood pressure up, just as screwing down the nozzle on a hose builds up pressure in the line. The heart must now work harder to force blood through. Over a period of time, the stepped-up pumping effort may cause the heart muscle to thicken and enlarge, much as the arm muscles do on a weight lifter. Eventually, the overworked circulatory system may break down, with resultant failure of the heart or kidneys, or the onset of stroke. The constant hammering of blood under high pressure on the walls of the arteries also accelerates the development of atherosclerosis and heart attacks.

How Blood Pressure Is Measured

Blood pressure is measured in millimeters of mercury with an instrument called a *sphygmomanometer*. The device consists of an inflatable cuff attached to a mercury meter. The physician wraps the cuff around the arm and inflates it with air from a squeeze-bulb. This drives the mercury column up towards the top of the gauge while shutting off blood flow through the brachial artery in the arm. With a stethoscope placed just below the cuff, the physician releases the air and listens for the first thudding sounds that signal the return of blood flow as the blood pressure on the wall of the artery equals

the air pressure in the cuff. He records this mercury meter reading. This number represents the *systolic* pressure, the force developed by the heart when it contracts.

By continuing to let air out, the physician reaches a point where he can no longer hear the pulsing sounds of flowing blood. He marks the gauge reading as the *diastolic* pressure, the pressure on the artery when the heart is relaxing between beats. Thus, two numbers are used to record blood pressure, the systolic followed by the diastolic.

Recorded when the patient is relaxed, normal systolic pressure for most adults is between 100 and 140, and diastolic between 60 and 90. Many factors, such as age and sex, account for the wide variations in normal readings from individual to individual. Systolic blood pressure, for example, tends to increase with age.

Normally, blood pressure goes up during periods of excitement and physical labor. Hypertension is the diagnosis when repeated measurements show a persistent elevated pressure—160 or higher for systolic and 95 or more for diastolic.

In addition to the sphygmomanometer reading in the examination for high blood pressure, the physician shines a bright light in the patient's eyes so that he can look at the blood vessels in the retina, the only blood vessels that are readily observable. Any damage there due to hypertension is usually a good index of the severity of the disease

and its effects elsewhere in the body.

An electrocardiogram and X ray may be in order to determine if and how much the heart has been damaged. The physician may also perform some tests of kidney function to ascertain whether hypertension, if detected, is of the essential or secondary kind, and if there has been damage to the kidneys as well.

Causes

About 85 percent of all hypertension cases are classified as *essential*. This simply means that no single cause can be defined. Rather, pressure is up because a number of factors—none of which has yet been firmly implicated—are operating in some complex interplay.

One theory holds that hypertension arises from excessive activity of the sympathetic nervous system, which helps regulate blood vessel response. This notion could help explain why tense individuals are susceptible to hypertension. Emotional reactions to unpleasant events or other mental stresses prompt the cardiovascular system to react as it might to exercise, including widespread constriction of small blood vessels and increased heart rate.

The theory suggests that repeated episodes of stress may ultimately affect pressure-sensitive cells called *baroreceptors*. Situated in strategic places in the arterial system, these sensing centers are thought to be preset to help maintain normal blood pressure, just as a thermostat works to keep a house at a preset temperature. Exposure to regularly recurrent elevated blood pressure episodes may bring about a resetting of the baroreceptors—or *barostats*—to a new, higher normal. Once reset, the barostats operate to sustain hypertension.

Symptoms

Essential hypertension usually first occurs when a person is in his thirties. In the early stages, one may pass through a transitional or pre-hypertensive phase lasting a few years in which blood pressure rises

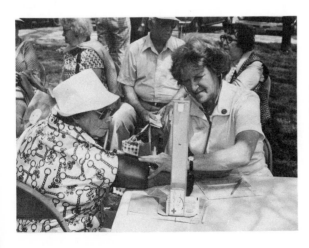

At a senior citizens' picnic, a nurse from the American Red Cross offers free blood pressure readings to help detect any hypertension problems.

above normal only occasionally, and then more and more often until finally it remains at these elevated levels.

Symptoms, if they exist at all, are likely to be something as nonspecific as headaches, dizziness, or nausea. As a result, without a physical examination to reveal its presence, a person may have the disease for years without being aware of it. That can be dangerous, since the longer hypertension is left untreated, the greater the likelihood that the heart will be affected.

About 15 percent of cases fall under the *secondary hypertension* classification, because they arise as a consequence of another known disorder. Curing the underlying disorder also cures the hypertension. Usually it is brought on by an obstruction of normal blood flow to the kidney because of atherosclerotic deposits in one or both of its major supply lines, the renal arteries. Many patients can be cured or substantially improved through surgery.

Treatment

The outlook is good for almost all patients with essential hypertension, whether mild or severe, because of the large arsenal of antihypertensive drugs now at the physician's disposal. Not all drugs will benefit all patients, but where one fails another or several in combination will almost invariably succeed. Even the usually lethal and hard-to-treat form of essential hypertension described as *malignant* is beginning to respond to new medications. *Malignant hypertension,* which may strike as many as five percent of hypertensive victims, does not refer to cancer, but rather describes the rapid, galloping way blood pressure rises.

Mild hypertension often may be readily treated with tranquilizers and mild sedatives, particularly if the patient is tense, or with one of a broad family of agents known as *diuretics*. These drugs flush the body of excess salt, which appears to have some direct though poorly-

understood role in hypertension.

Against more severe forms, there are a large number of drugs which work in a variety of ways to offset or curb the activity of the sympathetic nervous system so that it relaxes its hold on the constricted arterioles.

Rheumatic Fever and Rheumatic Heart Disease

Rheumatic heart disease is the possible sequel of rheumatic fever. Triggered by streptococcal attacks in childhood and adolescence, rheumatic fever may leave permanent heart scars. The heart structures most often affected are the valves.

Causes

The cause of rheumatic fever is still not entirely understood. It is known that rheumatic fever is always preceded by an invasion of bacteria belonging to the group A beta hemolytic streptococcus family. Sooner or later, everybody has a strep infection, such as a strep throat or scarlet fever. Most of us get over it without any complications. But in 1 out of every 100 children the strep infection produces rheumatic fever a few weeks later, even after the strep attack has long since subsided. The figure may rise to 3 per 100 during epidemics in closed communities, such as a children's camp.

The invasion of strep sparks the production of protective agents called antibodies. For some reason, in a kind of biological double-cross, the antibodies attack not only the strep but also make war on the body's own tissues—the very tissues they are called upon to protect.

Researchers are now suggesting the possible reason, although all the evidence is not yet in. According to a widely-held theory, the strep germ possesses constituents (*antigens*) which are similar in structure to components of normal, healthy cartilage and connective tissues— found abundantly in joints, tendons, and heart valves—in susceptible individuals. Failing to distinguish between them, the antibodies attack

both. The result: rheumatic fever, involving joint and valve inflammation and, perhaps, permanent scarring.

Prevention

The development of antibiotics has made rheumatic fever preventable. These drugs can knock out the strep before the germs get a chance to set off the inflammatory defense network sequences, but early detection is necessary. Among the symptoms of strep are a sore throat that comes on suddenly, with redness and swelling; rapidly acquired high fever; nausea and headaches. The only sure way to tell, however, is to have a throat swab taken by passing a sterile piece of cotton over the inflamed area. This culture is then exposed for 24 hours to a laboratory dish containing a substance that enhances strep growth. A positive identification calls for prompt treatment to kill the germs before the complications of rheumatic fever have a chance to set in.

Unfortunately, many strep infections may be mild enough to escape detection. The child may recover so quickly that the parents neglect to take the necessary precautions, but the insidious processes may still be going on in the apparently healthy child. This is a major reason why rheumatic fever is still with us, though in severe decline.

Symptoms

Rheumatic fever itself is not always easy to diagnose. The physician must detect at least one of five symptoms, derived by the American Heart Association from the work of the late Dr. T. Duckett Jones. The so-called Jones criteria include:

• Swelling or tenderness in one or more joints. Usually, several joints are involved, not simultaneously but one after the other in migratory fashion.

• Carditis or heart inflammation
• Heart murmur
• An unusual skin rash, which often disappears in 24 to 48 hours
• Chorea, or St. Vitus's dance, so-

called because of the uncoordinated, jerky and involuntary motions of the arms, legs, or face, which result from rheumatic inflammation of brain tissue. It may last six to eight weeks and even longer, but when symptoms disappear there is never any permanent damage and the brain and nervous system return to normal.

• Hard lumps, under the skin and over the inflamed joints, usually indicating severe heart inflammation.

Confirmation of rheumatic fever also requires other clinical and laboratory tests, to determine, for example, the presence of strep antibodies in the patient's blood. Rheumatic fever does not always involve the heart; even when it does, permanent damage is not inevitable. Nor does the severity of the attack have any relationship to the development of rheumatic heart disease.

The real danger arises when heart valve tissue becomes inflamed. When the acute attack has passed and the inflammation finally subsides, the valves begin to heal, with scar tissue forming.

Scar tissue may cause portions of the affected valve leaflets to fuse together. (*Leaflets* are the flaps of the heart valves.) This restricts leaflet motion, impeding the full swing action and thereby blood flow through the valve. This condition is called valvular *stenosis*. The leaflets may become shrunken or deformed by healing tissue, causing *regurgitation* or backspill because the valve fails to close completely.

Both stenosis and regurgitation are often present. Most susceptible are the *mitral valve,* which regulates flow from the upper to the lower left chambers of the heart, and the *aortic valve,* the gateway between the left ventricle and the general circulation. Rarely attacked are the two valves in the right chambers.

Treatment

During the acute stages of rheumatic fever, the patient is given heavy doses of antibiotics to rid the body of all strep traces, aspirin to

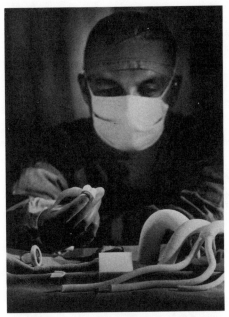

Materials used to repair damaged hearts *(left to right)*: mitral ball valve, aortic valve leaflet, aortic valve (in surgeon's hand), patching material, and artificial blood vessels.

control swelling and fever, and sometimes such hormones as ACTH and cortisone to reduce inflammation.

In the past, rheumatic fever spelled mandatory bed rest for months. Now the routine is to get the patient up and about as soon as the acute episode is over to avert the problem of psychological invalidism. The biggest restriction, especially for young people, is that no participation in competitive sports or other severely taxing exercises is allowed for two to three months while a close watch is kept on cardiac status.

The patient with valve damage can in many cases be treated medically, without the need for surgical intervention. He may, of course, have to desist from certain strenuous activities, but in all other ways he can lead a relatively normal life. Surgical relief or cure is available, however, for patients with severe damage or those who may, with age, develop progressive narrowing or leakage of the valves.

SURGERY: Stenotic valves can be scraped clear of excess scar tissues, thereby returning the leaflets to more normal operation. In some cases individually scarred leaflets are replaced with synthetic substitutes. The correction of severe valvular regurgitation requires replacement of the entire valve with an artificial substitute, or, as some surgeons prefer, with a healthy valve taken from a human donor dying of other causes.

Heart Murmurs and Recurrences of Rheumatic Fever

The prime sign that rheumatic heart disease has developed is a heart murmur—although a heart murmur does not always mean heart disease. The murmur may be only temporary, ceasing once the rheumatic fever attack subsides and the stretched and swollen valves return to normal. To complicate matters more, many heart murmurs are harmless. Such functional murmurs may appear in 30 to 50 percent of normal children at one time or another.

As many as three in five patients with rheumatic fever may develop murmurs characteristic of scarred valves—sounds of blood flowing through ailing valves that fail to open and close normally.

Anyone who has had an attack of rheumatic fever has about a 50-50 chance of having one again unless safeguards are taken. As a result, all patients are placed on a daily or monthly regimen of antibiotics. The preventive dose, although smaller than that given to quell an in-progress infection, is enough to sabotage any attempts on the part of the strep germs to mount an attack.

There is some encouraging evidence that rheumatic fever patients who escape heart damage the first time around will do so again should a repeat attack occur. On the other hand, those with damaged valves will probably sustain more damage with subsequent strep-initiated attacks.

Endocarditis

One of the additional bonuses of antibiotic therapy is that it has all but eliminated an invariably fatal complication to which rheumatic pa-

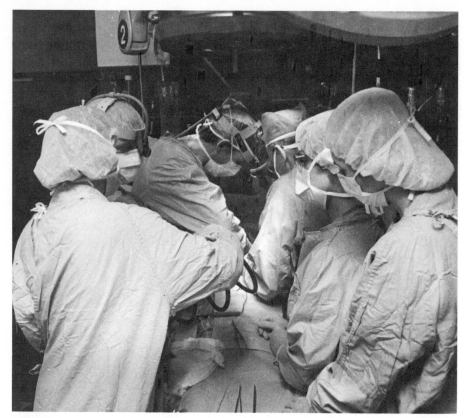

A corps of surgeons, cardiologists, nurses, and technicians is called upon during the hours-long surgery to replace the human heart with an artificial one.

that prevents blood from getting enough oxygen. Since blood low in oxygen is dark bluish red, it imparts a blue tinge to the skin and lips.

The cause of inborn heart abnormalities is not known in most cases. Some defects can be traced to maternal virus infection, such as German measles (rubella), during the first three months of pregnancy when the fetus' heart is growing rapidly. Certain drugs, vitamin deficiencies, or excessive exposure to radiation are among other environmental factors known to be associated with such defects.

Heart abnormalities may come singly or in combination. There may be, for example, a hole in the walls separating the right and left heart chambers, or a narrowing of a valve or blood vessel which obstructs blood flow, or a mixup in major blood vessel connections—or a combination of all of these.

Diagnosis

A skilled cardiologist often can make a reasonably complete diagnosis on the basis of a conventional physical examination, including visual inspection of the infant's general condition, blood pressure reading, X ray, blood tests, and electrocardio-

tients were especially vulnerable—an infection of the heart's inner lining, or *endocardium*, called *subacute bacterial endocarditis*. The scar tissue provides an excellent nesting site for bacteria to grow.

The responsible germs are found in almost everyone's mouth and usually invade the bloodstream after dental surgery. Fortunately, it is easy to prevent or cure because the germs offer little resistance to antibiotics. As a precaution, dentists are usually advised to give rheumatic fever patients larger doses of penicillin (or other antibiotics to those allergic to penicillin) before, during, and after dental work.

Congenital Heart Disease

There are some 35 recognized types of congenital heart malformations. Most—including all of the 15 most common types—can be either corrected or alleviated by surgery. The defects result from a failure of the in-

fant's heart to mature normally during development in the womb.

The term *blue baby* refers to the infant born with a heart impairment

The Jarvik-7 artificial heart is a result of over a decade's research by its inventor, Dr. Robert K. Jarvik. The hollow chambered, polyurethane plastic and aluminum device has the potential to be one of man's most rewarding medical successes.

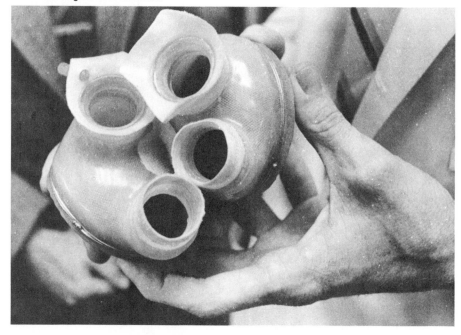

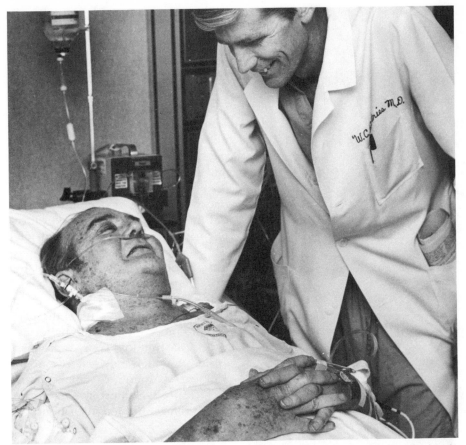

A surgeon explains to a possible artificial heart recipient the risks and procedures involved in the implantation of the device. Such operations are only performed on persons whose chances of survival without the surgery are nil.

often, however, since about one-third will die in the first month if untreated, and more than half within the first year.

Refinements in surgical techniques and post-operative care have given surgeons the confidence to operate on infants who are merely hours old with remarkable success. Specially adapted miniature heart-lung machines may also chill the blood to produce *hypothermia*, or body cooling. This slows metabolism and reduces tissue oxygen needs so that the heart and brain can withstand short periods of interrupted blood flow.

A good deal has been learned, too, about the delicate medical management required by infants during the surgical recovery period. All of this accounts for the admirable record of salvage among infants who would have been given up for lost only a few years ago.

gram. For more complex diagnosis, the physician may call for either *angiography* or *cardiac catheterization*. The former, a variation of coronary arteriography, allows direct X-ray visualization of the heart chambers and major blood vessels. In cardiac catheterization, a thin plastic tube or catheter is inserted into an arm or leg vein. While the physician watches with special X-ray equipment, the tube is advanced carefully through the vein until it reaches the heart chambers, there to provide information about the nature of the defect.

Advanced techniques known as computerized axial tomography (CAT), positron emission tomography (PET), and nuclear magnetic resonance (NMR) may also be used. Both the CAT and PET scanners require injection of a contrast fluid so that a "picture" can be taken. The CAT scanner takes X-ray images of "slices" of the patient's body with the aid of a computer. The PET scanner works on an electronic principle, with detectors located in a circle around the subject. Also computerized, NMR diagnoses by "seeing" through bones and revealing such details as the differences between healthy and diseased tissues.

Treatment

From these tests, the cardiologist together with a surgeon can decide for or against surgery. Depending on the severity of the disease, some conditions may require an immediate operation, even on days-old infants. In other conditions, the specialists may instead recommend waiting until the infant is older and stronger before surgery is undertaken. In a number of instances, the defect may not require surgery at all.

Open-heart surgery in infants with inborn heart defects carries a higher risk than does the same surgery in older children. Risks must be taken

Congestive Heart Failure

Heart failure may be found in conjunction with any disease of the heart—coronary artery disease, hypertension, rheumatic heart disease, or congenital defects. It occurs when the heart's ability to pump blood has been weakened by disease. To say the heart has failed, however, does not meant it has stopped beating. The heart muscle continues to contract, but it lacks the strength to keep blood circulating normally throughout the body. Doctors sometimes refer to the condition as cardiac insufficiency or *dropsy*, although the latter term is seldom heard anymore.

When the heart fails to pump efficiently, the flow slows down, causing blood returning to the heart through the veins to back up. Some of the fluid in the blood is forced out through the thin walls of smaller blood vessels into surrounding tissues. Here the fluid piles up, or congests.

The result may be swelling, or *edema*, which can occur in many

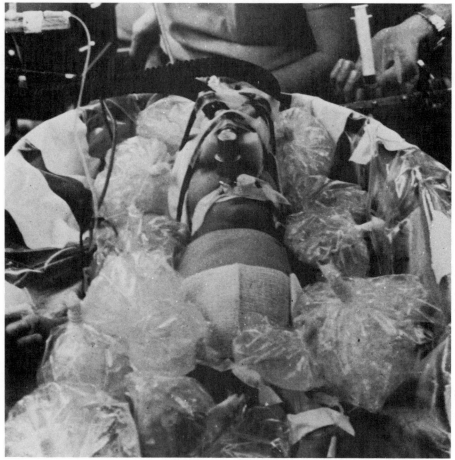

Crushed ice is used to lower an infant's body temperature (hypothermia) and slow metabolism so that blood flow can be briefly interrupted during open-heart surgery.

brain. Blackouts and convulsions may ensue.

For less serious slowdown, there are nervous system stimulants to keep the heart from lagging. In the case of *Stokes-Adams syndrome* — where the ventricles may not beat from four to ten seconds—drugs are not enough. An artificial electronic pacemaker, implanted in the body and connected to the heart by wires, has been successfully applied to many thousands of people throughout the world. This pacemaker fires electrical shocks into the ventricle wall to make it beat at the proper rate. Most devices are powered by tiny batteries which must be replaced on the average every three to five years, depending upon the particular composition of the batteries. Longer lasting fuel sources are also available which may last as long as 15 years. Atomic pacemakers are technically feasible but experience with them is limited at present.

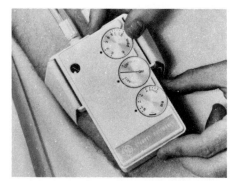

This cardiac pacemaker is designed to provide temporary external stimulation of the heart through internal electrodes. It may be used during heart surgery or before an internal pacemaker can be implanted.

parts of the body but is most commonly seen in the legs and ankles. Fluids sometimes collect in the lungs, interfering with breathing and making the person short of breath. Heart failure also affects the ability of the kidneys to rid the body of sodium and water. Fluid retained in this way adds to the edema.

Treatment

Treatment usually includes a combination of rest, drugs, diet, and restricted daily activity. *Digitalis*, in one of its many forms, is usually given to strengthen the action of the heart muscle. It also slows a rapid heartbeat, helps decrease heart enlargement, and promotes secretion of excess fluids. Care must be taken to find the right dose, since this will vary from person to person. When edema is present, diuretics are prescribed to speed up the elimination of excess salt and water. Many improved diuretics are available today. A sodium-restricted diet is generally necessary to reduce or prevent edema. Patients will also probably need bed rest for a while, with a gradual return to slower-paced activity.

Most important, however, is the adequate treatment of the underlying disease that led to heart failure in the first place.

Heart Block

Sometimes the scars resulting from rheumatic fever, heart attack, or surgical repair of the heart may damage the electrical network in a way that blocks normal transmission of the signal between the upper and lower chambers. The disruption, called *atrio-ventricular block*, may so severely slow down the rate at which the ventricles beat that blood flow is seriously affected, especially to the

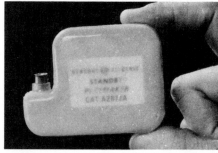

An implantable cardiac pacemaker suitable for patients with heart block or for those with normal heart rhythm who require occasional stimulus. It is powered by six silver mercury cells designed to last up to five years.

CHAPTER 17

Diseases of the Digestive System

Digestive Functions and Organs

The function of the digestive system is to accept food and water through the mouth, to break down the food's chemical structure so that its nutrients can be absorbed into the body, a process called *digestion*, and to expel undigested particles. This process takes place as the food passes through the entire *alimentary tract*. This tract, also called the *gastrointestinal tract*, is a long, hollow passageway that begins at the mouth and continues on through the esophagus, the stomach, the small intestine, the large intestine, the rectum, and the anus. The salivary glands, the stomach glands, the liver, the gall bladder, and the pancreas release substances into the gastrointestinal tract that help the digestion of various food substances.

Digestion

Digestion begins in the mouth where food is shredded by chewing and mixed with saliva, which helps break down starch into sugars and lubricates the food so that it can be swallowed easily. The food then enters the *esophagus*, a muscular tube that forcibly squeezes the food down toward the stomach, past the *cardiac sphincter*, a ring of muscle at the entrance of the stomach that opens to allow food into the stomach.

The stomach acts as a reservoir for food, churns the food, mixes it with gastric juices, and gradually releases the food into the small intestine. Some water, alcohol, and glucose are absorbed directly through the stomach into the bloodstream. Enzymes secreted by the stomach help break down proteins and fats into simpler substances. Hydrochloric acid secreted by the stomach kills bacteria and prepares some minerals for absorption in the small intestine. Some food may leave the stomach one minute after it enters, while other parts of a meal may remain in the stomach for as long as five hours.

The food passes from the stomach to the first section of the small intestine, the *duodenum*, where it is acted on by pancreatic enzymes that help break down fats, starches, proteins, and other substances. While the food is in the duodenum it is also digested by *bile*, which is produced by the liver and stored in the gall bladder. During a meal, the gall bladder discharges its bile into the duodenum. The bile promotes the absorption of fats and vitamins.

The semidigested food is squeezed down the entire length of the intestines by a wavelike motion of the intestinal muscles called *peristalsis*.

Digestion is largely completed as the food passes through 20 feet of small intestine, which absorbs the digested food substances and water and passes them into the bloodstream. The food nutrients are distributed by the bloodstream throughout the body and used by the body cells.

Those parts of the food that are indigestible, such as the skins of fruits, pass into the large intestine, or *colon*, along with bacteria, bile, some minerals, various cells, and mucus. This combination of substances makes up the *feces*, which are stored in the colon until *defecation*. Some water and salts in the feces are absorbed through the walls of the colon into the bloodstream. This conserves the body's fluids and dries the feces. The formation of a semisolid fecal mass helps precipitate defecation.

The Oral Cavity

The Salivary Glands

The smell of food triggers the salivary glands to pour saliva into the mouth; that is what is meant by "mouth-watering" odors. During a meal, saliva is released into the mouth to soften the food as it is chewed.

373

THE DIGESTIVE SYSTEM

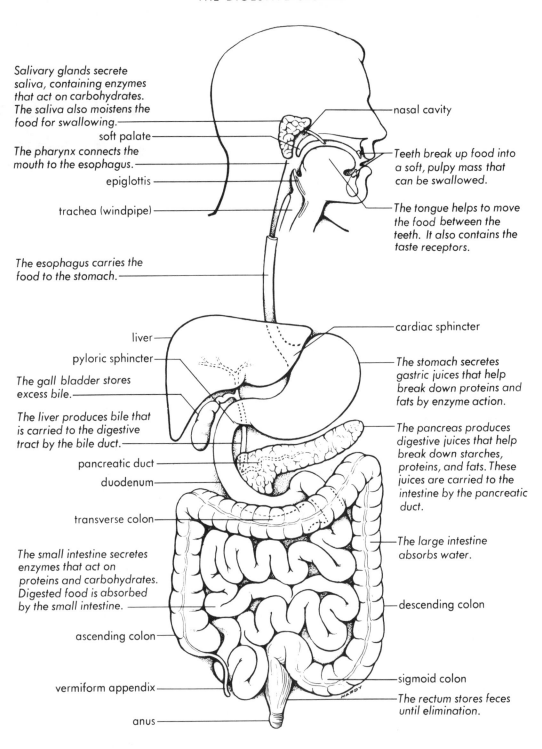

Salivary glands secrete saliva, containing enzymes that act on carbohydrates. The saliva also moistens the food for swallowing.

soft palate

The pharynx connects the mouth to the esophagus.

epiglottis

trachea (windpipe)

The esophagus carries the food to the stomach.

nasal cavity

Teeth break up food into a soft, pulpy mass that can be swallowed.

The tongue helps to move the food between the teeth. It also contains the taste receptors.

liver

pyloric sphincter

The gall bladder stores excess bile.

The liver produces bile that is carried to the digestive tract by the bile duct.

pancreatic duct

duodenum

transverse colon

The small intestine secretes enzymes that act on proteins and carbohydrates. Digested food is absorbed by the small intestine.

ascending colon

vermiform appendix

anus

cardiac sphincter

The stomach secretes gastric juices that help break down proteins and fats by enzyme action.

The pancreas produces digestive juices that help break down starches, proteins, and fats. These juices are carried to the intestine by the pancreatic duct.

The large intestine absorbs water.

descending colon

sigmoid colon

The rectum stores feces until elimination.

STONES: Stones will sometimes form in the salivary glands or ducts, blocking the ducts and preventing the free flow of saliva into the mouth. After a meal, the swollen saliva-filled glands and ducts slowly empty. The swelling may sometimes be complicated by infection. Surgical removal of the stones is the usual treatment; sometimes the entire gland is removed.

TUMORS: Tumors sometimes invade the salivary gland. An enlarged gland may press on the auditory canal and cause deafness, or it may result in stiffness of the jaw and mild facial palsy. The tumors can grow large enough to be felt by the fingers, and surgery is required to remove them.

INFLAMMATION OF THE PAROTID GLANDS: Inflammation of the upper (*parotid*) salivary glands may be caused by an infection in the oral cavity, by liver disease, or by malnutrition.

MUMPS: One of the commonest inflammations of the salivary glands, called *mumps*, occurs especially in children. It is a highly contagious virus disease characterized by inflammation and swelling of one or both parotid salivary glands, and can have serious complications in adults. See under *Alphabetic Guide to Child Care*, p. 60, for a fuller discussion of mumps.

Bad Breath (Halitosis)

Poor oral hygiene is the principal cause of offensive mouth odor, or *halitosis*. It can result from oral tumors, abscesses from decaying teeth, and gum disease or infection. The foul smell is primarily due to cell decay, and the odors are characteristic of the growth of some microorganisms.

When halitosis results from poor oral sanitation, the treatment is obvious—regular daily tooth brushing and the use of an antiseptic mouthwash. If the halitosis is due to disease of the oral cavity, alimentary tract, or respiratory system, the cure will depend on eradicating the primary cause.

Nonmalignant Lesions

The oral cavity is prone to invasion by several types of microorganisms that cause nonmalignant lesions. The most prominent are:

CANKER SORES: These are of unknown origin and show up as single or multiple small sores near the molar teeth, inside the lips, or in the lining of the mouth. They can be painful but usually heal in a few days.

FUNGUS INFECTIONS: *Thrush* is the most common oral fungus infection and appears as white round patches inside the cheeks of infants, small children, and sometimes adults. The lesions may involve the entire mouth, tongue, and pharynx. In advanced stages the lesions turn yellow. Malnutrition, especially lack of adequate vitamin B, is the principal cause. Fungus growth is also aided by the use of antibiotic lozenges, which kill normal oral bacteria and permit fungi to flourish.

TOOTH DECAY AND VITAMIN DEFICIENCIES: Lack of adequate vitamins in the daily diet is responsible for some types of lesions in the oral cavity. Insufficient vitamin A in children under five may be the cause of malformation in the crown, dentin, and enamel of the teeth. Lack of adequate vitamin C results in bleeding gums. Vitamin D insufficiency may lead to slow tooth development.

An inadequate and improper diet supports tooth decay, which in turn may be complicated by ulcers in the gums and abscesses in the roots of the decaying teeth. A diet with an adequate supply of the deficient vitamins will cause the symptoms to disappear. Infections, abscesses, cysts, or tumors in the mouth require the attention of a physician, dentist, or dental surgeon. See *The Teeth and Gums*, p. 252.

CHANCRES: These are primary syphilis lesions, which commonly develop at the lips and tongue. They appear as small, eroding red ulcers that exude yellow matter. They can invade the mouth, tonsils, and pharynx. Penicillin therapy is usually required.

The Esophagus

Varices

Varices (singular: *varix*) are enlarged and congested veins that appear in the esophagus due to increased blood pressure to the liver in patients with liver cirrhosis. This disease is most common in chronic alcoholics. Esophageal varices can be complicated by erosion of the mucous lining of the esophagus due to inflammation or vomiting. This causes hemorrhaging of the thin-walled veins, which can be fatal.

Bleeding esophageal varices may require hospitalization, immediate blood transfusions, and surgery.

Hiatus Hernia

The lower end of the esophagus or part of the stomach can sometimes protrude through the diaphragm. This *hiatus hernia*, sometimes referred to as a *diaphragmatic hernia*, can be due to congenital malformation; in adults, the principal cause is weakness of the muscles around the opening of the esophagus leading into the stomach.

In individuals who are obese and who have large stomachs, the stomach contents may be forced back into the lower esophagus, causing this area to herniate. Other causes include stooping, bending, or kneeling, which increases pressure in the stomach. Pregnancy may increase abdominal pressure in the same manner as obesity.

Typical symptoms are vomiting when the stomach is full, heartburn with pain spreading to the ears,

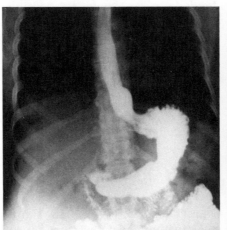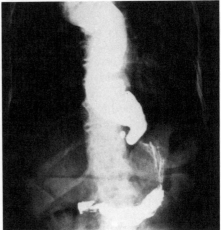

(Left) An X ray of a normal esophagus. *(Right)* The esophagus has been abnormally distended with food (achalasia) because of the failure of the cardiac sphincter to relax and allow food to enter the stomach.

neck, and arms, swallowing difficulty with the food sometimes sticking in the esophagus, and a swollen abdomen. The vomiting may occur at night, with relief obtained by getting up and walking about for a few minutes. Belching will relieve the distension, and *antacids* (acid neutralizers) may be prescribed to counter gastric hyperacidity.

Conservative treatment involves eating small portions at frequent intervals. Dieting and a reduction in weight cause the symptoms to disappear. When the symptoms are due to pregnancy, they disappear after delivery. When medical management is not successful, surgical repair of the hernia is necessary. See also *Hernias*, p. 380.

Achalasia

Achalasia is abnormal dilation of the lower esophagus caused by failure of the cardiac sphincter to relax and allow food to enter the stomach. Food collects in the esophagus and does not flow into the stomach. The patient feels as though the food is sticking in the middle of his chest wall. Small amounts of food may eventually pass into the stomach, and the mild pain or discomfort disappears.

If the condition persists, the pain may increase to become a continuous burning sensation at each meal, due to inflammation of the esophagus by accumulated food. If the patient lies down, some of this esophageal content will regurgitate and enter the pharynx. If the vomitus gets into the lungs, the end result may be *aspiration pneumonia*, a form of pneumonia caused by inhaling particles of foreign matter.

The disease is difficult to control, and the condition tends to return, so that surgery is often used to create a permanent opening between the esophagus and stomach.

Swallowing Difficulty

Difficulty in swallowing is called *dysphagia*, which should not be confused with *dysphasia*, a speech impairment. Dysphagia may be caused by lesions in the mouth and tongue, acute inflammatory conditions in the oral cavity and pharynx (mumps, tonsillitis, laryngitis, pharyngitis), lesions, cancers, or foreign bodies in the esophagus. Strictures in the esophagus—from esophageal ulcers or from swallowing corrosive liquids—will also impair swallowing.

Stomach and Intestines

Indigestion (Dyspepsia)

There are times when the gastrointestinal tract fails to carry out its normal digestive function. The resulting indigestion, or *dyspepsia*, generates a variety of symptoms, such as heartburn, nausea, pain in the upper abdomen, gases in the stomach (*flatulence*), belching, and a feeling of fullness after eating.

Indigestion can be caused by ulcers of the stomach or duodenum and by excessive or too rapid eating or drinking. It may also be caused by emotional disturbance.

Constipation

Constipation is the difficult or infrequent evacuation of feces. The urge to defecate is normally triggered by the pressure of feces on the rectum and by the intake of food into the stomach. On the toilet, the anal sphincter is relaxed voluntarily, and the fecal material is expelled. The need to defecate should be attended to as soon as possible. Habitual disregard of the desire to empty the bowels reduces intestinal motion and leads to constipation.

Daily or regular bowel movements are not necessary for good health. Normal bowel movements may occur at irregular intervals due to variations in diet, mental stress, and physical activity. For some individuals, normal defecation may take place as infrequently as once every four days.

SIMPLE CONSTIPATION: In simple constipation, the patient may have to practice good bowel movement habits, which include a trip to the toilet once daily, preferably after breakfast. Adequate fluid intake and proper diet, including fresh fruits and green vegetables, can help restore regular bowel movement. Laxatives can provide temporary relief, but they inhibit normal bowel function and lead to dependence. When toilet-training young children, parents should encourage but never force them to have regular bowel movements, preferably after breakfast.

CHRONIC CONSTIPATION: Chronic constipation can cause feces to accumulate in the rectum and *sigmoid*, the terminal section of the colon. The colonic fluid is absorbed and a mass of hard fecal material remains. Such impacted feces often prevent further passage of bowel contents. The individual suffers from abdominal pain with distension and sometimes vomiting. A cleansing enema will relieve the fecal impaction and related symptoms.

In the overall treatment of constipation, the principal cause must be identified and corrected so that normal evacuation can return.

Intestinal Obstructions

Obstruction to the free flow of digestive products may exist either in the stomach or in the small and large intestines. The typical symptoms of intestinal obstruction are constipation, painful abdominal distension,

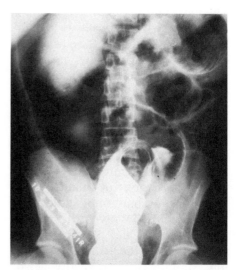

This X ray reveals volvulus of the colon, a looping or twisting of the bowel around itself which results in an intestinal obstruction.

and vomiting. Intestinal obstruction can be caused by the bowel's looping or twisting around itself, forming what is known as a *volvulus*. Malignant tumors can either block the intestine or press it closed.

In infants, especially boys, a common form of intestinal obstruction occurs when a segment of the intestine folds into the section below it. This condition is known as *intussusception*, and can significantly reduce the blood supply to the lower bowel segment. The cause may be traced to viral infection, injury to the abdomen, hard food, or a foreign body in the gastrointestinal tract.

The presence of intestinal obstructions is generally determined by consideration of the clinical symptoms, as well as X-ray examinations of the abdomen. Hospitalization is required, since intestinal obstruction has a high fatality rate if proper medical care is not administered. Surgery may be needed to remove the obstruction.

Diarrhea

Diarrhea is the frequent and repeated passage of liquid stools. It is usually accompanied by intestinal inflammation, and sometimes by the passing of mucus or blood.

The principal cause of diarrhea is infection in the intestinal tract by microorganisms. Chemical and food poisoning also brings on spasms of diarrhea. Long-standing episodes of diarrhea have been traced to inflammation of the intestinal mucosa, tumors, ulcers, allergies, vitamin deficiency, and in some cases emotional stress.

Patients with diarrhea commonly suffer abdominal cramps, lose weight from chronic attacks, or have vomiting spells. A physician must always be consulted for proper diagnosis and treatment; this is especially important if the attacks continue for more than two or three days. Untreated diarrhea can lead to dehydration and malnutrition; it may be fatal, especially in infants.

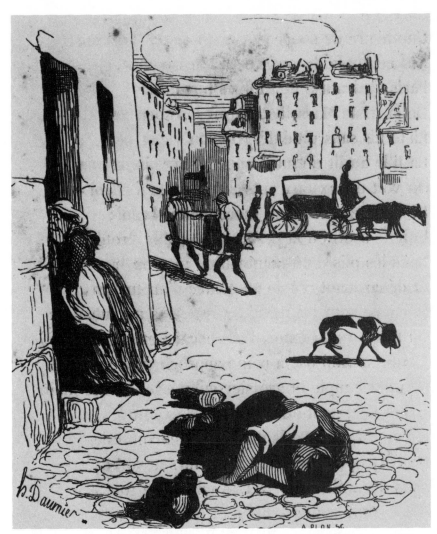

Cholera is an acute, infectious disease spread by bacteria that attack the intestinal system and cause vomiting and diarrhea. Extreme dehydration of body fluids can result, and before the discovery of antibiotics cholera epidemics claimed thousands of lives. In this 19th-century woodcut after a drawing by Daumier, a victim of the dreaded disease falls to the street, shunned by all, while in the background caskets are carried to burial.

Dysentery

Dysentery is caused by microorganisms that thrive in the intestines of infected individuals. Most common are *amoebic dysentery*, caused by amoebae, and *bacillary dysentery*, caused by bacteria. The symptoms are diarrhea with blood and pus in the stools, cramps, and fever. The infection is spread from person to person through infected excrement that contaminates food or water. The bacteria and amoebae responsible can also be spread by houseflies which feed on feces as well as on human foods. It is a common tropical disease and can occur wherever human excrement is not disposed of in a sanitary manner.

Dysentery must be treated early to avoid erosion of the intestinal wall. In bacillary dysentery, bed rest and hospitalization are recommended, especially for infants and the aged. Antibiotic drugs may be administered.

In most cases the disease can be spread by healthy human carriers who must be treated to check further spread.

Typhoid

Enteric fever or *typhoid* is an acute, highly communicable disease caused by the organism *Salmonella typhosa.* It is sometimes regarded as a tropical disease because epidemic outbreaks are common in tropical areas where careless disposal of feces and urine contaminates food, milk, and water supplies. In any location, tropical or temperate, where unsanitary living predominates, there is always the possibility that the disease can occur. Flies can transmit the disease, as can shellfish that live in typhoid-infested waters.

The typhoid bacilli do their damage to the mucosa of the small intestines. They enter via the oral cavity and stomach and finally reach the lymph nodes and blood vessels in the small bowel.

SYMPTOMS: Following an incubation period of about ten days, general bodily discomfort, fever, headache, nausea, and vomiting are experienced. Other clinical manifestations include abdominal pain with tenderness, greenish diarrhea (or constipation), bloody stools, and mental

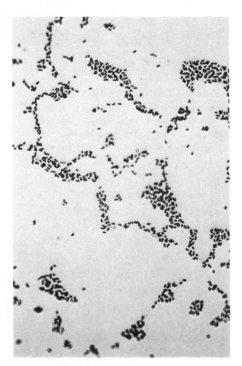

In spite of the existence of a vaccine to prevent the spread of cholera and of effective methods to treat the symptoms—replacement of fluid losses and the administration of antibiotics—the disease is still a threat to life in many parts of the world. Shown above are the bacterial organisms (greatly magnified) that cause one form of cholera.

confusion. It is not unusual for red spots to appear on the body.

If untreated, typhoid victims die within 21 days of the onset of the disease. The cause of death may be perforation of the small bowel, abdominal hemorrhage, toxemia, or other complications such as intestinal inflammation and pneumonia.

TREATMENT AND PREVENTION: A person can best recover from typhoid if he receives diligent medical and nursing care. He should be isolated in a hospital on complete bed rest. Diet should be restricted to highly nutritious liquids or preferably intravenous feeding. Destruction of the bacilli is achieved by antibiotic therapy, usually with Chloromycetin.

The best way to prevent the spread of typhoid is to disinfect all body refuse, clothing, and utensils of the person infected. Isolation techniques practiced in hospitals prevent local spread. Milk and milk products should always be pasteurized; drinking water should be chlorinated.

Human beings can carry the disease and infect others without themselves becoming ill; they are usually not aware that they are carriers. Within recent years, a vaccination effective for a year has been developed. People traveling to areas where sanitation practices may be conducive to typhoid should receive this vaccination. In such areas, it is usually a good practice to boil drinking water as well.

Foreign Bodies in the Alimentary Tract

Anyone who accidentally swallows a foreign body should seek immediate medical aid, preferably in a hospital. Foreign bodies that enter the gastrointestinal tract may cause obstruction anywhere along the tract, including the esophagus. For emergency procedures, see *Obstruction in the Windpipe*, p. 577.

Dental plates and large chunks of meat have been known to cause fatal choking. A foreign body in the esophagus may set off a reflex mechanism that causes the trachea to

close. The windpipe may have to be opened by means of a *tracheostomy* (incision in the windpipe) to restore breathing. If the object swallowed is long and sharp-pointed, it may perforate the tract.

Foreign bodies in the esophagus are usually the most troublesome. Small fish bones may stick to the walls of the esophagus; large pieces of meat may block the tract. X-ray studies aid the doctor in locating the swallowed object and in determining how best to deal with it.

Small objects like coins and paper clips may pass through the digestive tract without causing serious problems. Their progress may be checked by X rays of the abdomen. Examination of stools will indicate whether or not the entire object has been expelled. With larger objects, the problem of blockage must be considered. It is sometimes necessary for a surgeon to open the stomach in a hospital operating room and remove the foreign object.

Ulcers

A *peptic ulcer* is an eroded area of the mucous membrane of the digestive tract. The most common gastrointestinal ulcers are found in the lower end of the esophagus, stomach, or duodenum and are caused by the excessive secretion of gastric acid which erodes the lining membrane in these areas.

The cause of ulcers is obscure, but any factor that increases gastric acidity may contribute to the condition. Mental stress or conflict, excessive food intake, alcohol, and caffeine all cause the stomach to increase its output of hydrochloric acid.

The disease is sometimes considered to be hereditary, especially among persons with type O blood. Symptoms usually appear in individuals of the 20-to-40 age group, with the highest incidence in persons over age 45. Peptic ulcers of the stomach (*gastric ulcers*) and duodenal ulcers occur more frequently in men than in women. Ulcers are common in patients with arthritis and chronic lung disease.

SYMPTOMS: Early ulcer symptoms are gastric hyperacidity and burning abdominal pain which is relieved by eating, vomiting, or the use of antacids. The pain may occur as a dull ache, especially when one's stomach is empty, or it may be sharp and knifelike.

Other manifestations of a peptic ulcer are the following: nausea, associated with heartburn and regurgitation of gastric juice into the esophagus and mouth; excessive gas; poor appetite with undernourishment and weakness in older victims; black stools due to a bleeding ulcer.

The immediate goal of ulcer therapy is to heal the ulcer; the long-term goal is to prevent its recurrence. An ulcer normally heals through the formation of scar tissue in the ulcer crater. The healing process, under proper medical care, may take several weeks. The disappearance of pain does not necessarily indicate that the ulcer has healed completely, or even partially. The pain and the ulcerative process may recur at regular intervals over periods of weeks or months.

Although treatment can result in complete healing and recovery, some victims of chronic peptic ulcers have a 20-to-30-year history of periodic recurrences. For such patients, ulcer therapy may have to be extended indefinitely to avoid serious complications. If a recurrent ulcer perforates the stomach or intestine, or if it bleeds excessively, it can be quickly fatal. Emergency surgery is always required when perforation and persistent bleeding occur.

TREATMENT: The basic principles of ulcer therapy are diet, rest, and the suppression of stomach acidity. A patient with an active gastric ulcer is generally hospitalized for three weeks to make certain that he receives the proper diet and to remove him from sources of emotional stress, such as business or family problems. During hospitalization the healing process is monitored by X-ray examination. If there is no evidence of healing within three to four weeks,

surgery may be advisable. For patients with duodenal ulcers, a week or two of rest at home with proper diet may be sufficient.

Ulcer diets consist of low-residue bland foods taken in small amounts at frequent intervals, as often as once an hour when pain is severe. The preferred foods are milk, soft eggs, jellies, custards, creams, and cooked cereals. See *Minimal Residue Diet,* p. 223. Since ulcer diets often lack some essential nutrients, prolonged dietary treatment may have to be augmented with daily vitamin capsules. Antispasmodic medication may be prescribed to reduce contractions of the stomach, decrease the stomach's production of acid, and slow down digestion. Antacids, such as the combination of aluminum hydroxide and magnesium trisilicate, may be required after meals and between feedings. Spicy foods, alcohol, coffee, cola and other caffeine-containing drinks, large meals, and smoking should be strictly avoided.

In addition to common antacids, some new drugs have been introduced to help treat ulcers and other digestive disorders. Tagamet in particular, a brand name for the drug cimetidine, has been found to be effective in treating duodenal ulcers. It has also been used to prevent ulcer-related stomach, esophagus, and duodenal problems. The drug acts primarily to reduce secretions of gastric acid. But side effects have been reported, some of them serious. These include mental confusion, fever, slowed pulse, and others. Metiamide, another drug used to control the production of gastric acids in the digestive system, has been found to attack the leukocytes or white cells of the blood. Other problems have been reported with metiamide.

If the ulcer does not respond to medical therapy, or if pain persists, surgery may be the preferred treatment. Such surgery is elective surgery, a matter of choice, as opposed to the emergency surgery required by large, bleeding, or perforated ul-

cers. After the removal of the acid-producing section of the stomach, some patients may develop weakness and nausea as their digestive system adjusts to the reduced size of their stomach. A proper diet of special foods and fluids, plus sedatives, can alleviate the condition. The chances for complete recovery are good. For a full description of surgical treatment of peptic ulcers, see p. 324.

Diverticula

A *diverticulum* is an abnormal pouch caused by herniation of the mucous membrane of the digestive tract. The pouch has a narrow neck and a bulging round end. Diverticula are found in the esophagus, stomach, duodenum, colon, and other parts of the digestive tract.

The presence of diverticula in any segment of the digestive tract is referred to as *diverticulosis*. When diverticula become inflamed the condition is known as *diverticulitis*. The latter is a common form of disease of the sigmoid colon and is found in persons past the age of 45.

In mild cases, there may be no symptoms. On the other hand, a diverticulum may sometimes rupture and produce the same symptoms as an acute attack of appendicitis—

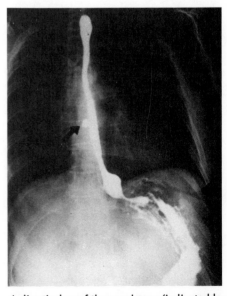

A diverticulum of the esophagus (indicated by the arrow) is an abnormal pouch caused by herniation of mucous membranes.

vomiting and pain with tenderness in the right lower portion of the abdomen. Other symptoms are intermittent constipation and diarrhea, and abdominal pain.

Diverticulosis is treated by bed rest, restriction of solid food and increase of fluid intake, and administration of antibiotics. Surgery is recommended when diverticulosis causes obstruction of the colon or creates an opening between the colon and the bladder, or when one or more diverticula rupture and perforate the colon. The outlook for recovery following surgery is good.

Hemorrhoids (Piles)

Hemorrhoids or *piles* are round, purplish protuberances at the anus. They are the results of rectal veins that become dilated and rupture. Hemorrhoids are very common and are often caused by straining due to constipation, pregnancy, or diarrhea.

Hemorrhoids may appear on the external side of the anus or on the internal side; they may or may not be painful. Rectal bleeding and tenderness are common. It is important to emphasize, however, that not all rectal bleeding is due to hemorrhoids. Small hemorrhoids are best left untreated; large painful ones may be surgically reduced or removed. *Prolapsed* piles—those that have slipped forward—are treated by gentle pressure to return the hemorrhoidal mass into the rectum. The rectal and anal opening must be lubricated to keep the area soft. Other conditions in the large bowel can simulate hemorrhoids and need to be adequately investigated.

Hernias

Hernias in the digestive tract occur when there is muscular weakness in surrounding body structures. Pressure from the gastrointestinal tract may cause a protrusion or *herniation* of the gut through the weakened wall. Such hernias exist in the diaphragmatic area (*hiatus hernias*, discussed above on p. 375), in the anterior abdomen (*ventral hernias*), or in the region of the groin

INGUINAL HERNIA

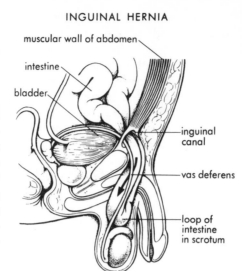

muscular wall of abdomen

intestine

bladder

inguinal canal

vas deferens

loop of intestine in scrotum

In this type of indirect hernia, a loop of small intestine has pushed through the weakened inguinal canal in the abdominal wall and descended into the scrotal sac.

(*inguinal hernias*). Apart from hiatus hernias, inguinal hernias are by far the most common.

One of the causes of intestinal obstruction is a *strangulated hernia*. A loop of herniated bowel becomes tightly constricted, blood supply is cut off, and the loop becomes gangrenous. Immediate surgery is required since life is threatened from further complications.

Except for hiatus hernias, diagnosis is usually made simple by the plainly visible herniated part. In men, an enlarged scrotum may be present in untreated inguinal hernias. The herniating bowel can be reduced, that is, manipulated back into position, and a truss worn to support the reduced hernia and provide temporary relief. In all hernias, however, surgical repair is the usual treatment.

Gastritis

Gastritis is inflammation of the mucosa of the stomach. The patient complains of *epigastric* pain—in the middle of the upper abdomen—with distension of the stomach, loss of appetite, nausea, and vomiting.

Attacks of acute gastritis can be traced to bacterial action, food poisoning, peptic ulcer, the presence of alcohol in the stomach, the ingestion of highly spiced foods, or overeating and drinking. Occasional gastritis, though painful, is not serious and may disappear spontaneously. The general treatment for gastritis is similar to the treatment of a gastric ulcer.

Enteritis

Enteritis, sometimes referred to as *regional entertitis*, is a chronic inflammatory condition of unknown origin that affects the small intestine. It is called regional because the disease most often involves the terminal ileum, even though any segment of the digestive tract can be involved. The diseased bowel becomes involved with multiple ulcer craters and ultimately stiffens because of fibrous healing of the ulcers.

Regional enteritis occurs most often in males from adolescence to middle age. The symptoms may exist for a long period before the disease is recognized. Intermittent bloody diarrhea, general weakness, and lassitude are the early manifestations. Later stages of the disease are marked by fever, increased bouts of diarrhea with resultant weight loss, and sharp lower abdominal pain on the right side. This last symptom sometimes causes the disease to be confused with appendicitis, since in both conditions there is nausea and vomiting. Occasionally in women there may be episodes of painful menstruation.

Treatment involves either surgical removal of the diseased bowel or conservative medical management and drug therapy. In acute attacks of enteritis, bed rest and intravenous fluids are two important aspects of treatment. Medical management in less severe occurrences includes a daily diet rich in proteins and vitamins, excluding harder foods such as fresh fruits and vegetables. Antibiotics are prescribed to combat bacterial invasion.

Colitis

Colitis is an inflammatory condition of the colon, of uncertain origin, and often chronic. It may result from a nervous predisposition which leads to bacterial or viral infection. The inflammation can cause spasms that damage the colon, or can lead to bleeding ulcers that may be fatal.

In milder forms, colitis first appears with diarrhea in which red bloody streaks can be observed. The symptoms may come and go for weeks before the effects become very significant. As the disease process advances, the diarrhea episodes become more frequent; more blood and mucus are present in the feces. These are combined with abdominal pain, nausea, and vomiting. Due to loss of blood the patient often becomes anemic and thin. If there are ulcer craters in the mucosa, the disease is called *ulcerative colitis*.

Hospitalization is necessary in order to provide proper treatment that will have a long-term effect. Surgery is sometimes necessary if an acute attack has been complicated by perforation of the intestines or if chronic colitis fails to respond to medical management.

Nonoperative treatment includes control of diarrhea and vomiting by drug therapy. Antibiotics are given to control infection and reduce fever, which always accompanies infection. A high protein and vitamin diet is necessary. But if the diarrhea and vomiting persist, intravenous feeding becomes a must. Blood transfusions may be required for individuals who have had severe rectal bleeding. Since there is no absolute cure, the disease may recur.

Appendicitis

The *vermiform appendix* is a narrow tubular attachment to the colon. It can become obstructed by the presence of undigested food such as small seeds from fruits, or by hard bits of feces. This irritates the appendix and causes inflammation to set in. If it is obstructed, pressure builds within the appendix due to increasing secretions, a situation that can result in rupture of the appendix. A ruptured appendix can be rapidly fatal if *peritonitis*, inflamma-

tion of the peritoneal cavity, sets in.

In most cases the onset of appendicitis is heralded by an acute attack of pain in the center of the abdomen. The pain intensity increases, shifts to the right lower abdomen with nausea, vomiting, and fever as added symptoms. Some individuals, however, suffer from recurrent attacks of dull pain without other signs of gastrointestinal disease, and these may not be significant enough to warrant immediate hospitalization.

Diagnosis of appendicitis is usually dependent on the above symptoms, along with tenderness in the appendix area, increased pulse rate, and decreasing blood pressure. The last two are very significant if the appendix ruptures and peritonitis sets in. Whenever these symptoms are observed, the patient should be rushed to the nearest hospital.

Immediate surgical removal of the diseased appendix by means of a small incision is necessary in all nonperforated acute cases. This type of operation (*appendectomy*) is no longer considered major surgery. If the appendix ruptures and peritonitis is evident, emergency major surgery is necessary to drain the infection and remove the appendix. In the absence of post-operative complications, the patient recovers completely. One of the major problems of appendicitis is early diagnosis to prevent dangerous complications.

Intestinal Parasites

Not all the diseases of man are caused by microscopic organisms. Some are caused by parasitic worms, *helminths*, which invade the digestive tract, most often via food and water. In recent years government health agencies have largely eliminated the prime sources of worm infection: unwholesome meat or untreated sewage that finds its way into drinking water. Nevertheless, helminths still exist. Drugs used to expel worms are called *vermifuges* or *anthelmintics*.

The following are among the major intestinal parasites:

TAPEWORMS (CESTODES): These ribbon-shaped flat worms are found primarily in beef, fish, and pork that have not been thoroughly cooked. There are several species ranging from inch-long worms to tapeworms that grow to about 30 feet and live for as long as 16 years.

Tapeworms attach themselves to intestinal mucosa and periodically expel their eggs in excreta. If such feces are carelessly disposed of, the eggs can reach drinking water and be taken in by fish or ingested by grazing cattle. The eggs hatch in the animal's large bowel and find their way into the bloodstream by boring through the intestinal wall. Once in the blood they eventually adhere to muscles and live a dormant life in a capsule.

People who eat raw or partially cooked meat and fish that are infested with tapeworms become infected. The worms enter the bowel, where they feed, grow, and produce eggs. When the egg-filled segments are excreted, the cycle begins anew. Tapeworm infection is usually asymptomatic. It is discovered when egg-laden segments in feces are recognized as such.

Medication must be given on an empty stomach, followed later by a laxative. This will dislodge the worms and enable the body to purge itself of them. A weekly check of stools for segments of the worms may be necessary to confirm that the host is free of the parasites.

HOOKWORMS: There are many species of these tiny, threadlike worms

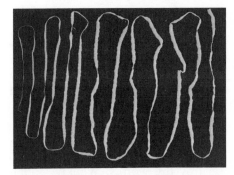

Some species of tapeworms, such as this specimen of the genus *Taenia*, can grow to about 30 feet. Tapeworm eggs are usually ingested with improperly cooked food.

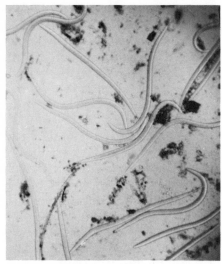

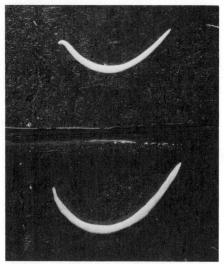

Hookworm eggs hatch into larvae (*left*, greatly enlarged) that can penetrate the skin of a bare foot. (*Right*, also much enlarged) Two adult hookworms: one *(top)* a variety with teeth resembling flat plates (genus *Necator*), the other *(bottom)* having hook-shaped teeth (genus *Ancylostoma*).

which are usually less than one centimeter long. They are found principally in tropical and subtropical areas of China, North Africa, Europe, Central America, and the West Indies, but they are by no means extinct in the United States.

The eggs are excreted in the feces of infected individuals, and if fecal materials are not well disposed of, the eggs may be found on the ground of unsanitary areas. In warm, moist conditions they hatch into larvae that penetrate the skin, especially the feet of people who walk around barefooted. The larvae can also be swallowed in impure water.

Hookworm-infected individuals, most often children, may experience an inflammatory itch in the area where the larvae entered. The host becomes anemic from blood loss, due to parasitic feeding of the worms, develops a cough, and experiences abdominal pain with diarrhea. Sometimes there is nausea or a distended abdomen. Diagnosis is confirmed by laboratory analysis of feces for the presence of eggs.

Successful treatment requires administration of anthelmintic drugs, preferably before breakfast, to destroy the worms. Weekly laboratory examination of the feces for evidence of hookworm eggs is a necessary precaution in ascertaining that

the disease has been eradicated. Untreated hookworm infestation often leads to small bowel obstruction.

TRICHINOSIS: This sometimes fatal disease is caused by a tiny worm, *Trichinella spiralis*, which is spread to man by eating improperly cooked pork containing the tiny worms in a capsulated form. After they are ingested the worms are set free to attach themselves to the mucosa of the small intestines. Here they mature in a few days and mate; the male dies and the female lays eggs that reach the muscles via the vascular system.

Trichinella organisms cause irritation of the intestinal mucosa. The infected individual suffers from abdominal pains with diarrhea, nausea, and vomiting. Later stages of the disease are marked by stiffness, pain, and swelling in the muscles, fever with sweating, respiratory distress, insomnia, and swelling of the face and eyelids. Death may result from complications such as pneumonia, heart damage, or respiratory failure. Despite government inspection of meats, all pork should be well-cooked before eating.

THREADWORMS (NEMATODES): These worms, also called pinworms, infect children more often than adults. Infection occurs by way of the mouth. The worms live in the bowel and sometimes journey through the anus,

where they cause intense itching. The eggs are laid at the anal opening, and can be blown about in the air and spread in that manner. The entire family must be medically treated to kill the egg-laying females, and soothing ointment should be applied at the rectal area to relieve the itching. Good personal hygiene, especially hand washing after toilet use, is an essential part of the treatment.

ROUND WORMS (ASCARIS): These intestinal parasites closely resemble earthworms. The eggs enter the digestive tract and hatch in the small bowel. The young parasites then penetrate the walls of the bowel, enter the bloodstream and find their way to the liver, heart, and lungs.

Untreated roundworm infestation leads to intestinal obstruction or blockage of pancreatic and bile ducts caused by the masses of roundworms, which usually exist in the hundreds. Ingestion of vermifuge drugs is the required treatment.

Food Poisoning

Acute gastrointestinal illnesses may result from eating food that is itself poisonous, from ingesting chemical poisons, or from bacterial sources.

Infant botulism was reported for the first time in 1976, in several cases in California. Unlike adults, infants can convert botulism spores to toxin.

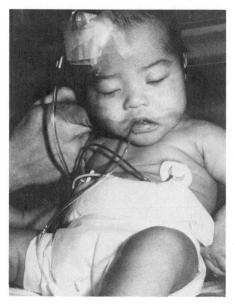

The bacteria can either manufacture *toxins* (poisonous substances) or cause infection. Improperly canned fish, meats, and vegetables may encourage the growth of certain toxin-manufacturing organisms that resist the action of gastric juice when ingested. A person who eats such foods may contract a type of food poisoning known as *botulism*. The symptoms include indigestion and abdominal pain, nausea and vomiting, blurred vision, dryness in the mouth and throat, and poor muscular coordination.

If the toxins become fixed in the central nervous system, they may cause death. Emergency hospitalization is required, where antitoxins are administered intravenously and other measures are taken to combat the effects of botulism.

Salmonella food poisoning is caused by a species of bacteria of that name and is spread by eating contaminated meat, or by eating fish, egg, and milk products that have not been properly cooked or stored or inadequately refrigerated. The organisms are also transmitted by individuals who handle well-prepared food with dirty hands. Victims suffer from vomiting, diarrhea, abdominal pain, and fever. This type of food poisoning can be fatal in children and the aged, especially if the latter are ailing. Medical treatment with hospitalization, administration of broad-spectrum antibiotics, and intravenous fluids (to replace body loss due to vomiting) is required.

Some people develop allergic reactions to certain foods and break out in severe rashes after a meal containing any of these foods. Among such foods are fruits, eggs, and milk or milk products. Vomiting or diarrhea may also occur. The best treatment is to avoid eating such foods and, when necessary, supplement the diet with manufactured protein and vitamins.

Liver Disease

Cirrhosis

Chronic disease of the liver with

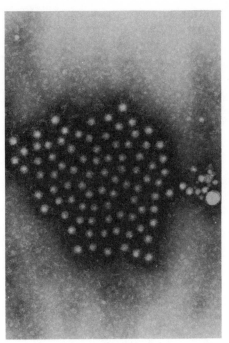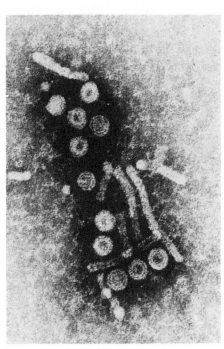

Antigens stimulate the development of antibodies that are specific against a particular disease. *(Left)* Antigens coated with antibodies against infectious hepatitis and *(right)* serum hepatitis antigens in filamentous form.

the destruction of liver cells is known as *cirrhosis*. A common cause is excessive intake of alcoholic beverages along with malnutrition. However, there are other predisposing factors, such as inflammation of the liver *(hepatitis)*, syphilis, intestinal worms, jaundice or biliary tract inflammation, and disorders in blood circulation to the liver.

Victims of cirrhosis are usually anemic and have an elevated temperature, around 100° F. Alcoholics very often lose weight, suffer from indigestion, and have distended abdomens.

Accurate diagnosis of cirrhosis depends on complex laboratory tests of liver function, urine, and blood. If liver damage is not too far advanced, treatment of the complications and underlying causes can aid the liver cells in the process of regeneration. In long-standing chronic disease, liver damage may be irreversible. Alcoholics who forgo alcohol may be restored to health, depending on the extent of liver damage, with a proper diet rich in proteins and vitamins.

Successful treatment of liver cirrhosis may require long hospitalization with drug therapy and blood

transfusions. During alcoholic withdrawal, the patient may require close medical observation and psychiatric help. If the patient's jaundice improves and his appetite returns, recovery in milder cirrhosis cases is possible.

Jaundice

In diseases of the liver and biliary tract, excessive bile pigment *(bilirubin)* is recirculated into the bloodstream. It enters the mucous membranes and skin, giving them the characteristic yellow pigmentation of the disease.

Gallstones or tumors that obstruct the free flow of bile are one cause of jaundice. Other causes include hepatitis, overproduction of bile pigments with resultant accumulation of bile within the liver, cirrhosis, and congenital closure of the bile ducts, the last a common cause of jaundice in infancy.

Apart from the typical yellow appearance of the skin, jaundice generates such symptoms as body itching, vomiting with bile (indicated by the green appearance and bitter taste of vomit), diarrhea with undigested fats present in the stools, and enlargement of the liver with pain and tenderness in the right upper abdomen.

Treatment of jaundice requires continued medical care with hospitalization. Surgery may be necessary to remove stones in the biliary tract or other obstructions. If there is bacterial infection, antibiotic therapy is necessary.

Hepatitis

Inflammation of the liver results in the disease known as *hepatitis*. The most common cause is an infectious process brought on by viruses, jaundice, or high fevers. Other causes of hepatitis include intestinal parasites, circulatory disturbances (such as congestive heart failure), hypersensitivity to drugs, damage to the liver or kidneys, or bacterial infection elsewhere in the body.

One common form of this disease is *infectious hepatitis*, a highly contagious viral infection that often attacks children and young adults, especially those who congregate in large groups. Infectious hepatitis has been known to break out as an epidemic in schools, summer camps, music festivals, and military installations.

The virus is spread by food and water contaminated by feces from infected individuals; good sanitation thus becomes a vital preventive factor. Whole blood used in transfusions can transmit the organisms if the donor is infected. This form of the disease is known as *serum hepatitis*. With the great increase in the use of blood transfusions in recent years in complex surgery, the danger of transmitting serum hepatitis by infected blood or infected syringes has become correspondingly greater. Drug addicts are particularly vulnerable to serum hepatitis from the use of shared, infected needles.

SYMPTOMS: The incubation period of infectious hepatitis lasts from one to six weeks—that of serum hepatitis is longer—followed by fever with headache, loss of appetite (especially for fatty foods), and gastrointestinal distress (nausea, vomiting, diarrhea, or constipation). As the disease progresses, the liver becomes enlarged and the patient jaundiced. There may be some pain in the right upper abdomen.

TREATMENT: Bed rest, preferably hospital isolation, is a necessary step in the initial treatment stages. Drug therapy with steroids may hasten the recovery process, which may take three to four weeks. When discharged from the hospital, the patient is usually very weak.

Untreated hepatitis causes severe liver damage and may result in coma due to liver failure. Sometimes death occurs. Several assaults on the liver reduce the regeneration process and promote cirrhosis. Persons who may have been exposed to the causative virus can receive temporary immunity if they are given an injection of gamma globulin, especially if there is an epidemic. Recent research directed toward the development of a vaccine against serum hepatitis has been very encouraging, and gives rise to the hope that some day widescale outbreaks of this disease may become a thing of the past.

Gall Bladder Disease

The biliary tract is very often plagued by the presence of stones, either in the gall bladder or in one of the bile ducts. Gallstones are mostly a mixture of calcium carbonate, cholesterol, and bile salts, and can occur either as one large stone, a few smaller ones, or several very small stones.

When fats from the daily diet enter the small intestines, the concentrated bile from the gall bladder is poured into the duodenum via the bile ducts. Bile is necessary if fats are to be digested and absorbed. If stones are present in the biliary tract, the gall bladder will contract, but little or no bile will reach the fats in the small bowel.

A sharp pain to the right of the stomach is usually the first warning sign of gallstones, especially if the pain is felt soon after a meal of fatty foods—eggs, pork, mayonnaise, or fried foods. The presence of stones very often causes inflammation of the gall bladder and such symptoms as occasional diarrhea and nausea with vomiting and belching. The abdominal area near the gall bladder is usually very tender.

Untreated gall bladder disease leads to several possible complications. The obstructed bile pigments may be recirculated in the bloodstream, causing jaundice. Obstruction of the ducts causes increased pressure and may also result in perforation of the gall bladder or ducts. Acute inflammation of the biliary tract is always a possibility due to the irritation caused by the concentrated bile.

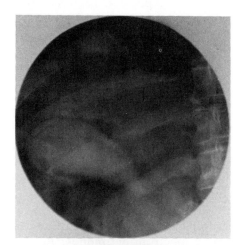

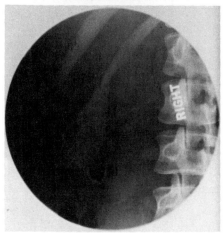

The normal gall bladder *(top)*, and a diseased gall bladder *(bottom)* filled with stones. The small stones are composed of calcium carbonate, cholesterol, and bile salts.

meals, or eating specific foods. Bland meals are vital in the treatment of peptic ulcers and should consist of unspiced soft foods and milk. Raw fruits and vegetables, salads, alcohol, and coffee do not belong in a bland diet. See under *Nutrition and Weight Control*, pp. 211–213, for further information on special diets.

X-ray examinations play an important role in diagnosis of gastrointestinal disorders, such as ulcers, diverticula, foreign bodies, malignant lesions, obstruction, achalasia of the esophagus, and varices.

Plain film radiographs are used in initial studies in cases where intestinal obstruction or perforation is suspected. Metallic foreign bodies are easily demonstrated on plain X rays of the digestive tract.

GI Series

By filling the digestive tract with *barium sulfate*, a substance opaque to X rays, a radiologist can locate areas of abnormality. Barium sulfate can be mixed as a thin liquid or paste and be swallowed by the patient during studies of the esophagus, stomach, and small intestines. The type of radiological examination which utilizes such a barium meal is known as a *GI (gastrointestinal) series*. The large bowel is examined with the barium mixture administered through the rectum like a standard enema, known as a *barium enema*. This procedure makes it possible to visualize the inner walls of the colon. For further information on diagnostic procedures, see Ch. 13, p. 289.

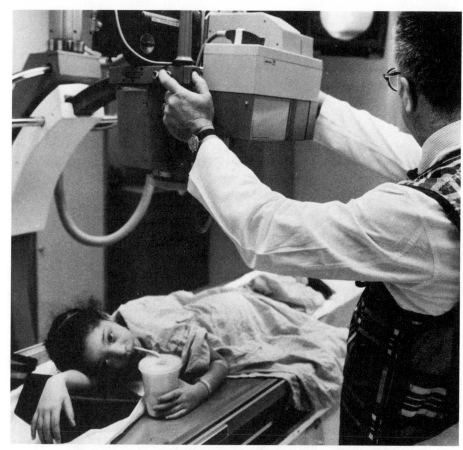

Barium sulfate, a substance opaque to X rays, is swallowed by patients during studies of the esophagus, stomach, and small intestines.

A gall bladder that is full of stones or badly diseased must be surgically removed for the patient's health to improve. In milder cases, other treatment and special diet can prevent attacks.

Treatment and Diagnosis of Gastrointestinal Disorders

Some medications used in treating gastrointestinal disorders, such as antacids and laxatives, can be purchased without prescription. Such medications should be taken only upon a physician's advice.

Treatment of gastrointestinal diseases may require low-residue diets—that is, a diet of foods that pass through the digestive tract very readily without a large amount of solid fecal residue. Included are low-fat meals, liquids, and finely crushed foods. Diagnostic tests may require overnight fasting, fat-free

CHAPTER 18

Diseases of
the Respiratory System

The human body cannot survive for more than a very few minutes in an environment that lacks oxygen. Oxygen is required for the normal functioning of all living body cells. This vital gas reaches the body cells via the bloodstream; each red blood cell transports oxygen molecules to the body tissues. The oxygen comes from the atmosphere one breathes, and it enters the bloodstream through the very thin membrane walls of the lung tissue, a fresh supply of oxygen entering the bloodstream each time a person inhales. As the red blood cells circulating through the walls of the lung tissue pick up their fresh supply of oxygen, they release molecules of carbon dioxide given off by the body cells as a waste product of metabolism. When a person exhales, the lungs are squeezed somewhat like a bellows, and the carbon dioxide is expelled from the lungs.

The automatic action of breathing in and out is caused by the alternate contraction and relaxation of several muscle groups. The main muscle of breathing is the *diaphragm,* a layer of muscle fibers that separates the organs of the chest from the organs of the abdomen. Other muscles of respiration are located between the ribs, in the neck, and in the abdomen. As the diaphragm contracts to let the lungs expand, the other muscles increase the capacity of the *thorax,* or chest cavity, when one inhales. The muscles literally squeeze the lungs and chest when an individual exhales.

Any disease of the muscles and bones of the chest wall or of the passages leading from the nose to the lung tissue—containing the small air sacs where the gases are actually exchanged—will interfere to some extent with normal function. As with any organ of the body, there is a great reserve built into the lungs that assures that small to even moderate amounts of diseased tissue can exist without compromising their ability to sustain life. However, when disease of the lungs, air passages, *thoracic* (rib) *cage,* or any combination of these parts decreases the capacity of the reserve areas, then the oxygen supply to all the organs and tissues of the body becomes deficient, and they become incapable of performing their vital functions.

Diseases of the thoracic cage are relatively uncommon. Certain forms of arthritis cause fixation of the bony cage and limit expansion when breathing. Various muscle and nervous system diseases weaken the muscles used to expand the chest for breathing.

Diseases of the *bronchi* or air passages tend to narrow those tubes and thereby limit the amount of air that can pass through to the tiny *alveoli* or air sacs. Other conditions affect the alveoli themselves, and, if widespread enough, allow no place for the oxygen and carbon dioxide to be exchanged.

The most common forms of lung disease are infections caused by vi-

THE DIAPHRAGM

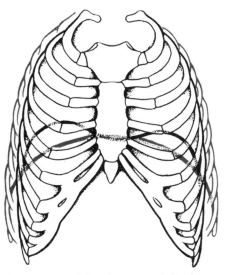

The positions of the rib cage and diaphragm are shown during inspiration of breath (expanded) and expiration (contracted). Volume of the chest area increases during inspiration as the diaphragm is stretched.

ruses, bacteria, or fungi. Infection is always a potential threat to the lung, since this organ is in constant contact with the outside air and therefore constantly exposed to infectious agents. It is only through elaborate defenses that the body is able to maintain normal functions without interference by these agents.

The major defenses are simply mechanical and consist mainly of the hairs in the nose and a mucous blanket coating the inside of the bronchi. The very small hairs (called *cilia*) in the breathing passage act as a filtering system; mucous membranes of the bronchi help to intercept small particles as they are swept along by the action of the cilia. Whenever these structures are diseased, as in chronic bronchitis, there is a much greater likelihood of acquiring infection.

The Common Cold, Influenza, and Other Viral Infections

The Common Cold

The common cold is the most prevalent illness known to mankind. It accounts for more time lost from work than any other single condition. The infection rate varies from one individual to another.

Surveys indicate that about 25 percent of the population experience four or more infections a year, 50 percent experience two or three a year, and the remaining 25 percent have one or no infections in a year. There is also some variation from year to year for each person, explained often by the amount of exposure to young children, frequent extreme changes in weather, fatigue, and other factors.

For years it has been felt that chilling plays a role in causing the common cold, and, although difficult to prove, there is almost certainly some truth to the idea. By some as yet unclear process, chilling probably causes certain changes in our respiratory passages that make them susceptible to viruses that otherwise

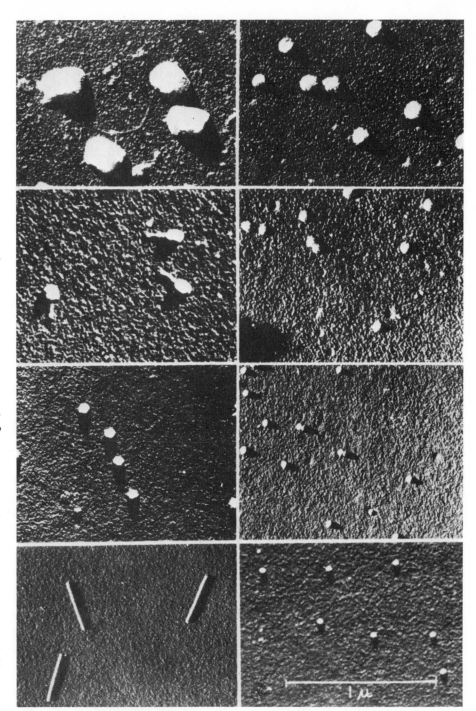

Micrographs (photographs of microscopic images) of viruses. The symbol μ in the lower righthand box is the Greek letter mu, which stands for micron, 1/1000th of a millimeter, or less than 4/10,000ths of an inch. One can gauge from this how small are the viruses shown here.

would be harmless.

The common cold affects only the upper respiratory passages: the nose, sinuses, and throat. It sometimes is associated with fever. Several viruses have been implicated as the cause for the common cold. But in the study centers that investigate this illness, isolation of a cold virus is only achieved in about one half of the cases. These viruses are not known to produce any other significant illnesses. Most likely they inhabit the nose and throat, often without producing any illness at all.

SYMPTOMS: The major part of the

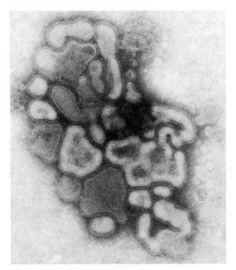

A photomicrograph of the influenza virus. Electron microscopy gave scientists their first clear look at this virus in 1960.

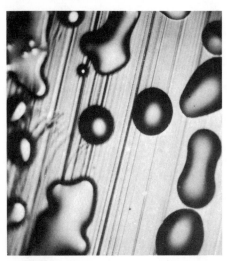

A photomicrograph of colonies of the pneumococcus bacteria, which can cause severe pneumonia.

ing activity, and late hours that can further lower the defenses and lead to complications.

COMPLICATIONS: Ear infection may develop due to blockage of the *Eustachian tube*, which leads from the back of the throat to the inner part of the ear. That complication is heralded by pain in the ear. Bronchitis and pneumonia may be recognized early by the development of cough and production of *sputum* (phlegm). *Sinusitis* develops when the sinus passages are obstructed so that the infected mucus cannot drain into the pharynx (as in postnasal drip). The pain develops near the sinus cavity involved. These com-

plications can and should be treated with specific drugs, and, if they develop, a physician should be consulted.

Influenza

A number of other viruses cause respiratory illness similar to the common cold, but are much more severe in intensity and with frequently serious, and even fatal, complications. The best known member of the group is the *influenza* (flu) virus. It can cause mild symptoms that are indistinguishable from those of the common cold, but in the more easily recognizable form it is ushered in by fever, cough, and what doctors refer

illness consists of about three days of nasal congestion, possibly a mild sore throat, some sneezing and irritation of the eyes (though not as severe as in hay fever), and a general feeling of ill health often associated with some muscle fatigue and aching. After three days the symptoms abate, but there is usually some degree of nasal congestion for another ten days.

Prevention is difficult, and there is no specific treatment. The natural defenses of the body usually are capable of resolving the infection. Attention should be paid to avoiding further chilling of the body, exhaust-

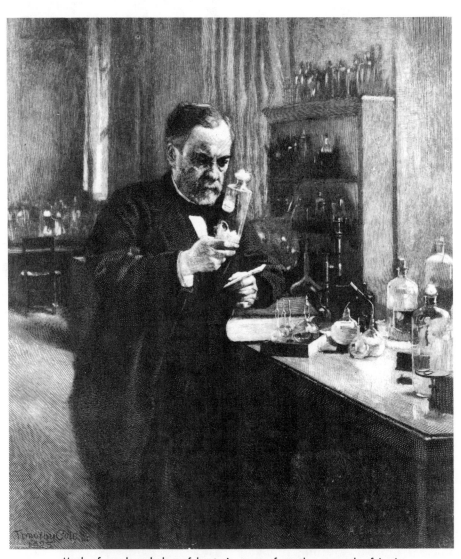

Much of our knowledge of bacteria comes from the research of Louis Pasteur (1822–1895). He proved that bacteria spread diseases, that heat can kill germs (pasteurization), and that an animal can be immunized against a disease by injecting it with weakened microbes (vaccination).

to as *malaise*—chills, muscle ache, and fatigue.

The symptoms of influenza appear quickly; they develop within hours and generally last in severe form from four to seven days. The disease gradually recedes over the following week. The severity of the local respiratory and generalized symptoms usually forces the influenza patient to stay in bed.

Not only is the individual case often severe, but an outbreak of influenza can easily spread to epidemic proportions in whole population groups, closing factories, schools, and hospitals in its wake. There have been 31 very severe *pandemics* (epidemics that sweep many countries) that have occurred since 1510. The most devastating of these pandemics occurred in 1918; it led to the death of twenty million people around the world. Rarely is death directly attributable to the influenza virus itself, but rather to complicating bacterial pneumonia or to the failure of vital organs previously weakened by chronic disease.

FLU SHOTS: Inoculation is fairly effective in preventing influenza, but is not long-lasting and has to be renewed each year. Unfortunately, there are several different types of influenza virus, and a slightly different vaccine is needed to provide immunity to each type of infection. Each recent epidemic in the United States has been the result of a different strain, and although there have been several months' warning before the epidemics started, it has been difficult to mass-produce a vaccine in time to use it before the epidemic developed.

TREATMENT: Once acquired, there is no cure for influenza, but the body defenses are usually capable of destroying the virus if given the necessary time and if the defenses are not depressed by other illness. Fluids, aspirin, and bed rest help relieve the symptoms. Special attention should be paid to sudden worsening of fever after seeming recovery, or the onset of sputum production. In elderly people more intensive medical care is often necessary, including hospitalization for some.

Pneumonia

Pneumonia might be defined as any inflammation of the lung tissue itself, but the term is generally applied only to infections of an acute or rapidly developing nature caused by certain bacteria or viruses. The term is generally not used for tuberculous or fungal infections. The most common severe pneumonia is that caused by the *pneumococcus bacterium*.

Pneumonia develops from inhaling infected mucus into the lower respiratory passages. The pneumococcus is often present in the nasal or throat secretions of healthy people, and it tends to be present even more often in the same secretions of an individual with a cold. Under certain conditions these secretions may be *aspirated*, or inhaled, into the lung. There the bacteria rapidly multiply and spread within hours to infect a sizable area. As with the common cold, chilling and fatigue often play a role in making this sequence possible. Any chronic debilitating illness also makes one very susceptible to pneumonia.

SYMPTOMS: Pneumonia develops very suddenly with the onset of high fever, shaking chills, chest pain, and a very definite feeling of total sickness or malaise. Within hours enough pus is produced within the lung for the patient to start coughing up thick yellow or greenish sputum which often may be tinged or streaked with blood. The patient has no problem in recognizing that he has suddenly become extremely ill.

Prior to penicillin the illness tended to last about seven days, at which time it would often suddenly resolve almost as quickly as it started, leaving a healthy but exhausted patient. But it also could frequently lead to death or to serious complications, such as abscess formation within the chest wall, meningitis, or abscess of the brain. Since penicillin is so very effective in curing this ill-

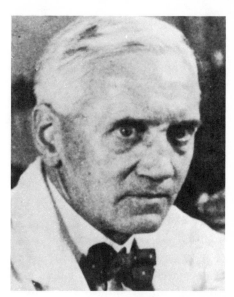

The bacteria-destroying capacity of the penicillin mold was discovered in 1929 by the Scottish bacteriologist, Sir Alexander Fleming (1881–1955). The subsequent development of penicillin to treat bacterial infections must surely be considered one of the great medical achievements of this century.

ness today, doctors rarely see those complications.

TREATMENT: The response of pneumococcal pneumonia to penicillin is at times one of the most dramatic therapeutic events in medicine. After only several hours of illness the patient presents himself to the hospital with a fever of 104 degrees, feeling so miserable that he does not want to eat, talk, or do anything but lie still in bed. Within four to six hours after being given penicillin he may have lost his fever and be sitting up in bed eating a meal. Not everyone responds this dramatically, but when someone does, it is striking.

PREVENTION: There is no guaranteed way to prevent pneumonia. The advice to avoid chilling temperatures, overexertion, and fatigue when one has a cold is directed principally toward avoiding pneumonia. Anybody exposed to the elements, especially when fatigued and wearing damp clothing, is particularly susceptible to pneumonia; this explains its frequent occurrence among army recruits and combat troops. The elderly and debilitated become more susceptible when exposed to extremes of temperature and dampness.

Pneumonia is not really a contagious illness except in very special circumstances, so that isolation of patients is not necessary. In fact, all of us carry the pneumococcus in our noses and throats, but we rarely have the constellation of circumstances that lead to infection. It is the added physical insults that allow pneumonia to take hold.

Other Kinds of Pneumonia

All bacteria are capable of causing pneumonia and they do so in the same manner, via the inhalation of infected upper airway secretions. Some diseases, such as alcoholism, tend to predispose to certain bacterial pneumonias. Usually these are not as dramatic as those caused by the pneumococcus, but they may be much more difficult to treat and thereby can often be more serious.

Far less severe are the pneumonias caused by certain viruses or a recently discovered organism that seems to be intermediate between a virus and bacterium. The term *walking pneumonia* is often applied to this type, because the patient is often so little incapacitated that he is walking about and not in bed. These pneumonias apparently occur in the same way as the bacterial pneumonias, but the difference is that the infecting agent is not capable of producing such severe destruction. These pneumonias are usually associated with only mild temperature elevation, scant amount of sputum production, and fewer general body symptoms. They should be suspected when coughing dominates the symptoms of a cold, especially if it turns from a dry or nonproductive cough to one that produces sputum. Antibiotic therapy tends to hasten recovery and prevent the complication of bacterial pneumonia.

Pleurisy

No discussion of pneumonia is complete without mention of *pleurisy*. This term refers to any inflam-

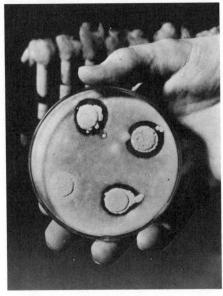

Disks of blotting paper soaked in antibiotic solution were placed on this Petri dish "seeded" with germs. The dark rings around the disks show the antibiotic inhibited bacterial growth.

mation of the lining between the chest wall and the lung. Infection is only one of the causes, but probably the most common, of inflammation of the *pleura*. Pleurisy is almost always painful, the pain being felt on inhaling and exhaling but not when the breath is quietly held for a brief period. It is a symptom that always deserves the attention of a physician and investigation of its cause. The same type of pain on breathing can often be mimicked by a strain of the

chest wall muscles, but the difference can usually be determined by a physician's examination. If not, a chest X ray will help to reveal the cause of the pain.

Tuberculosis

At the turn of the century *tuberculosis* was the leading cause of death in the world; now it is eighteenth. The change in status is due both to the discovery of antibiotics and to modern preventive measures. In this century most other infectious diseases have likewise decreased in incidence and severity for similar reasons. The general decline leaves tuberculosis still at the top of the list as the leading cause of death among infectious diseases. And tuberculosis remains a very serious health problem, accounting for 40,000 new illnesses every year in the United States. In contrast to a disease like influenza, doctors already have the tools with which to eliminate tuberculosis. But many factors, primarily social, make that a very distant possibility.

Tuberculosis is caused by one specific type of bacterium. Certain ethnic groups seem particularly susceptible to the disease, but the reasons are unclear. The American Indian and the Eskimo are two sus-

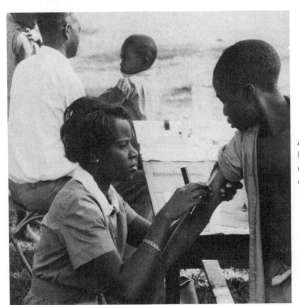

A technician from the World Health Organization vaccinates a young man in a campaign against tuberculosis in Uganda.

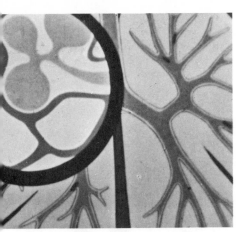

These photographs illustrate how tubercle bacilli infiltrate the air sacs of the lungs. Bacilli (dark, rodlike spots) have been breathed into the lungs.

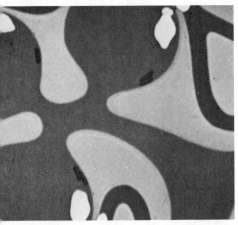

The tubercle bacilli have settled on the walls of air sacs of the lung. White cells from a nearby capillary move through the capillary wall into the air sacs.

ceptible groups. However, there is no recognized hereditary factor. The disease is different from many commonly known infections in several ways. Unlike pneumonia, tuberculosis is a chronic and painless infection, measured more in months than in days. Because of this pattern, it not only takes a long time to develop serious disease, but it also takes a long time to effect a cure.

Another very important difference between tuberculosis and many other infections is its ability to infect individuals without causing symptoms of illness, but then to lie dormant as a potential threat to that person for the rest of his life. The early stages of the disease do not produce any symptoms. Consequently a pa-

tient develops large areas of diseased tissue before he begins to feel sick. Screening procedures, therefore, are very important in detecting early disease in patients who feel perfectly healthy. Another is the skin testing of schoolchildren, which is carried out routinely in many communities today.

How Tuberculosis Spreads

Tuberculosis is contracted by inhaling into the lungs bacteria that have been coughed into the air by a person with advanced disease. It is, therefore, contagious, but not as contagious as measles, mumps, or chicken pox. Unlike those illnesses, it usually requires fairly close and prolonged contact with a tuberculous patient before the infection is passed on. Once the bacteria are inhaled, the body defenses are usually capable of isolating them into small areas within the tissues, thereby preventing any significant destruction or disease. However, though defenses are able to isolate the bacteria, they are not able to destroy all of them. Some bacteria persist in a state in which they are unable to break out and destroy tissue, but they always maintain the potential to do so at a time when the body defenses are impaired.

In about 20 percent of individuals the body defenses are not initially capable of isolating the tubercle bacilli. These individuals, mostly children, develop progressive tuber-

culosis directly following their initial contact. Others are successful in preventing actual disease at the time of initial contact, but they join a large group with the potential for active disease at some time in the future. Most of the new cases of active tuberculosis come from this second group; their defenses break down years after the initial contact and resultant infection.

Weight loss, malnutrition, alcoholism, diabetes, and certain other chronic illnesses are particularly likely to lead to deterioration of the defense mechanisms holding the tuberculosis organisms in check. Still other individuals develop active disease with no recognizable condition to account for the loss of defenses. In fact, the most likely age group to develop active disease as a result of breakdown of past infection is the 20- to 30-year-old group.

Once active disease has appeared it usually involves the chest, although it can develop anywhere in the body. There is gradual spread of inflammation within lung tissue until large areas are involved. Holes, or cavities, are formed as a result of tissue destruction. These contain large numbers of tuberculosis organisms and continue to enlarge as new tissue is destroyed at the edges. At any stage of this development organisms may find their way into the bloodstream and new foci of disease can spring up throughout the body. The sputum becomes loaded with

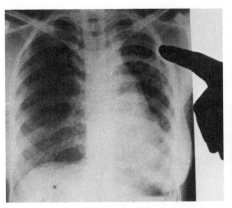
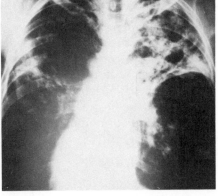

Lung-tissue destruction caused by tuberculosis results in cavities that show up as shadows on X-ray film. *(Left)* A physician points to such a shadow. *(Right)* Shadows on this X ray reveal advanced cavitary tuberculosis.

organisms that are coughed into the air and go on to infect other individuals. The infected sputum from one area of the lung may gain access to other areas and cause development of diseased tissue there as well.

Treatment

Before the modern era of drug treatment all these events followed an inexorable course to death in 85 percent of people with active tuberculosis. Only a lucky few were able to survive as cured, usually because their disease was found at an early stage. That survival was often at the expense of years confined to a sanatorium. Because of its almost uniform outcome and the required separation from family and home, tuberculosis was formerly looked upon with quite as much dread as cancer is today.

The sanatorium rest cure of tuberculosis was first developed in the mid-nineteenth century at a time when the cause of the disease was unknown. In 1882, Robert Koch first demonstrated the tuberculosis organism, thereby proving the disease was an infection. As the twentieth century progressed, general public health measures helped limit the number of new cases, and new surgical procedures were developed to treat the disease. These measures were effective enough to arrest tuberculosis in another 25 percent of cases, brightening somewhat the dismal outlook of the past century.

But the discovery of specific antibiotics in the 1940s made the real difference in tuberculosis. Because of drug treatment, surgery is rarely resorted to today, although it still may be helpful in certain patients. Now patients with tuberculosis can face a relatively bright future without having to be hospitalized for prolonged periods or enduring periods of endless disability.

Tuberculosis Control

People still contract tuberculosis, and people still die from it. Two of the principal causes of death are delayed therapy and interruptions in therapy, the latter leading to the development of tuberculosis organisms that are unaffected by drugs. Both of these causes are often under the control of the patient. The first can be avoided by seeing a physician whenever one develops a cough that lasts more than two weeks, especially when it is not associated with the typical symptoms of a cold at the outset. The other symptoms of developing tuberculosis are also seen in other illnesses, and should always lead one to recognize that he is sick and needs to consult his physician. These symptoms are weight loss, loss of appetite, fever, and night sweats. When tuberculosis is diagnosed, the patient must follow carefully the directions regarding medication, which is always continued for a long time after the patient has regained his feeling of well-being.

There are other ways, however, to attack tuberculosis, even before one becomes sick. Once a person has had contact with tuberculosis, even though he usually does not develop active disease, he produces antibodies against the bacteria. A person with such antibodies can be recognized by injecting under the skin specially prepared material from dead tuberculosis bacteria which gives rise to a reaction within the skin after two days. This material is called *tuberculin* and the test is known as the *tuberculin test*.

There are now many mass screening programs of tuberculin testing for schoolchildren, hospital personnel, and industrial groups. Those with positive skin test reactions are screened further for the presence of active disease. If they are found to be active cases, they are treated during what is usually an early and not very severe stage of the disease. The other people with positive tuberculin tests, without any evidence of active disease, are candidates for *prophylactic* (preventive) *therapy.* This therapy employs *isoniazid (INH)*, the most effective of many drugs for the treatment of tuberculosis and one that has virtually no side effects. Treatment for one year

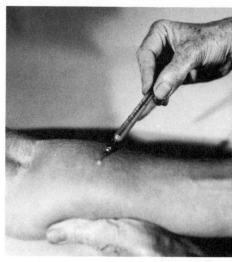

The tuberculin test is given to determine if antibodies are being produced against the tubercle bacilli, which may be present without active disease.

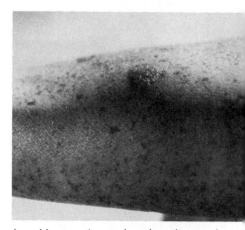

A positive reaction to the tuberculin test demands further screening for the presence of active disease. If none is found, preventive therapy is indicated.

has been shown to reduce greatly the chance of future progress from the merely infected state to the state of active disease.

The goal of prophylactic therapy is chiefly to prevent the far more serious development of active disease. But in addition, by preventing disease before it develops, physicians can prevent the infection of others, since the typical patient with tuberculosis has already infected some of those living with him before he becomes ill and seeks medical attention. The surface has just been scratched in this regard, however, as there are estimated to be 25 million people in the United States who would demonstrate reactions to tuberculin tests. Many of these people have never been tested and are not aware of the potential threat within them.

In most foreign countries the tuberculosis problem is much more serious. An estimated 80 percent of the populations of the countries of Asia, Africa, and South America would show positive tuberculin skin tests, with the number of active cases and deaths being proportionately high.

Sarcoidosis

Sarcoidosis (or *Boeck's sarcoid*), a disease that affects black people more often than whites, has symptoms closely resembling those of tuberculosis and other diseases. The most obvious symptom is the formation of skin nodules, often of the face, but the nodules, called *granulomas* (small tumors composed chiefly of granulation tissue), commonly occur in many other places as well, especially in the lungs and lymph nodes. They can occur also in the liver, bones, eyes, and other tissues.

Although sarcoidosis occurs all over the world, it is more common in temperate regions, and in the United States occurs more frequently in the southeastern states than elsewhere. Men and women are about equally affected. The onset of the disease occurs usually in the third or fourth decade of life.

Diagnosis and Treatment

The disease is diagnosed by an examination of chest X rays, which will show the proliferation of nodules in the lungs. Surgical biopsy and microscopic examination of skin tissue or tissue from a lymph node is usually necessary to confirm the presence of the disease.

There is no specific treatment for sarcoidosis, and in spite of its similarities in some respects to tuberculosis, no connection between the two disorders has been established. Steroids are sometimes used to treat the skin lesions, but in many cases the skin nodules clear up eventually without any treatment. About half of the patients, however, do not recover completely, and the disease becomes chronic—though of varying severity. Ultimately the granulomas can change into fibrous scars that may pose serious threats to the patient, depending upon where the scarring occurs. Respiratory distress, heart failure, and glaucoma, for example, can result from tissue changes in the lungs, heart, and eyes, respectively.

Respiratory Diseases Caused by Fungi

Two fungal diseases affecting respiration are of great importance in particular regions of the United States. They are both caused by types of fungi capable of growing within mammalian tissue, thereby infecting and destroying it. Both cause chronic diseases very similar to tuberculosis and may lead to death, though that is a far less common outcome— even when untreated—than in tuberculosis.

The spores of the fungi are inhaled from the air, and the response of the body is similar to that in tuberculosis in that most people become merely infected (the spores being contained by body defenses) while a few develop progressive disease. The body also produces antibodies, and consequently skin tests similar to the tuberculin test can identify infected individuals.

Histoplasmosis (named for a fungus called *histoplasma*) organisms are prevalent in the Midwest, generally in the areas of the Ohio, Mississippi, and Missouri Rivers. Largely unknown prior to World War II, histoplasmosis has been studied extensively since. Local epidemics have brought it to public attention on several occasions. The fungus grows readily in soil containing large amounts of bird (chickens, pigeons, starlings) or bat excrement. One of the better ways to assure exposure is to clean out an old chicken coop. The concentration of organisms may reach such high levels in bat caves that entry by spelunkers may prove fatal. In contrast to tuberculosis, the amount of exposure seems to play a very important role in determining the extent of disease. There also seem to be few cases of late break-

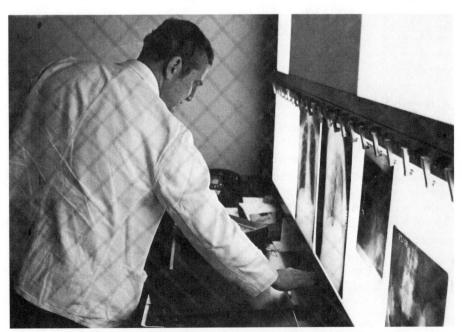

Sarcoidosis is diagnosed by examination of chest X rays, which reveal the presence of many small nodules, or granulomas, in the lungs.

down (the rule in tuberculosis). Most people develop the active disease, if at all, at the time of their initial exposure.

Coccidioidomycosis (for *coccidioides* fungus) also generates in the soil, in this case in California, the southwest United States, and Mexico. It grows best in hot, dry soil. The common names for this disease are *desert rheumatism* or *valley fever*. Infection and disease occur in a similar pattern to that of histoplasmosis. Skin testing of large population groups for both these fungi in the appropriate geographical areas indicates that the majority of exposed individuals quite adequately contain the initial infection and never develop any illness or active disease.

Because Americans travel into infected regions, these diseases are being seen more frequently in people who do not live where the fungi are found. Both conditions, fortunately, are often self-limited, even when active disease develops. For more severe cases there is a drug, *Amphotericin-B*, which is quite effective; however, since it is also quite toxic to the patient, it must be given in progressive doses starting with a small initial dose, to permit the body's tolerance to build up. It is hoped that less toxic agents will be found in the future that will be just as effective against the fungus.

Allergic Respiratory Diseases

Hay fever *(allergic rhinitis)* and *asthma* are two very common allergic diseases of the respiratory tract. The two have much in common as to age at onset, seasonal manifestations, and causation. Hay fever involves the *mucosa*, or lining, of the upper respiratory tract only, whereas asthma is confined to the bronchial tubes of the lower respiratory tract. Physicians usually distinguish two main types of asthma, allergic and infectious. The infectious type of asthma resembles bronchitis, with cough and much wheezing as well.

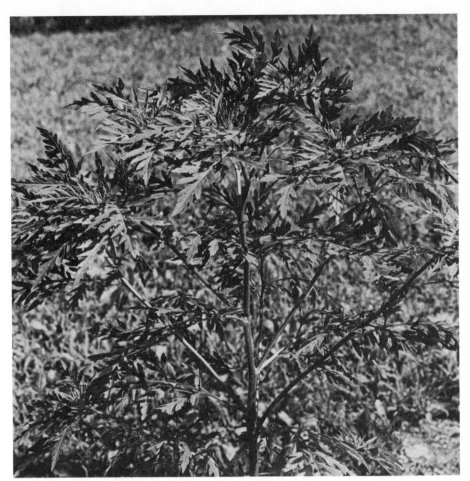

The pollen of the ragweed plant is one of the chief causes of hay fever, a late-summer allergy which affects the nasal passages and throat.

The discussion here will be confined to the allergic form of asthma.

In hay fever and asthma the allergenic substance causing the reaction is usually airborne, though it can be a food. In most cases the offender is pollen from a plant. The pollen is inhaled into the nostrils and alights upon the lining of the respiratory passages. In the allergic individual, antibodies react with the proteins in the pollen and cause various substances to be released from the tissue and blood cells in the immediate area. These substances, in turn, produce vessel engorgement in the area and an outpouring of mucus, plus certain irritating symptoms that result in a stuffy or runny nose and itchy eyes. The same reactions occur in the bronchial lining in asthma, but the substances released there also cause constriction of the bronchial muscle and consequent narrowing of

the passages. This muscular effect and the narrowing caused by greatly increased amounts of mucus in the passages are both responsible for the wheezing in asthma.

Hay Fever

Hay fever is never a threat to life, but in severe cases it can upset one's life patterns immensely. For unknown reasons it is more common in childhood, where it is often seen in conjunction with eczema or asthma. The tendency to develop hay fever, eczema, and asthma is hereditary. The transmission of the hereditary factors is complex, so that within a family group any number of individuals or none at all may exhibit the trait.

Most people with hay fever have their only or greatest difficulty in the summer months because of the airborne pollens from trees, grasses, flowers, and molds that are prevalent then. The most notorious of all pollens is the ragweed pollen. This weed pollinates around August 15 and continues to fill the air until late September. In many cities an official pollen count is issued every day, and those with severe difficulty can avoid some trouble by staying outside as little as possible on high-count days. *Antihistamine* drugs are used to counteract the nasal engorgement in hay fever. These drugs counteract the effects of *histamine,* which is one of the major substances released by the allergic reaction.

Allergic Asthma

Allergic asthma is the result of the allergic reaction taking place in the bronchial mucosal lining rather than in the nasal lining. A person may suffer from both asthma and hay fever. The common inciting factors are pollens, hair from pets (especially cats), house dust, molds, and certain foods (especially shellfish). When foods are responsible, the reaction initially occurs within the bloodstream, but the major effect is felt within the lung, which is spoken of as the target organ.

Most allergic asthma is seen in children. For unclear reasons it usually disappears spontaneously at puberty. In those who continue to have difficulty after puberty, the role of infection as a cause for the asthma usually becomes more prominent. Allergic asthma attacks start abruptly and can usually be aborted rather easily with medication.

People with asthma are symptom-free much of the time. When exposed to high concentrations of pollen they begin wheezing and producing sputum. Wheezing refers to the high-pitched squeaking sound that is made by people exhaling through narrowed bronchi. Associated with the wheezing and sputum is a distinct sensation of shortness of breath that varies in severity according to the nature of the attack. Milder at-

tacks of asthma often subside spontaneously, merely with relaxation. This is especially true when the wheezing is induced by nonspecific factors, such as a cloud of dust, cold air, or exercise. Asthmatic individuals have more sensitive air passages and they are more easily bothered by these nonspecific irritants.

TREATMENT: For more severe attacks of asthma there are several types of treatment. There are oral medications that dilate the bronchi and offset the effects of the allergic reaction. (Antihistamines, however, exert no effect on asthma and may even worsen the condition.) Also available are injectable medications, such as adrenaline, and sprays, that contain substances similar to adrenaline and that can be inhaled. Any or all of these methods may be employed by the physician. During times of high exposure it is often helpful to take one of the oral medications on a regular basis, thereby avoiding minor episodes of wheezing.

A recently discovered remedy for asthma is particularly useful to persons—primarily infants and small children—who cannot swallow tablets. The remedy comes in capsules containing tiny pellets of the drug theophylline. Once the capsule is twisted open, the pellets can be sprinkled on soft foods, including strained baby food, apple sauce, pudding, or hot or cold cereal. The pellets give relief for about 12 hours, long enough to protect children during sleep.

The best therapy for asthma and hay fever is avoidance of the allergen responsible for attacks. Obviously, cats and certain foods can be avoided more readily than pollens and other airborne substances. The first requisite, however, is to identify the offender. The most important method of identification is the patient's medical history. Sometimes the problem is easy, as when the patient states that he only has trouble during the ragweed season. At other times a great amount of detective work may be required. Skin testing is

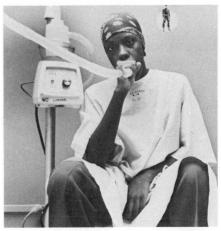

Patients with allergies receive inhalation therapy. Drafts of pure oxygen help force out air contaminated with dust and other allergens.

used to complement the history. The skin test merely involves the introduction under the skin (usually within a tiny scratch) of various materials suspected of being allergens. If the individual has antibodies to these substances he will form a hive at the site of introduction. That he reacts does not necessarily mean that his asthma is due to that test substance, because many people have reactions but no hay fever or asthma. The skin test results need to be interpreted in the light of the history of exposure.

If the substance so identified cannot be avoided, then hyposensitization may prove useful. This form of treatment is based on the useful fact that the human body varies its ability to react depending upon the degree and the frequency of exposure. In a hyposensitizing program, small amounts of pollen or other extract are injected frequently. Gradually the dose of extract is increased. By this technique many allergic individuals become able to tolerate moderate exposure to their offending material with few or no symptoms. Hyposensitization does not succeed in everyone, but it is usually worth attempting if other approaches are unsuccessful. For more information, See *Allergies and Hypersensitivities,* p. 283.

CHAPTER 19

Lung Disease

Two present-day problems of major proportions are not diseases in themselves, but both are detrimental to health. These are smoking and air pollution. The former is a habit that, in some users, can produce as serious results as narcotics or alcohol addiction. Knowledge of air pollution has grown with the increased public awareness of our environment. It is quite clear that there are many serious consequences produced by the products with which we foul our air. Both tobacco and air pollution are controllable: one by individual will, the other by public effort.

Smoking

Eighty-five million Americans smoke, and the vast majority of these people smoke cigarettes. This discussion will therefore center on cigarettes. The number of new smokers is increasing, which offsets the number of quitters, thereby producing a new gain in smokers each year. There was a temporary absolute decline in 1964 when the first U.S. Surgeon General's report on smoking outlined the many hazards, but that trend quickly reversed itself. The tobacco industry spends $280 million per year to promote smoking. The U.S. Public Health Service and several volunteer agencies spend $8 million in a contrary campaign to discourage smoking.

Dangers of Smoking

Scientists know much about the ways in which smoking produces health dangers. As they burn, cigarettes release more than 4,000 different substances into the atmosphere. Carried in the cigarette smoke, these substances enter the smoker's lungs or simply dissipate in the air. Three of the substances, carbon monoxide, "tar," and nicotine, are the primary threats to health.

Smoking has "mainstream" effects on the smoker who inhales. But there are "sidestream" effects as well. For example, persons who habitually breathe the smoke from others' cigarettes may be inhaling higher concentrations of possibly harmful chemicals than the smokers themselves. These nonsmokers may experience such unpleasant symptoms as watery eyes and headaches. If they have lung or heart diseases, suffer from asthma or some allergies, or wear contact lenses the nonsmokers may find that their symptoms are worsening.

Some of the direct effects of breathing tobacco smoke suggest its capacity for producing disease in the smoker. Smoking lowers skin temperature, often by several degrees, principally through the constricting effect of nicotine on blood vessels. Carbon monoxide levels rise in the blood when a person is smoking. Even a single cigarette may impair somewhat the smoker's ability to expel air from the lungs. Adverse changes in the activity of several important chemicals in the body can be demonstrated after smoking.

Smoking has been strongly implicated in bronchitis and emphysema, lung and other cancers, heart disease, and peripheral vascular disease. Cigarette smoking causes more "preventable" deaths in the United States than any other single factor. Of the five leading causes of American deaths, smoking is related to four. According to verified statistics, a smoker faces a 70 percent greater risk of dying prematurely than a nonsmoker of comparable age. Smoking-related diseases take six times as many American lives annually as automobile accidents.

A CAUSE OF CANCER: Lung cancer takes more American lives annually than any other type of cancer. Some 80 percent of all lung cancer deaths, over 90,000 in a typical year, may be attributed to cigarette smoking. On average, 7 in 10 lung cancer patients

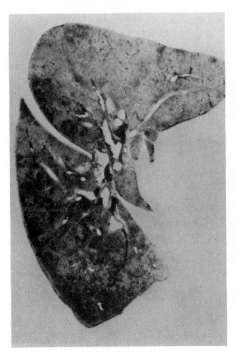
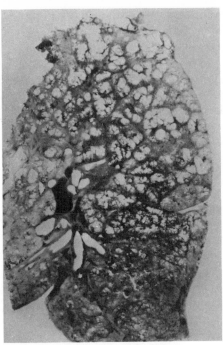

One of the effects of cigarette smoking is illustrated by these photographs. *(Left)* Normal lung tissue, with air sacs too fine to be visible. *(Right)* Lung tissue of a heavy smoker, showing numerous enlarged air sacs.

cer death in six in 1968, one-fourth of all such deaths occurred among women in 1979. Those figures suggest what later statistics have borne out: That lung cancer would soon— by 1985—replace breast cancer as the leading cause of cancer death among women.

Women were once thought to be less susceptible to smoking-related diseases than men. But later epidemiological studies have proved the opposite. When the earlier studies were conducted, women had simply not been smoking as long as men, or in such numbers. As the picture has changed, the statistics have changed. Like men, women smokers who experience other heart disease risk factors, including hypertension and high serum cholesterol levels, face a greatly increased risk of coronary heart disease.

THE DOSE-RESPONSE RELATIONSHIP: The number of cigarettes an individual smokes is one of the determinants of eventual damage even though individual susceptibility is also important. Thus a definite dose-response relationship exists

die within a year of diagnosis.

The cigarette smoker's risks are not confined to lung cancer. Such serious and sometimes fatal diseases as cancers of the mouth, pharynx, larynx, and esophagus may also be smoking-related. Of all cancer deaths, 30 percent are related to smoking. Smoking leads to 10 times as many cancer deaths as all other reliably identified cancer causes combined.

HEART DISEASE: Heart disease caused by smoking cigarettes takes more American lives than does cancer. But smoking is implicated in about 30 percent of all deaths resulting from coronary heart disease, the most common cause of American deaths. In 1982, about 170,000 U.S. citizens died of heart disease resulting from smoking.

In the middle 1980s, statistics showed that one living American in every 10 would die prematurely as a result of smoking-related heart disease. The smoker who refused to give up smoking after a heart attack was inviting a second attack to a significant degree. But the person who quit smoking would after some 10

years face a heart-disease risk about equal to that of a nonsmoker.

WOMEN AND SMOKING: Where women accounted for one lung can-

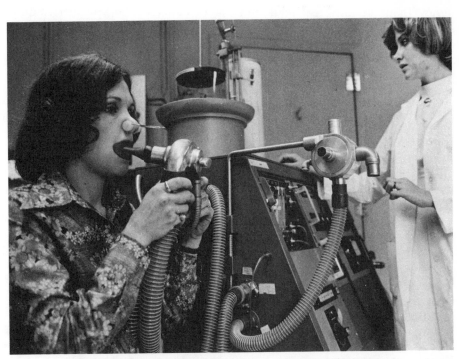

As the subject breathes into a tube, this lung-capacity machine registers changes in the volume of air and the speed of each breath. Smokers have been found to have impaired lung capacity compared to nonsmokers.

between smoking and disease. If a person smokes one pack a day for one year he has smoke one pack-year; if he smokes one pack a day for two years or two packs a day for one year, he has smoked two pack-years, and so on. Calculating by pack-years, it appears that 40 pack-years is a crucial time period above which the incidence of cancer of the lung, emphysema, and other serious consequences rises rapidly. Smoking three packs a day, it takes only about 13 years to reach this critical level.

Breaking the Smoking Habit

Obviously, the best way not to smoke is never to start. Unfortunately, young people are continuing to join the smoking ranks at a rapid rate. The teen-ager often is one of the hardest persons to convince of the hazards of smoking. He is healthy, suffers less from fatigue, headaches, breathlessness, and other immediate effects of smoking, and he often feels the need to smoke to keep up with his peers. Once he starts, it is not long before he becomes addicted. The addiction to cigarettes is very real. It is more psychological dependency than the physical addiction associated with narcotics, but there are definite physical addiction aspects to smoking that are mostly noted when one stops.

For most people it is quite a challenge to stop smoking. There are many avenues to travel and many sources now available to aid one on the way. They include smoking clinics that offer group support and medical guidance to those anxious to quit. The clinics vary in their format but basically depend on the support given the smoker by finding other individuals with the same problems and overcoming the problems as a group. The medical guidance helps people recognize and deal with withdrawal symptoms as well as helping them with weight control.

Withdrawal Symptoms

Withdrawal symptoms vary from person to person and include many symptoms other than just a craving for a cigarette. Many people who stop smoking become jittery and sleepless, start coughing more than usual, and often develop an increased appetite. This last withdrawal effect is especially disturbing to women, and the need to prevent weight gain is all too often used as a simple excuse to avoid stopping the cigarette habit or to start smoking again. The weight gained is usually not too great, and one generally stops gaining after a few weeks. Once the cigarette smoking problem is controlled, then efforts can be turned to weight reduction. Being overweight is also a threat to health, but ten extra pounds, even if maintained, do not represent nearly the threat that confirmed smoking does.

Despite all efforts, many individuals who would like to stop smoking fail in their attempts. The best advice for them is to keep trying. Continued effort will at least tend to decrease the amount of smoking and often leads to eventual abstinence, even after years of trying. If a three-pack-per-day smoker can decrease to one pack a day or less, he has helped himself even though he is still doing some damage. For prospective quitters it is important to remember that cigarette smoking is an acquired habit, and that the learning process can be reversed. The problem most people have is too little knowledge of the dangers and too much willingness to believe that disease and disability cannot strike them, just the other fellow.

Air Pollution

While 85 million Americans pollute the air they breathe individually with cigarettes, all 210 million of us collectively pollute the atmosphere we all breathe. Some people are obviously more responsible than others, but air, water, and land pollution is a disease of society and can only be solved through a concerted effort by the whole society. Pollution has always been a problem to man. As we have become more urbanized the problem has grown. It has now reached what many consider to be crisis proportions in our large cities and even in some of our smaller ones.

We have had ample warning. In 1948 a killer smog engulfed Donora, Pennsylvania, killing 20 persons and producing serious illness in 6,000 more. In 1952 a lingering smog over

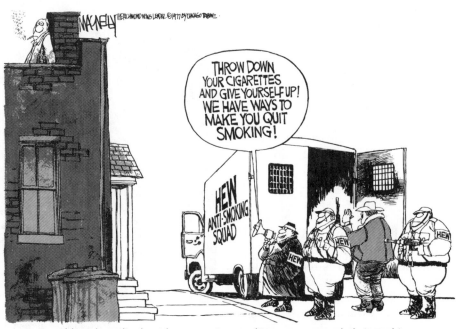

Although medical evidence against smoking seems overwhelming, this cartoonist pokes fun at antismoking crusaders for their militant stance.

London was blamed for 4,000 deaths in a few weeks. New York City has had several serious encounters with critical smog conditions that have accounted for many illnesses and deaths. The exteriors of many buildings in our cities are showing signs of vastly increased rates of decay due to the noxious substances in the air. It is estimated that air pollution costs the United States $11 billion a year in damage, illness, and in other ways. Even if all this loss of life and property were not a result it would clearly be more pleasant to live in a clean atmosphere than in a foul one.

Air pollution in any area varies greatly from day to day and even from hour to hour. The amount of air pollution depends mainly on the production of smoke and gases and the prevailing weather conditions. Pollutants include *particulate matter* in smoke that is first dispersed by the wind and then removed from the atmosphere by falling back to earth. Other major pollutants are organic gases and vapors, most of which are very toxic to humans in substantial concentrations. These include sulfur dioxide, nitrogen dioxide, carbon monoxide, ozone, and many others. These substances depend upon dilution in clean air to keep them from reaching toxic concentrations. That dilution depends principally upon the wind. When the air is stagnant these products do not disperse adequately in the atmosphere, and at these times many people suffer from burning eyes, increased cough, breathlessness, sore throat, and similar symptoms. To correct conditions at that point the only solution is to reduce emission of pollutants. Many large cities have developed staged plans for reducing emissions in a crisis.

Pollution and Disease

The diseases caused by air pollution are subtle and elusive. When pollution levels are significantly increased most people with moderate to severe chronic lung disease notice more symptoms, and some become quite ill. People with mild lung dis-

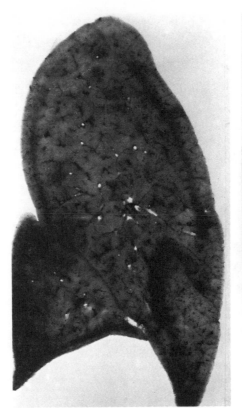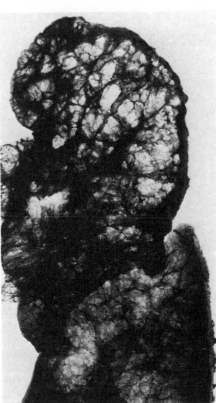

Inflated lung slices of *(left)* person with normal lungs and *(right)* person with emphysema, a disease in which the air sacs lose their elasticity.

ease but severe heart disease may find their heart problem to be much more bothersome. Studies show that many more persons die or are hospitalized for lung and related disorders during periods of high pollution than at other times. Evidence suggests that more lung cancer develops in and around large cities, but it is difficult to prove that this is solely due to air pollution. There even appear to be more common colds in high-pollution areas than in low ones.

For those people with lung disease who live in high-pollution areas there are several ways to reduce the irritation on particularly bad days. Staying indoors and exerting oneself as little as possible are two basic precepts. If one has an air conditioner or air filter system, he does even better by staying inside. These measures are aimed at reducing pollutant exposure and reducing the oxygen requirements of the body.

In the past decade efforts at controlling air pollution have increased

greatly. But the increased control is not yet keeping pace with the new production each year, which amounts to an added 12 million tons of pollutants. See also *Air Pollution,* p. 225, under *The Environment and Health.*

Emphysema and Bronchitis

Emphysema and chronic bronchitis are diseases that involve the whole lung. They can be of varying severity, and both are characterized by the gradual progression of breathlessness.

Because chronic bronchitis is almost invariably associated with pulmonary emphysema, the combined disorder frequently is called *obstructive-airway disease.* The disease involves damage to the lung tissue, with a loss of normal elasticity of the air sacs *(emphysema),* as well as damage to the *bronchi,* the main air passages to the lungs. In addition, chronic bronchitis is marked by a

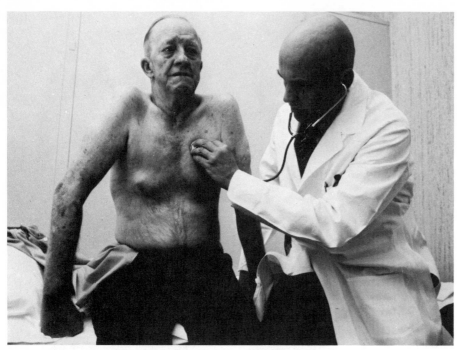

A patient with obstructive-airway disease may not realize he is sick until he becomes breathless with ordinary activity. By the time he sees a physician, the disease may be well established.

his fifties or sixties and little can be done to correct the damage. The time for prevention was in the previous 30 years when elimination of smoking could have prevented much or all of the illness.

Chronic cough and breathlessness are the two earliest signs of chronic bronchitis and emphysema. A smoker's cough is not an insignificant symptom. It indicates that very definite irritation of the bronchi has developed and it should be respected early. Along with the cough there is often production of phlegm or sputum, especially in the morning, due to less effective emptying of the bronchial tree during the relatively motionless period of sleep. Another early manifestation of disease is the tendency to develop chest infections along with what would otherwise be simple head colds. With these chest infections there is often a tightness or dull pain in the middle chest region, production of sputum, and sometimes wheezing.

Treatment

thickening of the walls of the bronchi with increased mucus production and difficulty in expelling these secretions. This results in coughing and sputum production.

The condition known as *acute bronchitis* is an acute process generally caused by a sudden infection, such as a cold, with an exaggeration of bronchitis symptoms. If a spasm of the bronchi occurs, accompanied by wheezing, the ailment is called infectious or nonallergic asthma.

Obstructive-airway disease is very insidious, and characteristically people do not, or will not, notice that they are sick until they suddenly are very sick. This is partly due to chronic denial of the morning cough and breathlessness, but also to the fact that we are fashioned in such a way as to have great reserve strength in our organs. As the disease progresses one starts using up his reserve for exertion. Since most people's life styles allow them to avoid exertion easily, the victim of this disease may have only rare chances to notice his breathlessness. Then, suddenly, within a period of a few months he becomes breathless with

ordinary activity because he has used up and surpassed all his reserve. He goes to a doctor thinking he has just become sick. Usually this event occurs when the patient is in

Once emphysema or bronchitis are diagnosed there are many forms

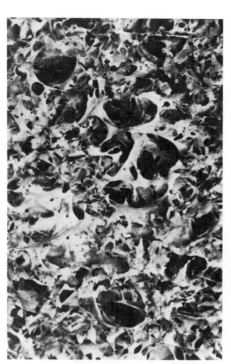

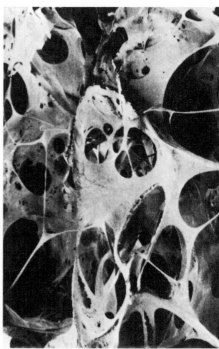

Photomicrographs of normal lung tissue (left), showing the many elastic air sacs that permit a normal flow of air, and (right) lung tissue of an emphysema patient, in which the air sacs have become permanently stretched.

of therapy that can help. Stopping smoking is the most important measure, and will in itself often produce dramatic effects. The more bronchitis the patient has the more noticeable the effect, as the bronchial irritation and mucus production decrease, cough lessens, and a greater sense of well-being ensues. The emphysema component does not change, as the damage to the air sacs is irreversible, but the progression may be greatly slowed. When chest infections develop they can be treated with antibiotics.

For more severe disease a program of breathing exercises and graded exertion may be beneficial. When these people develop heart trouble as a result of the strain on the heart, treatment to strengthen the heart is rewarding. For those with the most advanced stage of the disease new methods of treatment have been devised in recent years. One of the most encouraging is the use of controlled oxygen administration, a treatment that can sometimes allow a patient to return to an active working life from an otherwise helpless bed-and-chair existence. But it must be remembered that all these measures produce little effect if the patient continues to smoke.

Vaporizers, Nebulizers, IPPB

Mechanical methods have been developed to help control emphysema, bronchitis, acute and chronic asthma, and other respiratory disorders. These methods include the use of vaporizers, nebulizers, and intermittent positive pressure breathing (IPPB).

The vaporizer is a device that increases the moisture content of a home or room. In doing so, the vaporizer relieves the chronic condition that makes breathing difficult: the increased humidity loosens mucus and reduces nasal or bronchial congestion. One simple type of vaporizer or humidifier is the "croup kettle" or hot-steam type that releases steam into the air when heated on the stove or electrical unit. A more formal type of vaporizer is the electric humidifier that converts water into a spray. In dispersing the spray into the atmosphere, the vaporizer raises the humidity level without increasing the temperature.

The nebulizer also converts liquid into fine spray. But the nebulizer dispenses medications, such as isoproterenol hydrochloride, directly into the throat through a mouthpiece and pressure-injector apparatus like an atomizer. Used in limited doses according to a doctor's instructions, nebulization can relieve the labored or difficult breathing symptoms common to various respiratory diseases, among them asthma and bronchitis. The patient controls the dosage while using the nebulizer simply by employing finger pressure and obeying instructions.

In IPPB, a mask and ventilator are used to force air into the lungs and enable the patient to breathe more deeply. The ventilator supplies intermittent positive air pressure. The IPPB method of treatment has been used to help persons suffering from chronic pulmonary disease that makes breathing difficult. But IPPB may also be used with patients who cannot cough effectively; these patients include those who have recently undergone surgery. Newer IPPB units are highly portable; but they must be cleaned carefully with an antibacterial solution before use, and should always be used carefully to avoid producing breathing difficulties or aggravating heart problems.

Smoking and Obstructive Diseases

The problems encountered by patients with obstructive disease do not encompass merely that disease alone. Because of their smoking history these patients are also prone to develop lung cancer. All too often a person with a potentially curable form of lung cancer is unable to undergo surgery because his lungs will not tolerate the added strain of surgery. Patients with obstructive disease are also more prone to pneumonia and other infectious pulmonary conditions. When these develop in the already compromised lung, it may be impossible for the patient to maintain adequate oxygen supply to his vital tissues. If oxygen insufficiency is severe and prolonged enough, the patient dies from pulmonary failure.

Despite the emphasis placed on smoking as the predominant factor for the development of obstructive disease, there are people with the disease who have never smoked. For many of these individuals there is no

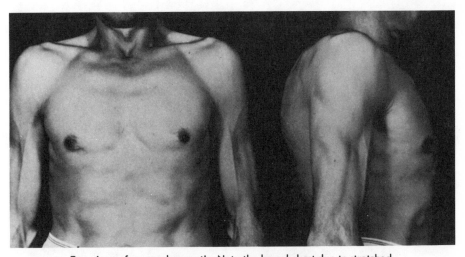

Two views of an emphysematic. Note the barrel chest due to stretched air sacs in the lung. Such lung-tissue damage is irreversible, but smoking aggravates the problem considerably. Stopping smoking will slow the progress of the disease and make the patient feel better.

known cause for their disease. However, a group of younger people with obstructive disease have been found to be deficient in a particular enzyme. (Enzymes are agents that are necessary for certain chemical reactions.) Individuals with this deficiency develop a particularly severe form of emphysema, become symptomatic in their third or fourth decade, and die at a young age. They may not smoke, but if they do, the disease is much more severe. Just how the enzyme deficiency leads to emphysema is not clear, but a great amount of research is being conducted on this new link to try to learn more about the causes of emphysema.

The Pneumoconioses

Pneumoconiosis is a chronic reaction of the lung to any of several types of inhaled dust particles. The reaction varies somewhat but generally consists of initial inflammation about the inhaled particle followed by the development of scar tissue. The pneumoconioses develop predominantly from various occupational exposures to high concentrations of certain inorganic compounds that cannot be broken down by the cells of the body. The severity of the disease is proportional to the amount of dust retained in the lung.

Silica is the most notorious of

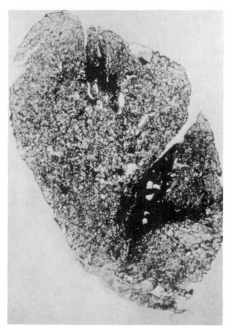

Lung tissue of a coal miner afflicted with pneumoconiosis (black lung), caused by inhaling coal dust over a period of many years.

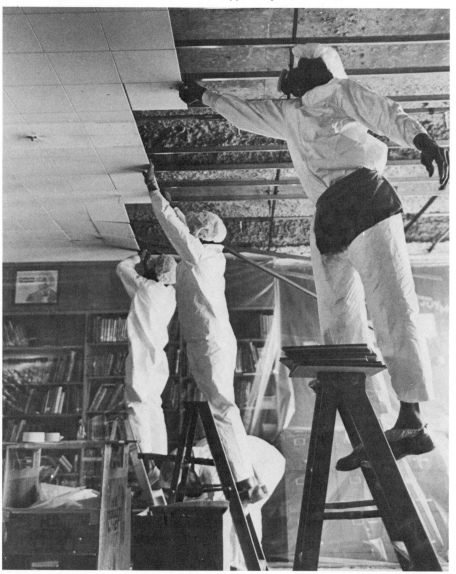

Wearing protective masks, workers remove asbestos insulation from the ceiling of a classroom. Asbestos dust apparently causes several diseases.

these substances. People who work in mining, steel production, and any occupation involved with chipping stone, such as manufacturing monuments, are exposed to silica dust. Many of the practices associated with these occupations have been altered over the years because of the recognition of the hazard to workers. Other important pneumoconioses involve talc and asbestos particles, cotton fibers, and coal dust. Coal dust has gained wide attention in recent years with the heightened awareness of *black lung*, a condition seen in varying degrees in coal miners. The attention has resulted in a federal black lung disease law under which more than 135,000 miners have filed for compensation.

Although there are individual differences in reaction to the varied forms of pneumoconiosis, the ultimate hazard is the loss of functioning lung tissue. When enough tissue becomes scarred, there is interference with oxygenation. Those people with pneumoconiosis who smoke are in great danger of compounding their problem by adding obstructive disease as well.

Prevention

Once the scarring has taken place there is no way to reverse the process. Therefore, the answer to the pneumoconioses is to prevent the exposure. Attention to occupational diseases in the United States has lagged about 30 years behind Europe, so that we are just now beginning to show concern about certain industrial practices condemned as hazardous in many European countries in the 1940s. New lung diseases caused by inhaled substances are discovered every year, and more will undoubtedly be found in the future. People in industries in which there is exposure to industrial dust should be aware of the potential danger and should be prepared to promote the maintenance of protective practices and the investigation of new ideas and devices. Where masks have been supplied, the workers should wear them, a practice too often neglected.

Pulmonary Embolism

Pulmonary embolism is a condition in which a part of a blood clot in a vein breaks away and travels through the heart and into the pulmonary circulatory system. Here the vessels leading from the heart branch like a tree, gradually becoming smaller until finally they form *capillaries*, the smallest blood vessels. Depending on its size, the clot will at some point reach a vessel through which it cannot pass, and there will lodge itself. The clot disrupts the blood supply to the area supplied by that vessel. The larger the clot, the greater is the area of lung that loses its blood supply, and the more drastic the results to the patient.

This condition develops most commonly in association with inflammation of the veins of the legs *(thrombophlebitis)*. People with varicose veins are particularly susceptible to thrombophlebitis. Because of constrictions produced by garters or rolled stockings, or just sitting with crossed legs for a long time, the sluggish blood flow already present is aggravated, and a clot may form in a vessel. Some people without varicose veins can also develop clots under the same conditions. The body often responds to the clot with the reaction of inflammation, which is painful. However, when there is no inflammatory response, there is no warning to tell that a clot has formed. In either situation there is always a chance that a piece may break off the main clot and travel to the lung. Of recent concern in this regard are studies that appear to link oral contraceptives with the incidence of clotting, thereby leading to pulmonary embolism. The number of women affected in this way by the use of oral contraceptives is small, but enough to be of concern.

The symptoms of pulmonary embolism are varied and may be minor or major. Most common are pleurisy—marked by chest pain during breathing—shortness of breath, and cough with the production of blood. Once the pulmonary embolism is diagnosed the treatment is simple in the less severe cases, which are the majority. But in cases of large clots and great areas of lung deprived of blood supply there may be catastrophic effects on the heart and general circulation.

Prevention

Certain preventive measures are worthwhile for all people. Stockings should not be rolled, because that produces a constricting band about the leg that impairs blood flow and predisposes to clot formation. Especially when taking long automobile or airplane rides one should be sure to stretch the legs periodically. Individuals with varicose veins or a history of thrombophlebitis should take these precautions more seriously. People who stand still for long periods during the day should wear elastic support stockings regularly and elevate their feet part of the day and at night.

When considering the use of oral contraceptives the physician must weigh the risks of developing clots from the drug against the psychological, social, and physical risks of pregnancy. The risk from oral contraceptives is lessened if the woman does not have high blood pressure. Any persistent pain in the leg, especially in the calf or behind the knee, deserves the attention of a physician. Anyone with varicose veins or anyone taking oral contraceptives should be especially attentive to these symptoms.

Pneumothorax

Another less common lung condition is spontaneous *pneumothorax* or collapse of a lung. This most commonly occurs in the second and third decade of life and presents itself with the sudden development of pain in the chest and breathlessness. The collapse occurs because of a sudden leak of air from the lung into the chest cavity.

The lung is ordinarily maintained in an expanded state by the rigid bony thorax, but if air leaks out into the space between the thorax and the lung, the lung collapses. This condition is rarely very serious but the patient needs to be observed to be sure that the air leak does not become greater with further lung collapse.

Treatment

Often a tube has to be placed in the chest, attached to a suction pump, and the air pumped out from the space where it has collected. When the air is removed the lung expands to fill the thoracic cage again. Some individuals tend to have several recurrences. Since the reason for the collapse is poorly understood, there is no satisfactory method of preventing these recurrences except by surgery. This is rarely required. In a person with a proven propensity for recurrence it is usually advisable to open the chest and produce scarring of the lung surface so that it becomes fixed to the thoracic cage. Although it is usually successful, even this procedure does not always solve this bothersome problem.

CHAPTER 20

Diseases of the Endocrine Glands

Glands are organs that produce and secrete substances essential for normal body functioning. There are two main types of glands: the *endocrine* and the *exocrine*. The endocrines or *ductless* glands send their secretions directly into the bloodstream. These secretions, which are biochemically related to each other, are called *hormones*. The exocrines, such as the sebaceous or sweat glands, the mammary or milk glands, and the lachrymal or tear glands, have ducts that carry their secretions to specific locations for specific purposes.

The exocrine glands are individually discussed elsewhere in connection with the various parts of the body where they are found. This section is devoted to diseases of the ductless glands, which include:

• The *pituitary,* which controls growth and the activity of the adrenal, thyroid and sex glands

• The *thyroid,* which controls the rate of the body's chemical activity or metabolism

• The *adrenals,* which affect metabolism and sex characteristics

• The *male gonads* or testicles; the *female gonads* or ovaries

• The *parathyroids,* which regulate bone metabolism.

Unlike the exocrine glands, which can function independently of each other, the endocrines form an inter-

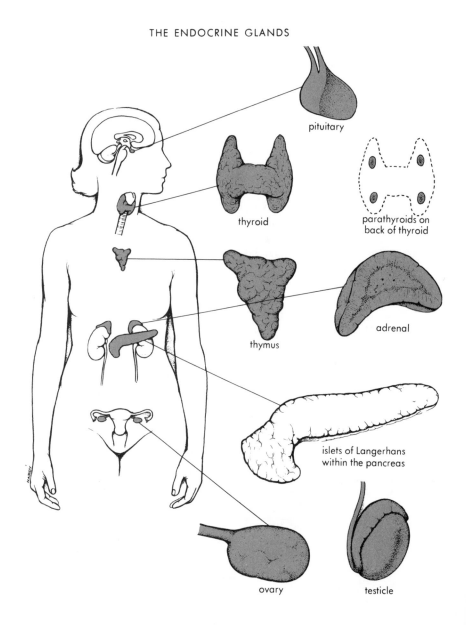

THE ENDOCRINE GLANDS

pituitary

thyroid

parathyroids on back of thyroid

thymus

adrenal

islets of Langerhans within the pancreas

ovary

testicle

related system. Thus a disorder in one of them is likely to affect the way the others behave. Glandular disorder can sometimes be anatomical, but it is usually functional. Functional disease can result in the production and release of too little or too much of a particular secretion.

When too much of a hormone is being secreted, the prefix *hyper-* is used for the condition, as in *hyperthyroidism*. When too little is being secreted, the prefix *hypo-* is used, as in the word *hypofunction*, to indicate that a gland operates below normal.

Abnormalities of the endocrine glands that cause changes in their functioning are responsible for a wide variety of illnesses. These illnesses are almost always accompanied by symptoms that can be recognized as distinctly abnormal. Prompt and accurate diagnosis can usually prevent the occurrence of irreversible damage. For many people with glandular disorders, treatment may have to be lifelong. They can feel well and function almost normally, but they must follow a program of regulated medication taken under a doctor's supervision.

Anterior Pituitary Gland

The anterior pituitary gland, also called the *hypophysis,* is located in the center of the brain. It produces two types of secretions: a growth hormone and hormones that stimulate certain other glands.

The anterior pituitary gland is subject to neurochemical stimulation by the *hypothalamus,* a nearby part of the brain. This stimulation results in the production of the hormones that promote testicular and ovarian functioning, and does not occur normally until around 12 years of age in girls and 14 in boys. The beginning of this glandular activity is known as the onset of *puberty.*

Puberty is sometimes delayed for no apparent reason until age 16 or 17. Since the hypothalamus is affected by emotional factors, all of the endocrine glands governed by the an-

terior pituitary can also be affected by feelings. Psychological factors can therefore upset the relationships in the glandular system and produce the physical symptoms of endocrine disorders.

It is extremely rare for the anterior pituitary to produce too much or too little of its hormones, but sometimes hypofunction may follow pregnancy because of thrombosis or changes in the blood vessels.

A truly hypofunctioning anterior pituitary gland can cause many serious disturbances: extreme thinness, growth failure, sexual aberration, and intolerance for normal variations in temperature. When appropriate diagnostic tests determine the deficiency, the patient is given the missing hormones in pill form.

Absence of the growth hormone alone is unknown. Most cases of *dwarfism* result from other causes. However, excess production of the growth hormone alone does occur, but only rarely. If it begins before puberty when the long bones are still growing, the child with the disorder will grow into a well-proportioned giant. When it begins after puberty, the head, hands, feet, and most body organs except the brain slowly enlarge. This condition is called *acromegaly.* The cause of both disorders is usually a tumor, and radiation is the usual treatment.

The thyroid, adrenal cortex, testicles, ovaries, and pancreatic glands are target glands for the anterior pituitary's stimulating hormones, which are specific for the functioning of each of these glands. Therefore, a disorder of any of the target organs could be caused either by an excess or a deficiency of a stimulating hormone, creating a so-called *secondary disease.* There are various tests that can be given to differentiate primary from secondary disorders.

The Thyroid Gland

The thyroid gland is located in the front of the neck just above its base. Normal amounts of *thyroxin,* the hormone secreted by the thyroid, are

necessary for the proper functioning of almost all bodily activities. When this hormone is deficient in infancy, growth and mental development are impaired and *cretinism* results.

Hypothyroidism

In adulthood, a deficiency of thyroxin hormone is caused primarily by a lack of sufficient iodine in the diet. In *hypothyroidism,* the disorder resulting from such a deficiency, the metabolic rate is slower than normal, the patient has no energy, his expression is dull, his skin is thick, and he has an intolerance to cold weather.

Treatment consists of increasing the amount of iodine in the diet if it is deficient, or giving thyroid hormone medication. Normal metabolic functioning usually follows, especially if treatment is begun soon after the symptoms appear.

Hyperthyroidism

An excess amount of thyroid hormone secretion is called *hyperthyroidism* and may relate to emotional stress. It causes physical fatigue but mental alertness, a staring quality in the eyes, tremor of the hands, weight loss with increased appetite, rapid pulse, sweating, and intolerance to hot weather.

Long-term treatment is aimed at decreasing hormone production with the use of a special medicine that inhibits it. In some cases, part of the gland may be removed by surgery; in others, radiation treatment with radioactive iodine is effective.

Hyperthyroidism may recur long after successful treatment. Both hypothyroidism and hyperthyroidism are common disorders, especially in women.

Other Thyroid Disorders

Enlargement of part or all of the thyroid gland occurs fairly often. It may be a simple enlargement of the gland itself due to lack of iodine, as in *goiter,* or it may be caused by a tumor or a nonspecific inflammation. Goiter is often treated with thyroxin, but it is easily prevented altogether by the regular use of iodized table and cooking salt. Treatment of other problems varies, but surgery is usually recommended for a tumor, especially if the surrounding organs are being obstructed.

The Adrenal Glands

The adrenals are paired glands located just above each kidney. Their outer part is called the *cortex*. The inner part is called the *medulla* and is not governed by the anterior pituitary. The cortex produces several hormones that affect the metabolism of salt, water, carbohydrate, fat, and protein, as well as secondary sex characteristics, skin pigmentation, and resistance to infection.

An insufficiency of these hormones can be caused by bacterial infection of the cortex, especially by *meningococcus;* by a hemorrhage into it; by an obstruction of blood flow into it; by its destruction because of tuberculosis; or by one of several unusual diseases.

In one type of sudden or acute underfunctioning of the cortex, the patient has a high fever, mental confusion, and circulatory collapse. Unless treated promptly, the disorder is likely to be fatal. When it persists after treatment, or when it develops

gradually, it is called *Addison's disease* and is usually chronic. The patient suffers from weakness, loss of body hair, and increased skin pigmentation. Hormone-replacement treatment is essential, along with added salt for as long as hypofunction persists.

The formation of an excess of certain cortical hormones (i.e., hormones produced in the adrenal cortex)—a disorder known as *Cushing's syndrome*—may be caused by a tumor of the anterior pituitary gland, which produces too much specific stimulating hormone; or by a tumor of one or both of the adrenal glands. It is a rare disease, more common in women, especially following pregnancy. Symptoms include weakness, loss of muscle tissue, the appearance of purple streaks in the skin, and an oval or "moon" face.

Treatment involves eliminating the over-producing tissue either by surgery or irradiation and then replacing any hormonal deficiencies with proper medication.

An excess of certain other cortical hormones because of an increase in cortical tissue or a tumor can result in the early onset of puberty in boys, or in an increase in the sexuality of females of any age. Surgical removal of the overproducing tissue is the only treatment.

The Adrenal Medulla

The medulla of the adrenal glands secretes two hormones: *epinephrine* (or *adrenaline*) and *nor-epinephrine.* Although they contribute to the proper functioning of the heart and blood vessels, neither one is absolutely indispensable. Disease due to hypofunction of the medulla is unknown. Hyperfunction is a rare cause of sustained high blood pressure. Even more rarely, it causes episodic or paroxysmal high blood pressure accompanied by such symptoms as throbbing headache, profuse perspiration, and severe anxiety. The disorder is caused by a tumor effectively treated by surgical removal. Cancer of the adrenal

medulla is extremely rare and virtually incurable.

Changes in hormone production can be caused by many intangible factors and are often temporary disorders. However, persistent or recurrent symptoms should be brought to a doctor's attention. The accurate diagnosis of an endocrine disease depends on careful professional evaluation of specific laboratory tests, individual medical history, and thorough examination. No one should take hormones or medicines that affect hormone production without this type of evaluation, since their misuse can cause major problems.

Male Sex Glands

The male sex glands or *gonads* are the two testicles normally located in the *scrotum*. In addition to producing sperm, the testicles also manufacture the male hormone called *testosterone*. This hormone is responsible for the development and maintenance of secondary sex characteristics as well as for the male *libido* or sexual impulse. Only one normal testicle is needed for full function.

Testicular Hypofunction

Hypofunction of one or both of the testicles can result from an abnormality in prenatal development, from infections such as mumps or tuberculosis, from injury, or from the increased temperature to which undescended testicles are exposed.

When hypofunction occurs before puberty, there is failure in the development of secondary sex characteristics. The sex organs do not enlarge; facial, pubic, and armpit hair fails to appear; and the normal voice change does not occur. Fertility and libido also fail to develop. A person with this combination of abnormalities is called a *eunuch.*

If the disorder is secondary to anterior pituitary disease, it is called *Froehlich's syndrome.* When it occurs after puberty, the body changes

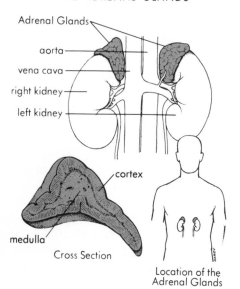

THE ADRENAL GLANDS

Adrenal Glands
aorta
vena cava
right kidney
left kidney

cortex

medulla

Cross Section

Location of the Adrenal Glands

are less striking, but there may be a loss of fertility and libido. The primary disease is usually treated by surgery, and testosterone may be given. If the disorder is secondary to anterior pituitary disease, the gonad-stimulating hormone should be administered.

Testicular hypofunction is rare because it results only when both testicles are damaged in some way. Although mumps may involve the testicles, it is rarely the cause of sterility, even though this is greatly feared. Even so, everyone should be immunized against mumps in infancy.

It is advisable to wear an appropriate athletic supporter to protect the testicles when engaged in strenuous athletics or when there is a possibility that they might be injured. However, nothing that restricts scrotal movement should be worn regularly, since movement is essential for the maintenance of constant testicular temperature.

A sudden decrease in sexual drive or performance may be caused by disease, trauma, or emotional factors. In certain cases administering male hormones may relieve the condition. However, a decrease in sexual drive is one of the natural consequences of aging. It is not a disease and should not be treated with testosterone.

THE TESTICLE

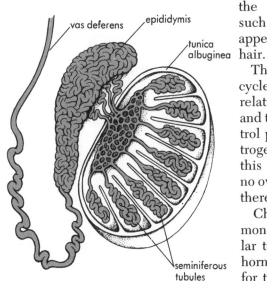

Testicular Hyperfunction

Testicular hyperfunction is extremely rare and is usually caused by a tumor. Before puberty, the condition results in the precocious development of secondary sex characteristics; after puberty, in the accentuation of these characteristics. Such a tumor must be removed surgically or destroyed by irradiation.

Cancer can develop in a testicle without causing any functional change. It is relatively uncommon. When it appears, it shows up first as a painless enlargement. The cancer cells then usually spread quickly to other organs and have a fatal result. Prompt treatment by surgery and irradiation can sometimes arrest the condition.

Since an undescended testicle may become cancerous, it should be repositioned into the scrotum by surgery or removed.

Female Sex Glands

The female gonads are the *ovaries,* situated on each side of and close to the uterus or womb. In addition to producing an *ovum* or egg each month, they manufacture the female hormones *estrogen* and *progesterone,* each making its special contribution to the menstrual cycle and to the many changes that go on during pregnancy. Estrogen regulates the secondary sex characteristics such as breast development and the appearance of pubic and axillary hair.

The periodicity of the menstrual cycle depends on a very complicated relationship between the ovaries and the anterior pituitary. Birth control pills, most of which contain estrogen and progesterone, interrupt this relationship in such a way that no ovum is produced and pregnancy therefore should not occur.

Changes in normal ovarian hormone function create problems similar to changes in normal testicular hormone function, except of course for the female-male differences. In

THE FEMALE REPRODUCTIVE SYSTEM

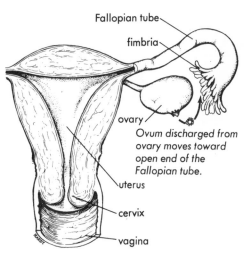

Ovum discharged from ovary moves toward open end of the Fallopian tube.

general, the diseases responsible for these changes are the same in males and females. However, changes in female hormone function are very often caused by emotional stress or by other unspecific circumstances.

Ovarian Hypofunction

Hypofunction of the ovaries may cause failure to menstruate at all or with reasonable regularity. A disruption of the menstrual cycle is an obvious indication to the woman past puberty that something is wrong. Less obvious is the reduction or complete loss of fertility that may accompany the disorder.

Both menstrual and infertility problems should be evaluated by a trained specialist, preferably a gynecologist, to find out their cause. If it should be hormonal deficiency, treatment may consist of replacement hormone therapy. In many cases, however, effective treatment consists of eliminating the emotional stress that has affected the stimulation relationship between the anterior pituitary and the ovaries, thereby inhibiting hormone production. Occasionally, hormone treatment for infertility causes several ova to be produced in the same month, increasing the possibility of a multiple pregnancy.

Menopause

All women eventually develop spontaneous ovarian hypofunction.

This usually happens between the ages of 45 and 50 and is called the *climacteric* or *menopause*. When it happens before the age of 35, it is called premature menopause.

Normal menopause results from the gradual burning out of the ovaries so that estrogen is deficient or absent altogether. Most women experience very few changes or symptoms at this time other than the cessation of menstruation, usually preceded by progressive irregularity and reduction of flow.

A few women become excessively irritable, have hot flashes, perspire a great deal, gain weight, and develop facial hair. Such women, as well as those who have premature menopause, are likely to benefit greatly from estrogen replacement therapy for a few years. However, because recent statistical studies have implicated sustained use of estrogen therapy as increasing the risk of uterine cancer in postmenopausal women, the American Cancer Society has cautioned doctors to supervise such women closely. At the present time, most physicians feel that the treatment should be given temporarily and only when menopause symptoms are causing special discomfort. See also p. 159.

Ovarian Hyperfunction

Hyperfunction of the ovaries after puberty is one cause of increased menstrual flow during or at the end of each cycle. This is called functional bleeding and is due to excess estrogen. The disorder is treated with progesterone, which slows down estrogen production. In cases where this treatment fails, it is sometimes necessary to remove the uterus by an operation called a *hysterectomy*.

Some diseases of the ovaries, such as infections, cysts, and tumors, do not necessarily cause functional changes, but they may call attention to themselves by being painful, or a doctor may discover them during a pelvic examination. Treatment may be medical, surgical, or by irradiation, depending on the nature of the disorder. See under *Women's Health*, p. 483, for fuller treatment of ovarian and other disorders affecting women.

A rather common cause of short-lived ovarian pain is connected with *ovulation*, which occurs about 14 days before the next expected menstrual period. This discomfort is called *mittelschmerz*, which is German for "middle pain," and can be treated with aspirin or any other simple analgesic.

The Pancreas

The pancreas, a combined duct and endocrine gland, is to some extent regulated by the anterior pituitary. See *Diabetes Mellitus*, p. 411, for a discussion of the pancreas and diabetes.

Posterior Pituitary Gland

The posterior lobe of the pituitary gland, the parathyroid glands, and the adrenal medulla are not governed by the anterior pituitary gland. The posterior pituitary produces a secretion called *antidiuretic hormone* which acts on the kidneys to control the amount of urine produced. A deficiency of this hormone causes *diabetes insipidus,* which re-sults in the production of an excessive amount of urine, sometimes as much as 25 quarts a day. (A normal amount is about 1 quart.) The natural consequence of this disorder is an unquenchable thirst. It is an extremely rare disease, the cause of which is often unknown, although it may result from a brain injury or tumor. Treatment involves curing the cause if it is known. If not, the patient is given an antidiuretic hormone.

The Parathyroid Glands

The parathyroid glands are located in or near the thyroid, usually two on each side. They are important in the regulation of blood calcium and phosphorus levels and therefore of bone metabolism. Hypofunction of these glands almost never occurs except when they have been removed surgically, usually inadvertently during a thyroid operation. In underfunctioning of the parathyroids, blood calcium levels fall and muscle spasm results. The patient is usually given calcium and replacement therapy with parathyroid hormone to correct the disorder.

Hyperfunction is rare and is slightly more common in women. A benign tumor or *adenoma* is the usual cause. The amount of calcium in the blood rises as calcium is removed from the bones, which then weaken and may break easily. The excess calcium is excreted in the urine and may coalesce into kidney stones, causing severe pain. Treatment for hyperfunction of the parathyroids consists of surgical removal of the affected glands.

CHAPTER 21

Diabetes Mellitus

A lot of people have diabetes and they live a long time with it. In the United States there are around four million *diabetics,* or people who have diabetes. About a third of them at any one time are undiagnosed. This figure constitutes about 2 percent of the population, and ranges from .01 percent of people under 24 years of age to 7 percent of those over 64.

Diabetes can develop at any age. Susceptibility gradually increases up to age 40, and then rapidly increases. After age 30 it more commonly affects women than men.

History of Diabetes

Diabetes has been known for several thousand years. Because people with this disease, when untreated, may urinate frequently and copiously, the Greeks named it diabetes, meaning "siphon." In the late seventeenth century the name *mellitus,* meaning sweet, was added. In early days, diagnosis was made by tasting the urine. The sweetness is caused by the presence of sugar *(glucose)* in the urine; its presence distinguishes diabetes mellitus from the much rarer *diabetes insipidus,* an entirely different problem. See under *Diseases of the Endocrine Glands,* p.

410, for a discussion of diabetes insipidus.

DISCOVERY OF INSULIN: Late in the nineteenth century, when diabetes was well recognized as an abnormality in carbohydrate metabolism, several scientists discovered that the experimental removal of certain cells, the *islets of Langerhans,* from the pancreas, produced diabetes in dogs. This observation led to the 1921 discovery and isolation of *insulin* by two Canadian doctors, Frederick Banting and Charles Best. Insulin is a hormone produced by these islets. Injection of insulin proved to be the first and remains the most effective means of treating diabetes. And so began a real revolution in improving the outcome of this disease. Previously death occurred in a few years for almost every diabetic. Often death was much quicker, especially for people who were under 30 years of age when they developed diabetes—since this age group tends to have a more severe form of the disease. Since 1921 new knowledge and techniques have made it possible to do more and more for diabetics.

An early pioneer in the treatment of diabetes with insulin was Dr. Elliott Joslin of Boston. Dr. Joslin realized that the diabetic patient needed to have a full understanding

of his disease so that he could take care of himself. He knew that the diabetic, with the chronic abnormality of a delicate and dynamic metabolic process, could not be cared for successfully solely by knowledgeable physicians. The patient and his family had to be informed about the disease and had to make day-to-day decisions about managing it.

In many ways this marked the beginning of what have become ever increasing efforts to educate patients about all their diseases, especially chronic ones. The results have been rather remarkable.

Characteristics of Diabetes

The fundamental problem in diabetes is the body's inability to metabolize glucose, a common form of sugar, fully and continually. This is a vital process in creating body cell energy. Glucose is a chemical derivative of the carbohydrate in foods after they have been ingested. Carbohydrates are mostly of plant origin and may be called starch, saccharide, sucrose, or simply sugar. Glucose is stored under normal conditions in the form of *glycogen,* or animal starch, in the liver and muscles for later use, at which time it is reconverted to glucose.

NEED FOR INSULIN: Insulin is necessary for both the storage and reconversion of glucose. The metabolic failure may come about because of an insufficiency of insulin, an inability of the body to respond normally to it for a number of complex chemical reasons, or a combination of both factors. In any event, the failure to metabolize glucose results in an abnormal accumulation of sugar in the bloodstream.

This failure is somewhat similar to starvation. A starved person eats no food, whereas the diabetic eats food but cannot use the carbohydrate in it and cannot get sufficient energy from the protein and fat content of food. After the starving person has used his previously stored glycogen, which the diabetic without insulin cannot do, the body has to metabolize its stored fat for energy. This results in a loss of weight and is often an early indication of diabetes.

A by-product of fat metabolism is the formation of *ketone bodies* (chemical compounds) which, when excessive, cause a condition known as diabetic *acidosis*. This can cause coma and death if not treated with insulin and the right kind of intravenous fluids. Before insulin was discovered, this was the way most diabetics died.

EXCESS URINE PRODUCTION: As glucose accumulates above normal levels in the diabetic's bloodstream it is filtered by his kidneys and remains in the urine. Additional amounts of urine are produced to contain the excess glucose. This situation results in copious and frequent urination which in turn causes dehydration and an often insatiable thirst. These are classically the first signs of the presence of diabetes.

This is diabetes described largely in terms of changes in carbohydrate metabolism. But protein and fat metabolism are also involved, as are almost invariably some changes in the nerves, muscles, eyes, kidneys, and blood vessels.

No one knows why diabetes develops. In some ways diabetes resembles premature aging, and the causes of diabetes, if known, might shed some light on the causes of aging.

The body's need to obtain energy from glucose and to convert glucose to glycogen and vice versa is continuous but always changing quantitatively. Meeting these needs requires constantly fluctuating amounts of effective insulin. Nondiabetics produce these amounts no matter what they eat or do, thus maintaining a steady state of metabolism. Diabetics, however, cannot achieve this steady state simply by taking insulin; they must also control their diets and their activities. They may have to change the amounts of their medications from time to time.

Diabetes is not an all-or-nothing phenomenon. It can be mild, moderate, or severe, and can fluctuate in degree in any one individual over a long period of time, or even from day to day. Very little is really known about the reasons for these differences and changes. It is known, however, that diabetes generally gets worse in the presence of illness, particularly infections (even colds). It is also affected adversely by hyperfunctioning diseases of the anterior pituitary, thyroid, and adrenal glands, by emotional and physical stress, and during pregnancy.

Diabetes Diagnosis

The diagnosis of diabetes is not ordinarily a difficult one. Especially in children, the symptoms of rapid weight loss, extreme hunger, generalized weakness, frequent and copious urination, and insatiable thirst make it easy to recognize. Finding glucose in the urine along with increased levels of glucose in the blood generally confirms the diagnosis. However, glucose in the urine does not always indicate the presence of diabetes. A few people with unusual kidney function have glucose in their urine with normal blood levels, a condition known as *renal glycosuria.*

Moreover, an adult with diabetes may not have such a definite set of symptoms for months or years after he has actually developed the disease. Instead he may have vague fatigue or persistent skin infections. A woman may have a persistent genital itch that a physician might suspect is due to diabetes. Proof is provided by urine and blood tests. Glucose in the urine at the time of a routine physical examination might provide the first clue. Once diagnosed, treatment should be begun.

Treatment of Diabetes

Diet

The diet of a diabetic, although a major part of his treatment, is similar to what a normal person of the same age should eat. However, some radical dietary changes may be ordered if the previous diet has not been a proper one. This is particularly true in regard to reducing the calories in food eaten by overweight diabetics.

Diet is the only treatment needed by many adult diabetics, particularly those who are obese when they develop the disease, provided they can lose and not regain their excess weight. Since obese people are more likely to develop diabetes, they should have urine or blood sugar tests yearly after the age of 40. But it is more important for them to make every effort to lose weight before they become diabetics.

INDIVIDUALIZED DIETS: Each diabetic's diet has to be individualized to a certain extent. This is done originally by the physician when the diagnosis is made and periodically thereafter. The physician must learn the eating habits, customs, and preferences of his diabetic patient. Since eating is so much a part of the patient's personality and has such great psychological importance, its pattern should be changed radically only when necessary.

Certain principles that may not involve major changes should be kept in mind. For example, the diet should conform to the patient's customary cultural and ethnic pattern. It should not make him feel weak and without energy. If it does, he needs more food and more insulin.

Some nonobese diabetics, especially elderly ones, need only to eliminate sugar, soft drinks, and pastry from their diets. A mild diabetic often needs only to reduce the amount of carbohydrate in his diet and replace it with fats and proteins. Alcohol can be a part of a diabetic's diet under certain circumstances, which he should discuss with his physician. Sugar-free foods and beverages enable a diabetic to enjoy some of life's minor luxuries.

Children should, if possible, have diets that are similar to those of their friends, although they must be helped to understand that they should avoid eating foods containing concentrated sugars, like soda pop, candy, jams, and jellies.

DIET GUIDES: Most physicians have available printed diet guides to help their patients adjust their diets as needed. These indicate the number of calories and amount of protein, carbohydrate, and fat per household measure in all foods. See also under *Nutrition and Weight Control*, p. 194, for additional reading on this subject.

When to eat is another matter, and this often necessitates some changes in eating habit patterns, especially for people taking insulin. Most important is regularity in relation to the patient's rest-activity time patterns. In general, almost half of the day's carbohydrates should be eaten at lunch, since this is usually when activity and energy expenditure are greatest. The remainder should be divided between breakfast and dinner.

Until recent years, insulin was prepared commercially in the United States from beef or pork pancreas. More recently, researchers have developed an insulin drug that is manufactured with a synthetic duplicate of human genes. Until this drug, called Humulin, appeared, diabetics who were allergic to insulin products made from animal cells had to resort to more complex drugs such as steroids. Unlike animal insulins, Humulin, the first consumer health product made with DNA (*deoxyribonucleic acid*), can be produced in unlimited quantities.

Insulin has to be given by injection, usually *subcutaneous injection*, just beneath the skin, because it is destroyed by gastric secretions when taken orally.

The method of preparation also determines the timing of its action, and it is classified into three basic types:

TYPE OF INSULIN	TIME (HOURS) OF ACTION AFTER INJECTION		
	Onset	Peak	Duration
Rapid	1/2–1	2–8	4–14
Intermediate	2–4	6–12	10–26
Prolonged	4–8	12–24	24–36

There are two or three different insulin preparations for each type—rapid, intermediate, and prolonged.

Ideally, insulin injected once a day should more or less mimic the normal insulin action of a nondiabetic. That is the purpose of the intermediate and long-acting insulins, with which a rapid insulin is sometimes combined. Many diabetics are able to take insulin only once a day, particularly when their diet and activity pattern is sufficiently constant. Others, however, require two or more injections. The usual time to take insulin is before breakfast. This should be the same time every day. Second injections are often taken at suppertime.

A diabetic's basic insulin dose has to be established initially according to the severity of his disease. The dose is determined largely by his blood and urine glucose levels, the physician's judgment, and trial and error. Once established, the dosage has to be assessed daily and adjusted as necessary on the basis of the amount of sugar in the urine, diet, activity, and other factors.

Many diabetics take the same dose daily for years; others need to readjust theirs constantly. The number of units taken per day varies greatly from person to person, but probably

INJECTION OF INSULIN DOSE

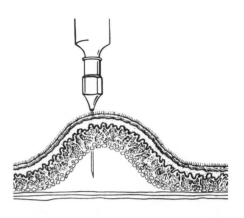

1. Wipe site of injection with cotton swab dipped in alcohol.
2. With one hand, pinch up skin at injection site. Place syringe perpendicularly to the skin and quickly insert needle for its entire length in order to insure injection of sufficient depth (see illustration). The more rapidly the needle is inserted, the less the pain will be. Stainless-steel needles are preferred.
3. Inject insulin dose.

SITES OF INSULIN INJECTIONS

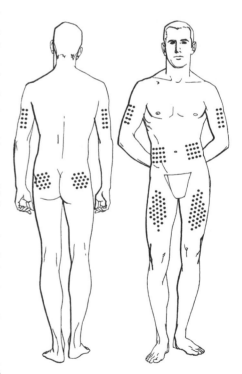

It is important to change the site of injection daily for best absorption of insulin.

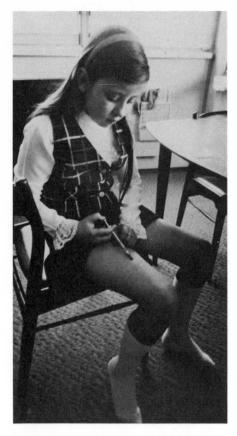

A girl with juvenile-onset diabetes gives herself the required daily injection of insulin.

most diabetics take between 10 and 40 units a day. The cost generally is less than one cent a unit. Insulin comes in ten-cc vials that must be refrigerated until first used. Thereafter they can be kept at room temperature.

SELF-MEDICATION: Most diabetics self-inject their insulin. One can learn the technique of self-injection by practicing injecting an orange before trying it on oneself. The needle should always be sharp. It is important to change the exact site of the injection from day to day. Too frequent use of the same site may impair insulin absorption. The specially calibrated syringe and the needle can be either presterilized and discarded after one use, or they can be reused after resterilization by boiling for five minutes.

Insulin Shock

When injected insulin is active in the body system it must be matched by a sufficient amount of blood sugar.

If not matched because of too much insulin, too much exercise, or too little ingested carbohydrate, the blood sugar level falls, a condition known as *hypoglycemia,* and the brain is deprived of an essential source of energy. This is most apt to occur at the time of the insulin's peak activity.

The first sign of an insulin reaction or *insulin shock* is usually mild hunger. Then come, and rather quickly, sweating, dizziness, palpitation, shallow breathing, trembling, mental confusion, strange behavior, and finally loss of consciousness. Prompt treatment is important. A lump of sugar or a piece of candy taken when symptoms first begin to appear will usually provide enough glucose to abort the reaction.

It is sometimes necessary to give intravenous glucose to counter insulin shock. This terminates the reaction almost immediately. Diabetics who use insulin should always have a lump or two of sugar or some candy with them and learn to recognize an oncoming insulin reaction. In general they should eat a small snack of glucose of some sort about the time their insulin activity reaches its peak.

Insulin reaction or shock can happen to any diabetic taking insulin. It is one of the liabilities of insulin therapy. Repeated and prolonged episodes of insulin reaction can be damaging to the brain. All diabetics, and especially those taking insulin, should have an identification bracelet or necklace indicating they have diabetes so that anyone examining them in an unconscious state can quickly realize the probable cause of their unconsciousness. This can be supplemented by a card in the wallet or purse with additional details. These are available from the Medic Alert Foundation, Turlock, California 95380, at a very modest cost. It is also vital that at least a few persons with whom the diabetic regularly associates know about his disease so that they can take prompt action if they see problems developing.

The Insulin Pump

Development of a pump for infusion of insulin into the body may offer a better method of treating diabetics with keto-acidosis, or ketosis (see "Diabetic Coma" p. 413). The pump method of continuous intravenous (IV) infusion has been used with moderate success in such cases.

Some advantages have been noted. A reduced amount of hypoglycemia has been reported, for example. Because the insulin is injected directly into the bloodstream, a smaller amount is required for control. Shots, or injections, under the skin have not been necessary while the patient has been receiving infusion treatment. Some medical men believe, however, that the older method of administering insulin by injection will remain useful. These doctors point out that better control of the treatment results when shots are given and the amount of urine glucose is monitored closely. Also, patients can observe how the insulin is given when the needle is used.

The insulin pump system generally includes a reservoir for the insulin; a peristaltic pump, one that impels the fluid by contracting and expanding; and a "power pack" containing batteries that activate the pump. The entire assembly, with associated tubings, typically weighs 525 grams or about 1.5 pounds. The system is rugged enough to withstand rough treatment under difficult weather and environmental conditions.

If widely accepted and used, the insulin pump system may answer a basic need for improved ways to introduce drugs into the body. Earlier methods, including the subcutaneous, or needle, technique, have been described as faulty because they are "nonphysiologic"—they do not deliver the drugs where they can be used immediately by the body.

Oral Drugs

Oral *hypoglycemic drugs* have

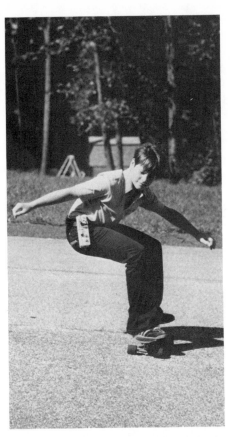

A portable insulin pump feeds the insulin directly into the bloodstream while allowing the diabetes patient to lead a normal active life.

been available since the late 1950s. They are mainly helpful in controlling mild diabetes that develops in people 45 and over. However, younger people can occasionally be maintained on these drugs rather than on insulin. They stimulate the release of *endogenous* (self-produced) *insulin* from the pancreas or foster insulin activity in other ways. Chemically composed of *sulfonylurea*, they are remotely related to sulfa drugs but are not true sulfas. An entirely different oral hypoglycemic agent is *DBI (phenformin)*. Some doctors urge that such drugs be prescribed only in cases that cannot be controlled effectively by other techniques.

For these drugs to work, some of the islet cells must be producing insulin or be capable of producing it. They either work well or not at all. The dose varies from one to eight tablets taken before meals and throughout the day. They cost a few cents a tablet. Insulin reactions do not occur although some diabetics take insulin also and are thereby vulnerable to insulin reactions. The decision about treating a given diabetic with these pills, insulin, or both, has to be left to the patient's physician.

Diabetic Coma

Prolonged *hyperglycemia*, or excess sugar in the blood, from insufficient insulin activity can cause *diabetic coma*. This condition involves the increasing buildup of ketone bodies, the by-product of fat metabolism, which creates an *acidotic* condition (chemical imbalance in the blood, marked by an excess of acid). When this has been present for several days, perhaps a week or longer, symptoms begin to develop that are similar to those associated with the onset of diabetes. They include excessive urination and thirst, dry and hot skin, drowsiness, and finally, coma. The earliest stage of the problem is called *diabetic ketosis;* a slightly later stage is known as *diabetic acidosis*. From the beginning there are increasing amounts of glucose as well as ketone bodies in the urine. The unconscious patient will have deep, labored breathing, and a fruity odor to his breath.

Diabetic acidosis resembles an insulin reaction, although they can be distinguished from one another. If you find a diabetic in coma and you do not know the cause, assume the cause is an insulin reaction and treat him initially with sugar. This will give immediate relief to an insulin reaction but will not affect diabetic acidosis.

Diabetic acidosis occurs for many reasons. The patient does not take his insulin or oral hypoglycemic drugs for several days. He may take too little insulin because he is confused about the dosage. He may overeat or underexercise for a number of days, perhaps because he feels ill or has a cold.

TREATMENT: In its early stages ketosis generally can be treated by the patient himself with directions from his physician, usually by telephone. The fundamentals of this treatment involve taking rapid-acting insulin—every diabetic should keep a bottle of this on hand—every three or four hours until the urine has less glucose and no longer contains ketone bodies. Ketone bodies can be tested in the urine along with glucose. If there is a treatable underlying cause for the acidosis, such as an infection, it should be treated as well. In the later stages, hospital treatment with larger amounts of insulin, often given intravenously, and specific intravenous fluid therapy is essential.

Diabetes Control

An occasional insulin reaction is almost unavoidable, but diabetic acidosis occurs mainly because the diabetes was not well controlled. Good control means feeling well with only small amounts of sugar, or none, in the urine. This is possible for most but not all diabetics. A few diabetics can never achieve good control for a variety of reasons relating largely to the vagaries of this disease.

Personal Glucose Tests

The amount of glucose in the urine provides a kind of barometer of diabetic control. The amount in the blood at a given point in time provides a better barometer but is more difficult to check for obvious reasons. Therefore all diabetics should test their urine daily and sometimes more often, particularly in the beginning or when they are having control problems.

The ordinary urine specimen contains urine collected in the bladder over a period of several hours or overnight. The glucose in it is an average indication of what the blood sugar has been during a previous period. To get an idea of the blood sugar level at the time of the urine test, the urine that has accumulated in the bladder must first be discarded. Then a second specimen of urine should be passed about a half

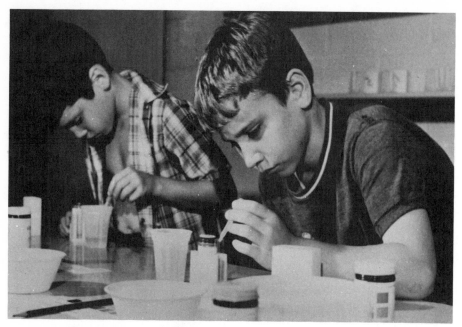

Testing their urine for sugar is a serious business for these young diabetics at summer camp. If the sugar level is up they report to the medical staff.

hour later and that specimen tested for glucose.

Several types of tests are available for this purpose. Some utilize chemically treated paper which, when dipped in urine, turns different colors to indicate varying amounts of glucose in the urine. Others use tablets that change to different colors when dropped into small amounts of urine. Adjustments in diet, activity, and insulin or oral hypoglycemic agents can be made on the basis of these test results. It costs a few cents to do each test.

Making Lifelong Adjustments

Once a diabetic has learned the fundamentals of his diet, his insulin or oral hypoglycemic agent medication, and has stabilized sufficiently his daily physical activities, he is well on his way to leading a normal life. There are, however, still a few psychological roadblocks.

First is the hard business of adjusting to the disease and coming to accept the fact that it can be lived with even though there is no cure. Initial depression is understandable and common. It does not persist. Then comes the often difficult task of regularizing one's life in terms of eating schedules, taking insulin, testing the urine, and exercising regularly.

Not many diabetics can maintain good control if they go to a Saturday night party, postpone their dinner time by four or five hours, and sleep until noon on Sunday. Maintaining one's usual schedule while traveling is another obstacle. The diabetic may feel that people treat him differently from the way they used to treat him or from the way they treat others. He will have to get used to seeing his physician frequently and regularly and having blood drawn to determine his blood sugar. He will have to spend a certain amount of money for insulin or oral hypoglycemic drugs, syringes and needles, urine-testing materials, special sugar-free foods, and medical care.

Self-pity and then rebellion against these factors are not unusual, especially in children. And with rebellion comes an increased likelihood of insulin reactions or diabetic ketosis. Some diabetics use their disease as a way to manipulate others and thus create trying interpersonal relationships. The good physician is aware of all of this and will give his patient the opportunity to verbalize his feelings.

Those with whom the diabetic lives—parents, siblings, spouse, and children—are also affected in various ways. The family's food style may be changed to some extent. Parents may have a sense of guilt about what they erroneously presume to be their part in the child's development of diabetes. They may have difficulty differentiating normal adolescent moods from those associated with the diabetic's fluctuating carbohydrate metabolism. They may become controlling and coddling or rejecting and resentful. Either reaction pattern will affect the child adversely. Parents should be helped to understand the disease as well as its effect on their child.

Juvenile Insulin Dependent Diabetes (JIDD)

Boys and girls develop diabetes in approximately equal numbers. For both sexes, the average age of onset is about 8 years. For both sexes, too, diabetes may be discovered in the first hours or days of life. More frequently, diabetes appears at the age of puberty.

In severe cases, the youthful victim of diabetes suffers from a critical shortage of insulin. Acidosis may occur. The child in this situation usually has what is known as juvenile insulin dependent diabetes (JIDD). Insulin therapy may be

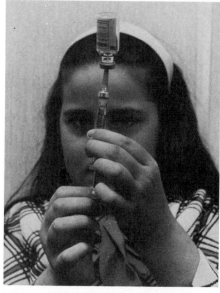

A ten-year-old diabetic who has mastered the technique of injecting herself with insulin prepares a syringe.

required throughout the young person's life.

Therapy need not adversely affect the child's activities, growth rate, or psychological or intellectual development. The young person on continuous insulin therapy can usually be allowed to eat as much as he or she wants; but if abnormally large quantities of food are consumed, or if hunger continues even after meals, a physician should be consulted.

What kind of diet is best for the child with juvenile insulin dependent diabetes? High-carbohydrate diets appear to meet this child's need best. But animal fats should be restricted; ice cream in particular should be avoided. Ice milk may serve as a substitute. The rule restricting the intake of animal fats also means that commercially baked cookies; candy containing fat, including chocolate mixtues; and similar foods are unsuitable.

Some kinds of candy, fruit juices, meat, and eggs may be included in the young JIDD child's diet. "Permissible" candy may contain honey, or it may be made from sorbitol. Some health-food shops stock sesame crunch that the diabetic child can enjoy. Because they contain protein and vegetable oil, nuts make good snack foods.

Fruit juices, meat, and eggs supply a number of nutrients that the diabetic child needs. Orange and grapefruit juices, for example, contain potassium, fructose, and vitamins C and A. Meat provides protein, and should be included in the diet. Eggs supply lecithin, which keeps cholesterol from building up in blood vessels, and amino acids, essential to body-building. Eggs should be soft- or hard-boiled or poached, not fried in butter or other kinds of fat.

Fresh fish, chicken, and turkey belong properly in the diabetic child's diet, as do peanut butter and jelly sandwiches. Peanut butter made from fresh-ground nuts is preferred, but cannot be obtained in all stores. For essential whole grains, the child should eat whole wheat bread, millet, oatmeal, and other cereals—but dried cereals should be ruled out. Fresh vegetables may be served if the child does not like cooked vegetables.

Adequate amounts of sugar and starches will usually prevent hypoglycemic reactions in the JIDD child. But where such a reaction does set in, the child should drink fruit juice or some kind of rapidly digestible carbohydrate. The prepared child always carries hard candy, or a box of raisins. Both help terminate hypoglycemic attacks.

Pregnancy and Diabetes

Pregnancy is a very special time in any woman's life, but it is particularly special for a diabetic and her unborn child. Diabetes is not a factor of any magnitude as far as conception is concerned, but pregnancy affects the diabetic's carbohydrate metabolism dramatically. In general there is an increase in blood glucose levels and an ever-increasing need for insulin. However, there can be periodic and unpredictable reductions in insulin need. Therefore, urine glucose and blood glucose need to be tested more frequently than under ordinary circumstances.

The urine should be tested three or four times a day and the blood glucose at every visit to the obstetrician. With good management during a diabetic's pregnancy, her baby has an excellent chance of being as normal and healthy as that of the non-diabetic mother.

Diabetes in Later Life

The association between aging and diabetes relates largely to a gradual loss of elasticity in the cells of the blood vessels, kidneys, eyegrounds (the inner sides of the backs of the eyeballs), and nerve tissues. These cellular changes may not become apparent for many years after the development of diabetes. However, occasionally they are present before or appear several years after the diabetes is recognized. This is particularly apt to be true in older people who develop diabetes.

The nerve-tissue changes can cause a diminished sensation to touch and pain and sometimes a loss of motor function of the extremities as well as sexual impotence. The eyeground changes damage the retina in various ways and can cause varying degrees of loss of vision. In about eight percent of cases this progresses to blindness.

The changes in the kidneys affect their filtration functions, causing *albuminuria,* a loss of protein from the blood serum into the urine and the development of high blood pressure in roughly 23 percent of diabetics. The vascular changes, which are rather diffuse, contribute to the specific organ changes noted above, and frequently cause a reduction in blood supply to the legs and heart muscle. This ultimately causes heart damage in perhaps 20 percent of diabetics. Medicine can do much to reduce the effects of these many changes but cannot cure them.

Some degree of prevention is possible, and good diabetic control generally is thought to contribute to a reduction and delay in the development of these complications. Since the nerve and vascular changes make the feet particularly vulnerable to infections that can be serious and even lead to amputation—gangrene occurs in about three percent of diabetics—proper and daily care of the feet is essential to prevent the development of infections. The older diabetic should be careful to keep his feet clean and dry and cut his toenails frequently and evenly. Some physicians recommend that diabetics have their toenails cut only by a podiatrist.

Early Detection

Anyone who does not have diabetes might very well wonder whether he or she is at all likely to get it, and, if so, what can be done to prevent it. One answer is clear. If you are obese, whatever your age, try to lose weight. This is especially important if you have grandparents, parents, brothers, sisters, or children who developed diabetes in middle age or earlier. It is important also if you are a mother who has had babies weighing nine or more pounds at birth.

A fairly simple laboratory test, called a *glucose tolerance test* (GTT), has been developed to identify a person who is prediabetic. The subject either swallows a drink containing 100 grams of glucose or is given the same amount intravenously. Thereafter his blood sugar is determined at set intervals over a three-to-six-hour period. If his blood sugar level remains abnormally high for too long, he is said to be a prediabetic or to have *chemical diabetes.*

All adults should have their urine tested at least once a year for the presence of sugar. Some adults and younger persons should have more frequent urine tests and perhaps periodic glucose tolerance tests. Both of these possibilities have to be determined individually by the attending physician.

Genetically, diabetes has many characteristics of a Mendelian recessive inherited disease. Theoretically the chances are one in four of a child developing diabetes if one parent has the disease; it is almost inevitable if both have it. These are obviously important factors for diabetics to consider before they have children, particularly when both prospective parents have diabetes.

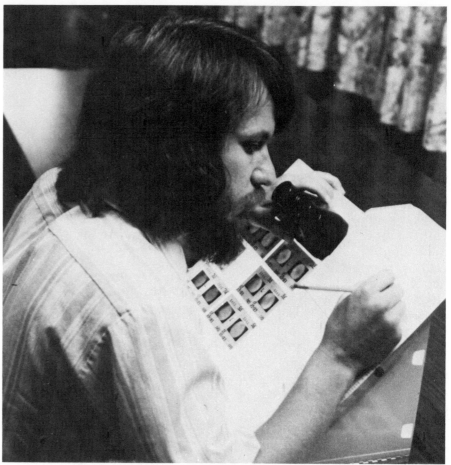

A researcher at the University of Wisconsin checks photographs of the *fundus* (the back of the eye) for early signs of diabetic retinopathy.

The person who develops diabetes today has a far better chance for a normal life than a patient of only a generation or two ago. The development of insulin therapy in the 1920s and oral hypoglycemic drugs in the late 1950s has made it possible for victims of a still very serious disease to add many active, productive years to their lives. Current research in the field of carbohydrate metabolism offers the promise of still more effective control of this insidious ailment in future years.

CHAPTER 22

Diseases of the Eye and Ear

Most people never experience any impairment of the senses of smell, taste, and touch. But it is indeed lucky and unusual to reach old age without having some problems connected with sight or with hearing or both.

The Eyes

All sensations must be processed in the brain by a normally functioning central nervous system for their proper perception. In addition, each sensation is perceived through a specific sense organ. Thus, sight is dependent on at least one functioning eye.

The eye is an optical system that can be compared to a camera, because the human lens perceives and the retina receives an image in the same way that a camera and its film does. Defects in this optical system are called errors in refraction and are the most common type of sight problem.

Myopia

Nearsightedness or *myopia* is a refractive error that causes faraway objects to be seen as blurred and indistinct. The degree of nearsightedness can be measured by testing each eye with a Snellen Test Chart. Normal vision is called 20/20. This means

that at 20 feet the eye sees an image clearly and accurately.

Eyesight of less-than-normal acuity is designated as 20/50 or 20/100 and so on. This means that what the deficient eye can see accurately at a distance of 20 feet or less, the normal eye can see accurately at 50 or 100 feet.

Myopia is the most common of all the refractive errors and usually results from an elongation of the eyeball. The cause of this abnormality is unknown, but it prevents the image from being focused on the retina. Those who are affected by myopia usually develop it between the ages of 6 and 15. They are likely to become aware of the condition when they can no longer see as well as they

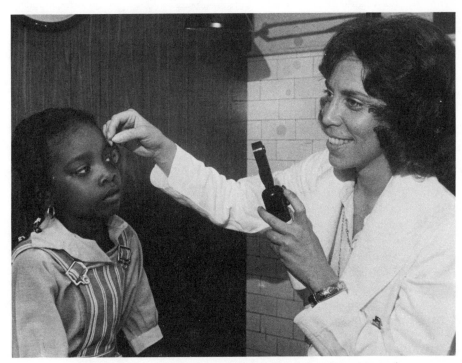

Children who become myopic usually develop the condition between the ages of 6 and 15. Eyeglasses can almost always correct myopia.

HOW EYEGLASSES CORRECT MYOPIA

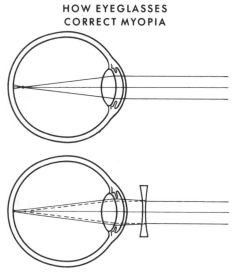

In a myopic or nearsighted eye *(top)*, parallel light rays from a viewed object come to a focus in front of, rather than on, the retina. *(Bottom)* A concave eyeglass lens diverges the rays so that they do not come to a focus and form an image until they have reached the retina.

used to in school or at the movies or as well as their friends can. Individually prescribed eyeglasses or contact lenses can correct the refractive error and produce normal vision.

Farsightedness and Astigmatism

The opposite of myopia is *hyperopia* or farsightedness, which results from a shortening of the eyeball. The two conditions may be combined with *astigmatism*, in which vertical and horizontal images do not focus on the same point, mainly because of some abnormality of the front surface of the cornea. Properly fitted glasses can correct all of these deficiencies.

Presbyopia

A fourth refractive error combines with the other three to make up about 80 percent of all visual defects. It is known as *presbyopia* or oldsight and results from an inability of the lens to focus on near objects. Almost everyone is affected by presbyopia some time after the age of 40, because of the aging of the lens itself or the muscles which expand and contract it. The condition is usually noticed when it becomes necessary to hold a book or newspaper farther

and farther away from the eyes in order to be able to read it. Although presbyopia is a nuisance, it can be easily corrected with glasses.

All these conditions represent variations in the sight of one or both eyes from what is considered the norm. Since seating distance from a school blackboard, the size of print, and the distance at which signs must be read are all based on what is considered to be normal vision, eye defects are handicaps, some mild and some severe.

Many people can function normally without glasses if the defects are minor. But since uncorrected refractive errors can cause headaches and general fatigue as well as eye aches and eye fatigue, they should receive prompt medical attention.

Color Blindness

Color blindness is a visual defect that occurs in about eight percent of men but is extremely rare in women. It is hereditary and usually involves an inability to differentiate clearly

between red, green, and blue. It is a handicap for which there is no known cure at the present time.

Glaucoma

Glaucoma is a serious problem that affects about two percent of those people who are over forty. It is caused not only by the aging process, but also and more importantly by anatomical changes inside the eye that prevent the normal drainage of fluid. The pressure inside the eye is therefore increased, and this pressure causes further anatomical change that can lead to blindness.

Glaucoma may begin with occasional eye pain or blurred vision, or it may be very insidious, cause no symptoms for years, and be discovered only at an eye examination. Glaucoma is the number one cause of blindness, and an annual check for its onset by a specialist is particularly recommended for everyone over forty. The test is quick, easy, and painless, and should symptoms appear, early treatment, either medical or surgical or both, can reduce the

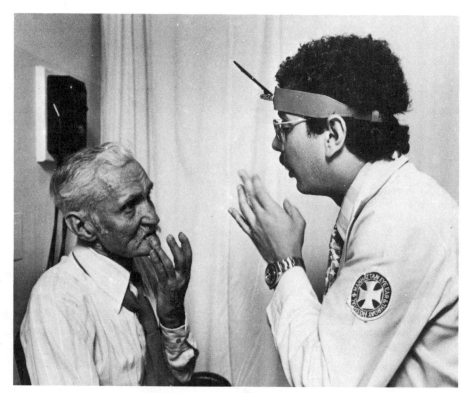

Some time after the age of 40, almost everyone is affected by the refractive error known as presbyopia, the inability of the lens to focus on near objects.

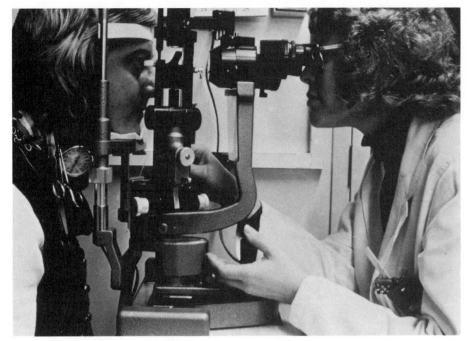

A patient being tested with a tonometer for elevated intraocular pressure. This is the initial test for glaucoma used by most ophthalmologists.

The symptoms of the onset of retinal separation are showers of drifting black spots and frequent flashes of light shaped like pinwheels that interfere with vision. These disturbances are usually followed by a dark shadow in the area of sight closest to the nose.

A retinal detachment is treated by surgical techniques in which the accumulated fluid is drained off and the hole in the tissue is sealed. About 60 percent of all cases are cured or considerably improved after surgery. The earlier the diagnosis, the more favorable is the outcome. Proper post-operative care usually involves several weeks of immobilization of the head so that the retinal tissue can heal without disturbance.

Trauma

Like any other part of the body, the eye can be injured by a major accident or *trauma*, although it is somewhat protected by the bones surrounding it. Trauma can cause most of the problems previously described. In addition, small objects

likelihood of partial or complete loss of sight.

Cataracts

Another serious eye problem is the development of *cataracts*. These are areas in the lens which are no longer transparent. The so-called *senile cataract* is common among elderly people because of degenerative changes in the lens. The condition causes varying degrees of loss of vision which are readily noticed by the patient. If the vision is reduced a great deal, the entire lens can be removed surgically and appropriate glasses or contact lenses can be provided.

Detached Retina

Among the most serious eye disorders is the condition known as *separated* or *detached retina*. It occurs when fluid from inside the eye gets under the retina (the inner membrane at the back of the eye, on which the image is focused) and separates it from its bed, thus breaking the connections that are essential for normal vision. The most common cause of the detachment is the formation of a hole or tear in the retina.

However, the condition may also develop following a blow to the head or to the eye, or because of a tumor, nephritis, or high blood pressure.

The Harvard University cyclotron, developed by physicists, treats an eye tumor by concentrating radiation in the very small area of the tumor.

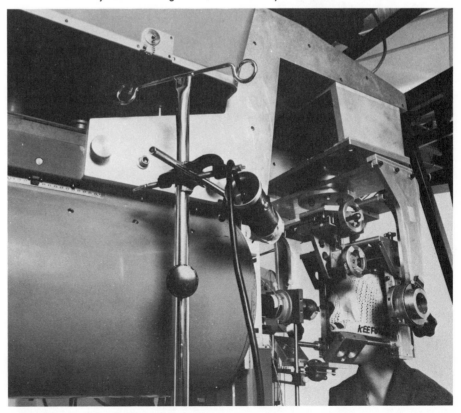

can get into the eye easily, and particles of soot and other wind-borne dirt can cause great discomfort. The tearing that results from the irritation usually floats foreign substances away, but occasionally they have to be removed by an instrument.

When a particle in the eye or under the eyelid is not easily dislodged and begins to cause redness, it should be removed by someone qualified to do so. The eye should never be poked at or into by untrained hands.

Leaving contact lenses in the eye for too long can cause discomfort which lasts for quite a while even after they have been taken out. Bacterial or viral infections of the outer surface of the eye such as *conjunctivitis* or *pinkeye*, or of the eyelids, are quite common and should be treated by a doctor if they are extensive or chronic.

Contact Lenses

Contact lenses, which are fitted directly over the iris and pupil of the eye in contact with the cornea (the tissue covering the outer, visible surface of the eye) are preferred by some people for the correction of vi-

sion defects. In some cases of severe astigmatism, nearsightedness, or following cataract surgery, contact lenses can be more effective than eyeglasses, but the chief reason for their popularity has been cosmetic. They are practically invisible. Hard plastic contact lenses adhere to the eye by suction: a partial vacuum is created between the inner surface of the lens and outer surface of the eyeball. Unfortunately, particles of dust can get under the lens and cause extreme discomfort. For this reason, many contact lens users habitually wear sunglasses when out of doors in sooty urban streets.

Soft plastic contact lenses are *hydrophilic* (literally, water-loving) and adapt their shape to the shape of the moist cornea, to which they adhere. Thus, they are more easily fitted, and patients seldom experience discomfort in adjusting to them. It is virtually impossible for dust particles to get underneath them. However, the soft lens must be sterilized daily; it scratches or tears easily; and it is limited to the correction of certain kinds of nearsightedness and farsightedness. It is also

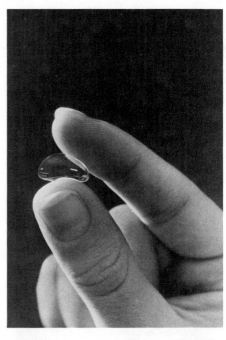

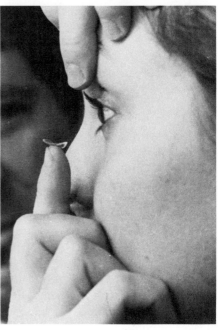

The "soft contact lens" (top), which contains 38.5 percent water, was said to be much more comfortable and easier to wear than the traditional hard lens. An even softer lens (bottom), 50 percent water, was introduced in 1981.

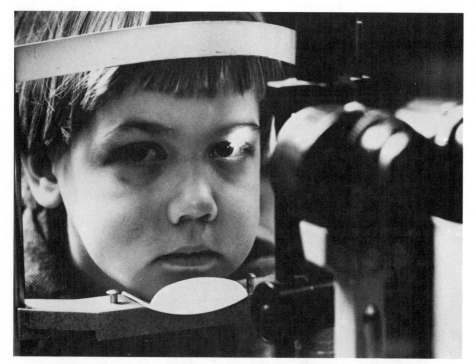

This child is being examined with a slit lamp microscope, which uses an intense light to facilitate microscopic study of the cornea and associated parts of the eye.

relatively expensive. Further technological improvements are likely to make it more widely applicable, however, and reduce the cost. The soft lens has already proved to be valuable therapeutically in the treatment of certain eye disorders, and some eye specialists believe that its potentialities have only begun to be explored. At present, neither soft nor hard lenses are recommended for 24-hour-a-day use; they should be removed before going to bed.

Diseases Which Affect Vision

In addition to the various disorders involving only the eye, there are a number of generalized diseases that affect vision. Among these are arteriosclerosis, diabetes mellitus, and hypertension or high blood pressure, which often cause abnormalities in the blood vessels of various parts of the eye. These abnormalities can lead to tissue changes which cause the patient to see spots or to notice that his vision is defective.

Diseases of the brain, such as multiple sclerosis, tumors, and abscesses, although rare, can result in double vision or loss of lateral or central vision. Any sudden or gradual changes in vision should be brought to a doctor's attention promptly, since early diagnosis and treatment is usually effective and can prevent serious deterioration.

The Ears

The ear, like the eye, is a complicated structure. Its major parts consist of the auditory canal, middle ear, and inner ear. Hearing results from the perception of sound waves whose loudness can be measured in decibels and whose highness or lowness of pitch can be measured by their frequency in cycles per second.

Sound waves usually travel through the auditory canal to the eardrum or *tympanic membrane,* vibrating it in such a way as to carry the vibrations to and along the three interlocking small bones in the middle ear to the inner ear. Here the vibrations are carried to the auditory nerve through a fluid-filled labyrinth called the communicating channel.

An abnormality at any of these points can produce a hearing deficiency. Normal hearing means the ability to hear the spoken voice in a relatively quiet room at a distance of about 18 feet. How well a person hears can be tested by an audiometer, which measures decibels and frequency of sound.

Wax Accumulation

A very common cause of hearing deficiency is the excessive accumulation of wax in the auditory canal, where it is continually being secreted. When the excess that blocks the passage of sound waves is removed—sometimes by professional instrumentation—hearing returns to normal. Anyone whose hearing is temporarily impaired in this way should avoid the use of rigid or pointed objects for cleaning out the accumulated wax.

Infection

Infections or other diseases of the skin that lines the auditory canal can sometimes cause a kind of local swelling that blocks the canal and interferes with hearing. Although such a condition can be painful, proper treatment, usually with antibiotics, generally results in a complete cure.

A major cause of hearing deficiency acquired after birth is recurrent bacterial infection of the middle ear. The infecting organisms commonly get to the middle ear through the *Eustachian tube,* which connects the middle ear to the upper throat, or through the eardrum if it has been perforated by injury or by previous infection.

The infection can cause hearing loss, either because it becomes chronic or because the tissues become scarred. Such infections are

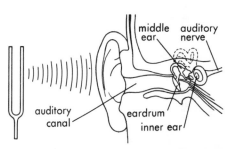

Sound waves pass through the auditory canal to the eardrum, whose vibrations are communicated to the three bones of the middle ear, then to the inner ear and auditory nerve.

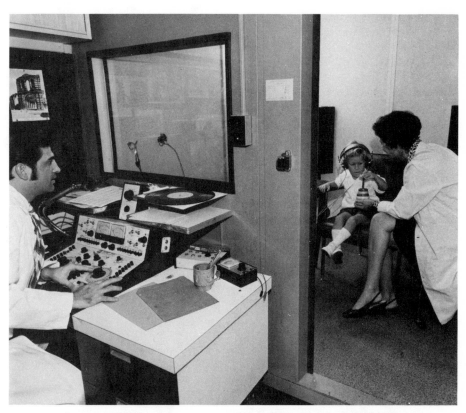

A young child's hearing tests are combined with games. Audiologist tells child, "Every time you hear a sound in your ear, put a ring on the stick."

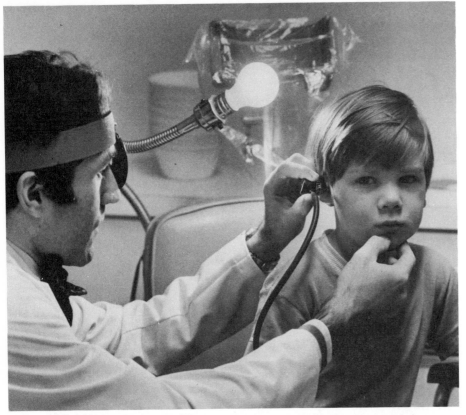

Anyone with an earache should seek medical attention promptly, since it might be caused by an infection that could cause permanent damage if left untreated.

otitis media and can cause permanent hearing damage.

Eustachian tube blockage is more commonly the result of swelling around its *nasopharyngeal* end because of a throat infection, a cold, or an allergy. Nose drops help to open up the tube, but sometimes it may be necessary to drain the ear through the eardrum or treat the disorder with other surgical procedures.

Otosclerosis

A very common cause of hearing loss that affects about 1 in 200 adults—usually women—is *otosclerosis*. This disorder is the result of a sort of freezing of the bones in the middle ear caused by an overgrowth of tissue. The onset of the disorder usually occurs before age 30 among about 70 percent of the people who will be affected. Only one ear may be involved, but the condition does get progressively worse. Although heredity is an important factor, the specific cause of

usually painful, but ever since treatment with antibiotics has become possible, they rarely spread to the mastoid bone as they used to in the past.

Disorders Caused by Pressure

The Eustachian tube usually permits the air pressure on either side of the eardrum to equalize. When the pressure inside the drum is less than that outside—as occurs during descent in an airplane or elevator, or when riding through an underwater tunnel, or during skin diving—the eardrum is pushed inward. This causes a noticeable hearing loss or a stuffy feeling in the ear which subsides as soon as the pressure equalizes again. Yawning or swallowing usually speeds up the return to normal.

When the unequal pressure continues for several days because the Eustachian tube is blocked, fluid begins to collect in the middle ear. This is called *serous* (or *nonsuppurative*)

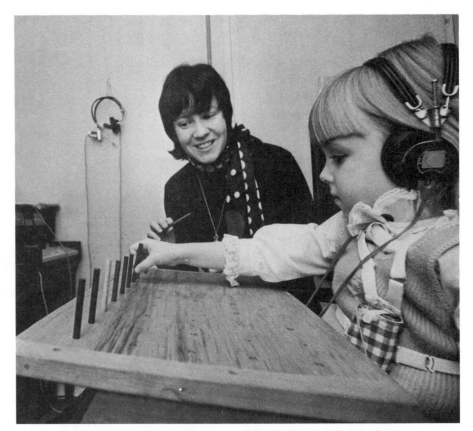

An audiologist measuring hearing ability. Doubts about hearing loss in a child should be brought to a doctor's attention as soon as possible.

otosclerosis is unknown. In some cases, surgery can be helpful.

Injury

A blow to the head, or a loud noise close to the ear such as the sound of a gunshot or a jet engine, especially when repeated often, can cause temporary and sometimes permanent hearing defects. Anyone who expects to be exposed to damaging noise should wear protective earmuffs. Injury to the auditory nerve by chemicals or by medicines such as streptomycin can also cause loss of hearing. For further information about the potential and actual dangers of noise, see *Noise Pollution* p. 232.

Ringing in the Ears

Sometimes people complain of hearing noises unrelated to the reception of sound waves from an outside source. This phenomenon is called *tinnitus* and occurs in the form of a buzzing, ringing, or hissing sound.

It may be caused by some of the conditions described above and may be relieved by proper treatment. In many cases, however, the cause is unknown and the patient simply has to learn to live with the sounds and ignore them.

Impairment of Balance

The *labyrinths* of the inner ear are involved not only in hearing but also in controlling postural balance. When the labyrinths are diseased, the result can be a feeling of *vertigo* or true dizziness. This sensation of being unable to maintain balance is quite different from feeling light-headed or giddy.

HOW A HEARING AID WORKS BY BONE CONDUCTION

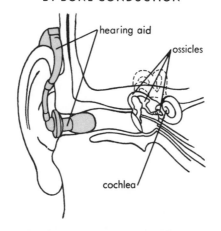

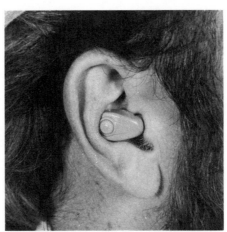

An inconspicuous hearing aid can be placed in the auditory canal, as shown above, for air conduction of sound waves, or it can be worn behind the ear for bone conduction.

Vertigo can be an incapacitating disorder. Sometimes it is caused by diseases of the central nervous system such as epilepsy or brain hemorrhage, but more often by inflammation sometimes caused by infection of the labyrinth. It can be sudden and recurrent as in *Ménière's disease,* or somewhat gradual and nonrecurrent.

It may or may not be accompanied by vomiting or hearing loss. Treatment for the condition varies depending on the cause.

Deafness

Deafness at birth or in a very young baby is an especially difficult problem because hearing is necessary for the development of speech. Although the deafness itself may be impossible to correct, its early recognition and management can usually prevent muteness from developing.

Many communities now have special schools for deaf children, and new techniques and machines are constantly being devised for helping them to learn how to speak, even if imperfectly. Any doubt about an infant's ability to hear should therefore be brought to a doctor's attention immediately.

Deafness at birth can be caused by a maternal infection such as rubella (German measles) during pregnancy. Since children are often the ones who spread this disease, youngsters should be immunized against it.

HEARING AIDS: Hearing loss that cannot be treated medically or surgically can often be compensated for by an accurately fitted hearing aid. This device, which now comes in many sizes, shapes, and types, converts sound waves into electrical impulses, amplifies them, and reconverts them into sound waves. A hearing aid can be placed in the auditory canal for air conduction of sound waves, or it can be worn behind the ear for bone conduction. See under *Hearing Loss*, p. 178, for further information about heating aids.

CHAPTER 23

Diseases of the Urinogenital System

The parts of the urinogenital tract that produce and get rid of urine are the same for men and women: the kidneys, ureters, bladder, and urethra. To understand some of the problems that can arise from diseases of the urinary tract, it is necessary to know a few facts about the anatomy and function of these parts.

The two kidneys are located on either side of the spinal column in the back portion of the abdomen between the last rib and the third lumbar vertebra of the spine. They are shaped like the beans named after them but are considerably larger.

Their function is to filter and cleanse the blood of waste substances produced in the course of normal living and, together with some other organs, to maintain a proper balance of body fluids. The kidneys do this job by filtering the fluid portion of the blood as it passes through them, returning the necessary solids and water to the bloodstream, and removing waste products and excess water, called *urine*. These products then flow into the *ureters*, the ducts that connect the kidneys and bladder.

The *bladder* holds the urine until voiding occurs. The duct from the bladder to the urinary opening is called the *urethra*. In the male, it passes through the penis; in the female, in front of the anterior wall of the vagina.

Symptoms of Kidney Disorders

Normal kidney function can be disrupted by bacterial or viral infection, by tumors, by external injury, or by congenital defects. Some of the common symptoms that may result under these circumstances are:

• *Anuria*—inability to produce or void urine
• *Dysuria*—pain, often of a burning quality, during urination
• Frequency—abnormally frequent urination, often of unusually small amounts
• Hesitancy—difficulty in starting urination
• Urgency—a very strong urge to urinate, often strong enough to cause loss of urine
• *Oliguria*—reduced production of urine
• *Polyuria*—voiding larger than normal amounts of urine
• *Nocturia*—frequent voiding at night
• *Hematuria*—voiding blood in the urine.

Since any of these symptoms may indicate a disease of the urinary tract, their appearance should be brought to the attention of a doctor without delay.

Kidney Failure

Kidney failure can occur gradually—either from kidney disease or as a secondary condition resulting from another disease—or suddenly, as from an infection.

Acute Kidney Failure

The sudden loss of kidney function over a period of minutes to several days is known as acute kidney failure. It may be caused by impairment of blood supply to the kidneys, by severe infection, by nephritis (discussed below), by poisons, and by various other conditions that injure both kidneys.

The body can function adequately throughout a normal lifespan with only one healthy kidney, but if both are impaired sufficiently over a short period of time, there will be symptoms of acute kidney failure: production of a decreased amount of urine *(oliguria)* sometimes with blood in it; fluid retention in body tissues, a condition known as *edema*; increasing fatigue and weakness; nausea and loss of appetite.

If damage to the kidneys hasn't been too severe, the patient begins to have a *diuresis*, or greater than

THE ANATOMY OF THE KIDNEY

The cortex is the darker, outer part of the kidney. The medulla, the inner part, includes the renal pyramids and the straight tubules associated with them.

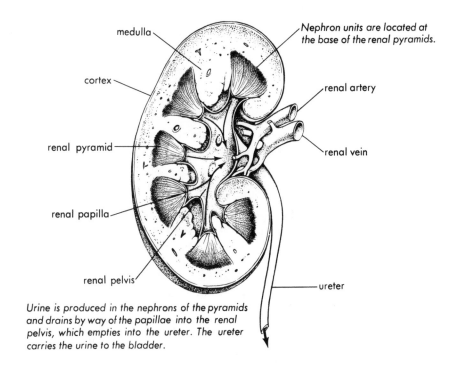

medulla

cortex

renal pyramid

renal papilla

renal pelvis

Nephron units are located at the base of the renal pyramids.

renal artery

renal vein

ureter

Urine is produced in the nephrons of the pyramids and drains by way of the papillae into the renal pelvis, which empties into the ureter. The ureter carries the urine to the bladder.

normal urine output. When this happens—usually after one or two weeks of reduced urine output—he is kept on a restricted diet and reduced fluid intake after recovery until normal kidney function returns.

CAUSES: Heredity is rarely a factor in acute kidney failure, although people born with one kidney or with congenital defects of the urinary tract may lack the normal reserve capacity to prevent it. It is also unusual for external injury to result in a loss of function in both kidneys. However, severe internal shock accompanied by a reduction of blood flow to the kidneys can cause acute kidney failure.

PREVENTION AND TREATMENT: Acute kidney failure can occur at any age. Prevention hinges on the proper control of its many causes. About 50 percent of patients with this disease may succumb to it; in cases of severe kidney failure involving widespread destruction of tissue, mortality may be almost 100 percent.

When acute kidney failure occurs as a complication of another serious illness, its prevention and treatment are usually managed by doctors in a hospital. If the patient is not already under a doctor's supervision when he has the characteristic symptoms, he should immediately be brought to a medical facility for diagnosis and treatment.

Chronic Kidney Failure and Uremia

Many progressive kidney diseases can eventually lead to a group of symptoms called *uremia*. Other diseases, such as severe high blood pressure, diabetes, and those leading to widespread damage of kidney tissue, can also cause uremia.

In this condition, as in acute kidney failure, waste products and excess fluid accumulate in the body and cause the symptoms of chronic kidney failure. Certain congenital defects in the urinogenital system such as *polycystic kidney disease*, in which cysts in the kidneys enlarge slowly and destroy normal kidney

tissue, may lead to uremia. Hereditary diseases such as hereditary nephritis may cause chronic kidney failure, but this is uncommon. Injury is also rarely the cause of uremia.

Although kidney failure is more likely to occur in older people because of the decreased capacity of the body to respond to stress, uremia can occur in any age group if kidney damage is severe enough. The onset of uremia may be so gradual that it goes unnoticed until the patient is weak and seems chronically ill. Voiding unusually large amounts of urine and voiding during the night are early symptoms.

Sleepiness and increasing fatigue set in as the kidney failure progresses, and there is a loss of appetite accompanied sometimes by nausea and hiccups. As the disease gets more serious, increasing weakness, anemia, muscle twitching, and sometimes internal bleeding may occur. High blood pressure is another characteristic symptom. Because of fluid retention, there will often be marked signs of facial puffiness and swelling of the legs.

Kidney damage that leads to chronic kidney failure is irreversible and the outlook for the victim of uremia is poor. The technique of dialysis (discussed below) has, however, prolonged many lives and continues to be a life-saving procedure for many.

Dialysis

An effective method of treatment of kidney failure developed in the 1960s is based on an artificial kidney that cleanses the patient's blood if his own kidneys are not functioning properly. The procedure, known as *dialysis* (or *hemodialysis*), removes dangerous waste products and excess fluids from the patient's bloodstream. It is the accumulation of waste products and fluids that probably causes the symptoms of acute kidney failure and that can be fatal if not reversed in one way or another.

DIALYSIS FOR CHRONIC KIDNEY FAILURE: For patients suffering chronic kidney failure or uremia, dialysis is a life-preserving but unfortunately expensive procedure. The patient must be dialyzed with the artificial kidney unit two or three times a week, usually for six to eight hours at a time. Although the technique does not cure uremia, it can keep the patient comfortable provided that his diet is carefully restricted and supervised.

DIALYSIS IN THE HOME: One approach that promises to be helpful in reducing the excessive cost is the development of home dialysis programs prepared with the cooperation of hospitals having departments specializing in kidney disease. Home dialysis is not suitable for everyone; the patient must be mature and stable enough to be relied on to undertake the procedure on schedule and in the prescribed manner. The overall costs of home dialysis, however, are about one-third those of in-hospital dialysis.

MEDICARE COVERAGE: Medicare coverage is now available for a part of the costs for dialysis maintenance for those suffering from permanent kidney failure, even if they are under 65 years of age. Coverage includes training in self-dialysis and the cost of dialysis equipment and applies to dialysis done in the home as well as

in hospitals or other approved facilities. For details of this coverage, see your local social security office or write for the free booklet, *Medicare Coverage of Kidney Dialysis and Kidney Transplant Services*, published by the Social Security Administration.

Kidney Transplant Surgery

Some people suffering from kidney disease may benefit greatly from the surgical transplant of a donor's kidney. The donor kidney may be taken from a live relative or from someone recently deceased. The organ is removed from the donor's abdomen, usually flushed with a salt solution, and then reattached to a large artery and vein in the recipient's abdomen and to his ureter.

The successfully transplanted kidney functions just as the patient's own did when he was healthy, removing wastes and excess fluids from his bloodstream and excreting the resulting urine through the bladder. The recipient of a kidney transplant must take special medication to prevent the rejection of the newly installed organ by his own body tissues. With proper medical care, recipients have lived for many years with their transplanted organs.

MEDICARE COVERAGE: Medicare coverage is now available for a part of the costs of kidney transplant surgery for those under 65 as well as those over 65. This coverage includes hospital charges for costs incurred by the donor. For details of this coverage, see your local social security office or write for the free booklet, *Medicare Coverage of Kidney Dialysis and Kidney Transplant Services*, published by the Social Security Administration.

Nephritis

Nephritis is a disorder characterized by inflammation of the *glomeruli* of the kidneys. The glomeruli are tiny coiled blood vessels through which the liquid portion of the blood is filtered as it enters the outer structure of the kidneys. There are about one million of these tiny blood vessels in each kidney. The fluid from the blood passes from them into many little ducts called *tubules*. Water and various substances are secreted into and absorbed from the liquid in the tubules. The final product of this passage of filtered fluid from the glomeruli through the tubules to the ureters and then to the bladder is urine. It contains the excess fluid and waste products produced by the body during normal functioning.

When the glomeruli become inflamed, the resulting disease is called *glomerulonephritis*. There are several forms of this disease. One type is thought to be caused by the body's allergic reaction to infection by certain streptococcal bacteria. Another type sometimes accompanies infection of the valves of the heart. The relationship between glomerulonephritis and strep infections is not fully understood at present, and the same may be said for nephritis, which is associated with allergic reaction to certain drugs and to heart valve infections.

Glomerulonephritis may occur ten days to two weeks after a severe strep throat infection. For this reason, any severe sore throat accompanied by a

A patient with chronic kidney failure undergoes dialysis in a hospital in Richmond, Va. Some patients are judged suitable for home dialysis.

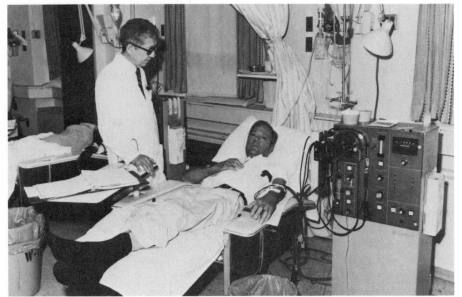

When the disease is suspected, the doctor examines a specimen of urine under a microscope and looks for red blood cells. These cells, which usually do not pass through the walls of the normal glomerulus in large numbers, do pass through the damaged walls of the inflamed blood vessels characteristic of nephritis. Evidence of decreased kidney function is also found by special blood tests.

Nephritis occurs in all age groups. Children under ten have an excellent chance of recovery, about 98 percent. In adults, from 20 to 50 percent of the cases may be fatal or may progress to chronic nephritis, which often leads to uremia and death.

Treatment

It is absolutely essential for anyone with a streptococcal infection, which may lead to acute glomerulonephritis, to receive prompt and proper treatment. Penicillin is considered the most effective antibiotic at present.

Once acute nephritis is present, the treatment consists of bed rest, some fluid restriction, and protein restriction if kidney failure occurs. If there is a total loss of kidney function, a specially restricted diet is prescribed. Complete lack of urine output—*anuria*—may last as long as ten days, but the patient can still make a full recovery if the treatment is right. Usually a gradual return of kidney function occurs over a period of several months.

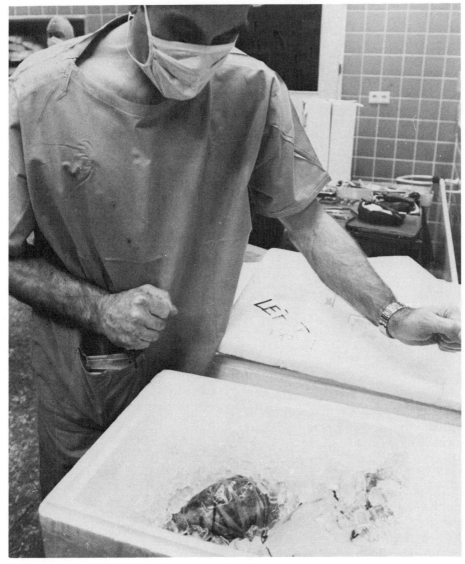

A human kidney, ready to be surgically transplanted in a patient whose kidneys are failing, can be kept on ice for 24 hours if properly wrapped.

high fever should be seen and diagnosed by a doctor. Prompt treatment with antibiotics may decrease the possibility of kidney involvement.

Nephritis Symptoms

The inflammation and swelling of the glomeruli cause a decrease in the amount of blood that the kidney is able to filter. As a result of the slowing down of this kidney function, the waste products of metabolism as well as excess fluid accumulate in the body instead of being eliminated at the normal rate.

In a typical case, a person will develop a severe sore throat with fever and a general feeling of sickness.

These symptoms will disappear, but after one or two weeks, there will be a return of weakness and loss of appetite. The eyes and the face may become puffy, the legs may swell, and there may be shortness of breath—all because of the retention of excess fluid in the body. The amount of urine is small and the color is dark brown, somewhat like coffee. Abdominal pain, nausea, and vomiting may occur, always accompanied by fatigue. In most cases, the blood pressure increases, leading to headaches.

Although there is a hereditary type of nephritis, the more common types of the disease have other causes.

Nephrosis

The *nephrotic syndrome*, commonly referred to as *nephrosis*, is a disease in which abnormal amounts of protein in the form of *albumin* are lost in the urine. Albumin consists of microscopic particles of protein present in the blood. These particles are important in maintaining the proper volume of fluids in the body, and they have other complicated functions as well. The loss of albumin in the urine affects the amount that remains in the blood, and it is this im-

THE NEPHRON

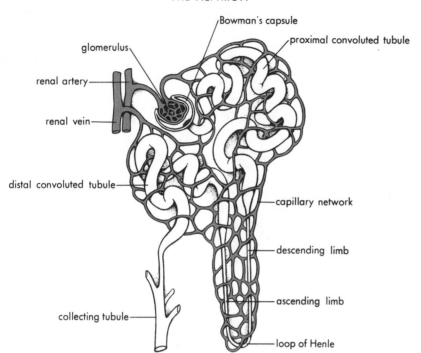

balance, together with other body changes, that results in the retention of excess fluid in the tissues, thus causing facial puffiness and swelling of the legs.

The disease is caused by damage to the glomeruli, but at the present time the exact nature of the damage is uncertain. It may be caused by an allergic reaction, by inflammation, or it may be a complication of diabetes. The nephrotic syndrome may also appear because of blood clots in the veins that drain the kidneys.

Although the disease is more common among children than among adults, it may affect a person of any age. The main symptom is painless swelling of the face, legs, and sometimes of the entire body. There is also loss of appetite, a tired, run-down feeling, and sometimes abdominal pain, vomiting, and diarrhea.

Recovery from nephrosis varies with age. Over 50 percent of child patients are completely free of kidney ailments after the first attack. Adults are more likely to develop some impairment of kidney function, or the disease may become chronic, with accompanying high blood pressure. In some people, protein loss

may continue over the years, although the kidneys function in an apparently normal manner without any visible symptoms.

Treatment

Treatment of the nephrotic syndrome has been greatly helped by the use of the adrenal hormones known as *steroids*. The treatment is effective for about two-thirds of child patients and for about one-fourth to one-third of adults. Some patients may relapse after therapy is completed, sometimes years after such therapy has been discontinued. For this reason, steroids are sometimes continued after initial treatment but in reduced dosage, to avoid some of the unpleasant side effects such as acne and facial swelling.

Unlike the dietary treatment for uremia, a high protein diet is used with nephrotic patients so that the protein loss can be replaced. Salt intake is usually restricted because salt contributes to fluid retention and may cause high blood pressure or heart failure. If fluid retention doesn't respond to steroid treatment, other medicines called *diuretics*, which increase urinary output, are used.

Anyone with unusual swelling of the face, limbs, or abdomen should see a physician promptly. Even though the swelling is painless, it may be the first sign of the onset of a serious kidney problem.

Infection in the Urinary Tract

Infection in the urinary tract is a common disorder that can be serious if the kidneys themselves are involved.

Cystitis

Infection of the bladder is called *cystitis*. The symptoms include a burning sensation when urine is passed, the frequent need to urinate, occasionally blood in the urine, and sometimes difficulty in starting to urinate. Cystitis is rarely accompanied by high fever.

The problem may be recurrent and is more usual with women than men, probably because the female urethra is shorter and closer to the rectum, permitting bacteria to enter the bladder more easily. These bacteria multiply in the urine contained in the bladder, causing irritation to the bladder walls and producing the symptoms described above.

Cystitis should be treated promptly because the infection in the bladder can easily spread to the kidneys, with serious consequences. Treatment usually consists of antibiotics after urine analysis and culture have determined the type of bacteria causing the infection. Cystitis and other kidney infections are especially common during pregnancy because of the body changes that occur at this time. At no time is cystitis itself a serious disease, but it must be diagnosed and treated promptly to avoid complications. For additional information on cystitis and other disorders of the female urinary system, see p. 494.

Other Causes of Infection

Infection of the bladder and kidneys may occur because of poor hygiene in the area of the urethra, especially in women. It is also caused by some congenital defects in the urinary tract or by the insertion of instruments used to diagnose a urinary problem.

Sometimes bacteria in the bloodstream can settle in and infect the kidneys. Patients with diabetes seem to be more prone to urinary infections—indeed to infections generally—than other people. Any obstruction to the flow of urine in the urinary tract, such as a kidney stone, increases the possibility of infection in the area behind the obstruction. Damage to the nerves controlling the bladder is another condition that increases the chances of infection in that area.

Pyelonephritis

Infection in the kidneys is called *pyelonephritis*. Although it sometimes occurs without any symptoms, a first attack usually causes an aching pain in the lower back, probably due to the swelling of the kidneys, as well as nausea, vomiting, diarrhea, and sometimes severe pain in the front of the abdomen on one or both sides, depending on whether one or both kidneys are involved. Fever may be quite high, ranging from 103 to 105 degrees, often accompanied by chills.

Although the symptoms of pyelonephritis may disappear in a few days without treatment, bacterial destruction of the kidney tissue may be going on. This silent type of infection can eventually disrupt normal kidney function and result in a chronic form of the disease, which in turn can lead to uremia. If the disease is not halted before this, it can be fatal.

Anyone with symptoms of acute pyelonephritis must have prompt medical attention. In order to diagnose the disease properly, the urine is analyzed and the number and type of bacteria in the urine are determined. The disease is brought under control by the right antibiotics and by administering large amounts of fluids to flush out the kidneys and urinary tract, thus decreasing the number of bacteria in the urine. In its

chronic form the disease is much more difficult to cure, since bacteria that are lodged deep in the kidney tissue do not seem to be susceptible to antibiotics and are therefore almost impossible to get rid of.

Kidney Stones

Another cause of infection in the bladder and kidneys is obstruction in the urinary tract by *kidney stones.* These stones, crystallizations of salts that form in the kidney tissue, may be quite small, but they can grow large enough to occupy a considerable part of one or both of the kidneys. The smaller ones often pass from the kidney through the ureters to the bladder, from which they are voided through the urethra. However, obstruction of the flow of urine behind a kidney stone anywhere in the urinary tract usually leads to infection in the urine. This type of infection may lead to attacks of acute pyelonephritis.

REMOVAL OF STONES: Unless the stone causes no symptoms of infection, it must be removed. Removal may be accomplished by flushing out the urinary tract with large fluid intake or by surgical methods. Any accompanying infection is treated with antibiotics.

Why kidney stones form in some people and not in others is not clearly understood. Because of metabolic disorders, certain substances may build up in the body. The increased excretion of these substances in the urine as well as excessive amounts of calcium in the blood may encourage kidney stone formation. People who have gout are also likely to develop them.

RENAL COLIC: Sometimes the formation and passage of stones cause no symptoms. However, when symptoms do occur with the passage of a kidney stone, they can be uncomfortably severe. The pain that results from the passage of a stone through the ureter, referred to as *renal colic*, is usually like an intense cramp. It begins in the side or back and moves toward the lower abdomen, the genital region, and the

inner thigh on the affected side. The attack may last for a few minutes or for several hours. Sometimes bloody urine may be passed accompanied by a burning sensation.

Kidney stones are more likely to form in middle-aged and older people than in young ones. A history of stones is sometimes found in several generations of a family, since the metabolic disorders encouraging their formation have a hereditary basis.

Treatment for an acute attack of renal colic usually relieves the pain several hours after the patient has taken medication and fluids. If they are not promptly treated, kidney stones may lead to serious infection and eventual impairment of function.

Tumors of the Urinary Tract

Benign and malignant tumors of the kidney are not common problems. However, anyone with pain in the midback, blood in the urine, or a mass in the abdomen should have the symptoms diagnosed. If a malignant tumor is discovered early enough, it can be removed with the affected kidney, and normal function can be maintained by the healthy kidney that remains.

Malignant kidney tumors are most often found in children or adults over 40, and more often in men than in women. A tumor of any type can usually be diagnosed by X-ray

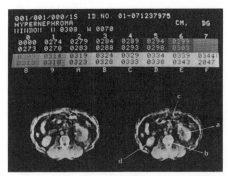

A computerized X ray (CAT scan) showing two adjacent sections of the abdomen of a patient with a tumor of the kidney. Structures shown include: *(a)* kidney tumor, *(b)* spine, *(c)* aorta, *(d)* normal kidney.

studies. Where this technique is inadequate, an operation is necessary to search for the suspected growth. About one-fourth of all patients with a malignant kidney tumor live for more than ten years after surgery.

A malignant tumor of the bladder is a serious problem since it obstructs kidney drainage and may cause death from uremia. The main symptom is the painless appearance of blood in the urine, although sometimes a burning sensation and a frequent need to urinate are also present. Treatment usually includes surgical removal of the bladder followed by radiation treatment of the affected area to destroy any malignant cells that remain after the operation.

Some malignant bladder tumors grow very slowly and do not invade the bladder wall extensively. Surgical treatment for this type, called *papillary tumors,* is likely to be more successful than for tumors of the more invasive kind. For a description of surgical treatment of the urinary tract, see p. 320.

The Prostate Gland

The *prostate gland,* which contributes to the production of semen, encircles the base of the male urethra where it joins the bladder. When it begins to enlarge, it compresses the urethra and causes difficulty in voiding. Urination may be difficult to start, and when the urine steam appears it may be thinner than normal.

Since urine may remain in the bladder, there is the possibility of local infection that may spread to the kidneys. If the kidneys become enlarged because of this type of obstruction, a condition of *hydronephrosis* is said to exist. This disease can cause impaired kidney function and lead to uremia.

Benign Prostatic Enlargement

Enlargement of the prostate gland occurs in about half the male population over 50, and the incidence increases with increasing age. The

THE MALE URINARY SYSTEM

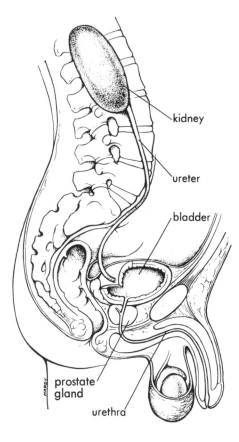

kidney

ureter

bladder

prostate gland

urethra

condition is called *benign prostatic enlargement* and must be treated surgically if sufficient obstruction is present. For temporary relief, a catheter can be inserted into the bladder through the urethra, allowing the urine to drain through the catheter and out of the body. If surgery is necessary, the entire prostate may be removed or only that part of it that surrounds the urethra.

Symptoms of benign prostatic enlargement are quite distinctive: increased difficulty in voiding; an urge to continue to urinate after voiding has been completed; burning and frequent urination, caused in part by infection from urine retained in the bladder.

The cause of benign prostatic enlargement is thought to be a change during the aging process in the hormones that affect prostate tissue, but the exact nature of the change and its effect is not clear. It is likely that hormone-containing medicines will eventually be developed that will

prevent or reverse prostate tissue growth.

Acute Prostatitis

Acute prostatitis occurs typically in young men. Symptoms include pain on urinating, sometimes a discharge of pus from the penis, pain in the lower back or abdomen indicating a tender and enlarged prostate, and fever. It is caused by a bacterial infection and usually responds promptly to antibiotics.

Cancer of the Prostate

Cancer of the prostate is a common type of malignancy in older men. It accounts for about 10 percent of male deaths from cancer in the United States. The disease may be present without any symptoms or interference with normal function and is therefore difficult to diagnose. A very high proportion of men over 80—probably more than 50 percent —has been found to have had cancer of the prostate at autopsy.

When symptoms are present, they are likely to be the same as those of benign prostatic enlargement. The disease can be diagnosed only by a biopsy examination of a tissue sample taken from the prostate during surgery. If malignancy is found, the gland is surgically removed when feasible to do so; the testes are removed too so that the level of male hormones in the body is lowered.

Male hormones increase the growth of malignant prostate tissue, but since female hormones slow it down, they may be administered after a diagnosis of prostate malignancy. If the tumor has spread to bone tissue, radiation treatment of the affected areas may slow down cancerous growth and relieve pain.

Men over 40 should have a rectal examination once a year, since tumors of the prostate and benign prostatic enlargement can often be diagnosed early in this way. For a description of prostate surgery, see p. 318.

Bedwetting

Enuresis, the medical term for bedwetting, is the unintentional loss of urine, usually during sleep at night. Infants do not have sufficiently developed nervous systems to control urination voluntarily until they are about two-and-a-half or three years old. Controlling urination through the night may not occur until after the age of three. A child who wets his bed recurrently after he has learned to control urination has the problem of enuresis.

There are many causes of enuresis. It may occur because of a delay in normal development or as a result of emotional stress. About 15 percent of boys and 10 percent of girls are bedwetters at the age of 5. By 9, about 5 percent of all children still have the problem, but most children outgrow it by the time they reach puberty.

Children who are bedwetters should be examined to rule out any physical abnormality in the urinary tract. Obstruction at the neck of the bladder where it joins the urethra or obstruction at the end of the urethra may cause uncontrollable dribbling of urine, but this usually occurs during the day as well as at night.

Disease of the nerves controlling the bladder, sometimes hereditary, can cause loss of urine. It can also occur in children who are mentally retarded or mentally ill, or because of an acute or chronic illness. In the latter cases, the problem disappears when the child regains his health.

EMOTIONAL PROBLEMS: If all physical abnormalities for bedwetting have been explored and eliminated as possible causes, the emotional problems of the child and his family should be examined. An understanding attitude rather than a hostile or punitive one on the part of the parents is extremely important in helping a child who is a bedwetter. He may be anxious about school or angry at a favored younger child, or he may feel insecure about parental acceptance. In such cases, an effort to bring the child's hidden feelings into the open and to deal with them sympathetically usually causes the problem to disappear.

Venereal Diseases

Venereal diseases are those which are transmitted by sexual contact. The most common are syphilis and gonorrhea, although several others are transmitted in the same way. Since they are highly contagious and can cause serious complications, the symptoms should be treated by a doctor without any delay. Additional information about venereal diseases may be found under *Women's Health*, p. 489.

Syphilis

Syphilis is caused by the type of microscopic organism known as a *spirochete*. The spirochete cannot survive outside the body for more than a brief period unless it is frozen. It is transmitted through the membranes of the reproductive system by direct sexual contact or through a break in the skin.

PRIMARY STAGE: Such transmission leads to an initial sore, usually an ulcerated area called a *chancre*, on

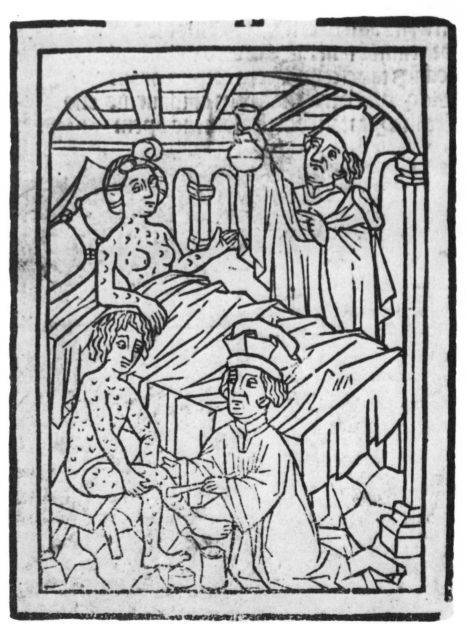

This 15th-century woodcut illustrates treatment of venereal disease patients who display the body rashes characteristic of secondary-stage syphilis.

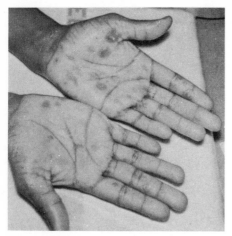

The onset of the secondary stage of syphilis is usually signaled by a rash that often covers the entire body, including the palms of the hands and the soles of the feet.

the penis, vagina, or any other area in contact with the spirochetes, including the fingers, lips, or breasts. The primary lesion, as the chancre is called, is usually a single one and not painful, although there are occasional exceptions. Any sore in the genital region should be examined by a physician. If the sore is actually a chancre, a specimen examined under a microscope will contain the spirochetes that cause syphilis. Certain blood tests also reveal the presence of the disease, but they require a waiting period before they turn positive.

SECONDARY STAGE: There are no symptoms when the spirochetes enter the body, but the chancre usually appears about three to six weeks later. It heals without treatment, sometimes leaving a scar. About six weeks after its appearance, there is usually a skin eruption that takes various forms. The rash signals the onset of the secondary stage of syphilis. The rash may consist of many small pigmented spots or wider areas of darkened pigmentation, often involving the entire body, including the palms, soles, and face. The rash may be accompanied by itching.

All the affected areas contain spirochetes and are therefore infectious. In addition to the rash, there are general symptoms of illness at this stage, such as sore throat, fatigue, headaches, fever, muscle pain, and sometimes temporary loss of scalp hair.

In some cases, the infected person does not experience either the primary or secondary phase of the illness, and there may be no history of symptoms until the onset of the third stage of syphilis, many years after the first contact with the spirochete. However, a blood test will be positive in almost all cases of secondary syphilis.

TERTIARY STAGE: The characteristic rash and other symptoms of secondary syphilis will also disappear without treatment in the same way as the chancre of the primary stage. Then a stage of latent syphilis may occur in which the spirochete is present for many years—sometimes for an entire lifetime—without doing further harm or causing further symptoms.

In many cases, however, the syphilis spirochetes seriously damage various organs, particularly the heart and brain. These late effects that appear years after the first untreated infection are called tertiary syphilis.

Neurosyphilis affects the brain and spinal cord, causing progressive loss of the mental faculties, eventual insanity, and death. Damage to the aorta, the main artery leading from the heart, can cause heart failure and the formation of an *aneurysm,* in which the wall of the aorta becomes weak and swollen. The rupture of such an aneurysm is likely to be fatal.

Although the devastating effects of tertiary syphilis are rarely seen today, they can result from lack of treatment or inadequate treatment of the early stages of the disease. Therefore, symptoms of primary or secondary syphilis, or knowledge of contact with a possible source of infection, makes medical attention absolutely essential.

Ninety percent of the deaths from syphilis are the result of the involvement of the heart and nervous system. Almost any part of the body may be involved in the tertiary stage, but even when the disease is this advanced, proper treatment can greatly improve the function of the damaged organ.

Children born of mothers having syphilis during pregnancy may have congenital syphilis at birth. These children require a great deal of special care if they are to survive the effects of this disease.

TREATMENT: Penicillin is extremely effective in killing the syphilis spirochete and should be called a wonder drug if only for this special role. However, proper and early treatment for the many forms of syphilis is a problem for many doctors, since the entire responsibility for seeking medical attention rests with the person exposed to the disease.

The possibility of catching or transmitting syphilis can be lessened by the use of a prophylactic condom. It is because of the widespread use of the contraceptive pill and the decreased use of the condom that the incidence of syphilis is presently on the rise. Even under these circumstances, without the protection afforded by the condom, washing the genital region thoroughly with soap and water after sexual relations will reduce the possibility of infection. Penicillin in the proper dosage immediately after suspected contact with syphilis will prevent infection altogether in most cases.

Gonorrhea

Gonorrhea is among the most common bacterial infectious diseases in the United States today. It is caused by a bacterium called the *gonococcus.* Infection with this organism causes the formation of pus composed of dead white blood cells and tissues on the lining of the genital tract. The urethra, the Fallopian tubes in women, the prostate in men, and other parts of the reproductive system of either sex may be subject to the infection, which causes a heavy white discharge from the penis and sometimes from the vagina.

In women, the infection may cause fever and low abdominal pain with or without the discharge. Since gonorrhea may occur without any symptoms at all, unsuspected damage to the female reproductive system can eventually lead to sterility. Infections of the joints and other parts of the body may occur if the gonococcus spreads through the bloodstream, but these complications are rare so long as penicillin is administered promptly.

The discharge from the urethra in the male usually occurs three to seven days after contact with an infected partner. Symptoms include a severe burning sensation during urination, a heavy white discharge, and occasional lower abdominal pain. A testicle may become swollen when infected.

The disease is diagnosed by a microscopic examination of the discharge. If the gonococcus is present, penicillin is administered. In cases where the gonococcus strain is resistant to this treatment, various other antibiotics are tested in the laboratory on a culture of the resistant bacteria. Immediate and adequate treatment is essential to prevent the complications of sterility and the spread of infection.

CHAPTER 24

Cancer

Cancer has always figured uniquely in the diseases of mankind. For centuries people spoke of it only in whispers, or not at all, as if the disease were not only dreadful but somehow shameful as well. Today, the picture is changing, and rapidly. This decade may see the time—undreamt of only scant years ago—when half of those stricken by cancer will survive its ravages. And much of the mystery that cloaked the disease in an awful shroud has been dissipated, although the last veils remain to be stripped away.

Of course, cancer remains a formidable enemy. More than a million Americans are under medical care for cancer; an estimated 385,000 will die of it each year. Of all Americans now alive, some 55 million—one in four—will be stricken; and some 36 million will die of the disease. Cancer is the greatest cause of lost working years among women and ranks third after heart disease and accidents in denying men working years.

But in context, the picture is not as bleak as it might seem. At the beginning of the century, survival from cancer was relatively rare. At the end of the 1930s, the five-year survival rate (alive after five years) was one in five or less. Ten years later it had shot up to one in four, and in the mid-fifties to one in three. This figure has remained relatively stable because the survival rate for some of the more widespread cancers has leveled off despite the best efforts of physicians to devise better forms of treatment. For such cancers, which include those of the breast, colon, and rectum, improvements will come through earlier detection and even prevention. Dr. Richard S. Doll, Pro-

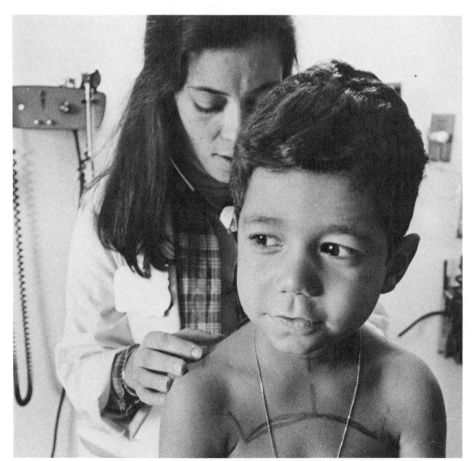

Cancer can strike at any age. A nurse examines a five-year-old boy being treated for a lymphoma at Memorial Hospital in New York City.

NORMAL CELLS

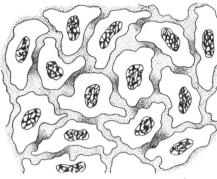

1. Cell surface bonding is strong.
2. Cells remain in place.
3. Electrical voltage level is high.
4. Cells divide at a low rate.

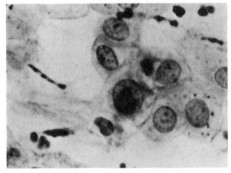

MALIGNANT CELLS

1. Cell surface bonding is very weak.
2. Cells spread and invade normal tissue.
3. Electrical voltage level is low.
4. Cells divide at a rapid pace.

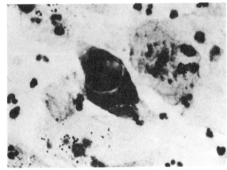

Cancer begins when body cells lose their normal development controls and begin to proliferate, often very rapidly and without any apparent limit.

fessor of Medicine at Oxford University, has said that we could prevent 40 percent of men's cancer deaths and 10 percent of women's simply by applying what we already know. For example, according to the American Cancer Society, the risk of death from lung cancer is 15 to 20 times greater among men who smoke cigarettes than among men who have never smoked. The relative risk of lung cancer among women smokers is five times that of women who have never smoked.

Considerable progress is being made on many fronts in the war against cancer. It ranges from advances in early detection to breakthroughs in treatment. The last 25 years have seen a 50 percent dip in the death rate from cervical cancer, mostly because of widening acceptance of the Pap test, which can detect the disease at a very early stage. At the same time, children with acute lymphocytic leukemia, which used to be invariably fatal in weeks

or months, have benefited from new therapies, with at least half now surviving three years, some more than five years, and a few on the verge of being pronounced cured. Similar advances in the treatment of a cancer

of the lymph system called *Hodgkin's disease* have improved the five-year survival rate from 25 percent at the end of World War II to about 55 percent today.

The mortality rates for some forms of cancer are dropping for no known reason. Stomach cancer, for example, produces only indigestion as an early symptom, so most patients do not get the benefit of early diagnosis. The result is a rather poor five-year survival rate. There are an estimated 23,000 new cases each year, and an estimated 14,600 deaths. Nevertheless, cancer of the stomach accounts for only 4 percent of all cancer deaths today, compared to 20 percent in the 1950s; nobody knows why.

What Is Cancer?

Cancer would surely be easier to detect and treat if it were a single entity with a single simple cause. But it is not. Experts agree that there are actually some 200 different diseases that can be called cancers. They have different causes, originate in different tissues, develop for different reasons and in different ways, and demand vastly different kinds of treatment. All have one fatal element in common, however; in every case, normal cells have gone wild and lost their normal growth and development controls.

A researcher at the National Cancer Institute studies viruses that cause leukemia in cats, hoping to shed light on the causes of human cancers.

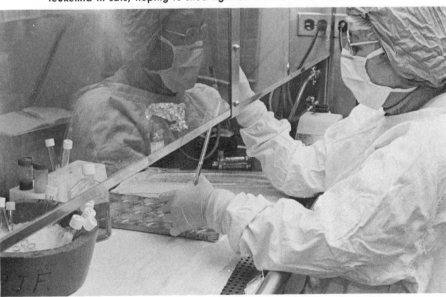

Initial Stages

The cancer may start with just one or a few cells somewhere in the body which undergo a change and become malignant, or cancerous. The cells divide and reproduce themselves, and the cancer grows.

Most cancers arise on the surface of a tissue, such as the skin, the lining of the uterus, mouth, stomach, bowel, bladder, or bronchial tube in the lung, or inside a duct in the breast, prostate gland, or other site. Eventually, they grow from a microscopic clump to a visible mass, then begin to invade underlying tissues. As long as the cells remain in one mass, however, the cancer is localized.

Later Stages

At some later phase, in a process called *metastasis,* some of the cancer cells split off and are swept into the lymph channels or bloodstream to other parts of the body. They may be captured for a while in a nearby lymph node (a stage called regional involvement), but unless the disease is arrested, it will rapidly invade the rest of the body, with death the almost certain result. Some cancers grow with an almost malevolent rapidity, some are dormant by comparison. Some respond to various therapies, such as radiation therapy; others do not. About half of the known types of cancer are incurable at almost any stage. Of the remaining half, it is obviously imperative to diagnose and treat them as early as possible.

How Cancers Are Classified

The cancers described above, arising in *epithelial* (covering or lining) tissue are called *carcinomas* as a group. Another class of malignant tumors, similar in most basic respects, is the *sarcomas,* which originate in connective tissue such as bones and muscles. A third group of cancers—*leukemia* and the *lymphomas*—are diseases of the blood-forming organs and the lymphatic system, respectively, and are not tumors. They arise and spread in a basically different way.

What Causes Cancer?

In its battle with cancer, medical science devotes constant attention to a search for those factors in our environment that can produce cancer in human beings. They include a large number of chemical agents such as those in tobacco smoke, and including asbestos fibers and other occupational chemical hazards; ionizing radiation such as that from X rays, nuclear bombs, and sunlight; injury or repeated irritation; metal or plastic implants; flaws in the body's immune reaction; genetic mistakes; parasites; and—many scientists believe—viruses.

It is this last factor that is generating perhaps the most interest among medical scientists today. It has been shown that viruses cause a variety of cancers in animals; yet they have never been proved responsible in human cancer, although they have been linked to at least six different ones. Recently, researchers discovered an enzyme in a virus believed to cause cancer and also in the tissues of leukemia patients. This enzyme may be the key to the mechanism by which a virus induces a malignant change in normal cells.

Scientists have also discovered that certain substances in the environment which by themselves may not stimulate the growth of a cancer can be dangerously activated to become carcinogenic by the presence of one or more other substances. Each of these potential cancer-causing agents is called a *co-carcinogen.* It is possible that some co-carcinogens are present in ordinary fruits and vegetables, in certain food additives, and in other substances such as the synthetic estrogen, diethylstilbestrol (DES). For more information on DES, see p. 503 under *Women's Health.*

MAJOR FORMS OF CANCER

The following material includes discussions of the major forms of cancer with the exception of those cancers that affect women only. Cancers affecting women are discussed under *Women's Health,* beginning on p. 500. See especially *Cancers of the Reproductive System,* p. 500, and *Cancer of the Breast,* p. 504.

For additional information on many kinds of tumors for which surgery may be indicated, see also under *Surgery,* p. 317.

Lung Cancer

Lung cancer kills more Americans than any other cancer. The average annual death toll for recent years is almost 70,000 men and over 20,000 women. It represents 22 percent of all cancers in men, 6 percent of all cancers in women. And there has been a steady increase in the incidence of lung cancer in both men and women over the last 35 years—especially so in men, among whom the mortality rate has gone up 15 times. In 1965, women accounted for 1 in 8 lung cancer mortalities; the figure now is almost 1 in 4. The current chances of being cured of this disease are no more than 10 percent where there is regional involvement.

CAUSES: Lung cancer is one of the most preventable of all malignancies. Most cases, the majority of medical experts agree, are caused by smoking cigarettes. The U.S. Public

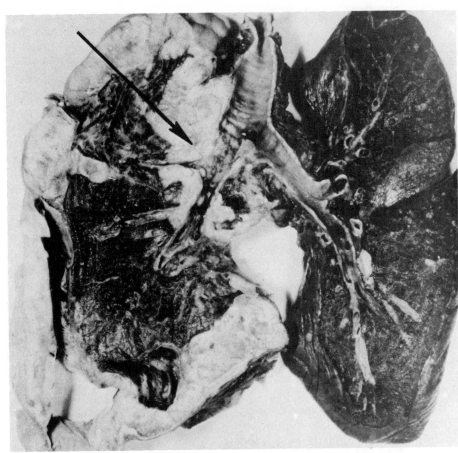

Although scientists do not yet understand exactly how smoking causes cancer, the cause-and-effect relationship has been established. Shown here are the lungs of a heavy smoker, with the arrow indicating the site of cancer.

the source of irritation—smoking—is removed. This is why a heavy smoker who has been puffing away for many years but then stops smoking has a better chance of avoiding lung cancer than one who continues smoking.

Until recently, the evidence linking cigarette smoking and lung cancer was purely statistical, although overwhelming. No one had succeeded in producing lung cancer in laboratory animals by having them smoke. However, lung cancer has been induced in dogs specially trained to inhale cigarette smoke, as reported by the American Cancer Society.

Cigarette smoking has also been implicated in other kinds of lung disease, including the often-fatal emphysema, and in cardiovascular diseases. To any sensible person, then, the options would seem clear: If you don't smoke, don't start. If you do smoke, stop. If you can't stop, cut down, and switch to a brand low in tars and nicotine—suspected but not proved to be the principal harmful agents in cigarette smoke.

DETECTION: If many lives could be

Health Service has indicted smoking as "the main cause of lung cancer in men." Even when other agents are known to produce lung cancers—uranium ore dust or asbestos fibers, for example—cigarette smoking enormously boosts the risk among uranium miners and asbestos workers. In fact, the incidence of lung cancer in such men is higher than the rate expected by merely adding the two probabilities together.

Various theories have been proposed to explain the mechanism by which smoking causes cancer in human beings; none has been proved. But it is known that the lungs of some cigarette smokers show tissue changes before cancer appears, changes apparently caused by irritation of the lining of the *bronchi*—the large air tubes in the lung. Physicians believe these changes can be reversed before the onset of cancer if

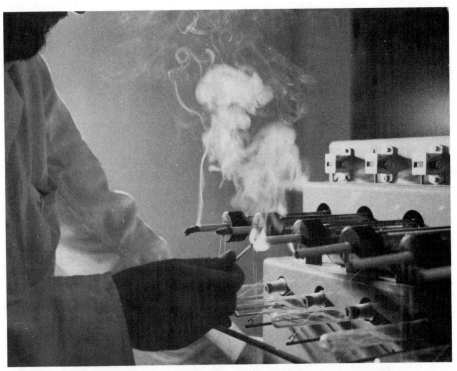

An automatic smoking machine used in cancer research. Suction stops when the thread near the butt end of each cigarette burns through.

saved by preventing lung cancer in the first place, others could be saved by early detection. By the time most lung cancers are diagnosed, it is too late even for the most radical approach to cure—removal of the afflicted lung. Experts estimate that up to five times the present cure rate of ten percent could be achieved if very early lung cancers could be spotted. They therefore recommend a routine chest X ray every six months for everyone over 45.

SYMPTOMS: Although some early lung cancers do not show up on an X-ray film, they are the ones that usually produce cough as an early symptom. For this reason, any cough that lasts more than two or three weeks—even if it seems to accompany a cold or bronchitis—should be regarded as suspicious and investigated in that light. Blood in the sputum is another early warning sign that must be investigated immediately; so should wheezing when breathing. Later symptoms include shortness of breath and pain in the chest, fever, and night sweats.

Colon-Rectum Cancer

Cancer of the colon (large intestine) and rectum is the second leading cause of cancer death in the United States. Each year it claims an estimated 50,000 lives, and produces about 100,000 new cases—more than any other kind of cancer except skin cancer. It afflicts men and women about equally. The five-year survival rate from this form of cancer, usually after surgery, is 71 percent where the cancer was localized and 43 percent where there was regional involvement. However, authorities now believe that this rate could be upped substantially through early diagnosis and prompt treatment.

SYMPTOMS: It is important, then, to be alert to the early symptoms of these cancers. Cancers of the colon often produce changes in bowel habits that persist longer than normal. The change may be constipation or diarrhea, or even both alter-

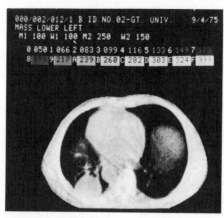

A computerized X ray (CAT scan) of the lungs, with the chest at the top, showing a cancer (lower left) invading the pleura and eroding the spinal column (bottom, center).

nating. Cancers of the colon also often produce large quantities of gas, which cause abdominal discomfort ranging from a feeling of overfullness to pain, intermittent at first and then coming as regular cramps.

Both colon cancer and rectal cancer may also cause bleeding. Sometimes such bleeding is evidenced in the stool or on the tissue (the most frequent first sign of rectal cancer); but if the bleeding is slight and occurs high enough up the colon, it may not be visible at all. After a period of weeks, however, the persistent bleeding causes anemia in the patient.

All such symptoms should be investigated promptly. Unfortunately, many persons tend to ignore them. Chronic constipation, for example, or gas, is easy to dismiss for the nuisance that it usually is. Even rectal bleeding, which demands immediate medical consultation, is ignored by hemorrhoid sufferers, who fail to realize that hemorrhoids and cancer, though unrelated, can and sometimes do exist in the same persons at the same time.

DETECTION: For these reasons, the key to successful and early diagnosis of colon and rectum cancer lies in making a *proctoscopy* part of the regular annual health checkup. In this procedure, performed in a doctor's office, a lighted tube called a *proctoscope* is passed into the rec-

tum. Through it, the doctor can examine the walls visually for signs of tumor. If the physician thinks it advisable to check the sigmoid colon also, the procedure is called a *proctosigmoidoscopy,* and a similar instrument called a *sigmoidoscope* is used. The American Cancer Society now recommends that everyone over age 40 have a proctoscopy or proctosigmoidoscopy in routine annual checkups.

THERAPY: The indicated treatment for colon-rectum cancer is surgical removal of the affected part of the bowel. Adjacent portions and related lymph nodes may also be removed, and if the surgeon sees that the cancer is widespread, he may have to perform extensive surgery. This may require that he create a *colostomy*—a temporary or permanent opening in the abdominal wall through which solid wastes may pass. Although this method of voiding the bowels is somewhat inconvenient at first, most colostomy patients adjust to it very easily and lead perfectly normal, active, and healthy lives. The wall of prudish silence that used to surround the disease and the colostomy is fortunately crumbling. An organization for colostomy patients called the United Ostomy Association keeps up with current information on diet, colostomy equipment, and other problems the members have in common.

Radiotherapy is sometimes used before the operation (occasionally to make surgery possible) and sometimes afterward to treat recurrence of the cancer. Various chemical agents have been found useful in treating colon-rectum cancer that has spread to the lymph nodes or more widely.

Skin Cancer

With 300,000 new cases predicted for each coming year, skin cancer is the largest single source of malignancy in the United States. There are an estimated 5,000 deaths from this disease per year.

SYMPTOMS: Experts believe that

many of these deaths could be avoided if only patients promptly reported to their doctors any sores that refuse to heal, or changes in warts or moles.

THERAPY: Fortunately, almost all skin cancers remain localized, and can either be removed surgically or with an electric needle, or treated by irradiation with X rays or radioactive sources.

CAUSES: Skin cancer is one of the easiest cancers to avoid entirely, for most are caused by prolonged and repeated exposure to ultraviolet radiation in sunlight; they usually appear after age 40. Fair-skinned individuals who burn readily, rather than tanning, are more vulnerable to this source of skin cancer than the rest of the population. Geographic location is also important. Skin cancer occurs more frequently in the southern belt of states, particularly in the brilliantly sunny Southwest.

Chemicals, too, can cause skin cancer. Before the relationship was discovered, the disease was an occupational hazard for many thousands of unprotected workers who dealt with arsenic and various derivatives of coal and petroleum.

MELANOMA: A *melanoma,* or so-called *black cancer,* is a malignant tumor that arises from a mole. Melanomas rarely occur before middle age; nearly three-fourths of the victims are women.

The moles may begin as flat, soft, brown, and hairless, but they can suddenly change into darker, larger growths that itch and bleed. They also can metastasize, spreading cancer cells to other parts of the body through the bloodstream and the lymphatic system.

Unlike other types of skin cancer that may be stimulated to grow by exposure to sunlight, melanomas tend to grow in skin areas usually not exposed to the sun, such as on the feet, in the genital area, or under the belt or collar.

A proposed cause of the change from a brown mole to a black cancer is chronic irritation by tight clothing or another source of friction against the skin. The proper therapy is removal of the mole before it develops into a true melanoma.

Oral Cancer

Cancers of the mouth and lips strike an estimated 24,000 persons in the United States each year and kill a shocking 8,500. Shocking because anyone with the aid of a mirror and a good light can see into his mouth and therefore spot even very small cancers early in their development. Six thousand of these deaths are among men; the disproportion may stem from the same source as the disproportion in lung cancer deaths between men and women—smoking.

SYMPTOMS: Any sore, lump, or lesion of the mouth or lips should be regarded as suspicious if it persists more than two weeks without healing, and a doctor or dentist should then be consulted without delay. The five-year survival rate for localized mouth cancers—when they are usually no larger than the little fingernail—is 67 percent—about two out of three. But if regional involvement occurs, the rate falls to 30 percent—fewer than one out of three.

DETECTION: Just as the Pap test screens for cervical cancer by scraping up sloughed-off cells which are then examined under a microscope, so one day your dentist may routinely scrape mouth cells to detect oral cancer. When more than 40,000 patients were screened over a five-and-one-half-year period at the Western Tennessee Cancer Clinic, about 230 cases of oral cancer were diagnosed, of which 35 percent would have been missed otherwise.

Right now, a weekly or monthly personal inspection of your mouth is the best detective method available. The American Cancer Society has materials explaining the best way to conduct such an examination.

THERAPY: Oral cancers are treated by surgical removal or by irradiation.

CAUSES: No one can pinpoint the causes of oral cancer definitely, but there are a number of leading suspects. They are smoking, in all its forms; exposure to wind and sun (for lip cancer); poor mouth hygiene; sharp or rough-edged teeth or improperly fitted, irritating dentures; dietary inadequacies; and constant use of very hot foods and liquids.

Stomach Cancer

Before World War II, cancer of the stomach was the most common type of cancer among men and women in the United States. The death rate from stomach cancer in the 1930s was about 30 per 100,000 population. In recent years, stomach cancer has declined in proportion to other forms of the disease, such as lung, breast, and uterine cancer. However, stomach cancer is still one of the more frequently diagnosed types of cancer and the death rate is relatively high, at nearly 10 per 100,000 population.

Today, men are twice as likely to be victims of stomach cancer as women. The disease is seldom found in persons under 30 years of age, but after that age the incidence increases steadily, reaching a peak before the age of 60 years. One of the disease's mysterious incidental factors is its peculiar geographical distribution, the highest rates of occurrence being in Japan, Chile, Iceland, northern Russia and the Scandinavian countries.

SYMPTOMS: Stomach cancer seems to develop slowly and insidiously, with initial symptoms that may be disregarded by the patient because they mimic ordinary gastric distress. The victim may experience a distaste for foods, particularly meats, and display a slow but progressive loss of weight. There may be sensations of fullness, bloating, or pain after meals. The same symptoms may be noted between meals and be aggravated by eating. The pain may vary from intermittent stomach aches to intense pain that seems to extend into the patient's back. The patient also experiences fatigue or weakness

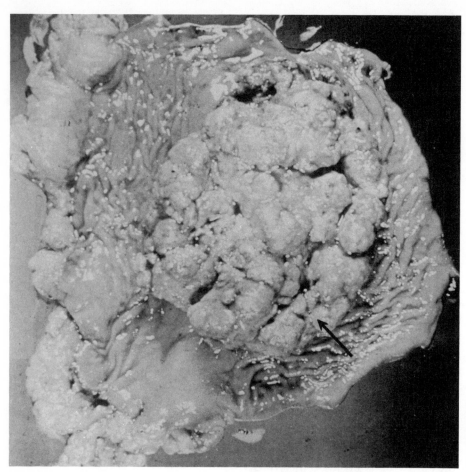

Stomach tissue showing an area of cancer (arrow). Cancer of the stomach often develops insidiously, with symptoms resembling indigestion.

cle tissue), or a *pseudotumor* (false tumor), such as an inflammatory fibroid growth. Such benign tumors produce symptoms ranging from gastric upset to internal bleeding and should be removed by surgery.

CAUSES: Many possible factors have been suggested as causes of stomach cancer. Dietary factors include hot foods and beverages, as well as fish and smoked foods. Food additives have been implicated despite the fact that the incidence of stomach cancer has been declining during the period in which the use of additives has been increasing. Cured meats and cheeses, preserved with nitrites to retard spoilage, reportedly foster the development of carcinogenic chemical compounds in the digestive tract.

On the other hand, the widespread

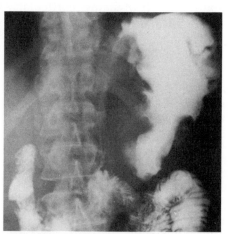

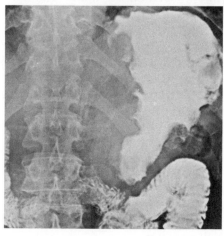

A high-resolution electron radiograph (below) clearly shows the irregular contours of the stomach wall, a sign of cancer. Details of the stomach are less clear on a conventional X-ray (top).

and anemia, and, as the cancerous condition progresses, may have periods of vomiting. The vomitus is dark, much like the color of coffee grounds, and there may be other signs of bleeding in the patient's stools.

DETECTION: X rays of the stomach and examination of the stomach interior by gastroscopy usually locate and define the cancerous area; they may also reveal another cause of the symptoms, such as a peptic ulcer. During the physical examination, the doctor may find a tissue mass and tenderness in the stomach area. The laboratory report usually will show signs of anemia from blood loss, the presence of blood in a stool sample, and the level of hydrochloric acid in the stomach; a lack of hydrochloric acid is found in more than half the stomach cancer patients. A biopsy study of the suspected tissue usually completes the diagnosis.

THERAPY: Unfortunately, because of the insidious nature of stomach cancer, the disease becomes easier to diagnose as it progresses. By the time cancer has been confirmed, the most expedient form of treatment is surgery to remove the affected area of the stomach. If the cancer is small and has not spread by metastasis to lymph nodes in the region, the chances are relatively good that the patient will survive five years or more; the odds against surviving five years without surgery are, by comparison, about 50 to 1 at best. Chemotherapy treatments may be used in cases where surgery is not feasible, but the use of medicines instead of surgery for stomach cancer is not a routine procedure and generally is not recommended.

Occasionally, a stomach tumor is found to be noncancerous. The tumor may be a polyp, a *leiomyoma* (a growth consisting of smooth mus-

use of refrigeration has been offered as an explanation for the declining incidence of stomach cancer, since refrigeration reduces the need for chemical food preservatives.

Beyond the influence of diet, medical epidemiologists have found that genetic factors may play a role in the development of stomach cancer. Statistical analysis of large population studies of stomach cancer shows a tendency for the disease to occur in persons with blood type A, or with below-normal levels of hydrochloric acid in the stomach, or with inherited variations in the stomach lining. There also seems to be a good possibility that stomach cancers evolve from noncancerous changes in the stomach lining, as from polyps or peptic ulcers.

Bladder Cancer

As with stomach cancer, the incidence of cancer of the bladder rises progressively with age and occurs much more frequently in men than in women. Extensive occurrence of bladder cancer is commonly associated with industrial growth, but internationally its incidence ranges from a high rate in England to a low one in Japan; in the United States, the highest incidence of bladder cancer is in southern New Jersey. A study by the Roswell Park Memorial Institute, a cancer research center in Buffalo, New York, found that per-

sons of Italian-American parentage were more likely to have bladder cancer than those of different parentage, and that women living in urban areas were more likely to develop the disease than their country cousins. American blacks have less bladder cancer than American whites.

Bladder cancer appears at an annual rate of about 30,000 new cases each year in the United States. Worldwide, it causes more than 7,000 deaths annually.

SYMPTOMS: A change in bladder habits is among the first signs of bladder cancer. The change might be the presence of pain while urinating, a noticeable difficulty in urinating, or a difference in the frequency of urination.

Another symptom of the disease is the appearance of blood in the urine. The degree of blood coloration is not necessarily related to the severity of the cancer; any sign of blood in the urine should be investigated. Nor should the absence of pain be allowed to minimize the seriousness of urinary bleeding as a symptom of a diseased bladder. Even without pain, the presence of blood can indicate a problem such as an obstruction to the urinary flow that can lead to uremia, a toxic condition caused by retention of urinary waste products in the system.

DETECTION: Cancer of the bladder is frequently diagnosed from common signs and symptoms, particularly the appearance of blood in the urine. A laboratory examination of the patient's urine may also reveal the presence of cancer cells that have been washed out of the bladder. The disease can be detected by a *pyelogram*—a kind of X-ray picture made by filling the urinary system with a fluid that makes tissue details appear in sharp contrast—and by examination of the membrane lining the bladder. The bladder lining may be examined by surgical biopsy or by *cystoscopy*, the viewing of the interior of the bladder by means of a device inserted in the urethra—or both.

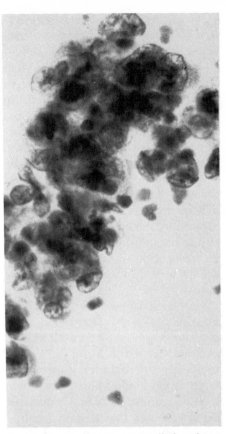

A photomicrograph of cancer cells found in a patient's urine specimen, indicating the presence of carcinoma of the bladder.

Examination of the bladder lining is needed to determine the type of tumor that may be the cause of the symptoms. One type, called a papillary tumor or *papilloma*, is relatively harmless and usually does not invade the wall of the bladder as does the more dangerous type, sometimes described as a solid lesion. The degree of invasion of the bladder tissues by the infiltrating mass determines the type of treatment recommended. However, any tumor found in the lining of the bladder must be removed because the papillary type can progress into a solid lesion if not treated.

THERAPY: The cure of a bladder tumor can be approached in several ways, the choice of treatments depending upon the size and type of growth, the location of the tumor, and so on. Chemotherapy, using drugs such as thiotepa, has been successful in treating papillary bladder tumors; the chemical is applied directly to the bladder lining. A kind of electric cautery known as *fulguration* also may be used to destroy the tissue growth; it may be employed by cystoscopy or as part of a surgical approach. Radiation therapy also may be used by implanting radium needles in the affected bladder tissue. Surgical excision of the cancerous area, with or without radiation, chemotherapy, or cautery may be the procedure chosen. In advanced cases of bladder cancer, the bladder may be removed and its function performed by the construction of a substitute organ from other tissues or by the relocation of the upper ends of the ureters at other urine-collecting points.

CAUSES: Cancer of the bladder may be caused by irritation from bladder stones or by toxic chemicals excreted from the kidneys. A high incidence of bladder cancer has been found among persons who are heavy cigarette smokers; a possible explanation is that certain carcinogenic tobacco-burning by-products are absorbed into the blood and excreted through the kidneys. The evidence includes studies showing that when such patients quit smoking, the carcinogens no longer appear in their urine.

Occupational factors have been associated with cancer of the bladder since 1895, when it was discovered that persons who worked with aniline chemical dyes were among those most likely to develop the disease. The incidence of the disease among chemical workers was found to be 30 times greater than that of the general population. The aniline dye workers developed bladder cancer at an average age 15 years younger than among the general population. The effect of the chemical dyes was verified by the development of cancer in the bladders of laboratory animals exposed to the dyes. In recent years, it has been found that many other chemicals can cause bladder cancer.

Besides the influence of industrial environmental factors, bladder cancer is associated with *schistosomiasis,* a disease occurring in Africa, Asia, South America, and other regions. Schistosomiasis develops after bathing or wading in water infested by a blood fluke. The organisms penetrate the skin and migrate to the intestines or urinary bladder, producing an inflammation that eventually leads to cancer. See under Ch. 29, p. 526, for a fuller description of the disease.

Cancer of the Prostate

Cancer of the prostate is one of the most common cancers among men and is second only to lung cancer as a lethal type of tumor for men. The death rate has been around 14 per 100,000. The incidence increases with advancing age from the fifth decade of life, when prostatic cancer cells are found in nearly 20 percent of all men examined, to those in their 70s, an age when 60 percent of the men have been found to have cancer cells in their prostate glands. Fortunately, only 15 percent of the men with evidence of latent carcinoma of the prostate ever develop clinical symptoms of cancer before death. But after the age of 75, there are almost as many deaths due to prostatic cancer as to lung cancer.

SYMPTOMS: Cancer of the prostate is a disease noted for its secondary symptoms. It usually is detected because a physician begins analyzing symptoms that could suggest other disorders. There may, for example, be blood in the urine, indicating a serious problem that could be located anywhere along the urinary tract. Because the prostate encircles the urethra, which is the outlet from the bladder, any prostatic problem can cause disturbances in the normal passage of urine, including increased frequency of urination or discomfort in urinating. However, these also could be the symptoms of ailments other than cancer of the prostate.

DETECTION: Diagnosis of prostatic cancer usually begins with an examination of the prostate through the wall of the rectum. This technique is a regular part of a physi-

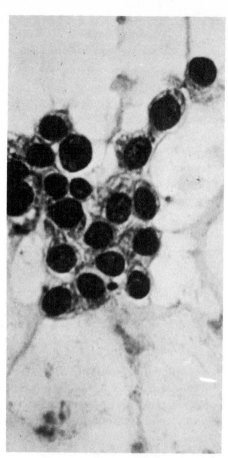

Cells indicating possible cancer of the prostate. Prostatic fluid smears are fixed and examined much as Pap smears are in women.

cal examination for men over the age of 40. If during the examination of the prostate the doctor feels a lump or hardened area, further tests are ordered. The presence of a lump in the prostate need not be evidence of cancer; about half the lumps and nodules are caused by fibrosis, calcium deposits, or other noncancerous bodies.

Additional tests may include examination by a cystoscope, which is inserted through the urethra to provide a view of the tissues of the area, plus a laboratory examination of tissue samples and prostatic fluid samples. A microscopic study of the samples may reveal the presence of cancer cells. The examination of prostatic cells for signs of cancer is similar to the technique used in the Pap test for cancer of the cervix in women.

In the search for evidence of cancer of the prostate, diagnostic clues may be found in blood chemistry tests and by the examination of a urinary pyelogram that could indicate obstructions from the prostate walls. Additional information may be forthcoming from an evaluation of the patient's medical history; low back pain complaints, for example, may be related to prostate disorders.

THERAPY: Surgery is the usual treatment for cancer of the prostate when the tumor is confined to the prostate gland. The surgical removal of the prostate may be supplemented by the administration of estrogens, or hormone therapy. If the cancer has spread to other areas, a frequent complication of prostatic cancer, an additional form of therapy could be the administration of radioactive drugs or some other form of radiation. An additional measure may be *orchiectomy*, the surgical removal of the testicles, performed because of the close physiological relationship between the testicles and the prostate.

CAUSES: Cancer of the prostate seems to be associated with activity of the sex hormones in men. It has been reported that all patients with prostatic cancer previously had a normal history of sex-hormone activity. The cancer symptoms begin to appear at a period of life when male sex-hormone activity is waning. Laboratory studies of the urine of patients show a decrease in levels of male sex hormones after the age of 40. As in female breast cancer, which also is related to sex-hormone activity, there are certain tissues of the body that appear to be more sensitive to influences of hormones. Changes in hormonal activity lead to increasing numbers of cells in those tissues and abnormal tissue growth.

Cancer of the Kidney

Cancer of the kidneys is most likely to occur in young children or in adults over the age of 40. The most common form of kidney cancer in children is known as *Wilms' tumor*. In adults, kidney cancer is usually in the form of a growth called *Grawitz's tumor,* or *hypernephroma,* a malignant growth that occurs chiefly among men.

Wilms' Tumor

Wilms' tumor, also called *nephroblastoma,* accounts for perhaps 25 percent of all cancers in children. About 90 percent of the cases develop before the age of seven years; it has been diagnosed in infants less than five months old.

SYMPTOMS: The symptoms can include fever, abdominal pain, weight loss, lack of appetite, blood in the urine, and an abdominal mass that may grow quickly to enormous size. The growth may be accompanied by symptoms of hypertension.

DETECTION: Examination of the patient may show the tumor to be on either the left or right kidney. In a small percentage of the cases both kidneys are affected. A biopsy usually is performed in order to verify the presence of cancer cells in the growth.

THERAPY: Treatment is most effective when the disease is diagnosed before the age of two years. Surgery, radiation, and chemotherapy may be employed. The choice of chemotherapeutic agents may be varied as follow-up examinations reveal side effects or tumor resistance to one of the previously administered medications.

The five-year survival rate for victims of Wilms' tumor is about 65 percent when surgery and other measures are employed at an early stage. If not controlled, the cancer cells from Wilms' tumor tend to spread by metastasis to the lungs, liver, and other organs.

CAUSE: Wilms' tumor is believed to be congenital in nature. Studies of the tumor cells indicate that it may develop from embryonic kidney tissue that fails to evolve as a normal part of that organ.

Grawitz's Tumor

In about half of the cases of Grawitz's tumor, the common adult kidney cancer, the disease manifests itself through a combination of three symptoms: abdominal mass, pain in the area of the kidneys, and blood in the urine. In the other half of the cases, the cancer has metastasized and is found in the brain, lung, liver, or bone.

DETECTION: The physician may get important information about the seriousness of the tumor through laboratory studies of blood and urine samples; these can indicate the presence of substances that appear in body fluids when cancer cells are active.

Information can also be obtained by angiogram studies. An angiogram is an X-ray picture of an organ that has been injected with a dye to make the blood vessels, which carry the dye, markedly visible. A kidney angiogram shows different dye patterns for a normal organ, a kidney with a cyst, or a kidney with a tumor. The diagnosis usually is confirmed by biopsy or surgical exploration.

THERAPY: Surgery and radiation treatment are the usual forms of therapy for adult kidney tumors and the chances of ten-year survival, even after removal of a cancerous kidney, are fairly good.

CAUSES: Causes of adult kidney tumors remain largely unknown but they have been thought to be associated with other disorders, such as infections or the presence of kidney stones.

Cancer of the Pancreas

Pancreatic cancer affects men about twice as frequently as women and accounts for about five percent of the cancer deaths. It is most likely to develop after the age of 40, and persons who are diabetic seem to be particularly susceptible to the disease.

SYMPTOMS: The pancreatic cancer patient complains of apparent digestive disorders, such as abdominal pain, nausea, loss of appetite, and perhaps constipation. The abdominal distress may improve or worsen after eating and the pain may increase when the patient lies on his back. He will suffer weight loss and there will be jaundice. Many victims of pancreatic cancer also complain of itching sensations. Abdominal pain is usually persistent.

DETECTION: Along with signs of jaundice and scratching, the examining physician will evaluate laboratory reports of urine, blood, and stool analyses. Glucose tolerance tests and bilirubin levels are helpful in defining the source of the disorder. Negative findings of X-ray studies of the gastrointestinal tract, kidney-bladder area, and gall bladder can suggest a pancreatic disorder; by their normal condition, the physician can conclude that the disease is elsewhere in the abdominal region.

THERAPY: Surgery is the usual treatment recommended for cancer of the pancreas; the precise location of the tumor within the pancreas may determine the exact surgical procedure to be undertaken. Removal of the tumor surgically has a more hopeful outcome if it is located at the head of the pancreas; cancers in the body or tail of the pancreas usually are not detected until the disease has spread to other parts of the body. Radiation and chemotherapy are not as effective in the treatment of pancreatic cancer as in controlling cancer in other organs.

Cancer of the Liver

Cancer of the liver is commonly found to be the result of metastasis from other parts of the body. Cancers that originate in the liver (primary cancers) account for less than two percent of the cancers reported in the United States. Primary cancers of the liver occur more frequently in men than in women and appear most frequently after the age of 40 years.

SYMPTOMS: Weakness, weight loss, and pain in the upper abdomen or right side of the chest are among the symptoms of liver cancer. A fever apparently unrelated to any infection also may mark the onset of liver cancer.

DETECTION: An enlarged liver with masses of abnormal tissue may be detected by an examining physician. Laboratory tests usually reveal alterations in metabolism that are associated with changes in the liver cells caused by the cancer growth. A biopsy test of the abnormal liver tissue may confirm the presence of cancer. A more direct approach is to perform exploratory surgery for examination of the liver.

THERAPY: If the tumor is located during exploratory surgery and the area can be excised, part of the liver is removed. Chemotherapy may also be used. The age of the patient and his general good health are important in making a successful recovery.

Researchers in 1985 announced a nonsurgical therapy for liver cancer involving the use of so-called "radiolabeled antibodies." To these molecules of antibodies, the body's defensive compounds, radioactive substances are attached. The antibodies then seek out the cancer cells, and the radioactivity helps them destroy the cancer. The procedure has been used experimentally on patients whose tumors were too large for surgical instruments.

CAUSES: While the exact cause of primary liver cancer is unknown, a large proportion of cases is associated with cirrhosis of the liver. In recent years, some types of liver cancer have been traced to exposure of industrial workers to chemicals known to be carcinogenic. The high incidence of primary liver cancer in Asia and Africa is related to *aflatoxins* in grains and legumes, such as peanuts; the aflatoxin molds grow rapidly in warm, moist climates where the foods are not protected against natural hazards of the environment.

Secondary cancers of the liver are the result of primary cancers in other body areas; the liver is vulnerable to metastasis from cancers in every organ except the brain because of the pattern of blood circulation that carries cancer cells through the body.

Cancer of the Brain

Cancers in the brain tissue frequently are the result of metatasis from other body organs. They travel through the bloodstream, primarily from cancers of the lung, kidney, gastrointestinal tract, and breast. They become implanted in both the cerebrum and cerebellum, and, although there is wide distribution of the cancer cells, they are centered mainly near the surfaces of the brain tissues. Primary brain tumors are more common among children than adults; in children, other cancer sites are not likely to have had time to develop to the stage of metastasis required for the transmission of malignant cells to the brain.

A cancer that seems to originate in the brain tissues is known as *glioblastoma multiforme,* a malignant growth that may strike at any age but is more likely to occur during middle age. The glioblastoma may develop in nearly any part of the brain structure, including the brain stem, and spread extensively into a large tumorous mass.

SYMPTOMS: Symptoms of brain cancer may be varied and misleading. They include headache, dizziness, nervousness, depression, mental confusion, vomiting, and paralysis. The symptoms sometimes are interpreted as those of a psychiatric disorder, and treatment of the organic disease may be postponed until too late.

DETECTION: Diagnosis may be difficult and the physician must evaluate the symptoms in terms of other findings from laboratory tests, X rays and other techniques. In some cases, cancer cells may be detected in samples of spinal fluid.

THERAPY: Treatment of brain cancers usually requires surgery or radiation or both, depending upon the type of tumor, its location, and other factors. Whether or not the brain tumor is a true cancer is not as important as early treatment, because any kind of abnormal tissue growth in the brain causes destructive pressure against vital tissues.

Cancer of the Larynx

Cancer of the larynx is chiefly a dis-

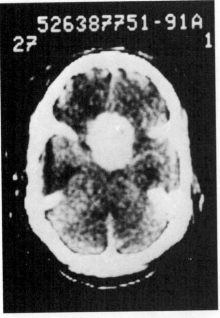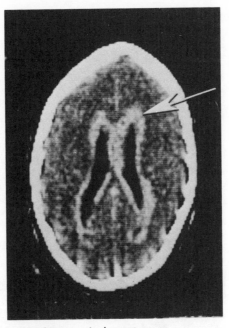

Two brain scans revealing tumors. *(Left)* The white mass in the center represents a tumor at the base of the brain. *(Right)* The arrow indicates a tumor surrounding the brain cavity that contains cerebrospinal fluid.

toms of intrinsic cancer of the larynx is hoarseness. Later the patient loses his ability to speak and experiences difficulty in breathing. The same series of symptoms occurs in cases of extrinsic cancer except that in extrinsic cancer there is an initial period of pain or discomfort in the throat before hoarseness begins. *Adenopathy*, or swelling of the lymph nodes in the area, also may be an early symptom of extrinsic cancer of the larynx.

DETECTION: Diagnosis of cancer of the larynx is relatively simple because the throat's interior can be examined by a doctor and tissue samples can be removed for biopsy study. Detection of extrinsic cancer may be complicated by the fact that it is more likely to metastasize than intrinsic forms.

THERAPY: In early cases of intrinsic cancer, treatment may require only radiation. Radiation also may be the therapy of choice for small lesions that appear in the middle of the vocal cords.

Surgery may be required for more serious cases, with radiation treatments before or after surgery, or both. The surgery, called a *laryngectomy*, may involve partial or total removal of the larynx. If a partial laryngectomy is performed, an effort is made to save as much of the vocal cords as possible. The voice will be changed after surgery, but it will be functional. The respiratory tract will be preserved. When total laryngectomy is required, the entire larynx is removed and the neck is dissected to determine if cancer cells have migrated to the lymph nodes in the neck. A new trachea is constructed by plastic surgery to permit normal or nearly normal respiration.

ease of men; about eight times as many men as women are stricken with this form of cancer, which usually makes its appearance around the age of 60. It is not one of the major types of cancer, with about 9,000 new cases appearing each year in the United States; but more than 35 percent of these cases are fatal. About 70 percent involve tumors on the vocal cords and are classed as *intrinsic* cancers of the larynx—that is, cancers originating within the larynx. The remainder of the cases involve tissues originating outside the vocal cords and are designated as *extrinsic*.

SYMPTOMS: One of the first symp-

Thyroid Cancer

Cancer of the thyroid gland is relatively uncommon, with fewer than three new cases per 100,000 population per year. The death rate is even less, about one thyroid-cancer death per year per 200,000 persons. One

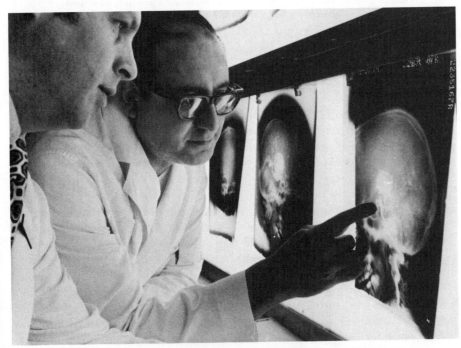

Physicians studying angiograms of the brain. These X-ray pictures are taken after dye has been injected into the blood vessels serving the brain.

reason for the low death rate is that many of the cancers are detected during examination or surgery for goiter or other throat symptoms.

SYMPTOMS: These include rapid growth of the thyroid gland, hoarseness, paralysis of nerves in the larynx, and enlarged lymph nodes in the neck and surrounding area. Diagnosis is aided by the rate at which suspected areas of cancer in the thyroid gland absorb radioactive iodine; the pattern of radioactive uptake helps pinpoint tissue abnormalities, including cysts and noncancerous tumors as well as cancerous growths.

THERAPY: Treatment may include surgery to remove the cancer and part of the surrounding tissue, plus removal of lymph nodes that may contain cancer cells that have metastasized from the thyroid tumor. In addition, surgeons may recommend removal of other lymph nodes that are in the path of drainage from the thyroid gland. Surgery usually is more successful in the treatment of young patients than in older persons. Radiation sometimes is used, either from an external source or by injection of large doses of radioactive chemicals.

CAUSES: Among causes of cancer of the thyroid gland is exposure of children and young adults to radiation therapy of the head and neck region; many such patients later develop thyroid cancer.

Hodgkin's Disease

Hodgkin's disease is one of the *lymphomas*—cancers of the lymphatic system. It occurs most commonly among young adults, although it can appear at any age. Men are more likely to be victims than are women.

SYMPTOMS: One of the first symptoms of Hodgkin's disease is a painless enlargement of a lymph node, usually in the area of the neck. The enlarged lymph nodes usually are firm and rubbery at first. The patient may experience a severe and

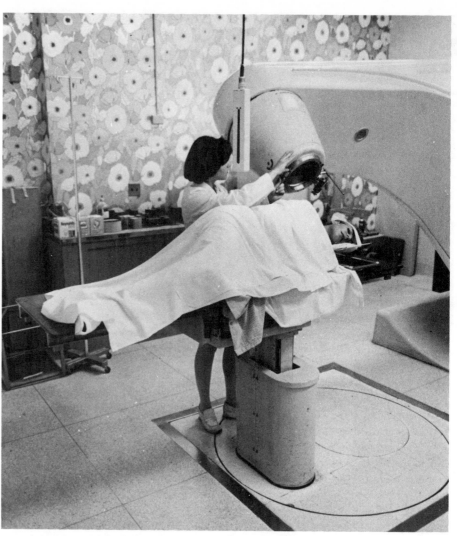

Radiation from the linear accelerator can be focused precisely on a tumor, causing a minimum of damage to surrounding tissues, especially the skin.

persistent itching for several weeks or months before the first enlarged lymph node appears.

Other symptoms may include shortness of breath, fever, weight loss, anemia, and some pressure or pain as the disease progresses and nerve tissue becomes involved. As the disease progresses, the lymph nodes that originally were separate and movable become matted and fixed, and sometimes become inflamed. Over a period of months to years, the disease spreads through other parts of the body.

THERAPY: The presence of Hodgkin's disease is ordinarily confirmed by removal of an affected lymph node for biopsy study. If the disease is limited to one or two localized areas the usual therapy is

radiation treatments. Surgical excision of the nodes may be employed in special cases, as when a mass of nodes threatens a vital organ. But intense radiation exposure is generally more effective than surgery in controlling the disease. Radiation treatments when properly applied may have a cure rate of as high as 95 percent at the site treated. In cases where the disease has spread over a large area of the body, the treatment of choice may be chemotherapy utilizing nitrogen mustard, steroid drugs, and other substances.

CAUSE: The cause of Hodgkin's disease is unknown. Experiments involving efforts to transmit the disease by injecting ground bits of excised nodes into animals have not been successful. The nodes also have failed to yield any bacteria that can be identified with the disease. However, because of the fever and other symptoms associated with the disorder, and because it appears to occur more frequently among members of the same family or community than in the population as a whole, it has been suggested that Hodgkin's disease is a viral disease that has a malignant effect on the human lymphatic system.

Leukemia

Because leukemia involves blood cells circulating through the body rather than a fixed mass of tissue, as in skin or stomach cancer, the classification of leukemia as a true cancer is occasionally challenged. However, leukemia cells, when studied under the microscope and in cell cultures, behave like cancer cells found in tumors. They have a nucleus and cytoplasm that are abnormal and tend to multiply in a prolific and erratic manner.

Medical scientists frequently refer to the disease in the plural, as leukemias, because there are at least ten different kinds of blood cells that have been identified with various forms of the disease. In addition, there are both acute and chronic forms of leukemia, such as *acute granulocytic leukemia* and *chronic lymphocytic leukemia*, named after the particular kind of white blood cells that are most affected.

Leukemia affects the blood-forming tissues, such as the bone marrow, resulting in an overproduction of white blood cells. The disease is particularly lethal to children under the age of 15; more than ten percent of the leukemia deaths each year are among children. The incidence by age group varies according to the specific type of leukemia, however; one variety of acute granulocytic leukemia can occur at any age, but chronic lymphocytic leukemia usually does not appear before the age of 40. Men are more likely than women to be the victims

of one of the various forms of leukemia.

SYMPTOMS: There are several symptoms that the different leukemias have in common. These include fever, weight loss, fatigue, bone pain, anemia as expressed in paleness, and an enlarged spleen or masses under the skin caused by an accumulation of leukemic cells. There may be skin lesions and, as the disease advances, a tendency to bleed. Infections may become more common and less responsive to treatment because of a loss of the normal blood cells needed to resist disease.

DETECTION: Diagnosis of leukemia from early symptoms may be difficult because they resemble those of mononucleosis and other infections. Biopsies of bone marrow and careful blood studies usually identify the disease.

THERAPY: Treatment usually is directed toward reducing the size of the spleen and the number of white cells in the blood, and increasing the level of blood hemoglobin to counteract the effects of anemia. Antibiotics may be included to help control infections when natural resistance to disease has been lowered. X-ray treatments, radioactive phosphorus, anti-cancer drugs, and steroid hormone medications are administered according to the needs of the individual patient and the type of leukemia being treated.

Acute leukemia may be fatal within a few weeks of the onset of symptoms. But chronic cases receiving proper treatment have been known to survive more than a quarter of a century with the disease. In recent years remission rates have improved, partly because of new drugs and methods of treatment. The new chemotherapeutic approaches include the following:

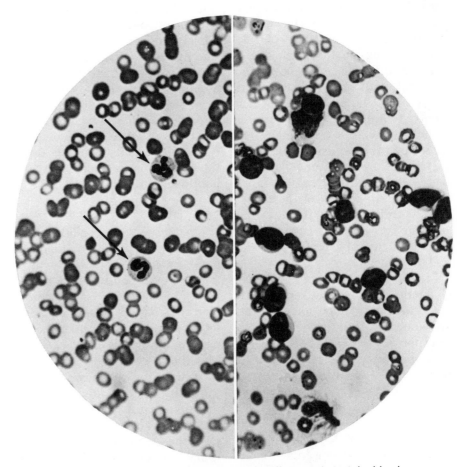

At left, normal blood, including two white cells (arrows). At right, blood from a leukemia patient, showing a fivefold increase in white cells.

• For acute leukemia in children, *methotrexate* has been used with increasing success. One of the antimetabolites, the family of drugs that interfere with development of essential cell components, methotrexate reduces the production in the blood of folic acid. In that way the drug competes with the cancer cells for the vital enzyme folic reductase—and inhibits the cancer's growth.

• In adults, chronic and acute forms of leukemia may be treated with *chlorambucil* or *cyclophosphamide.* Both drugs are types of nitrogen mustard. Both may produce side effects such as suppression of bone marrow, loss of hair, nausea, dizziness, and vomiting.

• In cases of acute leukemia in childhood, the *vinca*alkaloid drugs have proved valuable. These drugs, such as *vincristine*, are extremely powerful. They attack active cancer cells more directly than they attack normal cells. They may lead to such symptoms as headaches, convulsions, and loss of some muscular control.

Other drugs in the alkaloid and other drug families have been used to treat leukemia. The others include cytosine arabinoside, which works to prevent cell synthesis —including cancer cell synthesis; 6-Mercotopurine, which inhibits some metabolic process; and busulfan and similar drugs, which work against multiplication of the cancer cells. Antitumor antibiotics that prevent growth of cancer cells include Daunoribicin, Doxorubicin, and Bleomycin.

CAUSES: There is no general theory about the cause of leukemia. Animals, including mice and poultry, are known to be susceptible to a form of leukemia transmitted by virus, but there is no solid evidence that human leukemias are caused by viral infections. Survivors of nuclear explosions in Hiroshima and Nagasaki, as well as persons exposed to large doses of X rays, have developed leukemia at a higher-than-normal rate than other people. There is evidence that at least one type of acute leukemia may be due to an inherited genetic defect.

Other Cancers

Lymphosarcoma

Another of the cancers that involve the lymphatic system is called *lymphosarcoma*—a malignant lymphoma that tends to metastasize in lymphatic tissue. The most common first symptom is a swelling of the lymph nodes, and the diagnosis and treatment are similar to those of Hodgkin's disease. Lymphosarcoma can occur at any stage of life and make its appearance in any part of the body where there is lymphatic tissue, including the gastrointestinal tract, the tonsils, tongue, or the nasopharynx area.

Reticulum-cell Sarcoma

The lymphomas also include *reticulum-cell sarcoma*. (A sarcoma is a malignant tumor in the connective tissue. Reticulum cells are a particular kind of connective tissue.) The disease is marked by the invasion of normal tissue by increased numbers of reticulum cells or fibers. As in the treatment of leukemia, it is important to know which of the various types of cancer has affected the lymphatic system, because each of the lymphomas responds to a different therapeutic routine.

Myeloma and Multiple Myeloma

Myelomas, once considered rare but now reported in increasing numbers, are cancerous growths that seem to originate in the bone marrow. (*Myelos* is the Greek word for marrow.) The disease is seldom found in persons younger than 40; the average age at onset is about 65. Men are twice as likely as women to be victims of myelomas.

The disease is marked by bone destruction, mainly in the pelvis, ribs, and spine. The bones break easily, sometimes causing collapse of the spinal column and pressure on the spinal cord. There also may be anemia, kidney damage, and changes in the blood chemistry. When the myelomas occur at numerous sites in the bone marrow throughout the body, the disease is known as *multiple myeloma.*

Treatment

Various methods of treating lymphomas have evolved despite serious difficulties. Lymphomas appear in many different forms, and can change form in the process of spreading to another part of the body. Different types may be found in a single lymph gland.

Despite these difficulties, many chemotherapeutic agents have been found useful in treatment of lymphomas. To an extent, the preferred drugs fall in the same categories as those used in treating leukemia. The principal drugs, thus, include:

• Alkalyting agents such as nitrogen mustard, cyclyphosphamide, and chlorambucil

• Vinca alkaloids, among them vincristine and vinblastine

• Procarbazine (trade name: Natulan) which works like the alkalyting agents

• Antibiotics that work to reduce or eliminate tumors, including Adriamycin and actinomycin D

• The corticosteroids, combinations of agents including hormones, acids, and other body elements

These and other drugs have been used in various combinations in the treatment of lymphomas. One of the more successful has been named for the four drugs that are included in the protocol, or treatment series. The four are nitrogen mustard, vincristine (Oncovin), Procarbazine, and predaisone; the combination treatment is known as MOPP. The treatment is used at certain stages of lymphoma, and has encouraged medical specialists to consider lymphoma as potentially curable.

In addition to drug therapy, methods of treating lymphomas include irradiation therapy, or radiotherapy, and a combination of drugs and radiotherapy.

CHAPTER 25

Diseases of the Skeletal System

The bones and joints of the human body, although designed to withstand a great deal of stress, are subject to a variety of disorders which can affect people of all ages. Some skeletal deformities are the result of congenital defects, and can be treated by physical therapy or surgery with varying degrees of success. Arthritis and related joint diseases, caused by wear and tear over the years, probably affect more people than any other skeletal disorder.

Man's erect posture makes the spine especially vulnerable to problems of alignment, often causing considerable pain. Bone tissue can also be invaded by tumors, and by infections of the bone marrow. Also, stress to bones and joints can cause fractures or dislocations, which require prompt medical treatment to prevent deformity or loss of mobility.

CONGENITAL DEFECTS

As the fetus develops in the womb, its bony skeleton first appears as soft cartilage, which hardens into bone before birth. The calcium content of the mother's diet aids the fetus in bone formation and in the development of the normal human skeleton. Thus the basic skeletal structure of an individual is formed before his birth. In some instances, the bones of the fetus develop abnormally, and such defects are usually noticeable soon after delivery.

The causes of skeletal birth defects are not always known. Some may be due to hereditary factors; others have been traced to the mother's exposure to X rays, atomic radiation, chemicals, drugs, or to disease during pregnancy. Among the more common birth defects are extra fingers, toes, or ribs, or missing fingers, hands, toes, feet, or limbs. Sections of the spine may be fused together, often without causing serious problems later in life, although some fused joints can hinder the motion of limbs. The sections of the skull may unite prematurely, retarding the growth of the brain.

Defects of the Skull, Face, and Jaw

Various malformations of the skull, face, and jaw can appear at birth or soon after. They include *macrocephaly* (enlarged head) and *microcephaly* (very small head). Microcephaly is caused by the premature fusion of the cranial sutures in early childhood. If brain growth increases very rapidly during the first six months of life in infants whose skulls have fused prematurely, the brain cannot expand sufficiently within the rigid skull, and mental retardation results. Surgery is used to widen the sutures to permit normal brain development.

Cleft lip and *cleft palate* are common facial deformities and are visible at birth. These are longitudinal openings in the upper lip and palate. They result from failure of the area to unite in the normal manner during embryonic stages of pregnancy. They should be corrected at an early age. If surgery is performed in infancy there is a good chance that the child will mature with little or no physical evidence of the affliction and with no psychological damage as a result of it. See *Cleft Palate and Cleft Lip*, p. 69, for further information.

Defects of the Rib Cage

Every normal human being has 12 pairs of ribs attached to the spine, but some people are born with extra ribs on one or both sides.

Although such extra ribs are usually harmless, one that projects into the neck can damage nerves and the artery located in that area. In adults extra neck ribs may cause shooting pains down the arms, general periodic numbness in the arms and hands, weak wrist pulse, and possible diminished blood supply to the forearm. Surgery may be required to remove the rib and thereby relieve the pressure on the nerves or artery. Minor symptoms are treated by physiotherapy.

Congenital absence of one or more ribs is not uncommon. An individual may be born with some ribs fused together. Neither condition creates any serious threat to health.

Congenital Dislocation of the Hip

Dislocation of the hip is the most common congenital problem of the pelvic area. It is found more often in girls than in boys in a five to one ratio. Babies born from a breech presentation, buttocks first, are more likely to develop this abnormality than those delivered headfirst. The condition may be the result of inherited characteristics.

Clinical examination of infants, especially breech-born girls, may reveal early signs of congenital hip dislocation, with the affected hip appearing shorter than the normal side. If the condition is not diagnosed before the infant is ready to walk, the child may begin walking later than is normal. The child may develop a limp and an unsteady gait, with one leg shorter than the other.

Early diagnosis of this condition is important, followed by immediate reduction and immobilization by means of a plaster cast or by applying traction. Permanent deformity, dislocation, uneven pelvis, retarded walking, limping, and unsteady gait are possible complications if this condition remains untreated. Surgery is sometimes required.

ARTHRITIS AND OTHER JOINT DISEASES

Arthritis is probably the most common of all disabling diseases, at least in the temperate areas of the world. It has been estimated that ten percent of the population suffers from one of the many forms of arthritis. In the United States alone, more than 13 million persons each year seek professional medical care for arthritis. Of this number, some three million must restrict their daily activities and about 750,000 are so disabled by arthritis that they are unable to attend school, work, or even handle common household tasks.

Arthritis apparently is not associated with any stage of civilization; it has been diagnosed in the skeletons of prehistoric humans. There is even evidence that arthritic diseases afflict a variety of animals, including the dinosaurs that inhabited the earth more than 100 million years ago. Arthritis caused pain and suffering to such famous personages as Goethe, Henry VI, Charlemagne, and Alexander the Great.

Arthritis and *rheumatism* are terms sometimes used interchangeably by the layman to describe any abnormal condition of the joints, muscles, or related tissues. Many rheumatic or arthritic diseases have popular names, such as "housemaid's knee," "baseball finger," or "weaver's bottom." Doctors usually prefer to apply the term *arthritis* to disorders of the joints, especially joint disorders accompanied by inflammation. More than 75 different diseases of the joints have been identified; they are classified according to their specific signs, symptoms, and probable causes. The list includes bursitis, gout, and tendinitis in addition to the major disorders, rheumatoid arthritis and osteoarthritis.

Rheumatoid arthritis and osteoarthritis are examples of two types of arthritic ailment that are quite different diseases. Rheumatoid arthritis usually develops from unknown causes before the age of 45 and is marked by a nonspecific inflammation of the joints of the extremities; the inflammation is accompanied by changes in substances found in the blood. A victim of rheumatoid arthritis may develop limb deformities within a short period of time. Osteoarthritis, on the other hand, is most likely to produce symptoms after the age of 45. Here the cause is simply wear and tear on the cartilage cushions of the joints, mainly weight-bearing ones such as the hips and knees. Both kinds of joint disorders afflict millions of persons with painful and disabling symptoms.

Osteoarthritis

The most common form of arthritis is *osteoarthritis*, which is also known by the terms *hypertrophic arthritis* and *degenerative joint disease*. It can be said quite accurately that if you live long enough you will experience osteoarthritis. In fact, osteoarthritis is most common in areas of the world where people have the greatest longevity. The first signs of osteoarthritis may appear on X-ray

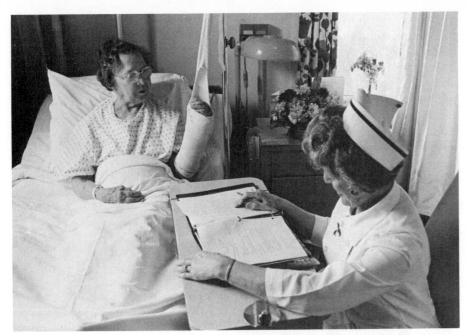

A nurse checks on the progress of an arthritis patient. Osteoarthritis is a function of age, resulting in part from wear and tear on the bones.

of the joints, a doctor frequently has little information to go on in making a diagnosis of this disease. In some cases, there may be enlargement of the joint and some tenderness. But few cases are marked by the excessive warmth, for example, associated with rheumatoid arthritis. There are no laboratory tests that can distinguish the disorder from other rheumatic or arthritic diseases.

Osteoarthritis seldom causes the degree of discomfort experienced by patients afflicted by rheumatoid arthritis; the disease is not as disabling for most patients, and even the stiffness associated with osteoarthritis is milder, usually lasting only a few minutes when activity is attempted, while the stiffness of rheumatoid arthritis may continue for hours.

Arthritis of the Hip

Although most cases of osteoarthritis are not seriously disabling, arthritis of the hip is a prominent cause of disability in older persons. It produces pain in the hips, the inner thigh, the groin, and very often in the knee. Walking, climbing steps, sitting, and bending become

pictures of persons in their 30s and 40s, even though they have not yet felt pain in the weight-bearing joints, the hips and knees, where discomfort usually appears first. Studies show that nearly everybody has at least the beginning signs or symptoms of osteoarthritis after they reach their 50s. It affects both men and women, although women may not experience symptoms until after they have reached the menopause.

CAUSES: A somewhat simplified explanation of the cause of osteoarthritis is this: the joints between the bones of a young person are cushioned and lubricated by cartilage pads and smooth lining membranes; normal wear and tear on the joints during a lifetime of activity gradually erodes the protective layers between the bones. In addition, the bones may develop small growths at the joints, a factor that aggravates the situation. There is evidence that heredity plays a role in the development of these bone growths, which are ten times more likely to occur in women than in men.

While hips and knees are among the most likely targets of osteoarthritis, the disease also can involve

the hands, the shoulders, or back. Weight-bearing joints are commonly involved when the patient is overweight and spends a great deal of time standing or walking.

SYMPTOMS: Except for the descriptions of aches and pains by victims of osteoarthritis and X-ray examination

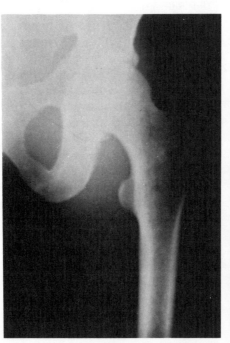
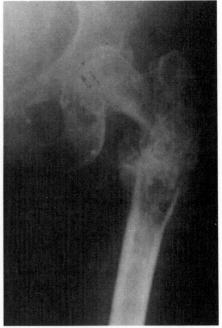

A normal hip (left) and a hip showing involvement of bone disease (right) as a result of complications from trauma. Osteoarthritis is a chronic disorder, found especially in older people.

very painful, since the joint is destroyed by degeneration of bone and cartilage. Stress and strain on the hip joint further aggravate the condition, which becomes worse with advancing age.

Surgery to replace the head of the femur or the entire hip joint with metal or plastic parts has brought relief from pain and restored mobility to some patients suffering from severe arthritis of the hip.

Small children sometimes suffer from transient arthritis of the hip, of unknown cause, manifested by pain, limitation of hip movement, and impeded walking. Since the condition usually disappears within six weeks, the only treatment is bed rest. Transient arthritis must not be mistaken for the more serious pyrogenic hip arthritis of children and adults, marked by high fever.

Spinal Arthritis

The aging process is the principal cause of spinal arthritis. Other contributing factors are disk lesions and injury. Spinal arthritis causes pronounced bone degeneration and disability. The sufferer experiences severe back pain radiating to the thighs as a result of interference of the nerve roots from *osteophytes,* or spurs, formed in the joints. In mild cases, physical therapy may be the only treatment required.

Treatment of Osteoarthritis

For most patients, osteoarthritis is not likely to be crippling or disabling. The effects generally are not more serious than stiffness of the involved joints, with occasional discomfort and some pain. When weight-bearing joints are involved, the basic remedies are weight control and adequate rest for the areas affected. In some instances, the patient may have to learn new postural adjustments; symptoms often appear in another joint after the first has been affected because the patient tends to favor the joint that first caused pain and shifts weight or muscle stress to the second joint.

Physical therapy and corrective exercises are helpful. The doctor may recommend the use of aspirin or another analgesic for the pain. Steroid drugs may be injected into an injured joint, but usually only for temporary relief. Surgery is sometimes recommended for removal of troublesome bone spurs or to correct a serious problem in a weight-bearing joint, where a metal cup or other device may be inserted as part of an artificial joint.

Rheumatoid Arthritis

Rheumatoid arthritis occurs at a much earlier age than osteoarthritis, appearing at any time from infancy to old age, but most commonly afflicting persons between the ages of 20 and 35. Women are three times as likely to be victims of rheumatoid arthritis as are men, although men seem to lose that advantage after the age of 50. All races seem to be equally vulnerable. Recent studies also suggest that two common beliefs about rheumatoid arthritis probably are untrue. The facts show that the disease is not hereditary and that it is not more prevalent in cold, damp climates.

Symptoms

Rheumatoid arthritis can begin as part of an acute illness, with high fever and intense inflammation of the joints, or it can develop insidiously with little or no discomfort except for fatigue, loss of appetite, weight loss, and perhaps a mild fever. Sometime later the victim becomes aware of aches and pains in the joints and muscles and seeks medical attention. Frequently, deformities develop before the patient realizes that rheumatoid arthritis may be the cause of swollen joints, pain, redness, or excessive warmth about the affected area.

The inflammation of a joint caused by rheumatoid arthritis may continue for weeks or it may last for a period of years. During inflammation, tendons become shortened and muscles lose their normal balance. The result is the deformity of joints

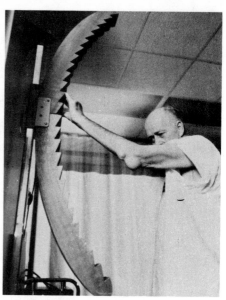

To help relieve his pain and to minimize the chances of disability from arthritis, a patient does progressive exercises, raising his arm each step on a "ladder."

commonly associated with rheumatoid arthritis, such as a swan-neck shape in the fingers. Muscular weakness develops and there is a loss of grip strength in the hands when that area is affected. Patients may be unable to make a tight fist.

A common symptom of rheumatoid arthritis is a stiffness that develops during periods of rest but gradually disappears when activity resumes. After a night's sleep, the stiffness may persist for a half hour or much longer. The stiffness may be due in part to the muscular weakness that accompanies the disease.

Although the effects of rheumatoid arthritis are most commonly observed in the hands or feet of patients, other body joints such as the elbows, shoulders, knees, hips, ankles, spine, and even the jawbones, may be involved. It is possible for all of a patient's joints to be involved, and the involvement often is symmetrical; that is, both hands will develop the symptoms at the same time and in the same pattern.

Probable Causes

The exact cause of rheumatoid arthritis is unknown, although a variety of factors have been associated with the onset of the disease. Emotional upsets, tuberculosis, venereal disease, psoriasis, and rheumatic fever are among conditions associated with the beginnings of the disease. Various viruses and other microorganisms have been isolated from the inflamed tissues of patients, but medical researchers have been unable to prove that any of the infectious agents is the cause. Efforts have also been made to transmit rheumatoid arthritis from a known victim to a normal volunteer by transfusions and injections of substances found in the victim's tissues, but without success in tracing the causative factor.

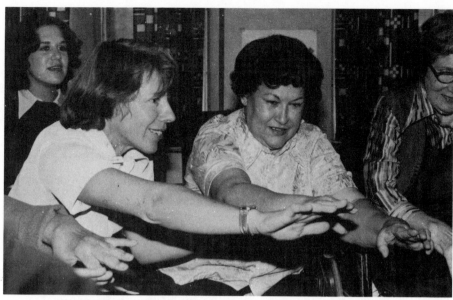

Exercise of an arthritic joint relieves its pain and stiffness. It also helps prevent the adjoining muscles from shrinking and weakening.

Treatment

The symptoms of rheumatoid arthritis intensify or abate spontaneously and unpredictably. Available methods of treatment do not cure the disease but relieve the symptoms so that the pain is reduced and some normal movement is facilitated. Proper nutrition, heat, rest, and exercise are also helpful. A number of drugs can reduce the inflammation of the joints, but they may have undesirable toxic side effects. Accordingly, before any drug therapy is embarked upon, the patient should seek the advice of a physician specializing in arthritic disorders.

ASPIRIN: The most common drug used to treat all kinds of arthritis is aspirin; it is also the most economical. Occasional side effects, such as irritation of ulcers or other gastrointestinal upsets, as well as a buzzing in the ears, can result from aspirin use, especially in massive doses; such complications can sometimes be avoided by the use of specially coated aspirin tablets. The size of the dose usually is started at a minimum level and gradually increased until the doctor finds a level that is most helpful to the patient but does not result in serious side effects.

Several other types of medication have been tried as alternatives to aspirin. One of the newer drugs, *indomethacin,* is about as effective as aspirin, but when taken in large doses it also seems to cause side effects, including nausea, heartburn, and headache.

Sulindac, a nonsteroidal anti-inflammatory drug (NSAI), made its appearance on the U.S. market in the late 1970s. Under the trade name Clinoril, sulindac came into wide use in the treatment of a variety of arthritic disorders. These included osteoarthritis, rheumatoid arthritis, gouty arthritis, and painful shoulder.

Sulindac both relieves pain and reduces fever while attacking inflammations. In those respects it resembles other anti-arthritis drugs such as fenoprofen (trade name: Nalfon), naproxen (trade name: Naprosyn), and tolmetin (trade name: Tolectin). Sulindac can be ingested on a twice-daily basis; but in use it was found to have adverse side effects, some of them serious.

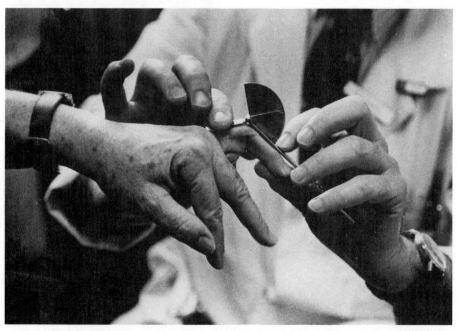

A common symptom of rheumatoid arthritis is stiffness in affected joints. Here, a testing device measures a patient's ability to flex his finger.

For example, some patients reported abdominal pains, nausea, and constipation. Diarrhea can also occur. Some side effects involved the central nervous system, and included dizziness, drowsiness, and headache.

Among other drugs used to treat arthritis, DMSO (dimethylsulfoxide) attracted widespread attention in the early 1980s. Research indicated that DMSO might have value as an anti-arthritic agent. The Arthritis Foundation of the United States indicated, however, that DMSO might serve as "a short-term analgesic for pain due to limited conditions." A liquid that arthritis sufferers rubbed on their skin, DMSO was reported to have such negative side effects as skin rashes and halitosis.

Many other drugs promising relief for victims of arthritis have made their appearance in recent years. For example, penicillamine (trade name: Cuprimine) was found to help patients with rheumatoid arthritis. Experiments with many other drugs—including aclofenac, flurbiprofen, and proquazone— were under way.

STEROIDS: The cortisone-type (steroid) drugs have proven effective in controlling severe cases of rheumatoid arthritis. They can be given orally or injected directly into the affected joints. However, these drugs generate a number of undesirable side effects, and withdrawal often results in a severe recurrence of the original symptoms. Thus, steroid drug therapy is a long-term process that can make the patient totally dependent on the medication. Some doctors are reluctant to inject steroid drugs into the joints because the effect is temporary and there is a danger of introducing infection by repeated use of the needle. In addition, some patients do not seem to respond to the steroid drugs and X-ray studies of the joints may show progressive destruction of the tissues despite the medications.

REST: Bed rest is recommended for acute cases and up to 10 hours of sleep per day is advised for mild cases of rheumatoid arthritis. The patient also should take rest periods during the day whenever possible, reducing fatigue and stress on the affected joints. As in severe cases of osteoarthritis, the patient should try to adjust his daily work habits to avoid strain on weight-bearing joints.

EXERCISE: Patients tend to avoid moving arthritic joints because of pain and stiffness. Exercise of an arthritic joint, however, helps prevent the adjoining muscles from shrinking and weakening. A program of physiotherapy—including hot packs and exercise—can be extremely helpful.

The exercise program should carry the joints through their normal range of movement. Exercises should be performed every day but not carried to the point of fatigue. In addition to exercises intended to prevent limitation of normal joint movement, isometric-type exercises should be used to maintain or increase muscle power in other parts of the body that might otherwise be neglected because of limited activity by the patient.

POSTURE: The patient should be encouraged to maintain proper posture as much as possible, through correct positioning of the body when standing, sitting, or reclining in bed. A sheet of thick plywood may be used under a mattress to prevent it from sagging. Chairs should be firm with straight backs. Pillows should be avoided whenever possible.

Crutches, canes, leg braces, and other devices may be needed by the patient in advanced stages of rheumatoid arthritis. In some cases, orthopedic surgery is recommended to help reconstruct the limbs and joints as a part of rehabilitation.

HEAT: Massages or vibrating equipment are not recommended as part of the therapy for rheumatoid arthritis patients. However, heat in the form of hot baths, hot compresses, or heating pads may be helpful. Paraffin baths are particularly helpful in treating hands or wrists.

DIET: While osteoarthritis patients are advised to lose as much weight as possible, rheumatoid arthritis patients tend to suffer from weight loss and nutritional deficiencies. Part of the cause may be a loss of appetite that is a characteristic of the disease and part may be due to the gastrointestinal problems that frequently accompany the disorder and which may be aggravated by the medications prescribed. Some doctors advise that rheumatoid arthritis patients include adequate amounts of protein and calcium in their diets as a preventive measure against a loss of bone tissue.

Juvenile Rheumatoid Arthritis

A form of arthritis quite similar to adult rheumatoid arthritis afflicts some children before the age of 16. Called *juvenile rheumatoid arthritis* or *Still's disease*, it includes a set of symptoms that nevertheless differentiate it from adult rheumatoid arthritis. In addition to the rheumatoid joint symptoms, the patient may have a high fever, rash,

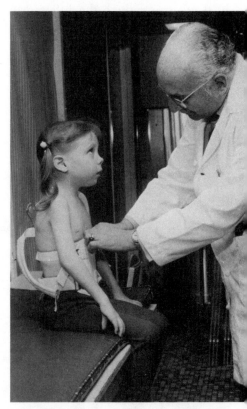

A pediatrician whose speciality is juvenile rheumatoid arthritis adjusts the back brace of one of his young patients.

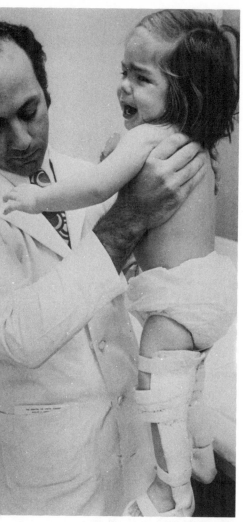

The pain of juvenile rheumatoid arthritis is very real to this toddler. The leg splints she wears help to prevent crippling.

pleurisy, and enlargement of the spleen. The onset of the disease may appear in the form of an unexplained childhood rash and fever, with arthritic symptoms developing as much as several weeks later. A possible complication is an eye inflammation that can lead to blindness if untreated.

Treatment

Juvenile rheumatoid arthritis is treated with aspirin or steroid drugs, or both, along with other kinds of therapy used for the adult version of rheumatoid arthritis. Steroid therapy is often more effective against rheumatoid arthritis in children than in adults. There may be a complete remission of the disease or the pa-

tient may experience rheumatoid symptoms into adult life.

Ankylosing Spondylitis

A kind of arthritis that affects the spine, causing a fusion of the joints, is known as *ankylosing spondylitis*. About 90 percent of the patients are young adult males. There is some evidence that it may be a hereditary disease.

Like other forms of arthritis, ankylosing spondylitis is insidious in its start. The patient may complain of a backache, usually in the lumbar area of the back. Some victims of the disease have claimed they were without pain but felt muscle spasms and perhaps tenderness along the lower part of the spine. Then stiffness and loss of motion spread rapidly over the back.

Along with fusion of the spine, the ligament along the spine calcifies like a bone. X-ray photographs of the spinal column may show the backbone to resemble a length of bamboo. A complication is that the spine is bent and chest expansion is limited by the fusion so that normal breathing is impaired.

Treatment of the disease consists of physical therapy and exercises to prevent or limit deformity and the

use of aspirin or other drugs to reduce pain.

Gout

Gout is an arthritic disease associated with an abnormality of body chemistry. There is an excessive accumulation of uric acid in the blood resulting from the chemical abnormality, and the uric acid, in the form of sharp urate crystals, may accumulate in the joints, where they cause an inflammation with symptoms like those of arthritis. A frequent target of the urate crystals is the great toe, which is why gout patients occasionally are pictured as sitting in a chair with one foot propped upon a pillow.

Primary Gout

There are two forms of gout, primary gout and secondary gout. Primary gout is presumed to be linked to a hereditary defect in metabolism and afflicts mostly men, although women may experience the disease after menopause. The painful inflammation may develop overnight following an injury or illness, or after a change in eating habits. The patient may suddenly feel feverish and unable to move because of the tenderness of the affected joint,

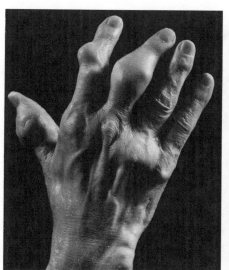
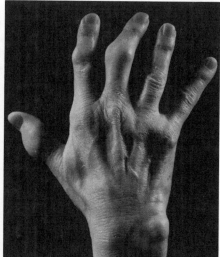

The hand of a gout patient is shown at left. Excess uric acid causes crystals to form around the joints, producing the swellings characteristic of this disease. At right, the same hand after treatment.

which becomes painfully swollen and red.

Although the great toe is a common site for the appearance of gout, it also may develop in the ankle, knee, wrist, hand, elbow, or another joint. Only one joint may be affected, or several joints might be involved at the same time or in sequence. The painful attack usually subsides within a week or so but it may return to the same joint or another joint after an absence of a few years. The inflammation subsides even if it is not treated, but untreated gout may eventually result in deformity or loss of use of the affected joint. During periods between attacks the patient may show no signs of the disease except for high blood serum levels of uric acid and the appearance of *tophi,* or *urate* (a salt of uric acid) deposits visible in X-ray photographs of the joints.

Secondary Gout

Secondary gout is related to a failure of the kidneys to excrete uric acid products or a variety of diseases that are characterized by overproduction of certain types of body cells. Failure of the kidneys to filter out urates can, in turn, be caused by various drugs, including aspirin and diuretics. Gout symptoms can also be caused by efforts to lose weight rapidly through a starvation diet,

since this speeds up the breakdown of stored body fats. Among diseases that may precipitate an attack of secondary gout are Hodgkin's disease, psoriasis, and some forms of leukemia.

Chronic Gouty Arthritis

A form of arthritis called *chronic gouty arthritis* is associated with patients who have abnormal levels of uric acid in their blood. While they may or may not be plagued by attacks of acute joint pain, the urate deposits apparently cause a certain amount of stiffness and soreness in various joints, especially during periods of stormy weather or falling barometric pressure. The tophi or urate crystals may spread to soft tissues of the body, such as bursae, the cartilage of the ear, and tendon sheaths. More than ten percent of gout patients eventually develop kidney stones formed from urate deposits in the kidney.

Treatment of Gout

Because gout was traditionally associated with certain meats that are rich in chemicals called *purines,* special diets were once a routine part of the treatment. In recent years, there has been less emphasis placed on maintaining a low-purine diet for gout patients. This change in therapy is mainly the result of the rel-

atively good success in maintaining proper uric-acid levels in gout patients with medications. However, adequate fluid intake is still recommended to prevent development of urate kidney stones.

Infectious Arthritic Agents

There are at least 12 types of arthritis and rheumatism that are associated with infections involving bacteria, viruses, fungi, or other organisms. One of these diseases is known as *pyrogenic arthritis.* The arthritis-causing organisms infect a joint and induce pain and fever and limitation of joint movement by muscle spasm and swelling. Treatment includes bed rest and antibiotics. If untreated, destruction of the joints is possible.

Gonococcal Arthritis

This disease is transmitted by the gonococcal bacteria associated with venereal disease. As in the venereal disease itself, the arthritic effects are more likely to be treated at an early stage in men than in women, since men are more likely to develop obvious infections of the urethra and thus seek medication from a physician. In females, the initial infection is likely to go unrecognized and untreated by antibiotics. The infection, meanwhile, may spread to body joints and produce acute attacks of arthritis. The symptoms tend to appear first in the wrists and finger joints; there may also be skin lesions that occur temporarily in areas near the joints.

Tuberculous Arthritis

As the name suggests, this disease is associated with tuberculosis and can be serious, leading to the destruction of involved joints. The infection spreads to the joints from other areas of the body. The early symptoms include pain, tenderness, or muscle spasm. In children and young adults the infection tends to settle in the spinal joints. If there is an absence of pain, the disease may go unnoticed until changes in pos-

In "Comfort in the Gout," a print from 1785, a gout patient elevates his foot to gain some relief from the pain concentrated in his big toe.

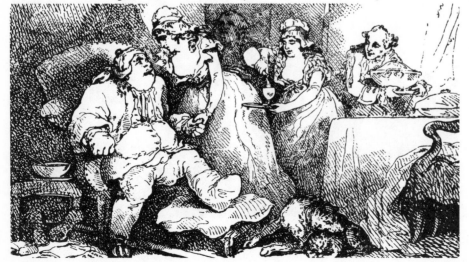

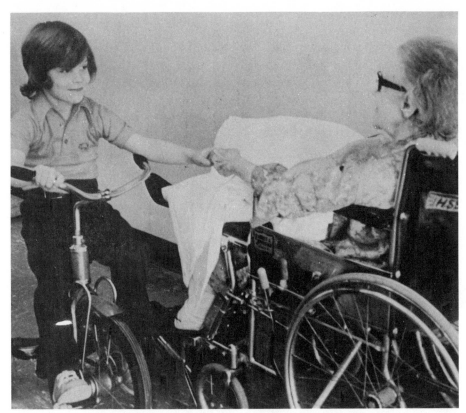

"How fast can you go?" Two victims of arthritis—one young, the other elderly—exchange an encouraging word during a physical therapy session.

ture or gait are observed. If untreated, the disease may progress toward spinal deformity. When detected early in the course of the disease, treatment with anti-tuberculosis drugs and physical therapy may control the disorder. In some cases, surgery may be required.

Rubella Arthritis

This form of arthritis derives from an infection involving the rubella virus. The arthritis symptoms may appear shortly after a rash appears, or they may be delayed until after the rash has faded. The onset of the arthritis effects may be accompanied by fever and a general feeling of illness; pain and swelling are most likely to occur in the small joints of the wrists, knees, or ankles. The doctor usually advises aspirin for the pain while it lasts, usually about a week. Eventually all signs and symptoms may subside without joint destruction.

Bacteria That Cause Arthritis

A type of bacteria that cause spinal meningitis also may cause symptoms of arthritis. The pain usually is not severe and may be limited to a few body joints. Antibiotics are administered to control the infection, although this form of the disease does not respond as rapidly to the medication as some of the other versions of arthritis caused by infection.

Several other kinds of bacteria may invade the joints and precipitate or aggravate arthritic symptoms. They include the increasingly common strains of bacteria that have become resistant to control by antibiotics. Patients who are being treated with steroid drugs or those whose resistance to infection has been lowered by disease are among the most vulnerable victims.

Fungal Arthritis

While fungal infections are relatively rare causes of arthritis, there are at least four kinds of fungus that have been identified as the responsible organisms in joint inflammations. The fungus seems to be carried by the bloodstream to the area of the joint where it causes an inflammation in the tissues surrounding the bony structures. The infection usually can be treated with special antibiotic remedies that destroy fungal organisms, but surgery is occasionally necessary to insure eradication of the source of the inflammation.

Psoriatic Arthropathy

Arthritis also may be associated with psoriasis (a chronic skin condition marked by bright red patches and scaling) in a disease known as *psoriatic arthropathy.* This variation of the disease is marked by a deep pitting of the nails along with a chronic arthritic condition. The disease may be mild or very destructive and the sacroiliac region of the spine may be involved. The uric acid levels associated with gout frequently are elevated in patients with psoriasis, so gout symptoms also can appear. Unfortunately, one of the medications commonly used in the treatment of rheumatoid arthritis and gout, chloroquine, cannot be used as therapy for psoriatic arthropathy symptoms because the drug aggravates the psoriasis. Otherwise, the treatment is quite similar to that used for rheumatoid arthritis —analgesics such as aspirin and steroid drugs. In severe cases, methotrexate may be administered to control both the joint and skin symptoms.

Other Arthritic Diseases

Two kinds of arthritis once associated with venereal diseases are no longer considered a hazard of intimate contact. One is syphilis-caused arthritis, which is a possible problem but actually quite rare because of improved control of syphilis. The second is *Reiter's syndrome,* a form of arthritis in which there is also involvement of urethritis, or inflammation of the urethra, and conjunctivitis, an inflammation of the eye. The disease also may be accompanied by skin lesions and a fever, pain in the heels, and a urethral discharge. Perhaps because Reiter's syndrome seems to affect young men and symptoms may be similar to those of gonococcal arthritis, it was once assumed that this form of arthritis was a kind of venereal disease. However, there is a lack of evidence that the disease is transmitted by sexual contact.

Rheumatic Fever

This generalized inflammatory disease, which affects the entire body with pain and swelling of the joints, sometimes is classified as a form of arthritis. Rheumatic fever usually follows a sore throat or tonsillitis caused by streptococcus bacteria; however, the disease is not regarded as a streptococcal infection by itself. A common effect of rheumatic fever is a scarring of the heart valves due to inflammation of that tissue. The heart-valve damage is permanent. The streptococcal infection itself can be controlled by antibiotic medications. For further information, see *Rheumatic Fever and Rheumatic Heart Disease*, p. 368.

Bursitis

The *bursa* is a fluid-filled sac located in the muscle near most joints. The fluid lubricates the joint, thereby providing smooth joint movement. Infection or injury may cause inflammation of the bursa. This condition is known as *bursitis* and can be very painful. The most commonly affected joints are the shoulder, knee, and hip.

Calcium deposits in the shoulder tendon or calcification of the bursa (*calcific bursitis*) leads to more painful shoulder problems. This may be similar to *interstitial calcinosis,* a condition in which calcium deposits are found in the skin and subcutaneous tissues of children. Recovery from calcific bursitis is achieved by medical care, minor surgery, and resting the inflamed joint. Radiation treatments can sometimes speed the recovery process.

Living With Joint Diseases

The control of arthritis requires skilled medical supervision over extended periods of time. The causes of the major forms of arthritis are still unknown, although various theories have been formulated to explain it based on metabolic, biochemical, and microscopic-tissue studies. Despite years of intensive research, it has not been possible to isolate a microorganism that is generally agreed to be a cause of rheumatoid arthritis. Viruses have been implicated in a number of arthritic diseases and may be a cause of rheumatoid arthritis; however, the evidence remains elusive, and the virus theory will remain a theory until the specific causative organism has been isolated and tested.

Whatever the mystery surrounding the causes of osteoarthritis and rheumatoid arthritis, severe crippling can be prevented in 70 percent of the cases if the patient seeks medical care early in the disease and receives proper medical treatment. The course of the disease varies from patient to patient and in many cases is confined to a few joints, causing little or no impairment of function. Commonly, however, there is a tendency toward relapse or continued inflammation.

The arthritis patient needs to develop a sense of coexistence with the disease, a tolerant attitude toward the problems of possible pain or disability without surrendering to arthritis. Millions of people have learned to live with arthritis and have found that it is possible to work, travel, raise families, and enjoy many of the recreational activities pursued by people not afflicted by the disease.

Joint Replacement

Over the years, various methods of replacing joints have evolved. Like artificial hips (see p. 1079), artificial knee, elbow, ankle, shoulder, toe, and finger joints are becoming more and more common. Technically known as arthroplasty, joint replacement both relieves pain, including the pain of arthritis, and improves function.

Materials used in joint replacement operations include metal, plastic, and ceramic components. Because of the tasks they perform in bodily movement, hip, knee, and ankle arthroplasties are undertaken much more often than those involving other parts. Developments in knee replacement surgery include a "cementless knee" that has a porous surface of chrome cobalt beads; aided by the beads, the patient's bone cells grow right into the knee replacement.

In each type of operation, the surgeon faces special problems. The elbow, for example, is not a simple hinge or joint but has three sections. Each involves one of the three arm bones that meet at that point: the humerus, the radius, and the ulna.

Surgical joint replacement techniques are continually evolving. In all cases, the patient faces some risks. Patients are also told usually that joint replacements do not really cure arthritis or osteoarthritis even though they normally relieve pain.

DEFECTS AND DISEASES OF THE SPINE

Spinal-Curve Deformities

When looked at from the side, the normal human spine follows a shallow S-shaped curve. If there is an exaggerated forward curvature of the spine, that condition is described as a *lordosis*. This type of spinal curvature is uncommon except in late pregnancy, and is caused by hip deformity or a defect in posture.

Kyphosis

Kyphosis is an exaggerated backward spinal curvature characterized by a humpback appearance. A person with this disorder develops an abnormal-looking thorax (or chest) due to the hump in the back, and may sometimes find it difficult to lie on his back. The condition is brought on by untreated fractures of a vertebral body, a spinal tumor, osteoporosis (described on p. 461), or spinal tuberculosis. If the principal cause is diagnosed and treated, recovery is possible.

Scoliosis

Scoliosis is a lateral curvature of the central part of the spine and appears mostly in children from birth and young adults up to age 15. Early diagnosis and proper orthopedic care are important. If scoliosis appears in early adulthood, the prognosis is better than if the disease starts in infancy. Growth of the curvature ends when the individual's skeletal development ceases.

Scoliosis creates an ugly spinal deformity, and this is usually the only symptom. Sometimes there may be an acute attack of sciatica. Treatment of scoliotic children requires hospitalization. In simple cases, a cast is applied from the chest to the waist to reduce the curvature. Fusion of the vertebral bodies with bone grafting to maintain the fusion may be necessary.

Spinal Tuberculosis

Chronic pulmonary tuberculosis can spread to the skeletal system, including the vertebral column. Spinal tuberculosis, also known as *Pott's disease*, affects one or more vertebrae in children and young adults. It is currently a relatively rare disease.

The diseased vertebrae may collapse due to pressure from the vertebrae above, resulting in a humpback deformity and possible paralysis of the lower limbs. The usual symptoms are back pain, stiffness, and limited movement. Antibiotics are administered to combat and cure the infection.

Spinal Infections

Fever-inducing microorganisms may reach the spine via the blood and lymph channels, resulting in spinal osteomyelitis or a general inflammation of the vertebrae. This results in bone destruction, pressure on the spinal cord, and paralysis of the legs. Successful treatment includes bed rest, drug therapy, and sometimes a body jacket (for immobilization) made from plaster of Paris.

Tumors

The spinal column is affected by both malignant and benign tumors. They can either destroy the bony makeup of the affected vertebra, apply pressure to the spinal cord with resultant paralysis, or interfere with the nerve roots.

Spinal tumors are generally destructive. Some, like *meningiomas* and *neurofibromas*, result in lack of control over bowel and bladder function in addition to the loss of functioning of the lower extremities. Malignant tumors of the spinal column may originate from cancer of the prostate, uterus, bladder, lungs, or breast.

The symptoms of spinal tumors are pain, deformity, weakness, and lower limb paralysis. Diagnosis requires careful study of the subjective symptoms, as well as special tests and radiological examinations. Treatment may involve radiation

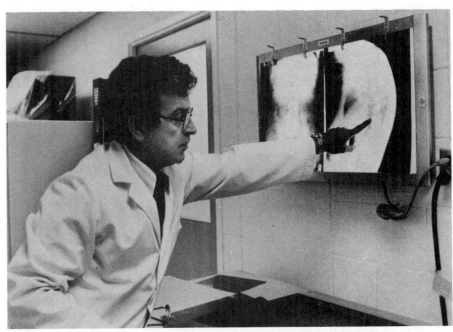

Diseases such as tuberculosis can have a destructive effect on the skeletal system. These X rays show bone losses in the spinal column.

therapy and chemotherapy; some tumors can be surgically removed. In many instances, the patient may be given analgesics to relieve the pain.

Back Pain and Its Causes

Most adults have experienced some form of back pain. Back pain is a serious physical impairment in persons of all ages, but it occurs more frequently in older persons.

Lumbago and Sciatica

Lumbago refers to general pain in the lower back. Technically, it is not a disease but a symptom that is accentuated by bending, lifting, turning, coughing, or stooping. Pain from neuritis of the sciatic nerve adds to one's misery, with pain shooting down the legs. This form of back pain is commonly known as *sciatica*, and, like lumbago, can be considered a symptom of some other condition. Treatment depends on the underlying cause of both.

Slipped and Herniating Disks

Between each two vertebrae is a fibro-cartilaginous disk that acts as a cushion. These disks are subjected to strain with every movement of the body, especially in the erect position. Increased pressure may cause a disk to protrude or herniate into the vertebral canal, causing what is referred to as a *slipped disk*. This condition can also be brought on by injury, degeneration due to aging, unaccustomed physical activity, or heavy lifting.

The herniating disk presses against nerves in the area, resulting in low back pain, sciatica, and in some instances, disabling muscle spasm. Back rest and a surgical corset may help milder forms of slipped disk by allowing natural healing to take place. Treatment may also include bed rest with intermittent traction to the legs for several weeks. Spinal fusion may be required in severe cases.

A severely herniated disk can be surgically removed to relieve pain and other symptoms. Disk removal is followed by fusion of the vertebral bodies on both sides of the removed disk. Fusion is accomplished by bridging the vertebral space with a bone graft. For a fuller description of surgical repair of a slipped disk, see under *Orthopedic Surgery*, p. 339.

Spondylolisthesis

A forward displacement of one vertebral body over another results in a painful condition known as *spondylolisthesis*. In mild cases there may be no symptoms at all. But in more advanced forms, there is severe low back pain when in the erect position and on bending, with the pain radiating to the legs. The displaced vertebra interferes with nerve roots in that area.

Mild cases require no treatment. Severe cases may require fusion of the vertebral segments with bone grafting; less severe symptoms can be relieved by a specially fitted corset.

Muscle Spasms and Strained Ligaments

Lack of physical exercise and unaccustomed bending can cause acute backache from undue muscle strain. Backache from strain on the ligaments is not uncommon in women following childbirth. The symptoms are similar to general low back pain. Physiotherapy with moist heat and massage helps restore muscular tone and relieve the pain. Muscle-relaxing drugs are sometimes prescribed.

Sacroiliac Pain

The *sacroiliac* joints in the lower back, where the *iliac* (hipbone) joins the sacrum, are a common location for osteoarthritic changes, rheumatoid arthritis, tuberculosis, and ankylosing spondylitis. The most common site of pain is in the lower lumbar region, radiating to the thighs and legs. X-ray diagnosis helps to pinpoint the cause of this particular form of back pain.

OTHER DISORDERS OF THE SKELETAL SYSTEM

Since bone consists of living cells, it is constantly changing as old cells die and new cells take their places. Any systemic disease during the growing period may temporarily halt the growth of long bones. As the aging process continues, dead bone cells are not replaced as consistently as in earlier life. The bony skeleton thus loses some of its calcium content, a process known as *decalcification* or *bone atrophy,* and the bones become fragile.

Pelvis and Hip Disorders

The hip joint presents most of the problems in the pelvic area. Symptoms may appear in early infancy in the form of congenital hip dislocation, in older children as tuberculous and transient arthritis, as slipped epiphysis in young adults (discussed below), and as osteoarthritis in adults and the aged. Early diagnosis of these conditions is very important in reducing the possibility of permanent deformity.

Diagnosis is achieved by physical examinations for signs of abnormal joint stability and mobility, postural changes, unstable and painful hip movement, fixed joint deformity, and pain in the lower back. Measurement of both lower limbs may indicate the presence of abnormal hip structure. X-ray examination of the pelvic area and both hips aids in diagnosis, as does blood analysis, which may yield evidence of early signs of gouty or arthritic conditions.

Slipped Epiphysis

This condition occurs in late childhood, between the ages of 9 and 18. The head of the *femur,* or thighbone, slips from its normal position, affecting one or both hips. The individual feels pain in the hip and knee, has limitation in joint movement, and walks with a limp. Usually there is evidence of endocrine disturbances.

Legg-Perthes' Disease

This is an inflammatory condition of unknown origin involving the bone and cartilage of the femoral head. It is found mostly in children between 4 and 12 years old and usually affects one hip. The symptoms are thigh and groin pain, joint movement limitation, and a walking impediment.

Successful treatment requires extended hospitalization with weight traction applied to the diseased hip, and limitation of body weight on the affected side. Untreated Legg-Perthes' disease leads to permanent hip joint deformity and possible osteoarthritis around middle age.

Coxa Vara

This hip deformity is due to a misshapen femur and causes shortening of the leg on the affected side; as a result, the person walks with a limp. The condition may be related to bone softening due to rickets, poorly joined fractures of the hip, or congenital malformation of the hip joint. Some cases may require surgical correction.

Any attack of persistent unexplained hip pains, limitation of movement, and walking impediments should be referred to the family doctor for further investigation. Early diagnosis is crucial in controlling and eradicating many of the crippling diseases of the pelvic area.

Other Bone Disorders

Osteoporosis

This metabolic disorder is marked by porousness and fragility of the bones. When the condition is associated with old age, it is referred to as senile *osteoporosis*. Its exact cause is not know, but protein deficiency, lack of gonadal hormones, or inadequate diet may be contributing factors.

Osteoporosis can originate in youth from improper metabolism of calcium or phosphorus, elements necessary for healthy bones. It can also result from a deficiency in the sex hormones, androgen and estrogen—which is why it often appears after menopause. Another cause is atrophy due to disuse and lack of stress and strain on the bones.

Osteogenesis Imperfecta

During the formation and development of bones, a process called *osteogenesis,* the bones may grow long and thin but not to the required width, becoming brittle so that they fracture easily. This condition is known as *osteogenesis imperfecta*. The individual may grow out of the condition in the middle twenties after suffering numerous fractures while growing up. A child thus afflicted cannot participate in games or other strenuous activities.

Paget's Disease

Paget's disease is characterized by a softening of the bones followed by an abnormal thickening of the bones. Its cause is unknown, and it manifests itself after the age of 30. It may cause pain in the thighs, knees, or legs, as well as backache, headache, and general fatigue. Symptoms include deafness, deformity of the pelvis, spine, and skull, and bowed legs. Although there is no known cure, Paget's disease is not usually fatal, but is eventually disabling.

Osteomyelitis

Osteomyelitis is an inflammation of the bone caused by fever-inducing bacteria or mold organisms. The invading microorganisms usually reach the bone through the bloodstream after entering the body through a wound or ulcer; the infection also can begin through a compound fracture or during surgery. The staphylococcus germ is most frequently the causative agent, and the most frequent site is the shaft of a long bone of a child. In adults, osteomyelitis usually occurs in the pelvis or spinal column.

SYMPTOMS: Symptoms are fever, chills, and pain, with nausea and vomiting, especially in younger patients. There also may be muscle spasms around the affected bone. The infected bone usually is sensitive to the touch but X rays may reveal no abnormality during the early stages. Redness and swelling sometimes appear in tissues above the inflamed bone, and as the disease progresses the patient may find that simply moving the affected limb is painful. The infection can involve a joint, producing misleading symptoms of arthritis.

CAUSES: Examination by a physician usually reveals signs of a recent wound, ulceration, or similar lesion that may have been accompanied by pus from the invading bacteria. Laboratory tests of the blood usually will show an abnormal number of white cells and the presence of the infectious microorganism. Signs of anemia also may be found.

TREATMENT: Treatment may include the use of antibiotics for a period of several weeks. In difficult cases, surgery may be required to drain abscesses or to remove dead bone tissue. Before the advent of antibiotic drugs, osteomyelitis could be a fatal disease; early and proper treatment with modern medications has virtually eliminated that risk.

Diet and Bone Disorders

A proper diet is necessary to maintain the health of the skeletal system. The body's retention of the bone-building minerals, phosphorus and calcium, depends on vitamin D, which is manufactured in the human skin through the action of the sun's ultraviolet radiation.

Rickets

An insufficient supply of vitamin D and a lack of exposure to sunlight leads to a vitamin-deficiency disease known as *rickets*. It can occur in infants and small children who live in northern latitudes and thus are not exposed to sufficient sunlight to permit their body to manufacture vitamin D. Rickets slows growth and causes bent and distorted bones and bandy legs. Symptoms first appear between the age of six months and the end of the first year. If rickets is recognized in time, it can be cured by a diet containing adequate vitamin D and by exposure to sunlight. If the disease is unchecked, the bones may develop permanent curves.

Bone Tumors

Benign and malignant tumors can occur in bone and bone marrow, although these growths are far less common than tumors of the body's soft tissues. Children and adolescents are more susceptible to bone tumors than adults. Since X rays cannot show whether a bone tumor is benign or malignant, surgical biopsy of the affected tissue is necessary in all cases.

Benign Tumors

These tumors usually take the form of an overgrowth of bone tissue, often near a joint, with many cysts or hollow spaces in the affected tissue.

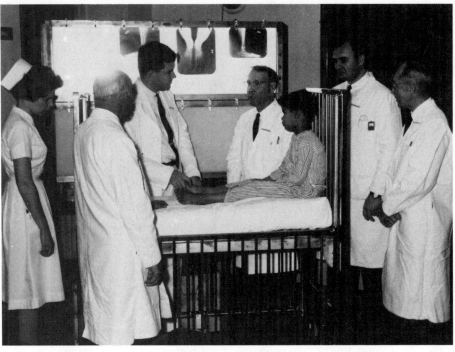

Children and adolescents are more susceptible to bone tumors than adults. Since X rays cannot show whether such a tumor is benign or malignant, surgical biopsy of the affected tissue is necessary in all cases.

These growths often cause pathological fractures, in which a bone breaks for no apparent reason. Swelling, pain, and limited mobility in the joint nearest the tumor are the most common symptoms. Treatment consists of surgical removal of the tumor, after which the surrounding bone gradually repairs itself as it does after a fracture.

Malignant Tumors

Bone cancers may be primary (originating in the bone tissue itself) or caused by metastasis of cancer cells from a site elsewhere in the body. The most common types of primary bone cancer are *osteogenic sarcoma*, a rapidly growing form of cancer that often spreads into nearby muscles; *chondrosarcoma*, which begins in cartilage at the end of a bone; and *Ewing's sarcoma*, a highly malignant cancer of the shafts of the long bones in children.

Bone cancer of the extremities is treated by amputation of the affected limb, followed by radiation therapy. If treatment is begun early enough and all the cancerous tissue is removed, the prognosis for survival is favorable.

INJURY TO BONES AND JOINTS: FRACTURES AND DISLOCATIONS

Bones can be broken or displaced when the body is subjected to a violent impact or when a limb is suddenly wrenched out of its normal position. Auto and bicycle accidents and accidents in and around the home account for many such injuries. See *Medical Emergencies*, p. 573, for information on accidents and how to provide treatment.

A *fracture* is a break in a bone as a result of injury or pathological weakness. Tumors, for example, can destroy bones to such an extent that a spontaneous fracture occurs due to pathological weakness. Osteoporosis (see p. 461) can also cause such fractures.

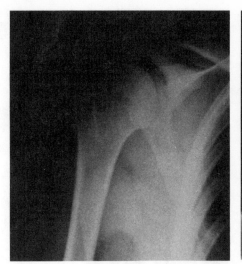

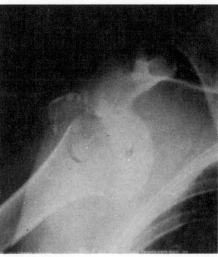

A *dislocation* is a displacement of any part, especially a bone. During this process the joint-capsule ligaments and muscle may be torn. The displaced bones must be reset by a bone specialist in their original position and immobilized until healing is complete. If this is not done, there is every possibility that the unhealed muscles will not provide the necessary support, thereby causing chronic spontaneous dislocation.

Injury *(trauma)* to bones and joints should not be dismissed lightly, especially if pain persists. If untreated, fractures and dislocations may heal with the bones out of alignment. Permanent deformity and joint degeneration are two possible complications.

Crush injuries, such as those occurring in some industrial and automobile accidents, may result in the clogging or blockage of blood vessels that supply blood to an extremity. When this happens, tissues below the blockage may die, and wounds do not heal due to lack of oxygenated blood and nutrition. If the fractures and wounds are not properly treated, *gangrene,* or the death of soft tissues, can sometimes result, requiring amputation just above the site of blockage and at a lo-

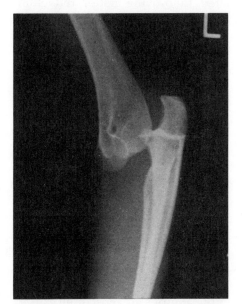

A dislocation at the elbow joint. Dislocated bones must be reset by a bone specialist in their original position and kept immobilized until they have healed completely.

A normal shoulder *(left)* and a fracture/dislocation of the shoulder joint *(right)*. Injuries in contact sports can be kept to a minimum if players wear the proper protective equipment at all times.

cation that will make the healing process possible.

Kinds of Fractures

Incomplete fractures are those which do not destroy the continuity of the bone. In a *complete fracture,* the bone is completely broken across. A *simple* or *closed fracture* is one in which the fragments are held together under the surface of the skin by the muscles and soft tissues. In a *compound* or *open fracture* one or both fragments pierce the skin, resulting in an open wound. In some cases the bony fragments can be seen protruding through the skin.

Comminuted fractures are the result of crushed bones. Several fragments appear at the trauma site. *Greenstick fractures* occur when one side of the bone is broken and the other bent. This type of fracture is more common in long bones, especially the forearms, clavicle, and legs of young children. *Stress fractures,* tiny cracks in the bone, can occur in the bones of the foot or leg of athletes who put these bones under repeated stress, such as ballet dancers and long-distance runners.

Healing of Fractures

When a bone breaks, new bone cells called *callus* are laid down at the ends of the fracture to unite the

fragments. This is the beginning of the healing process, the speed of which is dependent on the nature of the fracture.

Simple, incomplete, and greenstick fractures heal readily. Rest is usually sufficient to heal stress fractures. However, compound fractures have wounds and fragments to complicate the healing process. Cleaning and suturing the wound and administering antibiotics reduce the chance of infection and promote healing.

Comminuted fractures may have to be disimpacted and all fragments reset, usually by an orthopedic or general surgeon. Some very serious fractures of the extremities may require surgical insertion of metallic pins, nails, plates, wires, or screws to hold the fragments in proper position, thereby promoting rapid healing with minimal deformity. Such devices must be made from corrosion-free and rustproof metals since they may remain in the body for a few months or throughout the person's lifetime.

AGE AND THE HEALING PROCESS: The age of the fracture victim determines the speed of healing. In healthy, normal children, broken bones mend quickly because a rapid bone-cell manufacturing process is constantly in progress during the growth of the child. This is further advanced by proper diet, including daily intake of milk and milk products to provide the calcium required to build healthy bones.

In young adults, new bone cells do not develop as rapidly as in the growing child, but under normal circumstances, this will not present problems with the healing of fractures. Fractures in the aged heal slowly or not at all, depending on the age and health of the individual.

TREATMENT OF FRACTURES: Correction of a fracture or dislocation is called *reduction* and is usually performed by an orthopedic surgeon. Bones that are merely cracked do not require reduction; they heal with the aid of immobilization. More serious fractures require manipulation, pressure, and sometimes, as mentioned above, wires, pins, nails, and screws, to bring the fragments together so that they can unite.

Healing of fractures and dislocations following reduction requires

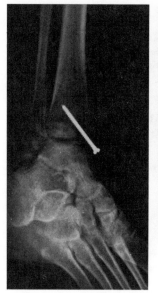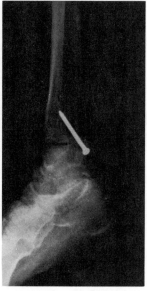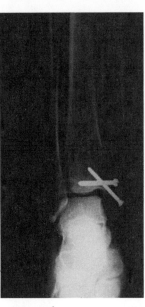

Surgical insertion of pins, nails, plates, wires, or screws may be required in certain serious fractures to hold fragments in proper position. Shown here are X rays of ankle fractures reset and secured by screws.

proper immobilization, which also reduces pain by preventing movement of the fragments. Immobilization is usually accomplished by the use of splints or plaster casts, or by applying *traction*. Traction subjects the fractured member to a pulling force by means of a special apparatus, such as a system of weights and pulleys.

After a fracture or dislocation is reduced and immobilized in a cast, the injury is X-rayed to insure that the immobilized reduction will heal without deformity. If the reduction is not satisfactory, the cast is removed, the fragments are remanipulated to provide better reduction, and a new cast or bandage is applied. Periodic X-ray rechecks help the doctor ascertain the degree of new bone formation as the healing continues. Casts are also checked to make sure there is not excess swelling of tissues and compression of blood vessels in the area.

How long a cast must remain depends on the extent of the injury and the rapidity of healing. A broken wrist may heal in four to six weeks while a fractured tibia may require four months of immobilization in a plaster cast.

Fracture of the Pelvis

Pelvic injuries are most often caused by falls in the home or on slippery streets, and by industrial or automobile accidents.

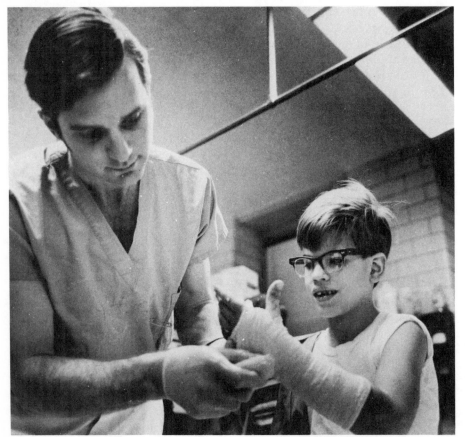

Broken bones usually mend quickly in normal, healthy children because of the rapid rate with which bone cells are constantly being manufactured.

The pelvis bears the entire weight of the body from the waist up and must bear the stress of general body motion during daily activity. The bony architecture of the pelvis does not readily permit the use of a plaster cast to immobilize a fracture. Consequently, fractures of the pelvis require bed rest for at least three weeks, depending on the nature of the injury and the age of the patient.

Simple fractures in children and young adults heal readily with complete bed rest and proper home care. Among the aged, the creation of new bone cells occurs more slowly, and this complicates the management of serious pelvic fractures in people over 65. Prolonged inactivity from extensive bed rest presents other health hazards for the aged, such as sluggish digestion and respiratory or vascular complications.

Fracture of the Hip

Falls are a major cause of hip fractures—the most common type of pelvic injury. Intense pain with limitation of hip movement and external rotation of the lower leg are indications of a hip fracture. When this occurs, a doctor should be contacted immediately. The patient should be placed flat in bed until medical ad-

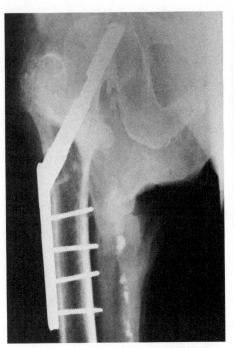 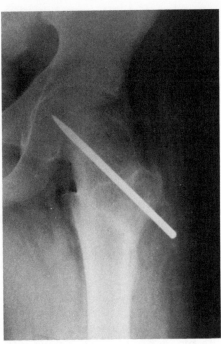

Immobilizing a fractured hip by the insertion of metal pins (as shown here) or with plates screwed to the bone helps speed recovery, enabling the patient to avoid the months of bed rest that would otherwise be necessary.

vice has been obtained. Proper diagnosis requires X-ray examinations.

Patients with hip fractures must be hospitalized. Although a hip fracture may be treated with traction, this method requires months of bed rest and is rarely used. The best method for treating such fractures is to nail the hip together with a metallic pin. The operation is performed by a surgeon, usually an orthopedist, who uses X-ray examinations during surgery to ascertain that the pin is in the correct position. Some hip fractures may also require a metallic plate screwed to the bone to help immobilize the fracture.

After plates and pins have been inserted, the patient can be out of bed within a day. This speeds recovery and prevents the complications of prolonged bed rest. Hip nails are usually left in the patient, depending on the nature of the fracture and the patient's age. Recuperation includes periodic medical checkups and X-ray examinations.

Hip Replacement

In recent years the technique of total hip replacement has become

well advanced. The technique can be used where the hip joint has been injured or severely weakened by disease.

Called "total prosthetic replacement of the hip," the operation involves removal of the upper portion of the large leg bone, the femur, and of the ball-like joint that holds it in the hip socket. A substitute piece shaped like the removed section of bone is attached to the femur. Care has to be taken during the operation to make certain the new part is firmly attached—by embedding the replacement part in the shaft of the bone. In addition, the surgeon tries not to destroy or damage the muscles and other tissues surrounding the hip. The replacement part is usually made of metal; a commonly used material is a durable cobalt-chromium alloy that produces no painful reactions in surrounding bones and tissues.

With modern techniques, hip replacement surgery can restore most patients to virtually normal levels of functioning. The implanted parts can carry weight and stand the strains of everyday use. Metal screws and a grouting agent,

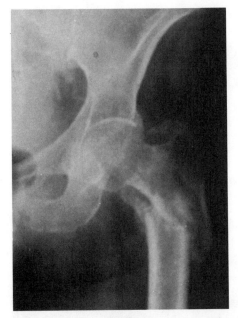

A healing fracture of the upper end of the femur, or thigh bone. Patients with hip fractures must be hospitalized.

or mortar of plastic cement or other material, help to join the metal implant to the leg bone. Patients may begin to walk one to three days after surgery. While they can later play golf or other nonstrenuous games, they are usually told to avoid more demanding activities, such as tennis or hand-ball, because of the danger that they might fall and injure the replacement hip.

Some patients have had successful hip replacement surgery on both their right and left sides. Later they were able to function with good mobility and without pain.

Pubic Fracture

Pubic fractures can cause ruptures of the bladder with urine leaking into the pelvic cavity. Routine urinalysis for the presence of blood cells is always necessary in cases of pelvic fractures. Surgical repair of the bladder may be required.

Skull Injury

Although the skull is very thick, it is not invulnerable. Head injuries can result from sports or playground accidents, falls, automobile or industrial accidents, or sharp blows to the head. Head injuries can cause linear or hairline skull fractures, depressed skull fractures (dents), brain injury due to fracture fragments or foreign bodies piercing the brain (as in the case of a bullet wound), or *concussion* with or without bone damage. The effects of concussion can show up as dizziness, nausea, irritability, the tendency to sleep deeply or lose consciousness, a weak pulse, and slowed respiration.

Any of these injuries can cause blood vessels to rupture and bleed. The resulting blood clots form what is known as a *subdural hematoma*, which may cause increased pressure on the brain. Patients with a subdural hematoma feel dizzy, slip slowly into unconsciousness, and may die unless immediate hospital care is available. Usually half of the body on the opposite side of the clot becomes paralyzed.

A depressed fracture can also apply pressure on the brain at the area of the depression. Surgery is required to relieve the pressure.

No skull injury should be treated lightly. A child may hit his head in a playground or in the backyard and conceal this from his parents, or a baby sitter may be afraid of losing her job if she reports such a fall. An alcoholic may slip on the street and strike his head on the sidewalk. Anyone who suffers a blow to the head or who falls on his head should be observed carefully for possible later complications. If such incidents are followed by vomiting, drowsiness, and headaches, immediate medical attention should be sought.

Facial Injury

A blow to the eye may fracture the upper or lower borders of the eye socket. It can also cause what is commonly known as a black eye, the blue-black appearance of which is due to bleeding under the skin. The swelling can be reduced by applying an ice pack to the area.

Fractures of the facial bones, jaw, and nose result from a direct blow to these areas. The impact may rupture blood vessels and cause bleeding in the sinuses. Fractures of the nose and jawbone may be severe enough to cause facial deformity. Dislocation of the jaw is a common problem caused by trauma. It may also occur spontaneously in certain individuals by an unusually wide-mouthed yawn or laugh. It is an uncomfortable rather than painful experience.

Serious facial injury requires hospitalization and surgical restoration. Skin lacerations may have to be sutured and the scars removed by plastic surgery; fractures of the jaw and mouth may require surgical wiring for stabilization and immobilization before healing can take place. In some instances both jaws may be wired together until healing takes place.

Injury to the Rib Cage

Accidents, athletic injuries, and fights account for most injuries to the rib cage. Any blow to the chest can cause rib fractures, which hurt when one coughs or inhales. Hairline and incomplete fractures are less serious

A smart driver buckles her seat belt, thus minimizing her chances of serious fractures in the event of a collision with another vehicle.

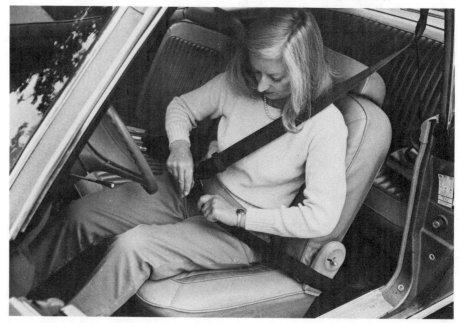

than complete fractures, where the fragments are usually sharp and pointed. Such fractured ribs can tear the lungs, causing air to leak into the pleural space, with possibly serious results. The lung can collapse as a result of being punctured. Punctured blood vessels can hemorrhage into the pleural space. The accumulated blood may have to be withdrawn before it reduces the capacity of the lungs to carry out their normal function.

Severe chest injuries—crush injuries with multiple fractures—require hospitalization. The patient must be confined to bed and kept under constant medical observation and treatment. If the lung has collapsed, it has to be reinflated. In simple rib fractures the chest may be strapped to immobilize the fragments and promote rapid healing. Generally, analgesics alone are enough to relieve pain.

Fractures of the sternum are caused by direct blows to the sternal area, as is usually the case with automobile accidents when the steering wheel hits the driver's chest. This injury can be avoided if the driver wears a shoulder-restraining belt, and if his car is equipped with a collapsible steering column.

Chest pains following a blow to the area of the sternum should be medically investigated by means of X-ray diagnosis for possible fracture. The fracture fragments may have to be wired together and remain in place until the injury has healed. For simple fractures, rest may be the only treatment required. The serious complication of a fractured sternum in a steering-wheel accident is contusion of the heart; it should be evaluated by means of an electrocardiogram.

Spinal Injury

Most spinal injuries originate from automobile accidents, industrial mishaps, falls, athletics, or from fights and beatings. Spinal injuries can create fractures that compress or sever the spinal cord, with resultant paralysis. A diving accident or headlong fall may cause a concussion and possible fractures of the cervical spine. Head-on collisions in the sports arena and automobile accidents are the chief causes of cervical spine fractures.

An individual who jumps from a considerable height and lands on his feet, especially on his heels, may easily fracture his spine. Sudden pain in the thoracic spine following a jump should receive immediate medical attention and investigation.

WHIPLASH: *Whiplash* injuries, the most common form of injury to the spine, occur most often during head-on and rear-end automobile accidents which suddenly jerk the neck and injure the cervical vertebrae. Accident victims thus injured may undergo months of agonizing headaches and pain in the neck. Immobilization of the neck by a surgical collar will reduce some of the pain and aid the healing process.

First Aid for Spinal Injuries

Victims of spinal injuries should be moved as little as possible. While waiting for professional help, the patient should be placed on his back and made as comfortable as possible. If an accident or explosion victim is wedged between debris, attempts should be made to free him, but his body should be kept flat with as little movement as possible. No attempt should be made to have the person sit up or stand before he has been examined by a physician. Unnecessary movement of victims of spinal injury can damage the spinal cord and cause permanent paralysis.

Decompression of Fractures

Anyone with a spinal injury should be taken to the emergency ward of the nearest hospital for X-ray examinations that will reveal possible fractures. If the fracture compresses against the spinal cord, the extremities may be paralyzed. In such cases, a neurosurgeon or an orthopedist may perform a delicate operation, lifting the fracture fragments away from the spinal cord, thereby relieving the pressure and reestablishing control and movement of the paralyzed extremities.

Fractures of the cervical spine can be decompressed by applying traction to the neck. Frequent X-ray rechecks are required to assess the degree of healing and new bone formation. Patients with fractured vertebrae undergo a lengthy rehabilitation with frequent medical rechecks and physical therapy. In some severe cases of spinal fractures that result in paralysis, the individual is never able to walk again.

CHAPTER 26

Diseases of the Muscles and Nervous System

We have the capacity to perceive our environment by receiving sensory messages—such as hearing, sight, touch, pain, and awareness of our posture—to associate all the incoming messages, store the information, and then call it back to our consciousness as needed. Another function of the nervous system is the control of the body by sending signals to the muscles to perform movements ranging from the broadest to the most delicate—from wielding a pickax to playing the flute. Further, many aspects of our behavior are not at all mysterious and can be explained in terms of a series of neuro-electrochemical events. In short, our day-to-day existence is a reflection of the state of our nervous system, the normal function of which can be disturbed in many ways.

DISEASES OF THE NERVOUS SYSTEM

If any part of the brain has developed abnormally, the usual function of that structure would be expected to be altered. Abnormalities present at birth are called *congenital* defects. If the nervous system does not receive a normal blood supply because of the obstruction of a blood vessel, or if there is a tear in the vessel with subsequent hemorrhage, the cells are deprived of blood and will die. These lesions are *vascular* or *cerebrovascular* accidents. Cerebral injury, or *trauma,* can destroy brain tissue, with consequent loss of normal function; infection of the nervous system may also permanently injure tissue. Finally, brain function can be altered by *metabolic, toxic,* or *degenerative* changes in normal body chemistry. It is not surprising, then, that such a beautifully or-

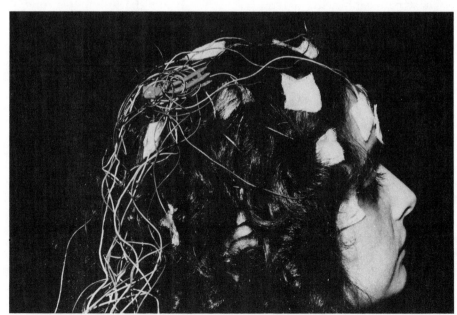

Electrodes are placed at various points on the head to take an electroencephalogram, a test that measures brain waves and pinpoints problems.

468

ganized nervous system is vulnerable to the hazards of living.

Diagnostic Tests

A patient who has been referred to a *neurologist*, a physician who specializes in diseases of the nervous system, will be asked to tell the history of the problem in great detail, for that history will describe the nature of the disorder; the neurological examination will help to localize the problem. After the neurological examination is completed, the physician may order radiographs (X-ray pictures) of the skull and spinal column and an electroencephalogram. The *electroencephalogram* (EEG), or brain wave recording, assists in localizing a brain abnormality or describing the nature of a convulsive disorder. A specific diagnosis is not based upon the EEG alone, but the EEG is used to corroborate the doctor's clinical impression of the disease process.

It may also be necessary to perform a *lumbar puncture (spinal tap)* in order to obtain a specimen of the *cerebrospinal fluid (CSF)*, the fluid that bathes the brain and spinal cord. This laboratory test is a benign, relatively painless procedure when performed by a skilled physician and is extremely useful in making a diagnosis. It entails a needle puncture under sterile conditions in the midline of the lower spine as the patient lies on his side or sits upright.

Occasionally, other more specialized diagnostic tests are used to better enable the physician to visualize the structure of the brain and the spinal cord. In a process called *ventriculography*, the cerebrospinal fluid is replaced by air introduced directly into the cavities *(ventricles)* of the brain. In *pneumoencephalography*, the air or other gas is inserted by means of a needle similar to that used in a lumbar puncture. In either case the outlines of the brain structure are photographed by X ray.

Another specialized neuroradiological test is the *angiogram*. A ma-

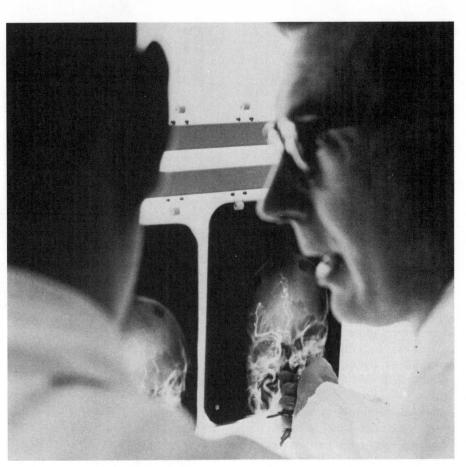

Doctors examine the angiogram of a head-injury patient. An opaque substance injected into the blood vessels makes them visible on X-ray film.

terial that is opaque to X rays is injected into the blood vessels that supply the brain. Since the vessels can be plainly seen on the X-ray film, any displacement of those vessels from the normal position is evident.

A more recent diagnostic tool is the *brain scanner* or *CAT scanner* (for *computerized axial tomography*). CAT scanning may in many cases make angiography, which can be painful and is not without risk, unnecessary. The scanner takes a series of computer-generated X-ray pictures of "slices" of the brain as it rotates about the patient. It can thus provide better pictures of parts of the brain (and of other internal areas of the body) than any older process.

More advanced than either the CAT scanner or radiography, *nuclear magnetic resonance* (NMR) uses neither X radiation, as does the CAT scanner, nor needle-injected contrast fluids. Instead, NMR uses

magnetic forces 3,000 to 25,000 times as strong as the earth's magnetic field. Taking three-dimensional "pictures" of various parts of the body, NMR "sees" through bones. It can differentiate between the brain's gray and white matter. NMR can also show blood moving through an artery or the reaction of a malignant tumor to therapy.

Another type of contrast study is called a *myelogram*. A radio-opaque liquid similar to that used in angiography is introduced through a spinal needle into the sac-enclosed space around the spinal cord. Any obstructive or compressive lesion of the spinal cord is thus seen on the radiograph and helps to confirm the diagnosis.

Each of these contrast studies helps the physician better understand the structures of the brain or spinal cord and may be essential for him to make a correct diagnosis.

Cerebral Palsy

The term *cerebral palsy* is not a diagnosis but a label for a problem in locomotion exhibited by some children. Definitions of cerebral palsy are many and varied, but in general refer to nonprogressive abnormalities of the brain that have occurred early in life from many causes. The label implies that there is no active disease process but rather a static or nonprogressive lesion that may affect the growth and development of the child.

SYMPTOMS: Included in the category of cerebral palsy are such problems as limpness (flaccidity), *spasticity* of one or all limbs, incoordination, or some other disorder of movement. In some patients, quick jerks affect different parts of the body at different times (*chorea*); in others, slow, writhing, incoordinated movements (*athetosis*) are most pronounced in the hands and arms. Incoordination of movement may also occur in muscles used for speaking and eating, so that speech becomes slurred, interrupted, or jerky; the patient may drool because incoordinated muscle action pre-

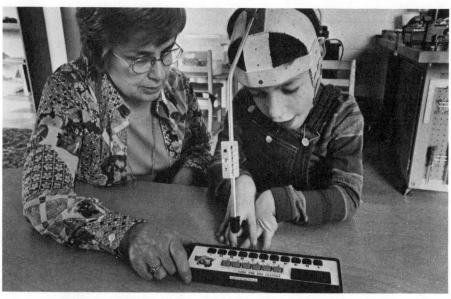

Cerebral palsy affects motor coordination. This child cannot operate a calculator by hand, but he can work it using a pointer on his head.

vents efficient swallowing of saliva. This does little to improve the physical appearance of the child and, unfortunately, he may look mentally subnormal.

The fact that a patient has an abnormality that is responsible for difficulty in locomotion or speech does not mean that the child is mentally retarded. There is some likelihood that he will be mentally slow, but patients in this group of disease states range from slow to superior in intelligence, a fact that emphasizes that each child must be assessed individually.

A complete physical examination must be completed, and to determine the patient's functional status complete psychological testing should be performed by a skilled psychologist.

TREATMENT: Treatment for cerebral palsy is a continuing process involving a careful surveillance of the patient's physical and psychological status. A physical therapist, under the doctor's guidance, will help to mobilize and maintain the function of the neuromuscular system. Occasionally, an orthopedic surgeon may surgically lengthen a tendon or in some way make a limb more functional. A speech therapist can provide additional speech training, and a vocational therapist can help the patient to find appropriate work. The key professional is the primary physician, usually the pediatrician, who with care and understanding guides the patient through the years.

Bell's Palsy

Bell's palsy is a paralysis of the facial

Positron-emission tomography (PET) is a sophisticated diagnostic system that measures very subtle physical and chemical changes in brain tissue.

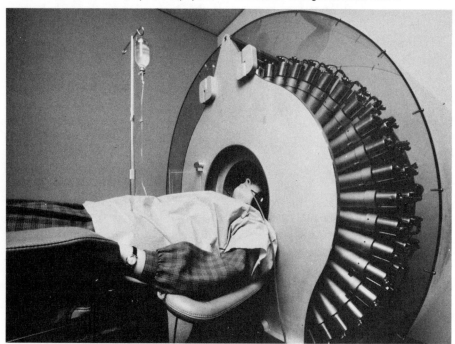

nerve that was first described by Sir Charles Bell, a Scottish surgeon of the early nineteenth century. It may affect men and women at any age, though it occurs most commonly between the ages of 30 and 50. The onset of the facial paralysis may be abrupt: the patient may awaken one morning unable to move one side of his face. He can't wrinkle one side of his forehead or raise the eyebrow; the eye will not close on the affected side, and when attempting to smile, the face is pulled to the opposite side. Occasionally the patient may experience discomfort about the ear on the involved side. There is no difficulty in swallowing, but since the muscles about the corner of the mouth are weak, drooling is not uncommon, and food may accumulate in the gutter between gum and lip.

Bell's palsy may affect the branch of the facial nerve that supplies taste sensation to the anterior part of the tongue, and the branch that supplies a small muscle in the middle ear (the *stapedius*) whose function it is to dampen loud sounds. Depending on the extent to which the facial nerve is affected, the patient may be unable to perceive taste on the side of the paralysis, and may be unusually sensitive to sounds, a condition known as *hyperacusis*.

The most probable causes of Bell's palsy are inflammation of the facial nerve as it passes through a bony canal within the skull or inflammation of that bony canal with subsequent swelling and compression of the nerve. It is not uncommon that the patient has a history of exposure to a cold breeze, such as sleeping in a draft or riding in an open car. Any patient who has a facial weakness should be carefully evaluated by a physician, preferably a neurologist, to be quite certain that there is no other neurologic abnormality. When the diagnosis of Bell's palsy is certain, some therapeutic measures can be taken.

TREATMENT: There is no specific treatment for Bell's palsy, but many physicians recommend massage, application of heat, and exercise of the weak muscles, either passive (by external manipulation) or active (by use). These therapeutic measures do not specifically influence the course of the facial nerve paralysis, but they are thought to be useful in maintaining tone of the facial muscles and preventing permanent deformity. Occasionally a V-shaped adhesive tape splint can be applied to the affected side of the face, from the corner of the mouth to the temple. Some physicians treat the condition with steroids such as cortisone, which may hasten recovery if begun at the onset of the illness.

In treating Bell's palsy, it is important to remember that when the eyelid does not close normally, the conjunctiva and cornea are not fully lubricated, and corneal lesions may develop from excessive dryness or exposure to the air. For this reason, some ophthalmic lubrication may be recommended by the doctor.

About 80 percent of the patients with Bell's palsy recover completely in a few days or weeks, and 10 to 15 percent recover more slowly, over a period of three to six months. The remaining 5 to 10 percent will have some residual facial deformity.

Parkinson's Disease

Patients with *Parkinson's disease,* or *parkinsonism,* are easily recognized because of the characteristic symptoms of tremor, rigidity, and a decrease of movement. This group of symptoms had another name, *shaking palsy,* long before it was scientifically described nearly a century and a half ago by an English physician, James Parkinson. It is associated with degeneration of nerve cells deep within the brain (*basal ganglia*) and the brain surface (*cerebral cortex*). It may follow encephalitis, a brain injury, or exposure to toxic substances, but in most cases, especially when the symptoms appear in a patient who is middle-aged or older, there is no known cause.

The tremor, or shaking, usually involves the fingers and the wrist, but sometimes the arms, legs, or head are involved to the extent that the entire body shakes. Characteristically, the tremor occurs when the patient is at rest. It stops or is much less marked during a voluntary muscle movement, only to start once again when that movement has been stopped. There is no tremor when the patient is asleep.

Early in the disease, the patient is aware that one leg seems a bit stiff; later, the arm does not swing normally at his side when he is walking. He moves about more slowly with stooped-over head and shoulders. Often he has difficulty in starting to walk, but once started he cannot stop unless he grabs at the wall or some other object. The face appears expressionless, the speech is slurred, and handwriting is small and uneven (*micrographia*) because of the rigidity and the tremor. Mental faculties are usually not impaired but, as might be expected in such a chronic disease in which the patient cannot move or communicate normally, mood disturbances are common.

TREATMENT: For many years parkinsonism was treated with drugs derived from belladonna. Many other remedies were tried, among them such toxic compounds as strychnine and cigarettes made from jimsonweed. In nearly all cases the results were less than gratifying. Neurosurgical procedures were then devised to produce very small destructive lesions in the brain, with subsequent lessening of the symptoms. The most gratifying improvements following surgery are usually seen in patients under 60 whose symptoms are confined primarily to one side of the body.

Today, three basic categories of drugs are used to relieve the symptoms of parkinsonism: anticholinergics, levodopa-containing compounds, and a single dopamine agonist.

The anticholinergic drugs include trihexyphenidyl hydrochloride (trade name: Artane), benztropine mesylate (trade name: Cogentin), diphenhydramine hydrochloride (trade name: Benadryl), biperiden (trade name: Akineton), and procyclidine hydrochloride (trade name: Kemadrin). All of these drugs reduce tremors and rigidity to a modest degree, but none affects bradykinesia, or slow movement. Patients using the drugs may experience such side effects as gingivitis or inflammation of the gums, constipation, mild dizziness, nausea, nervousness, and slightly blurred vision. More serious side effects could include urinary retention, confusion, and psychosis.

The levodopa-containing compounds reduce all the main symptoms of parkinsonism. One such compound combines levodopa, also known as L-dopa, with carbidopa (trade name: Sinemet). Levodopa is also sold alone under the trade names Larodopa and Dopar. Because L-dopa's effectiveness may dwindle after several years, physicians sometimes delay treatment until a patient shows more severe symptoms.

Side effects associated with L-dopa include nausea, involuntary movements, some mental changes, cardiac irregularities, and urinary retention. "End-of-dose" akinesia, the return of symptoms a few hours after taking medication, can be relieved in some cases by taking the patient off drugs entirely for three to seven days. The patient is usually hospitalized. During the "drug holiday" some patients take part in physical, occupational, and speech therapy programs.

The one drug in the dopamine agonist class, bromocriptine (trade name: Parlodel), stimulates the brain's dopamine receptors. Used in combination with L-dopa, bromocriptine reduces the end-of-dose response. But clincial studies have not established the drug's safety in long-term use (more than two years). Patients with histories of coronary or peripheral vascular disease should not take bromocriptine. Side effects may include confusion, nasal congestion, liver problems, and swelling of the feet.

One other drug used to treat Parkinson's disease, amantadine hydrochloride (trade name: Symmetrel), has brought rapid improvement when given along with L-dopa. But the drug may also produce such side effects as hypotension, urinary retention, depression, and congestive heart failure.

Epilepsy

Epilepsy is a common disorder of the human nervous system. In the United States, about five persons of every 1,000, or more than one million people, suffer from epilepsy.

Epilepsy affects all kinds of people, regardless of sex, intelligence, or standard of living. Among the more famous epileptics of history were Julius Caesar, Napoleon, Mohammed, Lord Byron, Dostoyevsky, Handel, Mendelssohn, and Mozart. The I.Q. range for epileptics is the same as that of the general population.

Unfortunately, epilepsy has been one of the most misunderstood diseases throughout its long history. Because of the involvement of the brain, epilepsy has commonly been associated with psychiatric disorders. Epilepsy differs strikingly from psychiatric disorders in being manifested in relatively brief episodes that begin and end abruptly.

Causes and Precipitating Factors

A single epileptic seizure usually occurs spontaneously. In some cases, seizures are triggered by visual stimuli, such as a flickering image on a television screen, a sudden change from dark to very bright illumination, or vice versa. Other patients may react to auditory stimuli such as a loud noise, a monotonous sound, or even to certain musical notes. A seizure is accompanied by a discharge of nerve impulses, which can be detected by electroencephalography. The effect is something like that of a telephone switchboard in which a defect in the circuits accidentally causes wrong number calls. The forms that seizures take depend upon the location of the nervous system disturbances within the brain and the spread of the nerve impulses. Doctors have found that certain kinds of epilepsy cases can be traced to specific areas of the brain where the lesion has occurred.

Epilepsy can develop at any age, although nearly 85 percent of all

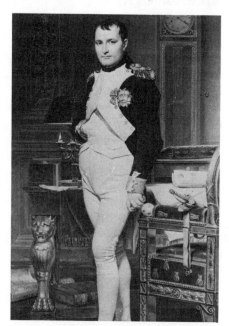 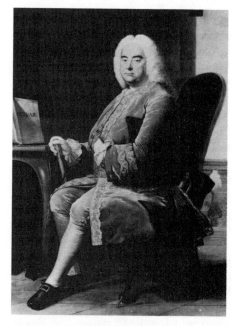

Epilepsy, a neurological condition, does not limit intelligence or ability. Famed epileptics in history have included France's Emperor Napoleon I (left) and classical composer George Frideric Handel (right).

cases appear before the age of 20 years. Hence, it is commonly seen as an affliction of children. There is no indication that epilepsy itself can be inherited, but some evidence exists that certain individuals inherit a greater tendency to develop the condition from precipitating causes than is true for the general population. According to the Epilepsy Foundation, studies show that if neither parent has epilepsy, the chances are one in 100 that they will have an epileptic child, but the chances rise to one in 40 if one parent is epileptic.

About 70 percent of epilepsy cases are *idiopathic*—that is, they are not attributable to any known cause. In the remaining 30 percent, the recurrent seizures are *symptomatic*— they are symptoms of some definite brain lesion, either congenital or resulting from subsequent injury. Since it can reasonably be assumed that some of the idiopathic cases are due to lesions that have not been identified, epilepsy is perhaps best regarded not as a specific disease but as a symptom of a brain abnormality due to any of various causes.

AURA PRECEDING A SEIZURE: Unusual sensory experiences have been reported to occur before a seizure by about half the victims of epilepsy. The sensation, which is called an *aura*, may appear in the form of an unpleasant odor, a tingling numbness, a sinking or gripping feeling, strangulation, palpitations, or a gastrointestinal sensation. Some patients say the sensation cannot be described. Others report feeling strange or confused for hours or even days before a seizure. Such an early warning is known as a *prodrome*.

The various types of epilepsy can be broadly grouped under four general categories: grand mal, petit mal, focal, and psychomotor. Only one feature is common to all types of epilepsy—the sudden, disorderly discharge of nerve impulses within the brain.

Grand Mal Seizure

The *grand mal* is a generalized convulsion during which the patient may initially look strange or bewildered, suddenly groan or scream, lose consciousness and become stiff *(tonic phase)*, hold the breath, fall to the ground unless supported, and then begin to jerk the arms and legs *(clonic phase)*. There may be loss of bowel and bladder control. The tongue may be bitten by coming between clenched jaws. The duration of the entire seizure, both the tonic and clonic phases, is less than two minutes—frequently less than one minute—followed by postconvulsive confusion or deep sleep that may last for minutes or hours.

FOLLOWING A SEIZURE: The patient may be able to resume normal activities shortly after the spell has ended. But after recovering from a long postconvulsive sleep, the patient may show a variety of signs or symptoms known as postconvulsive phenomena, which may include headache, mental confusion, and drowsiness.

VARIATIONS IN THE PATTERN: The sequence of events in grand mal seizures is not invariable. The tongue-biting and urinary and fecal incontinence do not occur as frequently in children as in adult patients. Children also may demonstrate a type of grand mal seizure in which the patient suddenly becomes limp and falls to the floor unconscious; there is no apparent tonic or clonic phase and the muscles do not become stiff. Other cases may manifest only the tonic phase, with unconsciousness and the muscles remaining in a stiffened, tonic state throughout the seizure. There also is a clonic type of seizure, which begins with rapid jerking movements that continue during the entire attack. In one very serious form of convulsive seizure known as *status epilepticus*, repeated grand mal seizures occur without the victim's becoming conscious between them.

Petit Mal Seizure

Petit mal seizures are characterized by momentary staring spells, as if the patient were suspended in the middle of his activity. He may have a blank stare or undergo rapid blinking, sometimes accompanied by small twitching movements in one part of the body or another— hands, legs, or facial muscles. He does not fall down. These spells, called *absence* or *lapse attacks*, usually begin in childhood before puberty. The attacks are typically very brief, lasting half a minute or less, and occur many times throughout the day. They may go unnoticed for weeks or months because the patient appears to be daydreaming.

Focal Seizure

Focal seizures proceed from neural discharges in one part of the brain, resulting in twitching movements in a corresponding part of the body. Usually, one side of the face, the thumb and fingers of one hand, or one entire side of the body is involved. The patient does not lose consciousness and may in fact remain aware of his surroundings and the circumstances during the entire focal convulsion. Focal convulsions in adults commonly indicate some focal abnormality, but this is less true in a child who may have a focal seizure without evidence of a related brain lesion.

With their knowledge of the nerve links between brain centers and body muscles, doctors are able to determine quite accurately the site of a brain lesion that is involved with a focal seizure.

JACKSONIAN EPILEPSY: One type of focal seizure has a distinctive pattern and is sometimes called a *Jacksonian seizure*, and the condition itself *Jacksonian epilepsy*. The attack begins with rhythmic twitching of muscles in one hand or one foot or one side of the face. The spasmodic movement or twitching then spreads from the body area first affected to other muscles on the same side of the body. The course of the twitching may, for example, begin on the left side of the face, then spread to the neck, down the arm, then along the trunk to the foot. Or the onset of the attack may begin at the foot and gradually spread upward along the trunk to the facial muscles. There may be a tingling or burning sensation and perspiration, and the hair may stand up on the skin of the areas affected.

Psychomotor Seizures

Psychomotor seizures, or *temporal lobe seizures,* often take the form of movements that appear purposeful but are irrelevant to the situation. Instead of losing control of his thoughts and actions, the patient behaves as if he is in a trancelike state. He may smack his lips and make chewing motions. He may suddenly rise from a chair and walk about while removing his clothes. He may attempt to speak or speak incoherently, repeating certain words or phrases, or he may go through the motions of some mechanical procedure, like driving a car, for example.

The patient in a psychomotor seizure usually does not respond to questions or commands. If physically restrained during a psychomotor episode, the patient may appear belligerent and obstreperous, or he may resist with great energy and violence. Usually, the entire episode lasts only a few minutes. When the seizure ends, the patient is confused and unable to recall clearly what has happened.

The aura experienced by victims of psychomotor seizures may differ from that of other forms of the disorder. The psychomotor epileptic may have sensations of taste or smell, but more likely will experience a complex illusion or hallucination that may have the quality of a vivid dream. The hallucination may be based on actual experiences or things the patient has seen, or it may deal with objects or experiences that only seem familiar though they are in fact unfamiliar. This distortion of memory, in which a strange experience seems to be a part of one's past life, is known as *déjà vu,* which in French means literally "already seen."

Other visual associations involved in various forms of epilepsy include those in which the patient experiences sensations of color, moving lights, or darkness. Red is the most common color observed in visual seizures, although blue, yellow, and green also are reported. The darkness illusion may occur as a temporary blindness, lasting only a few minutes. Stars or moving lights may appear as if visible to only one eye, indicating that the source of the disturbance is a lesion in the brain area on the opposite side of the head. Visual illusions before an epileptic attack may have a distorted quality, or consist of objects arranged in an unnatural pattern or of an unnatural size.

Auditory illusions, on the other hand, are comparatively rare. Occasionally a patient will report hearing buzzing or roaring noises as part of a seizure, or human voices repeating certain recognizable words.

Treatment of the Epileptic Patient

Usually the physician does not see the patient during a seizure and must rely on the description of others to make a proper diagnosis. Since the patient has no clear recollection of what happens during any of the epileptic convulsions, it is wise to have someone who has seen an attack accompany him to the doctor. First, the doctor begins the detective work to find the cause of the seizure. He will examine the patient thoroughly, obtain blood tests, an electroencephalogram, and a lumbar puncture, if indicated. However, even after all these studies, the doctor often can find no specific cause that can be eradicated. Efforts are then made to control the symptoms.

The treatment of epilepsy consists primarily of medication for the prevention of seizures. It is usually highly effective. About half of all patients are completely controlled and another quarter have a significant reduction in the frequency and severity of attacks. The medication, usually in tablet or capsule form, must be taken regularly according to the instructions of the physician. It may be necessary to try several drugs over a period of time to determine which drug or combination of drugs best controls the seizures. Phenobarbital and diphenylhydantoin (Dilantin) may be prescribed for the control of grand mal seizures and focal epilepsy, and the doctor may find that a combination of these drugs or others offers the best anticonvulsant control. Trimethadione frequently is administered to petit mal patients; primidone or phenobarbital may be prescribed for psychomotor attacks.

Surgery may be recommended when drugs fail to control the seizures. But this approach usually is used only as a last resort and is not always effective.

However, medicine and surgery are not the only treatments for epilepsy patients. Emotional factors are known to influence convulsive disorders. Lessening a patient's anger, anxiety, and fear can help to control the condition. An understanding family and friends are important, as are adequate rest, good nutrition, and proper exercise. The exercise program should not include vigorous contact sports, and some activities such as swimming should not be performed by the patient unless he is accompanied by another person who understands the condition and is capable of helping the epileptic during a seizure.

There is nothing permanent about epilepsy, although some patients may endure the symptoms for much of their lives. It is a disorder that changes appreciably and constantly in form and manifestations. Some experts claim that petit mal and psychomotor cases if untreated may progress to more serious cases of grand mal seizures. On the other hand, epilepsy that is given proper medical attention may eventually subside in frequency and severity of attacks. In many cases, seizures disappear or subside within a short time and treatment can be discontinued gradually.

While some effort has been made by medical scientists to determine if there is an "epileptic personality,"

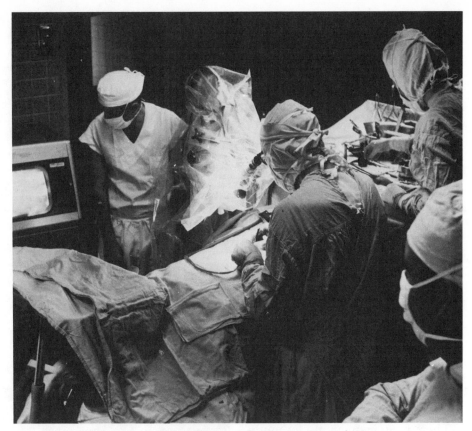

When drug treatment fails to control epileptic seizures, brain surgery may be performed as a last resort, but it is not always effective.

should be encouraged to participate in social and physical activities at school and in the neighborhood as long as they do not strain his capabilities. Finally, parents should not feel guilty about the child's condition and think that some action of theirs contributed to the child's condition. See *Epileptic seizures*, p. 595, for a description of what to do when a seizure occurs.

Further information about epilepsy, including causes, effects, treatment, rehabilitation, and laws regulating employment and driver permits, can be obtained from the Epilepsy Foundation of America, 1828 L Street, N.W., Washington, D.C. 20036, and from the U. S. Department of Health, Education and Welfare, Public Health Service, National Institutes of Health, Bethesda, Md. 20014.

Multiple Sclerosis

Multiple sclerosis is a disease involving the progressive destruction of myelin, the fatty material that covers the nerves of the body. The disease affects mainly the brain and spinal cord. It is termed *multiple* because there are distinct and separate areas of the nervous system involved, seemingly distributed in a random pattern.

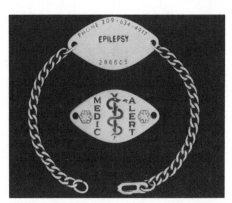

In order to avoid having an epileptic convulsion mistaken for some other disorder and treated improperly, some epileptics wear a bracelet or necklace that identifies their disease. These emblems are available for a slight charge from Medic Alert Foundation, Turlock, California 95380, a nonprofit organization.

evidence indicates there is no typical personality pattern involved. Whatever behavior patterns and emotional reactions are observed are the result of individual personality makeup rather than being directly related to epilepsy. Most epilepsy patients are capable of performing satisfactory work at various jobs; one study showed that only nine percent were partially dependent and four percent were incapable of holding a job. In some areas there may be restrictions on issuing driver's licenses to epileptics or other legal regulations that limit normal activities for epilepsy patients. As a result, some epileptics may conceal their condition or avoid medical treatment that might be reported to government agencies.

Because of ignorance and misinformation, some people regard epilepsy as frightening or mysterious, and patients may suffer unnecessarily and unjustly. In fact, behavioral abnormalities in patients with seizures are commonly the reflection of how they are viewed by others. The patient should be carefully observed by an understanding physician who watches not only for medical but for psychological problems.

When epilepsy has been diagnosed in a child, the parents must be instructed about the condition and the need for continuous careful medical supervision. If the child is old enough to understand, he also should learn more about the nature of the condition. Misbeliefs should be corrected. Both parents and child should understand that seizures are not likely to be fatal and that a brain lesion does not lead to mental deterioration. Parents and child should learn what actions should be taken in the event of a seizure, such as loosening clothing and taking steps to prevent injury. Natural concern should be balanced with an understanding that overprotection may itself become a handicap. The child

Incidence

The incidence of multiple sclerosis is puzzling. It occurs most frequently in the temperate geographic areas of the world; the high-risk regions generally are between 40 and 60 degrees of latitude on either side of the equator, where the incidence is about 40 cases per 100,000 population. Within the high-risk latitudes, however, there are countries in Asia where the disease is relatively rare, and in the Shetland and Orkney Islands to the north of Scotland the incidence of the disease is approximately five times that in the United States, Canada, and Northern Europe. Multiple sclerosis has never been found in certain black populations in Africa, but black persons living in the United States develop the disorder at about the same rate as white persons.

Multiple sclerosis rarely appears before the age of 15 or after 55. A person aged 30 years is statistically at peak risk of developing the disease. The typical patient, statistically speaking, is a woman of 45 who was born and raised in a temperate climate. Women are more susceptible to the disease than men by a ratio of 1.7 to 1, and women are more likely than men to experience the onset of symptoms before the age of 30.

Symptoms and Diagnosis

There are no laboratory tests that are specific for multiple sclerosis, although there are certain tests that may suggest the presence of the disease. Diagnosing the disorder depends to a large extent upon tests that rule out other diseases with similar signs and symptoms. The first symptom may be a transitory blurring of vision or a disturbance in one or more of the limbs, such as numbness, a tingling sensation, clumsiness, or weakness. There may be a partial or total loss of vision in one eye for a period of several days, sometimes with pain in moving the eye, or the patient may experience double vision or dizziness. In some cases, the patient may develop ei-

ther a lack of sensation over an area of the face or, paradoxically, a severe twitching pain of the face muscles. In more advanced cases, because of involvement of the spinal cord, the patient may have symptoms of bladder or bowel dysfunction and male patients may experience impotence.

When brain tissues become invaded by multiple sclerosis, the patient may suffer loss of memory and show signs of personality changes, displaying euphoria, cheerfulness, irritability, or depression for no apparent reason.

Multiple sclerosis is marked by periods of remission and recurrence of symptoms. Complete recovery can occur. About 20 percent of the patients may have to spend time confined to bed or wheelchair. In severe cases, there can be complications such as infections of the urinary tract and respiratory system.

Treatment

There is no known cure for multiple sclerosis, and treatment techniques generally are aimed at relieving symptoms, shortening the periods of exacerbation, and preventing complications that can be crippling or life-threatening. Most patients experience recurrences of symptoms that last for limited periods of days or weeks followed in cycles by periods of remission that may last for months or years, making it difficult to determine whether the therapy applied is actually effective or if the disease is merely following its natural fluctuating course. Because multiple sclerosis appears to be a disease that affects only humans, medical scientists are unable to use animals in experiments to develop effective remedies.

Among several types of medications now used are anti-inflammatory drugs such as adrenocorticotrophin (ACTH), a hormone that seems to reduce the severity and duration of recurrences. Cortisone and prednisone, two steroid hormones, also can be used and have an advantage over ACTH in that they can be taken by mouth rather than by intramuscu-

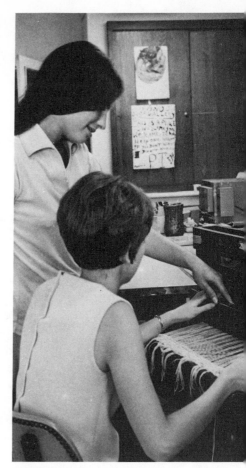

Physical therapy, such as weaving on a hand loom, can be of value in the treatment of multiple sclerosis and similar disorders.

lar injection. But not all patients react favorably to steroid drugs and serious side effects may be experienced. Several immunosuppressive drugs ordinarily used in the treatment of cancer and after organ transplants have been employed but they can be administered only in small doses for limited periods of time without undesirable side effects. Other therapies tested with varying effectiveness include vitamins and special diets.

Physical therapy and antispasmodic medications may be employed for patients suffering weakness or paralysis of the limbs. Bed rest during periods of exacerbation is important; continued activity seems to worsen the severity and duration of symptoms during those periods. Muscle relaxants and tranquilizers may be prescribed in some serious cases and braces could be required for patients who lose some limb functions.

Because of the lower incidence of multiple sclerosis in warmer climates, patients may be led to believe that moving to a "sunshine" state can have curative effects. But experience indicates that once the disease becomes established a change of climate does not change the course of the disorder. However, living in a warmer winter climate can lessen the impact of the physical handicaps faced by a multiple sclerosis patient.

Causes

The cause of multiple sclerosis has not been established. Multiple cases of the disease have been reported in only a small percentage of families but they occur often enough to suggest that the risk in brothers and sisters of patients is several times greater than the risk among the population at large. It is possible that patients with multiple sclerosis have inherited a specific susceptibility to the disease, a factor that could explain the vulnerability of members of the same family to acquire the disorder through one of several environmental causes, such as a virus or other infectious organism. Speculation about causes has covered dietary deficiencies, ingestion or inhalation of toxic substances, and occupation.

One widely entertained theory is that the disease is caused by a virus contracted at an early age. The virus presumably multiplies slowly, gradually attacking the myelin sheath that protects nerve fibers.

Infections of the Nervous System

Like any other organ system, the brain and its associated structures may be host to infection. These infections are usually serious because of the significantly high death rate and incidence of residual defects. If the brain is involved in the inflammation, it is known as *encephalitis;* inflammation of the brain coverings, or *meninges,* is called *meningitis.*

Encephalitis

Encephalitis is usually caused by a virus, and, since the symptoms are not specific, the diagnosis is usually made by special viral immunologic tests. Both sexes and all age groups can be afflicted. Most patients complain of fever, headache, nausea or vomiting, and a general feeling of malaise. The mental state varies from one of mild irritability to lethargy or coma, and some patients may have convulsions. The physician may suspect encephalitis after completing the history and the physical examination, but the diagnosis is usually established by laboratory tests that include examination of the cerebrospinal fluid (CSF), the EEG, and viral studies of the blood, CSF, and stool. Since there is no specific treatment for viral encephalitis at the present time, particular attention is paid to general supportive care.

Meningitis

Meningitis can occur in either sex at any time of life. The patient often has a preceding mild respiratory infection and later complains of headache, nausea, and vomiting. Fever and neck stiffness are usually pres-

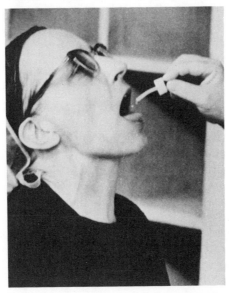

Public health officials were worried by an outbreak of polio in an Amish community in Pennsylvania in 1979. So they initiated a massive vaccination program to keep the disease from spreading.

ent early in the course of the disease, at which time the patient is commonly brought to the physician for examination. If there is any question of meningitis, a lumbar puncture is performed and the CSF examined. It is not possible to make a specific diagnosis of meningitis without examination of the cerebrospinal fluid.

Meningitis is usually caused by bacteria or a virus. It is important to learn what the infectious agent is in order to begin appropriate therapy. Bacterial infections can be treated by antibiotics, but there is no known specific treatment for viral (*aseptic*) meningitis. Meningitis is a life-threatening disease and, despite modern antibiotic therapy, the mortality rate varies from 10 to 20 percent.

Poliomyelitis

Poliomyelitis is an acute viral illness affecting males and females at any time of life, though most commonly before the age of ten. It is also called *polio, infantile paralysis,* or *Heine-Medin disease.*

Polio is caused by a virus that probably moves from the gastrointestinal tract via nerve trunks to the central nervous system, where it may affect any part of the nervous system. However, the disease most often involves the larger motor neurons (*anterior horn cells*) in the brain stem and spinal cord, with subsequent loss of nerve supply to the muscle. The neuron may be partially or completely damaged; clinical recovery is, therefore, dependent on whether those partially damaged nerves can regain normal function.

There are two categories of polio victims: asymptomatic and symptomatic. Those persons who have had no observed symptoms of the disease, but in whom antibodies to polio can be demonstrated, belong in the *asymptomatic* group. The *symptomatic* group, on the other hand, comprises patients who have the clinical disease, either with residual paralysis (paralytic polio) or without paralysis (nonparalytic polio).

SYMPTOMS: The symptoms of poliomyelitis are similar to those of other acute infectious processes. The patient may complain of headache, fever, or *coryza* (head cold or runny nose), or he may have loose stools and malaise. One-fourth to one-third of patients improve for several days only to have a recurrence of fever with neck stiffness. Most patients, however, do not improve, but rather have a progression of their symptoms, marked by neck stiffness and aching muscles. They are often irritable and apprehensive, and some are rather lethargic.

Whether or not the patient will have muscle paralysis should be evident in the first few weeks. Some have muscle paralysis with the onset of symptoms; others become aware of loss of muscle function several weeks after the onset. About half of the patients first notice paralysis during the second to the fifth day of the disease. Patients experience a muscle spasm or stiffness, and may complain of muscle pain, particularly if the muscle is stretched.

The extent of the muscle paralysis is variable, ranging from mild localized weakness to inability to move most of the skeletal muscles. Proximal muscles (those close to the trunk, like the shoulder-arm, or hipthigh) are involved more often than distal muscles (of the extremities), and the legs are affected more often than the arms. When the neurons of the lower brain stem and the spinal cord at the thoracic level and above are affected, the patient may have a paralysis of the muscles used in swallowing and breathing. This circumstance, obviously, is lifethreatening, and particular attention must be paid to the patient's ability to handle saliva and to breathe. If independent, spontaneous respiration is not possible, patients must be given respiratory assistance with mechanical respirators.

TREATMENT: There is no specific treatment for acute poliomyelitis. The patient should be kept at complete bed rest and given general supportive care, assuring adequate nutrition and fluid intake. Muscle spasm has been treated with hot as well as cold compresses, and no one method has been universally beneficial. Careful positioning of the patient with the musculature supported in a position midway between relaxation and contraction is probably of benefit, and skilled physical therapy is of great importance.

IMMUNIZATION: Since the early 1900s, attempts had been made to produce an effective vaccine against poliomyelitis, with success crowning the efforts of Dr. Jonas Salk in 1953. Today, vaccination is accomplished with either the Salk vaccine (killed virus), which is given intramuscularly, or the Sabin (live attenuated virus), given orally. There is little question that immunization with poliomyelitis vaccine has proven to be highly effective in eradicating the clinical disease within the community, and it is now a part of routine immunization for all children.

Dementia

Dementia is a term for mental deterioration, with particular regard to memory and thought processes. Such deterioration can be brought about in various ways: infection, brain injury, such toxic states as alcoholism, brain tumors, cerebral arteriosclerosis, and so forth.

The presenile dementias (*Alzheimer's disease*) represent a group of degenerative diseases of the brain in which mental deterioration first becomes apparent in middle age. Commonly, the first clue may be demonstrations of unusual unreasonableness and impairment of judgment. The patient can no longer grasp the content of a situation at hand and reacts inappropriately. Memory gradually fades and recent events are no longer remembered, but events that occurred early in life can be recalled. The patient may wander aimlessly or get lost in his own house. There is progressive deterioration of physical appearance and personal hygiene,

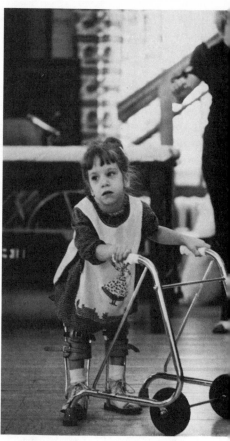

A child with legs weakened by polio uses a walker as an aid in her gait training in a hospital physical therapy program.

and, finally, the command of language deteriorates. Unfortunately, there is a relentless progression of the process, and the patient becomes confined to bed and quite helpless.

Whether the mental deterioration seen in some aged patients, senile dementia, is a specific brain degeneration or is secondary to cerebral arteriosclerosis is not yet settled. It does appear, however, that senile dementia is probably secondary to a degenerative process similar to that of Alzheimer's disease but occurring late in life.

Whether or not dementia can be halted depends upon its cause. If, for example, the dementia is secondary to brain infection or exposure to toxic material, eradication of the infectious agent or removal of the toxin may be of distinct benefit in arresting the dementing process. Unfortunately, there is no specific treatment for the brain degenerative processes.

MUSCLE DISEASES

When one hears the words "muscle disease", one may think only of muscular dystrophy and picture a small child confined to a wheelchair. But there are many diseases other than muscular dystrophy in which muscle is either primarily or secondarily involved, and many of these diseases do not have a particularly bad prognosis. Muscle diseases may make their presence known at any time, from early infancy to old age; no age group or sex is exempt.

Any disease of muscle is called a *myopathy*. The hallmark of muscle disease is weakness, or loss of muscle power. This may be recognized in the infant who seems unusually limp or *hypotonic*. Often the first clue to the presence of muscle weakness is a child's failure to achieve the developmental milestones within a normal range of time. He may be unusually clumsy or have difficulty in running, climbing stairs, or even walking. Occasionally a teacher is the first one to be aware that the child cannot keep up with classmates and reports this fact to the parents. The onset of the muscle weakness can be so insidious that it may go unnoticed or be misinterpreted as laziness until there is an obvious and striking loss of muscle power.

This is true in the adult as well who at first may feel tired or worn out and then realize that he cannot keep up his previous pace. Often his feet and legs are involved in the beginning. He may wear out the toes of his shoes and may then recognize that he must flex his ankles more to avoid tripping or dragging the toes. Or he finds that he must make a conscious effort to raise the legs in climbing stairs; he may even have to climb one step at a time. Getting out of bed in the morning may be a chore, and rising from a seated position in a low chair or from the floor may be difficult or impossible. Those with arm involvement may recognize that the hands are weak; if the shoulder muscles are involved, there is often difficulty in raising the arms over the head. The patient may take a long time in recognizing the loss of muscle power because the human body can so well compensate or use other muscles to perform the same motor tasks. If the weakness is present for a considerable length of time, there may be a wasting, or a loss of muscle bulk.

Diagnostic Evaluation of Muscle Disease

In evaluating patients with motor weakness, the physician must have a complete history of the present complaints, past history of the patient, and details of the family history. A general physical and neurological examination is required, with particular reference to the motor, or musculoskeletal, system. In most cases, the physician will be able to make a clinical diagnosis of the disease process, but occasionally the examination does not reveal whether the nerve, the muscle, or both are involved. In order to clarify the diagnosis, some additional examinations may be required, mainly determination of serum enzymes (a good indicator of loss of muscle substance), a muscle biopsy, and an electromyogram.

SERUM ENZYMES: Enzymes are essential for the maintenance of normal body chemistry. Since the normal concentration in the blood serum of some enzymes specifically related to muscle chemistry is known, the determination of concentrations of these enzymes can provide additional evidence that muscle chemistry is either normal or abnormal.

MUSCLE BIOPSY: The first step is the surgical removal of a small segment of muscle, which is then prepared for examination under the microscope. The examination enables the physician to see any abnormality in the muscle fibers, supporting tissue, small nerve twigs, and blood vessels. The muscle biopsy can be of great value in making a cor-

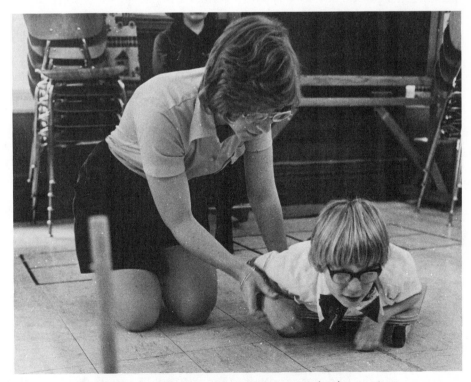

Rehabilitative physical therapy to encourage motor development is an essential part of the treatment of muscle diseases in all age groups.

rect diagnosis, but occasionally, even in good hands, there is not sufficient visible change from the normal state to identify the disease process.

ELECTROMYOGRAPH (EMG): This is a technique for studying electrical activity of muscle. Fine needles attached to electronic equipment are inserted into the muscle to measure the electrical activity, which is displayed on an *oscilloscope*, a device something like a television screen. It is not a particularly painful process when performed by a skilled physician, and the information gained may be important in establishing a diagnosis.

Muscular Dystrophy

Muscular dystrophy (MD) is defined as an inborn degenerative disease of the muscles. Several varieties of MD have been described and classified according to the muscles involved and the pattern of inheritance. There is no specific treatment for any form of MD, but the patient's life can be made more pleasant and probably prolonged if careful attention is paid to good nutrition, activity without overfatigue, and avoidance of infection. Physical therapists can be helpful in instructing the patient or the parents in an exercise program that relieves joint and muscle stiffness. Sound, prudent, psychological support and guidance cannot be overemphasized.

Duchenne's Muscular Dystrophy

In 1886, Dr. Guillaume Duchenne described a muscle disease characterized by weakness and an increase in the size of the muscles and the supporting connective tissue of those muscles. He named the disease *pseudohypertrophic* (false enlargement) *muscular paralysis,* but it is now known as *Duchenne's muscular dystrophy.*

Duchenne's MD is observed almost entirely in males. However, it is inherited, like many other sex-linked anomalies, through the

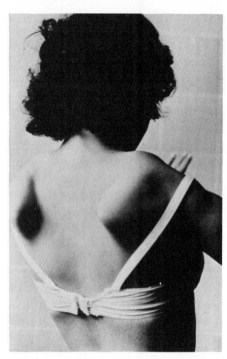

A patient with facio-scapulo-humoral muscular dystrophy. Muscles of the face and shoulders have become wasted. Note the protruding scapulae (shoulder blades).

maternal side of the family. The mother can pass the clinical disease to her son; her daughters will not demonstrate the disease but are potential carriers to their sons. More than one-quarter of the cases of Duchenne's MD are sporadic, that is, without any known family history of the disease. There are rare cases of Duchenne's MD in females who have *ovarian dysgenesis*, a condition in which normal female chromosomal makeup is lacking.

The disease process in Duchenne's MD may be apparent during the first few years of life when the child has difficulty in walking or appears clumsy. The muscles of the pelvis and legs are usually affected first, but the shoulders and the arms soon become involved. About 90 percent of the patients have some enlargement of a muscle or group of muscles and appear to be rather muscular and strong; however, as the disease progresses, the muscular enlargement disappears. Most patients progressively deteriorate and at the age of about 10 to 15 are unable to walk. Once the child is confined to a

wheelchair or bed, there is a progressive deformity with muscle contracture, with death usually occurring toward the end of the second decade. A small percentage of patients appear to have a remission of the disease process and survive until the fourth or fifth decade. Despite herculean attempts to unravel the riddle of muscular dystrophy, the problem is yet unsolved.

A benign variety of MD, *Becker type,* begins at 5 to 25 years of age and progresses slowly. Most of the reported patients with Becker type are still able to walk 20 to 30 years after the onset of the disease.

Facio-scapulo-humoral Muscular Dystrophy

This type of muscular dystrophy affects males and females equally and is thought to be inherited as a dominant trait. The onset may be at any age from childhood to adult life, but is commonly first seen in adolescence. There is no false enlargement of the muscles. The muscles affected, as indicated by the name of the disease, are those of the face and shoulders, usually with abnormal winging of the *scapula* (either of the large, flat bones at the backs of the shoulders). There is also a characteristic appearance of lip prominence, as if the patient were pouting. Occasionally there is an involvement of the anterior leg muscles, and weakness in raising the foot. The disease progresses more slowly than Duchenne's type, and some patients can remain active for a normal life span.

Limb-girdle Muscular Dystrophy

This type of muscular dystrophy is less clearly delineated than the others. Males and females are equally affected and the onset is usually in the second or third decade, but the process may start later. It is probably inherited as a recessive trait, but many cases are sporadic. It may first affect the muscles of the pelvis or the shoulder, but in 10 to 15 years both pelvis and shoulder girdles are usually involved. The disease varies considerably from patient to patient; sometimes the disease process appears to be arrested after involvement of either the pelvis or the shoulder, and the course thereafter may be a benign one. Most, however, have significant difficulty in walking by middle age.

Other Varieties of Muscular Dystrophy

These include ocular, oculopharyngeal, and a distal form (involving the muscles of the hands or feet).

OCULAR MD: This type involves the muscles that move the eye as well as the eyelids; occasionally, the small muscles of the face and the shoulder girdle are affected.

OCULOPHARYNGEAL MD: This type involves not only the muscles that move the eye and the eyelids but may also affect the throat muscles, so that patients have difficulty in swallowing food (dysphagia).

DISTAL MD: This type is rare in the United States but has been reported in Scandinavia. Both sexes can be affected. Usually after the fifth decade, the patient recognizes weakness of the small muscles of the hands and the anterior leg muscles that assist in raising the toes. The disease is relatively benign and progresses slowly.

The Myotonias

This is a group of muscle diseases characterized by *myotonia*, a continuation of muscle contraction after the patient has voluntarily tried to relax that contraction. It is best observed in the patient who holds an object firmly in his hand and then tries to release his grasp suddenly, only to realize that he cannot let go quickly. There are two major members of this group of diseases and several other less common variants.

TREATMENT: As in the case of muscular dystrophy, there is no specific treatment for myotonia. Some drugs, such as quinine, have limited value in decreasing the abnormally prolonged muscular contractions, but as yet no treatment has been completely effective.

Myotonia Congenita

This condition is usually present at birth, but is recognized later in the first or second decade of life when the child complains of stiffness or when clumsiness is noted. A child with this condition appears very muscular and has been called the "infant Hercules." The unusual muscular development persists throughout life, but the myotonia tends to improve with age.

Myotonic Dystrophy

The other major variety of myotonia, *myotonic dystrophy*, is a disease in which many organ systems in addition to muscle are involved. Both males and females are affected equally, and the onset may occur at any time from birth to the fifth decade. It is not unusual for a patient to recognize some clumsiness, but he may not be aware that he has a muscle disease. The myotonia may range from mild to severe. There is a striking similarity in the physical appearance of patients with myotonic dystrophy, the features of which include frontal baldness in the male, wasting and weakness of the temporal muscles (that control closing the jaws), muscles of the forearm, hands, and anterior leg muscles. Other physical abnormalities include cataracts in about 90 percent of the patients, small testicles, and abnormality of the heart muscle. Thickening and other bony abnormalities have been seen in the skull radiogram and, with time, many patients become demented.

Polymyositis

Polymyositis is a disorder of muscular and connective tissues affecting both sexes, males more commonly than females. It can occur at any age, although usually after the fourth decade. It is characterized by muscle weakness with associated muscle wasting; about half of the patients complain of muscle pain or tenderness. The disease may begin suddenly, but often follows an earlier mild, febrile illness. Changes in the skin are common, including a faint red-violet discoloration, particularly about the eyelids, and these changes are often associated with mild swelling. There may be a scaly rash. Some patients have ulcerations over the bony prominences. About one-quarter of the patients with polymyositis complain of joint stiffness and tenderness and an unusual phenomenon in which the nail beds become blue (*cyanotic*) after minor exposure to cold.

TREATMENT: The treatment involves the administration of cortisone preparations, which may be required for many years. General supportive care, including appropriate physical therapy, is recommended.

Myasthenia Gravis

Myasthenia gravis is characterized by muscle weakness and an abnormal muscle fatigability (pathologic fatigue); patients are abnormally weak after exercise or at the end of the day. The disease affects males and females at any period, from infancy to old age, but it is most common during the second to the fourth decades. There is no complete explanation for myasthenia gravis, but it is believed that there is some defect in the transmission of a nerve impulse to the muscle (*myoneural junction defect*). The disease may occur spontaneously, during pregnancy, or following an acute infection, and there appears to be a curious association with diseases in which there is an immunologic abnormality, such as tumors of the thymus gland, increased or decreased activity of the thyroid gland and rheumatoid arthritis.

Usually there is an insidious onset of generalized weakness or weakness confined to small groups of muscles. Normal muscle power may be present early in the day, but as the hours pass the patient notices that one or both eyelids droop *(ptosis)* or he may see double images *(diplopia)*. If he rests and closes his eyes for a short time, the ptosis and the diplopia clear up, only to return after further muscle activity. The weakness can also be seen in the trunk or the limbs, and some patients have involvement of the muscles used in speaking, chewing, or swallowing (*bulbar* muscles). Some are weak all the time and have an increase in that weakness the longer they use their muscles. The muscles used in breathing may be affected in patients with severe myasthenia, and these patients must be maintained on a respirator for varying periods of time.

TREATMENT: Myasthenia gravis is treated with drugs that assist in the transmission of the nerve impulse to the muscle. Medication is very effective, but the patient should be carefully observed by the physician to determine that the drug dose and the time of administration are adjusted so that the patient may have the benefit of maximal muscle power. Sur-

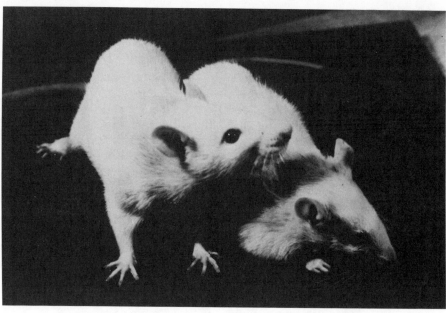

On the left, a healthy rat; on the right, one showing the characteristic weakness of myasthenia after being immunized with receptor protein.

gical removal of the thymus gland, *thymectomy*, may prove of benefit to some patients in lessening the symptoms of muscle weakness; however, not all patients have clinical improvement of the disease after thymectomy, and patients must be selected very carefully by the physician. Myasthenia gravis is another chronic disease in which long-term careful observation by the physician is most important in obtaining an optimal medical and psychological outcome.

CHAPTER 27

Women's Health

The special health matters that are related to a woman's reproductive system belong to the branch of medicine known as *gynecology*. *Obstetrics* is a closely related specialty associated with pregnancy and childbirth. The distinction is something of a technicality for most patients, since obstetricians usually are quite capable of handling gynecological cases and vice versa. The practice of obstetrics and gynecology is commonly combined in a medical service identified by the contraction *Ob-Gyn*. However, there are medical matters that are specifically concerned with female reproductive organs and related tissues but have little to do with obstetrics. For a discussion of obstetrics, see *Infertility, Pregnancy, and Childbirth*, p. 127.

The Gynecological Examination

What should a woman expect on her first visit to a gynecologist? First, the gynecologist will interview her, asking about her family, her medical history, and any fears or apprehensions she may have about her personal health. The woman's answers and comments are written into her medical records for future refer-

ence. The information can contain important clues that may help in diagnosing any present or future disorders.

A sample of urine and a sample of blood are usually obtained for laboratory tests. During the ensuing physical examination, the woman lies on a special examination table with her feet in metal stirrups and her knees apart. A nurse will be present to assist the doctor. While lying in the *lithotomy position*, the woman's abdomen will be palpated for lumps or other abnormalities. The

breasts also will be palpated for possible lumps. Then an external inspection of the vulva and surrounding areas is made by the doctor, followed by internal inspection, in which a speculum is used to spread apart the sides of the vagina so that the cervix is exposed. A digital examination (using the fingers) is made of the walls of the vagina and rectum and the neighboring tissue areas, in a search for possible growths or other abnormal conditions. And a sample of cells and secretions from the cervix is taken for a

DES, a synthetic hormone, was given to thousands of pregnant women in the 1950s, apparently causing many of their daughters to get cancer.

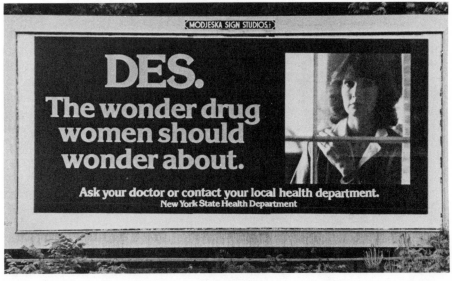

Pap smear test (described in detail on p. 501).

In addition to the examination of the breasts and reproductive system, the gynecologist usually conducts a general physical examination, recording information about height, weight, blood pressure, heart and lung condition, and so on. The routine physical examination, like the medical history, provides additional clues which, when added to the results of the examination of the breasts and reproductive system, will give a complete picture of the patient's gynecological health.

Following the examination, the gynecologist discusses his appraisal of the woman's condition and answers questions. He will discuss whatever treatment she needs. Medications can be explained at this time, including reasons why certain drugs can or should not be taken. If any surgery or further testing is recommended, those aspects of the health picture also should be discussed in some detail. Any important information that might be misunderstood or forgotten should be jotted down for future reference.

Results of some laboratory tests and the Pap smear are not usually available for several days. But the doctor or nurse will contact the patient when the results are available and advise if she should return in the near future for follow-up testing. The woman also should discuss arrangements for future checkups or Pap smear tests rather than wait until signs or symptoms of a serious disorder warrant an immediate visit. In the event of some possible future physical complaint, the fact that the woman has established some basic medical records with her gynecologist will be of help in making a proper diagnosis and establishing the best course of treatment.

MENSTRUAL DISORDERS

Among the health concerns of women that specifically belong to gynecology are menstrual disorders. Normally, the first menstrual period (menarche) occurs about age 12 or 13, or sometimes earlier or later. Periods are generally irregular for the first year or two, and then they tend to recur at intervals of 24 to 32 days. Each period begins about two weeks after ovulation, or the release of an egg cell (ovum) from the ovary —unless, of course, the ovum happens to be fertilized in the interval and pregnancy interrupts the whole process.

The menstrual flow, which lasts from three to seven days, is composed mainly of serum, mucus, and dead cells shed from the lining (endometrium) of the uterus. The loss of blood is minimal, usually from two to four ounces. The volume of flow, as well as the time schedule, tends to be fairly regular for most women. When one's menstrual pattern varies noticeably from the expected pattern, and in the absence of pregnancy, it may be a sign of a physical or emotional disorder.

Amenorrhea

Failure to menstruate is called *amenorrhea*. Amenorrhea is a natural effect of pregnancy and of nursing a baby. In an older woman, it may be a sign of menopause. But if a nonpregnant or nonnursing woman after menarche and before menopause (say between the ages of 17 or 18 and 52) fails to menstruate for two or more periods, she should bring it to the attention of a doctor —unless, of course, she has undergone a hysterectomy or other surgical or medical treatment that eliminates menstruation.

Primary Amenorrhea

When menarche has not occurred by the age of 16 or 17, the absence of menstruation is called *primary amenorrhea*. In such a case, a physical examination may show that an imperforate hymen or a closed cervix is obstructing the flow of menses, or a congenital defect may be interfering with menstruation. In almost all cases, menarche can be started with a bit of minor surgery, by treatment of any existing systemic disease, or by the injection of sex hormones; or it will start spontaneously later.

Secondary Amenorrhea

When menstrual periods cease after menarche, the condition is known as *secondary*, or *acquired*, *amenorrhea*. Secondary amenorrhea may involve missing a single menstrual period or many periods in consecutive months. Among possible causes of interrupted menstruation are certain medications, drugs of abuse, emotional stress, normal fluctuations in ovarian activity in the first few years after menarche, and a number of organic diseases. Medicines that can disrupt normal menstrual activity include tranquilizers and other psychotropic (mind-affecting) drugs that apparently influence hormonal activity in the brain centers, amphetamines, and oral contraceptives. When a particular medication is found to be the cause of amenorrhea, the medical treatment may be judged to be more important than maintaining normal menstrual cycles. When the use of oral contraceptives is followed by amenorrhea for six or more months, normal menstrual activity may resume eventually, but it can often be started sooner by a prescribed medication. Among drugs of abuse known to cause amenorrhea are alcohol and opium-based drugs.

Just as the mind-altering effects

of psychotropic drugs involve the hypothalamus and pituitary glands in the brain, which control the hormones that regulate menstrual functions, emotional stress seems to have a parallel influence on the incidence of amenorrhea. *Anorexia nervosa,* a disorder associated with emaciation due to an emotional disturbance, also can result in an interruption of menstruation.

Other factors contributing to secondary amenorrhea are measles, mumps, and other infections; cysts and tumors of the ovaries; changes in the tissues lining the vagina or uterus; premature aging of the ovaries; diabetes; obesity; anemia; leukemia; and Hodgkin's disease. In many cases, normal or near-normal menstrual function can be restored by medical treatment, such as administration of hormones, or by surgery, or both. In one type of amenorrhea, marked by adhesion of the walls of the uterus, curettage (scraping of the uterus) is followed by insertion of an intrauterine contraceptive device (IUD) to help hold the uterine walls apart.

Menorrhagia

Almost the opposite of amenorrhea is *menorrhagia,* an excessive menstrual flow. The causes of menorrhagia are as varied as those associated with amenorrhea. They include influenza and other infectious diseases, emotional stress, polyps of the cervical or uterine tissues (see p. 498), hypertension, congestive heart failure, leukemia, and blood coagulation disorders. Menorrhagia may occur during the early stages of a young woman's reproductive life soon after reaching puberty, and medical treatment may be necessary to control the excessive loss of blood. In some cases, dilation and curettage is recommended in addition to the administration of hormones and other medications, such as iron tablets to correct anemia resulting from the loss of red blood cells.

DILATION AND CURETTAGE: *Dilation and curettage,* generally referred to as *D and C,* is a procedure in which

the cervix is dilated and the cavity of the uterus is cleaned out by a scoop-like instrument, a curette. The same procedure is sometimes used to abort an embryo or to remove a tumor or a polyp.

Although it takes only a few minutes to perform a D and C, the procedure is done in a hospital while the patient is anesthetized. There is no afterpain, only a dull discomfort in the lower pelvic region similar to menstrual awareness.

A physical examination is usually made to determine if there are tumors anywhere in the reproductive organs. Except where tumors are found to be a causative factor, most women will resume normal menstrual cycles after treatment of menorrhagia with medications and D and C. For women beyond the age of 40, the doctor may recommend a hysterectomy to prevent recurrence of excessive menstrual blood loss.

Polymenorrhea and Metrorrhagia

These medical terms refer to two other ways in which menstrual periods may depart from typical patterns. *Polymenorrhea* is abnormally frequent menstruation, so that men-

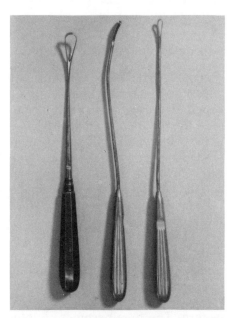

Two types of curettes are shown above. The middle and right instruments are the same, seen from different angles.

strual periods occur at intervals of less than 21 days. This short interval may be the natural established pattern for some women. If it is not, the cause may be physical or emotional stress. *Metrorrhagia* is marked by menstrual bleeding that occurs erratically at unpredictable times. It may be the result of a cyst in the lining of the uterus, a tumor in the reproductive tract, polyps, or some hormonal imbalance, including a disorder of the thyroid gland.

Dysmenorrhea

Abdominal or pelvic pain occurring just before or along with the onset of menstruation is known as *dysmenorrhea.* The symptoms include severe colicky abdominal cramps, backache, headache, and, in some cases, nausea and vomiting. As with amenorrhea, there are two general types of dysmenorrhea, primary and secondary.

Primary Dysmenorrhea

This type includes all cases in which no organic disorder is associated with the symptoms, which are presumed to be due to uterine contractions and emotional factors. More than 75 percent of all cases are of this type. Primary dysmenorrhea generally begins before age 25, but it may appear at any time from menarche to menopause. It frequently ends with the birth of the first child.

Since primary dysmenorrhea by definition occurs in the absence of organic disease, the diagnosis can be made only after a careful medical history is compiled and a special study of the reproductive organs is made to insure that no disorder has been overlooked. In some cases, oral contraceptives may be prescribed because of the effect such drugs have in suppressing ovulation; the contraceptives prevent the natural production of the hormone progesterone, which is responsible for certain tissue changes associated with the discomfort of dysmenorrhea. Analgesic drugs to relieve pain and medications that help to relax muscles may be prescribed. However, medication is often less beneficial than emotional support—including the easing of any stress at home, school, or work, and reassurance about the worries sometimes associated with menstruation.

Secondary Dysmenorrhea

This condition comprises all menstrual pain that is due to or associated with an organic disease of the reproductive organs, such as endometriosis (see p. 499) to cite just one example. Secondary dysmenorrhea can occur at any age.

Edema and Premenstrual Tension

Primary dysmenorrhea is often associated with fluid accumulation in the tissues (edema) and sensations of bloating and pelvic heaviness that increase with physical activity. But those symptoms subside after the menstrual flow begins. Although physical activity may aggravate some cases of dysmenorrhea, exercise can be helpful for other patients. Simple exercises that include twisting and bending the trunk often produce beneficial results if performed two or three times a day. During menstrual periods, most women are able to work, play, bathe, swim, and carry on as usual with all their physical activities.

Premenstrual fluid retention and premenstrual tension very often coexist. Premenstrual tension produces greater discomfort in some women than menstruation itself. About half of all women experience the effects at some time during their reproductive years, particularly after the age of thirty. Typical symptoms are anxiety, agitation, insomnia, and depression. A women may appear irritable, sometimes moody or sullen, or aggressive for about a week or ten days before the start of a menstrual period. Some women experience headaches, a bloated feeling, nausea and vomiting, and diarrhea or constipation. Seemingly unrelated conditions, ranging from mental illness to obesity, tend to be aggravated at this time. Many women develop unusual appetites, and weight gain can be as much as eight pounds, due mostly, however, to fluid retention in the tissues. This fluid is quickly lost through urination once the menstrual flow has begun.

Treatment of premenstrual tension is similar to that recommended for dysmenorrhea. In order to alleviate edema, the doctor may recommend a low-salt diet and a diuretic, particularly for the days between ovulation and the beginning of a menstrual period. The woman may also be encouraged to divide her daily food intake into numerous small meals rather than three square meals a day. A greater proportion of the calorie allowance might be shifted to proteins instead of carbohydrates. Oral contraceptives that suppress ovulation may be prescribed. Although tranquilizers may be prescribed for a woman who displays agitation as an effect of premenstrual tension, women who show signs of depression and self-pity would benefit more from stimulants and encouragement toward a more active life style.

Minor Menstrual Problems

BLOOD CLOTS: There is not usually any cause for alarm if blood clots are expelled during menstruation. Ordinarily, the menstrual flow is completely liquefied, but a few clots tend to appear when the flow is profuse. However, if many clots appear and the flow seems excessive, medical advice is recommended, since these conditions may be a sign of fibroid tumors in the uterus. See p. 499.

ORAL CONTRACEPTIVES: Women on combination birth-control pills can expect to see a changed menstrual pattern. The flow becomes slighter than before and very regular. For a discussion of oral contraceptives, see *Birth Control*. p. 146.

ODOR: The menstrual flow of a healthy woman generally has a mild odor which develops when it is exposed to the air or to the vulva. Some women are concerned about this odor, although it usually is not offensive. When it is, it tends to be associated with inadequate bathing. Detergents are added to some commercial tampons and pad products, and special deodorants have been developed to mask the odor. However, such materials produce allergic reactions in some women, and they can have the unfortunate effect of masking an odor that may be the sign of an abnormal condition.

ONSET OF MENOPAUSE: Menstrual irregularities almost always precede the natural cessation of menstrual function. For a full discussion of menopause, see p. 159.

Postmenopausal Bleeding

Bleeding that occurs after the final cessation of menstrual activity should be seen as an urgent signal to seek medical advice. The bleeding may be painless or painful and may range from occasional spotting that is brownish or bright red to rather profuse bleeding that continues for several days or more. The various signs and symptoms should be noted carefully because they can help suggest to the doctor the possible cause of bleeding. Bleeding after the menopause is often a sign of cancer of the cervix or the lining of the uterus, but there is a wide variety of other possible causes, including polyps, ulcers, hypertensive heart disease, an ovarian tumor, or infection. In many cases, the problem can be treated by dilation and curettage or withdrawal of any hormone medications, such as estrogens prescribed for menopausal symptoms, or both. In these cases, if D and C and treatment and discontinuance of hormone therapy fail, the doctor may advise a hysterectomy.

INFECTIONS OF THE REPRODUCTIVE TRACT

Vaginal and other reproductive tract infections are among the most common gynecological problems, and among the most stubborn to treat successfully.

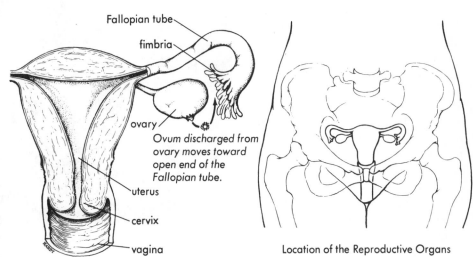

THE FEMALE REPRODUCTIVE SYSTEM

Fallopian tube

fimbria

ovary

Ovum discharged from ovary moves toward open end of the Fallopian tube.

uterus

cervix

vagina

Location of the Reproductive Organs

Leukorrhea

A whitish, somewhat viscid discharge from the vagina, which is known medically as *leukorrhea,* may be quite normal, especially if it is not continual but occurs only intermittently—prior to menstruation, for example, or associated with sexual excitation. It may also be increased when oral contraceptives are used.

Constant leukorrhea, on the other hand, often is a sign and symptom of an abnormality. Leukorrhea due to disease can occur at any age. It is generally associated with an infection of the lower reproductive tract. The discharge may occur without any discomfort, but in some cases there is itching, irritation, and dyspareunia—the medical term for painful intercourse (see p. 499).

Laboratory tests of vaginal secretions may be needed to help identify the precise cause of the discharge. Leukorrhea can result from vaginal ulcers; a tumor of the vagina, uterus, or Fallopian tubes; gonorrhea; or infection by any of various disease organisms of the vulva, vagina, cervix, uterus, or tubes. It may also be due to an abnormality of menstrual function, or even emotional stress.

Treatment, of course, depends on the cause. If the discharge is due to an infection, care must be taken to avoid being reinfected or transmitting the disease organism through sexual contact or possibly contaminated underclothing, etc. The condition may be particularly difficult to control if the woman is pregnant or suffers from some chronic disorder, such as diabetes.

Moniliasis

Moniliasis, also known as *candidiasis,* is an infection by a yeastlike fungus that is capable of invading mucous membrane and sometimes skin in various parts of the body. Inside the mouth, the organism causes thrush, most commonly in babies. When the organism invades the vaginal area it causes a scant white discharge of a thick consistency resembling that of cottage cheese. There is itching, burning, and swelling of the labial and vulvar areas. The symptoms tend to worsen just before the menstrual period. The occurrence of the disease is thought by some to be enhanced by oral contraceptives. Antibiotic therapy, too, generally favors the moniliasis organism, which is unaffected by the antibiotics that destroy many of the benign organisms that regularly share the same environment.

Moniliasis is treated with suppositories, creams, and other medications. The woman's partner should be treated at the same time to prevent a cycle of infection and reinfection of both partners, because the fungus will otherwise spread to the genital tissues of the man.

Trichomoniasis

A type of leukorrhea that consists of a copious yellow to green frothy and fetid discharge is caused by infection by the *trichomonas* organism. The organism causes an irritating itching condition that tends to set in or worsen just after a menstrual period. The condition is diagnosed by a test similar to a Pap smear, made with a specimen taken from the vagina. Trichomonas organisms, if present, are easy to identify under a microscope; they are pear-shaped protozoa with three to five whiplike tails.

The organism favors warm moist areas, such as genital tissues, but it can also survive in damp towels and wash cloths, around toilet seats, and on beaches and the perimeters of swimming pools. Thus it can spread from one member of a family to other members and from one woman to other women. *Trichomoniasis* is not technically a venereal disease, but it can be transmitted by sexual contact. When one partner is infected with trichomoniasis, both must be treated at the same time and a condom must be worn during intercourse.

Several drugs are available for

treating trichomoniasis, including tablets taken orally and suppositories inserted in the vagina. The tablets usually are taken three times daily for ten days, after which an examination is made to determine if any trichomonas organisms are still present. The oral medication may be continued for several months if the infection resists the drug—some studies show that the organism appears to survive in about ten percent of treated cases. There are douches available in drugstores for removing the discharge, but women are advised to consult their physicians before experimenting with home remedies or over-the-counter products that may be offered as douche treatments for trichomoniasis. The substances contained in some douches can aggravate the condition or irritate the vaginal tissues.

Herpes Simplex Virus Type 2

In recent years, doctors have become aware of a viral infection that is acquired by contact with the mucous membranes of an infected person. The mucous membrane of the mouth and lips, the genitals, or the rectum may be affected. The causative agent is known as *Herpes simplex virus*

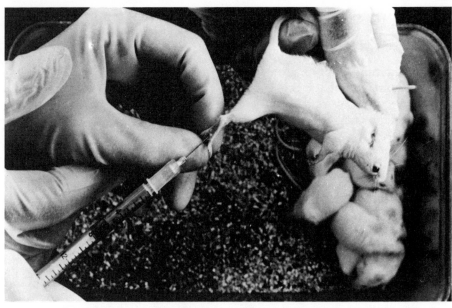

In a laboratory study, a researcher injects a mouse's foot with HSV-2 virus, which will remain in a latent state in the animal's nervous system.

Type 2, or *HSV-2*. It is similar to but not the same as the virus that causes fever blisters, or cold sores, which is Type 1 (HSV-1). Information about the incidence of Type 2 is not well documented. The virus is associated with some spontaneous abortions, stillbirths, and deaths of newborn babies. If the mother is infected at the time of delivery, the virus can be transmitted to the baby as it passes through the vagina. The central

nervous system, including the brain, may be damaged by the virus if the baby becomes infected. To avoid exposure to the virus, a Caesarian delivery is recommended when the mother is infected.

SYMPTOMS: Patients with their first HSV-2 infection usually complain of intense itching, painful blisterlike eruptions, and ulcerated patches with a discharge. Other symptoms may include genital pain and vaginal bleeding. Fever, swelling, difficult urination, and a general feeling of ill health and lack of appetite may accompany the infection. Diagnosis of HSV-2 is verified through biopsies and smears examined microscopically, cultures, and the presence of HSV-2 antibodies.

Symptoms may subside after a few weeks but recurrences are common, though they are less painful and of shorter duration. There is no known cure for the viral infection.

TREATMENT: Treatment was once limited to applications of anesthetic creams, steroid ointments, and other medications to relieve symptoms. No drug has been found to attack the viruses while they are "hibernating" in cells at the base of the spine. But one antiviral drug, *acyclovir*, has been found to reduce

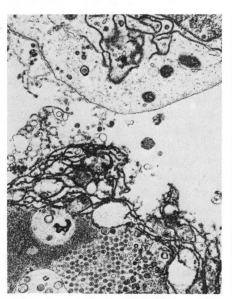
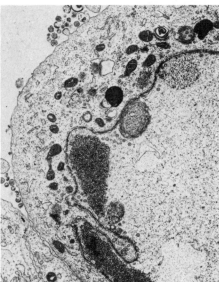

The Herpes simplex virus Type 2, greatly magnified under an electron microscope. This virus can cause serious damage to a newborn baby if the mother is infected with it at the time of delivery.

recurrent outbreaks and to block flareups for up to several months.

Taken orally in pill form, acyclovir in tests has brought relief, but not cures, to hundreds of subjects. The drug is ingested daily. Researchers have discovered that the capsules kill or neutralize the herpes viruses only when they are active. Because of evidence that the virus may be related to the subsequent development of cervical cancer, women sufferers should have Pap smear tests at intervals of six months instead of the usual twelve.

VENEREAL DISEASES

The name of Venus, the goddess of love, is preserved in the term *venereal disease* in recognition of the fact that the venereal diseases are commonly transmitted by sexual contact during intercourse. Although the term can be applied to any infection that is transmissible through sexual activity, such as moniliasis or trichomoniasis, *venereal disease* is usually confined to syphilis, gonorrhea, and three lesser infections that are of concern to public health authorities and are reportable by law in the United States—lymphogranuloma venereum, chancroid, and granuloma inguinale. Although doctors are required to report all infectious cases that come to their attention, there are no reliable figures on the number of people who are in urgent need of treatment but fail to seek it, either through indifference or ignorance. It is generally agreed that the number is very high. See also p. 431 for additional information about venereal diseases.

Syphilis

Potentially the most devastating of the venereal diseases, syphilis was once known as the great pox, so-called in comparison with the less-dreaded scourge, smallpox. Its gravity was greatly lessened by the discovery of penicillin, which provided the first quick and effective cure for the early stages of the disease. At the time of the introduction of antibiotics, more than 100,000 new cases of syphilis were reported each year. The incidence then dropped dramatically to about 6,000 cases a year, but the rate began rising during the

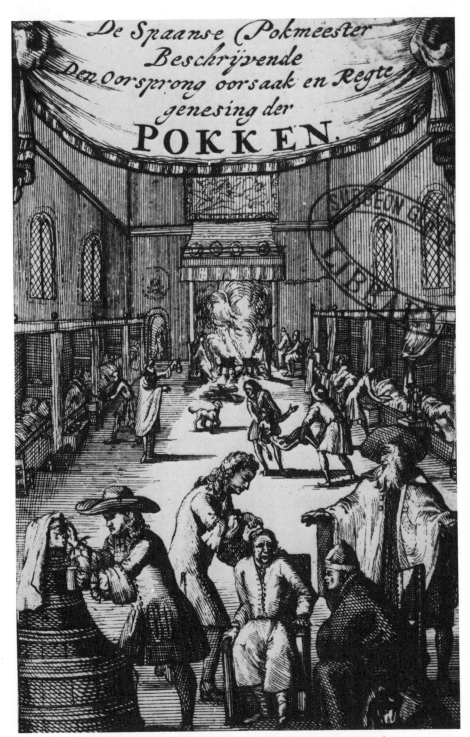

This 17th-century Dutch engraving depicts doctors treating syphilis in a venereal-disease ward. ("Pokken" means "pox" in Dutch.)

1960s and 1970s. A partial explanation for the increased incidence may be that the widespread use of oral contraceptives led to a reduced use of the condom during intercourse. There also is some evidence that oral contraceptives subtly alter vaginal secretions, thereby providing a climate that allows the organisms to thrive. Nearly 25,000 infectious syphilis cases were reported in the United States in the mid-1970s, leaving an untreated reservoir, according to the American Social Health Association, of probably more than 450,000 persons.

Primary Syphilis

Syphilis is caused by a spirally shaped bacterium belonging to a group of spiral organisms known as *spirochetes*. Sexual intercourse is the usual path of transmission, since the organism is too fragile to survive long exposure on contaminated objects. It is killed by heat, dryness, ordinary antiseptics, and soap, but it can tolerate cold and survive freezing. It is thought to be capable of penetrating intact mucous membrane, such as the inner surface of the mouth, or skin that may be intact but is more commonly marked by a lesion.

Once inside the body, the spirochetes can spread to almost any organ, producing inflammation and tissue destruction. Syphilis sometimes is called the great imitator of diseases because it produces signs and symptoms resembling a wide variety of organic disorders. Even the initial manifestation of syphilis can be misleading. The first sign is a painless chancre, or ulcer, which may be small, single or multiple, and look like almost any other ulcer. Syphilitic chancres in women occur mostly on the external genital areas, in the vagina, or on the cervix, but they may appear on the breasts, lips, or in the mouth. Ordinarily, chancres heal completely and leave no scar. This primary stage, the first sign of infection, may occur at any time from about ten days to three months after a

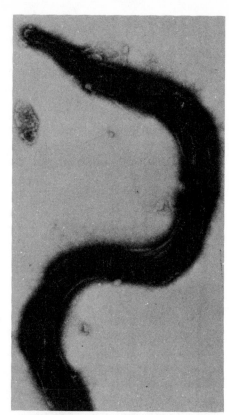

A *Treponema* spirochete, which causes syphilis, enlarged about 40,000 times. Note the spiral shape of the organism.

communicable contact with an infected person or object. The usual interval is about three weeks.

Secondary and Latent Stages

About six weeks after the appearance of the chancre, whether or not the patient was aware of it, secondary-stage lesions develop in most untreated cases. These secondary lesions take the form of a rash or almost any other kind of skin eruption. The skin lesions may appear on the trunk of the body, on the face, the arms and legs, or the palms of the hands and soles of the feet. The lesions may or may not cause itching. It is possible for a patient to develop a primary chancre without the later appearance of the secondary-stage skin symptoms.

A latent phase of many years' duration follows untreated secondary syphilis. The only clue to the presence of syphilis in the body during the latent period is the presence of the organism responsible as revealed by a blood test.

Tertiary Syphilis

If syphilis is not treated during the primary, secondary, or latent stages, it can progress to late syphilis, which usually involves chronic destructive effects in the central nervous system, the heart, bones, liver, stomach, or other tissues. The skin, mucous membranes, and other organs may develop rubbery tumors called *gummas*. A gumma lesion can occur in the throat and affect the larynx or the respiratory tract. The gummas frequently have the appearance of malignant tumors; biopsies are needed to determine whether the growths are caused by cancer or by syphilis.

One of the most dangerous effects of untreated syphilis is an invasion of the circulatory system, resulting in an aneurysm (dilated part) of the aorta just above the heart, with damage to the aortic valve that causes a decrease in blood flow to the coronary arteries. A ruptured aneurysm can produce a fatal hemorrhage. While gummas may respond to antibiotic treatment in the late stage of syphilis, damage to the heart valve and arteries may not be reversible.

GENERAL PARESIS: Similarly, permanent tissue damage to the brain and nerves can result from syphilitic invasion of the central nervous system—the chronic, progressive form of syphilis known as *general paresis*. The damage evolves in an insidious manner, and early symptoms may include headaches, a tendency to forget things, or difficulty in concentrating. Mental effects may progress from memory loss to psychotic symptoms of delusions of grandeur.

TABES DORSALIS: Syphilis involving deterioration of the sheaths of spinal nerves (demyelination) and other destructive changes in the spinal cord is known as *tabes dorsalis*. The patient may become incoordinated in movement. Tremors of the hands and fingers may be noticed, as well as tremors of the lips and tongue. Vision may be affected, and sensory effects can range from sharp sudden pains to a loss of feeling. The patient may lose control of bladder function or the ability to walk.

Congenital Syphilis

The latent syphilitic condition is not uncommon, and it is a period of great danger to the fetus if an infected woman, especially a recently infected woman, becomes pregnant at this time. The fetus can acquire syphilis through the placenta and be born with congenital syphilis. Or it can be stillborn or die shortly after birth. Some of the signs of syphilis in an infant born with the congenital form of the disease are similar to those of secondary syphilis. Others are very different, more closely resembling tertiary syphilis. Because of the hazards to the child, most doctors test the mother's blood for the presence of the spirochete during the first three months of pregnancy and again during the last three months; syphilis acquired during pregnancy is especially likely to affect the fetus. Treatment of the mother has the added benefit of treating the fetus. Treatment begun before the eighteenth week of pregnancy prevents syphilis from developing; treatment begun after the eighteenth week cures the fetus of syphilis.

Treatment of Syphilis and Public Health

Therapy for primary or secondary syphilis usually consists of injections of penicillin, or an alternative antibiotic if the patient is allergic to penicillin. The dosage of penicillin may vary according to the stage of the disease. A single injection might be administered for a patient in the primary or secondary stage, while the patient having latent syphilis might require daily doses of antibiotics for one to two weeks.

Patients are usually interviewed regarding their past contacts with other individuals, who may have become infected. If they can be lo-

cated, they may be advised to receive a penicillin injection or other antibiotic as a protective measure, regardless of whether or not blood tests reveal the presence of the syphilis spirochete. Further blood tests at regular intervals thereafter are also recommended for exposed as well as infected persons to assess their status.

VD CLINICS: Free venereal disease (VD) clinics are available to both men and women in many parts of the United States. Any person who has become infected with syphilis, who thinks he or she may have been exposed to syphilis, or who has signs or symptoms of syphilis can receive a checkup to determine if there is cause for concern. The clinics make blood tests on a small sample of blood taken from a pricked finger. This blood test sometimes is called a Wasserman test, an STS (for serological test for syphilis), or by other names, depending upon the screening technique used. A positive test reaction would be followed by a more detailed series of tests and examinations. A screening test for syphilis is required in most of the United States in order to obtain a marriage license.

Information about the nearest VD clinic can usually be obtained from a county medical society, a local health department, or a local hospital. Many towns have a "hot line" available for persons who want to obtain venereal-disease information by telephone. A toll-free number, 800-523-1885, has been established to permit persons anywhere in the United States to get information about nearby venereal disease clinics.

Gonorrhea

Of the estimated total of nearly three million cases of venereal disease treated each year in the United States, more than half involve *gonorrhea*. Gonorrhea is a primary infection of the lining of the urino-genital tract, rectum, and pharynx

caused by a spherical pus-producing bacterium called a gonococcus. The common vernacular name for the disease is *clap* or *GC*.

Like syphilis, gonorrhea is not invariably acquired through sexual contact. One example is the spread of the gonococcus germ to the eyes of a baby born to an infected mother. However, the usual route of transmission of gonorrhea is by sexual contact. The several strains of the gonococcus organism differ in virulence. Unlike its response to many other kinds of infectious diseases, the human body apparently does not produce antibodies after exposure to gonorrhea; therefore, a person does not acquire a natural protection from the disease organism after being infected.

Women often carry the disease without symptoms and transmit it to others. In fact, women without symptoms have been described as the major reservoir of gonorrhea. Women quite frequently learn of their infection only because of the development of symptoms in the male partner or because an infected man has reported the identities of women with whom he has had sexual contact.

Symptoms and Complications

In men, the symptoms may begin suddenly with a profuse puslike discharge from the penis, accompanied by a frequent urge to urinate, though urination is painful. The gonococcus germ may spread into the prostate gland, the seminal vesicles, and the epididymis, a portion of the seminal ducts just above the testis. In a woman a gonorrheal infection is much more insidious, often without any symptoms.

However, some women do have symptoms of gonorrhea. They may include irritation or inflammation of the urethra, a vaginal discharge, and possibly serious complications such as pelvic inflammatory disease, with lower abdominal pain, nausea and vomiting, chills, fever, and involvement of the Fallopian tubes. If untreated at an early stage, the gonorrheal infection can result in scarring and sealing of the Fallopian tubes. This complication, called *salpingitis*, can be caused by other infections as well. It was more commonly a result of gonorrhea before the development of effective antibiotic medications; it was also, and still is, a cause of female sterility.

Because of changing sexual attitudes in recent years, gonorrheal infections and complications that were once associated with young heterosexual adults now occur frequently in young teen-agers and male homosexuals. Prepubertal girls —girls who have not begun to menstruate—may acquire gonorrhea through sexual activity but, because of their immature reproductive systems, they seldom develop the complications of salpingitis or pelvic inflammatory disease that affect mature women who are not treated at an early stage.

GONORRHEAL ARTHRITIS: *Gonorrheal arthritis*, once a complication associated mainly with untreated male patients, is now reported to be more common in women than in men. It is also found more frequently now than in past years among male homosexuals. Gonorrheal arthritis may be marked at the onset by fever, pains in one or more joints of the body, and, in many cases, a rash about the hands and feet. The knee joint is most commonly involved, but the pain may be felt in the wrists, ankles, elbows, hips, or shoulders. In more than half the cases, the inflammation also affects the tendons. If untreated, the arthritis of gonorrhea can destroy the joints, resulting in permanent disability.

Diagnosis and Treatment

Most cases of gonorrhea can be treated effectively with penicillin or other antibiotics. A single injection of penicillin is the recommended therapy for most cases, but when complications occur larger doses may have to be given for a period of from one to two weeks. Penicillin is the treatment used to eradicate gonococcal infection of the eyes, a problem that once accounted for more than ten percent of the cases of blindness in children. The spread of gonorrhea to the eyes is possible, although unlikely, in adults. The main symptom is a puslike discharge accompanying inflammation of the cornea.

Since there are no blood tests for gonorrhea infections, diagnosis depends on testing samples of the puslike discharge or other body fluids. For most men, it is a fairly simple procedure to obtain a sample of a suspicious discharge from the penis, place it on a microscope slide, stain it, and examine it for the presence of gonococci. It is more difficult to obtain a reliable sample of an infected secretion from most women. The doctor or clinic technician may take a sample of the secretions in the vagina and culture them in a special way. Sometimes the diagnosis is made from a culture taken from the rectum, urethra, or pharynx, where the disease organism may be found. Because syphilis and gonorrhea are sometimes acquired at the same time, doctors treating patients for gonorrhea frequently take a blood sample to test for the syphilis spirochete.

Even if the gonococcus is identified, antibiotic treatment is not a surefire guarantee of a cure, because some gonococci may not be reached by the antibiotic medication; also, some strains of the disease have in recent years shown an immunity to the antibiotics used. The recommended personal controls are the use of a condom by the man during intercourse and the use of penicillin medication immediately following any suspected exposure to the disease. Other prophylactic measures that are effective in lessening the risk of one partner's contracting gonorrhea from the other include, for both partners, bathing before intercourse and urinating both before and afterwards. Abstinence in the presence of a penile discharge and during menstruation are also recommended.

Lymphogranuloma Venereum

This disease, also known as *LGV* and *lymphogranuloma inguinale*, is a venereal disease that produces a primary lesion like a small blister, which ruptures to form a small ulcer. It is caused by a virus that is spread by sexual intercourse, although sexual contact is not necessary for transmission of the disease. It can be acquired by contact with the fluid excreted by a lesion.

The primary lesion usually appears in the genital area within one to three weeks after contact with an infected person. It may appear only briefly or be so small as to go unnoticed. But the disease spreads to neighboring lymph nodes, where the next sign of the disorder appears ten days to a month later. The swelling of the lymph nodes (forming *buboes*) is often the first symptom to be noted by the patient; the lymph nodes become matted together and hard, forming channels (or *fistulas*) through which pus drains to the surface of the skin. Enlargement of the lymph nodes may produce painful swelling of the external genitalia. The lymph-node involvement may spread to the anal region, leading to rectal constriction and painful bowel movements.

Since the lesions of lymphogranuloma venereum may resemble those of syphilis, chancroid, or certain nonvenereal diseases, doctors usually make a number of tests to determine whether or not the condition is, in fact, LGV. Therapy includes administration of antibiotics and sulfa drugs for a period of about a week up to a month, depending on the severity of the infection.

Chancroid

Chancroid, or *soft chancre*, is a venereal disease transmitted by a bacterium that causes a tender, painful ulcer. The ulcer, which may erode deeply into the tissues, follows the formation of a primary pustule at the site of infection. The pustule appears within five days after contact with an infected person. While essentially a venereal disease, like other venereal diseases it is transmissible without sexual intercourse. Doctors, for example, have been known to develop a soft chancre on a finger after examining an infected patient. Doctors usually do tests to make sure that the lesion is not a syphilitic chancre. Although the disease can spread from the genital region to other parts of the body, the soft chancre generally is self-limiting. Therapy consists of administration of sulfa drugs or tetracycline.

Granuloma Inguinale

Granuloma inguinale, also called *granuloma venereum,* is not the same, in spite of the similarity in name, as lymphogranuloma venereum. It is an insidious, chronic venereal disease that produces lesions on the skin or mucuous membrane of the genital or anal regions. The first sign of the infection may be a painless papule or nodule that leaves an ulcer with a reddish granular base. If untreated, the lesions tend to spread to the lower abdomen and thighs. In time, the sores produce a sour, pungent odor. Antibiotics such as streptomycin and tetracycline are prescribed. Relapses may occur and cure may be slow, especially in cases of long standing.

EXTERNAL VENEREAL MALADIES

The three conditions described below—two of them related to viruses and the third a parasitic infestation—may generally be considered sources of discomfort and disfigurement rather than threats to general health. All three are transmissible by other means besides sexual contact.

Warts

Venereal warts, known medically as *condyloma acuminatum,* are caused by a virus that proliferates in the warmth and moisture of the anal and genital regions. They occur within the vagina and rectum as well as externally about body openings and on the external genitalia of both men and women. Although generally harmless, venereal warts may be contagious and cause varying amounts of discomfort. Syphilitic lesions or other disorders of the genital region may simulate the warts, so it is important that the necessary tests be made to rule out more serious disorders. Discharges, as from gonorrhea or other infections, tend to aggravate the discomfort of venereal warts and encourage their spread.

In some cases, drugs may be used to remove the warts. They also may be removed by *cryosurgery,* a technique employing liquid nitrogen to freeze and destroy the virus-affected cells forming a wart. However, removing the wart may not completely remove the virus, which can be the "seed" of additional warts at the same site. Many doctors recommend that venereal warts be left alone unless they are a source of discomfort to the patient.

Molluscum Contagiosum

Another viral disease transmitted during sexual intercourse is known by the medical term *molluscum contagiosum.* The disease can also be transmitted by ordinary person-to-person contact, as between members of a family or children in a classroom. The virus causes raised lesions containing a waxy, white material. The lesions, which may be very small or as large as an inch in diameter, occur on the skin or mucous membranes, commonly in the anal or genital area but sometimes on the face or torso. The lesions may last for several months or several years, then disappear spontaneously, or they may be removed by medications or surgery.

Pubic Lice

Infestations of pubic lice constitute a unique kind of venereal disease. Pubic lice, known popularly as *crabs,* are a species somewhat larger than body and head lice but still almost invisible to the naked eye. These whitish, oval parasites usually remain in the hair of the anal and genital regions, but they may sometimes be found attached to the skin at the base of any body hair, including the eyelashes and scalp. A very few pubic lice in the anal and genital areas can cause intense irritation and itching. The itching results in scratching which, in turn, produces abrasions of the skin. The lice may also produce patches of bluish spots on the skin of the inner thighs and lower abdomen. Another sign of their presence is the appearance of tiny brown specks deposited by the lice on the inside of undergarments.

Pubic lice are commonly spread by sexual contact, but they can be acquired from toilet seats, clothing, towels, bedclothes, combs, or any article of intimate use. Creams or ointments containing various parasiticides are available for disinfestation. They are applied every night for several nights, but overuse should be avoided because of the danger of injury to the tender tissues of the genital and anal region. Some doctors recommend soaking the infested part of the body several times daily in a mild solution of potassium permanganate. Lice on the eyebrows and eyelashes may have to be removed individually with a pair of tweezers. Clothing and other contaminated materials must be carefully cleaned to prevent reinfestation.

Complications of an infestation of pubic lice include intense itching (known medically as *pruritus*) and secondary infections from scratch-ing. These may require special medical care and administration of antibiotics, corticosteroid creams, or other appropriate remedies.

DISORDERS OF THE URINARY SYSTEM

Both men and women are subject to disorders of the urinary system, but there are a few disorders that affect women chiefly or women only, for reasons related to anatomical structure. See also *Diseases of the Urino-genital system*, p. 424.

Inflammation of the Bladder

Any inflammation of the bladder is known medically as *cystitis*. Factors such as urinary tract stones, injury, and obstructions to the normal flow of urine can aggravate or cause cystitis in either sex. Cystitis due to infectious organisms, however, is much more common in women than men. This is understandable in view of the relative shortness of the

female urethra—the tube through which urine is discharged from the bladder and through which infectious organisms can reach the bladder from the outside. In addition, the anus and the vagina, both of which may frequently be sources of infection, are situated relatively close to the external opening of the female urethra.

In women generally, the symptoms of cystitis may include a burning sensation around the edges of the vulva. There is usually a frequent urge to urinate and difficulty or pain *(dysuria)* associated with urination. Urinary retention and dehydration, which are generally under the control of the individual, can contribute to the spread of infection once it begins. The lining of the urinary bladder is relatively resistant to infection by most microorganisms as long as the normal flow of liquids through the urinary tract is maintained. In cases that do not yield quickly to copious fluid intake, there are medications that may be prescribed to cure the infection. Where urinary frequency or difficulty is accompanied by the appearance of blood in the urine, a doctor should be consulted immediately.

HONEYMOON CYSTITIS: One type of cystitis tends to occur mostly in young women during the first few weeks of frequent sexual activity, to which it is attributed. This so-called honeymoon cystitis may result in swelling of the urethra and the neck of the bladder, making urination difficult. The inflammation of these tissues can in turn make them more susceptible to infection. A treatment recommended specifical-

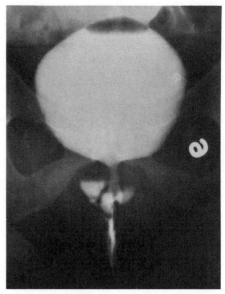

An X-ray photograph of a urethral diverticulum, visible as a spreading light area just below the balloon-shaped bladder.

ly for honeymoon cystitis is to drink large quantities of water or other fluids and to empty the bladder before and after engaging in sexual intercourse. Adequate lubrication, such as petroleum jelly, is also important. Medical care should be sought if the condition persists.

Urethral Disorders

The urethra is perforce involved in the inflammation of cystitis, since it is the route by which infectious organisms reach the bladder. In addition, there are disorders that are essentially confined to the urethra.

Urethral Caruncle

Urethral caruncle is a rather uncommon urinary-tract disorder that tends to be confined to women after the menopause. A *caruncle* (not to be

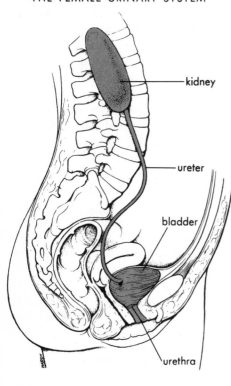

THE FEMALE URINARY SYSTEM

kidney

ureter

bladder

urethra

confused with *carbuncle*) is a small, red, fleshy outgrowth. It may be visible near the opening of the urethra. A caruncle growing from the cells of the urethra may be a sign of a bacterial infection, a tumor, or any of several other possible conditions. Symptoms may include vaginal bleeding, pain, tenderness, painful sexual intercourse (dyspareunia), a whitish, viscid discharge, and difficulty in urinating. A doctor should be consulted when such symptoms are present. A tissue biopsy and Pap smear may be taken to diagnose the condition. Caruncles are easily treated and of no long-term consequence.

Urethral Diverticulum

Another disorder of the urethra is a *urethral diverticulum,* or outpocketing of the urethra. The problem can be due to a developmental malformation, an injury, inflammation, a cyst, a urinary stone, or a venereal disease. Stones are a common cause, and in some patients there may be more than one diverticulum. The symptoms may include discomfort and urinary difficulty as well as dyspareunia. The disorder can be diagnosed with the help of X-ray photographs of the region of the urethra and bladder after they have been filled with a radiopaque substance that flows into any diverticula that may be present.

Treatment of a urethral diverticulum includes antibiotics to stop infection, medications to relieve pain and discomfort, and douches. In some cases, surgery is needed to eliminate the diverticula.

STRUCTURAL ANOMALIES

Various kinds of injury may be sustained by the female reproductive system and other abdominal organs, chiefly as a result of childbearing. The structural damage can generally be repaired by surgical measures.

Fistula

An abnormal opening between two organs or from an organ to the outside of the body is known as a *fistula.* Fistulas may involve the urinary and reproductive systems of a woman. Damage to the organs during pregnancy or surgery, for example, can result in a fistula between the urethra and the vagina, causing urinary incontinence. A similar kind of fistula can develop between the rectum and the vagina as a result of injury, complications of pregnancy, or surgery. Disorders of this sort must be repaired surgically.

Prolapsed Uterus

The uterus normally rests on the floor of the pelvis, held in position by numerous ligaments. Damage to the ligaments and other supporting tissues permits the uterus to descend, or *prolapse,* into the vagina. There are various degrees of prolapse, ranging from a slight intrusion of the uterus into the vagina to a severe condition in which the cervix of the uterus protrudes out of the vaginal orifice. Prolapse of the uterus resembles a hernia but is not a true hernia because the opening through which the uterus protrudes is a normal one.

Backache and a feeling of heaviness in the pelvic region may accompany the condition. Many women complain of a "dragging" sensation. An assortment of complications may involve neighboring organ systems; bleeding and ulceration of the uterus are not uncommon. Coughing and straining can aggravate the symptoms.

Like the various types of hernia, a prolapsed uterus does not improve without treatment, but tends instead to worsen gradually. The only permanent treatment is surgical repair. In mild cases, a woman may get relief from symptoms through exercises intended to strengthen the muscles of the pelvic region. Supporting devices, such as an inflatable, doughnut-shaped pessary, are available as temporary methods of correcting a prolapse. Preventive exercises may be recommended for childbearing women who want to

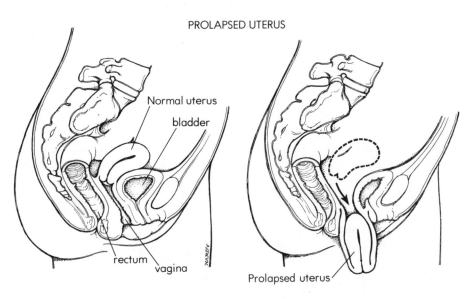

PROLAPSED UTERUS

Normal uterus
bladder
rectum
vagina

Prolapsed uterus

avoid weakened muscles and ligaments leading to prolapse.

Tipped Uterus

The uterus may be out of its normal position without being prolapsed. A malpositioned uterus may be "tipped" forward, backward, or otherwise be out of alignment with neighboring organs. A malpositioned uterus may cause no symptoms, or it may be associated with dysmenorrhea or infertility. If a malpositioned uterus causes pain, bleeding, or other problems, the condition can be corrected surgically, or a pessary support may relieve the symptoms. Displacement of the uterus occasionally is the result of a separate pelvic disease that requires treatment.

Hernias of the Vaginal Wall

The wall of the vagina may be ruptured in childbirth, especially in a multiple delivery or birth of a larger-than-average baby. The kind of hernia depends on the exact site of the rupture and what organ happens to lie against the vaginal wall at that point. The condition may be further complicated by a prolapsed uterus. Careful examination of the patient and X-ray pictures may be necessary to determine whether just one or several of the urinary, reproductive, and gastrointestinal organs in the pelvic cavity are involved.

CYSTOCELE: *Cystocele* is a hernia involving the bladder and the vagina. Structurally, part of the bladder protrudes through the wall of the vagina. The symptoms, in addition to a feeling of pressure deep in the vagina, may be urinary difficulties such as incontinence, a frequent urge to urinate, and inability to completely empty the bladder. Residual urine in the bladder may contribute to infection and inflammation of the bladder. Treatment includes surgery to correct the condition, pessaries if needed to support the structures, and medications to control infection.

RECTOCELE: A hernia involving the

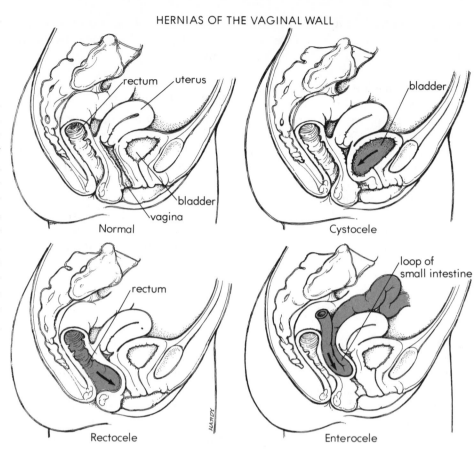

HERNIAS OF THE VAGINAL WALL

Normal — rectum, uterus, bladder, vagina

Cystocele — bladder

Rectocele — rectum

Enterocele — loop of small intestine

tissues separating the vagina and the rectum, behind the vagina, is called a *rectocele*. The symptoms are a feeling of fullness in the vagina and difficulty in defecating. Enemas or laxatives may be needed to relieve constipation because straining, or even coughing, can aggravate the condition. Surgery is the only permanently effective treatment. Special diets, laxatives, and rectal suppositories may be prescribed pending surgery.

ENTEROCELE: A herniation of the small intestine into the vagina is called an *enterocele*. Some of the symptoms are similar to those of other hernias involving the vaginal wall, and in addition, a patient with an enterocele may experience abdominal cramps shortly after eating. An enterocele can be dangerous as well as uncomfortable, since a segment of the small bowel can become trapped and obstructed, requiring emergency surgery.

Varicose Veins

Varicose veins of the vulva, vagina,

and neighboring areas are another possible effect of pregnancy, although the legs are more often affected. Obesity, reduced physical activity during pregnancy, and circulatory changes associated with pregnancy can contribute to the development of varicose veins. The symptoms generally are limited to discomfort although there can be bleeding, particularly at the time of childbirth. Varicose veins that occur in the vulva and vagina during pregnancy and cause discomfort can be treated surgically during the early months of pregnancy. Some drugs and supportive therapy can be used to help relieve symptoms. But many doctors recommend that surgical stripping of veins be delayed until after the pregnancy has been terminated. A complication of untreated varicose veins can be development of blood clots in the abnormal blood vessels. For a discussion of varicose veins of the legs during pregnancy, see p. 133. See also p. 356.

BENIGN NEOPLASMS

The word *neoplasm* refers to any abnormal proliferation of tissue that serves no useful function. There are numerous kinds of neoplasms, but just two main groups—cancerous, or *malignant*; or noncancerous, or *benign*. In ordinary speech the word *benign* suggests some positive benefit, but a benign neoplasm, though noncancerous, may in fact be harmful to health or at least worrisome. Benign neoplasms that are of particular concern to women are discussed below.

Cysts

A *cyst* is a sac containing a gaseous, fluid, or semisolid material. (Certain normal anatomical structures, like the urinary bladder, are technically known as cysts—hence the term *cystitis* for inflammation of the bladder.) Abnormal, or neoplastic, cysts can develop at several sites within the urinary and reproductive systems.

Vaginal Cysts

A cyst may develop in a gland at the opening of the vagina as a result of infection with a venereal or other disease. Such a cyst can block the flow of secretions from the gland and produce swelling and pain. Dyspareunia, or painful intercourse, is sometimes a symptom. A vaginal gland cyst usually is treated with antibiotics and hot packs. In some cases, it may be necessary for a doctor to make an incision to drain the cyst.

Ovarian Cysts

Cysts in the ovaries may be caused by a malfunction of physiological process or by a pathological condition. Some pathological cysts are malignant. The cysts in the ovaries generally are filled with fluid that may range in color from pale and clear to reddish brown, depending upon the source of the fluid. Some cysts are too small to be seen with the naked eye, whereas others may

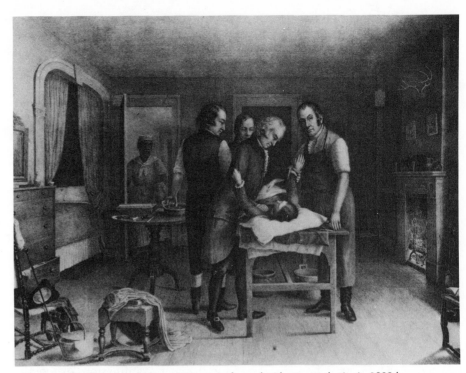

The first recorded ovariotomy, performed without anesthetics in 1809 by the American surgeon Ephraim McDowell. A 20-pound tumor was removed from the patient, who recovered and survived for another 30 years.

be four or five inches in diameter when symptoms begin to cause discomfort. There are several different kinds of ovarian cysts.

FOLLICULAR CYST: A *follicular,* or *retention,* cyst, is a physiological cyst and is one of the most common types. It develops in an old follicle in which an ovum for some reason has failed to break out of its capsule during the ovulation process. Ordinarily, the contents of such a follicle are resorbed, but sometimes a cyst develops. It rarely grows larger than about two inches in diameter. It may rupture but usually disappears after a few months. The symptoms may include pain with some uterine bleeding and dyspareunia. Treatment consists of warm douches, analgesics, and hormone therapy designed to restore normal ovarian activity. If the symptoms persist or the cyst continues to increase in size, or if serious complications occur, the doctor may recommend exploratory surgery.

Occasionally such cysts, whether or not they rupture, produce symptoms that mimic those of appendicitis, with severe abdominal pain. The abdomen may become so tender that a doctor cannot palpate the organs in order to distinguish between an ovarian cyst and appendicitis, particularly if the right ovary is involved. The symptoms occur at the time that ovulation would be expected. If the doctor cannot be certain that the cause of the abdominal pain is indeed a cyst, for which surgery is not needed, he may recommend surgery anyway—just to be on the safe side.

Multiple follicular cysts, involving the ovaries on both sides (*bilateral polycystic ovaries*) can result in a syndrome (or group of symptoms) that includes infertility, obesity, and abnormal growth of body hair. All of these effects are related to a disruption of normal sex-hormone activity; they generally occur in young women, from teen-agers to those in their 20s. The therapy includes both medical and surgical efforts to restore normal menstrual function, a diet to control obesity, and the use of various depilatory techniques to remove unwanted body hair.

CORPUS LUTEUM CYST: This kind of cyst may develop in the ovary following ovulation or during the early part of a pregnancy. The corpus luteum is a small, temporary gland that forms in the empty follicle after the ovum has been released from the ovary. Its function is to produce the hormone progesterone, which is important in preparing the endometrium, the lining of the uterus, to receive a fertilized ovum. However, the corpus luteum also can be overproductive of a brownish fluid which fills the former follicular space, causing it to swell to a diameter of two or three inches. The cyst causes symptoms of pain and tenderness and may also result in a disruption of normal menstrual cycles in a woman who is not pregnant.

Most corpus luteum cysts gradually decrease in size without special treatment, except to relieve the symptoms. There may, however, be complications such as torsion, or painful twisting of the ovary, or a rupture of the cyst. A ruptured corpus luteum cyst can result in hemorrhage and peritonitis, requiring immediate surgery.

CHOCOLATE CYST: So called because of their brownish-red color, chocolate cysts consist of misplaced endometrial tissue growing on the ovary instead of in its normal position lining the uterus. Chocolate cysts are among the largest of the ovarian cysts, ranging up to five or six inches in diameter. They cause symptoms associated with a variety of disorders of the reproductive system, including infertility, dyspareunia, and dysmenorrhea. Surgery usually is a favored method of therapy, the precise procedure depending upon the amount of ovarian tissue involved. A small chocolate cyst can be cauterized but a large cyst may require removal of a portion of the ovary. See also *Cancer of the Ovary,* p. 504.

Cysts of the Breast

Cysts may form in the milk glands or the ducts leading from the glands. They are caused by imbalances in ovarian hormones and they tend to develop in mature women approach-

ing the menopause. The cysts tend to fluctuate in size, often enlarging just before or during menstruation, and there may be a discharge from the nipple. Pain and tenderness are usually present, although painless cysts are sometimes discovered only when a woman examines her breasts for possible lumps. Cysts may be almost microscopic in size or as large as an inch or more in diameter. It is not uncommon for more than one cyst to occur at the same time in one breast or both.

A medical examination is recommended when any kind of lump can be felt in the breast tissue. This is particularly important for women who have passed menopause. The doctor frequently can determine whether a lump is a result of a cyst or cancer by the patient's history and by physical examination, especially when repeated at intervals of several weeks. Mammography and biopsy study of a small bit of tissue are used to confirm the diagnosis.

Women who are troubled by breast cysts may be helped by wearing a good brassiere at all times, even during sleep, to protect tender areas. The only medications available are those that relieve pain and discomfort—symptoms that usually subside when the menopause is reached.

OTHER NONCANCEROUS MASSES: A benign lump in the breast can be caused by either a fat deposit or an abscess. A fatty mass frequently forms if an injury to the breast damages adipose tissue. Because of a similarity of the symptoms to those of breast cancer, a biopsy is usually required to distinguish the lesion from a cancer. The involved tissue may in any case be removed surgically.

An abscess of the breast as a result of an infection, although a rare problem, may produce a lump that requires treatment with antibiotic medications or by an incision to drain the pus. Breast infections leading to abscesses are most likely to occur in nursing mothers but can also develop in women who are not

lactating. When an infection develops in a breast being used to nurse a baby, nursing has to be discontinued temporarily while the infection is treated. See also *Cancer of the Breast,* p. 504.

Polyps

A *polyp* is a strange-looking growth, even for an abnormal growth of tissue. It has been described as having the appearance of a tennis racket or a small mushroom. Polyps are found in many parts of the body, from the nose to the rectum. Usually they are harmless. But a polyp can result in discomfort or bleeding and require surgical excision. A polyp on the breast, for example, can become irritated by rubbing against the fabric of a brassiere. Although polyps generally are not cancerous, it is standard procedure to have the polyp tissue, like any excised tissue, tested in the laboratory. If malignant cells accompany a polyp, they are usually found at the base of the growth, which means that some of the tissue around the polyp must be excised along with the growth itself. Once a polyp is removed it does not grow again, although other polyps can occur in the same region.

CERVICAL POLYP: Polyps in the cervix are not uncommon, occurring most frequently in the years between menarche and menopause. A cervical polyp may be associated with vaginal bleeding or leukorrhea; the bleeding may occur after douching or sexual intercourse. In some cases, the bleeding is severe. Cervical polyps can usually be located visually by an examining physician and removed by minor surgery.

ENDOMETRIAL POLYP: Endometrial polyps, which develop in the lining of the uterus, usually occur in women who are over 40, although they can develop at any age after menarche. They are frequently the cause of nonmenstrual bleeding. They tend to be much larger than polyps that grow in other organs of the body: an endometrial polyp may be rooted high in the uterus with a stem reaching all the way to the cervix. Such a polyp is usually located and removed during a D and C procedure. As in the case of a cervical polyp, the growth and a bit of surrounding tissue are studied for traces of cancer cells.

Benign Tumors

Tumors are rather firm growths that may be either benign or malignant. In practice, any tumor is regarded with suspicion unless malignancy is ruled out by actual laboratory tests. Even a benign tumor represents a tissue abnormality, and if untreated can produce symptoms that interfere with normal health and activity.

Fibromas

Among the more common of the benign tumors is the *fibroma*, commonly known as a *fibroid tumor,* composed of fibrous connective tissue. About one of every 20 ovarian tumors is a fibroma, and a similar growth in the uterus is the most common type of tumor found in that organ. Fibromas also occur in the vulva.

OVARIAN FIBROMA: Ovarian fibromas are usually small, but there are instances in which they have grown to weigh as much as five pounds. A large fibroma can be very painful and produce symptoms such as a feeling of heaviness in the pelvic area, nausea, and vomiting. The growth may crowd other organs of the body, causing enlargement of the abdomen and cardiac and respiratory symptoms. The only treatment is surgical removal of the tumor, after which there is usually a quick and full recovery.

UTERINE FIBROMA: Fibroid tumors of the uterus can also grow to a very large size, some weighing many pounds. Like ovarian fibromas, they can press against neighboring organs such as the intestine or the urinary bladder, producing constipation or urinary difficulty. More commonly, there is pain and vaginal bleeding, along with pelvic pressure and enlargement of the abdomen. It is pos-

sible in some cases for a fibroid tumor to grow slowly in the uterus for several years without causing serious discomfort to the patient. If the tumor obstructs or distorts the reproductive tract, it may be a cause of infertility.

Treatment of fibroid tumors varies according to their size, the age of the patient and her expectations about having children, and other factors. If the tumor is small and does not appear to be growing at a rapid rate, the doctor may recommend that surgery be postponed as long as the tumor poses no threat to health. For an older woman, or for a woman who does not want to bear children, a hysterectomy may be advised, especially if symptoms are troublesome. If the patient is a young woman who wants to have children, the doctor is likely to advise a *myomectomy*, a surgical excision of the tumor, since a fibroid tumor of the uterus can cause serious complications during pregnancy and labor. It can result in abortion or premature labor, malpresentation of the fetus, difficult labor, and severe loss of blood during childbirth. While fibroid tumors of the uterus are not malignant, special tests are made of the endometrial tissue as part of any myomectomy or hysterectomy to rule out the possibility that cancer cells may be involved in the disorder.

Endometriosis

Endometriosis is the medical term for a condition in which endometrial tissue, the special kind of tissue that lines the uterus, grows in various areas of the pelvic cavity outside the uterus. Endometrial cells may invade such unlikely places as the ovaries (the most common site), the bladder, appendix, Fallopian tubes, intestinal tract, or the supporting structure of the uterus. The external endometrial tissue may appear as small blisters of endometrial cells, as solid nodules, or as cysts, usually of the ovary, which may be four inches or more in diameter, like the chocolate cysts of the ovaries. Such a mass

of sometimes tumorlike endometrial cells is called an *endometrioma.*

The misplaced endometrial tissue causes problems because it goes through menstrual cycles just as the endometrium does within the cavity of the uterus. The endometrial tissue proliferates after ovulation and may cause almost constant pain, wherever it is located, for a few days before the start of menstruation. The symptoms subside after the menstrual flow begins. The effects may include dyspareunia, rectal bleeding, backache, and generalized pain in the pelvic region as sensitive tissues throughout the pelvic cavity are irritated by monthly cycles of swelling and bleeding.

Since infertility is associated with endometriosis, which can become progressively worse, young women who want to bear children are sometimes encouraged to begin efforts to become pregnant as early as possible if they show signs or symptoms of the disorder. Treatment includes hormone medication and surgery to remove the lesions of endometriosis or the organ involved. For patients with extensive spread of endometrial tissue outside the uterus the doctor may recommend removal of one or both ovaries. Destruction of the ovaries surgically or by radiation therapy may be employed to eliminate the menstrual cycle activity that aggravates the symptoms of endometriosis. These procedures cause sterility and premature menopause, but some women prefer this to the discomfort of endometriosis. The hormone therapy inhibits the ovulation phase of the menstrual cycle. Without ovulation, the endometrial tissue does not proliferate. For this reason, pregnancy often eliminates or eases the symptoms of endometriosis during parturition and for a period of time thereafter.

Dyspareunia

Dyspareunia, or painful intercourse, is often associated with endometriosis and is attributed to irritation of nerve fibers in the area of the cervix from the pressure of sexual activity. There are many other possible causes of painful intercourse, some functional and some organic in nature. In addition to endometriosis, the problem may be due to a vaginal contracture, a disorder involving the muscles of the pelvic region, inflammation of the vagina or urethra, prolapsed or malpositioned uterus, *cervicitis* (inflammation of the cervix), or a disorder of the bladder or rectum. A cause of dyspareunia in older women may be a degeneration of the tissues lining the vagina, which become thin and dry. Temporary therapy for dyspareunia may include water-soluble lubricants, anesthetic ointments, steroid hormones, analgesics, and sedatives. In appropriate cases, surgery is effective in correcting an organic cause of painful sexual intercourse. Functional or psychogenic (of psychological origin) causes of dyspareunia usually require psychological counseling for the patient and her sexual partner.

Backache

Still another effect of endometriosis that can mimic symptoms of other disorders is backache. When endometrial tissue invades the pelvic region, there may be a fairly constant pain in the back near the tailbone or the rectum. Usually the backache subsides only after the cause has been eliminated. Temporary measures include those advised for other kinds of backache: sleeping on a firm mattress, preferably reinforced with a sheet of plywood between springs and mattress; application of dry heat or warm baths; sedatives to relieve tension, and analgesics to relieve the pain.

A backache that radiates down the back and into a leg, following the path of a sciatic nerve, can be due to a disorder of the ovaries or uterus. An ovarian cyst or infection of the Fallopian tubes can produce a backache that seems to be centered in the lumbosacral area of the spinal column. Such backaches, sometimes called gynecologic backaches, tend to occur most frequently during a woman's childbearing years and affect women who have had several children more often than women who have not been pregnant. Tumors also can produce backache symptoms. X-ray pictures, myelograms, and laboratory studies may be required in order to rule out the possibilities that the back pain may be caused by a tumor, a herniated or "slipped" disk, or a deformity of the spinal column that might have been aggravated by one or more pregnancies. Most backaches, however, relate to poor posture or muscle tension. Anxiety or other kinds of emotional stress can aggravate the symptoms. See also *Backaches*, p. 268, and *Back Pain and Its Causes*, p. 460.

CANCERS OF THE REPRODUCTIVE SYSTEM

Cancer of the Cervix

The cervix of the uterus is the second most common site of cancers affecting the reproductive system of women. As compared with all cancers affecting women, it rates third, after breast cancer and colon and rectum cancer. It has been estimated that about 20,000 cases of cervical cancer are found among American women each year, and approximately 7,500 deaths every year are due to this disease.

Though it is not considered a venereal disease, cancer of the cervix seems to be closely related to past sexual activity. Statistically, women who began sexual intercourse at an early age or who have had many partners are much more likely to have cervical cancer than women who have never engaged in sexual activity or who have had one or very

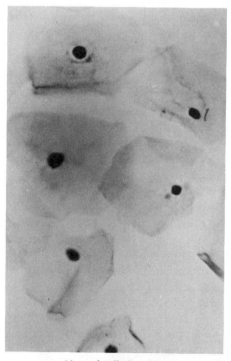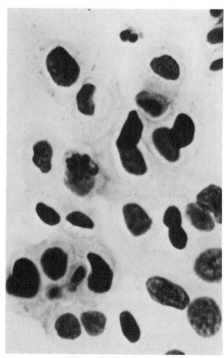

Normal cells from the cervix *(left)* contrasted with cancer cells *(right)*.

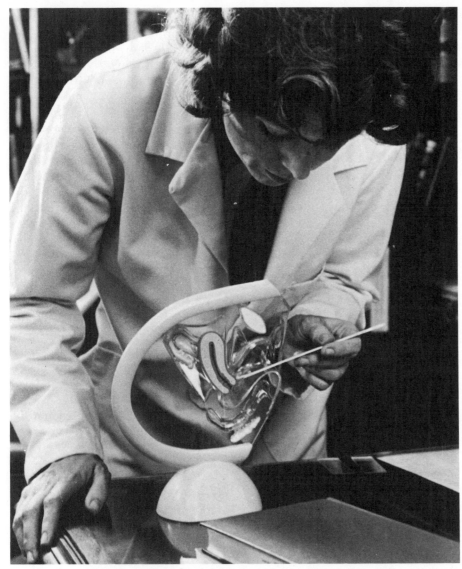

A demonstration of the technique of taking Pap test smears from the cervix, using a plastic model of the female reproductive system.

smear test before it becomes invasive.

Diagnostic Methods

PAP SMEAR TEST: The *Pap smear* test (named for Dr. George Papanicolaou, who developed the technique in 1928) is a quick and simple method of detecting cancerous cells in secretions and scrapings from mucous membrane. It requires the collection of small samples of cells from the surface of the cervix and from the cervical canal. Such samples are obtained by inserting a plastic spatula or a cut wooden tongue depressor into the vagina, into which a speculum has been placed previously. The device is scraped gently over the areas of the cervix in which a cancer is most likely to develop, or from any other surface of the cervix that appears abnormal during visual inspection. The doctor may collect also a sample of vaginal secretions, which may contain possibly cancerous cells not only from the cervix but from the ovaries and uterus as well. (This is the only way a Pap smear test can be done if a woman has had a complete hysterectomy and has no cervix.) All cell samples are placed (smeared) on microscope slides and treated with a chemical preservative. The slides are sent to a laboratory for study and a report is made to the examining physician, usually within a few days, on the findings.

The laboratory report may classify the cell samples as negative (normal), suspicious, or positive. If the findings are negative, the woman will be advised to return in one year for another Pap smear test. If the findings are suspicious, the woman usually will be asked to return for a second test either immediately or within six months. A report of suspicious findings generally indicates the presence of unusual or abnormal cells, which may be due to an infection or inflammation as well as to a cancerous condition. If a specific disease organism is found in a sample—such as a trichomonas organism, for example—the laboratory

few sexual partners. There is also statistical evidence that intercourse with uncircumcised men increases the probability of cervical cancer and that the incidence of cancer of the penis is increased in men whose sexual partners have developed cancer of the cervix, and vice versa. Studies also indicate that cancer of the cervix is less likely to occur when the male partner habitually wears a condom. However interesting these statistical associations may be, the actual causes of cervical cancer are still unknown. Current medical thinking suggests that there is no causal relationship between

cervical cancer and the use of oral contraceptives.

PREINVASIVE STAGE: The earliest signs of cervical cancer tend to appear between the ages of 25 and 45. At this early, *preinvasive* stage, the cancer is described as *in situ*—confined to its original site. If the cancer is not treated at this stage, the disease spreads and becomes a typical invasive cancer within five to ten years. Signs of bleeding and ulceration usually do not appear until this has occurred. However, because of the relatively slow growth of cervical cancer in the early stage, the disease usually can be detected by a Pap

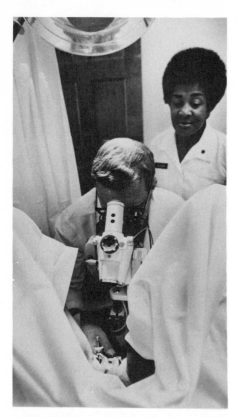

A doctor uses a colposcope, a magnifying instrument, to make a biopsy test for possible cervical cancer. The test is said to be virtually painless and does not require hospitalization.

report includes that information.

OTHER DIAGNOSTIC TESTS: A positive Pap smear is one containing cells that are probably or definitely cancerous. When a report of positive findings is returned by the laboratory, the doctor immediately arranges for further studies. These involve examination of the cervix visually by a special microscopic technique known as *colposcopy* and the removal of small tissue samples. These studies are usually done in the doctor's office. In some cases a biopsy is necessary. This requires that the woman enter a hospital where she can receive an anesthetic. The biopsy sample is taken when possible from the same location on the cervix as the Pap smear that resulted in positive findings. Other tests, including X-ray films of the chest and bones, can be made during the hospital stay to determine whether the cancer, if verified by biopsy, has extended to nearby areas or spread to other areas of the body by metastasis.

Treatment ordinarily is not started until all of the studies have verified that there is cancer in the tissues of the cervix; other disorders such as cervicitis, venereal infection, and polyps can mimic symptoms of cervical cancer.

Therapy

The kind of treatment recommended for a case of cervical cancer generally depends upon several factors, such as the stage of cancer development and the age and general health of the patient. For a young woman who wishes to have children despite cancer in situ, which is limited to the cervix, surgeons may excise a portion of the cervix and continue watching for further developments with frequent Pap smears and other tests. The treatment of choice for cervical cancer in the early stage, however, is surgical removal of the body of the uterus as well as the cervix—a procedure called a *total hysterectomy*. This is the usual treatment for women over the age of 40 or for those who do not wish to have children. Sometimes more extensive surgery is necessary.

Radiation treatment may be advised for women who are not considered to be good surgical risks because of other health problems. Radiation may be recommended along with surgery for women with advanced cervical cancer in order to help destroy cancer cells that may have spread by metastasis to other tissues.

The five-year cure rate for cervical cancer is about 99 percent when treatment is started in the early preinvasive stage. The chances of a cure drop sharply in later stages, but the five-year cure rate is still as high as 65 percent if treatment is started when the cancer has just begun to spread to the vagina or other nearby tissues.

Cancer of the Body of the Uterus

Cancer of the body of the uterus, or *endometrial cancer*, is less common than cancer of the cervix. Cervical cancer primarily affects women before middle age; endometrial cancer occurs more frequently among women beyond the menopause, with its highest rate occurring among women between the ages of 60 and 70. A statistical association has been found between the increased use of estrogen hormones and the increasing rate of cancer of the uterus among middle-aged women since the 1960s. It has been suggested that the uterine lining (endometrium) in some women is particularly sensitive to the effects of estrogens.

Diagnostic Methods

Early symptoms usually include bleeding between menstrual periods or after menopause, and occasionally, a watery or blood-stained vaginal discharge. Most patients experience no pain in the early stages although pain is a symptom in advanced uterine cancer or when the disease is complicated by an infection. Unfortunately, there is no simple test, like the Pap smear for cervical cancer, that provides a good diagnostic clue to the presence of endometrial cancer. The Pap smear does occasionally pick up cells sloughed off by the endometrium, and laboratory tests can tell if they might be malignant. But a doctor who is suspicious of symptoms of endometrial cancer must depend upon more direct methods to confirm or rule out the disease. The usual method is a D and C, during which a small sample of uterine lining will be removed for biopsy, or a sample may be withdrawn by suction (aspirated) from the uterine cavity. Aspiration can be done in the doctor's office with local anesthesia of the cervix or with no anesthesia. There is little or no discomfort following aspiration.

Therapy

If the diagnostic D and C is done when the abnormal bleeding associated with uterine cancer first begins, the chances of a cure are very good. The first step, if the general

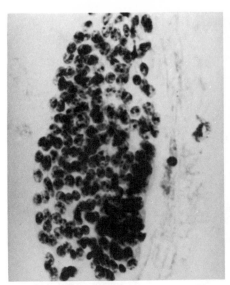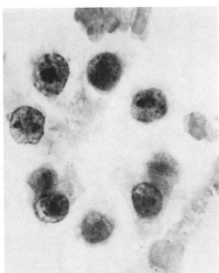

(Left) Normal cells from the lining of the uterus. *(Right)* Uterine cells taken in an aspiration smear, showing a rosettelike pattern indicating cancer.

health of the patient permits surgery, is complete removal of the uterus, ovaries, and Fallopian tubes—a procedure called a *radical hysterectomy.* Radiation may also be administered to control the spread of cancer cells in the pelvic region.

Since 90 percent of the women affected by endometrial cancer are past childbearing age, removal of the reproductive organs is usually less traumatic for them than it would be if they were young women with hopes of raising families. For premenopausal women, the natural ovarian hormones that are lost with the ovaries may be artificially replaced by prescription in order to ease the sudden transition to a menopausal condition.

A hysterectomy should not affect a woman's normal sexual activity. Sexual relations usually can be resumed about six to eight weeks after the operation, or when the incision has healed. If the incision is made through the pubic region or vagina, there should be little or no visible scar.

A number of possible causes of uterine cancer have been suggested. High blood pressure, diabetes, and obesity are believed to increase the risk of developing endometrial cancer. There is some evidence that the disease tends to occur in families,

particularly among women who experience a greater-than-average degree of menstrual difficulty.

Estrogen and Cancer

There is a higher incidence of cancer of the uterus among women who have tumors of the ovary that produce estrogen as well as among women whose menopause begins later than the usual age (and hence who have produced estrogen naturally for a longer-than-usual period). Because of the statistical associations between uterine cancer and estrogen-producing tumors, as well as other factors, the American Cancer Society has cautioned that doctors should exert "close supervision of women on estrogen, with an awareness that sustained use [of estrogens] may stimulate dormant factors in the body and lead to development of endometrial cancer."

Among the conditions for which estrogen has been prescribed for women of middle age and beyond are uncomfortable effects of menopause, such as itching and irritation caused by dryness of the vagina. However, there are available hormone creams that help relieve dryness of the vaginal tissues; the creams may contain estrogen, but not enough to cause concern about their possible carcinogenic properties.

Diethylstilbestrol

An estrogenlike synthetic compound has definitely been implicated in the development of a type of cancer *(adenocarcinoma)* which primarily affects epithelial tissue. The synthetic hormone known chemically as diethylstilbestrol (DES) or stilbestrol was taken for the most part in the late 1940s and through the 1950s by pregnant women, primarily for the treatment of such complications as bleeding and threatened miscarriage. Around 1971, doctors became aware that some of the daughters whose mothers had taken DES during their pregnancy had developed an unusual cell formation in vaginal tissue, vaginal and cervical cancers, and some anatomical abnormalities. Cancers have been discovered in daughters as young as seven years of age. An unknown but substantial number of women in the United States alone received DES while pregnant, but only about 200 of their daughters have been found to be afflicted with cervical or vaginal cancers. The National Cancer Institute has urged that all mothers and daughters who may have been ex-

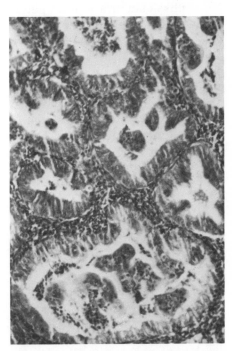

This photomicrograph shows invasive adenocarcinoma of the endometrium, or lining of the uterus.

posed to DES during the mother's pregnancy arrange to be examined by a physician for possible effects of the drug.

The use of DES for pregnant women has been discontinued, although the compound is still available for treating certain cases of breast cancer and menopausal symptoms in nonpregnant women.

Cancer of the Ovary

Cancer of the ovary is not as common as cervical and endometrial cancers, but ovarian cancer does account for nearly one out of every six malignant tumors of the female reproductive system. The disease is responsible for a greater number of deaths because an ovarian cancer can remain symptomless until it has spread. There are several different kinds of malignant tumors of the ovary; some originate in the ovaries and others are caused by cells that have metastasized from a cancer at some other site, such as the uterus.

There are no age limits for cancer of the ovary, although most cases are detected in women between 50 and 70. A physician at a routine pelvic examination may notice a lump or other abnormal growth in the abdominal region. The symptoms reported by patients usually include abdominal discomfort or digestive problems, possibly because ovarian cancers often grow large enough to press on neighboring organs and cause urinary difficulties, constipation, or other digestive disorders. A

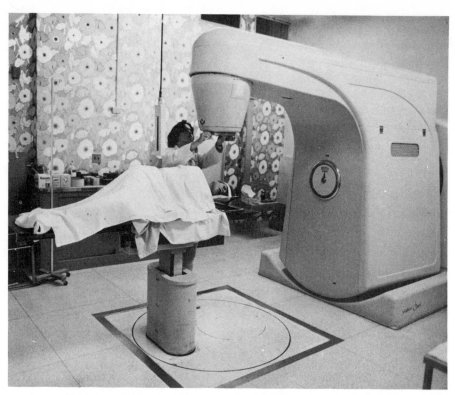

The linear accelerator treats cancer by delivering a concentrated dose of radiation to the tumor, with minimal effect on surrounding tissues.

clue is given in some cases by endometrial bleeding as a result of abnormal hormone production by the affected ovary. However, the more common kinds of ovarian cancers do not produce hormones. Occasionally, cancer cells from an ovarian tumor will be found in a Pap smear sample. But there are no direct, simple tests for cancer of the ovary.

Treatment for ovarian cancer varies with the individual case. As with cancer at other sites, surgery is generally necessary. The extent of the surgery depends upon the type of lesion and other factors. In an advanced case of an older woman, total hysterectomy along with removal of the ovaries and Fallopian tubes would be the treatment of choice. But if the patient is a young woman and the cancer is not extensive, the surgeon may excise the affected ovary and leave the remainder of the reproductive system intact. Radiation and chemotherapy are commonly applied in addition to surgery. The cure rate for ovarian cancers depends upon the type of tumor and the stage at which treatment started; the five-year survival chances range upward to about 65 percent.

CANCER OF THE BREAST

Cancer of the breast is one of the oldest and best-known types of cancer. It is described in an ancient Egyptian papyrus of 5,000 years ago. The hormonal factors involved in the physiology of breast cancer have been studied by doctors for more than 100 years. But it remains the most common of cancers affecting woman. It kills more women than any other kind of cancer, and more people of both sexes (a minuscule number are men) than only two other cancers—lung cancer and cancer of the colon and rectum. About 90,000 women in the United States develop breast cancer each year, and more than a third die of the disease. Nearly everyone knows a friend or relative who has been stricken by breast cancer. Yet the cause of breast cancer is still unknown.

Breast cancer is less common in the Orient than in America and Western Europe, but Asian women who move to America seem to increase their risk of developing breast cancer—indicating that there may be a dietary factor or some other environmental influence. Women whose female relatives have had breast cancer are more likely to be victims than women from families in which breast cancer is not present. The disease appears to be linked statistically also to women who do not have children before their 30s or who do not have any children; to mothers who do not nurse their babies; to women who reach the menopause later than normal; and to women who began menstruation earlier in life than normal. There is increasing evidence also that ovarian activity may play an important role in the development of breast cancer. Women with ovarian tumors and women who use supplementary estrogen have been shown by some studies to be at increased risk, while the process of having many children and nursing them, which suppresses estrogen hormone activity, is associated with a decreased risk of developing breast cancer.

Cancer of the breast may occur as early as the teens, but this is rare. It is generally not found before the age of 30, and the incidence peaks around the time of menopause. Then there is a second period after the age of about 65 when the incidence of breast cancer rises again.

Breast cancer usually begins in the ducts of the milk glands; the first noticeable sign is a lump in the breast. The lump may appear anywhere in the breast, but the most common site is the upper, outer quadrant. Such lumps are not necessarily or even usually cancerous, but a biopsy (described below) must be performed to check the tissue involved.

In a typical case of breast cancer, a small tumor half an inch in diameter, large enough to be detected during careful self-examination, can grow to a cancer two inches in diameter in six months to a year. The lump generally causes no pain; pain is rarely associated with early breast cancer. If the tumor is allowed to grow unchecked, it may cause pulling of the skin from within. This effect may appear as a flattening of the breast or a dimpling of the skin, or a sinking, tilting, or flattening of the nipple. Less frequently, the tumor begins in a duct near the nipple, causing irritation of the skin of the nipple and a moist discharge. In such cases a scab eventually forms at that site. In time, cancer cells spread to the nearby

SELF-EXAMINATION OF THE BREASTS

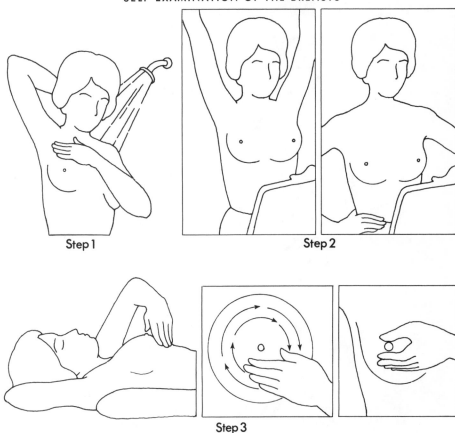

Step 1   Step 2   Step 3

Self-examination of the breasts as recommended by the American Cancer Society. *(Step 1)* Examine breasts during a shower or bath; hands glide easier over wet skin. With fingers flat, move the left hand gently over every part of the right breast, then the right hand over the left breast. Check for any lump, hard knot, or thickening. *(Step 2)* Before a mirror, inspect the breasts with arms at the sides, then with arms raised. Look for any changes in the contour of each breast, a swelling, dimple of skin, or changes in the nipple. Then rest palms on hips and press down firmly to flex the chest muscles. Left and right breasts will not match exactly—few women's breasts do. But regular inspection will show what is normal for you. *(Step 3)* While lying down with a pillow or folded towel under the right shoulder and with the right hand behind the head, examine the right breast with the left hand. With fingers flat, press gently in small circular motions around an imaginary clock face. Begin at 12 o'clock, then move to 1 o'clock, and so on around back to 12. A ridge of firm tissue in the lower curve of each breast is normal. Next, move in an inch toward the nipple and keep circling to examine every part of the breast, including the nipple. This requires at least three more circles. Then repeat the procedure slowly on the left breast with the pillow under the left shoulder and left hand behind the head. Notice how the breast structure feels. Finally, squeeze the nipple of each breast gently between thumb and index finger. Any discharge, clear or bloody, should be reported to a doctor immediately.

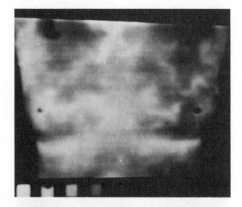

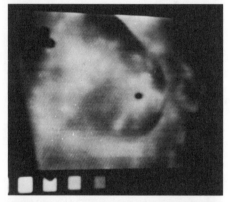

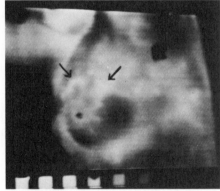

Thermograms, pictures of heat radiation of body tissues, can sometimes reveal the presence of a breast tumor that could not be discovered by touch. The tissue of tumors has a distinctively higher temperature than normal tissue. *(Top)* A typical thermogram, with lightest shades reflecting warmest areas. The other thermograms show an abnormal pattern of temperature elevation in both breasts. Arrows point to a hot quadrant and a dilated vein produced by the lesion.

lymph nodes and the danger becomes very serious of metastasis to any part of the body.

Detection of Breast Cancer

Fortunately, breast cancer can be treated effectively if it is detected early enough. Some 95 percent of breast cancers are discovered by the patient herself when she notices a lump. In all too many cases the discovery is made by chance and the lump may be quite large. The cure rate for breast cancer could be greatly improved if all women made a routine of monthly self-examination and then consulted a physician immediately if they found the least indication of a thickening or lump. Most such lumps are benign, but it is most important that the ones that are malignant be identified without delay.

The American Cancer Society and the National Cancer Institute recommend that every woman follow a prescribed method of self-examination just after the menstrual period, continuing every month after the menopause. The procedure consists of carefully looking at and feeling the breasts, and takes only a few minutes. A detailed description of the proper procedure is available in pamphlet form from the Superintendent of Documents, U.S. Government Printing Office, Washington, D.C. 20402 for 40 cents. Ask for Public Health Service Publication No. 1730. A film entitled "Breast Self-Examination," produced by the American Cancer Society and the National Cancer Institute, is also available.

If a tumor can be detected as even a small lump it must have been developing for some time. There is a truism about breast cancer to the effect that a cancer that is undetectable is curable—leaving unspoken the implication that a cancer that is detectable may not be curable. In recent years, methods of early detection have been refined to the point that tumors once undetectable can now be detected before any lump becomes palpable.

THERMOGRAPHY: One early warning detection technique involves the use of *thermography,* which is based on the fact that tumor cells produce slightly more heat than normal tissue. Hence a device that is sufficiently heat-sensitive can detect and pinpoint the location of an incipient tumor. A harmless tumor, too, would have a higher-than-normal temperature. Further tests would be needed to determine the true cause of the "hot" tissue reading.

MAMMOGRAPHY: *Mammography* is an X-ray technique developed specifically for examination of breast tissue. A tumor shows up on a mammogram as an opaque spot because of mineral concentrations associated with the growth. However, like thermography, mammography cannot determine whether a tumor is benign or malignant or if the opaque spot on the film is due to some other mineral-rich tissue rather than a tumor. The examining physician uses mammography only as one among other diagnostic tools.

Mammography has been widely used by cancer detection centers throughout America in past years. Since 1976, the National Cancer Institute and the American Cancer Society have cautioned doctors and patients about the routine use of mammography, particularly for women under 50 years of age and if older types of X-ray equipment are used. Studies have shown that exposure of the breasts to X rays, especially at the dosages produced by the older equipment, and perhaps even by the newer low-intensity equipment, increases the chances of breast cancer by about one percentage point. This means that a woman at low risk who has, say, a six percent chance of developing breast cancer would increase her risk to seven—by a factor of almost 17 percent—by exposure to X-ray mammography. A woman originally at higher risk would suffer a smaller-percentage increment. Hence cancer experts continue to approve the use of X-ray mammography only for high-risk groups— women who have a history of breast cancer or who have had lumps in their breasts, women above the age of 50, and younger women in the high-risk categories outlined above.

XERORADIOGRAPHY: *Xeroradiography* is a method that, like mammography, uses X rays, but it entails only about half the exposure to radiation. The pictures are developed by xerography, the process made familiar by Xerox copying machines. The picture consists of dots in varying shades of blue. The process produces a sharp picture, making interpretation simpler and more accurate than is possible with X-ray photographs. When performed by experienced medical technicians, xeroradiography can detect from 85 to 95 percent of all breast cancers, including those too small to be located by palpation. The xeroradiography examination and the doctor's examination of the breast usually take only about 20 minutes.

BIOPSY: When a doctor believes there is good evidence of a cancer in a breast as a result of thermography, xeroradiography, mammography, palpation of lumps, and other factors, the next step is a biopsy study. The suspected lesion is located for the biopsy procedure and the exact position and extent of the planned incision is marked on the

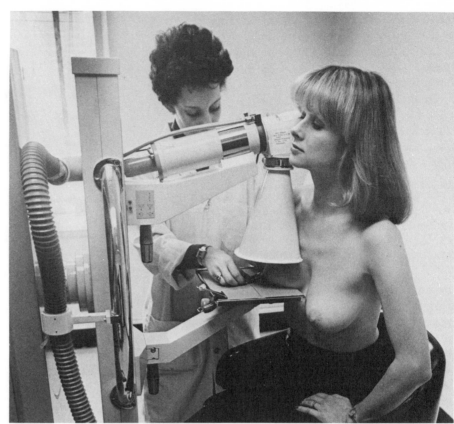

A complete checkup for possible breast cancer involves thermography (recording the heat generated by the breast) and mammography (X rays).

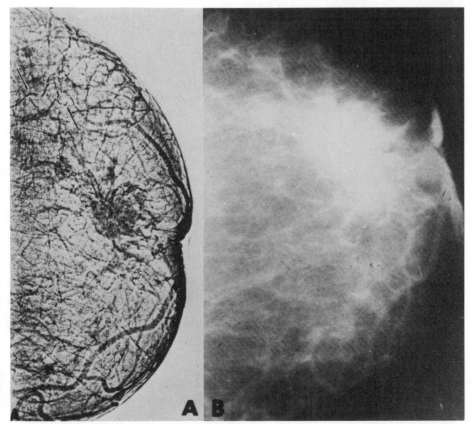

A comparison between a xeroradiogram *(left)* and a mammogram *(right)* of the same breast. The specklike area of cancer shows more clearly in the xeroradiogram.

skin. The patient is then wheeled into the operating room and the tissue sample is excised while the patient is anesthetized. An entire nodule of breast tissue is removed for microscopic examination of the tissue cells. It is sent to the pathology department, which usually reports within 90 minutes whether the tissue is noncancerous or malignant. Provisional preparations are made for a mastectomy. If the lesion is not cancerous—and between 60 and 80 percent of biopsies of breast lumps are not—the patient is taken back to the recovery room and reassured that the tumor was benign. The incision made for the biopsy leaves an almost indiscernible scar.

THE TWO-STEP PROCEDURE: Because of the psychological and physical problems associated with breast cancer, approaches to surgery have changed drastically in recent years. The patient today has a choice: if she desires, she can request that the test and operation take place in two separate stages. To make that choice, the woman simply does not sign a form granting permission to perform both the biopsy and the *mastectomy*, or breast removal, on the same day.

In many cases, it may be necessary to perform both operations on the same day. In such cases, experts say, the woman should insist that her surgeon refer her for pre-surgical *staging*.

Staging involves administration of various tests that are carried out before a mastectomy. The tests show whether the cancer has already spread, or metastasized, to other parts of the body outside the breast and local lymph node regions. Staging is widely regarded as a necessary procedure in all cases of breast cancer. A mastectomy has the single purpose of preventing the spread of cancer; the patient has to know, for her own peace of mind, whether it has already spread.

A two-step procedure involves other choices. Where the biopsy is to be carried out separately, the patient may ask to have it done under local anesthesia as an outpatient. That possibility can be explored with the surgeon. If a general anesthetic appears preferable, the patient may have to spend a night in the hospital. But the *diagnostic biopsy*—involving surgical removal of the entire tumor—and mastectomy can still be performed separately. After a biopsy specimen is removed, the specimen may be subjected to an estrogen-receptor assay. The assay tells the surgeon whether or not the cancer depends on the female hormone estrogen for its growth. That information provides a clue to possible future treatment.

Following the biopsy, the patient receives the pathologist's report on whether the finding is positive or negative. If positive, precise information will usually be given on the type of cancer and where it is located in the breast. Then the patient may want to obtain a second opinion on the permanent-section pathology report and slides. The

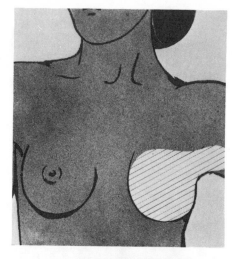
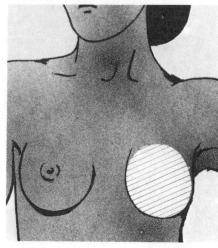

The striped areas show the tissue removed in a radical (above) and a simple (below) mastectomy, including the axillary lymph nodes in the former case.

second opinion is also given by a pathologist. It helps materially in making decisions on appropriate surgery.

Mastectomy

If the lesion is malignant, the surgeon proceeds with the mastectomy. Depending on the seriousness of the case and the procedure recommended by the surgeon and pathologist, the operation may be a *simple mastectomy*, a *radical mastectomy*, a *modified radical mastectomy*, or any of a number of other forms of breast operation. In the United States until recently, radical mastectomy was the usual procedure for breast cancer treatment. Today, at least seven different types of mastectomy, some more widely

accepted than others, may be performed. All may be recommended in different cases depending on the type of cancer, its invasive potential, or ability to spread, and other factors. The seven:

• *Wedge excision*, *lumpectomy*, or *segmental resection*: the tumor is removed along with some surrounding tissue

• *Simple mastectomy*: the breast alone is removed

• *Simple mastectomy* accompanied by *low axillary dissection*: the breast is removed along with some of the underarm nodes or glands

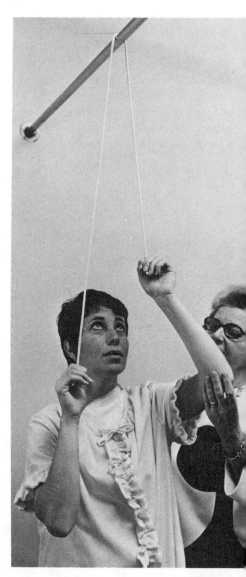

A mastectomy patient doing muscle-strengthening exercises in the American Cancer Society's "Reach to Recovery" program.

• *Modified-radical mastectomy* accompanied by *full axillary dissection*: the breast is removed along with all the lymph glands under the arm

• *Halsted-type radical mastectomy*: the breast is removed along with all the underarm lymph glands and the chest muscles

• *Radical mastectomy with internal mammary node biopsy*: the same procedure as the Halsted-type radical mastectomy, except that the lymph nodes that lie under the ribs, next to the breastbone, are also sampled for biopsy

• *Super-radical mastectomy*: the same as the above, but all of the internal mammary nodes are removed

Most patients have deep concern about many aspects of breast surgery, including the cosmetic effects. For that reason, it is important to select the appropriate type of surgery. The rates of survival appear to depend as much on timely use of pre- and post-operative radiotherapy and post-operative chemotherapy as on the type of operation. But the kind of operation may determine whether the patient will be able to function normally in a relatively short period of time.

Post-Operative Chemotheraphy and Immunotherapy

Immunotherapy after breast surgery has also become more common (see "Relief from Allergies" "Immunotherapy") p. 288. Immunotherapy, or immunization therapy, seeks to strengthen the patient's own body defenses against cancer. In one form of immunotherapy, a vaccine known as *BCG (bacille Calmette-Guerin)* is

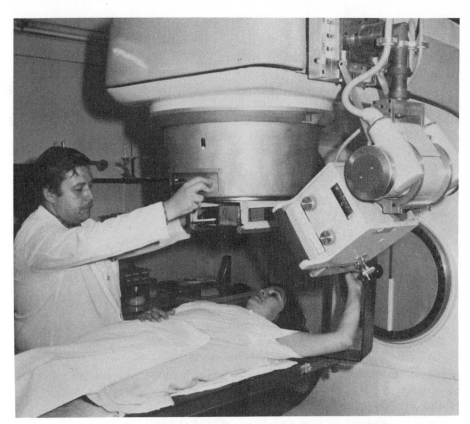

Radiation therapy is frequently used to treat breast cancer patients, sometimes in combination with surgery and other times with drugs.

administered. The vaccine, ordinarily used to prevent tuberculosis, stimulates the production of antibodies that are believed to destroy cancer cells. Immunotherapy, it should be noted, was still somewhat experimental in the early 1980s.

Other Therapeutic Measures

In some cases of breast cancer, surgeons may recommend excision of the ovaries in addition to removal of breast tissue. Because of the relationships between ovarian function and breast cancer, some doctors believe that elimination of estrogen production by means of surgery or radiation can increase the chances of long-term cure.

Radiation therapy frequently is recommended for cases of breast cancer when the disease is so far advanced that surgery is not feasible, or when the patient's health is too poor to risk surgery. In addition, radiation treatment may be effective in reducing the pain in bones or areas of the central nervous system that may have been invaded by metastasized cancer cells. Radiation also may be used in addition to chemotherapy in certain cases because X rays, or similar radiation, can reach areas where chemical medications cannot penetrate. When administered immediately after surgery, radiation appears to reduce by as much as 50 percent the chances of recurrence of breast cancer.

CHAPTER 28

Home Care of the Sick

Patients suffering from serious illnesses or from certain communicable diseases should be hospitalized. Home care facilities do not normally include the expensive and delicate medical equipment required for the complete care of these diseases.

If, however, the physician in charge of a case decides that his patient does not need hospitalization and that adequate home nursing care can be provided, the well-being of the patient can be greatly enhanced by his being cared for in the comfortable and familiar surroundings of his own home.

When the decision to treat a patient at home is made, it must be understood that the doctor's orders regarding rest, exercise, diet, and medications have to be rigorously adhered to. Nursing responsibilities assigned to the patient and whoever else is tending to the patient's recovery should be carried out as conscientiously as they would be if the patient's care were entrusted to a team of medical professionals in a hospital environment.

The physician in charge of a case should, of course, be notified of any significant changes in the condition of the patient. The doctor should be contacted if, for example, the patient complains of severe pain, pain of long duration, or pain that apparently is not directly related to an injury or surgical procedure. The location and characteristics of the pain should be noted, and the doctor will want to know whether the pain is affected by changing the position of the patient or if it seems to be related to the intake of food or fluids.

In addition to being informed of such potentially dangerous developments, the doctor should get daily or frequent reports on the patient's progress. The easiest and best way to see that this is done is to keep a written record of the following functions, symptoms, and conditions of the patient:

1. Morning and evening body temperature, pulse rate, and respiration rate.

2. Bowel movements—frequency, consistency of stools, presence of blood.

3. Urination—amount, frequency, presence of burning sensation, color.

4. Vomiting or nausea.

5. The amount and kind of solid foods and liquids taken by the patient.

6. Hours of sleep.

7. Medications given. Medications should be administered only on the instructions of the physician.

8. Patient's general appearance. This includes any unusual swelling, skin rash, or skin discoloration.

9. General mental and psychological condition of the patient, such as signs of irritability or despondency.

Checking the Pulse and Respiration

The pulse and respiration are usually checked in the morning and again in the evening; the doctor may recommend other times as well.

Pulse

The home nurse should learn how to measure the pulse rate in beats per minute. A watch with a second hand or a nearby electric clock will help count the passage of time while the pulse beat is counted. The pulse can be felt on the inner side of the wrist, above the thumb; the pulse also can be checked at the temple, the throat, or at the ankle if for some reason the wrist is not conveniently accessible.

The patient should be resting quietly when the pulse is counted; if the patient has been physically active the pulse count probably will be higher than normal, suggesting a possible disorder when none actually exists. Temperature extremes, emotional upsets, and the digesting of a meal also can produce misleading pulse rates.

510

What is a normal pulse rate? The answer is hard to define in standard or average terms. For an adult male, a pulse rate of about 72 per minute is considered normal. The pulse of an adult woman might range around 80 per minute and still be normal. For children, a normal pulse might be one that is regularly well above 100 per minute. Also, a normal pulse may vary by a few beats per minute in either direction from the average for the individual. The home nurse with a bit of practice can determine whether a patient's pulse is significantly fast or slow, strong or weak, and report any important changes to the doctor.

Respiration

The patient's respiration can be checked while his pulse is taken. By observing the rising and falling of the patient's chest, a close estimate of the rate of respiration can be made. An average for adults would be close to 16 per minute, with a variation of a few inhalations and exhalations in either direction. The rate of respiration, like the pulse rate, is higher in children.

Sometimes the respiration rate can be noted without making it obvious to the patient that there is concern about the information; many persons alter their natural breathing rate unconsciously if they know that function is being watched.

Body Temperature

A fever thermometer, available at any drugstore, is specially shaped to help the home nurse read any tiny change in the patient's temperature, such changes being measured in tenths of a degree. Instead of being round in cross-section like an ordinary thermometer, a fever thermometer is flat on one side and ridge-shaped on the other. The inner surface of the flat side is coated with a reflective material and the ridge-shaped side actually is a magnifying lens. Thus, to read a fever thermometer quickly and properly, one looks at the lens (ridged) side.

How to Take the Temperature

The usual ways of taking temperature are by mouth (oral) or by the rectum (rectal), and fever thermometers are specialized for these uses. The rectal thermometer has a more rounded bulb to protect the sensitive tissues in the anus. Normal body temperature taken orally is 98.6° F. or 37° C. for most people, but slight variations do occur in the normal range. When the temperature is taken rectally, a normal reading is about 1° F. higher—99.6° F. or about 37.5° C.—because rectal veins in the area elevate the temperature slightly.

Before a patient's temperature is taken, the thermometer should be carefully cleaned with soap and water, then wiped dry, or sterilized in alcohol or similar disinfectant. The thermometer should then be grasped firmly at the shaft and shaken briskly, bulb end downward, to force the mercury down to a level of 95° F. or lower—or 35° C. or lower if the thermometer is calibrated according to the Celsius temperature scale. See the chart *Body Temperature in Degrees* for comparative values of the Fahrenheit and Celsius scales.

BODY TEMPERATURE IN DEGREES		
Fahrenheit		**Celsius**
105.5		40.8
105		40.6
104.5		40.3
104		40
103.5		39.7
103		39.4
102.5		39.2
102		38.9
101.5		38.6
101		38.3
100.5		38.1
100		37.8
99.5		37.5
99		37.2
98.6	Normal Range	37.0
97.8		36.6

If the temperature is taken orally, the thermometer should be moistened in clean fresh water and placed well under the tongue on one side. If the temperature is taken rectally, the thermometer should be dipped first in petroleum jelly and then inserted about one inch into the opening of the rectum. If an oral thermometer is used in the rectum, special care should be taken to make sure that the lubrication is adequate and that it is inserted gently to avoid irritating rectal tissues. Whichever method is used, the thermometer should be left in place for at least three minutes in order to get an accurate reading.

If circumstances preclude an oral or rectal temperature check, the patient's temperature may be taken under the arm; a normal reading in that area is about 97.6° F. or 36.5° C.

Above-Normal Temperature

If the patient's temperature hovers around one degree above his normal reading, the home nurse should note the fact and watch for other signs of a fever that would indicate the presence of an infection or some other bodily disorder. A mild fever immediately after surgery or during the course of an infectious disease may not be cause for alarm. Also, the normal body temperature of a mature woman may vary with hormonal changes during her menstrual cycle. But when oral temperatures rise above 100° F. the change should be regarded as a warning signal. A rise of as much as three degrees above normal, Fahrenheit, for a period of several hours or more, could be critical, and a physician should be notified immediately.

Sleep

Another item to be checked each day for the at-home medical records is the patient's sleeping habits. While there is no standard number of hours of sleep per day preferred for healthy individuals, a regular pattern of sleep is very important during recovery from disease or injury, and an obvious change from such a pattern can suggest tension, discomfort, or other problems. Typical daily sleep periods for most adults range from seven to nine hours, while children and infants may sleep as much as 12 to 20 hours per day and be considered normal; sleep in the form of naps should be included in total amounts per day.

Making the Patient Comfortable

A good deal of the patient's time at home will be devoted to sleep or rest, most or all of it in bed. The bed should give firm support to the body; if the mattress does not offer such support, place a thick sheet of plywood between the springs and mattress. Pillows can be placed under the head and shoulders of the patient to raise those parts of the body from time to time. When the patient is lying on his back, a small pillow can be slipped under the knees to provide support and comfort. A small pillow can also be placed under the small of the back if necessary. Additional pillows may be placed as needed between the ankles or under one foot or both feet.

If the pressure of bed clothing on the feet causes discomfort, a bridge made from a grocery carton or similar box can be placed over the feet but beneath the blankets. To help maintain muscle tone and circulation in the feet and legs, a firm barrier can be placed as needed at the foot of the bed so the patient can stretch his legs and push against the barrier while lying on his back.

Changing Position

Helping the patient change position in bed is an important home-nursing technique. Unless a definite effort is made to help the patient change positions at regular intervals the sick person may tend to curl up into a sort of fetal position, with the hips and knees flexed and the spine curved. While this position may be preferred by the patient in order to increase body warmth or to relieve pain, the practice of staying in one position for long periods of time can lead to loss of muscle tone and even deformities.

Moving or positioning the patient in bed should, of course, be done according to directions outlined by the doctor for the specific medical problem involved. Body movements should not aggravate any injury or other disorder by placing undue strain or stress on a body part or organ system that is in the healing stage. At the same time, the patient should be stimulated and encouraged to change positions frequently and to use as much of his own strength as possible.

If the patient is likely to need a very long period of bed rest, and the family can afford the modest expense, it may be wise to purchase or rent a hospital-type bed. The basic hospital bed is higher from the floor than ordinary beds, making the tasks of changing bed linens, taking temperatures, etc., easier for the home nurse. More sophisticated hospital beds have manual or electrical controls to raise the head and foot of the bed.

Helping the Patient Sit Up

The patient can be helped to a sitting position in bed by placing one arm, palm upward, under the patient's shoulder while the patient extends an arm around the nurse's back or shoulders. The nurse also may slip both hands, palms facing upward, under the patient's pillow, raising it along with the patient's head and shoulders. The same procedures can be used to help move a patient from one side of the bed to the other if the patient is unable to move himself.

When the patient has been raised to a sitting position, he should try to brace his arms behind him on the bed surface with elbows straightened. If the patient feels dizzy or faint as a result of the effort, he can be lowered to the back rest position again by simply reversing the procedure.

When the patient is able to support himself in a sitting position, he should be encouraged to dangle his legs over the side of the bed, and—when his strength permits—to move to a chair beside the bed and rest for a while in a seated position.

Bathing the Patient

A patient who is unable to leave the bed will require special help in bathing. When bath time comes, the nurse will need a large basin of warm water, soap, a washcloth, and several towels, large and small. A cotton blanket also should be used to replace the regular blanket during bathing, and pillows should be removed from the bed unless they are

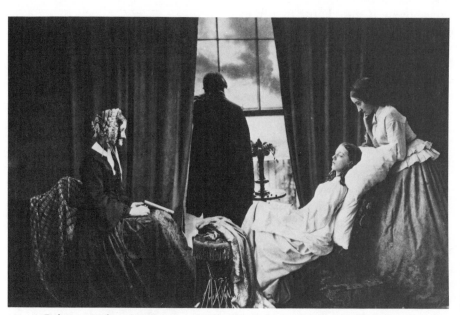

Today, as in the past, many terminally ill people are choosing to die at home in the care of a loving family rather than in an impersonal hospital setting.

necessary at the time.

One large towel should be placed under the patient's head and another should be placed on top of the bath blanket, with part of the towel folded under the bath blanket. This preliminary procedure should help protect the bed area from moisture that may be spilled during the bathing procedure.

The bath should begin at the area of the eyes, using only clear water and brushing outward from the eyes. Soapy water can be applied to the rest of the face, as needed, with rinsing afterward. After the face, bathing and rinsing are continued over the chest and abdomen, the arms and hands, the legs and feet, and the back of the body from the neck downward to the buttocks. The external genitalia are washed last.

During the washing procedure, the nurse uses firm strokes to aid circulation and checks for signs of pressure areas or bed sores. Skin lotions or body powders may be applied, and a back rub given, after washing. The teeth may be brushed and the patient may want to use a mouth wash. After the personal hygiene routine is completed, a fresh pair of pajamas can be put on. If bed linen needs to be changed, the bathing period provides a good opportunity for that chore.

Changing the Bed Linen

Changing the bed linen while the patient is in bed can be a challenge for any home nurse. However, there are a few shortcuts that make the task much easier. First, remove all pillows, or all but one, as well as the top spread if one is used. Loosen the rest of the bedding materials on all sides and begin removing the sheets from the head of the bed, top sheet first. By letting the patient hold the top edge of the blanket, or by tucking the top edges under his shoulder, the blanket can remain in place while the top sheet is pulled down, under the blanket, to the foot of the bed. If the top sheet is to be used as the next bottom sheet, it can be folded and

placed on the side with the top spread.

Next, the patient must be moved to one side of the bed and the bottom sheet gathered in a flat roll close to the patient. Then the clean bottom sheet is unfolded on the mattress cover and the edges, top, and bottom, tucked under the mattress. The rest of the clean sheet is spread over the empty side of the bed and pushed in a flat roll under the soiled sheet next to the patient's back.

The next step is to roll the patient from one side of the bed onto the clean sheet that has been spread on the other side. The soiled bottom sheets can be pulled out easily and the new bottom sheet spread and tucked in on the other side.

The new top sheet can be pulled up under the blanket, which has been used to cover the patient throughout the change of bed linens. Finally, the top spread and pillows can be replaced, after the pillow cases have been changed. A special effort should be made, meanwhile, to keep the mattress cover and bottom sheet of the patient's bed as flat and smooth as possible and to allow room for the feet to move while the sheets are firmly tucked in at the foot of the bed.

The home nurse should handle the soiled linens carefully if the patient is being treated for an infectious disease; they should never be held close to the face.

Bowel Movements and Urination

If the patient is expected to remain bedridden for a long period of time, the home nurse should acquire a bedpan and perhaps a urinal from a drugstore. A sheet of oilcloth, rubber, or plastic material should also be provided to protect the bed during bowel movements and urination.

If the patient is unable to sit up on a bedpan because of weakness, his body can be propped up with pillows. If he is capable of getting out of bed but is unable to walk to the bath-

room, a commode can be placed near the bed and the patient can be helped from the bed to the commode and back. Another alternative is to use a wheelchair or any chair with casters to move the patient between the bedroom and bathroom.

Administering an Enema

Occasionally, the doctor may recommend an enema to help the patient empty his bowels or to stimulate the peristaltic action associated with normal functioning of the intestinal tract.

Since enemas are seldom an emergency aspect of home nursing, there usually is time to purchase disposable enema units from a drugstore. The disposable enema contains about four or five ounces of prepared solution packaged in a plastic bag with a lubricated nozzle for injecting the fluid into the patient's rectum. The entire package can be thrown away after it has been used, thus eliminating the need to clean and store equipment. The alternative is to use a traditional enema bag filled with plain warm water or a prescribed formulation.

An enema is best administered while the patient is lying on his side with his knees drawn up toward his chest. When using the disposable enema unit, the home nurse simply squeezes the solution through the lubricated nozzle that has been inserted into the rectum. When using an enema bag, the home nurse should lubricate the nozzle before insertion. After insertion of the nozzle, the enema bag should be held or suspended above the patient so that, upon the opening of the valve which controls the flow of the enema, the liquid will flow easily into the patient's rectum.

Feeding the Patient

It may be necessary at times for the home nurse to feed a patient unable to feed himself. An effort should be

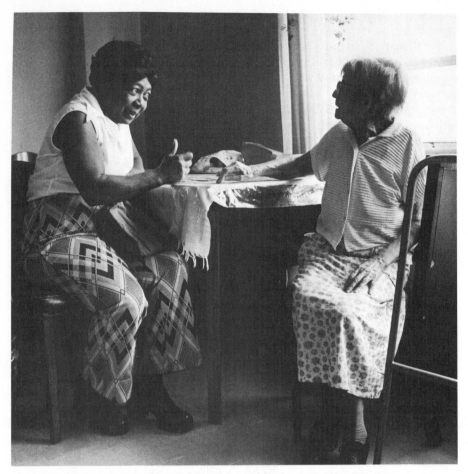

This disabled widow gets regular assistance from a volunteer worker, herself a senior citizen, as part of the federal program called ACTION.

made to serve meals to the patient in an attractive and, when possible, colorful manner. The bedding should be protected with towels or plastic sheeting and the patient made as comfortable as possible with his head raised.

Liquids should be offered in a spoon filled about two-thirds full with any drops on the bottom of the spoon carefully wiped off. The spoon should be held so that the area between the tip and the side touch the patient's lower lip. Then the spoon is tilted toward the tip so the liquid will run into the patient's mouth. The process takes time, and much patience is required of the nurse. The patient may be slow to swallow and in no hurry to finish the meal.

If the patient can take liquids through a glass tube or plastic straw, the home nurse should see to it that the end of the tube inserted in the container of liquid is always below the surface of the fluid so that the patient will swallow as little air as possible.

A patient who can drink liquids from a spoon or tube may be able to drink from a cup. In making the step from tube or spoon to cup, the home nurse can help the patient by holding the cup by its handle and letting the patient guide the cup to his lips with his own hands.

The nurse should always make sure the patient is fully alert before trying to put food or liquid into his mouth; a semiconscious person may not be able to swallow. The nurse also should test the temperature of the food; cold foods should be served cold and warm foods should be served warm. But foods should never be too hot or too cold for the patient. Finally, the dishes, tubes, or

other devices used to feed the patient should be carefully cleaned before storing them.

Ice Bags and Hot-Water Bottles

Ice bags and hot-water bottles frequently are used in home nursing to relieve pain and discomfort. The temperature of the water in a hot-water bottle or bag should be tested before it is placed near a patient's body. The maximum temperature of the water should be about 130° F., and preferably a few degrees cooler. The hot-water container should never be placed directly against the skin of a patient; it must be covered with soft material, such as a towel, to protect the patient against burns. A patient who is receiving pain-killing medications could suffer serious tissue damage from a hot-water bottle without feeling severe pain.

When ice is the preferred method of relieving pain, it can be applied in a rubber or plastic bag sealed to prevent leakage and covered with a soft cloth. Cold applications to very young and old persons should be handled cautiously and with medical consultation, particularly if ice packs are to be applied to large body areas for long periods of time; individuals at both age extremes can lack the normal physiological mechanisms for coping with the effects of cold temperatures.

Steam Inhalators

If the at-home patient suffers from a respiratory ailment that is relieved by steam inhalation, there are several devices to provide the relief he needs. One, is the commercial electric inhalator which boils water to which a few drops of a volatile medication are added to provide a pleasantly moist and warm breathing environment. If a commercial inhalator is not available, a similar apparatus can be made by fashioning a cone from a sheet of newspaper and placing the wide end of the cone over the top and spout of a teapot containing freshly boiled water. The narrow end of the cone will direct the hot water vapor toward the face of the patient. If a medication is to be added, it can be applied to a ball of cotton placed in the cone; the steam or water vapor will pick up the medication as it passes through the cone.

If medicated vapor is intended for a small child or infant, the end of the cone can be directed into a canopy or tent made of blankets placed over a crib or the head of a bed. This arrangement should produce an effective respiratory environment for the child while keeping his body safely separated from the hot teakettle.

Still another method of providing steam inhalation for a patient requires only an old-fashioned washstand pitcher and bowl plus a grocery bag. An opening is cut in one corner of the bottom of the bag which is placed upside down over the pitcher filled with hot steaming water and, if needed, a medication. The patient simply breathes the hot moist air seeping through the opening in the bag. The pitcher of steaming water is placed in a bowl or basin as a safety precaution.

Improvising Sickroom Devices

With a bit of imagination, many sickroom devices can be contrived from items already around the house. A criblike bed railing can be arranged, for example, by lining up a series of ordinary kitchen chairs beside a bed; if necessary, they can be tied together to prevent a patient from falling out of bed. The bed itself can be raised to the level of a hospital bed by placing the bed legs on blocks built from scrap lumber. Cardboard boxes can be shaped with scissors and tape into bed rests, foot supports, bed tables, or other helpful bedside aids.

Plastic bags from the kitchen can be used to collect tissues and other materials that must be removed reg-

ularly from the sickroom. Smaller plastic bags may be attached to the side of the bed to hold comb, hairbrush, and other personal items.

Keeping Health Records

The family that keeps good records of past injuries and illnesses, as well as immunization information and notes on reactions to medications, has a head start in organizing the home care of a member who suddenly requires nursing. The file of family health records should include information about temperatures and pulse rates taked during periods of good health; such data can serve as benchmark readings for evaluating the information recorded during periods of illness. Also, if each member of the family can practice taking temperatures and counting pulse and respiration rates during periods of good health, the family will be better able to handle home nursing routines when the need arises.

Home Care Equipment Checklist

Following is a convenient checklist of basic supplies needed for home care of the sick:

1. Disinfectants for soaking clothing and utensils used by the sick. Not all disinfectants are equally effective for every purpose. For clothing and food utensils, corrosive or poisonous disinfectants are to be avoided. Antiseptics do not kill bacteria; they only retard their growth. Among the common disinfectants that can be used in the home are:

• Alcohol, 75 percent by weight, used for disinfecting instruments and cleaning the skin

• Lysol for decontaminating clothing and utensils

• Soap with an antibacterial agent for scrubbing the hands

• Carbolic acid (phenol) for disinfecting instruments and utensils. It is corrosive, poisonous, and very effective if used in 5 percent solution

• Cresol in 2.5 percent solution for disinfecting sputum and feces. It is

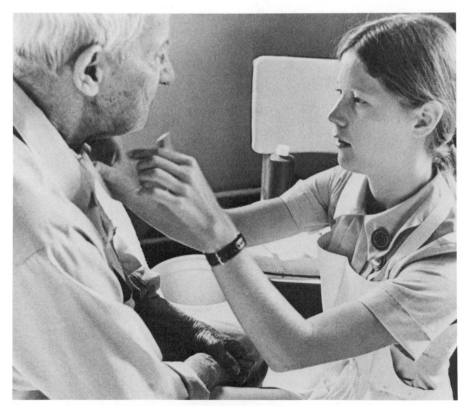

Visiting nurse services in many cities provide home nursing care for patients who do not need hospitalization but do need medical attention.

less poisonous than phenol and can be obtained as an alkali solution in soap

• Boric acid, a weak antiseptic eyewash

• Detergent creams, used to reduce skin bacteria.

2. Disposable rubber gloves, to be used when handling patients with open wounds or contagious diseases, as well as for cleaning feces.

3. Paper napkins and tissues for cleaning nasal and oral discharges.

4. Rectal and oral thermometers. The former is used primarily for infants, while the latter is used for adults and older children. Thermometers should always be thoroughly disinfected after use by soaking in isopropyl alcohol, and they should be washed prior to reuse.

5. Eating and drinking utensils to be used only by the patient. Disposable utensils are preferable.

6. Urinal, bedpan, and sputum cup for patients who cannot go to the toilet. After use, they should be thoroughly disinfected with cresol and washed with liquid soap containing an antibacterial agent.

7. Personal toilet requisites: face cloths and towels, toilet soap, washbasin, toothbrush and toothpaste, comb, hairbrush, razor, and a water pitcher (if running water is not accessible to the patient).

8. Measuring glass graduated in teaspoon and tablespoon levels for liquid medication.

9. Plastic waste-disposal bags that can be closed and tied.

CHAPTER 29

Other Diseases of Major Importance

This chapter discusses a number of diseases of major importance that are not dealt with elsewhere: acquired immune deficiency syndrome (AIDS), a disease characterized by a defect in the body's natural immune system; plague, of great historical importance but fortunately now uncommon in the United States; two infectious diseases—tularemia and Rocky Mountain Spotted Fever; and seven major tropical diseases that afflict millions of people in the warmer regions of the world and that occasionally occur elsewhere—malaria and yellow fever, leishmaniasis, trypanosomiasis, filariasis, schistosomiasis, and leprosy.

AIDS

First reported widely in 1981, AIDS has become a priority of the U.S. Public Health Service. People with AIDS (PWAs) are susceptible to a variety of unusual or rare illnesses called "opportunistic diseases." These include a parasite-caused form of pneumonia, and Kaposi's sarcoma, a rare type of cancer that attacks the blood vessel walls. In the great majority of the reported AIDS cases, PWAs have included members of the following adult groups:

• Males who have had sex with more than one male partner since 1979, and males whose sole male sexual partner has had sex with more than one male since 1979;

• Past or present abusers of intravenous drugs;

• Hemophiliacs;

• Sexual partners of persons in these groups.

Nearly half of all diagnosed PWAs have died. Others may live one to three years. But no treatment has successfully restored the immune system of an AIDS patient to normal functioning. While the specific causes of AIDS are unknown, researchers have found evidence of several viral infections in the blood of sufferers. Three such infections are cytomegalovirus (CMV), Epstein-Barr virus (EBV), and human T-cell leukemia virus III (HTLV-III). Research has focused on the last as the probable cause of AIDS.

Symptoms

Some PWAs have recalled specific symptoms before a diagnosis of AIDS was made. The symptoms may be confusing, however, because they often resemble those of flu or even the common cold. They may include swollen glands, or enlarged lymph nodes, in the neck, armpits, or groin; night sweats; fever; unexplained weight loss; diarrhea; fatigue; and loss of appetite. Physicians suggest that persons showing such symptoms over a period of time should seek medical advice. AIDS appears to have an incubation period ranging from a few months to two or more years.

Prevention

To prevent the spread of AIDS, the U.S. Public Health Service has recommended that persons at risk of contracting the disease use extreme caution. To avoid spreading AIDS to other people, including family members and close contacts, these persons should:

517

• Forgo donations of blood or plasma, sperm, body organs, or other tissues.

• Limit sexual contacts and be frank with sexual partners about steps taken to prevent the spread of the virus.

• Avoid practices in which exchange of body fluids, including semen, takes place.

• Refrain from sharing toothbrushes, razors, or other implements that could become contaminated with blood.

• If a drug user, limit drug use, do not let others use needles you have used, and do not leave needles or other items where others might use them.

• If a woman who has had a positive antibody test (see below) or who is the sexual partner of a man with a positive antibody test, avoid or postpone pregnancy. The disease can be transmitted from mother to unborn child in the mother's uterus.

The U.S. Public Health Service has reported that no evidence indicates that the AIDS virus can be transmitted through casual kissing or other casual social contacts. But persons who have had positive antibody tests should let their doctors and dentists know about the test results. The physician and dentist can then cooperate in preventing the spread of the virus—if the patient has become infected. In general, all persons should avoid sexual contact with persons at risk; avoid sex, whether homosexual or heterosexual, with multiple partners; and take routine but thorough care in handling blood. There is no risk of contracting AIDS through blood donations because needles and other supplies are used only once and then discarded. The risk of contracting AIDS through blood transfusion is also insignificant since the implementation of blood-screening procedures.

Treatment

Although there is no known cure, a blood test—called the ELISA test —has been developed to identify the presence of antibodies to the AIDS virus in human blood. The presence of antibodies does not necessarily mean the person will become ill with AIDS. Nor does the absence of antibodies mean the person does not have the disease. This person could, for example, have the virus in an incubational stage. A positive test does mean the individual should undergo a follow-up test called the "Western blot." This test will ensure that the results of the ELISA test are accurate.

Doctors have had some success in treating the various illnesses that attack AIDS patients. Antibiotics have been used to treat *Pneumocystis carinii*. Interferon, a virus-fighting protein that the body produces naturally, has been used to treat PWAs with Kaposi's sarcoma. Some attempts to repair the immunologic deficiencies of AIDS patients have relied on natural and genetically produced preparations of interleukin, or Interleukin-2, one of the elements of the human body's immune system. Clinical studies of suramin and other antiviral agents have also shown some promise. But researchers and physicians believe treatments are needed for all stages of AIDS infections.

Plague

Bubonic plague, one of the many diseases transmitted to humans through direct or indirect contact with animals, usually is listed among the scourges of past centuries. At least three great epidemics of bubonic plague have been recorded, including the Black Death of the 14th century when the disease claimed at least 50 million lives. The most recent worldwide epidemic of the plague occurred in the 1800s. While recent cases of the plague in North America have been relatively rare, the disease organism is still carried by rodents, including squirrels, rats, and rabbits; and cases of the plague still occur in the western United States. Increased activity in western areas by hunters, campers, and other outdoor enthusiasts has resulted in a higher incidence of the disease among humans in recent years. The disease also is fairly common in Asia, Africa, and South America.

Symptoms

The infection is transmitted from animals to man through the bite of a flea carrying the disease organism. Symptoms usually develop in several days but may take as long as two weeks after the flea bite. The victim experiences chills and fever, with the temperature rising above 102° Fahrenheit. He may feel headaches, a rapid heart beat, and find it difficult to walk. Vomiting and delirium also are among the symptoms of plague. There may be pain and tenderness of the lymph nodes, which become inflamed and swollen; the enlarged lymph nodes are known as *buboes*, a term that gives its name to the type of plague involved. The buboes occur most frequently in the legs and groin because the flea bites are most likely to introduce the disease through the legs; children may develop buboes in glands of the neck and shoulder areas.

The site of the flea bite may or may not be found after the symptoms develop. If present, it may be marked by a swollen, pus-filled area of the skin.

Diagnosis of plague can be confirmed by laboratory tests that might include examination of the bacteria taken in samples from buboes or other diseased areas of the body, inoculation of laboratory animals with suspected disease organisms, and studies of the white blood cells of the patient.

Complications can include pneumonia and hemorrhages, with bleeding from the nose or mouth or through the gastrointestinal or urinary tracts, and abscesses and ulcerations. The pneumonic form of plague can be transmitted from one person to another like colds or other infectious diseases; in other words, plague organisms are spread by being exhaled by one person and inhaled by another.

Treatment and Prevention

As in other infectious diseases, early treatment is most effective. Antibiotics are administered every day for a period of one to two weeks and buboes are treated with hot, moist applications. The buboes may be drained if necessary after the patient has responded to antibiotic medications. Antibiotics have reduced the fatality rate from plague infections from a high of 90 percent to a maximum of about 10 percent. Vaccines are available but are of limited and temporary value. Prevention requires eradication of rats and other possibly infected rodents (some 200 species are known to carry the disease), use of insecticides to control fleas, and avoiding contact with wild animals in areas where plague is known to exist. Domestic animals also should be protected from contact with possibly infected wild animals.

Tularemia

An infectious disease known as *tularemia*, sometimes called rabbit fever, is transmitted from animals to humans who come in contact with the animal tissues. It also can be transmitted through the bites of ticks or flies or by drinking contaminated water. Like the plague-disease organism, tularemia can be transmitted by inhalation of infected particles from the lungs of a diseased person, although such occurrences are rare.

Symptoms

Within a couple of days to perhaps two weeks after exposure to the tularemia germ, the patient develops chills and a fever with temperatures rising to 103°F. or higher. Other symptoms include headache, nausea and vomiting, extreme weakness, and drenching sweats. Lymph nodes become enlarged and a pus-filled lesion develops at the site of the infection. Usually only one pustular papule develops on a finger or other

skin area, marking the point of the insect bite or contact with infected animal tissues; but there may be several such sores in the membranes of the mouth if that is the point of infection. It is not uncommon for the eyes or lungs to become involved.

Laboratory tests, along with a record of contact with wild animals or game birds, eating improperly cooked meats, being bitten by deer flies or ticks, or drinking water from ponds or streams, usually helps verify the cause of the symptoms as tularemia. In some cases the contact with the disease organism can be made through bites or scratches of infected dogs or cats, but most frequently the disease in humans originates through handling of the meat or fur of wild animals or by camping or hiking in areas where the disease is endemic.

TREATMENT: Treatment includes bed rest and administration of antibiotics. Adequate fluid intake is important and oxygen may be required. Aspirin usually is given also, to relieve headache and muscle aches. Hot compresses are applied to the enlarged lymph node areas; it may be necessary to drain the swollen, infected nodes. If the disease is complicated by pneumonic tularemia or infection of the eye, the patient usually is hospitalized. Success of the therapy depends upon early and adequate treatment. The disease is rarely fatal when properly treated with antibiotics, but it can be lethal if the symptoms are ignored. Anyone who develops the symptoms of tularemia after handling wild animals or being exposed to biting insects or contaminated water in rural or rugged country should seek immediate medical help.

Hunters, campers, hikers, and others venturing into the great outdoors should protect their bodies against invasion by ticks by wearing long-sleeved shirts and long trousers with cuffs securely fastened. Regular checks should be made of the scalp, groin, and armpits for ticks. Any ticks found should be detached quickly and the bite area cleansed

with soap and water, followed by an alcohol cleansing. If the head of the tick breaks off, it can be removed by the same techniques used to remove a splinter from the skin. Raw water from ponds and streams should be boiled or disinfected with chemicals before using. Rubber gloves should be worn while dressing the meat of wild game or birds, and the meat should be thoroughly cooked. On the positive side, once the disease occurs, the recovered patient develops immunity to tularemia.

Rocky Mountain Spotted Fever

The name of an increasingly common tick-borne disease, *Rocky Mountain spotted fever*, is misleading because humans are most likely to become infected in regions far from the Rocky Mountains. The disease, also known as *tick fever*, has become most prevalent in rural and suburban areas of the southern and eastern United States. It is caused by a rickettsial organism transmitted by a tick bite. Wild rodents are a reservoir of the infected ticks that carry the disease.

Symptoms

Rocky Mountain spotted fever may be relatively mild or dangerously severe. The symptoms of headache, chills, and fever may begin suddenly and persist for a period of two or three weeks. Fever temperatures may reach 104° F. and may be accompanied by nausea and occasional vomiting. Headaches have been described in some cases as excruciating, with the pain most intense along the forehead. Muscles of the legs, back, and abdomen may ache and feel tender. The most serious cases seem to develop within a few days after a tick bite, milder cases usually are slower to develop. A rash usually develops a few days after the onset of other symptoms and is most likely to be concentrated on the forearm, ankles, feet, wrists, and hands. If untreated, Rocky Mountain spotted fever symptoms may abate in about two weeks but the infection can be fatal, particularly in persons over the age of 40.

Treatment

Treatment includes administration of antibiotics and, in some cases, steroid hormones. Careful nursing care and adequate intake of protein foods and liquids also are needed.

Preventive measures are similar to those recommended to guard against tularemia. Wear adequate protective clothing that forms a barrier against tick invasion of the skin surfaces, check the scalp and other hairy body areas regularly for ticks, and remove and destroy any ticks found. In addition, ground areas known to be inhabited by wood ticks should be sprayed with an effective insecticide safe for humans; insect repellents also should be applied to clothing and exposed skin surfaces when venturing into wooded or brushy areas. Ticks may become attached to dogs and other animals and care should be used in removing them from the pets because the disease organism can enter the body through minor cuts and scratches on the skin. A vaccine is available for protection of persons who are likely to use possibly infested tick areas for work or recreation. Immunity usually is established by two inoculations, about a month apart, and booster shots as needed.

TROPICAL DISEASES

Most people living in the temperate climates of North America and Europe are spared the ravages of some of the most lethal and debilitating diseases known to mankind. They include malaria, which probably has killed more people than any other disease in history, yellow fever, leishmaniasis, trypanosomiasis, filariasis, schistosomiasis, and leprosy.

While many persons probably have never heard of some of these diseases and at least a few doctors might have trouble in diagnosing the symptoms, they affect hundreds of millions of people each year and could pose a threat to persons living in any part of the world. They are generally classed as tropical diseases, but so-called tropical or exotic diseases have been prevented from spreading into temperate regions partly because of alert medical care and preventive measures by public health experts. Malaria, for example, has been found as far north as the Arctic Circle, as far south as the tip of South America, and at one time was a disease of epidemic proportions in such northern cities as Philadelphia and London. These diseases have altered the course of history, ending the life of Alexander the Great as he tried to conquer the world, nipping in the bud plans of Napoleon to retake Canada from the English, defeating French efforts to build the Panama Canal, and contributing to the black-slave trade between Africa and the Americas.

The major tropical diseases are caused by a variety of organisms, including viruses, protozoa, and worms. Some are transmitted by insect bites, some by contact with contaminated water, and others, like leprosy, are spread by means that remain a mystery despite centuries of medical experience with millions of cases of the disease. Space does not permit detailed discussion of all tropical diseases; only those regarded by medical authorities as among the most significant to world health are described in this chapter.

Malaria

Malaria, one of the most common diseases in the world, gets its name from an Italian word for "bad air" because of a belief in ancient times

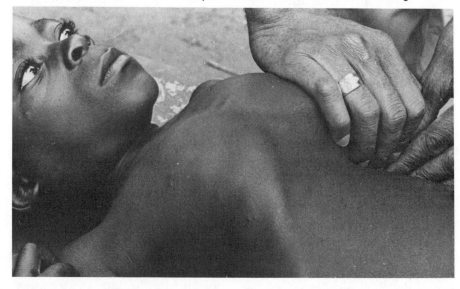

A young man in Africa is checked for spleen enlargment, a symptom of malaria. The disease is rampant wherever water sanitation is lacking.

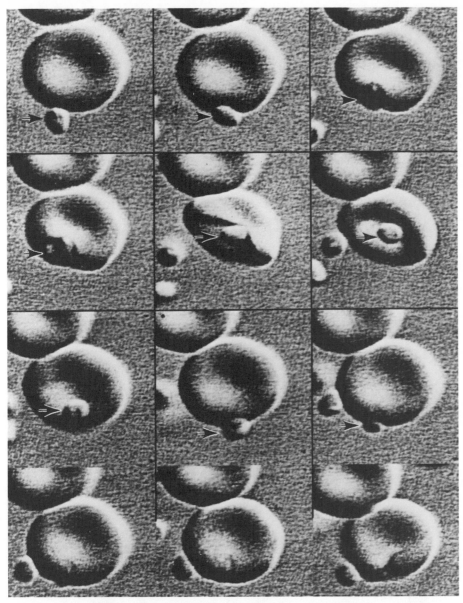

This microscopic sequence, from upper left to lower right, shows the attachment, invasion, and distortion of a red blood cell by a malaria parasite (arrow).

plasmodia, or protozoa, that cause the infection do not produce the same specific effects. However, the general symptoms common to all forms of malaria are fever, chills, headache, muscle pains, and, in some cases, skin disorders such as cold sores, hives, or a rash. A malaria attack may begin with a severe chill that lasts from twenty minutes to an hour, followed by a fever lasting from three to eight hours with temperature rising to more than 104° Fahrenheit. The fever usually is accompanied by profuse sweating, and the afflicted person is left exhausted by the cycle of chills and fever. The attacks become more or less successively milder, less frequent, and more irregular, and finally cease, although there may be relapses.

One kind of malarial organism seems to cause attacks that occur every other day while another type produces attacks that appear quite regularly on every third day; still another type of malaria plasmodium seems to cause a fever that is continuous. While the liver seems to be a favored target organ, other body systems can be involved, with related complications. If the organism reaches the brain, the patient may suffer convulsions, delirium, partial paralysis, or coma. If the organism invades the lungs, there may be coughing symptoms and blood-stained sputum. In some cases, there may be gastrointestinal symptoms with abdominal pain, vomiting or diarrhea.

Medical examination of malaria patients frequently reveals signs of anemia, an enlarged spleen, liver abnormalities, and edema, or swelling due to fluid accumulation. Blood studies may show the malaria parasites in the blood, damaged red blood cells, and an abnormal white blood cell count. The four species of malaria organism are distinctive enough to be identified in laboratory tests.

that a mysterious substance in the air was the cause of the ailment. It is now known that the disease is caused by any of at least four parasites carried by Anopheles mosquitoes. According to the World Health Organization (commonly abbreviated WHO), some 200 million persons are affected by the disease, including one-fourth of the adult population on the continent of Africa. WHO estimates that at least one million children die each year of malaria. The disease was relatively rare in the United States until the 1960s when hundreds of cases began

to appear among military personnel who apparently contracted the disease in southeast Asia but did not develop symptoms until they returned to the U.S.; the disease later occurred in soldiers who had never left the United States, apparently transmitted by domestic Anopheles mosquitoes that had become infested with the malaria parasites.

Symptoms

The symptoms of malaria differ somewhat among various patients because the four known kinds of

Treatment

Treatment includes administra-

HOW MALARIA IS TRANSMITTED

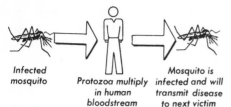

Infected mosquito | Protozoa multiply in human bloodstream | Mosquito is infected and will transmit disease to next victim

A mosquito infected with malaria protozoa bites a human. The protozoa produce daughter cells within the human bloodstream. These cells are transmitted to another mosquito that bites the infected human. This mosquito will infect the next human it bites, thus perpetuating the malaria cycle.

tion of antimalarial drugs such as quinine, chloroquine, or primaquine. Newer antimalarial drugs are sometimes used in combinations because of the development of drug-resistant strains of the organism in South America and Asia. There is no vaccine that protects against malaria.

Causes

The protozoa that cause malaria are carried by the Anopheles mosquito, but humans are the intermediate host. This means that both infected humans and infected mosquitoes are needed to continue the life cycle of the organism. The disease therefore can be controlled if Anopheles mosquito populations are eradicated and humans are not carrying the protozoa in their blood. When these organisms get into human blood, they invade the red blood cells and multiply until the blood cells rupture to release offspring called daughter cells. When the mosquito bites a human for a blood meal, the daughter cells enter the mosquito stomach where they complete their life cycle and migrate to the mosquito's salivary gland to be injected into the next human, and so on. It takes from ten days to six weeks following a mosquito bite for the first malaria symptoms to develop, the time differences varying with the species of protozoa involved. The malaria mosquito in recent years has developed resistance to insecticides and areas of infestation have spread

in some countries where irrigation for farming has been expanded.

Yellow Fever

Yellow fever, which sometimes produces symptoms similar to those of malaria, also is transmitted by a mosquito. But yellow fever is a virus disease carried by the Aedes mosquito. Yellow fever also can be harbored by other animals, while the malaria organism that affects humans is not transmitted between humans and lower animals. Like malaria, yellow fever has in past years spread deeply into North America with cases reported along the Gulf Coast, the Mississippi River Valley, and as far north as Boston. A vaccine is available for protection against yellow fever.

Leishmaniasis

Leishmaniasis is similar to malaria in that the disease organisms are protozoa transmitted to humans by an insect bite, but the insect in this case is the sandfly. There are several forms that leishmaniasis can take. The kind considered most lethal, with a mortality rate of up to 95 percent of untreated adults, is known as *kala-azar*, a term derived from the Hindi language meaning black disease. Kala-azar also is known as *black fever, dumdum fever,* and *visceral leishmaniasis*. It occurs from China through Russia and India to North Africa, the Mediterranean countries of Europe, and in parts of Central and South America. Kala-azar has appeared in the United States in cases contracted overseas.

Symptoms

The symptoms may not appear for a period of from ten days to more than three months after the bite of a sandfly, although the disease organism may be found in blood tests before the first symptoms occur. Symptoms include a fever that

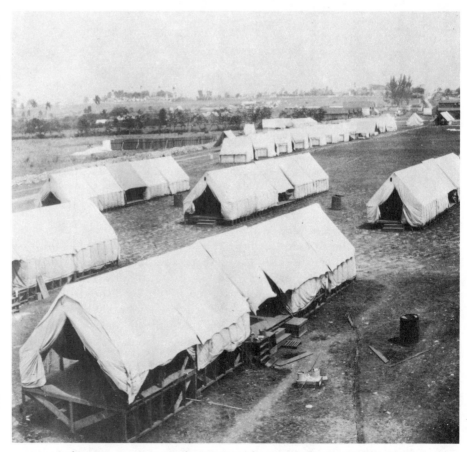

In this camp near Havana, the American physician Walter Reed (1851–1902) conducted research leading to the discovery of the cause of yellow fever.

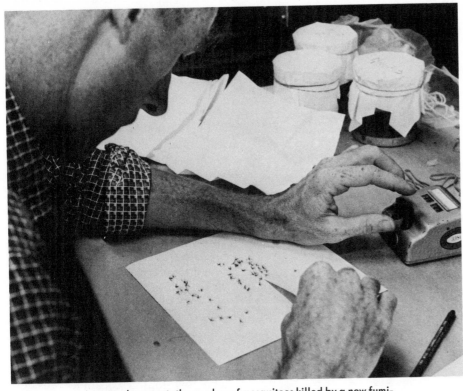

A researcher counts the number of mosquitoes killed by a new fumigant insecticide being tested at a disease-control laboratory.

America, more than ten percent of the population suffer from the disfiguring effects of leishmaniasis. Diagnosis usually is confirmed by medical tests that identify the leishmaniasis organism in the patient's tissues.

OLD WORLD CUTANEOUS LEISHMANIASIS: A milder form, sometimes known as Old World cutaneous leishmaniasis, occurs from India westward to the Mediterranean countries and North Africa. An ulcer appears at the site of a sandfly bite, usually several weeks after the bite, but it heals during a period of from three months to a year. A large pitted scar frequently remains to mark the site of the ulceration but the invading organism does not spread deeply into the body tissues as in the severe types of leishmaniasis.

Treatment

Therapy for leishmaniasis cases includes administration of various medications containing antimony, along with antibiotics for the control of secondary infections. Bed rest, proper diet, and, in severe cases, blood transfusions, also are advised.

Causes

The leishmaniasis organisms in-

reaches a peak twice a day for a period of perhaps several weeks, then recurs at irregular intervals while the patient experiences progressive weakness, loss of weight, loss of skin color, and a rapid heart beat. In some cases, depending upon the type of infection, there may be gastrointestinal complaints and bleeding of the mucous membranes, particularly around the teeth. There also can be edema, an accumulation of fluid in the tissues that conceals the actual loss of body tissue. Physical examination shows an enlarged spleen and liver plus abnormal findings in blood and urine tests.

AMERICAN CUTANEOUS LEISHMANIASIS: The American cutaneous form of leishmaniasis usually begins with one or more skin ulcers resulting from sandfly bites, with the skin of the ear the target site of the insect in many cases. The skin lesion may enlarge, with or without secondary infection by other disease organisms, and spread into the lymphatic system of the body. From the lymph system, the infecting protozoa may invade the mouth and nose,

producing painful and mutilating skin ulcers and other destructive changes in the tissues. Bacterial infections and respiratory problems can lead to the death of the patient. In some areas of Central and South

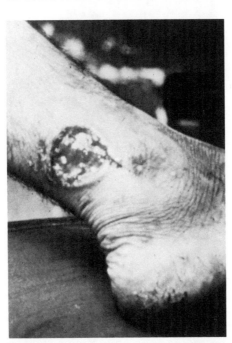

A leg ulcer, showing the tissue destruction characteristic of the cutaneous form of leishmaniasis, which is transmitted by insect bites.

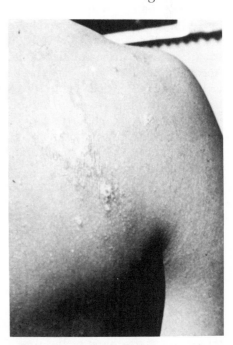

A healed lesion (large light area) and new papules forming on the back of a patient afflicted with leishmaniasis.

jected into the human body by the sandfly bite multiply through parasitic invasion of the tissue cells, particularly blood cells that usually resist infection. They may invade the lymph nodes, spleen, liver, and bone marrow, causing anemia and other symptoms. In populated areas, sandflies can be eradicated by insecticides. Unfortunately, rodents and other wild and domestic animals serve as a reservoir for the leishmaniasis protozoa and tend to perpetuate the disease in rural and jungle areas of warm climates.

Trypanosomiasis

Trypanosomiasis is a group of diseases caused by similar kinds of parasitic protozoa. The diseases, which include two kinds of African *sleeping sickness* and *Chagas' disease* of Central and South America, affect about 10 million people. The sleeping sickness forms of trypanosomiasis are transmitted by species of the tsetse fly, while Chagas' disease is carried by insects known as assassin bugs or kissing bugs. Besides affecting humans, the trypanosomiasis organisms infect other animals, including cattle, horses, dogs, and donkeys, and have made an area of nearly four million square miles of Africa uninhabitable. According to the World Health Organization, the African land devastated by trypanosomiasis contains large fertile areas capable of supporting 125 million cattle, but domestic animals cannot survive the infestation of tsetse flies.

Sleeping Sickness

The two kinds of African sleeping sickness, Gambian and Rhodesian, are similar. Gambian, or mid-African sleeping sickness, is transmitted by a tsetse fly that lives near water; Rhodesian, or East African sleeping sickness, is carried by a woodland species of tsetse fly that uses antelopes as a reservoir of the infectious organism. The most likely victims of tsetse fly bites are young men,

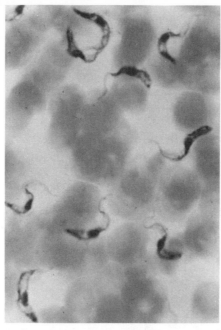

A photomicrograph of parasitic protozoa of the trypanosome type, which can cause sleeping sickness and Chagas' disease.

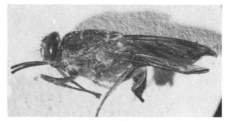
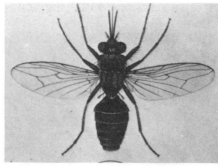

Two views of the tsetse fly, which has spread sleeping sickness over large areas of Africa. In addition to causing illness and death in humans, sleeping sickness also causes destruction of domestic animals, especially cattle.

probably because they are more likely to be exposed to the insects.

SYMPTOMS: The symptoms of trypanosomiasis infections from tsetse fly bites can vary considerably according to various factors such as the general health of the victim. A small area of inflammation, called a

chancre, appears at the site of the tsetse fly bite about two days after the incident; some patients complain of pain and irritation in the area around the bite for several weeks, but others have no symptoms. Then, for a period of perhaps several months, episodes of fever occur, with temperatures rising to 106° Fahrenheit. The bouts of fever may be accompanied by skin rashes, severe headaches, and heart palpitations. Loss of appetite and weight follow, with insomnia, an inability to concentrate, tremors, and difficulty in speaking and walking. There also may be signs of anemia and delayed reaction to a painful stimulus. Eventually, the protozoa can invade the central nervous system, producing convulsions, coma, and death.

Sleeping sickness, which may progress gradually, gets its name from the appearance of the patient, who develops a vacant expression and drooping eyelids, along with blurred speech, general lethargy, and occasional periods of paralysis.

GAMBIAN AND RHODESIAN VARIETIES: A major difference between the Gambian and Rhodesian forms of African sleeping sickness is that the Rhodesian variety, which has similar symptoms, is more acute and progresses more rapidly than the Gambian. The fever temperatures are higher, weight losses are greater, the disease more resistant to treatment, and the span of time from first symptoms to death much shorter. Even with intensive treatment, Rhodesian sleeping sickness patients have only a 50–50 chance of survival, while 90 to 95 percent of the Gambian sleeping sickness patients recover when properly treated for the disease.

TREATMENT: Several chemotherapeutic agents are available for treatment of Gambian and Rhodesian sleeping sickness; they include suramin, pentamidine, and tryparsamide given by injection. Good nutrition, good nursing care, and treatment of secondary infections are additional therapeutic measures.

Chagas' Disease

Chagas' disease, or American trypanosomiasis, is a primary cause of heart disease from Mexico through much of South America. The protozoan infection is rare in the United States, but cases have been reported. The first symptoms may be edema, or fluid accumulation of the face in the area of the eyelids, conjunctivitis, hard reddish nodules on the skin, along with the fever and involvement of the heart, brain, and liver tissues. The assassin or kissing bugs by which the disease is spread tend to bite the face, especially around the lips or eyelids, accounting for the swelling of those facial areas. The bite may be painful, or if the victim is sleeping at the time, it may not be noticed at all.

SYMPTOMS: The protozoa multiply rapidly at the site of the bug bite, frequently producing symptoms resembling those of leishmaniasis—intermittent fever, swollen spleen, and enlarged liver, after signs of an insect bite. After several days, the trypanosomiasis organisms spread from the site of infection into other tissues, especially the heart and brain, where they cause tissue destruction, inflammation, and often death.

TREATMENT: There is no specific treatment for Chagas' disease and, except for experimental drugs, most therapeutic measures are intended to treat the symptoms.

Like the African sleeping sickness forms of trypanosomiasis, the American type can involve reservoirs of wild and domestic animals; the disease has been found in cats and dogs as well as in opossums and armadillos. Persons traveling in endemic areas should use preventive measures that are appropriate, such as insect sprays and repellents. Efforts to eradicate large areas of insects carrying the trypanosomiasis organisms have been futile; in some instances it has been found to be more effective to move villages away from the insects than to try to remove the insects from the villages.

Filariasis

The species of mosquitoes that transmit malaria and yellow fever, diseases caused by protozoa and viruses, also transmit *filariasis*, caused by a parasitic worm—a nematode or roundworm. Filariasis affects 300 million people living in tropical and subtropical areas of the world. The worm invades the subcutaneous tissues and lymph system of the human body, blocking the flow of lymph and producing symptoms of inflammation, edema, abcesses, and, in one form of the disease, blindness. Filariasis is not unknown to Americans; some 15,000 soldiers contracted the disease during World War II fighting in the Pacific Theater, and cases have been reported along the Carolina coast area. But most of the victims of filariasis live in a region extending from Africa through Asia to the islands of New Guinea and Borneo.

Symptoms

Symptoms of filariasis can develop insidiously during an incubation period that may last from three months to a year after infection. There can be brief attacks of a low-grade fever, with chills and sweating, headache, nausea, and muscle pain. The patient also may feel sensitive to bright lights. Signs and symptoms more specifically related to filariasis are the appearance of red, swollen skin areas with tender spots that indicate the spread of the thread-like worms through the lymphatic system. Most likely sites for the first signs of filariasis are the lymph vessels of the legs, with later involvement of the groin and abdomen, producing the swollen lower frontal effect known as *elephantiasis*. Diagnosis of the disease is confirmed by finding the tiny worms in the lymph; the infecting organism also may be found in blood tests, but only at certain times. The worms of one form of the disease are only 35 to 90 millimeters long in the adult stage, and those of a second type of the disease are only half that size. Larvae, or embryos, of the worms may be only 200 microns (one-fifth of a millimeter) in size.

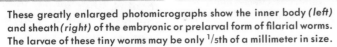

These greatly enlarged photomicrographs show the inner body (left) and sheath (right) of the embryonic or prelarval form of filarial worms. The larvae of these tiny worms may be only 1/5th of a millimeter in size.

Treatment

An oral medication, diethylcarbamazine, is available to kill the larvae, in the system; the drug has only limited value in destroying the adult worms. The drug is taken orally for three weeks but courses may have to be repeated over a period of two years because relapses can occur. Other therapeutic measures include bed rest during periods of fever and inflammation, antibiotics to control secondary infections, and, occasionally, surgery to remove damaged tissues that may interfere with normal working activities following recovery.

Onchocerciasis

The type of filariasis that causes blindness is transmitted by a species of blackfly that introduces or picks up the worm larvae while biting. As in mosquito-transmitted filariasis, the worms work their way through the skin to the lymphatic system but tend to migrate to eye structures. Blackfly filariasis, also called *onchocerciasis*, occurs most frequently in Africa and from southern Mexico to northern South America. More than one million cases of onchocerciasis have been found in the upper basin of the Volta River of Africa, with thousands of patients already blinded by the infection.

Loiasis

A third variation of filariasis is called *loiasis*. It is carried from man to monkey or from monkey to man by a biting fly. The larvae develop into adult worms that migrate under the skin and sometimes through the eye. Migration of a worm through the skin causes swelling, irritation, and redness. The disease is treated with drugs to kill the larvae, as well as by antihistamines, and occasionally surgery to remove the adult worms.

Control of filariasis requires eradication of the flies and mosquitoes that transmit the parasitic worms and perhaps the wild animals that can serve as reservoirs. As in the examples of other tropical diseases, it frequently is easier to separate the humans from the areas infested by the insects than to eradicate the insects.

Schistosomiasis

A worm of a different sort—the trematode, a flatworm of the class *Trematoda*, which includes the flukes—is responsible for *schistosomiasis*. This disease occurs in various forms in Africa, Asia, South America, and the Caribbean, including Puerto Rico. About 200 million people are infected with schistosomiasis, also called *bilharziasis*.

Life Cycle of the Fluke Parasite

The process of infection by one kind of fluke involves free-swimming larvae that penetrate the skin of a human who has entered waters containing the organism. The larvae follow the human bloodstream to the liver where they develop into adult worms. The adult worms then move into the blood vessels of the host and lay eggs. Some of the eggs find their way into the intestine or urinary bladder and are excreted with the urine or feces of the

HOW SCHISTOSOMIASIS IS TRANSMITTED

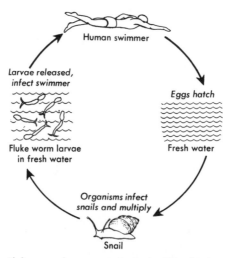

Human swimmer

Larvae released, infect swimmer

Eggs hatch

Fluke worm larvae in fresh water

Fresh water

Organisms infect snails and multiply

Snail

Fluke worm larvae penetrate the skin of a human swimmer, develop into worms, and lay eggs in the human bloodstream. Some of the eggs are eventually excreted in urine or feces, hatch in fresh water, and infect a snail, where the larvae multiply. Completing the life cycle, the larvae return to water, where they are ready to infect the next swimmer.

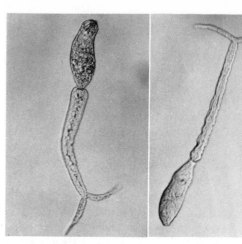

Free-swimming larvae of the parasite that causes schistosomiasis. These larvae are so tiny that they can penetrate the skin of swimmers.

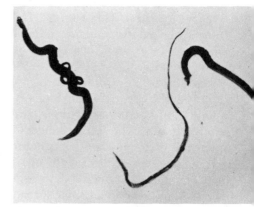

Adult *Schistosoma* worms. From right to left: a male, female, male-and-female. These worms lay eggs in the blood vessels of the host.

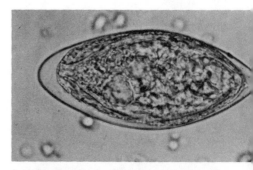

A photomicrograph of a *Schistosoma* egg. The presence of these eggs in the human bloodstream can cause severe intestinal symptoms.

host. If they find their way to fresh water, the eggs hatch and the released organisms find their way to the body of a snail. Inside the snail they multiply into thousands of new larvae over a period of one or two months, after which they return to the water and invade the skin of another human. In this manner the fluke worm continues its life cycle, infecting more humans who venture into the contaminated waters.

Symptoms

Skin rashes and itching, loss of appetite, abdominal discomfort, and diarrhea are among early symptoms of schistosomiasis infections. There also may be fever and generalized aches and pains. During a period of from one to two or more months after the initial infection, more severe symptoms may occur due to a growing number of adult worms and eggs in the body, which produce allergic reactions. Those symptoms may include diarrhea, abdominal pain, coughing spells, and high fever and chills. Medical examination may reveal a tender and enlarged liver plus signs of bleeding in the intestinal tract. Complications may result from obstruction by masses of worms and eggs or by rupturing of the walls of body organs during migration of the organisms. Diagnosis usually can be confirmed by examination of the victim's stools or of the lining of the rectum for the presence of eggs of the fluke worms.

Treatment

Therapy may consist of administration of antimony-based drugs, tartar emetic, measures to relieve the symptoms, and, when deemed necessary, surgery. In some cases, a medication may be administered to flush the eggs of the fluke worm through a specific part of the circulatory system during a surgical procedure in which a filter is inserted in a vein to trap the eggs; thousands of fluke worms can be removed by this technique. Some of the medications used in treating schistosomiasis can have serious side effects and are used cautiously. However, the alternative may be prolonged emaciation of the victim with a bloated abdomen and early death by cancer or other causes related to the infection. The female fluke worm has been known to continue depositing eggs during a life span of 30 years, causing frequent

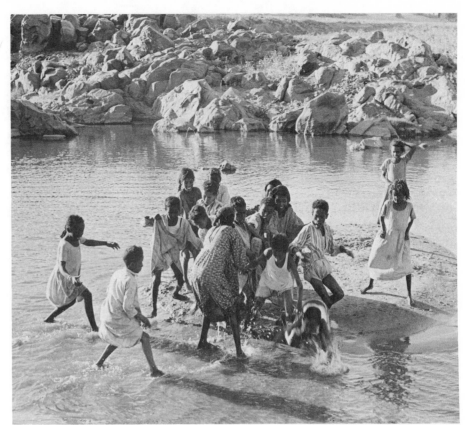

This scene of happy frolicking near the Aswan Dam in Egypt is a nightmare to public health experts trying to stop the spread of schistosomiasis.

recurrence of acute symptoms.

Other Forms of Schistosomiasis

There are several other forms of schistosomiasis that cause variations in symptoms. One kind involves the liver and central nervous system, resulting in death of the victims within as little as two years after infection. Another form seems to involve the urinary bladder, causing frequent, painful, and blood-tinged urination with bacterial infection as a complication.

SWIMMER'S ITCH: A mild form of schistosomiasis is known by the popular name of *swimmer's itch*. It can occur anywhere from Asia to South America and as far north as Canada and western Europe, affecting bathers in both fresh water and sea water. As in the severe forms of schistosomiasis, snails are the intermediate hosts and wild animals and birds provide a reservoir of the organism. The effects are treated as a skin allergy, and shallow local wa-

ters used for swimming are treated with chemicals to eradicate the snails. Careful drying and examination of the skin after swimming in possibly infected waters can control to some degree the invasion of the skin by fluke larvae. A chemical skin cream that tends to repel fluke larvae also is available as a protective measure.

Leprosy

More than 10 million people are victims of *leprosy*, an infectious disorder also known as *Hansen's disease*. Although leprosy is more common in tropical regions, where up to ten percent of some population groups may be affected, the disease also occurs in several northern countries including the United States, where the disease is found in coastal states from California through Texas and Louisana, and from Florida to New York. Ancient medical writings indicate that leprosy was known in China and India about 3,000 years ago but did not spread to the eastern Mediterranean until A.D. 500 or 600 Thus, the disease described in the Bible as leprosy probably was not the same disease known today by that name.

Symptoms

The manifestations of leprosy resemble those of several other diseases, including syphilis, sarcoidosis, and vitiligo, a skin disease marked by patches where pigmentation has been lost. The lesions of leprosy, which may begin as pale or reddish areas of from one-half inch to three or four inches in diameter, appear on body surfaces where the temperature is cooler than other body areas. These cooler surfaces include the skin, nose and throat, eyes, and testicles. The early cosmetic symptoms are followed gradually by a loss of feeling in the affected areas due to involvement of the nerve endings in those tissues. At first the patient may notice a loss of ability to distinguish hot and cold sensations in the diseased area. Then there may be a loss of tactile sensation. Finally, there is a loss of pain sensation in the affected tissues.

A case of leprosy may progress into one of two major forms, *tuberculoid leprosy* or *lepromatous leprosy,* or a combination of the two forms. The advanced symptoms can include more severe nerve damage and muscular atrophy with foot drop and contracted hands, plus damage to body areas from burns and injuries which are not felt but which can become infected. Damage to nose tissues can lead to breathing difficulties and speech problems. Crippling and

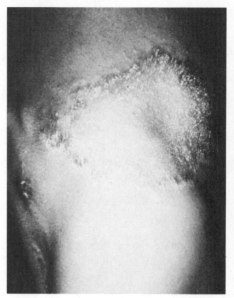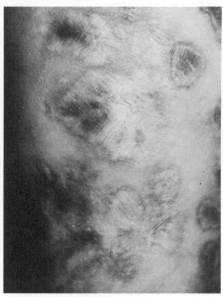

Lesions of tuberculoid *(left)* and lepromatous leprosy *(right)*. In these advanced stages of the disease, nerve damage and resulting loss of sensation, muscular atrophy, crippling, and blindness are not uncommon.

blinding are not uncommon in untreated causes of leprosy, and death may occur as a result of secondary infections.

Treatment

A number of different sulfone drugs have been found effective against the mycobacterium that apparently causes leprosy, but the drugs also produce side effects such as fever and anemia. When intolerance to sulfones occurs, other medications are offered, including thiourea, mercaptan, and streptomycin. Steroid hormones are used to help control adverse reactions.

Causes

The disease organism, *Mycobacterium leprae,* or Hansen's bacillus, is believed to enter the skin or the respiratory system of the victim, probably during childhood. It rarely infects adults except under unusual circumstances, as through skin tattooing. Some medical scientists believe the infection may be transmitted through an insect bite since the disease organism has been found in insects. However, the true process of leprosy infection remains unknown, and efforts to cultivate the mycobacterium in laboratory tissue cultures have been futile, although the disease can be induced in the footpads of experimental animals. Doctors have not found it necessary to isolate patients with the disease except during the period when treatments begin. Regular and thorough skin examinations of persons who have been in contact with leprosy patients and early detection and treatment of the disease by specialists are the recommended means of control.

CHAPTER 30

Mental and Emotional Disorders

The ability to adapt is central to being emotionally fit, healthy, and mature. An emotionally fit person is one who can adapt to changing circumstances with constructive reactions and who can enjoy living, loving others, and working productively. In everyone's life there are bound to be experiences that are anxious or deeply disturbing, such as the sadness of losing a loved one or the disappointment of failure. The emotionally fit person is stable enough not to be overwhelmed by the anxiety, grief, or guilt that such experiences frequently produce. His sense of his own worth is not lost easily by a setback in life; rather, he can learn from his own mistakes.

Communication and Tolerance

Even the most unpleasant experiences can add to one's understanding of life. Emerging from a crisis with new wisdom can give a sense of pride and mastery. The emotionally fit person can listen attentively to the opinions of others, yet if his decision differs from that being urged by friends and relatives, he will abide by it and can stand alone if necessary, without guilt and anger at those who disagree.

Communicating well with others is an important part of emotional fitness. Sharing experiences, both good and bad, is one of the joys of living. Although the capacity to enjoy is often increased by such sharing, independence is also essential, for one person's pleasure may leave others indifferent. It is just as important to appreciate and respect the individuality of others as it is to value our own individual preferences, as long as these are reasonable and do not give pain to others.

Ways of Expressing Disagreement

Communication should be kept open at all times. Anger toward those who disagree may be an immediate response, but it should not lead to cutting off communication, as it so frequently does, particularly between husbands and wives, parents and children.

Emotional maturity enables us to disagree with what another says, feels, or does, yet make the distinction between that person and how we feel about his thoughts and actions. To tell someone, "I don't like what you are doing," is more likely to keep the lines of communication open than telling him "I don't like you." This is particularly important between parents and children.

It is unfortunately common for parents to launch personal attacks when children do something that displeases them. The child, or any person to whom this is done, then feels unworthy or rejected, which often makes him angry and defiant. Revenge becomes uppermost, and communication is lost; each party feels misunderstood and lonely, perhaps even wounded, and is not likely to want to reopen communication. The joy in a human relationship is gone, and one's pleasure in living is by that much diminished.

Function of Guilt

The same principles used in dealing with others can be applied to ourselves. Everyone makes mistakes, has angry or even murderous thoughts that can produce excessive guilt. Sometimes there is a realistic reason for feeling guilty, which should be a spur to take corrective action. Differentiate clearly between thoughts, feelings, and actions. Only actions need cause guilt. In the privacy of one's own mind, anything may be thought as long as it is not acted out; an emotionally fit person can accept this difference.

Role of the Subconscious

Emotional disorders are similar to other medical diseases and can be treated by doctors or other professionals just as any other disease can be treated. Fortunately, this truth is widely accepted today, but as recently as 200 years ago it was believed that the emotionally ill were evil, possessed by the devil. Their illness was punished rather than treated. The strange and sometimes bizarre actions of the mentally ill were feared and misunderstood.

Freud and Psychoanalysis

Although we have penetrated many of the mysteries of the mind, much remains to be discovered. Significant steps toward understanding mental functioning came about through the work of Sigmund Freud. Building upon the work of others before him and making his own detailed observations, Freud demonstrated that there is a subconscious part of the mind which functions without our awareness.

He taught that mental illness resulting from subconscious memories could be cured by *psychoanalysis*, which brings the memories out into consciousness. He believed that dreams are a major key to the subconscious mind and that thoughts, dreams, fantasies, and abnormal fears follow the rules of cause and effect and are not random. This is called *psychic determinism*, meaning that emotional disorders can be understood by exploring the subconscious. *Psychiatrists* help the patient understand how his mind works and why it works that way—often the first step toward a cure.

Does psychic determinism rule out will power as a function of the mind? No, because the subconscious is only one part of the mind. Although it has an important influence, there are other forces influencing behavior and thought: the *id,* or instinctive force, the *superego,* or conscience, and the *ego,* or decision-maker. The more we know about how our minds work, what underlies our wishes and thoughts, the more control we can exercise in choosing how to behave in order to achieve our goals.

Role of Sexuality

Freud discovered that young children and even babies are aware of the sensations, pleasurable and painful, that can be experienced from all parts of the body. The sexual organs have a rich supply of nerves; the baby receives pleasure when these organs are touched, for example, during a bath or a diaper change. The child learns that when he touches these organs he obtains a pleasant feeling; therefore he repeatedly touches and rubs them (*infantile masturbation*).

This concept, that the child derives pleasure from his body and sex

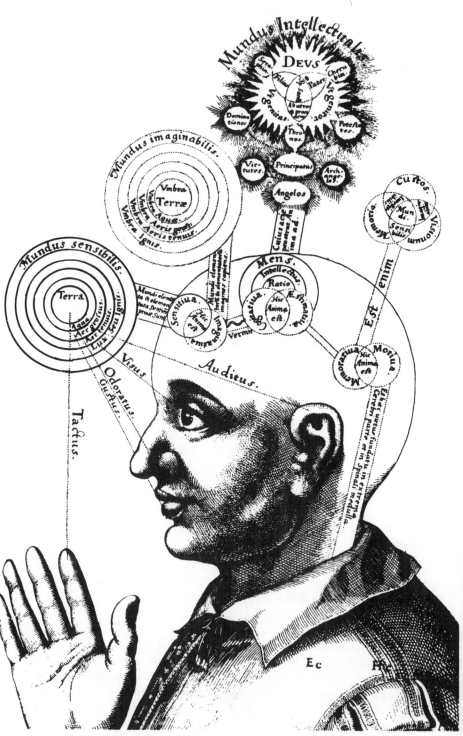

This 17th-century etching depicts the artist's visualization of the mind as the seat of the intellect, the imagination, and the senses.

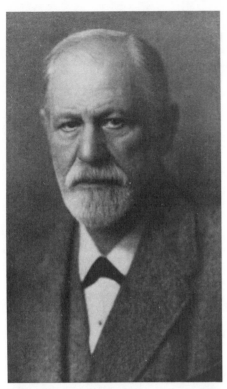

Sigmund Freud (1856–1939) was the founder of psychoanalysis, a system for treating mental illness that teaches, in part, that memories stored in the subconscious mind can cause mental illness.

organs, is called *infantile sexuality*. It does not mean that the baby has adult sexual ideas or wishes. These do not develop until puberty. It does mean that parents have the responsibility to see to it that children learn early that sex is associated with tenderness and love between man and woman. Even young children are aware of what their parents do and how they treat each other.

Types of Mental Illness

Although there is considerable disagreement about the classification of mental disorders, a convenient system used by many doctors divides mental illnesses into two general categories, organic and functional.

Some types of mental illness show little or no evidence of changes in brain tissue: these are called *functional* disorders. Another group of mental illnesses does involve some definable impairment of brain tissue due to disease, injury, the introduction of poisonous substances, mal-

function of the body's metabolic processes, nutritional problems, or inherited defects. These are *organic* disorders. Organic brain damage may be *congenital*—that is, existing at or prior to birth—or *acquired*. Examples of congenital defects are *hydrocephalus*, an accumulation of fluid within the skull of a newborn infant that destroys brain tissue; *phenylketonuria* (PKU), a type of mental retardation associated with an inability of the child's body to metabolize a protein substance; and *Down's syndrome* (also called *Mongolism*), a form of retardation which occurs more frequently in children of older mothers and which is marked by certain physical features such as eyes that resemble those of Oriental people. Some examples of acquired defects are cerebrovascular accidents such as stroke; injuries to the brain, as from a fall or from the introduction of poisonous substances such as lead, arsenic, or mercury; and arteriosclerosis, resulting in senile psychosis in aged people.

This chapter will deal only with functional mental illness. Organic disorders are treated in the chapters on diseases of particular systems of the body (Ch. 15–26) and often in other sections as well. If you are in doubt about where to find information about a particular disorder, consult the index.

Who Is Mentally Ill?

Most people occasionally experience spells of anxiety, blue moods, or temper tantrums, but unless the psychological suffering they endure or inflict upon others begins to interfere with their job or marriage, they seldom seek professional guidance. There is no exacting scientific standard for determining when an eccentric pattern of behavior becomes a mental illness. Norms vary from culture to culture and within each culture, and, as every student of history and every parent know, norms also change from generation to generation.

Just how can a determination be made as to who is mentally ill? No temperature reading, no acute pain, no abnormal growth can be looked for as evidence of a serious problem. Yet there are warning signs, and among the common ones are these:

• Anxiety that is severe, prolonged, and unrelated to any identifiable reason or cause

• Depression, especially when it is followed by withdrawal from loved ones, from friends, or from the usual occupations or hobbies that ordinarily afford one pleasure

• Loss of confidence in oneself

• Undue pessimism

• A feeling of constant helplessness

• Uncalled-for or unexplainable mood changes—for example, an abrupt switch from happiness to unhappiness when nothing has happened to warrant it

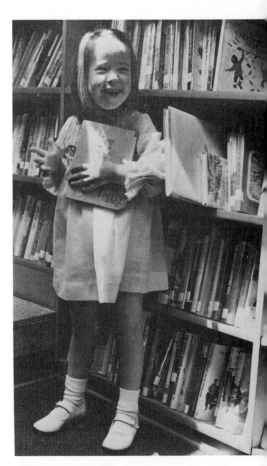

A warm, supportive family life and good medical care will help the child with Down's syndrome lead a productive life. Many Down's children are cheerful and happy.

• Rudeness or aggression that is without apparent cause or which is occasioned by some trivial incident

• An unreasonable demand for perfectionism, not only in oneself but in one's loved ones, friends, business associates, and even from things or situations

• Habitual underachievement, especially if one is adequately equipped to do the work one is called upon to perform

• The inability to accept responsibility, often manifested by a recurrent loss of employment

• Phobias

• Unreasonable feelings of persecution

• Self-destructive acts

• Sexual deviation

• A sudden and dramatic change in sleeping habits

• Physical ailments and complaints for which there are no organic causes.

If one or more of these warning signs occur frequently or in severe form, a mental illness may be present, and professional help should be sought to evaluate the underlying problem.

TYPES OF FUNCTIONAL MENTAL ILLNESS

Functional mental disorders may be broken down into four general categories: neuroses; psychophysiological (or psychosomatic) disorders; personality or character disorders; and psychoses.

Neurosis

A *neurosis* (or *psychoneurosis*) is characterized primarily by emotional rather than physical symptoms—although physical symptoms may be present. The neuroses are usually categorized according to the type of reaction that the patient exhibits in his attempt to resolve the underlying emotional conflict. All of them involve anxiety as a prominent symptom.

Anxiety Reaction

The *anxiety reaction* is probably the most widespread of all the neurotic response patterns. Although, as noted above, all the neuroses share anxiety as a symptom, the most common and outstanding characteristic of the anxiety reaction is a feeling of dread or apprehension that is not related to any apparent cause. The anxiety is caused by conflicts of which the patient himself is unaware but which may be stimulated by thoughts or events in his present life. For example, the junior executive who is constantly apprehensive that his employer will ridicule his work and dismiss his ideas may be ex-

pressing an anxiety reaction to a childhood fear that equated ridicule with abandonment or mutilation.

While anxiety reaction symptoms are primarily mental or emotional—the patient feels inadequate or ineffectual, or behaves irrationally—anxiety is always accompanied by physiological changes such as sweating and heart palpitations. Fatigue and feelings of panic are also common symptoms.

Conversion Reaction

The *conversion reaction* (or *conversion hysteria*) describes a type of neurotic behavior in which the patient, instead of coming to grips with his underlying psychic conflict, manages to convert it into physical symptoms involving functions over which he ordinarily exerts complete control. Sometimes the physical symptoms are unimportant, but often they are markedly dramatic. For example, the soldier who becomes deaf to the sound of explosions even though there is no organic defect that would account for a loss of hearing has effectively obliterated a sensation that evokes associations too painful to acknowledge.

Obsessive-Compulsive Reaction

A person beset by persistent, unwanted ideas or feelings (*obsessions*), who is impelled to carry out certain acts (*compulsions*) ritualisti-

cally, no matter how irrational they are, is reacting to a psychic conflict in an *obsessive-compulsive* manner. The obsession may involve a feeling of violence or sexuality directed toward a member of his own family. Usually the feeling will never lead to any overt action of the type imagined, but the idea is nevertheless persistent and painful.

Obsessive-compulsive patients are typically exceptionally meticulous and conscientious, often intelligent and gifted in their work. But they expend an enormous amount of energy and time in observing compulsive acts. For example, they may take a dozen or more showers every day because they are obsessed with the idea that they are dirty or carrying a contagious disease. By performing an apparently harmless compulsive act, the patient is temporarily relieved of the obsession.

Depressive Reaction

Most people have blue moods from time to time in their lives. Indeed, when faced with a personal tragedy like the death of a loved one, a normal healthy individual may well undergo a period of depression. A person suffering from the *depressive reaction*, however, has persistent feelings of worthlessness and pessimism unrelated to events that might depress a normal person. An inability to cope with problem situations is gradually magnified into an inability to cope with anything at all. Attempts to mask the crisis by putting on a "front"—feigning cheerfulness and optimism—give way to episodes of total hopelessness. Suicide is often considered and sometimes attempted. Threats of suicide from a depressed person should always be regarded seriously.

Common physical symptoms accompaning depression are fatigue, loss of appetite, and insomnia.

Phobic Reaction

A *phobic reaction* is the result of an individual's attempt to deal with an anxiety-producing conflict, not by facing up to the actual source of that conflict but by avoiding something else. The substitute—whether it be an animal, closed places, or whatever—is responded to with the intense anxiety that is really felt for the true source of anxiety. This process is known as *displacement,* and the irrational fears or dreads are known as *phobias.*

Thus, a person who had been regularly punished as a child by having been forcibly confined in a closet might be unable to deal with the anxiety of the experience consciously. The anxiety might be displaced and emerge later in life in the form of terror of crowded or confined places—*claustrophobia.*

Phobias can involve almost anything one encounters in life—including things that go on in one's body and one's mind. Some of the most common phobias have to do with disease—*bacteriophobia,* for example, the fear of germs.

Scores of phobias exist, ranging alphabetically from *acrophobia,* the fear of heights, to *xenophobia,* the fear of strangers. Other well-known examples are *ailurophobia,* the fear of cats; *cynophobia,* the fear of dogs; *algophobia,* the fear of pain; *agoraphobia,* the fear of open spaces; *erythrophobia,* the fear of blushing; *mysophobia,* the fear of dirt and contamination; *nyctophobia,* the fear of the dark; and *lyssophobia,* the fear of becoming insane.

Dissociative Reaction

The *dissociative reaction* involves a basic disruption of the patient's personality. The dissociative reaction permits a person to escape from a part of his personality associated with intolerable anxiety. The escape is made in various ways: by forgetfulness or absent-mindedness, dream states (including sleepwalking), amnesia, and—most seriously—the adoption of multiple personalities, in which the patient behaves like one person at certain times and like an altogether different person at other times.

Psychophysiological Disorders

It has been estimated that one-half or more of the patients of a general practitioner either do not have any organic illness or do not have any organic disease that could account for the severity or extent of the symptoms described. These patients are obviously not inventing their symptoms. The symptoms—whether they be itching, constipation, asthma, or heart palpitations—are real enough. But in many cases they

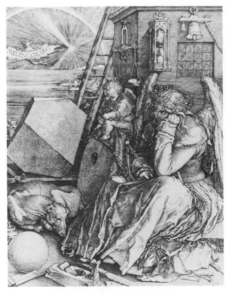

"Melancholia," an engraving by the renowned artist Albrecht Durer, depicts very graphically the emotional condition we now call depression.

are either wholly or partly of psychological origin—*psychogenic* is the medical term.

The psychological and physiological aspects of humans are so closely interwoven that the problem of *psychophysiological* (or *psychosomatic*) disorders must be considered with attention to both aspects. Consider how many physiological changes in normal people can be induced by psychological states: sweating, blushing, gooseflesh, sexual arousal, weeping, the feeling of "a lump in the throat," etc. It should hardly be surprising, then, that when someone has a physical illness there are profound concomitant psychological factors that can materially affect the physiological disease.

In many cases, however, as noted above, there is no detectable organic disease. Anxiety and other disturbing emotions such as rage are sometimes dealt with by the individual by constructing a pattern of defense that involves physiological reactions. Confronted with an emotional conflict that cannot be handled consciously, the individual may channel his feelings inward and deal with it by the formation of troublesome physical symptoms. It must be stressed that this strategy is not consciously engineered by the patient and that the symptoms are genuinely experienced.

Psychophysiological disorders affect many parts of the body, but certain organs and tissues seem more vulnerable than others. The digestive tract, for example, is frequently beset by disorders that are psychophysiological, including diarrhea, constipation, regional enteritis (inflammation of the intestine), ulcerative colitis (ulcers and inflammation of the colon), and peptic ulcers. Hypertension is frequently associated with psychogenic causes. Muscle cramps, recurrent stiff necks, arthritis, backaches, and tension headaches are other common complaints. Many skin conditions such as hives and eczema can be triggered by or are aggravated by psychological factors.

The symptoms of a psychophysiological illness appear to have no logical relation to the conflict that is responsible for them, nor do they relieve the underlying anxiety.

Personality or Character Disorders

Another group of mental illnesses is the *personality* or *character disorders,* so called because they appear to stem from a kind of defect in or arrested development of the personality. Unlike neurotic patients, individuals with personality disorders do not especially suffer from anxiety, nor is their behavior markedly eccentric. But when observed over a period of time, the personality problem becomes evident.

Personality disorders fall into various categories including:

• the *passive-dependent* individual, who needs excessive emotional support and reassurance from an authority figure;

• the *schizoid* individual, who is withdrawn from and indifferent to other people;

• the *paranoid* individual, who is exquisitely sensitive to praise or criticism and often suspicious of expressed or implied attitudes toward him, and who often is subject to feelings of persecution;

• the *cyclothymic* (or *cycloid*) individual, who is subject to sharply defined moods of elation or depression, seemingly without relation to external circumstances;

• the *sociopathic* individual, who is characteristically lacking in a sense of personal responsibility or of morality. Formerly called the *psychopathic* personality, the sociopath may be disposed to aggressive, hostile, sometimes violent behavior and frequently engages in self-destructive behavior such as alcoholism or addiction to drugs. See Ch. 31, p. 540, and Ch. 32, p. 552, for further information about alcoholism and drug addiction, respectively. Sociopathic behavior also includes sexual deviation.

Psychosis

The chief distinction between *psychosis* and neurosis is that a psychosis represents a more complete disintegration of personality and a loss of contact with the outside world. The psychotic is therefore unable to form relationships with people. Most people who suffer from nonpsychotic mental disorders are seldom, if ever, hospitalized, and then usually for very brief periods. But many psychotics are so crippled by their illness that they are hospitalized repeatedly or for protracted periods of time.

Schizophrenic Reaction

Schizophrenia, the most common and destructive of the psychotic reactions, is characterized by withdrawal from external reality, inability to think clearly, disturbances in affective reaction (capacity to feel and express emotion), and a retreat into a fantasy life—all of these resulting in a progressive deterioration of the patient's ordinary behavioral patterns.

SIMPLE SCHIZOPHRENIA: The patient with *simple schizophrenia* experiences a gradual loss of concern and contact with other people, and a lessening of the motivation needed to perform the routine activities of everyday life. There may be some personality deterioration, but the presence of hallucinations and delusions is rare.

HEBEPHRENIC SCHIZOPHRENIA: This form of schizophrenia is marked by delusions, hallucinations, and regressed behavior. Hebephrenics babble and giggle, and often react in inappropriately childish ways. Their silly manner can make them seem happier than other schizophrenics, but this disorder often results in severe personality disintegration— more severe, in fact, than in other types of schizophrenia.

CATATONIC SCHIZOPHRENIA: In *catatonic schizophrenia* there are dramatic disturbances of the motor functions. Patients may remain in a fixed position for hours, days, or even weeks. During this time their muscles may be rigid, their limbs held in awkward positions. They may have to be fed, and their urinary and bowel functions may be abnormal. This stuporous state may be varied by an occasional period of frenzied but purposeless excitement.

PARANOID SCHIZOPHRENIA: The *paranoid schizophrenic* is preoccupied with variable delusions of persecution or grandeur. Men working with pneumatic drills on the street, for example, are really sending out super-sonic beams designed to destroy his brain cells; the water supply is being poisoned by visitors from other planets; any mechanical malfunction, as of a telephone or an elevator, is part of a deliberate plot of harassment or intimidation.

Paranoid schizophrenia is often marked by the presence of hallucinations, by disturbances in mental processes, and by behavioral deterioration. The disorder is regarded as particularly serious—hard to deal with and likely to become permanent.

Paranoid Reaction

The patient with this disorder suffers from delusions, usually of persecution, sometimes of grandeur. In this respect, *paranoia* is very similar to paranoid schizophrenia. However, in paranoid schizophrenia the delusions are often variable, and usually there is a breakdown of the patient's behavioral patterns.

A case of true paranoia, by contrast, is characterized by an invariable delusion around which the patient constructs and adheres to a highly systematized pattern of behavior. When the delusion is of such a nature that its persistence does not engender a conflict between the patient and his surrounding social structure, the patient may never be suspected of mental illness, perhaps merely of eccentricity. If, however, the delusion does provoke conflict, the patient may react with destructive hostility, and hospitalization or some other kind of professional treatment will be necessary.

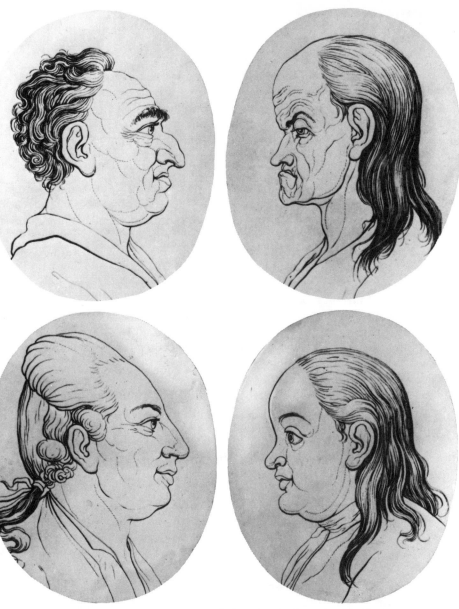

In medieval times, temperament was believed to be determined by the predominance of one or the other of four basic body liquids, or *humors:* yellow bile, black bile, blood, and phlegm. These 18th-century drawings depict representatives of each type. The person with an excess of yellow bile, thought to be secreted by the liver, was said to have a *choleric* disposition *(upper left)*, characterized by a hot temper and irritability. Too much black bile was supposed to cause a *melancholic* temperament *(upper right)*, marked by gloominess and depression. An excess of blood resulted in a *sanguine* disposition *(lower left)*—associated then as now with a ruddy complexion and cheerful temperament. Finally, an excess of phlegm caused one to be *phlegmatic (lower right)*, marked by a slow or sluggish disposition.

food and sleep and ends in a state of total collapse.

In a mild depressive phase, the individual feels dull and melancholy, his confidence begins to drain away, and he becomes easily fatigued by daily routines. When the depressive phase is more severe, the patient starts to retreat from reality, gradually entering into a state of withdrawal that is very much like a stupor. At this point he hardly moves or speaks. He may be unable to sleep. Eventually he begins to question his value as a human being and is crushed by feelings of guilt. He may refuse to eat. Symptoms may progress to the point where an attempt at suicide is a real possibility.

Although the manic-depressive psychosis may alternate from one of its phases to the other, one or the other phase is usually dominant for a prolonged period of time. Depression is more often dominant than mania. Manic-depressive patients often recover spontaneously for periods of time, but relapses are fairly common.

Depressive Reaction

The *depressive reaction* is a disorder connected with aging and its attendant changes in sexual functioning; it usually occurs at the time of the menopause in women, in the middle or late 40s, and somewhat later in men. Formerly called *involutional melancholia*, it is characterized, as that name suggests, by a sense of hopeless melancholy and despair.

Patients begin to feel that life has passed them by. They experience real physical symptoms such as loss of vigor, and develop various hypochondriacal complaints. Their interests become narrower, and they begin to retreat from the world.

As the melancholy deepens, there are periods of senseless weeping, bouts of intense anxiety, feelings of worthlessness, and growing concern—coupled with delusions—about dying and death. The depth of the depression is overwhelming, and the danger of suicide greater than in any other psychosis.

Manic-Depressive Reaction

This disorder, also called an *affective reaction,* is characterized by two phases—*mania* and *depression.* Patients are governed by one phase or another or by the alternation of both.

The manic phase may be mild and bring elation and a general stepping up of all kinds of activity. The patient tends to talk endlessly and in an associative rather than a logical way. If the disorder is more severe, he may act or dress bizarrely; he may be a whirlwind of activity and become so excited and agitated that he forgoes

TREATMENT OF EMOTIONAL PROBLEMS AND MENTAL DISORDERS

When should help be sought for an emotional problem? Sometimes individuals themselves realize that they need help and seek it without urging. They may have symptoms such as anxiety, depression, or troublesome thoughts that they cannot put out of their mind. But many others who need help do not know it or do not want to know that they need it. They usually have symptoms that disturb others rather than themselves, such as irritability, impulsive behavior, or excessive use of drugs or alcohol that interferes with their family relationships and work responsibilities.

Other people in need of psychological guidance are those who have a physical disease that is based on psychological factors. They react to stress internally rather than externally. Instead of displaying anger, they feel it inside. We are all familiar with headaches or heartburn caused by tension; more serious diseases clearly associated with emotional factors are asthma, certain skin disorders, ulcerative colitis, essential hypertension, hyperthyroidism, and peptic ulcer. Other physical symptoms that may be related to psychological factors are some types of paralysis, blindness, and loss of memory.

In all these situations the patient's enjoyment of life is curtailed. He has no feeling of control over what he does and little or no tolerance for himself and others. Such an existence is completely unnecessary today, with the many agencies and specialists capable of effectively treating these problems.

Mental Health Professionals

Who can help those with emotional problems? Confusion about the different professions in the mental health field is understandable. To add to the muddle, self-appointed counselors without professional training and experience have set themselves up in this field, so it is necessary to know whom to consult to obtain the best help possible.

Psychiatrists

Psychiatrists are medical doctors; that is, they have graduated from a medical school, served internships and afterwards residencies specializing in emotional disorders. They are specialists in the same way that a surgeon or an eye doctor is a specialist. Most are members of the American Psychiatric Association. They are experienced in treating medical illnesses, having done so for many years before being certified as specialists in emotional disorders. Generally they can be relied upon to adhere to the ethical and professional standards of the medical field.

The American Psychiatric Association, 1700 18th Street, N.W., Washington, D. C. 20009, can supply the names of members. The American Board of Psychiatry and Neurology, 1603 Orrington Avenue, Evanston, Illinois 60201, examines and certifies psychiatrists who pass its tests, so that the term "board certified" means that the psychiatrist has passed its tests. If a family doctor is consulted about an emotional problem, he will often refer the patient to a psychiatrist, just as he would to any other specialist.

Psychologists

Psychologists have gone to college, majored in psychology, and sometimes have advanced degrees, for example, a doctorate in psychology. They are not medical doctors and may get a degree in psychology without ever working with a human being, e.g., by working in animal behavior, experimental psychology, or other fields. They may or may not have clinical training, but many acquire this training and experience with human beings. There is no guarantee that a psychologist has this background, however, without looking into the qualifications of each individual.

Psychotherapists

Psychotherapy is the general term for any treatment that tries to effect a cure by psychological rather than physical means. A psychotherapist may be as highly trained as a psychiatrist, or he may be a psychologist, or may even have no training at all. Anyone can set up an office and call himself a psychotherapist, psychoanalyst, marriage counselor, family therapist, or anything else he desires. It is up to the patient to check on the training and background of a therapist. Any reputable therapist should be pleased to tell patients his credentials and qualifications for helping them. A psychoanalyst, for example, may be a psychiatrist with several years of additional training in psychoanalysis, or may be someone whose qualifications consist of a college psychology courses.

Social Workers

Social workers are another group of trained persons who may also counsel those with emotional problems. They may work either with individuals, families, or groups after meeting the educational requirements for the profession, which include a bachelor's degree and two years of professional training leading to a master's degree in social work.

Professionals should be associated with recognized groups of their peers, or perhaps with a medical center or hospital. Generally a person with emotional problems should consult a psychiatrist first, who will then either treat the problem or be in a good position to advise what is necessary and who can best be available for treatment.

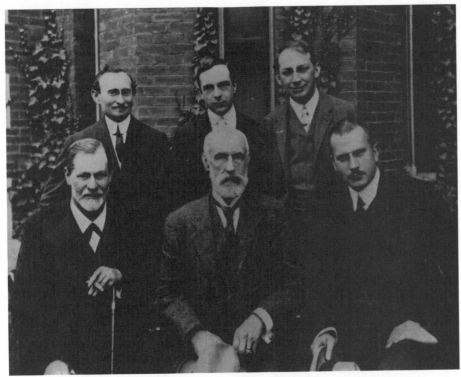

A 1909 photo taken of Sigmund Freud and colleagues who were major figures in the history of psychology. From left to right: seated, Freud, G. Stanley Hall, Carl G. Jung; standing, A. A. Brill, Ernest Jones, Sandor Ferenczi.

Types of Therapy

Functional mental illnesses are treated by a variety of tools, among them psychotherapy and chemotherapy (treatment with drugs), and —much less often—electroshock treatment.

Psychotherapy

As noted above, psychotherapy applies to various forms of treatment that employ psychological methods designed to help patients understand themselves. With this knowledge, or insight, the patient learns how to handle his life—with all its relationships and conflicts—in a happier and more socially responsible manner.

The best known form of psychotherapy is psychoanalysis, developed by Freud but modified by many others, which seeks to lift to the level of awareness the patient's repressed subconscious feelings. The information about subconscious conflicts is explored and interpreted to explain the causes of the patient's emotional upsets.

The technique employs a series of steps beginning with *free association,* in which the patient is encouraged to discuss anything that comes to mind, including things that the patient might be reluctant to discuss with anyone else but the analyst. Other steps include dream analysis and *transference,* which is the redirection to the analyst of repressed childhood emotions.

Group therapy is a form of therapeutic treatment in which a group of approximately six to ten patients, usually under the guidance of a therapist, participate in discussions of their mental and emotional problems. The therapist may establish the direction of the discussion or may remain mostly silent, allowing the patients' interaction to bring about the special cathartic benefits of this technique.

Family therapy is much like group therapy, with an individual family functioning as a group. It is felt that the family members may be better able to discuss the problems of relating to each other within the context of a group than they would be on an individual basis with a therapist.

Psychodrama is a therapeutic technique in which a patient or a group of patients act out situations centered about their personal conflicts. The psychodrama is "performed" in the presence of a therapist and, sometimes, other people.

Children are sometimes enrolled in programs of *play therapy* in which dolls, doll houses, and other appropriate toys are made available so that they can express their frustrations, hostilities, and other feelings through play. This activity, carried on under the observation of a therapist, is considered a form of catharsis in that it often prevents the repression of hostile emotions. In the case of a maladjusted child, it can also act as a helpful diagnostic tool—revealing the source of the child's emotional problem.

Chemotherapy

The relationship between body chemistry and mental illness has been studied for over half a century. The result of this study is the therapeutic technique known as *chemotherapy,* the treatment of disease with drugs or chemicals.

EARLY USES OF CHEMICAL AGENTS: Sedatives to provide treatment of mental diseases were used during World War I for soldiers suffering from shell shock. *Sodium amytal,* one of the early chemicals used, offered a prolonged restful sleep, after which the army patients could tolerate some form of psychotherapeutic treatment.

In the 1930s, doctors introduced *insulin shock therapy* as a method for treating psychotic patients. The patients received injections of insulin in doses large enough to produce a deep coma, after which they were revived by doses of sugar. As with the use of sodium amytal, the insulin treatment was accompanied by psychotherapy for most effective results.

PRESENT-DAY USES OF CHEMICAL

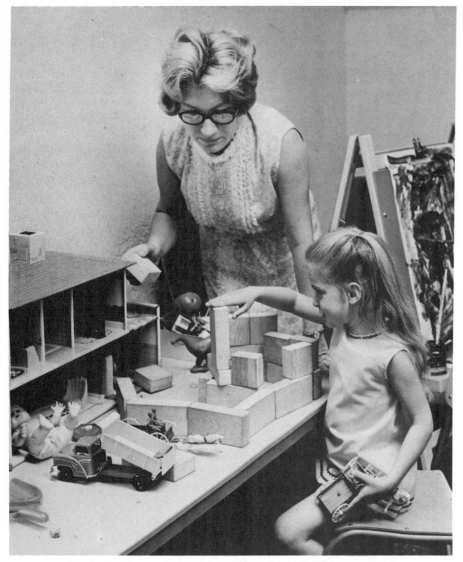

Play therapy is a psychoanalytic technique in which children, under the observation of a therapist, can express their inner feelings through play.

Electroshock Treatment

Electroshock is a form of therapy in which a carefully regulated electric current is passed through a patient's head, thereby producing convulsions and unconsciousness.

Electroshock is primarily a treatment for the manic-depressive psychosis; to a lesser extent the therapy is used on schizophrenic patients. It often shortens depressed periods, and sometimes the patient seems totally free of the symptoms of his disorder. Unfortunately, the remission may be temporary; electroshock does not prevent further attacks. Also, transitory memory impairment often occurs.

Because of the recent advances in the techniques of chemotherapy, electroshock is used much less frequently than it was in the past.

Facilities Available for the Mentally Ill

The last decade has seen a number of hopeful changes in the facilities for treatment of mental disorders in the United States. The great majority of severely ill mental patients used to be cared for in county or state mental hospitals, many of which were crowded and able to offer custodial care but very little in the way of therapeutic programs. The picture has changed, however, and the extent and quality of care in these hospitals is expanding and improving.

Patients with mental illnesses are also being treated in greater numbers at general hospitals. As a matter of fact, more patients who need hospitalization for such illnesses are being admitted to general hospitals than to public mental hospitals.

Treatment for the mentally or emotionally disturbed is also provided in other facilities, including private mental hospitals, mental health clinics, and various social agencies.

Among the new facilities for treating mental illness is one which permits many patients who would formerly have been hospitalized, per-

AGENTS: More recently, the control of mental illness has taken a giant step forward with the development of *tranquilizers* and *antidepressants*. Tranquilizers counteract anxiety, tension, and overexcitement; they are used to calm patients whose behavior is dangerously confused or disturbed. Antidepressants help to stimulate the physiological activity of depressed patients, thereby tending to relieve the sluggishness that attends depression.

The treatment of the manic-depressive psychosis has been facilitated with the use of salts derived from lithium, a metal. Lithium salts seem to control the disease without producing the undesirable emotional and intellectual effects that resulted from the previous treatment with tranquilizers and antidepressants. The medication has been found to be particularly effective in treating patients with frequent manic episodes; it is also said to be effective as a preventive measure against future manifestations of mania or depression. Lithium may have adverse side effects and must be administered carefully.

Chemotherapy does not usually cure mental illness. It does, however, improve the patient's mental state, thereby enabling him to cope more effectively with problems.

haps for the rest of their lives, to be served by community mental health centers. These centers offer both in-patient and out-patient care. The services they provide go beyond diagnosis and treatment to include rehabilitation, thus making it possible for more and more of today's mental patients to live at home, function in a job situation, and be a part of their own community.

Results of Treatment

What can be expected from treatment? Does a person who has been through treatment emerge bland, uncaring about others, with absolutely no problems, and without guilt for his misdeeds? Absolutely not. What treatment can do, said Freud, is to change neurotic misery into common unhappiness. There will always be things in life that are disappointing or otherwise upsetting. No treatment can eliminate such problems. After successful treatment, however, one should be better able to handle these stresses with flexible and constructive responses and to see his own difficulties in relation to the problems of others.

To feel emotionally fit is to have a capacity for enjoying life, working well, and loving others. Fear, shame, and guilt about undergoing needed treatment should not prevent anyone from reaching that potential.

CHAPTER 31

Alcohol

Alcoholic beverages have an ancient history. Long before man began to keep records of any kind, they were valued as food, medicine, and ceremonial drinks. When people nowadays have a beer with dinner, or toast newlyweds with champagne, or share wine at a religious festival, they are observing traditions that have deep roots in the past.

The consumption of alcoholic beverages has always been a fact of American life. Most Americans drink, either occasionally or often. Most drinkers are usually in control of what they are doing and are none the worse for their habit. However, of the estimated 90 million drinkers in this country, about 9 million have some kind of problem with alcohol.

Some people have the idea that anyone with an alcohol problem is sinful, or has a weak character, or wants to thumb his nose at the law. Scientists have come to believe that *alcoholism* is a disease and should be treated as such. In 1956, the American Medical Association officially termed alcoholism an illness and a medical responsibility.

In the following pages, alcohol is examined as the neutral spirit that it truly is. Some people have a sickness involving food; others can't be trusted with a car. Alcohol too can be properly used or hopelessly abused.

What Is Alcohol?

The alcohol in beverages is chemically known as *ethyl alcohol*. It is often called *grain alcohol*. It is produced by the natural process of *fermentation:* that is, when certain foods such as honey, fruits, grains, or their juices remain in a warm place, airborne yeast organisms begin to change the sugars and starches in these foods into alcohol. Although ethyl alcohol is in itself a food in the sense that its caloric content produces energy in the body, it contains practically no essential nutriments.

Methyl alcohol, also called *wood alcohol* because it is obtained by the dry distillation of maple, birch, and beech, is useful as a fuel and solvent. It is poisonous if taken internally and can cause blindness and death. Other members of the same family of chemicals, such as *isopropyl alcohol*, are also used as rubbing alcohols—that is, they are used as cooling agents and skin disinfectants, and they too are poisonous if taken internally.

How Alcoholic Beverages Evolved

FERMENTATION: In all times and places, man has made use of those local products that lend themselves to fermentation. One of the earliest alcoholic beverages was probably mead, made from honey. Wines originated from fruits and berries, beers from grains. Palm leaves, bananas, cactus, corn, sugar cane, and rice are among the natural products that provide fermented drinks for social and religious occasions.

DISTILLATION OF ALCOHOL: Distilled alcoholic beverages appear to be the result of a process discovered in the Arab world some time around the year 800. *Distillation* consists in separating the compound parts of a substance by boiling them until they become vapors. The vapors are then condensed into separate liquids. Since alcohol has a lower boiling point than water, it can be separated from water in this way. Soon after the process of distillation was discovered, it was applied to wine to make brandy and to the various beers based on rye, corn, and barley to make whiskies.

The earliest distilled beverages were produced during the Middle Ages by monks. The different monasteries guarded their secret formulas involving medicinal herbs and spices—as the makers of Benedictine and Chartreuse continue to do—and sold their products to physicians.

Still later, the nobility worked out

complicated routines for the use of alcoholic beverages to enhance the taste of foods, such as directions concerning which wine complemented which food and what time of day suited a particular beverage. The poor at this time usually drank the fermented beverages that came easily to hand.

Changes in Drinking Habits

The Europeans who came to the New World brought their drinking customs with them. Even the most rigid Puritans took the view that since drinking was sanctioned by the Scriptures, moderate drinking was no sin. But as the early settlers began to move westward, established drinking habits changed.

For the frontiersmen, barrels of wine and beer were too heavy to transport. Corn "likker" and rum—more potent and easily carried in small jugs—became the favored drinks of the pioneers. Saloons began to spring up and public drunkenness became more and more of a problem.

The temperance movement was born out of a need to reestablish moderation in drinking—not total abstention. Eventually, however, it was instrumental in imposing Prohibition on the whole country. The era of Prohibition lasted for about 12 years. By the time it came to an end in 1933, it was obvious that when the majority of the population want to drink alcoholic beverages, the law is not likely to stop them.

Present-Day Drinking Trends

On a per capita basis, Americans drink twice as much wine and beer as they did a century ago, and half as much distilled spirits. Where the drinking takes place has changed, too. There's less hard drinking in saloons and more social drinking at home and in clubs. The acceptance of drinking in mixed company has made it more a part of social situations than it used to be.

Here are some facts about the current consumption of alcoholic beverages in the United States:

• Drinking is more common among men than among women, but the gap keeps closing.

• It is more common among people who are under 40.

• It is more common among the well-to-do than the poor.

• There are more drinkers among the educated than among the uneducated.

• Drinking is more common in metropolitan areas than in rural areas.

• Beyond the age of 45, the number of drinkers steadily declines.

Teen-Agers and Alcohol

One fact emerges clearly and consistently from all the surveys of teenage drinking in all parts of the country: the drinking behavior of parents is more closely related to what children do about drinking than any other factor. It is more influential than their friends, their neighborhood, their religion, their social and economic status, or their local laws.

Depending on the part of the country investigated, from 71 percent to 92 percent of the nation's teen-agers have tasted an alcoholic beverage at one time or another. The older the teen-ager who drinks, the more often he does so. After 17, the percentage of young people who drink is the same as that of the adult percentage.

Most high school students drink only on holidays or special family occasions. College students drink at their own parties. Solitary drinking is rare, and so is drinking in parked cars. Most youngsters have beer, and less often, wine in their own homes or in the homes of friends. Only about one in ten drinks away from

An exhibition at the Museum of the City of New York emphasizes the serious social consequences that result from the disease alcoholism.

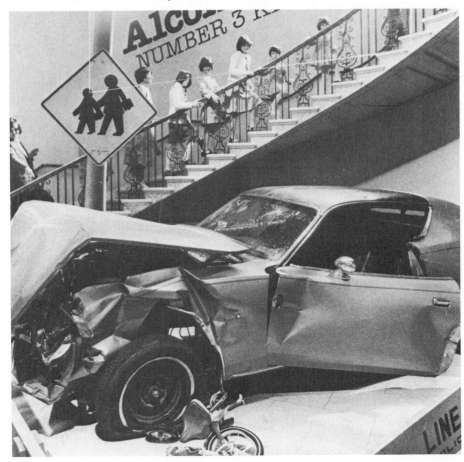

home against parental wishes. However, the rebels drink more and get drunk more often than those who drink with their parent's consent.

It is not true that high school students who drink occasionally are more likely to be delinquent or maladjusted. They play as important a role in all student activities as do the abstainers. In the group with grades over 90 percent, half drink and half don't. The statistics connected with automobile accidents involving teen-agers show that alcohol is negligible as a cause compared to faulty judgment and faulty cars.

In general, drinking is an activity connected with growing up. For boys, it represents manhood, for girls, sophistication. Since adult drinking is a widespread custom, teen-agers adopt the established patterns as they progress towards maturity.

Young Problem Drinkers

Teen-age drinking behavior studied in many different states shows that 2 to 5 out of every 100 young people who drink are misusing alcohol. This is the group that drinks in defiance of parental or school authority. It includes young people from families with mixed feelings about drinking and from families where adults drink heavily but forbid their children to do so until they are 21.

Constituents of Alcoholic Beverages

The way any alcoholic drink affects the body depends chiefly upon how much alcohol it contains. The portion of alcohol can range from less than 1/20th of the total volume—in the case of beer—to more than one half—in the case of rum. It is a general rule that distilled drinks have a higher alcohol content than fermented ones.

The five basic types of beverages are beers, table wines, dessert or cocktail wines, cordials and liqueurs, and distilled spirits. The labels of beers and wines usually indicate the percentage of alcohol by volume. The labels of distilled spirits indicate *proof*.

PROOF: The proof number is twice the percentage of alcohol by volume. Thus a rye whisky which is 90-proof contains 45 percent alcohol; 80-proof bourbon is 40 percent alcohol and so on. The word *proof* used in this way comes from an old English test to determine the strength of distilled spirits. If gunpowder soaked with whisky would still ignite when lighted, this was "proof" that the whisky contained the right amount of alcohol. The amount, approximately 57 percent, is still the standard in Canada and Great Britain. Any distilled beverage containing less is labeled "under-proof."

Many alcoholic beverages contain additional substances such as minerals, sugars, and vitamins. The list below describes the contents of the best-known beverages.

BEERS: Light beer, known as lager or pilsner, dark beer, ale, stout, and porter vary in alcohol content from 3 percent to 8 percent. Beers are also rich in carbohydrates.

TABLE WINES: Red and white table wines have an alcohol content of about 12 percent. Although the age and origin of a particular type of wine affects its aroma, taste, and especially its price, the physiological effect on the wine drinker is essentially the same. Red table wines are higher in acids, potassium, and vitamins such as riboflavin; white table wines, including champagne, have a higher content of sugar, sodium, and thiamine. The sugar content can range from as little as 0.2 percent in a dry red wine to 10 percent in a vintage sauterne. Some kosher wines contain enough added sugar to bring the content up to 20 percent.

COCKTAIL AND DESSERT WINES: In aperitif drinks such as sherry and vermouth, and in such dessert wines as port and marsala, the alcohol content ranges from about 15 percent to 20 percent. The amount of sugar can be as low as 0.1 percent in dry sherry or as much as 20 percent in marsala.

These wines are lower in iron, potassium, and sodium than are table wines, but higher in various vitamin B compounds.

OTHER FERMENTED DRINKS: Hard apple cider contains from 4 percent to 14 percent alcohol; mead or honey wine from 10 percent to 20 percent, and sake, the Japanese rice wine, about 15 percent.

LIQUEURS AND CORDIALS: These are usually very sweet, containing as much as 50 percent sugar, and are flavored with fruit, herbs, and spices. Alcohol content can reach as much as 30 percent.

BRANDY: The oldest of the distilled spirits, brandy is still made from grape wine and usually has an alcohol content of 50 percent. Apple brandy, known as applejack in the United States and as calvados in France, may be 55 percent alcohol.

WHISKY: Whisky-making probably began in Ireland as early as the 12th century, spread to Scotland, and eventually reached Canada and the United States. The technique for preparing all types of whisky is essentially the same. Production begins with a strong beer derived from a fermented grain such as rye, corn, or barley. The beer is distilled, and the distillate is stored in charred oak barrels. Scotch, Irish, Canadian, rye, and bourbon whiskies range from 80- to over 100-proof.

RUM: The basic ingredient in rum is fermented molasses or sugar-cane juice, and the distillate may be flavored with a dessert wine, spices, or fruit extract. Caramel or burnt sugar is often added for color. Rums range from 80-proof to as much as 150-proof.

GIN AND VODKA: These are made from any fermentable carbohydrate and are essentially redistilled alcohol with some flavor added. Since the product is bottled without aging, it is the least expensive of the distilled spirits. It ranges from 80- to 100-proof.

How Alcohol Affects the Body

The overall effects of alcoholic bev-

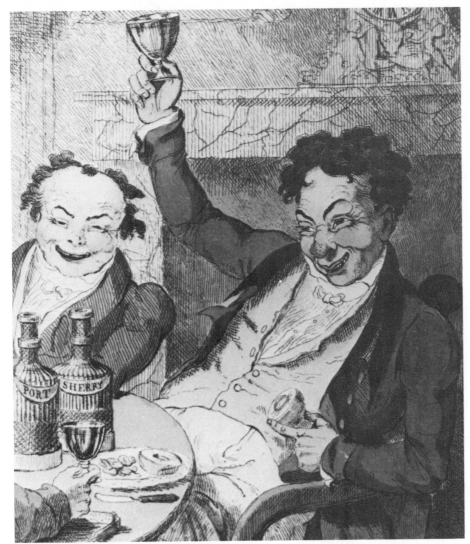

The conviviality often associated with drinking has been romantically celebrated in graphic representations, songs, stories, and legends.

cocktails or highballs in quick succession without any food, a marked change sets in. Depending on individual and group behavior patterns, the drinker becomes either much noisier or much quieter; his speech gets sloppier or more precise, and his general attitude is likely to be either unusually affectionate or unusually hostile.

If the concentration of alcohol in the bloodstream reaches 0.12 percent, there is a noticeable lack of coordination in standing or walking, and if it goes up to 0.15 percent, the physical signs of intoxication are obvious, and they are accompanied by an impairment of mental faculties as well.

A concentration of as much as 0.4 percent can cause a coma, and of 0.7 percent, paralysis of the brain centers that control the activities of the lungs and heart, a condition which can be fatal.

Alcohol affects the brain and nervous system in this way because it is a depressant and an anesthetic. In small amounts, it acts as a sedative. In larger amounts, it depresses the brain centers that control behavior. In still larger amounts, it causes paralysis, unconsciousness, and death.

How Alcohol Moves Through the Body

Although it is negligible in nourishment, alcohol is an energy-producing food like sugar. Unlike most foods, however, it is quickly absorbed into the bloodstream through the stomach and small intestines without first having to undergo complicated digestive processes. It is then carried to the liver, where most of it is converted into heat and energy. From the liver, the remainder is carried by the bloodstream to the heart and pumped to the lungs. Some is expelled in the breath and some is eventually eliminated in sweat and urine. From the lungs, the alcohol is circulated to the brain, where it affects the central nervous system in the manner already described.

People who use good judgment when drinking rarely, if ever, get

erages on the body and on behavior vary a great deal depending on many factors. Although the concentration of alcohol in the drink is the chief factor, other significant factors are: how quickly the drink is consumed; the other components of the drink; how much the person has eaten before or while drinking; his weight, physical condition, and emotional stability.

One factor remains constant: if the bloodstream that reaches the brain contains a certain percentage of alcohol, there are marked changes in reaction. As the percentage increases, the functioning of the brain and central nervous system is increasingly affected. As the alcohol is gradually metabolized and eliminated, the process reverses itself.

Alcohol Concentration in the Blood

If at any given time the blood contains a concentration of about $3/100$ of one percent (0.03 percent), no effects are observable. This amount will make its way into the bloodstream after drinking a highball or cocktail made with one and one-half ounces of whisky, or two small glasses of table wine, or two bottles of beer. It takes about two hours for this amount of alcohol to leave the body completely.

Twice that number of drinks produces twice the concentration of alcohol in the bloodstream—0.06 percent—with an accompanying feeling of warmth and relaxation. By the time the drinker has had three

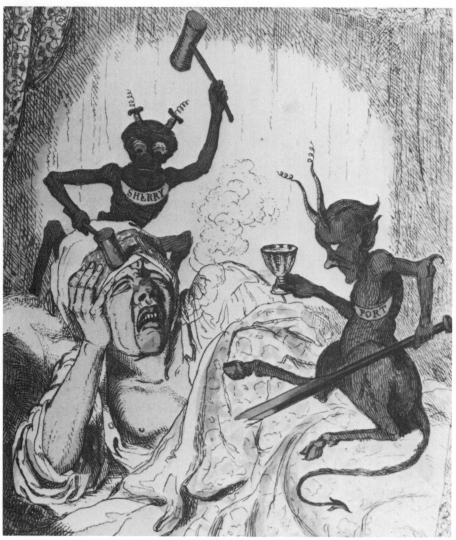

The other side of a jolly evening of drinking (see the illustration on page 543) is "the morning after"— the physical and emotional hangover.

The Hangover

The feeling of discomfort that sometimes sets in the morning after excessive drinking is known as a hangover. It is caused by the disruptive effect of too much alcohol on the central nervous system. The symptoms of nausea, dizziness, heartburn, and a feeling of apprehension are usually most acute several hours after drinking and not while there is still any appreciable amount of alcohol in the system.

Although many people believe that "mixing" drinks—such as switching from whisky drinks to wine—is the main cause of hangovers, a hangover can just as easily be induced by too much of one type of drink or by pure alcohol. Nor is it always the result of drinking too much, since emotional stress or allergy may well be contributing factors.

Some aspects of a hangover may be caused by substances called *congeners*. These are the natural products of fermentation found in small amounts in all alcoholic beverages. Some congeners have toxic properties that produce nausea by irritating certain nerve centers.

In spite of accumulated lore about hangover remedies, there is no certain cure for the symptoms. Neither raw eggs, oysters, alkalizers, sugar, black coffee, nor another drink has any therapeutic value. A throbbing head and aching joints can be relieved by aspirin and bed rest. Stomach irritation can be eased by bland foods such as skim milk, cooked cereal, or a poached egg.

drunk. The safe and pleasurable use of alcoholic beverages depends on the following factors:

THE CONCENTRATION OF ALCOHOL IN THE BEVERAGE: The higher the alcohol content in terms of total volume, the faster it is absorbed. Three ounces of straight whisky—two shot glasses—contain the same amount of alcohol as 48 ounces (or 4 cans) of beer.

SIPPING VS. GULPING: Two shots of straight whisky can be downed in two minutes, but the same amount diluted in two highballs can be sipped through an entire evening. The former makes trouble, and the latter makes sense, because during the elapsed time, the body has a chance to keep getting rid of the alcohol.

ADDITIONAL COMPONENTS OF THE DRINK: The carbohydrates in beer and wine slow down the absorption of alcohol into the blood. Vodka mixed with orange juice travels much more slowly than a vodka martini.

FOOD IN THE STOMACH: The alcohol concentration in two cocktails consumed at the peak of hunger before dinner can have a nasty effect. Several glasses of wine with a meal or a brandy sipped after dinner get to the bloodstream much more slowly and at a lower concentration. The sensible drinker doesn't drink on an empty stomach. The wise host or hostess doesn't prolong the cocktail hour before dinner.

Alcohol and General Health

As a result of new studies of the effect of alcohol on the body, many myths have been laid to rest. In general, it is known that in moderate quantities, alcohol causes the following reactions: the heartbeat quickens slightly, appetite increases, and gastric juices are stimulated. In other words, a drink makes people "feel good."

Tissue Impairment

Habitual drinking of straight whisky can irritate the membranes that line the mouth and throat. The hoarse voice of some heavy drinkers is the result of a thickening of vocal cord tissue. As for the effect on the stomach, alcohol doesn't cause ulcers, but it does aggravate them.

It used to be thought that drinking was the direct cause of cirrhosis of the liver. It now appears that this disease, as well as many deficiency diseases formerly attributed to alcohol, are caused by some form of malnutrition. Laboratory experiments have shown that a daily intake of twenty bottles of a sweet carbonated soft drink is as likely to cause liver impairment as the consumption of a pint of whisky a day.

There is no evidence to support the belief that port wine or any other alcoholic beverage taken in moderation will cause gout. Studies in California show that 60 percent of all patients with this disease had never drunk any wine at all.

The moderate use of alcoholic beverages has no proven permanent effect on brain or nerve tissue. Laboratory scientists, however, continue to investigate the possibility of a direct link between alcohol consumption and brain and nerve tissue damage. While it is true that brain damage has been observed in chronic alcoholics, the impairment is generally attributed to the absence from the diet of essential proteins and vitamins.

Alcohol and Immunity to Infection

Moderate drinkers who maintain proper health habits are no more likely to catch viral or bacterial diseases than nondrinkers. Heavy drinkers suffering from malnutrition have conspicuously lower resistance to infection. However, it has been shown by recent research that even well-nourished heavy drinkers have a generally lower immunity to infection than normal. When the blood-alcohol level is 0.15 percent or above, the alcohol appears to paralyze the activities of disease-fighting white blood cells.

Alcohol and Life Expectancy

It is difficult to isolate drinking in itself as a factor in longevity. A study made some time ago reports the shortest life span for heavy drinkers, a somewhat longer one for those who don't drink at all, and the longest for moderate drinkers. In this connection, it has been pointed out that those who drink sensibly are likely to have equally good judgment in other health matters.

Alcohol and Sex Activity

Alcohol in sufficient quantity depresses the part of the brain that controls inhibitions; this liberating effect has led some people to think that alcohol is an aphrodisiac. This is far from the truth, since at the same time that alcohol increases the sexual appetite, it decreases the ability to perform. In excessive amounts, it unfortunately causes enough impairment of judgment, particularly among the young, to be the indirect cause of many unwanted pregnancies. There is no proof, however, that drinking even in large quantities can cause sterility or defective children.

Alcohol as an Irritant

There are many otherwise healthy people who can't drink alcoholic beverages of any kind, or of a particular kind, without getting sick. In some cases, the negative reaction may be psychological in origin. It may be connected with a disastrous experience with drunkenness in the teen years, or with an early hatred for a drinker in the family. Some people can drink one type of beverage but not another because of a particular congener, or because of an allergy to a particular grain or fruit.

People suffering from certain diseases should never drink any alcoholic beverages unless specifically told to do so by the doctor. Among these diseases are peptic ulcers, kidney and liver infections, and epilepsy.

Alcoholic Beverages as Medicine

At practically all times and in many parts of the world today, alcoholic beverages of various kinds have been and are still used for medicinal purposes. This should not be taken to mean that Aunt Sally is right about the curative powers of her elderberry wine, or that grandpa knows best when he says brandy is the best cure for hiccups.

European doctors prescribe wine, beer, and occasionally distilled spirits—each in specific doses—for their value in treating specific disorders. American doctors did the same until the Prohibition era. During that time, such prescriptions were seriously abused in the same way that prescriptions for amphetamines and barbiturates are currently abused. Today an American physician may recommend a particular alcoholic beverage as a tranquilizer, a sleep-inducer, or an appetite stimulant.

Use of Alcohol With Other Drugs

Alcoholic beverages should be avoided by anyone taking barbiturates or other sedatives. See under *Drug Use and Abuse*, p. 556, for a discussion of barbiturates.

Alcohol and Driving

Recent studies of traffic accidents indicate that considerably more than half of those that are fatal are the result of drunken driving.

Although small amounts of alcohol affect reflex responses, there appears to be no deterioration in response and judgment when the blood-alcohol content is below 0.05 percent. According to the law in most states, a blood-alcohol content beyond 0.15 percent is legal ground for prosecution. In most European countries, this limit is set at 0.10 percent.

For many people, coordination, alertness, and general driving skills are impaired at blood-alcohol levels below the legal limit. There are some people who become dangerous drivers after only one drink. Attempts are constantly being made, but so far with less than perfect success, to educate the public about the very real dangers of drunken driving.

Alcohol Problems

The obvious proof that a deep confusion exists about the place of alcoholic beverages in American life is the fact that only one amendment to the Constitution has ever been repealed: the Prohibition Amendment. The conflict continues to express itself in the bewildering range of laws in different states.

LOCAL LAWS: In some parts of the U.S., it is illegal to buy a drink in a public place. In others, only state-operated stores can sell distilled beverages by the bottle. In some states, bars can't have a liquor license unless they also prepare and serve food.

Often the local laws governing such matters are enacted through the support of interests that would seem to be opposed to each other. In many areas with dry statutes, church and temperance groups have voted with bootleggers to defeat the legal sale of alcoholic beverages.

Alcohol education is required in all states. Yet teachers are rarely given guidelines to make the education effective. Are they supposed to encourage complete abstinence? Should the problem be thrown at the physical education department with a chart that shows liver damage? Should there be open discussions on the social and psychological causes of problem drinking?

Until comparatively recently, people with drinking problems had few places to turn for help. When they got obstreperous in public, they were put in jail. When they deteriorated physically, they were put in a hospital. And when their brains were sufficiently affected, they were sent off to a state or private asylum.

CHANGING ATTITUDES: The situation has changed somewhat over the past 30 years. The concern of gov-

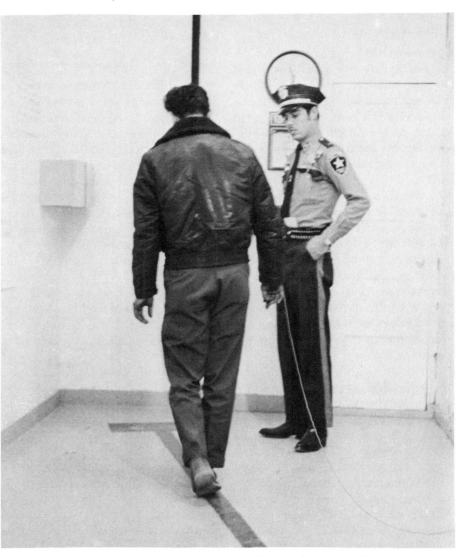

Alcohol impairs driving skills. The ability to walk in a straight line is used as a test of intoxication for drivers in some states.

ernment agencies, of the medical profession, and of industry has led to efforts to create a broad and effective program for dealing with problem drinking, for educating the public, and for shaping a national policy about the use of alcoholic beverages.

What Is Problem Drinking?

The National Institute of Mental Health, under the jurisdiction of the U.S. Department of Health, Education and Welfare, established a commission to study the problems related to alcohol. In its report, the commission, which was composed of specialists in medicine, psychiatry, and sociology, defined problem drinking as "the repetitive use of beverage alcohol causing physical,

psychological, or social harm to the drinker or to others."

The commission further defined alcoholism as "the condition in which an individual has lost control over his alcoholic intake in the sense that he is consistently unable to refrain from drinking or to stop drinking before getting intoxicated."

Specialists have pointed out that excessive use of beverage alcohol is the most important drug abuse problem in the United States today. Of the approximately 90 million Americans who drink, 1 out of 10 has problems related to drinking. Of the nine million who need some help with problem drinking, about half are addictive alcoholics, and of this number, only about 5 percent are homeless, jobless or skid row alcoholics. Most people with drinking problems are otherwise respectable members of society.

Alcoholism as a Disease

The American Medical Association, the World Health Organization, and more recently the courts, now recognize the type of alcoholism involving loss of control over drinking behavior as a disease. More specifically, it has come to be considered a complex illness best described as a drug dependency.

The leadership of the medical profession points out that although the liquor industry is expanding and the per capita consumption of alcoholic beverages is increasing, there is no reason to assume an increase in alcoholism. It is also true that some ethnic groups have a conspicuously higher rate of addictive alcoholism than others. The rate among Irish-Americans is high and so is the rate among white Anglo-Saxon Protes-

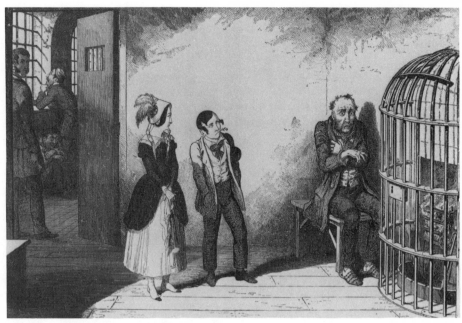

This 19th-century lithograph by George Cruikshank shows a hopeless alcoholic confined to an institution and being visited by his son and daughter.

tants; the rate is low among Italian-Americans, and lower still among the Chinese and Jews in this country. Recent studies suggest, however, that changing cultural habits among some groups with traditionally low rates of alcohol abuse may call for a re-examination of these statistical conclusions. Their rates may be climbing relative to the higher-incidence groups.

Possible Causes of Alcoholism

Before examining some of the complicated factors that lead to the development of alcoholism, a few popular misconceptions should be disposed of. Alcohol doesn't cause alcoholism any more than sugar causes diabetes. Alcoholism isn't caused by a particular beverage. Nor is it an inherited illness.

PHYSIOLOGICAL CAUSES: Although several physiological factors seem to be involved in the progression of alcoholism, no single one can be pointed to as the cause of the disease. Among the theories now being investigated are the following: abnormal sugar metabolism; disorder of the endocrine glands; dietary deficiencies.

PSYCHOLOGICAL CAUSES: Up to this point, there is no conclusive evidence that there is such a thing as an alcoholic or a prealcoholic personality. Common traits of emotional im-

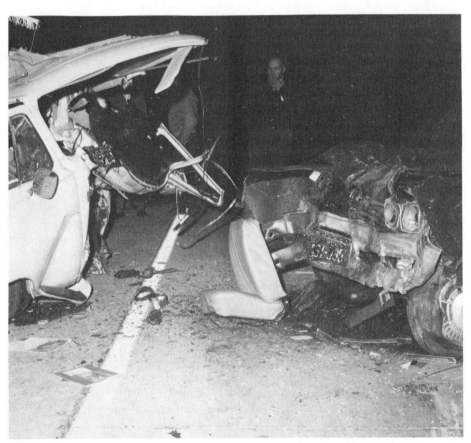

Recent studies of traffic accidents indicate that considerably more than half of those that are fatal are the result of drunken driving.

maturity and strong dependency needs have been observed in patients. However, it is still not certain whether these conditions forerun or follow excessive alcohol use. The neurotic patterns that alcoholics share with each other they also share with nonalcoholics suffering from personality disturbances.

Many psychiatrists believe that emotional traumas and deprivation suffered in childhood can eventually cause certain poorly adjusted adults to seek relief through alcohol from such feelings as anxiety, hostility, extreme guilt, and a deep sense of inferiority.

SOCIOLOGICAL FACTORS: Practically all studies of alcoholism in this country indicate that ethnic groups vary dramatically in their rate of problem drinkers. A great deal of attention has therefore been focused recently on *learned attitudes* towards alcoholic beverages and how they affect drinking patterns.

It has been found that in low-incidence groups, the attitude toward drinking is clearly defined, understood by all the members of the group, and drunkenness is consistently disapproved of and viewed as unacceptable. In these groups, alcoholic beverages are introduced to children in the home with no emotional overtones and are used in family situations, at meals, or for religious celebrations.

In the high-incidence groups, there is usually a great deal of conflict about alcohol. The basic rules aren't clearly defined, and there are no clear-cut standards for acceptable and unacceptable drinking behavior. In such groups, drinking is more often looked on as a way of drowning one's sorrows; solitary drinking is therefore more common.

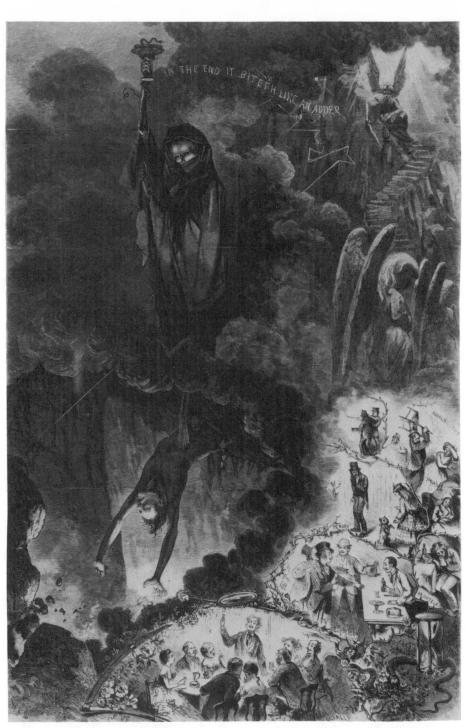

Attitudes toward problem drinking are changing, but it was only a hundred years ago that this engraving called "The Drunkard's Progress" reflected a prevalent feeling of hopelessness about the alcoholic's moral degeneration.

Recognizing the Danger Signals of Problem Drinking

Because different groups have different standards about drinking and drunkenness, it is extremely important for families to have a clear idea of some of the recognizable symptoms of problem drinking. A man or woman—or a teen-ager—with several of the following symptoms needs professional help before the situation becomes unmanageable:

• Using alcohol as a way of handling problems or escaping from them

• An increasing use of alcohol with repeated occasions of unintended intoxication

• Sneaking drinks or gulping them rapidly in quick succession

• Irritation, hostility, and lying when the subject of excessive drinking is mentioned

• Marital, financial, and job problems that can be traced to alcohol

• A noticeable deterioration in appearance, health, and social behavior

• Arrests for drunkenness or drunken driving

• Persistent drinking in spite of such symptoms as headaches, loss of appetite, sleeplessness, and stomach trouble.

Symptoms of Chronic Alcoholism

Excessive drinking over a long period is often accompanied by nutritional deficiencies that show up in liver disorders, anemia, and lowered resistance to infection. Chronic alcoholism is often accompanied by disorders of the central nervous system. There may be tremors of the hands; eye function may deteriorate; bladder control may suffer. Changes in behavior result from a decrease in inhibition control: excessive cheerfulness quickly turns into weeping; moods of self-hatred alternate with moods of hostility to others. The attention span grows shorter, and there are increasing lapses of memory.

DELIRIUM TREMENS: Chronic alcoholics occasionally suffer from episodes of hallucination during which they may "see things" and hear accusing voices. Such episodes are different from the acute disorder known as *delirium tremens,* or the *DTs.* This mental and physical disturbance is accompanied by nausea, confusion, the sensation that something is crawling on the skin, and hallucinations involving fantastic, brightly-colored animals. The condition is caused by rapid lowering of blood alcohol levels in very heavy drinkers, usually at a time of withdrawal from alcohol.

Delirium tremens is a medical emergency requiring prompt treatment and sometimes hospitalization.

Where to Go for Help With an Alcohol Problem

Resources for the diagnosis and treatment of problem drinkers are more readily available than they used to be. Detailed information about agencies that treat alcoholism in a particular community will be supplied by the Alcohol and Drug Problems Association of North America, 1130 17th Street, N. W., Washington, D.C. 20036.

ALCOHOL INFORMATION CENTER: Although more help is available in metropolitan than in rural areas, many places now have their own Alcoholism Information Center, listed in phone directories under that name.

BUSINESS: Many large business and industrial firms as well as unions have medical programs that can help in identifying an alcohol problem. Some group health insurance plans provide coverage for long-term treatment as well as for hospitalization.

ALCOHOLICS ANONYMOUS: One of the oldest agencies offering help is Alcoholics Anonymous. Founded in the 1930s, it now has chapters throughout the United States. Its program has been successful with those problem drinkers willing to seek help on their own.

FAMILY DOCTOR: Family doctors have been alerted to the need for dealing with alcohol problems as part of their regular medical practice. They should be called on for individual care as well as for information about special alcoholism programs in the community.

Some Methods of Treatment

The kind of treatment to which a problem drinker will respond depends on many factors: the extent of his dependence on alcohol, his general health, his attitudes toward treatment, and the cooperation of his family, friends, and community.

It is only in recent years that general hospitals have begun to admit people suffering from alcoholism in the same routine way that they admit other sick people. A study at Massachusetts General Hospital indicates that when an alcoholic patient is received with courtesy and sympathy, he is much more likely to cooperate in the prescribed treatment.

Currently, various medicines are being used to help the patient break his drinking pattern. Tranquilizers are used to reduce tensions and to get the patient calm enough to begin some form of psychotherapy.

The purpose of exploring the patient's past is to dig up buried conflicts and try to resolve them so that he can accept himself without self-hatred and face his real problems as a sober adult. It is customary to include the patient's family in the therapeutic sessions from time to time.

A MODEL TREATMENT PROGRAM: An outstanding example of team treatment of alcoholics is being practiced at a state clinic in Georgia. Because the director of the project felt that an alcoholic was a person sick in body, mind, and soul, he consolidated the services of medical doctors, psychiatrists, and clergymen of various faiths. The program has been described as follows:

After physical evaluation, the patient undergoes psychiatric, social, and vocational screening in an attempt to determine his recovery potential. Medical management and treatment prescription is begun immediately and continued throughout the contact. A series of orientation procedures follows: the patient sees appropriate films, attends personal interviews and counseling sessions, and participates in group meetings. Each week, there are 69 group meetings together with 16 staff group meetings. A network of occupational, recreational, and vocational activities designed to aid self-expression is woven into the program. The patients themselves form a therapeutic community, earlier members sponsoring the newer and more frightened. This "acceptance attitude therapy" is an important factor in orienting and strengthening the new patient. After leaving the clinic, all patients are urged to attend group meetings regularly for at least two years in the outpatient clinic, or at a local chapter of Alcoholics Anonymous or at a community-based clinic, and to continue indefinitely if possible.

Chances for Recovery

The word "cure" is rarely used in connection with alcoholics, since a cure implies complete control over alcohol intake. Even the arbitrary goal of permanent abstention is achieved by only a small number of treated patients.

Leading therapists consider that treatment has been successful when the patient can reestablish and maintain a good family life, a good work record, and a respectable place in his community by controlling his drinking most of the time. There is no doubt that the sooner a problem drinker is treated, the greater his chances for recovery.

Help With Family Problems

Alcoholics usually disrupt family life in one way or another. In some cases, they remain alcoholics because of an unhealthy family situation. It is therefore recommended that family members seek help and support from outside agencies that can take a detached view of the problem.

Mental health clinics, family service agencies, and church-sponsored groups are among the community organizations that can be called on for assistance. Relatives and friends of alcoholics can join one of the Al-Anon Family Groups that work with Alcoholics Anonymous. The Alateen Groups are specifically set up for the children of problem drinkers.

Laws to Cure Alcohol Problems

Neither here nor in any European country has it been possible to eliminate the use of alcoholic beverages by the enactment of national laws. As for the various state laws, they bear practically no relation to the extent and nature of the use and abuse of alcohol. Regulations aimed at controlling the legal minimum drinking age are extremely difficult to enforce and may even be irrelevant. Neither France nor Italy has a minimum drinking age. France has

one of the highest rates of alcohol problems of any European country and Italy has one of the lowest.

Since 1882, when Vermont voted to make alcohol education compulsory in the public schools, every state has enacted a similar law. Yet even though this education has consisted chiefly of stressing the dangers of alcohol, a majority of the students grew up to be drinking adults. The reason for the failure of a negative approach to drinking has been summarized by Dr. Robert Straus, Professor of Behavioral Science at the University of Kentucky, a leading figure in the field of alcohol studies. This is what he says:

It is as if driver-education classes in schools would be concerned only with the gorier aspects of speeding and reckless driving. This might frighten a few students, but it would not produce many who know how to handle an automobile safely. With the emphasis placed solely on alcoholism, alcohol might similarly frighten a few students, but it would not produce many who knew about drinking, or how to handle alcohol safely.

Alcohol Education

As research in all areas connected with problem drinking goes forward, new ways are being examined to enlighten the American people about the differences between a safe and sensible approach to alcohol and a damaging one.

At Home

Since most basic attitudes are instilled in the home, each family has the responsibility for clear thinking and clear-cut behavior about alcoholic beverages. Those people who abstain completely out of religious or moral principle obviously hope that their children will do the same. To present drinking, however, simply as an evil or a sinful activity may only succeed in making it more attractive, especially to teen-agers. If total abstention is recommended, it should be for reasons that make sense to youngsters, particularly if

they are exposed to other attitudes in the homes of friends whom they respect.

On the other hand, no one should be made to feel inferior because he doesn't drink. Alcoholic beverages aren't essential to good health or the good life. They in no way add to anyone's masculinity, sophistication, or social status.

In families where drinking is part of the pattern, it appears that the most wholesome attitudes result from a clear agreement about the acceptable and unacceptable use of alcoholic beverages. If children are taught that drinking is first and foremost a social activity, they are less likely to see alcohol as a solution to personal misery.

Groups with especially low rates of alcohol problems have clear standards not only about drinking but also about drunkenness. Children in these groups get the idea that drunkenness is never sanctioned and never excused. Someone who is drunk isn't laughed at or argued with. The consensus, clearly stated and frequently implied, is that anyone who gets drunk simply doesn't know how to behave and therefore there must be something wrong with him.

New Approaches

"It is a historical medical fact that almost no condition has been eradicated by treating casualties."—Dr. M. E. Chafetz, Director of Clinical Services, Massachusetts General Hospital.

Many educators are trying to present a more realistic and sensible picture of drinking than the negative one that was presented in the past. Some schools are considering alcohol education as part of courses where it is relevant: not only in health, hygiene, and safety, but also in history, geography, science, and literature.

A current government pamphlet prepared especially for teen-agers is an excellent starting point for classroom discussions. It is called "Thinking About Drinking" and is a lively presentation of the latest findings in alcohol research. It can be ordered by mail by writing to the Superintendent of Documents, U.S. Government Printing Office, Washington, D. C. 20401. The pamphlet is officially referred to as Children's Bureau Publication No. 456.

Whether in politics, sex education, or alcohol education, it is the duty of teachers to put aside personal bias so that young people can trust them as a source of information and reliable guidance. A presentation of alcohol that clarifies its use as food, that discusses standards of behavior, and that encourages young people to think about what's really good for them achieves better results in the long run than scare tactics and horror stories.

In the Community

Wherever possible, guidelines should be agreed on for drinking at parties and in public. Hosts should never press additional drinks on guests who have had enough already. They should never permit a guest who is "high" to drive his own car home.

Alcohol education programs for community presentation are available on request from the National Institute on Alcohol Abuse and Alcoholism, Rockville, Maryland 20852. Such programs can be presented by committees including doctors, ministers, educators, social workers, and young people. Meetings should encourage questions and discussion so that prejudices and misconceptions about drinking can be handled by authorities who know the facts.

Hopefully, general enlightenment will eventually lead to a code of behavior about alcohol that has wide acceptance. Such a code will go a long way toward eliminating a great deal of personal misery and a major national health problem.

CHAPTER 32

Drugs

The drug problem is obviously concerning more and more people these days. Most of the adults who are upset about drugs have young people and the so-called dangerous drugs in mind. But many authorities think we should really examine our whole American society for the "pill-happy" context in which the drug explosion is taking place.

For example, Dr. W. Walter Menninger of the Menninger Foundation has said:

> . . . in recent years, the American people have annually consumed nearly 2.5 billion gallons of alcoholic beverages, 34 million pounds of aspirin, nearly 10 million pounds of vitamins, nearly three million pounds of tranquilizers and barbiturates—and the medicine cabinets in American homes have never been so full.

We are constantly bombarded by television commericals promising us instant relief from even minor pain, as if brief discomfort were somehow immoral. Dr. Joel Fort, former Consultant on Drug Abuse to the World Health Organization, called us—

> a drug-prone nation . . . the average "straight" adult consumes three to five mind-altering drugs a day, beginning with the stimulant caffeine in coffee, tea, and Coca Cola, going on to include alcohol and nicotine, often a tranquilizer, not uncommonly a sleeping pill at night and sometimes an amphetamine the next morning. . . .

What Is a Drug?

Some people are surprised to hear aspirin, coffee, tobacco, and whisky described in the same context as marihuana. The definition of a drug varies with the user; however, here is the one accepted by pharmacologists: a drug is any substance that changes body form or function. In the much narrower medical sense, a drug is a substance used to diagnose, treat, or prevent illness. The drugs we take for medical purposes fall into two broad categories: over-the-counter and prescription (or *ethical*) drugs.

Over-the-Counter Drugs

Over-the-counter drugs are sold and consumed by us in enormous quantities—from headache remedies to cold nostrums, laxatives to tonics, acne ointments to vitamins. Many physicians think that Americans indulge in far too much self-diagnosis and self-dosing, with the risk that serious conditions may go undetected and untreated, and even be aggravated by the medicine being used.

In general, good practice is to use over-the-counter drugs as seldom as possible, for short-term, minor illness, being careful to choose medicines of proven effectiveness: taking a couple of aspirins for a headache is a good example. The

U.S. Public Health Service offers these guidelines:

> Self-prescribed drugs should never be used continuously for long periods of time . . . a physician is required for: abdominal pain that is severe or recurs periodically; pains anywhere, if severe, disabling, persistent, or recurring; headache, if unusually severe or prolonged more than one day; a prolonged cold with fever or cough; earache; unexplained loss of weight; unexplained and unusual symptoms; *malaise* lasting more than a week or two.

The Food and Drug Administration (FDA), a branch of the Public Health Service, is responsible for establishing the safety and usefulness of all drugs marketed in this country, both over-the-counter and prescription. You can be assured that over-the-counter drugs are safe for you to use, provided you take them in strict accordance with the label instruction, which will tell you the appropriate dose, among other things, and carry warnings against prolonged or improper use, such as "discontinue if pain persists" or "do not take if abdominal pain is present." This labeling information is regulated by the FDA.

From time to time the FDA decides that a particular over-the-counter product is useless for its advertised function and seeks to have it removed from the market or its advertising changed. An example is the ruling that mouthwashes are ineffective in eliminating that most dread of all maladies—bad breath. However, the fact that a patent remedy may be useful in some cases doesn't mean that it is necessary, or even good, for you personally. Your own doctor should tell you whether you really need vitamins and tonics; buffered aspirin or a combination of aspirin with other ingredients; cough drops and syrups; reducing tablets; hemorrhoid ointments; and other over-the-counter favorites.

Prescription Drugs

Prescription drugs are in theory at the opposite pole from over-the-counter drugs. They require medical supervision for safe use and so may only be sold, by law, to persons holding a doctor's prescription. A prescription drug is a uniquely personal product; it must be used only by the one for whom it was prescribed. It is meant to be taken in consultation with your doctor.

The label may or may not carry direction, size of dose, name of drug, warnings—at the option of the physician. Therefore, you must make sure you understand exactly how your doctor wants you to take the medication. If the labeling is skimpy, write down what you need to know. Some drugs cannot be refilled without a new prescription. Even if it can be refilled, do not do so without checking first with your doctor. You may no longer need it, and it may do you harm.

Similarly, it is a good idea to keep only those medicines you are currently taking. Destroy old prescriptions; they may decompose in time. Resist the powerful temptation to play doctor by passing on the unused part of one of your medications to a friend who you feel certain has the same thing wrong with him that you did. Also resist treating one child with another child's prescription without the doctor's approval.

Some drugs have undesirable side effects in some individuals, even though they have been judged safe for general use. The reason they are marketed is that their special therapeutic properties far outweigh the potential for adverse reactions. Your doctor may warn you in advance of the possibility of such reactions. If you think you are having a reaction that is not normal—gastric distress following a drug taken for muscle pain, for example—call your doctor immediately. If you can't reach him, discontinue the drug until you get his advice.

A few individuals are aware that they are allergic or have severe reactions to certain drugs, such as penicillin, or vaccines made from poultry eggs. These persons should of course alert their doctor and pharmacist to their allergies.

The problem of selecting the right drug for your case is not an easy one; 90 percent of prescriptions written today are for drugs that didn't exist ten years ago. You can help your doctor by taking them exactly as ordered.

DRUG USE AND ABUSE

Among the drugs that may be prescribed for you are some that possess a tremendous capability for abuse. They include: *stimulants*, such as amphetamines; *depressants*, such as sleeping pills and tranquilizers; and *narcotic* painkillers, such as morphine and codeine. When abused—that is, when taken in any way other than according to a doctor's strict instuction for medical use—they constitute the worst part of our burgeoning national drug problem.

The remainder of this chapter will discuss the use and abuse of these drugs as well as others for which medical use is limited or experimental, such as marihuana, or for which there is no present medical use, such as the hallucinogens.

Stimulant Drugs

The Amphetamines

The *amphetamines*, first synthesized in the 1920s, are powerful stimulators of the central nervous system.

The major forms of the drug are: amphetamine (Benzedrine), the more powerful dextroamphetamine (Dexedrine), and methamphetamine (Methedrine, Desoxyn). The general street name given to these drugs is "speed," which some abusers restrict to Methedrine.

LEGITIMATE USE OF AMPHETAMINES: The legitimate use of amphetamines in medicine and their great capacity for abuse both stem from the same property—the ability to speed up the body's systems, and especially the central nervous system.

Doctors prescribe amphetamines mostly to curb the appetite of patients who are dieting and to counteract mild depression. More rarely, they use it to treat *narcolepsy*—a disease in which the patient is overwhelmed by bouts of sleep—and to counteract the drowsiness caused by sedatives. Amphetamines and an amphetaminelike drug (Ritalin) are also used to treat certain hyperactive children who—probably because of mild brain damage—are extremely excitable and easily distracted. For reasons imperfectly understood, the drug calms them instead of stimulating them. For all these uses, amphetamines are called for in approximately eight percent of all prescriptions written in this country, according to one estimate.

AMPHETAMINE ABUSE: The consumption of amphetamines, however, is far greater than the prescription books indicate. Some ten billion tablets are produced in this country annually, enough for 50 doses for every man, woman, and child. Of this amount, probably half is diverted into illicit channels. Underground laboratories manufacture even more, especially methamphetamine.

Who uses this enormous quantity of drugs, and why? The student cramming for an exam, the housewife trying to get through the day without collapsing from exhaustion, the businessman who has tossed and turned all night in a strange hotel bedroom and needs to be alert for an important conference the next morning.

EFFECTS: For many of these people, the drugs are obtained legally, by prescription. There is no question whatever that used judiciously, amphetamines can bring the desired results without any problems to the user or the society. They can improve performance, both mental and physical, over a moderate period of time, by delaying the deterioration in performance that fatigue normally produces. This has been especially useful when an individual has been temporarily required to carry out routine duties under difficult circumstances and for extended time. Thus some astronauts have used amphetamines, under long-range medical supervision, while in space. There is also no question that for some people amphetamines can bring feelings of self-confidence, well-being, alertness, and an increased ability to concentrate and perform at the peak of their powers.

But some individuals may have completely different reactions to amphetamines, including an increase in tension ranging from the merely uncomfortable to an agonizing pitch of anxiety. Some experi-

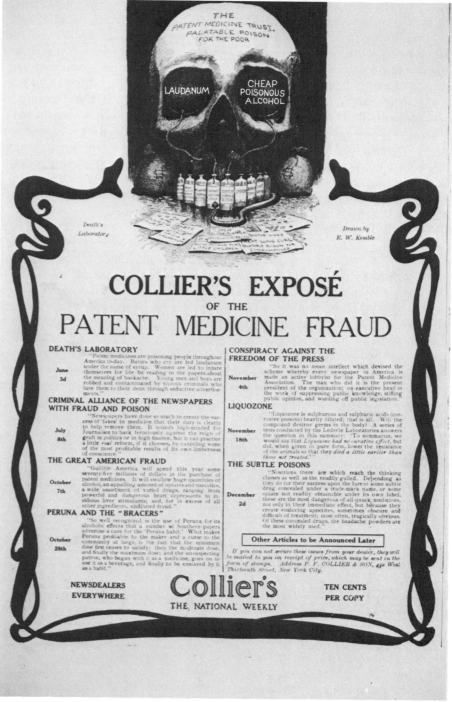

An ad for a magazine series on fraudulent over-the-counter drugs stresses that "gullible Americans will spend this year (1905) some $75 million."

ence unpleasant physical symptoms that are generally linked only to fairly high doses. These include dry mouth, sweating, palpitations, and a rise in blood pressure.

Moreover, since the drugs merely defer the effects of fatigue, the benefits are fleeting, and the let-down from amphetamines can be both severe and dangerously inconvenient,

especially for someone like a long-haul truck driver. Some authorities believe that many truck accidents derive from the effects of amphetamine abuse.

Also, the feelings of self-confidence about improved performance are often highly deceptive. Because of certain freak effects of amphetamines, performance may actually have deteriorated sharply or vanished entirely. Stories abound of students who have crammed all night for a final and then written what they thought to be a masterly paper, only to learn that their examination book is blank, or written all on one dense line.

Most serious, the repeated use of amphetamines may lead to an utterly different kind of drug experience and an exceedingly dangerous one. Amphetamine users quickly develop tolerance to the drug. Even those who use amphetamines as appetite suppressants or minor mood elevators usually find that after a few days or weeks the dose must be increased to attain the same results. Psychological dependence, for some individuals, can build rapidly, with the results that the user becomes "hooked"—dependent on the drug. Fortunately, newspapers, magazines, and television news reports gave a great deal of publicity to amphetamine abuse in the 1970s. As a result, many physicians became extremely cautious about prescribing these drugs. Still, the black market in amphetamines remained strong.

SPEED FREAK: The *speed freak* may be someone who started using amphetamines as diet or pep pills, or someone out for kicks from the beginning. Whatever the origin, greatly increased tolerance and iron-strong psychological dependence compel him to take large quantities of the drugs. Pill-popping and snorting (sniffing powdered amphetamine) have, for most speeders, been superseded by injecting large doses of a methamphetamine, usually Methedrine, directly into a vein.

The speed freak uses a hypodermic because the Methedrine thus given has an immediate, electric effect on his body. He experiences an almost instant *rush*—a surge of powerful physical feelings that make his skin tingle, make him feel suddenly a hundred times more alive.

The price for this gorgeous rush is a stiff one by any standard. The heavy user cannot sleep, sometimes going for ten days or two weeks with only a kind of half-sleep. During this time he tends to be suspicious without cause, aggressive, and frantically active. If the "run" (the time on an amphetamine high) is a long one, if the dose is large, or if the speed freak is a chronic user, then his belligerence may phase into confusion and fear, or paranoia with delusions and hallucinations. High-dose users are apparently regularly skirting incidents of murder or mayhem. But death from overdose is actually rare.

During his high, the user is obviously not capable of much meaningful activity; his life is riveted to the sensations of the drug. In fact, one of the hallmarks of a methamphetamine binge is the "hangup" in which the user repeats some action over and over again—like a phonograph needle stuck in a groove. He may shower all day long, or mindlessly dismantle and reassemble the same piece of equipment, or sing the same song or note endlessly.

At the end of his run is the crash: depression, extreme fatigue, debilitated physical condition (he has probably been unable to eat or sleep), irritability. There is a great temptation to ease the descent of the crash by using barbiturates to come down from the high, or simply to take more stimulants and get back into the next run as soon as possible.

Some experts believe that this reaction is actually a set of withdrawal symptoms; most disagree, and hold that amphetamines do not create true physical dependence, as the barbiturates and narcotics do.

PROLONGED AMPHETAMINE ABUSE: But prolonged amphetamine abuse is in itself harmful to the body, unlike heroin abuse (short of fatal overdoses). It has caused permanent brain damage in experimental animals, and may do so in human users. One researcher has said: "Speed is a hundred times more dangerous than heroin." Recovery usually follows, however, if the speeder can stop.

The U.S. Food and Drug Administration and the Bureau of Narcotics and Dangerous Drugs reacted to the situation in April, 1973 by recalling all diet drugs that contained amphetamines. The specific targets were amphetamines designed for injection and diet drugs that combined amphetamines with tranquilizers or vitamins. The FDA said that combination diet pills were not effective in controlling obesity and that the injectable type was too subject to abuse. The federal agencies also ordered a substantial cutback in the legitimate production of amphetamines and methamphetamines.

Amphetaminelike Stimulants

Several drugs, although chemically unrelated to the amphetamines, have very similar effects on the body: they are strong stimulants of the central nervous system. The two most important ones in this country are methylphenidate (Ritalin), mentioned above, and phenmetrazine (Preludin). Preludin has been widely touted as a diet pill. Both drugs seem to be as prone to abuse and as dangerous as the amphetamines.

Cocaine

Cocaine is the principal active ingredient of the coca plant, whose leaves are chewed by millions of Andean Indians as a mild stimulant. Cocaine itself is a powerful stimulant to the central nervous system.

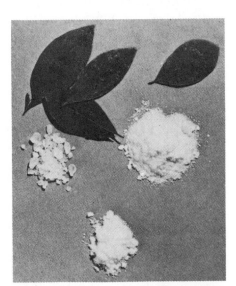

Cocaine, shown here with leaves of the coca plant from which it is derived, resembles moth flakes when in its crystalline form.

In its crystalline form, cocaine is a white powder that looks like moth flakes. It is called *snow, coke* and by a dozen or more other names. A cocaine user is a *snowbird.* Generally, he sniffs it or injects it into a vein, with results similar to those from amphetamines. Snowbirds, however, don't seem to develop tolerance, and thus don't need to increase the dosage. An overdose of cocaine can kill the user by depressing heart and lung functions.

A classic recipe for many years has been the speedball, a combination of heroin and cocaine that is injected. The shot yields a sudden rush in the genitals or lower abdomen (from the cocaine) followed by a long daze (from the heroin). Because cocaine is costly and often hard to get, many addicts have been switching to combinations of heroin and methamphetamine.

Depressant Drugs

Depressant drugs are those that depress the central nervous system; they have a sedative, or calming effect. Apart from alcohol—probably the most widely used and abused depressant—they consist mainly of barbiturates, which are both *sedative* and *hypnotic* (sleep-producing), and those, called *tranquilizers,* that can calm without producing sleep. Some 14 to 18 percent of all prescriptions written by physicians in this country are for sedatives and tranquilizers. By far the largest number of these prescriptions call for barbiturates.

Barbiturates

The *barbiturates,* hypnotic and sedative derivatives of barbituric acid, have been used by physicians for almost 75 years.

LEGITIMATE USE OF BARBITURATES: In legitimate medical practice, barbiturates are prescribed for any of the following reasons: to overcome insomnia, to reduce high blood pressure, to treat mental disorders, to alleviate anxiety, to sedate patients both before and after surgery, and to control the convulsions accompanying epilepsy, tetanus, and the administration of certain other drugs. The Food and Drug Administration has conducted a survey showing that during one representative year a million pounds of barbiturates were made available—enough to furnish 24 doses to every living soul in the country.

The barbiturates have widely varying effects, but they can usually be sorted according to how long-lived their action is: long-acting, short-acting, and ultra-short-acting. (The last category includes the shot the dentist gives you intravenously for instant oblivion: thiopental or Pentothal.) When barbiturates are abused, it is generally the short-acting variety, because these drugs also start their action quickly.

BARBITURATE ABUSE: Who abuses barbiturates, and why? Basically, barbiturate abusers fall into four categories, with some overlap.

The "silent abuser" takes sleeping pills first simply to get some sleep, probably with a doctor's prescription, then to deal with tension and anxiety. These users are usually middle-aged or older, do not take any other drugs, and confine their problem to the privacy of their own homes. For them, barbiturates produce a state of intoxication very close to that from an alcoholic binge, with slurred speech, confusion, poor judgment and coordination, and sometimes wild emotional swings, from combative irritability to elation. These users eventually wind up getting their drugs primarily through illicit channels. They may become so trapped in the cycle of sedation and hangover that they literally spend their lives in bed in a kind of permanent half-sleep, interrupted only to rise for more drugs, and, occasionally, food.

The second group of abusers takes barbiturates, strangely enough, for stimulation. This effect appears in some long-time users of the drug who have developed a high tolerance to it. In others, the drug gives an apparent boost because it releases inhibitions. This may be the kind of sensation sought by such a group as high school students.

A third group, probably consisting mostly of young people who are into the drug scene and taking a variety of drugs, uses barbiturates to counter the effects of an amphetamine spree, to come down from a high. This establishes a vicious cycle of dependence that has been called a seesaw of stimulation and sedation. Some drug abusers take the barbiturate-amphetamine combination in the same swallow to obtain their effects simultaneously; the combination is known as a set-up.

Finally, heroin (and other narcotics) users may use barbiturates for two reasons: as a substitute when heroin is temporarily unavailable, or combined with heroin to prolong its effect. In one hospital surveyed, 23 percent of the narcotics users said they were also dependent on barbiturates.

DANGERS OF BARBITURATE ABUSE: Contrary to popular belief, barbiturate abuse is far more dangerous than the abuse of narcotics. Indeed, many physicians hold barbiturates to be the most perilous of all drugs. Chronic abuse brings psychological dependence and increased tolerance. The continued use of large doses in turn leads to physical dependence of a particularly anguishing kind.

Abrupt withdrawal from barbiturates is far more dangerous than cold-turkey withdrawal from heroin. It begins with anxiety, headache, muscle twitches, weakness, nausea, and sharp drops in blood pressure. If the user stands up suddenly he may faint. These symptoms develop after one day of withdrawal. Later, delirium and convulsions resembling epileptic seizures can develop. If the withdrawal is not performed under medical supervision, an absolute must with barbiturates, these convulsions may be fatal. By contrast, withdrawal from narcotics may be unpleasant, but does not involve convulsions. A supervised withdrawal from barbiturates may take as long as two months.

Even discounting the hazards of withdrawal, abuse of barbiturates is extremely dangerous. Unintentional overdose, which is often fatal, may occur very easily. If someone takes a regular dose to achieve sleep and then remains awake, or awakens shortly thereafter, he may be so confused that he will continue to take repeated normal doses until he is severely poisoned or dead. Fatal reactions are also possible if he mixes barbiturates and alcohol. Each drug reinforces the depressant or toxic effect of the other, often with deadly effects on respiration. Moreover, tolerance does not increase the lethal dose of barbiturates, as it does with narcotics. Every year there are some three thousand deaths from barbiturate overdose, accidental or intentional. More deaths result from the misuse of barbiturates than from any other drug.

Other Drugs of the Barbiturate Type

Other depressants that are chemically unrelated to the barbiturates but have similar effects are glutethimide (Doriden), ethchlorvynol (Placidyl), ethinamate (Valmid), and methyprylon (Noludar). These, too, when abused, bring tolerance and psychological and physical dependence, as well as withdrawal symptoms.

Tranquilizers

Current since the early 1950s, these drugs, unlike the barbiturates, can allay anxiety without inducing sleep. The tranquilizers fall into two groups, major and minor, depending on their influence on *psychoses,* severe mental disorders.

The minor tranquilizers are generally ineffective in dealing with such mental disease, but are used in treating emotional tension and sometimes as muscle relaxants. It is this group that is subject to abuse, for unlike the major tranquilizers—reserpine and phenothiazine, for example—their use induces tolerance and physical dependence as well as psychological dependence.

They include meprobamate (Miltown, Equanil), chlordiazepoxide (Librium), and diazepam (Valium).

TRANQUILIZER ABUSE: Abuse of tranquilizers has been on the increase since the 1960s. By mid-1975 the situation had gotten out of hand. It was reported that 3 billion (yes, *billion*) tablets of Valium had been produced during the preceding year and over 1 billion tablets of Librium. No one, the federal authorities seemed to feel, needed that much tranquilizing. In 1976 the National Institute of Drug Abuse reported that alcohol and Valium were responsible for more drug-related illnesses during the preceding year than any other drugs. It was estimated that Valium was taken by approximately 65 million Americans; it was the nation's leading prescription drug.

To curb such enormous overproduction and overuse, in July, 1975 the federal government placed Valium and Librium, along with several other drugs, under federal control. From then on, anyone requiring a prescription for these drugs was limited to five prescription refills within a six-month period following the initial prescription. If more of the medication was required after that, a new prescription had to be written.

DANGERS OF TRANQUILIZER ABUSE: Abuse of tranquilizers results in a set of symptoms similar to those caused by barbiturate abuse. As mentioned above, prolonged use of tranquilizers induces psychological dependence and increased tolerance, which can in turn lead to physical dependence. Abrupt withdrawal can result in symptoms like those described for barbiturate withdrawal, including convulsions and delirium.

Narcotic Drugs

Narcotics are drugs that relieve pain and induce sleep and stupor by depressing the central nervous system. Legally, they include *opium* and its derivatives *(morphine, codeine, heroin)* and the so-called synthetic opiates, such as *meperidine,* and *methadone.* (Federal law classifies cocaine as a narcotic, but it bears no resemblance to these drugs; it is actually a stimulant.)

Opium

The seedpods of the opium poppy, *Papaver somniferum,* produce a brownish gummy resin that yields narcotic effects when it is eaten or smoked. Opium has been used extensively in many lands and many cultures; not until relatively recently did its addictive characteristics become known. Of the more than two dozen active compounds, called *alkaloids,* that can be isolated from opium, the two most important are morphine and codeine.

Morphine

Morphine, the first alkaloid to be extracted from a plant, was isolated from opium in 1805 and later synthesized in pure form. In the illicit drug market it appears as a white powder called *M, dreamer,* or *Miss Emma.* Its more formal name stems from Morpheus, god of dreams, son of the god of sleep. It is a remarkably effective painkiller. It is also addicting.

During the Civil War, Army physicians believed that by injecting morphine with the recently developed hypodermic syringe, they could avoid addiction in their patients. They were wrong, and 45,000 soldiers left the Army with the soldiers' disease, *morphinism.* The civilian population was also being exposed to opiates, mostly in the form of uncontrolled patent medicines. In the years following the war, perhaps one and one-quarter million Americans, four percent of the population, were snared in some variety of opiate abuse. Then, at the end of the century, a substance was synthesized from morphine (by adding acetic acid to it) that seemed at first to cure addiction both to opium and to morphine. The name of the wonder drug—heroin.

Heroin

Today the problem of narcotics

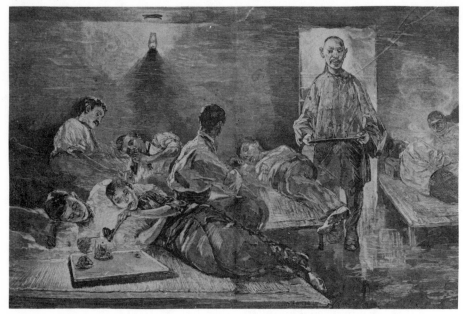

Opium, whether smoked or eaten, has been used as a narcotic in many cultures. This engraving shows an opium den in New York City in the 1880s.

abuse focuses on heroin. (There are still some morphine abusers, mostly doctors and nurses.) Called *H*, *horse, junk, smack,* and *scag*, heroin (or diacetylmorphine) is several times more powerful than morphine.

EFFECTS: All of the opiates produce a dulling of the senses to external events, a feeling of well-being, a reduction of fear, hunger, tension, anxiety, and pain. Heroin offers one an immediate escape from any and all problems. Because the drug depresses the central nervous system, the user also becomes sleepy and lethargic; "nodding" is one of the symptoms of heroin abuse. Some possible side effects are nausea, flushing, constipation, slowing of respiration, retention of urine, and eventually, malnutrition through loss of appetite.

The degree to which heroin's agreeable effects are felt depends in part on how the user takes it. Sniffing is the mildest form of abuse, followed by skin-popping (subcutaneous injection), and then by mainlining (injecting directly into a vein), which is the mode used by almost all those dependent on heroin.

DEPENDENCE ON HEROIN: A high and rapid tolerance to heroin is one of its hallmarks, with the regular user re-

quiring ever-larger doses to produce the same degree of euphoria. In the chronic user, it produces both psychological and physical dependence. The former is far more important, and its shackles are the harder to break. With the need to take larger doses, the cost of the habit increases, and the addict's life becomes increasingly centered on the desperate cycle of obtaining enough money for the drug (often by criminal means), injecting it, relaxing for a few hours, and then starting again.

The addict may be driven as much by the need to avoid withdrawal symptoms, or even the thought of them, as by the search for escape. Yet, strangely, the addict may fear a greatly exaggerated monster. It is true that withdrawal for a heavy, chronic heroin user can be difficult and painful, with anxiety, sweating, muscle aches, vomiting, and diarrhea. But the experience is more likely to be no worse than recovering from a bad cold.

The explanation is that heroin as sold today on the street is "cut" or diluted with milk sugar, quinine, or baking soda. A *bag* or *deck* of it may contain a mere 1 to 5 percent heroin. On this kind of habit, most addicts will have very mild withdrawal

symptoms.

Unfortunately, pushers sometimes begin selling decks of more than 30 percent pure heroin. For the unwary addict, the tremendously more potent doses can spell grave illness or death. In New York City, where perhaps half of the nation's heroin addicts are concentrated, more than 900 persons have died from heroin abuse in a single year, 224 of them nineteen or younger.

The notion that one shot of heroin inevitably leads to addiction is a myth; many have certainly experimented with the drug without becoming addicted, and there are even some individuals who "joy-pop" (shoot on weekends or occasionally for kicks), or take a certain amount every day, without developing tolerance or physical dependence. Nevertheless, the majority of people who use heroin regularly do apparently become addicted, and although some of these may be able to

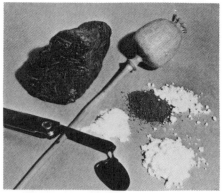

An opium poppy and derivatives: crude and smoking opium, codeine, heroin, morphine.

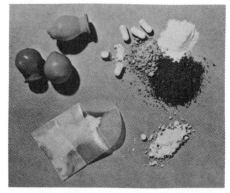

Forms of heroin. The heroin sold on the streets is usually greatly diluted, but varies so much in potency that addicts risk grave illness and death from accidental overdoses.

that can be produced from gum opium or can be converted from morphine. Called *schoolboy* in the streets, it has much milder effects than either morphine or heroin, and is an ingredient in some popular nonprescription cough syrups.

Synthetic Opiates

Prescription pain-relievers such as Demerol, Dilaudid, Pantopon, and other synthetic opiates can become addicting if used indiscriminately. They occasionally appear on the drug scene. With the increased availability of methadone in treatment clinics, methadone is increasingly used illicitly, often in combination with alcohol or other drugs, and especially when heroin is in short supply.

The Hallucinogens: LSD and Others

LSD (lysergic acid diethylamide) is one of a group of drugs legally classed as *hallucinogens*—agents that cause the user to experience hallucinations, illusions, and distorted perceptions.

LSD

LSD is a colorless, tasteless, odorless compound, as plain-looking as water. What makes it truly remarkable is its potency. A single effective dose requires, on the average, only 100 millionths of a gram. A quantity of LSD equivalent to two aspirin tablets would furnish 6,500 such doses.

LSD may not be made legally except for use in certain well-supervised experiments. Doctors are using it to treat alcoholism and some mental disease, without convincing results. But on the illicit market it is provided in vials of liquid, or as capsules or tablets. It is consumed in sugar cubes, candy, cookies, on the surface of beads, even in the mucilage of stamps and envelopes. One dose is enough to provoke a 4 to 18 hour *trip*—a hallucinogenic experience.

It is this trip that made LSD, at least for a while in the 1960s, a focus

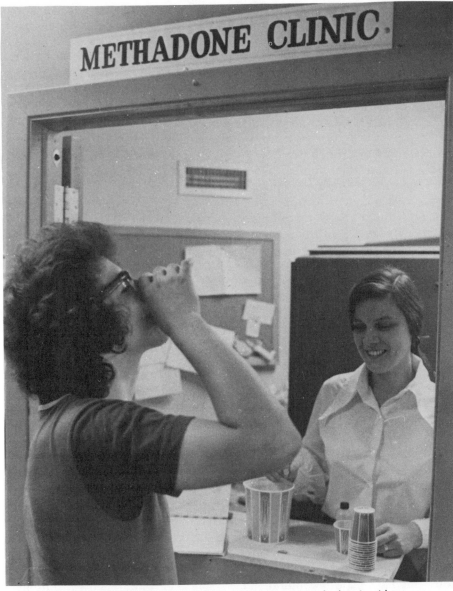

Methadone, a synthetic opiate that satisfies the craving for heroin without producing euphoria, is used in maintenance programs for heroin addicts.

break the habit themselves, most need some kind of help. For reasons not yet determined, many addicts who reach maturity, about age 35, spontaneously get off the heroin treadmill without treatment.

TREATMENT FOR HEROIN ADDICTS: There is little agreement among experts on what kinds of therapy for heroin addiction stand most chance of success. One of the most promising yet controversial methods is the substitution of controlled doses of *methadone*. Called *Dolly* after its trade name Dolophine, methadone is a synthetic opiate that does not produce the euphoria of heroin. The substitution is designed to allow the addict to lead a stabilized life, but he is still addicted—to methadone.

Other forms of treatment concentrate on group psychotherapy, often in live-in communities modeled after the West Coast's *Synanon*. Some experts believe that only a multi-pronged attack, combining chemical treatment, psychiatry, user communities, and rehabilitation by social services, will prove effective. As of now, the five-year cure rate for heroin addicts is only about one-third that for alcoholics.

Codeine

Codeine is a modest pain-reliever

of almost idolatrous interest. Many, including well-known public figures, claimed that LSD and other psychedelic drugs were consciousness-expanding. That is, they were supposed to enhance the tripper's appreciation of everything in the world around him, increase his creativity, open the doors to mind-bending mystical or religious experiences, and perhaps bring about profound changes, hopefully for the better, in his personality.

Indeed, some trippers reported just such results—although several studies suggest the improvements are illusory. In many groups, it became a distinction to be an *acid-head*, a user of lysergic acid. The people who flocked to the LSD banner were mostly from the educated white middle class, including large numbers of high school and college students. One authority estimates that something under one percent of the total population have experimented with LSD.

Today, the peak popularity of this drug is past, although it is still an important part of the drug scene. The reason: as more and more people experienced the drug, and as more intensive research was carried out, disquieting things came to the surface—dangers, previously unsuspected, of LSD use.

EFFECTS: When an individual takes LSD, he is prepared for a certain amount of minor physical discomfort: a rise in temperature, pulse, and blood pressure; the sensation of hair standing on end; some nausea, dizziness, and headache. About an hour after the drug is first taken, the psychedelic part of the trip begins, with striking impact on the senses. Vision is affected the most profoundly. Walls may seem to sway and buckle. Colors become more intense, more beautiful; those in a painting may seem to merge and stream. Flat objects become three-dimensional. The other senses also seem to become more acute.

On a bad trip, all these sensations can add up to a terrifying experience. The hallucinations can be horrible as well as bizarre. Deep depression, anxiety, and fright can alternate with insight and ecstasy. A tripper may panic because he fears he is losing his mind.

Some bad trips have ended in the psychiatric ward, with the tripper suffering from a severe mental disorder, a *psychosis*. This sometimes results from an effect peculiar to LSD: a severe distortion of a person's body image (his mental picture of his own body). If a tripper sees himself without a head, for example, his panic may be extreme. Sometimes these psychotic episodes, or breaks, clear up within a day or two. Sometimes they last for months or years.

Certain trips have ended even more badly. Convinced that they could literally float through the air, trippers have waltzed through high windows and fallen to their deaths. Others have walked in front of trains or cars, apparently in the belief that they were invulnerable.

It is impossible to say how frequent or rare these adverse reactions are in LSD users, because the overwhelming majority of trips are made illegally and thus without professional supervision. It seems likely that those whose emotional balance is already precarious are those most prone to develop psychotic reactions. But many experts contend that the drug's effect on any given person is completely unpredictable. One reason is that no one really knows exactly how LSD works inside the body to affect the mind and how it can be so potent in such microscopic amounts. The upshot is that abusing LSD, according to a former FDA Commissioner, is something like playing "chemical Russian roulette."

LSD does not cause physical dependence, although tolerance does develop; psychological dependence doesn't seem to be severe. Apparently, no one has died as a result of a lethal dose of LSD.

RESEARCH ON HAZARDS: Some recent research suggests that the drug may have toxic effects on some cells of the human body. One set of studies indicates that there may be a link between LSD use and breaks in chromosomes that could conceivably lead to leukemia or to birth defects in trippers' children. As of now, however, there is no conclusive scientific evidence on which to base a final judgment.

One long-term study is more definite. Dr. Cheston M. Berlin, of George Washington University, followed 127 pregnancies in women who had taken LSD before or during the pregnancy. The study turned up this statistic: children of LSD users are 18 times more likely to have birth defects than the average. Dr. Berlin said that although his study does not prove conclusively that LSD causes birth defects, "we are more suspicious than ever before."

Other Hallucinogens

Many other substances, both natural and synthetic, are being used as hallucinogens. Most of them produce effects similar to those of LSD, but are less potent. Here is a list of some in common use:

MESCALINE: Mescaline is the active ingredient of *peyote*, a Mexican cactus that has been used by American Indians for centuries to attain mystical states in religious ceremonies. Users consume cactus "buttons" either ground or whole; mescaline itself may be had as a powder or a

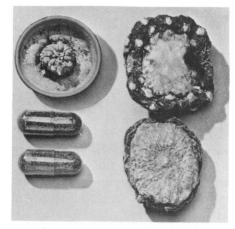

Mescaline is the active ingredient in the peyote cactus. Users consume the buttons either whole or ground to produce trance states.

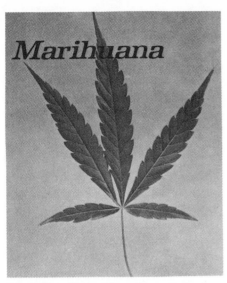

Marihuana

The Indian hemp (*Cannabis sativa*), from whose flowering tops and leaves marihuana is obtained, is a tall, weedy plant that grows freely in many parts of the world.

liquid. Mescaline can also be synthesized in the laboratory.

PSILOCYBIN AND PSILOCIN: Psilocybin and psilocin come from the Aztec hallucinatory mushroom, *Psilocybe mexicana*, which grows in southern Mexico and has been eaten raw by the natives from about 1500 B.C. Both derivatives can be made in the laboratory.

DMT: DMT, or dimethyltryptamine, has been called the businessman's high, because its effects may last only 40 to 50 minutes. It can be smoked (tobacco or parsley is soaked in the liquid) or injected, which results in a powerful wave of exhilaration. It is an ingredient of various plants native to South America, and has long been used by Indian tribes in the form of intoxicating drinks or snuff, often very dangerous. In the United States, however, DMT is synthesized from tryptamine in the laboratory.

DOM OR STP: DOM or STP is a synthetic compound originally developed by the Dow Chemical Company as a possible agent for the treatment of mental disorders, but never released. When manufactured illicitly, it was given the name STP, so the story goes, for Serenity, Tranquillity, Peace. It is powerful, produces vivid hallucinations, and seems to last as long as LSD. But it is also extremely poisonous. It can bring on fever, blurred vision, difficulty in swallowing, and occasionally death from convulsions. It can also cause manic psychoses lasting for days.

Marihuana

Marihuana may be, after alcohol, the most widely used drug in our country. One estimate is that 40 million Americans have tried it. It is certainly the most controversial. We are in the midst of a great debate over whether marihuana (commonly called *pot* or *grass*) is a dangerous drug or only a mild intoxicant.

In 1970, for example, the U.S. Department of Agriculture issued a booklet on marihuana that called abuse of the drug a "major menace . . . [that] frequently leads to dangerous forms of addiction and dependencies." Just a few days later, Dr. Roger O. Egeberg, then Assistant Secretary of Health, Education and Welfare and thus the senior federal health official, said that on the available evidence, "marihuana is not a narcotic, its use does not lead to physiological dependence under ordinary circumstances, and . . . there is no proof that it predisposes an individual to go on to more potent and dangerous drugs."

Marihuana is a Mexican-Spanish word originally applied to a poor grade of tobacco, and only later meaning a smoking preparation made from the hemp plant. The Indian hemp (*Cannabis sativa*) is a tall, weedy plant related to the fig tree and the hop. It grows freely in many parts of the world and provides drug preparations of one kind or another (the general term is cannabis) to some 300 million people. But the quality and strength of these drugs depend on where the plant is grown, whether it is wild or cultivated, and especially on how the preparation is made.

Drugs are obtained almost solely from the female plants. (The males produce the fiber for hemp.) When the female plants are ripe, in the heat of the summer, their top leaves and especially the clusters of flowers at their tops produce a minty, sticky, golden-yellow resin, which eventually blackens. It is this resin that contains the active principles of the drug. And obviously, the pure resin of carefully cultivated plants is the most potent form of cannabis. It is available in cakes, called *charas* in India, and as a brown powder, called *hashish* in the Middle East.

A small but increasing quantity of hashish is smuggled here. But it is the weakest form of cannabis, made from the tops, leaves, and often stems of low-resin plants, that is smoked in this country as marihuana. Some experts have ranked hashish from four to ten times as powerful as marihuana.

Scientists have not yet succeeded in establishing exactly what substances in the cannabis plant produce its drug effects in man, nor how. Three of the resin's ingredients are chemical compounds called cannabinol, cannabidiol, and tetrahydrocannabinol (*THC*), the last actually a group of related substances. THC is probably the most important active principle in the hemp plant, but most chemists believe it is not the only one.

EFFECTS: What happens when a marihuana cigarette is smoked? If the smoker is a novice, if he doesn't know what to expect, or how to inhale properly, nothing at all may be noticeable, apart from the lingering sweetish smell of burning rope that the reefer exudes. If he is insecure about smoking, he may experience a feeling of panic, usually controllable with some reassurance. More serious reactions have been reported among marihuana smokers, including *toxic psychosis*—psychosis caused by a toxic agent—with confusion and disorientation; but these are rare. Also, experimenters using large doses of marihuana, hashish, and THC have induced what they termed hallucinations and psychotic reactions in their subjects.

For the experienced smoker, however, the usual reaction is to feel about half way between elation and sleepiness, with some heightened or altered perceptions (of sound and color, for example), and a greatly slowed-down sense of time. The smoker can usually control the extent of his high and does not feel tempted to smoke beyond the point he wishes to reach. He often experiences mild headache or nausea.

SPECIAL PROPERTIES OF MARIHUANA: Marihuana seems to be in a class by itself as a drug. It resembles both stimulants and depressants in some of its actions. It certainly has psychedelic effects, but it is far less potent than the hallucinogens and differs from them in other important ways. (A standard text on pharmacology lists it as a "miscellaneous" drug.) It is not a narcotic. It does not produce physical dependence, nor does its use entail tolerance; some users, in fact, find that with regular use they need less marihuana to produce the desired high. There seems, in general, to be slight to moderate psychological dependence among regular users—less, in some experts' opinion, than among regular users of alcohol or tobacco.

None of these general observations can be presented as gospel; there simply have not been enough scientific studies performed to say we know very much positively about marihuana.

CONTINUING RESEARCH: The most serious indictment of marihuana as a dangerous drug stems from recent research at St. John's University in New York. When pregnant mice and rats "smoked" marihuana, some 20 percent of their offspring had birth defects such as cleft palate. Moreover, the defects were transmitted to the next two generations, indicating genetic damage. Drug experiments on rodents cannot be regarded as conclusive as far as human drug use is concerned, but they do suggest the need for further study of the effects of marihuana on human beings.

MEDICAL USE OF MARIHUANA: Recent studies have shown that marihuana can be effective in reducing the pressure of fluids within the eyes of patients suffering from glaucoma. In October, 1976, the Food and Drug Administration approved a plan for the use of marihuana in the treatment of such patients.

THE LEGAL OUTLOOK: In the light of the continuing widespread illicit use of marihuana and the lack of any firm evidence that the drug was seriously harmful, some states passed laws in the mid-1970s to decriminalize the possession of small amounts. The debate as to whether marihuana should be legalized still goes on. Few argue that all penalties should be dropped for major suppliers so long as marihuana remains illegal; but many people apparently agree that sending a young person to prison for smoking a marihuana cigarette while his or her parents can down three martinis every evening doesn't make much sense.

CHAPTER 33

Eye Disorders

NEW DIRECTIONS IN DIAGNOSIS AND TREATMENT

Of all of man's senses, sight is without doubt the most important. Without the senses of hearing, taste, or smell, most persons find ways to live, work, and play in relatively normal ways. Loss of the sense of touch or the sense of balance (vestibular sense) might indicate serious problems. But even in such cases medical science can usually provide remedies. By contrast, loss of sight, or blindness, can mean that the victim faces a complete, permanent change of lifestyle (see "The Sense Organs," p. 40).

In the world of the 1980s, fortunately, research has recorded so many advances in eye testing and treatment that few persons need fear a total loss of sight. Eye problems remain, of course; and, for various reasons, some of these problems have become more common. As the population of the United States ages, for example, eye problems afflict more and more individuals. But medical science has more than kept pace with such changes. Researchers have discovered new ways to treat such age-old problems as nearsightedness, cataracts, and glaucoma. New testing techniques and devices have led to new treatments and taken the guesswork out of many established methods.

The revolution in our understanding of the eye and its disorders and diseases has given new hope to millions of persons with eye problems. The contact lens, only a little over 40 years old, has appeared in so many new forms that they are difficult to catalog. Congenital eye defects, caused perhaps by German measles in the mother or by mother-father Rh factor conflict, can be prevented. Doctors can even treat some potential eye problems while a fetus is still in the womb.

The ways in which the eye functions are well-known. So are the common eye disorders (see *The Eyes*, p. 417). We also know that man "sees" with the brain. The unconscious person, or the person who has suffered brain death, can no longer use the intricate process called vision. This is true even if the eyes appear to be functioning.

Against that background, the revolution in eye care, testing, and treatment underscores the importance of knowledge about our eyes. It has become more than ever necessary to know what can go wrong with our eyes and what can be done to treat them when problems arise. Early detection of eye difficulties may make it possible to save the sight of one or both eyes. Fear of what a doctor may find has been

known to cause many persons to delay visits to their eye specialists. But knowledge can often eliminate fear.

Of primary importance, the persons who deal with the eyes and their problems should be familiar. In addition to the *ophthalmologist* and the *optometrist*, three other types of specialists help with eye problems and care. The *optician* uses highly developed skills in filling special lens prescriptions. The *orthoptist* and *ophthalmic assistant* usually help the ophthalmologist, working in the latter's office or laboratory to relieve the ophthalmologist of time-consuming duties (see *The Sense Organs—Eye, Ear, Nose*, p. 301).

The Eye Examination

What can you expect when you go to have your eyes examined? Despite the many advances in eye problem diagnosis and treatment, the basic examination remains relatively simple.

The eye doctor, or ophthalmologist, starts on the outside of your eye. Using a wall chart he gauges the *visual acuity* of each eye—the ability to see clear, sharp images. Next, the specialist probably checks for *color vision*. The patient is mere-

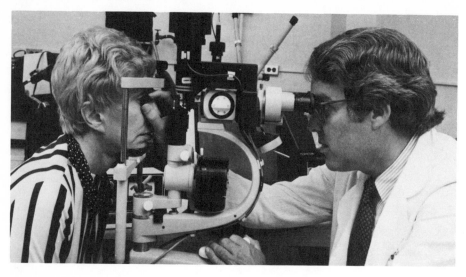

Ophthalmologists employ powerful argon lasers to treat glaucoma, detached retinas, diabetic retinal damage, and senile macular degeneration. Light rays are directed at the retina and the extreme heat produced by the laser destroys and welds abnormal tissue.

ly asked to distinguish colors. At one phase of the basic examination the ophthalmologist screens the person being tested for *peripheral vision field*. He does this by having the patient cover one eye and look with the other at an object across the room. While the patient stares, the doctor brings an object into the peripheral field from above, from either side, or from below. The results tell the examiner whether the patient is seeing with the peripheral portion of the retina.

Using a biomicroscope mounted on a small table, the ophthalmologist examines the conjunctiva, the eyelids, the cornea, and the lens of each eye. Other parts of the eye that undergo examination—visual or mechanical—include the iris, the tear ducts, and the white of the eye.

The doctor can now "work into" the eye. The retina, orange-red in color, provides many clues in disease detection. To check it, the doctor dilates the eyes with drops. He can then look into the back of the eye for signs of blood pressure problems, diabetic retinopathy, narrowed vessels that could indicate hardening of the arteries, and other disorders. He examines the optic nerve, the hundreds of thousands of tiny fibers that carry visual images to the brain.

Only after such basic tests have been conducted may the ophthalmologist recommend special tests. He makes such a recommendation if he finds evidence of serious problems that call for medical or surgical attention.

TESTING, DIAGNOSTIC, AND TREATMENT DEVICES AND PROCEDURES

Using our eyes and brains, we see. Examining and testing our eyes, doctors can look into our bodies for signals indicating a wide range of eye and other problems. An eye examination may tell the ophthalmologist that the patient has glaucoma, for example. But the same examination, conducted thoroughly, may show that the blood vessels of the patient's retina have been damaged by diabetes or hypertension.

Some testing, diagnostic, and treatment devices and procedures are itemized below. Some of the items on the list are new, some established.

ARGON, OR ARGON-GAS, LASER PHOTO COAGULATION. A somewhat experimental method of treating patients, argon lasers utilize the needlelike beam of an argon-gas laser to weld a torn or detached section of tissue back onto the retina. The lasers have other uses, including treatment of glaucoma.

CONTACT LENSES. New technology in contact lenses has created an entire range of new types of lenses. Some of the new developments:

• In the early 1980s, bifocal soft lenses were being used to correct for both distance and near vision. The new products make it unnecessary to use reading glasses or half-glasses for close work.

• Extended wear lenses, special soft lenses that can be worn night and day for up to a month or more, answer a need for lenses that will not get lost or mislaid. Thinner and more water-absorbent than standard soft lenses, the extended wear lenses permit freer tear-flow and thus are more comfortable for the wearer. They should only be worn with medical supervision.

• Silicon lenses come in both hard and soft types. Both are gas permeable, or oxygen permeable, meaning they provide greater comfort for the eye because they allow movement of air to and around the eye. Both are very durable as well.

• Tinted lenses that can change the color of nearly all but the darkest eyes have the additional advantage of extreme thinness. They reduce glare for persons whose eyes are sensitive to light. They can also be found more easily if dropped.

• For persons over 40 especially, invisible monocles are growing in popularity. Actually a contact lens worn in only one eye, the monocle corrects farsightedness. It offers an alternative to bifocal lenses; in effect, one eye is prepared for reading while the other remains adapted to distance vision.

Some of the special medical or postsurgical uses to which the various kinds of special lenses can be put will be noted in later pages.

CRYOPROBE. Used in cataract surgery, the needlelike cryoprobe enables the surgeon to free the lens, which can then be removed intact.

DIRECT OPHTHALMOSCOPE. The direct ophthalmoscope has for years been used to examine the central part of the retina, the rear wall of the eye. A companion instrument, the *binocular indirect ophthalmoscope,* has proved even more effective in the detection of detached or torn retinal tissue.

ELECTROOCULOGRAM OR ELECTRORETINOGRAM. Two electrodiagnostic techniques, both methods enable the ophthalmologist to identify various retinal conditions. Both instruments also serve in diagnoses of problems of the choroid and the optic nerve.

FLUORESCEIN ANGIOGRAPHY. The X-ray technique called angiography or *arteriography* helps the examiner locate retinal lesions and various kinds of degeneration. The test utilizes fluid that is injected into the blood stream. In the angiogram the fluid shows in the picture, providing an interior view of the eye.

KERATOPROSTHESIS. Relatively new and experimental in the early 1980s, keratoprosthesis involves implantation of a plastic cornea. The procedure offers an alternative to the standard corneal transplant.

LASER-DOPPLER VELOCIMETRY. The relatively new Laser-Doppler velocimetry test resembles closely the industrial process used to measure the flow of gas or liquid through pipes. Among the disorders that measurement by laser from outside the eye (noninvasive) can reveal are abnormal blood vessel growth; narrowed vessels; capillary damage, an early sign of diabetes; damage to nerve tissue as a result of pressure inside the eye, a possible sign of glaucoma or a tumor; and slow constriction of blood vessels.

OCULAR SCREENING SYSTEM. Using a 35 mm camera and a strobe light, the Ocular Screening System has been hailed as an eye testing method that is particularly effective with very young children. From a distance of 21 feet, the strobe unit flashes light into the subject's eyes. The retina reflects the flashing light back at the camera, which records the picture on color film. Healthy eyes have pupils that look red. They also show identical images. Unhealthy eyes have differently colored pupils and different images. The differences may be signs of amblyopia, tumors, cataracts, crossed eyes, or other problems. A computer is used to interpret test results.

PHACOEMULSIFICATION. A method of flushing out cataracts, phacoemulsification employs an ultrasonic probe that vibrates at a rate of about 40,000 times a second. This controversial technique sucks out the emulsified materials from the interior of the eye while irrigating the chamber.

PHOROPTER. An established method of testing for refractive error, the multiple-lens phoropter indicates whether a patient is farsighted, nearsighted, or astigmatic. The phoropter's lenses make possible billions of lens combinations.

RETINOSCOPE. Used with children or others who cannot give reliable

The extremely small size of these plastic intraocular lenses is emphasized by their comparison with a standard-size paper clip. (Left) The surgical insertion of plastic lenses into the eye provides some cataract patients with an alternative to postoperative glasses.

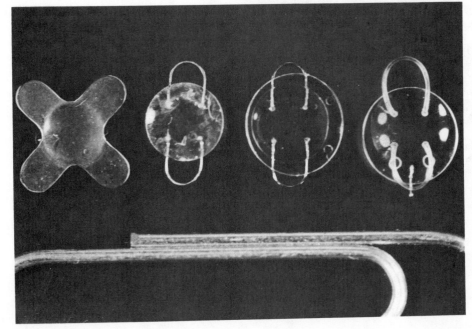

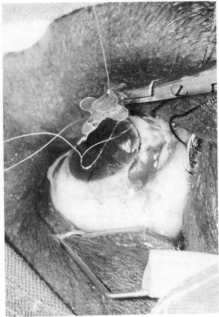

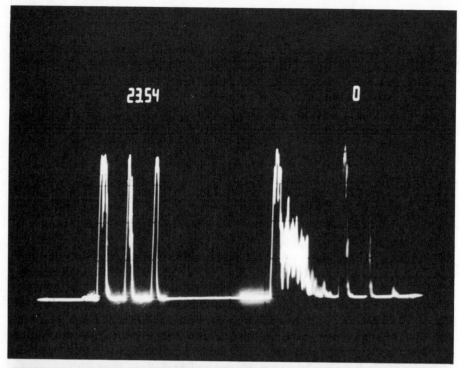

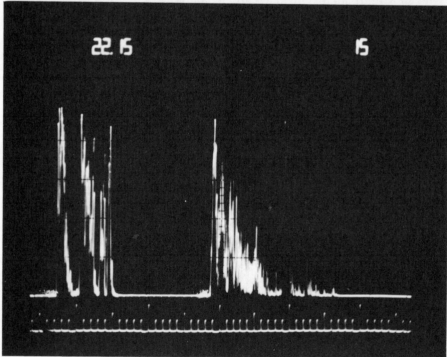

The above ultrasound scans show a detached retina. Ultrasonography helps the ophthalmologist pinpoint the exact position of the detached retina and provides specific information for a correct treatment.

and the iris, lens, and vitreous.

VISUAL FIELD TEST. A simple, well-established test procedure, the visual field test helps in detection of normal or abnormal blind spots. The examiner simply has the patient fix his gaze on one spot. By holding objects at different places in the subject's field of vision, the doctor can determine the total field of vision and the blind spots.

TONOMETER. The instrument that measures the pressure inside the eye, the tonometer is critically important in the detection of glaucoma. An *applanation tonometer* can be used with a slit lamp to measure the pressure painlessly. With a *Schiotz tonometer*, the patient lies down during testing. Unlike other types of pressure testing, the *air-blast tonometer* makes corneal anesthesia unnecessary.

ULTRASOUND. A special new procedure, ultrasound may be used where the examiner's view in the inner eye is obstructed. This may occur with cataracts or vitreous bleeding. A transducer produces sound waves at a pitch too high to be heard by humans; reflections of the waves off parts of the eye aid in diagnosis.

Still other special methods may be recommended. Where ordinary X rays cannot detect foreign bodies or growths in the eye, *computerized axial tomography* (CAT) scans may be used. In a sophisticated new measuring test, a dye is injected into the patient's arm. Doctors look for leakage of the dye into the eye fluid, or vitreous. Because they have poor control over their blood sugar, diabetics may show more leakage than nondiabetics. Many other tests and diagnostic procedures are in development; many will undoubtedly come into use in future years.

Eye Banks

The eye bank of the 1980s, serving its special purpose in the treatment of eye problems, bears little resemblance to the first eye bank, established on Staten Island, N.Y., in 1944 (see *Cornea Transplant,*

responses to questions, the retinoscope also identifies refractive error. The instrument throws a series of light streaks into the patient's eye. The movements of the reflected images show the presence or absence of refractive error.

SLIT-LAMP BIOMICROSCOPE. In eye tests, while the patient rests his or her chin on a firm base, the doctor examines the interior sections of the eye with the biomicroscope. Areas of particular concern are the cornea; the anterior or forward chamber;

p. 334). Usually associated with a university or major medical center, the modern eye bank plays a role in every phase of the task of obtaining viable corneal tissue. The very complex modern bank coordinates at least the following activities:

• obtaining consent to tissue donation after death.

• surgically removing eyes.

• transporting eyes to the bank facility.

• evaluating the processing of donor corneas.

Because basic changes take place in the cornea soon after death, eyes must be removed within 12 hours after the donor dies. Most banks prefer to take the eyes within six hours. Often, delays result because the bank cannot obtain consent quickly enough. Once frozen, the eye can be preserved for a year or more.

The staff of an eye bank, including the medical director, an executive director, technicians, and others, functions according to strict protocols. These are established by the Eye Bank Association of America. Seventy-one eye banks belonged to the Association in the early 1980s. In each, the staff checks every donor cornea to make sure it can survive after transplantation. Staff members may use such new techniques as *vital staining* to evaluate an eye both anatomically and biomedically. To the extent possible, a cornea is age-matched to a suitable recipient.

Cornea transplants have become so common that the nation's eye banks cannot come close to meeting national needs. According to one estimate, some 100,000 Americans experience severe corneal problems each year; yet, only about 10,000 operations are performed annually.

DISORDERS AND NEW TREATMENT METHODS

The revolution in eye disorder diagnosis and treatment led to new ways to treat such common problems as nearsightedness, cataracts, and glaucoma. Research also brought new knowledge about more serious diseases and problems. Some of the more widely used techniques, with the eye problems they help to control, are described below.

Refractive Problems, Treatments

The most common eye problems result from differences in the total length of the eyeball or from slight variations in the curvature of the cornea, the front window of the human eye. These differences cause refractive problems, or problems having to do with the distribution of light in the eye. In the normal eye the light rays coming from a distance focus on the retina. Because some eyes are shorter from front to back, the rays focus behind the retina, which is too close to the cornea. The individual then suffers from farsightedness, or *hyperopia* (also hypermetropia).

Three other refractive problems are nearsightedness, or myopia; astigmatism, the result of a flaw or irregularity in the cornea; and old sight, or presbyopia. Nearsightedness occurs among persons whose eyes are longer; the light rays focus in front of the retina because it is too far back. Astigmatism, which can accompany either far- or nearsightedness, makes things look somewhat blurred. In presbyopia, a problem among older people, the eye gradually loses it ability to focus and, consequently, to perform tasks like reading. The old sight victim can usually correct the problem with spectacles.

The development of advanced contact lenses in the 1930s marked a major advance in the treatment of refractive problems. In recent years research has led to many other developments. Most of these help nearsighted persons primarily.

Two other methods of treating refractive problems remained experimental in the early 1980s. Radial keratotomy involves a 15-minute operation during which a surgeon makes tiny cuts on the surface of the cornea. The incisions change the cornea's shape, curing the patient's nearsightedness. In orthokeratology, patients suffering from nearsightedness receive new pairs of hard contact lenses every six weeks. The lenses become progressively flatter, and thus change the shape of the cornea and relieve myopia. Some scientists and doctors reported that these "ortho-k" lenses did not change the cornea's shape permanently.

Color Blindness

In recent years color blindness afflicted some 9 million American males and 500,000 females. These persons had difficulty seeing or distinguishing certain colors. Many found that they were handicapped for jobs in the electronics, aviation, computer, chemical, and many other industries. In children, color blindness has been known to affect the ability to learn.

The X-Chrom contact lens has been found to correct color blindness almost entirely. A ruby-red lens, the X-Chrom is worn on only one eye. That eye sends messages to the brain to correct for color errors made by the other eye. The wearer may perceive some colors at once, and recognizable colors may become instantly more brilliant. Because the color blind person has to learn slowly to recognize the entire range of unfamiliar shades and colors, the lens has to be worn continuously for six months or more.

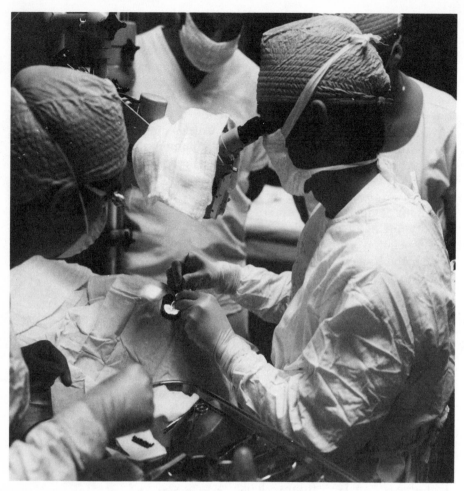

Several methods of treatment for glaucoma have been perfected in the past few years. Conventional surgery is still performed in advanced cases.

Glaucoma

While rare among young people, glaucoma occurs with increasing frequency among persons 40 and older. The disorder can cause blindness. But patients who are found to have glaucoma early and who follow their doctors' instructions can usually retain their eyesight throughout their lives.

Glaucoma involves a progressive loss of sight. It begins when the fluid (aqueous humor) that circulates through the eye cannot, for any reason, flow out. For example, drainage through the eye's tiny outflow channels may be partially blocked. Pressure then builds up inside the eye, damaging the sight nerves in the retina and optic nerve. The rate of visual loss is usually slow, but varies from person to person. Periodic eye checkups are

the best defense against advanced glaucoma.

In diagnosis, three-dimensional photography has been used successfully where eye pressure tests with a tonometer, a pressure-measuring device, have proved inadequate. The photographs show early glaucoma in the optic disc, a part of the optic nerve. A fluorescent dye may be injected into the body and allowed to circulate before the picture is taken. Minimal discoloration of the optic disc may then indicate abnormalities. A computer may be used to analyze the photos.

New methods of treating glaucoma have replaced the medications that were once commonly used. Where miotics, or drugs in drop form that cause contraction of the pupil, were once prescribed almost exclusively, more doctors have

begun to use *timolol maleate* (Timoptic). This drug reduces the inside pressure by inhibiting the production of eye fluid. Timoptic has been found to cause fewer side effects than other antiglaucoma drugs.

Miotics may also be used with *epinephrine* and other pills. Again, the effect is to reduce pressure inside the eye.

Marijuana has been found useful as an alternative to other pressure-reducing drugs. A marijuana compound, nabilone, has been used in research and clinical treatment to treat early glaucoma. The drug works without producing the typical marijuana "high."

Surgery may be recommended if glaucoma is far advanced. In *filtering surgery*, a doctor may create a tiny drainage channel that enables the fluid to flow out. Filtering surgery is successful in about eight cases out of ten. In *peripheral iridectomy*, the patient first takes drugs to control the pressure inside the eyeball. A surgeon then removes a small piece of the iris, the aperture near the front of the eye, to permit fluid to flow from the rear eye chamber to the front.

Glaucoma may occur as a side effect of diabetes. In one form of treatment, the doctor makes a small incision in the side of the eye. He then inserts a tiny plastic valve. When pressure rises inside the eye, the valve opens, allowing fluid to drain away.

Laser therapy offers a modern alternative to drugs and other methods of treating glaucoma. Basically, the laser beam directed into the eye is intended to ease the flow of fluid from the eye's center. In acute glaucoma, which may occur suddenly, emergency laser therapy may be used instead of surgery. Laser treatment has also been found to be effective in patients for whom eye drops were ineffective in reducing pressure.

Cataracts

Another form of eye disorder that

becomes more common with aging, cataracts involve clouding of the lens of the eyeball. In ancient times many persons thought the gradual clouding was caused by water that leaked down over the pupil, making it white. The image of falling water led to the name "cataract." Cataracts may develop slowly. They may also progress a little, then stop (see "Cataract," p. 334).

Many cataract victims never need surgery. On the advice of qualified doctors, many others undergo the relatively simple surgical procedure that removes cataracts. Patients who have cataract surgery sometimes experience difficulty in seeing afterward. Diagnosis may show that some of the remaining cells have come back to life, forming a new membrane where the cloudy lens was. To prevent secondary surgery, doctors have recently begun to use a *cryo extractor* to freeze parts of the eye in the surgery area. A standard item of hospital equipment, the extractor clears the eye of tissue that could cloud the eye later on.

Newer forms of cataract treatment include the *intraocular lens implant*. The implant involves surgical insertion of plastic lenses that replace the removed defective lenses. In many cases the artificial lenses work so well that neither eyeglasses nor contact lenses are needed.

Among the newer approaches to cataract therapy, *microsurgery* offers yet another option. In this kind of surgery, the cornea is removed; a donor cornea is frozen and then placed on a lathe. Using precision controls, a doctor reshapes the cornea, or cornea disc, to the proper contours. The donor cornea is then placed in the patient's eye.

Microsurgery remained partly experimental in the early 1980s. But researchers believed it held great potential, especially for patients afflicted with the condition called *monocular aphakia*, or loss of vision due to lens loss or deterioration. The microsurgical procedure involved four steps or stages:

1. Using a *microelectrokeratome*, a kind of electrically operated block plane, the surgeon shaves off the outer layer of the patient's cornea.

2. A disc of corneal tissue from a donor is frozen on the optical lathe. The feezing agent is carbon dioxide. The liquid CO_2 circulates through the lathe.

3. A computer is used to set the measurements for reshaping the frozen segment of cornea. The surgeon operates the lathe during the actual cutting or shaving process.

4. The final step involves suturing the newly shaped cornea segment into the patient's eye.

Following cataract surgery, the extended wear contact lens may prove to be the most convenient type of lens. Wearing it for weeks at a time, sleeping and awake, the patient need not worry about losing or mislaying the lens.

Acting on the finding that ultraviolet (UV) light can cause cataracts, researchers have also developed *ultraviolet eyeglasses*. These screen out ultraviolet light so that it cannot reach the eye. The glasses have plastic lenses made with an absorbent dye that is mixed into the plastic in the manufacturing process.

Thus far, the UV-absorbing glasses have had two main uses. They have helped persons who had cataracts removed and were then fitted with the special glasses. The patients who wore the glasses in tests had better vision than others who did not wear them after cataract surgery. In a second use, the glasses appeared to promise relief for persons who had early indications of cataract growth. The UV lenses may prevent further development of cataracts in such persons.

Detached Retina

"I felt as if a curtain were being drawn across my eyes," reported a victim of detached retina. Actually, a hole or tear appeared in the patient's retina, the membrane that stretches across the back of the eyeball. Because the retina serves as the film of the camera that is the eye, the hole or tear can cause sudden loss of vision in the affected eye and even blindness. Victims may see flashes of light, or find black spots floating in front of their eyes, or experience periodic losses of sight (see "Retinal Detachment or Disease," p. 335).

Detached retina can be cured. But prompt action is important. Among new techniques, intense heat (*diathermy*) may be used to close the hole or tear in the retina. Intense cold (*cryosurgery* or *cryotherapy*) may serve a similar purpose. Both methods help to restore the damaged tissue to its normal place in the eye. Where severe detachment occurs, diathermy and cryotherapy may be used in combination with surgery. The doctor in such cases repositions the retinal tissue by surgical means.

Lasers have also proved useful in the treatment of detached retina. *Laser therapy* may be recommended where the retina has developed a hole. The laser beam has the effect of reattaching the tissue.

Diabetic Retinopathy

Diabetes has various side effects. One, *diabetic retinopathy*, involves loss of vision that results when

Ophthalmologists use cryoprobes for a number of surgical techniques. Here, the cryoprobe freezes the crystalline lens to a temperature of approximately −30 degrees C. to facilitate its extraction during cataract surgery.

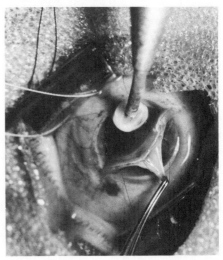

blood vessels at the back of the eye become clogged. The vessels may swell and bleed. The victim may experience impaired vision. The same disorder may occur when fragile new blood vessels multiply in the eye of the diabetic (*neovascularization*). The blood vessels may appear on the retina of the optic nerve, or in the vitreous cavity. The blood vessels may rupture, causing partial or total loss of vision.

Laser therapy has become the most widely used method of treating diabetic retinopathy. The laser beam seals off the hemorrhaging blood vessels. Laser therapy, a painless form of treatment, may also be used to slow the growth of new blood vessels and to aid the functioning of the *macula lutea*, the tiny area at the center of the retina that helps keep vision clear.

Shooting powerful beams of light, the laser may also be used in *scatter photocoagulation*. In this process, instead of burning the new blood vessels by direct exposure, the laser creates hundreds of burns on the retina. As many as 2,000 tiny burns may be made, with the result that the extra blood vessels solidify and then disappear. The patient may experience some reduction of the field of vision after scatter photocoagulation, but the loss is rarely bothersome.

Early detection of diabetic problems of the retina increases the chances of successful therapy. Thus regular eye examinations are important to the diabetic. Where vision has been totally lost, an operation called a *vitrectomy* may be recommended. The vitrectomy, which can help persons with persistent vitreous hemorrhaging, employs a fine grinding or nibbling device. The device, guided into the eye's vitreous cavity by a microscope, grinds up and flushes out blood residue and debris.

Macular Degeneration of the Retina

Macular degeneration (or *senile macular degeneration*) of the retina

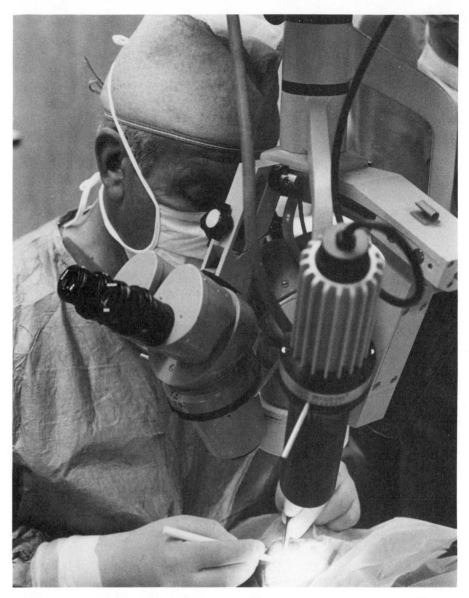

Advancements in microsurgery have enabled ophthalmogists to perform previously impossible surgical repairs and reconstructions.

results in an inability to see clearly. The victim's vision may become distorted or blurred. Vague early symptoms may include progressive difficulty in reading fine print. The sufferer may also find it difficult to recognize people's faces. As the macula, the part of the retina that makes clear vision possible, degenerates, eyeglasses usually become necessary. Magnification spectacles help many persons to use what vision they retain.

Macular degeneration rarely results in total blindness. Usually, victims retain side vision. But they may have difficulty performing tasks, like driving, reading, and doing housework, that normally require central vision.

Laser therapy for macular degeneration of the retina holds great promise, physicians believe. Where abnormal blood vessels develop under the retina, with bleeding and discharges of fluids that disturb the macula, laser therapy may be appropriate. The purpose is to destroy the new vessels. If the macula has already been destroyed, however, laser therapy cannot help. The same is true if the degeneration has causes other than the growth of abnormal blood vessels.

Retinitis Pigmentosa

An inherited disease, *retinitis pigmentosa* usually appears first in children or adolescents. Over time, the disease leads to night blindness, an inability to see well in the dark. Total blindness may follow in some cases. A promising new treatment calls for the injection of large doses of Vitamin B_6. Early evidence has shown that the vitamin raises the levels of an enzyme that the body needs for healthy retinal functioning.

In tests, a number of patients were given the vitamin injections. The drug was particularly effective in patients suffering from the disorder *gyrate atrophy*. In this retinal problem, one very similar to retinitis pigmentosa, portions of the lining (*epithelium*) of the retina waste away.

Blindness

Artificial vision may eventually offer the totally blind person an opportunity to see again — if indistinctly. In the surgical procedure that restores partial sight, a surgeon implants electrodes in the visual cortex of the patient's brain. Connected to light-sensitive implants within the eye, the electrodes are said to restore at least some vision — for some people. What does the newly sighted person see? The images have been compared to the grainy black-and-white photographs that were sent back from the moon during early lunar flights.

A virus, *herpes simplex*, can cause corneal blindness. In fact, herpes ranks as the second leading cause of such blindness in the United States. It affects an estimated 300,000 persons a year.

The treatment of virus blindness involves drugs that are applied directly to the cornea. The drugs usually eliminate the active infection, but they may not prevent later attacks. The virus lies dormant in the nerves at the base of the brain, returning to the cornea if the individual experiences emotional or physical stress. The repeated invasions of the cornea may lead to corneal scars. Vision may be impaired.

A new drug that in tests has been found more effective than old remedies acts only on cells invaded by the virus infection. The drug, Aciclovir (ACV), is injected. Activated by an enzyme produced by the virus, the drug attacks the virus while avoiding healthy cells.

EXAMINING AND TREATING CHILDREN

Research has shown that children go through a critical period insofar as vision is concerned. Babies or young children who do not see clearly may actually turn off the sight of one eye. As early as the first year after birth one eye may stop receiving and passing on visual information. The vision centers in the infant's brain may then stop functioning. *Amblyopia*, or lazy eye, may become well advanced and, often, untreatable.

At birth children may have other visual disorders. Crossed eyes or squint-eye (strabismus) may produce the same effect as amblyopia: in order to avoid double vision, the infant may stop using one eye (see "Crossed Eyes (Strabismus)," p. 333). The visual acuity of the faulty eye will gradually deteriorate. Such tumors as *retinoblastoma* may affect one or both eyes. Congenital cataracts may make it necessary to remove one eye's lens.

When a baby is born with a disorder like strabismus or amblyopia, in which the two eyes suffer from major differences in vision, doctors face the problem of identifying the disorder. They know that the first two years are important, and that disorders or diseases that are not treated in that period may become incurable. Amblyopia should, for example, be treated in the youngster's first six to eight years. But many children with eye problems look perfectly normal. The question arises: how to test young people who can neither talk nor read?

To detect amblyopia early, researchers have developed what is

Researchers at the Massachusetts Institute of Technology have devised an ingenious test called the preferential viewing procedure which helps doctors determine early eye disorders in infants and young children.

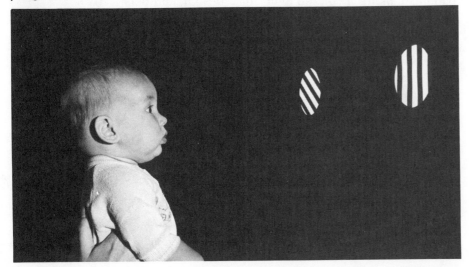

called the *preferential viewing procedure.* The method works on the principle that a baby's eyes, shown two patches of light on a wall in a dark room, will turn toward the one that has the most edges. The two patches are different; one is totally blank, the other has vertical black and white bars or stripes. As the test proceeds, the bars in the one patch become thinner and thinner. At some point the infant stops looking at them. At this point, it is assumed, the baby cannot tell the difference between the two patches. The tester has a measure of the baby's visual acuity.

Other methods of detecting and treating eye problems in infants have come under study. The *Ocular Screening System,* already mentioned, has proved initially to be a safe, simple, and reliable approach. Eye surgery to remove cataracts has been undertaken on infants who were only a few hours old as well as on older children. The results have generally been good. A drug, *Oculinum,* has been found to correct strabismus without surgery

In experiments, Oculinum has been injected into the eye muscle that is drawing the eye up, down, or to one side. As that muscle relaxes, the muscle on the other side of the affected eye works to straighten it. In weeks the muscles that control both eyes have begun to work together. The eyes become properly aligned.

The old cure for strabismus? A patch might be placed over the good eye so that the other would have to work, thus preventing laziness. The system is still used. Surgery and glasses offer two other alternatives.

In another relatively new treatment technique *biofeedback* principles come into play to help the young strabismus patient. Hooked up to an electronic device, the patient observes signals that reflect his control and use of the lazy eye. Signals include flashing lights, movements of a needle, and a steady tone. Initial biofeedback therapy has been found to teach the patient to achieve better use of the defective eye without a signal.

THE EYE GYM

The so-called eye gym represents a final contribution to modern methods of treating eye disorders. While some doctors question the value of eye exercises, many developmental ophthalmologists teach and use *vision training.* Such training in the world's first eye gym, in San Diego, California, is designed to help people who suffer from blurred vision, crossed eyes, visual discomfort, eye fatigue, and other problems related to inefficient vision.

The eye gym offers an integrated eye training program. People working out at the gym may follow the exercise routine devised by New York ophthalmologist William H. Bates. In one of the four phases of this Bates Method of Vision Improvement, exercisers swing or rotate their bodies from left to right and back. The eyes remain relaxed. In another sequence patients may do specially created exercises that help the eyes to work together. A typical two-eye or *binocular* exercise, for example, requires that the patient, using a pencil seen only by the right eye, trace a picture seen only by the left. A third routine has patients looking at colored lights for 20 minutes in syntonics or color balance therapy.

Persons of all ages use the eye gym. Special exercises for persons 40 and older reportedly delay the loss of flexibility in the eye that creates a need for bifocal glasses. Children old enough to read may work out on a trampoline while reading sentences in time with each bounce. People of various ages may engage in developmental art to learn better eye-hand coordination. According to some participants, they also develop awareness of shape, design, and perspective.

CHAPTER 34

Medical Emergencies

Anyone attempting to deal with a medical emergency will do so with considerably more confidence if he has a clear notion of the order of importance of various problems. Over and above all technical knowledge about such things as tourniquets or cardiac massage is the ability of the rescuer to keep a cool head so that he can make the right decisions and delegate tasks to others who wish to be helpful.

Cessation of Breathing

The medical emergency which requires prompt attention before any others is cessation of breathing. No matter what other injuries are involved, artificial respiration must be administered immediately to anyone suffering from respiratory arrest.

To determine whether a person is breathing naturally, place your cheek as near as possible to the victim's mouth and nose. While you are feeling and listening for evidence of respiration, watch the victim's chest and upper abdomen to see if they rise and fall. If respiratory arrest is indicated, begin artificial respiration immediately.

Time is critical; a human body has only about a four-minute reserve supply of oxygen in its tissues, although some persons have been re-

vived after being submerged in water for 10 minutes or more. Do not waste time moving the victim to a more comfortable location unless his position is life-threatening.

If more than one person is available, the second person should summon a doctor. A second rescuer can also assist in preparing the victim for artificial respiration by helping to loosen clothing around the neck, chest, and waist, and by inspecting the mouth for false teeth, chewing gum, or other objects that could block the flow of air. The victim's tongue must be pulled forward before artificial respiration begins.

Normal breathing should start after not more than 15 minutes of artificial respiration. If it doesn't, you should continue the procedure for at least two hours, alternating, if possible, with other persons to maintain maximum efficiency. Medical experts have defined normal breathing as 8 or more breaths per minute; if breathing resumes but slackens to a rate of fewer than 8 breaths per minute, or if breathing stops suddenly for more than 30 seconds, continue artificial respiration.

Mouth-to-Mouth and Mouth-to-Nose Artificial Respiration

Following is a description of the

techniques used to provide mouth-to-mouth or mouth-to-nose artificial respiration. These are the preferred methods of artificial respiration because they move a greater volume of air into a victim's lungs than any alternative method.

After quickly clearing the victim's mouth and throat of obstacles, tilt the victim's head back as far as possible, with the chin up and neck stretched to insure an open passage of air to the lungs. If mouth-to-mouth breathing is employed, pull the lower jaw of the victim open with one hand, inserting your thumb between the victim's teeth, and pinch the nostrils with the other to prevent air leakage through the nose. If using the mouth-to-nose technique, hold one hand over the mouth to seal it against air leakage.

Next, open your own mouth and take a deep breath. Then blow forcefully into the victim's mouth (or nose) until you can see the chest rise. Quickly remove your mouth and listen for normal exhalation sounds from the victim. If you hear gurgling sounds, try to move the jaw higher because the throat may not be stretched open properly. Continue blowing forcefully into the victim's mouth (or nose) at a rate of once every three or four seconds. (For infants, do not blow forcefully; blow

573

MOUTH-TO-MOUTH RESPIRATION

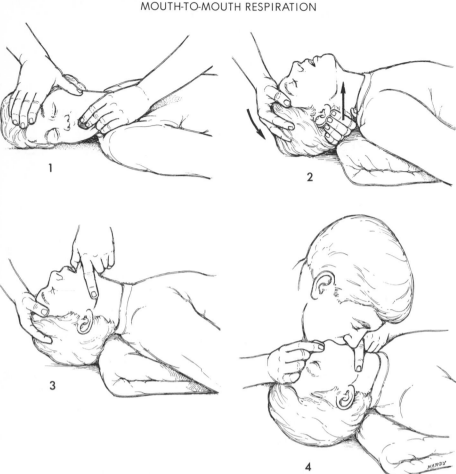

(1) Clear the victim's mouth and throat of obstructions. (2) Tilt the head back as far as possible, with the chin up and neck stretched taut. (3) Insert your thumb between the victim's teeth to pull his lower jaw open. Keep his head pushed back. (4) Pinch the nostrils shut. Open your mouth, take a deep breath, and, placing your mouth firmly against the victim's, blow forcefully. Repeat every 3 or 4 seconds.

only small puffs of air from your cheeks.)

If the victim's stomach becomes distended, it may be a sign that air is being blown into the stomach; press firmly with one hand on the upper abdomen to push the air out of the stomach.

If you are hesitant about direct physical contact of the lips, make a ring with the index finger and thumb of the hand being used to hold the victim's chin in position. Place the ring of fingers firmly about the victim's mouth; the outside of the thumb may at the same time be positioned to seal the nose against air leakage. Then blow the air into the victim's mouth through the finger-thumb ring. Direct lip-to-lip contact can also be avoided by placing a piece of gauze or other clean porous cloth over the victim's mouth.

Severe Bleeding

If the victim is not suffering from respiration failure or if breathing has been restored, severe bleeding is the second most serious emergency to attend to. Such bleeding occurs when either an artery or a vein has been severed. Arterial blood is bright red and spurts rather than flows from the body, sometimes in very large amounts. It is also more difficult to control than blood from a vein, which can be recognized by its dark red color and steady flow.

EMERGENCY TREATMENT: The quickest and most effective way to stop bleeding is by direct pressure on the wound. If heavy layers of sterile gauze are not available, use a clean handkerchief, or a clean piece of material torn from a shirt, slip, or sheet to cover the wound. Then place the fingers or the palm of the hand directly over the bleeding area. The pressure must be *firm and constant* and should be interrupted only when the blood has soaked through the dressing. *Do not remove the soaked dressing.* Cover it as quickly as possible with additional new layers. When the blood stops seeping through to the surface of the dressing, secure it with strips of cloth until the victim can receive medical attention. This procedure is almost always successful in stopping blood flow from a vein.

If direct pressure doesn't stop arterial bleeding, two alternatives are possible: pressure by finger or hand on the pressure point nearest the wound, or the application of a tourniquet. No matter what the source of the bleeding, if the wound is on an arm or leg, elevation of the limb as

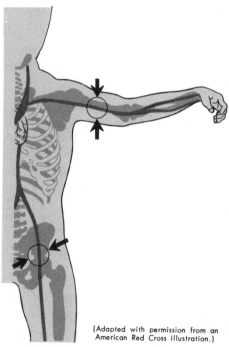

(Adapted with permission from an American Red Cross illustration.)

Two major pressure points: in the arm, the brachial artery; in the leg, the femoral artery. Continue to apply direct pressure and elevate the wounded part while utilizing pressure points to stop blood flow.

high as is comfortable will reduce the blood flow.

TOURNIQUETS: A tourniquet improperly applied can be an extremely dangerous device, and should only be considered for a hemorrhage that can't be controlled in any other way.

It must be remembered that arterial blood flows away from the heart, and that venous blood flows toward the heart. Therefore, while a tourniquet placed on a limb between the site of a wound and the heart may slow or stop arterial bleeding, it may actually increase venous bleeding. By obstructing blood flow in the veins beyond the wound site, the venous blood flowing toward the heart will have to exit from the wound. Thus, the proper application of a tourniquet depends upon an understanding and differentiation of

arterial from venous bleeding. Arterial bleeding can be recognized by the pumping action of the blood and by the bright red color of the blood.

Once a tourniquet is applied, it should not be left in place for an excessive period of time, since the tissues in the limb beyond the site of

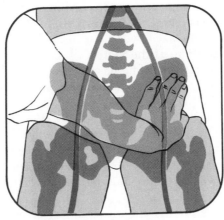

the wound need to be supplied with blood.

Shock

In any acute medical emergency, the possibility of the onset of shock must always be taken into account, especially following the fracture of a large bone, extensive burns, or serious wounds. If untreated, or if treated too late, shock can be fatal.

Shock is an emergency condition in which the circulation of the blood is so disrupted that all bodily functions are affected. It occurs when blood pressure is so low that insufficient blood supply reaches the vital tissues.

Types of Circulatory Shock and Their Causes

• *Low-volume shock* is a condition brought about by so great a loss of blood or blood plasma that the remaining blood is insufficient to fill the whole circulatory system. The blood loss may occur outside the body, as in a hemorrhage caused by injury to an artery or vein, or the loss may be internal because of the blood loss at the site of a major fracture, burn, or bleeding ulcer. Professional treatment involves replacement of blood loss by transfusion.

• *Neurogenic shock,* manifested by *fainting,* occurs when the regulating capacity of the nervous system is impaired by severe pain, profound fright, or overwhelming stimulus. This type of shock is usually relieved by having the victim lie down with his head lower than the rest of his body.

• *Allergic shock,* also called *anaphylactic shock,* occurs when the functioning of the blood vessels is disturbed by a person's sensitivity to the injection of a particular foreign substance, as in the case of an insect sting or certain medicines.

• *Septic shock* is brought on by infection from certain bacteria that release a poison which affects the proper functioning of the blood vessels.

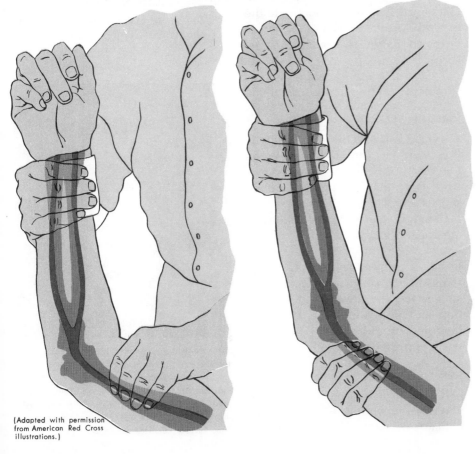

(Top) Use the femoral artery for control of severe bleeding from an open leg wound. Place the victim flat on his back, and put the heel of your hand directly over the pressure point. Apply pressure by forcing the artery against the pelvic bone. *(Bottom)* Use the brachial artery for control of severe bleeding from an open arm wound. Apply pressure by forcing the artery against the arm bone. Continue to apply direct pressure over the wound, and keep the wounded part elevated.

(Adapted with permission from American Red Cross illustrations.)

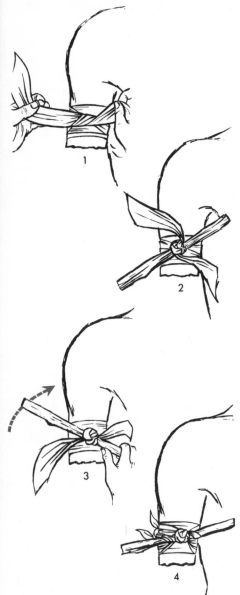

Severe arterial bleeding can be controlled by the correct application of a tourniquet. (1) A long strip of gauze or other material is wrapped twice around the arm or leg above the wound and tied in a half-knot. (2) A stick, called a windlass, is placed over the knot, and the knot is completed. (3) The windlass is turned to tighten the knot and finally, (4) the windlass is secured with the tails of the tourniquet. Improper use of a tourniquet can be very dangerous.

• *Cardiac shock* can be caused by any circumstance that affects the pumping action of the heart.

SYMPTOMS: Shock caused by blood loss makes the victim feel restless, thirsty, and cold. He may perspire a great deal, and although his pulse is fast, it is also very weak. His breathing becomes labored and his lips turn blue.

EMERGENCY TREATMENT: A doctor should be called immediately if the onset of shock is suspected. Until medical help is obtained, the following procedures can alleviate some of the symptoms:

1. With a minimum amount of disturbance, arrange the victim so that he is lying on his back with his head somewhat lower than his feet. (*Exception:* If the victim's breathing is difficult, or if he has suffered a head injury or a stroke, keep his body flat but place a pillow or similar cushioning material under his head.) Loosen any clothing that may cause constriction, such as a belt, tie, waistband, shoes. Cover him warmly against possible chill, but see that he isn't too hot.

2. If his breathing is weak and shallow, begin mouth-to-mouth respiration.

3. If he is hemorrhaging, try to control bleeding.

4. When appropriate help and transportation facilities are available, quickly move the victim to the nearest hospital or health facility in order to begin resuscitative measures.

5. *Do not* try to force any food or stimulant into the victim's mouth.

Cardiac Arrest

Cardiac arrest is a condition in which the heart has stopped beating altogether or is beating so weakly or so irregularly that it cannot maintain proper blood circulation.

Common causes of cardiac arrest are heart attack, electric shock, hemorrhage, suffocation, and other forms of respiratory arrest. Symptoms of cardiac arrest are unconsciousness, the absence of respiration and pulse, and the lack of a heartbeat or a heartbeat that is very weak or irregular.

Cardiac Massage

If the victim of a medical emergency manifests signs of cardiac arrest, he should be given cardiac massage at the same time that another rescuer is administering mouth-to-mouth resuscitation. Both procedures can be carried on in the moving vehicle taking him to the hospital.

It is assumed that he is lying down with his mouth clear and his air passage unobstructed. The massage is given in the following way:

1. The heel of one hand with the heel of the other crossed over it should be placed on the bottom third of the breastbone and pressed firmly down with a force of about 80 pounds so that the breastbone moves about two inches toward the spine. Pressure should not be applied directly on the ribs by the fingers.

2. The hands are then relaxed to allow the chest to expand.

3. If one person is doing both the cardiac massage and the mouth-to-mouth respiration, he should stop the massage after every 15 chest compressions and administer two very quick lung inflations to the victim.

4. The rescuer should try to make the rate of cardiac massage simulate restoration of the pulse rate. This is not always easily accomplished, but

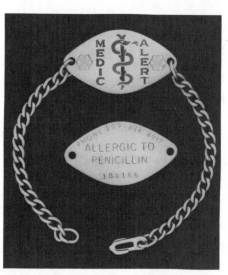

Some people are so severely allergic to certain medications that exposure to them can produce unconsciousness and, if not treated promptly, even death. To alert others, emblems identifying the allergy are available for a slight charge from the nonprofit Medic Alert Foundation, Turlock, California 95380.

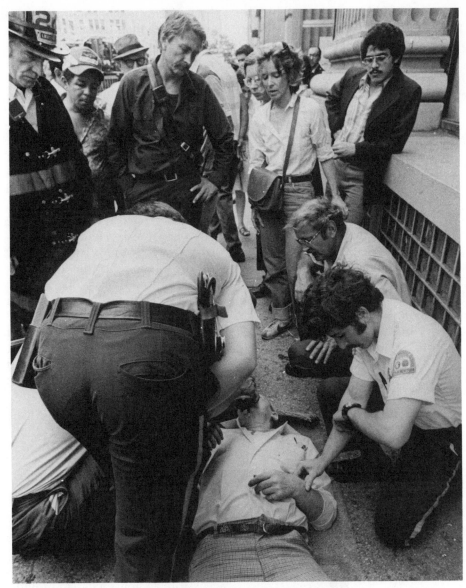

Trained paramedical personnel administer life-giving first-aid treatment to a heart attack victim.

at the back of the throat or at the opening of the trachea, or windpipe. The victim cannot breathe or speak. He may become pale or turn blue before collapsing. Death can occur within four or five minutes. But the lungs of an average person may contain at least one quart of air, inhaled before the start of choking, and that air can be used to unblock the windpipe and save the victim's life.

Finger Probe

If the object can be seen, a quick attempt can be made to remove it by probing with a finger. Use a hooking motion to dislodge the object. Under no circumstances should this method be pursued if it appears that the object is being pushed farther downward rather than being released and brought up.

BACK BLOWS FOR TREATMENT OF STRANGULATION

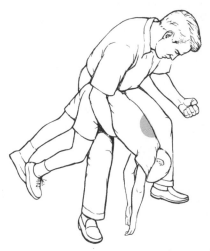

Children may be placed over the knee and struck sharply between the shoulders.

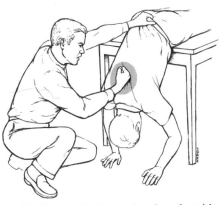

Adults may be placed over the edge of a table, supported by grasping the waist, and struck sharply between the shoulders with the fist.

compression should reach 60 times per minute.

The techniques for administering cardiac massage to children are the same as those used for adults, except that much less pressure should be applied to a child's chest, and, in the case of babies or young children, the pressure should be exerted with the tips of the fingers rather than with the heel of the hand.

CAUTION: Cardiac massage can be damaging if applied improperly. Courses in emergency medical care offered by the American Red Cross and other groups are well worth taking. In an emergency in which car-diac massage is called for, an un-trained person should seek the immediate aid of someone trained in the technique before attempting it himself.

Obstruction in the Windpipe

Many people die each year from choking on food; children incur an additional hazard in swallowing foreign objects. Most of these victims could be saved through quick action by nearly any other person, and without special equipment.

Food choking usually occurs be-cause a bite of food becomes lodged

Back Blows

Give the victim four quick, hard blows with the fist on his back between the shoulder blades. The blows should be given in rapid succession. If the victim is a child, he can be held over the knee while being struck; an adult should lie face down on a bed or table, with the upper half of his body suspended in the direction of the floor so that he can receive the same type of blows. A very small child or infant should be held upside down by the torso or legs and struck much more lightly than an adult.

The Heimlich Maneuver

If the back blows fail to dislodge the obstruction, the Heimlich ma-neuver should be given without delay. (Back blows may loosen the object even if they fail to dislodge it completely; that is why they are given first.) The lifesaving technique known as the *Heimlich maneuver* (named for Dr. Henry J. Heimlich) works simply by squeezing the volume of air trapped in the victim's lungs. The piece of food literally pops out of the throat as if it were ejected from a squeezed balloon.

To perform the Heimlich ma-neuver, the rescuer stands behind the victim and grasps his hands firm-ly over the victim's abdomen, just below the victim's rib cage. The res-cuer makes a fist with one hand and places his other hand over the clenched fist. Then, the rescuer forces his fist sharply inward and upward against the victim's dia-phragm. This action compresses the lungs within the rib cage. If the food does not pop out on the first try, the maneuver should be repeated until the air passage is unblocked.

When the victim is unable to stand, he should be rolled over on his back on the floor. The rescuer then kneels astride the victim and per-forms a variation of the Heimlich maneuver by placing the heel of one open hand, rather than a clenched fist, just below the victim's rib cage. The second hand is placed over the first. Then the rescuer presses up-ward (toward the victim's head) quickly to compress the lungs, re-peating several times if necessary.

The Heimlich maneuver has been used successfully by persons who were alone when they choked on food; some pressed their own fist into their abdomen, others forced the edge of a chair or sink against their abdomen.

Poisoning

In all cases of poisoning, it is impera-tive to get professional assistance as soon as possible.

Listed below are telephone num-bers for Poison Control Centers throughout the United States. These health service organizations are accessible 24 hours a day to provide information on how best to counter-act the effects of toxic substances.

In the event of known or suspected poisoning, call the center nearest you immediately. Give the staff member to whom you speak as much information as possible: the name or nature of the poison ingested, if you know; if not, the symptoms man-ifested by the victim.

If for any reason it is impossible to telephone or get to a Poison Control Center (or a doctor or hospital), fol-low these two general rules:

1. If a strong acid or alkali or a pe-troleum product has been ingested, dilute the poison by administering large quantities of milk or water. Do not induce vomiting.

2. For methanol or related prod-

THE HEIMLICH MANEUVER

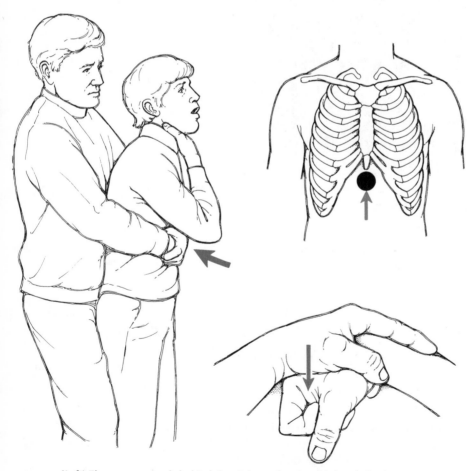

(Left) The rescuer stands behind the victim and grasps his hands firmly over the victim's abdomen just below the rib cage *(top right)*. The position of the rescuer's hands and the direction of thrust are shown at the bottom right.

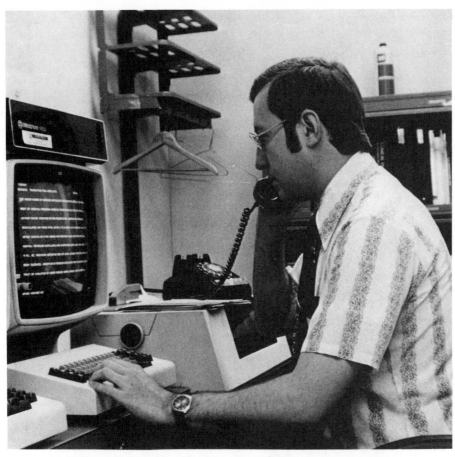

National Clearinghouse for Poison Control Centers uses a computer terminal for quick viewing of information about a particular product.

Practically all hospitals have emergency rooms for the prompt treatment of accident cases. If the victim is in good enough physical condition, he can be placed in a prone position in a family station wagon for removal to a hospital. However, under no circumstances should a person who has sustained major injuries or who has collapsed be made to sit upright in a car. First aid must be administered to him on the spot until a suitable conveyance arrives.

Every family should find out the telephone number of the nearest Poison Control Center (see p.580) and note it on the emergency number card.

Reaching a Doctor

Emergencies are usually best handled in a hospital since they are likely to require oxygen, blood transfusions, or other services only a hospital can provide. However, there are many situations in which a doctor's guidance on the phone can

(continued on p.584)

ucts such as window cleaners, antifreeze, paint removers, and shoe polish, induce vomiting—preferably with syrup of ipecac.

Calling for Help

Every household should have a card close by the telephone—if possible attached to an adjacent wall—that contains the numbers of various emergency services. In most communities, it is possible to simply dial the operator and ask for the police or fire department. In many large cities, there is a special three-digit number that can be dialed for reaching the police directly.

An ambulance can be summoned either by asking for a police ambulance, by calling the nearest hospital, or by having on hand the telephone numbers of whatever private ambulance services are locally available. Such services are listed in the classified pages of the telephone directory.

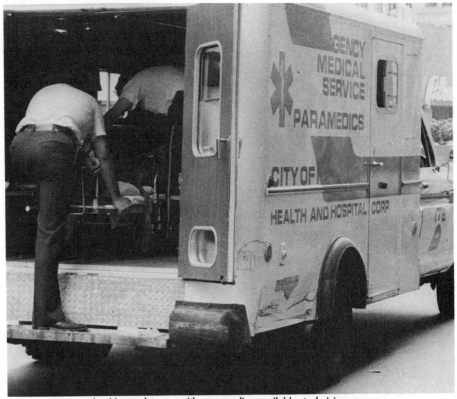

In cities and towns with paramedics available, technicians can speed poisoning victims to the nearest poison control center.

POISON CONTROL CENTERS

This list of poison control and information centers is compiled by the American Association of Poison Control Centers. State or regional control centers and other centers with a 24-hour poison control staff are listed in boldface (darker) type. All centers are listed by state and are grouped alphabetically by city or town. CAUTION: These numbers occasionally change and smaller centers are not available at all hours of the day. If you do not get an answer from the number you call after several rings, call your local police or fire emergency number in case of a crisis in your home.

ALABAMA

Alabama Poison Center*
Druid City Hospital
809 University Blvd., E.
Tuscaloosa 35401
(800) 462-0800 (statewide)
(205) 345-0600

Birmingham
Children's Hospital
1600 Seventh Ave., S.
35233
(800) 292-6678 (local)
(205) 933-9201
939-9201
939-9202

ALASKA

Anchorage
Anchorage Poison Center
Providence Hospital
3200 Providence Dr. 99504
(907) 563-3393

Fairbanks
Fairbanks Poison Control
Center
Fairbanks Memorial
Hospital
1650 Cowles St. 99701
(907) 456-7182

ARIZONA

**Arizona Regional Poison
Control System***
Tucson
(800) 362-0101

Flagstaff
Flagstaff Hospital and
Medical Center of Northern
Arizona
1215 N. Beaver St. 86001
(602) 779-0555

Phoenix
St. Luke's Hospital Medical
Center
525 N. 18th St. 85006
(602) 253-3334

Tucson
Arizona Poison and Drug
Information Center*
University of Arizona
Arizona Health Sciences
Center
85724
(800) 362-0101
(602) 626-6016

Yuma
Yuma Regional Medical
Center
Avenue A & 24th St. 85364
(602) 344-2000

ARKANSAS

**Statewide Poison Control
Drug Information Center**
University of Arkansas for
Medical Sciences
College of Pharmacy
4301 W. Markham St.
Little Rock 72201
(800) 428-8948 (statewide)
**(501) 666-5532 (Pulaski
County)**

El Dorado
Warner Brown Hospital
Emergency Room
460 W. Oak St. 71730
(501) 863-2266

Fort Smith
St. Edward Mercy
Medial Center
Emergency Room
7301 Rogers Ave. 72904
(501) 452-5100, ext. 2041

Sparks Regional Medical
Center
Emergency Room
1311 S. Eye St. 72902
(501) 441-5011

Harrison
Boone County Hospital
Emergency Room
620 N. Willow St. 72601
(501) 365-2000

Helena
Helena Hospital
Emergency Room
Hi-Way 49 Bypass 72342
(501) 338-6411, ext. 340

Osceola
Osceola Memorial Hospital
Emergency Room
611 W. Lee Ave. 72370
(501) 563-7182
563-3174

Pine Bluff
Jefferson Regional Medical
Center
Emergency Room
1515 W. 42nd Ave. 71601
(501) 541-7100

CALIFORNIA

Los Angeles
**Los Angeles County
Medical Association**

**Regional Poison
Information Center**
1925 Wilshire Blvd. 90057
(213) 484-5151 (public)
**664-2121 (MDs and
hospitals)**

Orange
**University of California
Poison Control Center**
Irvine Medical Center
101 City Drive S., Rte. 78
92668
(714) 634-5988

Sacramento
**UCDMC Regional Poison
Control Center***
2315 Stockton Blvd. 95817
**(800) 852-7221 (Northern
Calif.)**
(916) 453-3692

San Diego
**San Diego Regional
Poison Center***
University of California, San
Diego,
Medical Center
225 Dickinson St. 92103
(619) 294-6000

San Francisco
**San Francisco Bay Area
Regional Poison Center***
San Francisco General
Hospital
Room 1 E 86
1001 Potrero Ave. 94110
(415) 666-2845

San Jose
**Central-Coast Counties
Regional Poison Control
Center**
Santa Clara Valley Medical
Center
751 S. Bascom Ave. 95128
(800) 662-9886
(408) 299-5112

Fresno
Fresno Community Hospital
Regional Poison Control
Center
Fresno & R Sts. 93715
(209) 445-1222

Oakland
Children's Hospital Medical
Center of Northern
California
51st & Grove Sts. 94609
(415) 428-3248

Redding
Redding Medical Center
1450 Liberty St. 96099
(916) 243-4043

COLORADO

**Rocky Mountain Poison
Center***
645 Bannock St.
Denver 80204-4507
(800) 332-3073
(303) 629-1123

CONNECTICUT

**Connecticut Poison
Control Center**
University of Connecticut
Health Center
Farmington 06032
(203) 674-3456
674-3457

Bridgeport
Bridgeport Hospital
267 Grant St. 06602
(203) 384-3566

St. Vincent's Medical
Center
2800 Main St. 06606
(203) 576-5178

Danbury
Danbury Hospital
95 Locust Ave. 06810
(203) 797-7300

Farmington
Connecticut Poison Control
Center
University of Connecticut
Health Center
Farmington 06032
(203) 674-3456
674-3457

Middletown
Middlesex Memorial
Hospital
28 Crescent St. 06457
(203) 347-9471

New Haven
Hospital of St. Raphael
1450 Chapel St. 06511
(203) 789-3464

Yale-New Haven Hospital
Department of Pediatrics
Pediatric Emergency Room
789 Howard Ave. 06504
(203) 785-2222

Norwalk
Norwalk Hospital
Department of
Emergency Medicine
Maple St. 06856
(203) 852-2160

Waterbury
St. Mary's Hospital
Emergency Room
56 Franklin St. 06702
(203) 574-6011

DELAWARE

**Poison Information
Center**
Medical Center of Delaware
Wilmington Division

501 W. 14th St.
Wilmington 19899
(302) 655-3389

DISTRICT OF COLUMBIA

**National Capital Poison
Center***
Georgetown University
Hospital
3800 Reservoir Rd.
Washington 20007
(202) 625-3333

FLORIDA

Bradenton
Manatee Memorial Hosp
206 Second St. E. 3350
(813) 748-2121

Ft. Lauderdale
Broward General Medica
Center
Poison Control Center
Emergency Department
1600 S. Andrews Ave.
33316
**(305) 463-3131, ext. 195
1956**

Ft. Myers
Lee Memorial Hospital
2776 Cleveland Ave. 339
(813) 334-5334
334-5287

Ft. Walton Beach
Humana Hospital of Ft.
Walton Beach
1000 Mar-Walt Dr. 3254
(904) 863-7606

Gainesville
Shands Hospital
University of Florida 326
(904) 392-3389

Inverness
Citrus Memorial Hospital
502 Highland Blvd. 3265
(904) 726-2800

Jacksonville
St. Vincent's Medical
Center
1800 Barrs St. 32203
(904) 387-7500
387-7499 (TTY)

Leesburg
Leesburg Regional Medic
Center
600 E. Dixie 32748
(904) 787-9900

Melbourne
James E. Holmes Region
Medical Center
1350 S. Hickory St. 3290
(305) 676-7199

Naples
Naples Community Hosp
350 Seventh St. N. 3394
(813) 262-3131

cala
Munroe Regional Medical
Center
131 S.W. 15th St. 32670
(904) 351-7607

rlando
Orlando Regional Medical
Center
Orange Memorial Division
1414 S. Kuhl Ave. 32806
(305) 841-5222

unta Gorda
Medical Center Hospital
809 E. Marion Ave. 33950
(813) 637-2529

ockledge
Wuesthoff Memorial
Hospital
110 Longwood Ave. 32955
(305) 636-4357

arasota
Memorial Hospital
1901 Arlington St. 33577
(813) 953-1332

allahassee
Tallahassee Memorial
Regional Medical Center
1300 Miccosukee Rd.
32308
(904) 681-5411

ampa
**Tampa Bay Regional
Poison Control Center**
Tampa General Hospital
Davis Island 33606
(800) 282-3171
(813) 251-6995

itusville
Jess Parrish Memorial
Hospital
951 N. Washington Ave.
32780
(305) 268-6260

Vest Palm Beach
Good Samaritan Hospital
Flagler Dr. at Palm Beach
Lakes Blvd. 33402
(305) 655-5511, ext. 4333

Vinter Haven
Poison Control Center
Winter Haven Hospital
200 Avenue F, N.E. 33880
(813) 299-9701

GEORGIA

**Georgia Poison Control
Center***
Grady Memorial Hospital
80 Butler St., S.E.
Atlanta 30335
(800) 282-5846
(404) 589-4400
     525-3323 (TTY)

Albany
Phoebe Putney Memorial
Hospital
417 Third Ave. 31705
(912) 883-1800, ext. 4150

Augusta
University Hospital
1350 Walton Way 30902
(404) 724-5050

Columbus
The Medical Center
Emergency Dept.
710 Center St. 31902
(404) 571-1080

Macon
Regional Poison Control
Center
Medical Center of Central
Georgia
777 Hemlock St. 31201
(912) 744-1427
     744-1146
     744-1000

Rome
Floyd Medical Center
Regional Poison Control
Center
Emergency Dept.
Turner McCall Blvd. 30161
(404) 295-5500

Savannah
Savannah Regional EMS
Poison Center
Department of Emergency
Medicine
Memorial Medical Center
31403
(912) 355-5228

Thomasville
John D. Archbold Memorial
Hospital
Poison Control
900 Gordon Ave. 31792
(912) 228-2000

Valdosta
South Georgia Medical
Center
Emergency Dept.
2501 N. Patterson St.
31601
(912) 333-1110

Waycross
Memorial Hospital
Emergency Dept.
410 Darling Ave. 31501
(912) 283-3030

HAWAII

Hawaii Poison Center*
Kapiolani-Children's Medical
Center
1319 Punahou St.
Honolulu 96826
(800) 362-3585
(808) 941-4411

IDAHO

**Mid-Plains Poison Control
Center***
Omaha, Neb.
(800) 228-9515

Boise
Idaho Emergency Medical
Poison Center
State House

450 W. State St., 1st Fl.
83706
(800) 632-8000
(208) 334-2241

Idaho Falls
Idaho Falls Consolidated
Hospitals
Emergency Dept.
900 Memorial Dr. 83401
(208) 522-3600

Pocatello
Idaho Drug Information
Service and Poison Control
Center
Pocatello Regional Medical
Center
777 Hospital Way 83202
(800) 632-9490
(208) 234-0777

ILLINOIS

**Chicago Area Poison
Resource Center**
Rush-Presbyterian-St.
Luke's Medical Center
1753 W. Congress Pkwy.
Chicago 60612
(800) 942-5969
(312) 942-5969

Peoria Poison Center
St. Francis Hospital Medical
Center
530 N.E. Glen Oak Ave.
Peoria 61637
(800) 322-5330
(309) 672-2334

**Central and Southern
Illinois
Regional Poison
Resource Center***
St. John's Hospital
800 E. Carpenter St.
Springfield 62769
(800) 252-2022
(217) 753-3330

INDIANA

Indiana Poison Center*
1001 W. 10th St.
Indianapolis 46202
(800) 382-9097
(317) 630-7351

Anderson
Community Hospital
1515 N. Madison Ave.
46012
(317) 646-5143

St. John's Medical Center
2015 Jackson St. 46014
(317) 646-8222

Angola
Cameron Memorial Hospital
416 E. Maumee St. 46703
(219) 665-2141, ext. 146

Crown Point
St. Anthony Medical Center
Main at Franciscan Rd.
46307
(219) 738-2100, ext. 1311

Columbus
Bartholomew County
Hospital
2400 E. 17th St. 47201
(812) 376-5277

East Chicago
St. Catherine Hospital
4321 Fir St. 46312
(219) 392-7203

Elkhart
Elkhart General Hospital
600 East Blvd. 46514
(800) 382-9097
(219) 294-2621

Evansville
Deaconess Hospital
600 Mary St. 47710
(812) 426-3333

Welborn Memorial Baptist
Hospital
401 S.E. Sixth St. 47713
(812) 426-8249

Fort Wayne
Lutheran Hospital
3024 Fairfield Ave. 46807
(219) 458-2211

Parkview Memorial Hospital
2200 Randalia Dr. 46805
(219) 484-6636, ext. 6000

St. Joseph's Hospital
700 Broadway 46802
(219) 425-3765

Frankfort
Clinton County Hospital
1300 S. Jackson St. 46041
(317) 659-4731

Gary
Methodist Hospital of Gary
600 Grant St. 46402
(219) 886-4710

Goshen
Goshen General Hospital
200 High Park Ave. 46526
(219) 533-2141

Hammond
St. Margaret Hospital
25 Douglas St. 46320
(219) 932-2300, ext. 4350

Indianapolis
Indiana Poison Center*
Principal Information Center
for Indiana
1001 W. 10th St. 46202
(800) 382-9097
(317) 630-7351

Kendallville
McCray Memorial Hospital
Hospital Dr. 46755
(219) 347-1100

Kokomo
Howard Community
Hospital
3500 S. LaFountain St.
46902
(317) 453-8444

Lafayette
Lafayette Home Hospital
2400 South St. 47902
(317) 447-6811

Poison Control Center
St. Elizabeth Hospital
Medical Center
1501 Hartford St. 47904
(317) 423-6271

LaGrange
LaGrange Hospital
Rte. 5 46761
(219) 463-2143

LaPorte
LaPorte Hospital
State & Madison Sts.
46350
(219) 326-1234

Lebanon
Witham Memorial Hospital
1124 N. Lebanon St. 46052
(317) 482-2700, ext. 241

Madison
King's Daughters' Hospital
112 Presbyterian Ave.
47250
(812) 265-5211, ext. 154

Marion
Marion General Hospital
Wabash & Euclid Aves.
46952
(317) 662-4693

Muncie
Ball Memorial Hospital
2401 University Ave. 47303
(317) 747-4321

Portland
Jay County Hospital
505 W. Votaw St. 47371
(219) 726-7131

Richmond
Reid Memorial Hospital
1401 Chester Blvd. 47374
(317) 983-3148

Shelbyville
Major Hospital
150 W. Washington St.
46176
(317) 392-3793

Terre Haute
Union Hospital
1606 N. Seventh St. 47804
(812) 238-7000, ext. 7523

Valparaiso
Porter Memorial Hospital
814 LaPorte Ave. 46383
*(219) 464-8611, ext. 301,
302*

Vincennes
Good Samaritan Hospital
520 S. Seventh St. 47591
(812) 885-3344

IOWA

**Mid-Plains Poison Control
Center***
Omaha, Neb.
(800) 228-9515

**University of Iowa
Hospitals and Clinics
Poison Control Center***

Iowa City 52242
(800) 272-6477
(319) 356-2922

Des Moines
Variety Club Poison and
Drug Information Center
Iowa Methodist Medical
Center
1200 Pleasant St. 50308
(800) 362-2327
(515) 283-6254

Fort Dodge
Trinity Regional Hospital
Kenyon Rd. 50501
(515) 573-7211
        573-3101 (night)

Waterloo
Allen Memorial Hospital
Emergency Dept.
1625 Logan Ave. 50703
(319) 235-3893

KANSAS

**Mid-American Poison
Center**
University of Kansas
Medical Center
39th & Rainbow Blvd.
Kansas City 66103
(800) 332-6633
(913) 588-6633

**Mid-Plains Poison Control
Center***
Omaha, Neb.
(800) 228-9515

Atchison
Atchison Hospital
1301 N. Second St. 66002
(913) 367-2131

Dodge City
Dodge City Regional
Hospital
3001 Avenue A 67801
(316) 225-9050, ext. 381

Emporia
Newman Memorial Hospital
12th & Chestnut Sts. 66801
(316) 343-6800, ext. 545

Fort Riley
Irwin Army Hospital
Emergency Room 66442
(913) 239-7776
        239-7777
        239-7778

Fort Scott
Mercy Hospital
821 Burke St. 66701
(316) 223-2200, ext. 135

Great Bend
Central Kansas Medical
Center
3515 Broadway 67530
(316) 792-2511, ext. 115

Hays
Hadley Regional Medical
Center
201 E. Seventh St. 67601
(913) 628-8251

Lawrence
Lawrence Memorial
Hospital
325 Maine St. 66044
(913) 749-6100, ext. 162

Salina
St. John's Hospital
139 N. Penn St. 67401
(913) 827-3187
        827-5591, ext. 112

Topeka
Northeast Kansas Poison
Center
St. Francis Hospital and
Medical Center
1700 W. Seventh St. 66606
(913) 295-8094

Stormont-Vail Regional
Medical
Center
10th & Washburn Sts.
66606
(913) 354-6100

Wichita
Wesley Medical Center
550 N. Hillside 67214
(316) 688-2277

KENTUCKY

Fort Thomas
St. Luke Hospital of
Campbell County
Northern Kentucky Poison
Center
85 N. Grand Ave. 41075
(800) 352-9900
(606) 572-3215

Lexington
Central Baptist Hospital
Poison Control Center
1740 S. Limestone St.
40503
(606) 278-3411, ext. 1663

Drug Information Center
University of Kentucky
Medical Center 40506
(606) 233-5320

Louisville
**Kentucky Regional
Poison Center of Kosair-
Children's Hospital***
40232
(800) 722-5725
(502) 589-8222

Murray
Murray-Calloway County
Hospital
Poison Control Center
803 Poplar St. 42071
(502) 753-7588

Owensboro
Owensboro-Daviess County
Hospital
Emergency Room

811 Hospital Ct. 42301
*(502) 926-3030, ext. 180,
174, 391*

Paducah
Western Baptist Hospital
Poison Control
2501 Kentucky Ave. 42001
*(502) 575-2105—days
    (8 a.m. to 8 p.m.)*
*(502) 575-2199—nights
    (8 p.m. to 8 a.m.)*

Prestonburg
Poison Control Center
Highlands Regional Medical
Center 41653
*(606) 886-8511, ext. 132,
160*

South Williamson
Williamson Appalachian
Regional Hospital
Central Pharmaceutical
Service
Emergency Dept.
2000 Central Ave. 41503
(606) 237-1010

LOUISIANA

**Louisiana Regional
Poison Control Center***
1501 Kings Hwy.
Shreveport 71130
(800) 535-0525
(318) 425-1524

Monroe
St. Francis Medical Center
309 Jackson St. 71201
(318) 325-6454

MAINE

**Maine Poison Control
Center**
at Maine Medical Center
22 Bramhall St.
Portland 04102
(800) 442-6305
(207) 871-2381 (ER)

MARYLAND

Maryland Poison Center*
University of Maryland
School of Pharmacy
636 W. Lombard St.
Baltimore 21201
(800) 492-2414
(301) 528-7701

Cumberland
Tri-State Poison Center
Sacred Heart Hospital
900 Seton Dr. 21502
(301) 722-6677

MASSACHUSETTS

**Massachusetts Poison
Control System**
300 Longwood Ave.
Boston 02115

(800) 682-9211
(617) 232-2120
    277-3323 (TTY)

MICHIGAN

Poison Control Center*
Children's Hospital of
Michigan
3901 Beaubien
Detroit 48201
(800) 572-1655
(800) 462-6642
(313) 494-5711

**Blodgett Regional Poison
Center***
Blodgett Memorial Medical
Center
1840 Wealthy, S.E.
Grand Rapids 49506
(800) 632-2727
(616) 774-7854

Battle Creek
Community Hospital
Pharmacy Dept.
183 West St. 49016
(616) 963-5521

Flint
Poison Information Center
Hurley Medical Center
1 Hurley Plaza 48502
(800) 572-5396
(313) 257-9111

Kalamazoo
Great Lakes Poison Center
Bronson Methodist Hospital
252 E. Lovell St. 49001
(800) 442-4112
(616) 383-6409

Midwest Poison Center
Borgess Medical Center
1521 Gull Rd. 49001
(800) 632-4177
(616) 383-7070

Lansing
St. Lawrence Hospital
1210 W. Saginaw St. 48915
(517) 372-5112
        372-5113

Marquette
Upper Peninsula Regional
Poison Center
Marquette General Hospital
420 W. Magnetic St. 49855
(800) 562-9781
(906) 228-9440

Pontiac
Poison Information Center
St. Joseph Mercy Hospital
900 Woodward Ave. 48053
(313) 858-7373
        858-7374

Saginaw
Saginaw Region Poison
Center
Saginaw General Hospital
1447 N. Harrison St. 48602
(517) 755-1111

MINNESOTA

Hennepin Poison Center*
Hennepin County Medical
Center
701 Park Ave.
Minneapolis 55415
(612) 347-3141

**Minnesota Poison Control
System***
St. Paul-Ramsey Medical
Center
640 Jackson St.
St. Paul 55101
(800) 222-1222
(612) 221-2113

MISSISSIPPI

**Regional Poison Control
Center**
University Medical Center
2500 N. State St.
Jackson 39216
(601) 354-7660

Hattiesburg
Forrest County General
Hospital
400 S. 28th St. 39401
(601) 264-4235

MISSOURI

**Cardinal Glennon
Children's Hospital
Regional Poison Center***
1465 S. Grand Blvd.
St. Louis 63104
(800) 392-9111
(314) 772-5200

**Mid-Plains Poison Control
Center***
Omaha, Neb.
(800) 228-9515

Kansas City
Children's Mercy Hospital
24th at Gillham Rd. 64108
(816) 234-3000

MONTANA

**Rocky Mountain Poison
Center***
Denver, Colo.
(800) 525-5042

NEBRASKA

**Mid-Plains Poison Control
Center***
Children's Memorial
Hospital
8301 Dodge St.
Omaha 68114
*(800) 642-9999 (outside
    Omaha)*
(402) 390-5400 (Omaha)
*(800) 228-9515 (Idaho,
    Iowa, Kan., Mo., S. Dak.*

NEVADA

as Vegas
Southern Nevada Memorial
Hospital
1800 W. Charleston Blvd.
89102
(702) 385-1277

Sunrise Hospital Medical
Center
3186 S. Maryland Pkwy.
89109
(702) 732-4989

eno
St. Mary's Hospital
235 W. Sixth St. 89520
(702) 789-3013

Washoe Medical Center
77 Pringle Way 89520
(702) 785-4129

NEW HAMPSHIRE

**New Hampshire Poison
Center**
NH-Dartmouth Hitchcock
Medical Center
2 Maynard St.
Hanover 03756
(800) 562-8236
(603) 646-5000

NEW JERSEY

**New Jersey Poison
Information and
Education System***
Newark Beth Israel Medical
Center
201 Lyons Ave.
Newark 07112
(800) 962-1253
(201) 926-8005

NEW MEXICO

**New Mexico Poison and
Drug Information Center***
University of New Mexico
Albuquerque 87131
(800) 432-6866
(505) 277-4261

NEW YORK

**Binghamton
Southern Tier Poison
Center**
Binghamton General
Hospital
Mitchell Ave. 13903
(607) 723-8929

**uffalo
Western New York Poison
Center**
Children's Hospital
219 Bryant St. 14222
(716) 878-7654
878-7655

Dunkirk
Brooks Memorial Hospital
10 W. Sixth St. 14048
(716) 366-1111

**East Meadow
Long Island Regional
Poison Control Center***
Nassau County Medical
Center
2201 Hempsted Tnpk.
11554
(516) 542-2324
542-2325
542-2323 (TTY)

Elmira
Arnot Ogden Memorial
Hospital
Roe Ave. & Grove St.
14901
(607) 737-4100

St. Joseph's Hospital
Health Center
555 E. Market St. 14901
(607) 734-2662

Jamestown
Women's Christian
Association Hospital
207 Foote Ave. 14701
(716) 487-0141
484-8648

**New York
New York City Poison
Center***
455 First Ave. 10016
(212) 340-4494
764-7667

**Nyack
Hudson Valley Poison
Center**
Nyack Hospital
N. Midland Ave. 10960
(914) 353-1000

**Rochester
Finger Lakes Poison
Center**
LIFE LINE
University of Rochester
Medical Center 14620
(716) 275-5151
275-2700 (TTY)

Schenectady
Ellis Hospital Poison Center
1101 Nott St. 12308
(518) 382-4039
382-4309

**Syracuse
Syracuse Poison
Information Center**
Upstate Medical Center
750 E. Adams St. 13210
(315) 476-7529
473-5831

Troy
St. Mary's Hospital
1300 Massachusetts Ave.
12180
(518) 272-5792

Utica
St. Luke's Memorial

Hospital Center
P.O. Box 479 13503
(315) 798-6200
798-6223

Watertown
Watertown Poison
Information Center
House of the Good
Samaritan Hospital
Washington & Pratt Sts.
13602
(315) 788-8700

NORTH CAROLINA

**Duke Poison Control
Center***
Duke University Medical
Center
Durham 27710
(800) 672-1697
(919) 684-8111

Asheville
Western NC Poison Control
Center
Memorial Mission Hospital
509 Biltmore Ave. 28801
(704) 255-4490

Charlotte
Mercy Hospital
2001 Vail Ave. 28207
(704) 379-5827

Greensboro
Moses H. Cone Memorial
Hospital
Triad Poison Center
1200 N. Elm St. 27420
(800) 722-2222
(919) 379-4105

Hendersonville
Margaret R. Pardee
Memorial Hospital
Fleming St. 28739
*(704) 693-6522, ext. 555,
556*

Hickory
Catawba Memorial Hospital
Fairgrove Church Rd.
28601
(704) 322-6649

Jacksonville
Onslow Memorial Hospital
Western Blvd. 28540
(919) 577-2555

Wilmington
New Hanover Memorial
Hospital
2131 S. 17th St. 28401
(919) 343-7046

NORTH DAKOTA

**North Dakota Poison
Information Center**
St. Luke's Hospitals
Fifth St. N. & Mills Ave.
Fargo 58122
(800) 732-2200
(701) 280-5575

OHIO

**Central Ohio Poison
Control Center***
Children's Hospital
700 Children's Dr.
Columbus 43205
(800) 682-7625
(614) 228-1323

**Southwest Ohio Regional
Poison Control System
Drug and Poison
Information Center***
University of Cincinnati
Medical Center
Bridge Medical Science
Bldg.
231 Bethesda Ave.
Cincinnati 45267
(800) 872-5111
(513) 872-5111

Akron
Children's Hospital Medical
Center of Akron
281 Locust St. 44308
(800) 362-9922
(216) 379-8562

Cleveland
Greater Cleveland Poison
Control Center
2119 Abington Rd. 44106
(216) 231-4455

Dayton
Children's Medical Center
1 Children's Plaza 45404
(800) 762-0727
(513) 222-2227

Lorain
Lorain Community Hospital
3700 Kolbe Rd. 44053
(216) 282-2220

Mansfield
Mansfield General Hospital
335 Glessner Ave. 44903
(419) 526-8200

Springfield
Community Hospital
2615 E. High St. 45505
(513) 325-1255

Toledo
Poison Information Center
Medical College of Ohio
Hospital
3000 Arlington Ave. 43614
(419) 381-3897

Youngstown
Mahoning Valley Poison
Center
St. Elizabeth Hospital
Medical Center
1044 Belmont Ave. 44501
(216) 746-2222
746-5510 (TTY)

Zanesville
Bethesda Poison Control
Center
Bethesda Hospital
2951 Maple Ave. 43701
(614) 454-4221

OKLAHOMA

**Oklahoma Poison Control
Center**
Oklahoma Children's
Memorial Hospital
Oklahoma City 73126
(800) 522-4611
(405) 271-5454

Ada
Valley View Hospital
1300 E. Sixth St. 74820
(405) 332-2323, ext. 200

Lawton
Comanche County
Memorial Hospital
3401 Gore Blvd. 73502
(405) 355-8620

McAlester
McAlester Regional
Hospital
1 Clark Bass Blvd. 74501
(918) 426-1800, ext. 7705

Ponca City
St. Joseph Medical Center
Emergency Room
14th St. & Hartford Ave.
74601
(405) 765-0584

OREGON

**Oregon Poison Control
and Drug Information
Center**
University of Oregon Health
Sciences Center
3181 S.W. Sam Jackson
Park Rd.
Portland 97201
(800) 452-7165
(503) 225-8968

PENNSYLVANIA

Allentown
Lehigh Valley Poison
Center
Allentown Hospital
17th & Chew Sts. 18102
(215) 433-2311

Altoona
Keystone Region Poison
Center
Mercy Hospital
2500 Seventh Ave. 16603
(814) 946-3711

Bloomsburg
Bloomsburg Hospital
549 E. Fair St. 17815
(717) 784-4241

Bradford
Bradford Hospital
Emergency Room
Interstate Pkwy. 16701
(814) 368-4143, ext. 274

Bryn Mawr
Bryn Mawr Hospital
Bryn Mawr Ave. 19010
(215) 896-3577

Chester
Sacred Heart Medical
Center
Ninth & Wilson Sts. 19013
(215) 494-4400

Clearfield
Clearfield Hospital
809 Turnpike Ave. 16830
(814) 765-5341

Coaldale
Coaldale State General
Hospital
Seventh St. 18218
(717) 645-2131

Coudersport
Charles Cole Memorial
Hospital
RD 3, Rte. 6 16915
(814) 274-9300

Danville
Susquehanna Poison
Center
Geisinger Medical Center
N. Academy Ave. 17821
(717) 271-6116

Doylestown
Doylestown Hospital
595 W. State St. 18901
(215) 345-2283

Erie
Hamot Medical Center
201 State St. 16550
(814) 452-4242

Metro Health Center
252 W. 11th St. 16501
(814) 454-2120

Millcreek Community
Hospital
5515 Peach St. 16509
(814) 864-4031, ext. 442

Northwest Poison Center
Saint Vincent Health Center
232 W. 25th St. 16544
(814) 452-3232

Gettysburg
Gettysburg Hospital
147 Gettys St. 17325
(717) 334-9155

Greensburg
Westmoreland Hospital
532 W. Pittsburgh St.
15601
(412) 832-4355

Hanover
Hanover General Hospital
300 Highland Ave. 17331
(717) 637-3711

Hershey
Capital Area Poison

Center
Milton S. Hershey Medical
Center
University Dr. 17033
(717) 534-6111
534-6039

Jeannette
Jeannette District
Memorial Hospital
600 Jefferson Ave. 15644
(412) 527-9300

Jersey Shore
Jersey Shore Hospital
Thompson St. 17740
(717) 398-0100, ext. 225

Johnstown
Conemaugh Valley
Memorial Hospital
1086 Franklin St. 15905
(814) 535-5351

Lee Hospital
320 Main St. 15901
(814) 533-0109

Mercy Hospital
1020 Franklin St. 15905
(814) 535-5353

Lancaster
Lancaster General Hospital
555 N. Duke St. 17604
(717) 295-8322

St. Joseph's Hospital
250 College Ave. 17604
(717) 299-4546

Lansdale
North Penn Hospital
Medical Campus Dr. 19446
(215) 368-2100

Lebanon
Good Samaritan Hospital
Fourth & Walnut Sts. 17042
(717) 272-7611

Lehighton
Gnaden Huetten Memorial
Hospital
11th & Hamilton Sts. 18235
(215) 377-1300, ext. 552

Lewistown
Lewistown Hospital
Highland Ave. 17044
(717) 248-5411

Muncy
Muncy Valley Hospital
Water St. 17756
(717) 546-8282

Nanticoke
Nanticoke State General
Hospital
W. Washington St. 18634
(717) 735-5000, ext. 261

Philadelphia
Philadelphia Poison
Information
321 University Ave. 19104
(215) 922-5523
922-5524

Philipsburg
Philipsburg State General
Hospital
Locklomond Rd. 16866
(814) 342-3320, ext. 293

Pittsburgh
Pittsburgh Poison Center*
Children's Hospital
125 De Soto St. 15213
(412) 681-6669—
(emergency)
647-5600—(admin./
consultation)

Reading
Community General
Hospital
145 N. Sixth St. 19601
(215) 375-9115

Sayre
Robert Packer Hospital
Guthrie Sq. 18840
(717) 888-6666

Sellersville
Grand View Hospital
Lawn Ave. 18960
(215) 257-5955

State College
Centre Community Hospital
Orchard Rd. 16803
(814) 238-4351

Titusville
Titusville Hospital
406 W. Oak St. 16354
(814) 827-1851

Tunkhannock
Tyler Memorial Hospital
RD 1 18657
(717) 836-2161, ext. 180

Wilkes-Barre
NPW-Medical Center
1000 E. Mountain Blvd.
18704
(717) 826-7762

York
Memorial Osteopathic
Hospital
325 S. Belmont St. 17403
(717) 843-8623

York Hospital
1001 S. George St. 17405
(717) 771-2311

PUERTO RICO

Poison Control Center
Centro Médico
Rio Piedras 00936
(809) 754-8535

RHODE ISLAND

Rhode Island Poison
Center
Rhode Island Hospital
593 Eddy St.
Providence 02902
(401) 277-5906

SOUTH CAROLINA

Palmetto Poison Center
University of South Carolina

College of Pharmacy
Columbia 29208
(800) 922-1117
(803) 765-7359

SOUTH DAKOTA

Mid-Plains Poison Control
Center*
Omaha, Neb.
(800) 228-9515

Aberdeen
Dakota Midland Poison
Control Center
57501
(605) 773-3361

Rapid City
Rapid City Regional Poison
Center
353 Fairmont Blvd. 57701
(800) 742-8925
(605) 341-8222

Sioux Falls
McKennan Hospital Poison
Center
800 E. 21st St. 57101
(800) 952-0123
843-0505
(605) 336-3894

TENNESSEE

Chattanooga
T. C. Thompson Children's
Hospital
910 Blackford St. 37403
(615) 778-6100

Columbia
Maury County Hospital
1224 Trotwood Ave. 38401
(615) 381-4500, ext. 405

Cookeville
Cookeville General Hospital
142 W. Fifth St. 38501
(615) 526-4818

Jackson
Jackson-Madison County
General Hospital
708 W. Forest Ave. 38301
(901) 424-0424, ext. 525

Johnson City
Johnson City Medical
Center Hospital
Poison Control Center
400 State of Franklin Rd.
37601
(615) 461-6572

Knoxville
Memorial Research Center
and Hospital
1924 Alcoa Hwy. 37920
(615) 544-9400

Memphis
Southern Poison Center
Le Bonheur Children's
Medical Center
848 Adams Ave. 38103
(901) 528-6048

Nashville
Vanderbilt University

Hospital
1161 21st Ave. S. 37232
(615) 322-6435

TEXAS

Texas State Poison
Center
University of Texas Medical
Branch
Eighth & Mechanic Sts.
Galveston 77550
(800) 392-8548
(409) 765-1420 (Galveston)
(713) 654-1701 (Houston)
(512) 478-4490 (Austin)

Abilene
Hendrick Hospital
N. 19th & Hickory Sts.
79601
(915) 677-7762

Amarillo
Amarillo Emergency
Receiving Center
Amarillo Hospital District
1501 Coulter Dr. 79106
(806) 376-4292

Beaumont
Baptist Hospital
of Southeast Texas
College & 11th Sts. 77701
(409) 833-7409

Corpus Christi
Memorial Medical Center
2606 Hospital Blvd. 78405
(512) 881-4559

Dallas
North Central Texas Poison
Center
75235
(214) 920-2400

El Paso
El Paso Poison Control
Center
R. E. Thomason General
Hospital
4815 Alameda Ave. 79905
(915) 533-1244

Fort Worth
Cook Poison Center
W. I. Cook Children's
Hospital
1212 W. Lancaster St.
76102
(817) 336-6611

Harlingen
Valley Baptist Medical
Center
2000 Peace St. 78550
(512) 421-1860
421-1859

Laredo
Mercy Regional Medical
Center
1515 Logan St. 78040
(512) 724-6247

obock
lethodist Hospital
615 19th St. 79410
306) 793-4366

dland
lidland Memorial Hospital
200 W. Illinois Ave. 79701
15) 685-1558

essa
ledical Center Hospital
oison Control Center
ourth & Allegheny Sts.
9760
15) 333-1231

inview
entral Plains Regional
ospital
601 Dimmitt Rd. 79072
306) 296-9601

n Angelo
hannon West Texas
lemorial Hospital
20 E. Harris Ave. 76903
15) 655-5330

ler
ledical Center Hospital
000 S. Beckham St.
5701
214) 597-8884

co
lillcrest Baptist Medical
enter
000 Herring Ave. 76708
817) 753-1412

chita Falls
Vichita Falls General
lospital
600 Eighth St. 76301
817) 322-6771

UTAH

ntermountain Regional
Poison Control Center*
0 N. Medical Dr.
alt Lake City 84132
800) 662-0062
801) 581-2151

VERMONT

rmont Poison Center

Medical Center Hospital
Burlington 05401
(802) 658-3456

VIRGINIA

Alexandria
Alexandria Hospital
4320 Seminary Rd. 22314
(703) 379-3070

Arlington
Arlington Hospital
1701 N. George Mason Dr.
22205
(703) 558-6161

Blacksburg
Montgomery County
Hospital
Rte. 460, S. 24060
(703) 951-1111, ext. 140

Charlottesville
Blue Ridge Poison Center
University of Virginia
Hospital
22903
(800) 552-3723 (TTY:
Va. only)
(800) 446-9876 (TTY:
out of state)
(804) 924-5543

Danville
Danville Memorial Hospital
142 S. Main St. 24541
(804) 799-2222

Falls Church
Poison Control Center
Fairfax Hospital
3300 Gallows Rd. 22046
(703) 698-2900

Hampton
Hampton General Hospital
3120 Victoria Blvd. 23661
(804) 722-1131

Harrisonburg
Rockingham Memorial
Hospital
Emergency Room

235 Cantrell Ave. 22801
(703) 433-9706

Lexington
Stonewall Jackson Hospital
Spotswood Dr. 24450
(703) 463-1492

Lynchburg
Lynchburg General-
Marshall Lodge Hospitals
Tate Springs Rd. 24504
(804) 528-2066

Nassawadox
Northampton-Accomack
Memorial Hospital 23413
(804) 442-8700

Newport News
Riverside Hospital
500 J. Clyde Morris Blvd.
23601
(804) 599-2050

Norfolk
Tidewater Poison Center
150 Kingsley Lane 23505
(804) 489-5288

Petersburg
Petersburg General
Hospital
Apollo & Adams Sts. 23803
(804) 861-2992

Portsmouth
U.S. Naval Hospital 23708
(804) 398-5898

Reston
Access Emergency Center
11900 Baron Cameron Ave.
22091
(703) 437-5992

Richmond
**Central Virginia Poison
Center**
Medical College of Virginia
23298
(804) 786-4780

Roanoke
Southwest Virginia Poison
Center
Roanoke Memorial Hospital
Belleview at Jefferson St.
24033
(703) 981-7336

Staunton
King's Daughters' Hospital
1410 N. Augusta St. 24401
(703) 885-6848

Waynesboro
Waynesboro Community
Hospital
501 Oak Ave. 22980
(703) 942-4096

WASHINGTON

Seattle
Seattle Poison Center*
Children's Orthopedic
Hospital and Medical
Center
4800 Sand Point Way, N.E.
98105
(206) 526-2121
(800) 732-6985 (statewide)

Spokane
Spokane Poison Center
Deaconess Medical Center
800 W. Fifth Ave. 99210
(509) 747-1077 (TTY)
(800) 572-5842 (statewide)
541-5624 (N. Idaho
and W. Montana)

Tacoma
**Mary Bridge Poison
Information Center**
Mary Bridge Children's
Health Center
311 S. L St. 98405
(800) 542-6319 (statewide)
(206) 594-1414

Yakima
**Central Washington
Poison Center**
Yakima Valley Memorial
Hospital
2811 Tieton Dr. 98902
(800) 572-9176 (statewide)
(509) 248-4400

WEST VIRGINIA

**West Virginia Poison
System**
West Virginia University
School of Pharmacy
3110 McCorkle Ave., S.E.
(800) 642-3625
(304) 348-2971
348-4211

WISCONSIN

Green Bay
Green Bay Poison Center
St. Vincent Hospital
835 S. Van Buren St.
54305
(414) 433-8100

Madison
**Madison Area Poison
Center**
University Hospital and
Clinics
600 Highland Ave. 53792
(608) 262-3702

Milwaukee
Milwaukee Poison Center
Milwaukee Children's
Hospital
1700 W. Wisconsin Ave.
53233
(414) 931-4114

WYOMING

Wyoming Poison Center
DePaul Hospital
2600 E. 18th St.
Cheyenne 82001
(307) 777-7955

be extremely helpful and reassuring.

Since there are times when the family physician may not be available by phone, it's a good idea to ask for the names and phone numbers of doctors who can be called when your own doctor can't be reached. In many communities, it is also possi-ble to get the services of a physi-cian by calling the County Medical Society.

A family on vacation in a remote area or on a cross-country trip by car can be directed to the nearest medi-cal services by calling the telephone operator. If the operator can't pro-vide adequate information promptly, ask to be connected with the nearest headquarters of the State Police.

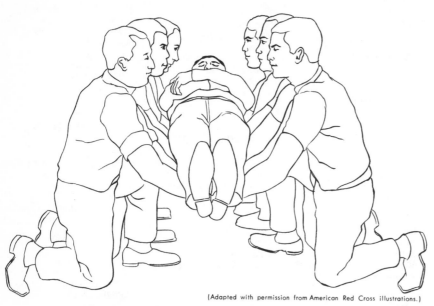

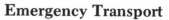
(Adapted with permission from American Red Cross illustrations.)

How to lift an injured or unconscious person to place him on a stretcher. Three bearers on each side of the victim kneel on the knee closer to the victim's feet. The bearers work their hands and forearms gently under the victim to about the midline of the back. On signal, they lift together as shown; on a following sig-nal, they stand as a unit, if that is necessary. In lowering the victim to a stretcher or other litter, the procedure is reversed.

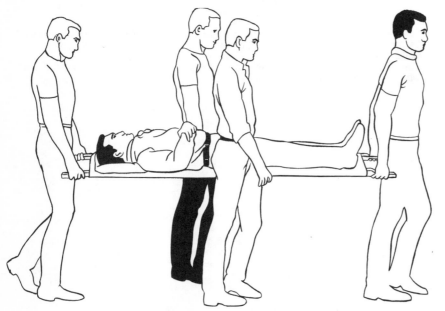

The proper way to carry a victim on a stretcher. One bear-er is at the head, one at the foot, and one at either side of the stretcher. The victim should be carried feet first.

Emergency Transport

In the majority of situations, the transfer of an injured person should be handled only by experienced res-cue personnel. If you yourself must move a victim to a doctor's office or hospital emergency room, here are a few important rules to remember:

1. Give all necessary first aid be-fore attempting to move the victim. Do everything to reduce pain and to make the patient comfortable.

2. If you improvise a stretcher, be sure it is strong enough to carry the victim and that you have enough people to carry it. Shutters, doors, boards, and even ladders may be used as stretchers. Just be sure that the stretcher is padded underneath to protect the victim and that a blan-ket or coat is available to cover him and protect him from exposure.

3. Bring the stretcher to the vic-tim, not the victim to the stretch-er. Slide him onto the stretcher by grasping his clothing or lift him—if enough bearers are available—as shown in the illustration.

4. Secure the victim to the stretch-er so he won't fall off. You may want to tie his feet together to minimize his movements.

5. Unless specific injuries prevent it, the victim should be lying on his back while he is being moved. How-ever, a person who is having difficulty breathing because of a chest injury might be more comfort-able if his head and shoulders are raised slightly. A person with a se-vere injury to the back of his head should be kept lying on his side. In any case, place the patient in a com-fortable position that will protect him from further injury.

6. Try to transport the patient feet first.

7. Unless absolutely necessary, don't try to put a stretcher into a pas-senger car. It's almost impossible to get the stretcher or injured person

into a passenger car without further injuring him. If there is no ambulance, a station wagon or truck makes a good substitute.

8. When you turn the patient over to a doctor or take him to an emergency room of a hospital, give a complete account of the situation to the person taking charge. Tell the doctor what you've done for the patient and what you suspect might cause further problems.

ALPHABETIC GUIDE TO MEDICAL EMERGENCIES

Abdominal wound

Abdominal wounds can result from gunshots during hunting or working with firearms, from falling on a knife or sharp object at home or work, or from a variety of other mishaps ranging from automobile accidents to a mugging attack. Such a wound can be a major emergency requiring surgery and other professional care. Call a doctor or arrange for quick transportation to a hospital as quickly as possible.

EMERGENCY TREATMENT: If there is severe bleeding, try to control it with pressure. Keep the victim lying on his back with the knees bent; place a pillow, coat, or a similar soft object under the knees to help hold them in the bent position. If abdominal organs are exposed, do not touch them for any reason. Cover the wound with a sterile dressing. Keep the dressing moistened with sterile water or the cleanest water available. Boiled water can be used to moisten the dressing, but be sure it has cooled before applying.

If the victim is to be moved to a hospital or doctor's office, be sure the dressing over the wound is large enough and is held in place with a bandage. In addition to pain, you can expect the victim to experience nausea and vomiting, muscle spasms, and severe shock. Make the victim as comfortable as possible under the circumstances; if he complains of thirst, moisten his mouth with a few drops of water, but do not permit him to swallow the liquid.

Abrasions

EMERGENCY TREATMENT: Wash the area in which the skin is scraped or rubbed off with soap and water, using clean gauze or cotton. Allow the abrasion to air-dry, and then cover it with a loose sterile dressing held in place with a bandage. If a sterile dressing is not available, use a clean handerchief.

Change the dressing after the first 24 hours, using household hydrogen peroxide to ease its removal if it sticks to the abrasion because of clotted blood. If the skinned area appears to be accompanied by swelling, or is painful or tender to the touch, consult a doctor.

Acid burns

Among acids likely to be encountered at work and around the home are sulphuric, nitric, and hydrochloric acids. Wet-cell batteries, such as automobile batteries, contain acid powerful enough to cause chemical destruction of body tissues, and some metal cleaners contain powerful acids.

EMERGENCY TREATMENT: Wash off the acid immediately, using large amounts of clean, fresh, cool water. Strip off or cut off any clothing that may have absorbed any of the acid. If possible, put the victim in a shower bath; if a shower is not available, flood the affected skin areas with as much water as possible. However, do not apply water forcefully since this could aggravate damage already done to skin or other tissues.

After as much of the acid as possible has been eliminated by flooding with water, apply a mild solution of sodium bicarbonate or another mild alkali such as lime water. However, caution should be exercised in neutralizing an acid burn because the chemical reaction between an acid and an alkali can produce intense heat that would aggravate the injury; also, not all acids are effectively neutralized by alkalis—carbolic acid burns, for example, should be neutralized with alcohol.

Wash the affected areas once more with fresh water, then dry gently with sterile gauze; be careful not to break the skin or to open blisters. Extensive acid burns will cause extreme pain and shock; have the victim lie down with the head and chest a little lower than the rest of the body. As soon as possible, summon a physician or rush the victim to the emergency room of a hospital.

Aerosol sprays

Although aerosol sprays generally are regarded as safe when handled according to directions, they can be directed accidentally toward the face with resulting contamination of the eyes or inhalation of the fumes. The pressurized containers may also contain products or propellants that are highly flammable, producing burns when used near an open flame. When stored near heat, in direct sunlight, or in a closed auto, the containers may explode violently.

EMERGENCY TREATMENT: If eyes are contaminated by spray particles, flush the eye surfaces with water to remove any particles of the powder mist. Then carefully examine eye surfaces to determine if chemicals appear to be imbedded in the surface of the cornea. If aerosol spray is inhaled, move the patient to a well-ventilated area; keep him lying down, warm, and quiet. If breathing fails, administer artificial respiration. Victims of exploding containers or burning contents of aerosol containers should be given appropriate emergency treatment for bleeding, burns, and shock.

The redness and irritation of eye injuries should subside within a short time. If they do not, or if particles of spray seem to be imbedded in the surface of the eyes, take the victim to an ophthalmologist. A doctor should also be summoned if a victim fails to recover quickly from the effects of inhaling an aerosol spray, particularly if the victim suffers from asthma or a similar lung disorder or from an abnormal heart condition.

Alkali burns

Alkalis are used in the manufacture of soap and cleaners and in certain household cleaning products. They combine with fats to form soaps and may produce a painful injury when in contact with body surfaces.

EMERGENCY TREATMENT: Flood the burned area with copious amounts of clean, cool, fresh water. Put the victim under a shower if possible, or otherwise pour running water over the area for as long as is necessary to dilute and weaken the corrosive chemical. Do not apply the water with such force that skin or other tissues are damaged. Remove clothing contaminated by the chemical.

Neutralize the remaining alkali with diluted vinegar, lemon juice, or a similar mild acid. Then wash the affected areas again with fresh water. Dry carefully with sterile gauze, being careful not to open blisters or otherwise cause skin breaks that could result in infection. Summon professional medical care as soon as possible. Meanwhile, treat the victim for shock.

Angina pectoris

Angina pectoris is a condition that causes acute chest pain because of interference with the supply of oxygen to the heart. Although the pain is sometimes confused with ulcer or acute indigestion symptoms, it has a distinct characteristic of its own, producing a feeling of heaviness,

strangling, tightness, or suffocation. Angina is a symptom rather than a disease. It may be treated with nitroglycerin or one of the newer beta-blocker or calcium channel blocker drugs.

See ANGINA PECTORIS in Index.

An attack of acute angina can be brought on by emotional stress, overeating, strenuous exercise, or by any activity that makes excessive demands on heart function.

EMERGENCY TREATMENT: An attack usually subsides in about ten minutes, during which the patient appears to be gasping for breath. He should be kept in a semireclining position rather than made to lie flat, and should be moved carefully only in order to place pillows under his head and chest so that he can breathe more easily. A doctor should be called promptly after the onset of an attack.

Animal bites/rabies

Wild animals, particularly bats, serve as a natural reservoir of rabies, a disease that is almost always fatal unless promptly and properly treated. But the virus may be present in the saliva of any warm-blooded animal. Domestic animals should be immunized against rabies by vaccines injected by a veterinarian.

Rabies is transmitted to humans by an animal bite or through a cut or scratch already in the skin. The infected saliva may enter through any opening, including the membranes lining the nose or mouth. After an incubation period of about ten days, a person infected by a rabid animal experiences pain at the site of infection, extreme sensitivity of the skin to temperature changes, and painful spasms of the larynx that make it almost impossible to drink. Saliva thickens and the patient becomes restless and easily excitable. By the time symptoms develop, death may be imminent. Obviously, professional medical attention should begin promptly after having been exposed to the possibility of infection.

EMERGENCY TREATMENT: The area

around the wound should be washed thoroughly and repeatedly with soap and water, using a sterile gauze dressing to wipe fluid away from—not toward—the wound. Another sterile dressing is used to dry the wound and a third to cover it while the patient is taken to a hospital or doctor's office. A tetanus injection is also indicated, and police and health authorities should be promptly notified of the biting incident.

If at all possible the biting animal should be identified—if a wild animal, captured alive—and held for observation for a period of 10 to 15 days. If it can be determined during that period that the animal is not rabid, further treatment may not be required. If the animal is rabid, however, or if it cannot be located and impounded, the patient may have to undergo a series of daily rabies vaccine injections lasting from 14 days for a case of mild exposure to 21 days for severe exposure (a bite near the head, for example), plus several booster shots. Because of the sensitivity of some individuals to the rabies vaccines used, the treatment itself can be quite dangerous.

Recent research, however, has established that a new vaccine called HDCV (human diploid cell vaccine), which requires only six or fewer injections, is immunologically effective and is not usually accompanied by any side effects. The new vaccine has been used successfully on people of all ages who had been bitten by animals known to be rabid.

Appendicitis

The common signal for approaching appendicitis is a period of several days of indigestion and constipation, culminating in pain and tenderness on the lower right side of the abdomen. Besides these symptoms, appendicitis may be accompanied by nausea and a slight fever. Call a doctor immediately and describe the symptoms in detail; delay may result in a ruptured appendix.

EMERGENCY TREATMENT: While awaiting medical care, the victim may find some relief from the pain and discomfort by having an ice bag placed over the abdomen. Do not apply heat and give nothing by mouth. A laxative should not be offered.

Asphyxiation

See GAS POISONING.

Asthma attack

EMERGENCY TREATMENT: Make the patient comfortable and offer reassurance. If he has been examined by a doctor and properly diagnosed, the patient probably has an inhalant device or other forms of medication on his person or nearby.

The coughing and wheezing spell may have been triggered by the presence of an allergenic substance such as animal hair, feathers, or kapok in pillows or cushions. Such items should be removed from the presence of the patient. In addition, placing the patient in a room with high humidity, such as a bathroom with the shower turned on, may be helpful.

Asthma attacks are rarely fatal in young people, but elderly persons should be watched carefully because of possible heart strain. In a severe attack, professional medical care including oxygen equipment may be required.

Back injuries

In the event of any serious back injury, call a doctor or arrange for immediate professional transfer of the victim to a hospital.

EMERGENCY TREATMENT: Until determined otherwise by a physician, treat the injured person as a victim of a fractured spine. If he complains that he cannot move his head, feet, or toes, the chances are that the back is fractured. But even if he can move his feet or legs, it does not necessarily mean that he can be moved safely, since the back can be fractured without immediate injury to the spinal cord.

If the victim shows symptoms of shock, do not attempt to lower his head or move his body into the usual position for shock control. If it is absolutely essential to move the victim because of immediate danger to his life, make a rigid stretcher from a wide piece of solid lumber such as a door and cover the stretcher with a blanket for padding. Then carefully slide or pull the victim onto the stretcher, using his clothing to hold him. Tie the body onto the stretcher with strips of cloth.

Back pain

See SCIATICA.

Black eye

Although a black eye is frequently regarded as a minor medical problem, it can result in serious visual problems, including cataract or glaucoma.

EMERGENCY TREATMENT: Inspect the area about the eye for possible damage to the eye itself, such as hemorrhage, rupture of the eyeball, or dislocated lens. Check also for cuts around the eye that may require professional medical care. Then treat the bruised area by putting the victim to bed, covering the eye with a bandage, and applying an ice bag to the area.

If vision appears to be distorted or lacerations need stitching and antibiotic treatment, take the victim to a doctor's office. A doctor should also be consulted about continued pain and swelling about the eye.

Black widow spider bites

EMERGENCY TREATMENT: Make the victim lie still. If the bite is on the arm or leg, position the victim so that the bite is lower than the level of the heart. Apply a rubber band or similar tourniquet between the bite and the heart to retard venom flow toward the heart. The bite usually is marked by two puncture points. Apply ice packs to the bite. Summon a doctor or carry the patient to the nearest hospital.

Loosen the tourniquet or constriction band for a few seconds every 15 minutes while awaiting help; you should be able to feel a pulse beyond the tourniquet if it is not too tight. Do not let the victim move about. Do not permit him to drink alcoholic beverages. He probably will feel weakness, tremor, and severe pain, but reassure him that he will recover. Medications, usually available only to a physician, should be administered promptly.

Bleeding, internal

Internal bleeding is always a very serious condition; it requires immediate professional medical attention.

In cases of internal bleeding, blood is sometimes brought to the outside of the body by coughing from the lungs, by vomiting from the stomach, by trickling from the ear or nose, or by passing in the urine or bowel movement.

Often, however, internal bleeding is concealed, and the only symptom may be the swelling that appears around the site of broken bones. A person can lose three or four pints of blood inside the body without a trace of blood appearing outside the body.

SOME SYMPTOMS OF INTERNAL BLEEDING: The victim will appear ill and pale. His skin will be colder than normal, especially the hands and feet; often the skin looks clammy because of sweating. The pulse usually will be rapid (over 90 beats a minute) and feeble.

EMERGENCY TREATMENT: Serious internal bleeding is beyond the scope of first aid. If necessary treat the victim for respiratory and cardiac arrest and for shock while waiting for medical aid.

Bleeding, minor

Bleeding from minor cuts, scrapes, and bruises usually stops by itself, but even small injuries of this kind should receive attention to prevent infection.

EMERGENCY TREATMENT: The injured area should be washed thoroughly with soap and water, or if possible, held under running water. The surface should then be covered with a sterile bandage.

The type of wound known as a puncture wound may bleed very little, but is potentially extremely dangerous because of the possibility of tetanus infection. Anyone who steps on a rusty nail or thumbtack or has a similar accident involving a pointed object that penetrates deep under the skin surface should consult a physician about the need for anti-tetanus inoculation or a booster shot.

Blisters

EMERGENCY TREATMENT: If the blister is on a hand or foot or other easily accessible part of the body, wash the area around the blister thoroughly with soap and water. After carefully drying the skin around the blister, apply an antiseptic to the same area. Then sterilize the point and a substantial part of a needle by heating it in an open flame. When the needle has been thoroughly sterilized, use the point to puncture the blister along the margin of the blister. Carefully squeeze the fluid from the blister by pressing it with a sterile gauze dressing; the dressing should soak up most of the fluid. Next, place a fresh sterile dressing over the blister and fasten it in place with a bandage. If a blister forms in a tender area or in a place that is not easily accessible, such as under the arm, do not open it yourself; consult your doctor.

The danger from any break in the skin is that germs or dirt can slip through the natural barrier to produce an infection or inflammation. Continue to apply an antiseptic each day to the puncture area until it has healed. If it appears that an infection has developed or healing is unusually slow, consult a doctor. Persons with diabetes or circulatory problems may have to be more cautious about healing of skin breaks than other individuals.

Blood blisters

Blood blisters, sometimes called hematomas, usually are caused by a sharp blow to the body surface such as hitting a finger with a hammer while pounding nails.

EMERGENCY TREATMENT: Wash the area of the blood blister thoroughly with soap and water. Do not open it. If it is a small blood blister, cover it with a protective bandage; in many cases, the tiny pool of blood under the skin will be absorbed by the surrounding tissues if there is no further pressure at that point.

If the blood blister fails to heal quickly or becomes infected, consult a physician. Because the pool of blood has resulted from damage to a blood vessel, a blood blister usually is more vulnerable to infection or inflammation than an ordinary blister.

Boils

Boils frequently are an early sign of diabetes or another illness and should be watched carefully if they occur often. In general, they result from germs or dirt being rubbed into the skin by tight-fitting clothing, scratching, or through tiny cuts made during shaving.

EMERGENCY TREATMENT: If the boil is above the lip, do not squeeze it or apply any pressure. The infection in that area of the face may drain into the brain because of the pattern of blood circulation on the face. Let a doctor treat any boil on the face. If the boil is on the surface of another part of the body, apply moist hot packs, but do not squeeze or press on the boil because that action can force the infection into the circulatory system. A wet compress can be made by soaking a wash cloth or towel in warm water.

If the boil erupts, carefully wipe away the pus with a sterile dressing, and then cover it with another sterile dressing. If the boil is large or slow to erupt, or if it is slow to heal, consult a doctor.

Bone bruises

EMERGENCY TREATMENT: Make sure the bone is not broken. If the injury is limited to the thin layer of tissue surrounding the bone, and the function of the limb is normal though painful, apply a compression dressing and an ice pack. Limit use of the injured limb for the next day or two.

As the pain and swelling recede, cover the injured area with a foam-rubber pad held in place with an elastic bandage. Because the part of the limb that is likely to receive a bone bruise lacks a layer of muscle and fat, it will be particularly sensitive to any pressure until recovery is complete.

Botulism

The bacteria that produce the lethal toxin of botulism are commonly present on unwashed farm vegetables and thrive in containers that are improperly sealed against the damaging effects of air. Home-canned vegetables, particularly string beans, are a likely source of botulism, but the toxin can be found in fruits, meats, and other foods. It can also appear in food that has been properly prepared but allowed to cool before being served. Examples are cold soups and marinated vegetables.

EMERGENCY TREATMENT: As soon as acute symptoms—nausea, diarrhea, and abdominal distress—appear, try to induce vomiting. Vomiting usually can be started by touching the back of the victim's throat with a finger or the handle of a spoon, which should be smooth and blunt, or by offering him a glass of water in which two tablespoons of salt have been dissolved. Call a doctor; describe all of the symptoms, which also may include, after several hours, double vision, muscular weakness, and difficulty in swallowing and breathing Save samples of the food suspected of contamination for analysis.

Prompt hospitalization and injection of antitoxin are needed to save most cases of botulism poisoning. Additional emergency measures may include artificial respiration if regular breathing fails because of paralysis of respiratory muscles. Continue artificial respiration until professional medical care is provided. If other individuals have eaten the contaminated food, they should receive treatment for botulism even if they show no symptoms of the toxin's effects, since symptoms may be delayed several days.

Brown house (or recluse) spider bites

EMERGENCY TREATMENT: Apply an ice bag or cold pack to the wound area. Aspirin and antihistamines may be offered to help relieve any pain or feeling of irritation. Keep the victim lying down and quiet. Call a doctor as quickly as possible and describe the situation; the doctor will advise what further action should be taken at this point.

The effects of a brown spider bite frequently last much longer than the pain of the bite, which may be comparatively mild for an insect bite or sting. But the poison from the bite can gradually destroy the surrounding tissues, leaving at first an ulcer and eventually a disfiguring scar. A physician's treatment is needed to control the loss of tissue; he probably will prescribe drugs and recommend continued use of cold compresses. The victim, meanwhile, will feel numbness and muscular weakness, requiring a prolonged period of bed rest in addition to the medical treatments.

Bruises/contusions

EMERGENCY TREATMENT: Bruises or contusions result usually from a blow to the body that is powerful enough to damage muscles, tendons, blood vessels, or other tissues without causing a break in the skin.

Because the bruised area will be tender, protect it from further injury. If possible, immobilize the injured body part with a sling, bandage, or other device that makes the victim feel more comfortable; pillows, folded blankets, or similar soft materials can be used to elevate an arm or leg. Apply an ice bag or cold water dressing to the injured area.

A simple bruise usually will heal without extensive treatment. The swelling and discoloration are due to blood oozing from damaged tissues. However, severe bruising can be quite serious and requires medical attention. Keep the victim quiet and

watch for symptoms of shock. Give aspirin for pain.

Bullet wounds

Bullet wounds, whether accidental or purposely inflicted, can range from those that are superficial and external to those that involve internal bleeding and extensive tissue damage.

EMERGENCY TREATMENT: A surface bullet wound accompanied by bleeding should be covered promptly with sterile gauze to prevent further infection. The flow of blood should be controlled as described on p.574. *Don't* try to clean the wound with soap or water.

If the wound is internal, keep the patient lying down and wrap him with coats or blankets placed over and under his body. If respiration has ceased or is impaired, give mouth-to-mouth respiration and treat him for shock. Get medical aid promptly.

Burns, thermal

Burns are generally described according to the depth or area of skin damage involved. First-degree burns are the most superficial. They are marked by reddening of the skin and swelling, increased warmth, tenderness and pain. Second-degree burns, deeper than first-degree, are in effect open wounds, characterized by blisters and severe pain in addition to redness. Third-degree burns are deep enough to involve damage to muscles and bones. The skin is charred and there may be no pain because nerve endings have been destroyed. However, the area of the burn generally is more important than the degree of burn; a first or second-degree burn covering a large area of the body is more likely to be fatal than a small third-degree burn.

EMERGENCY TREATMENT: You will want to get professional medical help for treatment of a severe burn, but there are a number of things you can do until such help is obtained. If burns are minor, apply ice or ice water until pain subsides. Then wash the area with soap and water. Cover with a sterile dressing. Give the victim one or two aspirin tablets to help relieve discomfort. A sterile gauze pad soaked in a solution of two

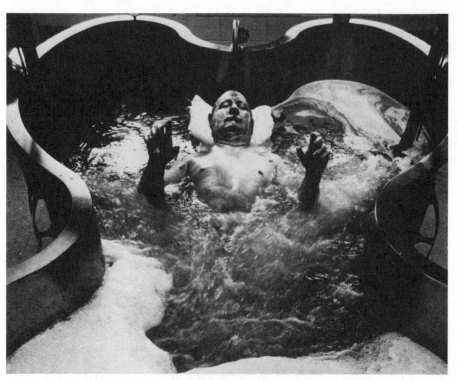

Hydrotherapy—therapy involving the use of water, as in this whirlpool bath—is one of the methods of treating burn patients.

tablespoons of baking soda (sodium bicarbonate) per quart of lukewarm water may be applied.

For more extensive or severe burns, there are three first-aid objectives: (1) relieve pain, (2) prevent shock, (3) prevent infection. To relieve pain, exclude air by applying a thick dressing of four to six layers plus additional coverings of clean, tightly-woven material; for extensive burns, use clean sheets or towels. Clothing should be cut away —never pulled—from burned areas; where fabric is stuck to the wound, leave it for a doctor to remove later. Do not apply any ointment, grease, powder, salve, or other medication; the doctor simply will have to remove such material before he can begin professional treatment of the burns.

To prevent shock, make sure the victim's head is lower than his feet. Be sure that the victim is covered sufficiently to keep him warm, but not enough to make him overheated; exposure to cold can make the effects of shock more severe. Provide the victim with plenty of nonalcoholic liquids such as sweetened water, tea, or fruit juices, so long as he is conscious and able to swallow.

To prevent infection, do not permit absorbent cotton or adhesive tape to touch the wound caused by a burn. Do not apply iodine or any other antiseptic to the burn. Do not open any blisters. Do not permit any unsterile matter to contact the burn area. If possible, prevent other persons from coughing, sneezing, or even breathing toward the wound resulting from a burn. Serious infections frequently develop in burn victims from contamination by microorganisms of the mouth and nose.

LONG-TERM TREATMENT: A highly effective method of treating serious burns involves, first, removal of samples of uninjured skin from victims' bodies. Laboratory workers then "grind up" the healthy skin samples and separate them into groups of cells. Placed in flasks and bathed in a growth-stimulating solution, the cells grow rapidly; while the colonies are small, they double in size every 17 hours. New skin appears. The procedure can be repeated until enough has been grown to cover the burned areas.

Because the "test-tube skin" is developed from samples of a victim's own skin, the body does not reject it. It can be grafted onto a burned area in patches until the entire burn is covered. The new skin has no hair follicles or sweat glands, and is thinner than normal skin. But it offers hope to some 10 to 15 percent of the those persons who are hospitalized with burn injuries.

See also CHEMICAL BURNS OF THE EYE.

Carbuncles

Carbuncles are quite similar to boils except that they usually develop around multiple hair follicles and commonly appear on the neck or face. Personal hygiene is one factor involved in the development of carbuncles; persons apparently susceptible to the pustular inflammations must exercise special care in cleansing areas in which carbuncles occur, particularly if they suffer from diabetes or circulatory ailments.

EMERGENCY TREATMENT: Apply moist hot packs to the boil-like swelling. Change the moist hot packs frequently, or place a hot-water bottle on the moist dressing to maintain the moist heat application. Do not handle the carbuncle beyond whatever contact is necessary to apply or maintain the moist heat. The carbuncle should eventually rupture or reach a point where it can be opened with a sterile sharp instrument. After the carbuncle has ruptured and drained, and the fluid from the growth has been carefully cleaned away, apply a sterile dressing.

Frequently, carbuncles must be opened and drained by a physician.

Cat scratch fever

Although the scratch or bite of a house cat or alley cat may appear at first to be only a mild injury, the wound can become the site of entry for a disease virus transmitted by apparently healthy cats. The inflammation, accompanied by fever, generally affects the lymph nodes and produces some aches and pains as well as fatigue. Although the disease is seldom fatal, an untreated case can spread to brain tissues and lead to other complications.

EMERGENCY TREATMENT: Wash the scratch thoroughly with water and either soap or a mild detergent. Apply a mild antiseptic such as hydrogen peroxide. Cover with a sterile dressing.

Watch the area of the scratch carefully for the next week or two. If redness or swelling develop, even after the scratch appears healed, consult your doctor. The inflammation of the scratch area may be accompanied by mild fever and symptoms similar to those of influenza; in small children, the symptoms may be quite serious. Bed rest and antibiotics usually are prescribed.

Charley horse

A charley horse occurs because a small number of muscle fibers have been torn or ruptured by overstraining the muscle, or by the force of a blow to the muscle.

EMERGENCY TREATMENT: Rest the injured muscle and apply an ice pack if there is swelling. A compression dressing can be applied to support the muscle. Avoid movement that stretches the muscle, and restrict other movements that make the victim uncomfortable. If pain and swelling persist, call a doctor.

During the recovery period, which may not begin for a day or two, apply local heat with a hot water bottle or an electric heating pad, being careful not to burn the victim. A return to active use of the muscle can begin gradually as pain permits.

Chemical burns of the eye

EMERGENCY TREATMENT: Flush the victim's eye immediately with large quantities of fresh, clean water; a drinking fountain can be used to provide a steady stream of water. If a drinking fountain is not available, lay the victim on the floor or ground with his head turned slightly to one side and pour water into the eye from a cup or glass. Always direct the stream of water so that it enters the eye surface at the inside corner and flows across the eye to the outside corner. If the victim is unable, because of intense pain, to open his eyes, it may be necessary to hold the lids apart while water pours across the eye. Continue flushing the eye for at least 15 minutes. (An alternate method is to immerse the victim's face in a pan or basin or bucket of water while he opens and closes his eyes repeatedly; continue the process for at least 15 minutes.)

When the chemical has been flushed from the victim's eye, the eye should be covered with a small, thick compress held in place with a bandage that covers both eyes, if possible; the bandage can be tied around the victim's head. NOTE: Apply nothing but water to the eye; do not attempt to neutralize a chemical burn of the eye and do not apply oil, ointment, salve, or other medications. Rush the victim to a doctor as soon as possible, preferably to an ophthalmologist.

Chemicals on skin

Many household and industrial chemicals, such as ammonia, lye, iodine, creosote, and a wide range of insecticides can cause serious injury if accidentally spilled on the skin.

EMERGENCY TREATMENT: Wash the body surface which has been affected by the chemical with large amounts of water. Do not try to neutralize the chemical with another substance; the reaction may aggravate the injury. If blisters appear, apply a sterile dressing. If the chemical is a refrigerant, such as Freon, or carbon dioxide under pressure, treat for frostbite.

If the chemical has splashed into the eyes or produces serious injury to the affected body surface, call a doctor. The victim should be watched closely for possible poisoning effects if the chemical is a pesticide, since such substances may be absorbed through the skin to produce internal toxic reactions. If there is any question about the toxicity of a chemical, ask your doctor or call the nearest poison control center.

Chigger bites

EMERGENCY TREATMENT: Apply ice water or rub ice over the area afflicted by bites of the tiny red insects. Bathing the area with alcohol, ammonia water or a solution of baking soda also will provide some relief from the itching.

Wash thoroughly with soap, using a scrub brush to prevent further infestation by the chiggers in other areas of the body. Rub alcohol over the surrounding areas and apply sulfur ointment as protection against mites that may not have attached themselves to the skin. Continue applications of ice water or alcohol to skin areas invaded by the insects. Clothing that was worn should be laundered immediately.

Chilblains

EMERGENCY TREATMENT: Move the victim to a moderately warm place and remove wet or tight clothing. Soak the affected body area in warm —but not hot—water for about 10 minutes. Then carefully blot the skin dry, but do not rub the skin. Replace the clothing with garments that are warm, soft, and dry.

Give the victim a stimulant such as tea or coffee, or an alcoholic beverage, and put him to bed with only light blankets; avoid the pressure of heavy blankets or heavy, tight garments on the sensitive skin areas. The victim should move the affected body areas gently to help restore normal circulation. If complications develop, such as marked discoloration of the skin, pain, or blistering and splitting of the skin, call a doctor.

Cold sores/fever blisters

EMERGENCY TREATMENT: Apply a soothing ointment or a medication such as camphor ice. Avoid squeezing or otherwise handling the blisters; moisture can aggravate the sores and hinder their healing. Repeated appearances of cold sores or fever blisters, which are caused by the herpes simplex virus, may require treatment by a physician.

Concussion

See HEAD INJURIES.

Contusions

See BRUISES.

Convulsions

EMERGENCY TREATMENT: Protect the victim from injury by moving him to a safe place; loosen any constricting clothing such as a tie or belt; put a pillow or coat under his head; if his mouth is open, place a folded cloth between his teeth to keep him from biting his tongue. Do not force anything into his mouth. Keep the patient warm but do not disturb him; do not try to restrain his convulsive movements.

Send for a doctor as quickly as possible. Watch the patient's breathing and begin artificial respiration if breathing stops for more than one minute. Be sure that breathing actually has stopped; the patient may be sleeping or unconscious after an attack but breathing normally.

Convulsions in a small child may signal the onset of an infectious disease and may be accompanied by a high fever. The same general precautions should be taken to prevent self-injury on the part of the child. If placed in a bed, the child should be protected against falling onto the floor. Place him on his side—not on his back or stomach—if he vomits. Cold compresses or ice packs on the back of the neck and the head may help relieve symptoms. Immediate professional medical care is vital because brain damage can result if treatment is delayed.

See also EPILEPTIC SEIZURES.

Cramps

See MUSCLE CRAMPS.

Croup

Croup is a breathing disorder usually

caused by a virus infection and less often by bacteria or allergy. It is a common condition during childhood, and in some cases, may require brief hospitalization for proper treatment.

The onset of a croup attack is likely to occur during the night with a sudden hoarse or barking cough accompanied by difficulty in breathing. The coughing is usually followed by choking spasms that sound as though the child is strangling. There may also be a mild fever. A doctor should be called immediately when these symptoms appear.

EMERGENCY TREATMENT: The most effective treatment for croup is cool moist air. Cool water vaporizers are available as well as warm steam vaporizers. Another alternative is to take the child into the bathroom, close the door and windows, and let the hot water run from the shower and sink taps until the room is filled with steam.

It is also possible to improvise a croup tent by boiling water in a kettle on a portable hot plate and arranging a blanket over the back of a chair so that it encloses the child and an adult as well as the steaming kettle. A child should never be left alone even for an instant in such a makeshift arrangement.

If the symptoms do not subside in about 20 minutes with any of the above procedures, or if there is mounting fever, and if the doctor is not on his way, the child should be rushed to the closest hospital. Cold moist night air, rather than being a danger, may actually make the symptoms subside temporarily.

Diabetic coma and insulin shock

Diabetics should always carry an identification tag or card to alert others of their condition in the event of a diabetic coma—which is due to a lack of insulin. They also should advise friends or family members of their diabetic condition and the proper emergency measures that can be taken in the event of an onset of diabetic coma. A bottle of rapid-acting insulin should be kept on hand for such an emergency.

EMERGENCY TREATMENT: If the victim is being treated for diabetes, he probably will have nearby a supply of insulin and a hypodermic apparatus for injecting it. Find the insulin, hypodermic syringe, and needle; clean a spot on the upper arm or thigh, and inject about 50 units of insulin. Call a doctor without delay, and describe the patient's symptoms and your treatment. The patient usually will respond without ill effects, but may be quite thirsty. Give him plenty of fluids, as needed.

If the victim does not respond to the insulin, or if you cannot find the insulin and hypodermic syringe, rush the victim to the nearest doctor's office.

Insulin shock—which is due to a reaction to too much insulin and not enough sugar in the blood—can be treated in an emergency by offering a sugar-rich fluid such as a cola beverage or orange juice. Diabetics frequently carry a lump of sugar or candy which can be placed in their mouth in case of an insulin shock reaction. It should be tucked between the teeth and cheek so the victim will not choke on it.

If you find a diabetic in a coma and do not know the cause, assume the cause is an insulin reaction and treat him with sugar. This will give immediate relief to an insulin reaction but will not affect diabetic coma.

Diarrhea

EMERGENCY TREATMENT: Give the victim an antidiarrheal agent; all drugstores carry medications composed of kaolin and pectin that are useful for this purpose. Certain bismuth compounds also are recommended for diarrhea control.

Put the victim in bed for a period of at least 12 hours and withhold food and drink for that length of time. Do not let the victim become dehydrated; if he is thirsty, let him suck on pieces of ice. If the diarrhea appears to be subsiding, let him sip a mild beverage like tea or ginger ale; cola syrup is also recommended.

Later on the patient can try eating bland foods such as dry toast, crackers, gelatin desserts, or jellied consomme. Avoid feeding rich, fatty, or spicy foods. If the diarrhea fails to subside or is complicated by colic or vomiting, call a physician.

Dizziness/vertigo

Emotional upsets, allergies, and improper eating and drinking habits—too much food, too little food, or foods that are too rich—can precipitate symptoms of dizziness. The cause also can be a physical disorder such as abnormal functioning of the inner ear or a circulatory problem. Smoking tobacco, certain drugs such as quinine, and fumes of some chemicals also can produce dizziness.

EMERGENCY TREATMENT: Have the victim lie down with the eyes closed. In many cases, a period of simple bed rest will alleviate the symptoms. Keep the victim quiet and comfortable. If the feeling of dizziness continues, becomes worse, or is accompanied by nausea and vomiting, call a physician.

Severe or persistent dizziness or vertigo requires a longer period of bed rest and the use of medicines prescribed by a doctor. While recovering, the victim should avoid sudden changes in body position or turning the head rapidly. In some types of vertigo, surgery is required to cure the disorder.

Drowning

Victims of drowning seldom die because of water in the lungs or stomach. They die because of lack of air.

EMERGENCY TREATMENT: If the victim's breathing has been impaired, start artificial respiration immediately. If there is evidence of cardiac arrest, administer cardiac massage. When the victim is able to breathe for himself, treat him for shock and get medical help.

Drug overdose (barbiturates)

Barbiturates are used in a number of drugs prescribed as sedatives, although many are also available through illegal channels. Because the drugs can affect the judgment of the user, he may not remember having taken a dose and so may take additional pills, thus producing overdose effects.

EMERGENCY TREATMENT: If the drug was taken orally, try to induce vomiting in the victim. Have him drink a glass of water containing two tablespoons of salt. Or touch the back of his throat gently with a finger or a smooth blunt object like the handle of a spoon. Then give the victim plenty of warm water to drink. It is important to rid the stomach of as much of the drug as possible and to dilute the substance remaining in the gastrointestinal tract.

As soon as possible, call a doctor or get the victim to the nearest hospital or doctor's office. If breathing fails, administer artificial respiration.

Drug overdose (stimulants)

Although most of the powerful stimulant drugs, or pep pills, are available only through a doctor's prescription, the same medications are available through illicit sources. When taken without direction of a supervising physician, the stimulants can produce a variety of adverse side effects, and when used frequently over a period of time can result in physical and psychological problems that require hospital treatment.

EMERGENCY TREATMENT: Give the victim a solution of one tablespoon of activated charcoal mixed with a small amount of water, or give him a glass of milk, to dilute the effects of the medication in the stomach. Then induce vomiting by pressing gently on the back of the throat with a finger or the smooth blunt edge of a spoon handle. Vomiting also may be induced with a solution made of one teaspoonful of mustard in a half glass of water. Do not give syrup of ipecac to a victim who has been taking stimulants.

As soon as possible call a doctor or get the victim to the nearest hospital or doctor's office. If breathing fails, administer artificial respiration.

Earaches

An earache may be associated with a wide variety of ailments ranging from the common cold or influenza to impacted molars or tonsillitis. An earache also may be involved in certain infectious diseases such as measles or scarlet fever. Because of the relationship of ear structures to other parts of the head and throat, an infection involving the symptoms of earache can easily spread to the brain tissues or the spongy mastoid bone behind the ear. Call a doctor and describe all of the symptoms, including temperature, any discharge, pain, ringing in the ear, or deafness. Delay in reporting an earache to a doctor can result in complications that require hospital treatment.

EMERGENCY TREATMENT: This may include a few drops of warm olive oil or sweet oil held in the ear by a small wad of cotton. Aspirin can be given to help relieve any pain. Professional medical treatment may include the use of antibiotics.

Ear, foreign body in

EMERGENCY TREATMENT: Do not insert a hairpin, stick, or other object in the ear in an effort to remove a foreign object; you are likely to force the object farther into the ear canal. Instead, have the victim tilt his head to one side, with the ear containing the foreign object facing upward. While pulling gently on the lobe of the ear to straighten the canal, pour a little warmed olive oil or mineral oil into the ear. Then have the victim tilt that ear downward so the oil will run out quickly; it should dislodge the foreign object.

Wipe the ear canal gently with a cotton-tipped matchstick, or a similar device that will not irritate the lining of the ear canal, after the foreign body has been removed. If the emergency treatment is not successful, call a doctor.

Electric shocks

An electric shock from the usual 110-volt current in most homes can be a serious emergency, especially if the person's skin or clothing is wet. Under these circumstances, the shock may paralyze the part of the brain that controls breathing and stop the heart completely or disorder its pumping action.

EMERGENCY TREATMENT: It is of the utmost importance to break the electrical contact *immediately* by unplugging the wire of the appliance involved or by shutting off the house current switch. *Do not touch the victim of the shock while he is still acting as an electrical conductor.*

If the shock has come from a faulty wire out of doors and the source of the electrical current can't be reached easily, make a lasso of dry rope on a long sturdy dry stick. Catch the victim's hand or foot in the loop and drag him away from the wire. Another way to break the contact is to cut the wire with a dry axe.

If the victim of the shock is unconscious, or if his pulse is very weak, administer mouth-to-mouth respiration and cardiac massage until he can get to a hospital.

Epileptic seizures

Epilepsy is a disorder of the nervous system that produces convulsive seizures. In a major seizure or *grand mal*, the epileptic usually falls to the ground. Indeed, falling is in most cases one of the principal dangers of the disease. Then the epileptic's body begins to twitch or jerk spasmodically. His breathing may be labored, and saliva may appear on his lips. His face may become pale or bluish. Although the scene can be frightening, it is not truly a medical emergency; the afflicted person is in no danger of losing his life.

EMERGENCY TREATMENT: Make the person suffering the seizure as comfortable as possible. If he is on a hard surface, put something soft under his head, and move any hard or dangerous objects away from him. *Make no attempt to restrain his movements, and do not force anything into his mouth.* Just leave him alone until the attack is over, as it should be in a few minutes. If his mouth is already open, you might put something soft, such as a folded handerchief, between his side teeth. This will help to prevent him from biting his tongue or lips. If he seems to go into another seizure after coming out of the first, or if the seizure lasts more than ten minutes, call a doctor. If his lower jaw sags and begins to obstruct his breathing, support of the lower jaw may be helpful in improving his breathing.

When the seizure is over, the patient should be allowed to rest quietly. Some people sleep heavily after a seizure. Others awake at once but are disoriented or confused for a while. Treat the episode in a matter-of-fact way. If it is the first seizure the person is aware of having had, advise him to see his physician promptly.

Eye, foreign body in

EMERGENCY TREATMENT: Do not rub the eye or touch it with unwashed hands. The foreign body usually becomes lodged on the inner surface of the upper eyelid. Pull the upper eyelid down over the lower lid to help work the object loose. Tears or clean water can help wash out the dirt or other object. If the bit of irritating material can be seen on the surface of the eyeball, try very carefully to flick it out with the tip of a clean, moistened handkerchief or a piece of moistened cotton. Never touch the surface of the eye with dry materials. Sometimes a foreign body can be removed by carefully rolling the upper lid over a pencil or wooden matchstick to expose the object.

After the foreign object has been removed, the eye should be washed with clean water or with a solution made from one teaspoon of salt dissolved in a pint of water. This will help remove any remaining particles of the foreign body as well as any traces of irritating chemicals that might have been a part of it. Iron particles, for example, may leave traces of rust on the eye's surface unless washed away.

If the object cannot be located and removed without difficulty, a small patch of gauze or a folded handkerchief should be taped over the eye and the victim taken to a doctor's office—preferably the office of an ophthalmologist. A doctor also should be consulted if a feeling of irritation in the eye continues after the foreign body has been removed.

Fever

EMERGENCY TREATMENT: If the fever is mild, around 100° F. by mouth, have the victim rest in bed and provide him with a light diet. Watch closely for other symptoms, such as a rash, and any further increase in body temperature. Aspirin usually can be given.

If the temperature rises to 101° or higher, is accompanied by pain, headache, delirium, confused behavior, coughing, vomiting, or other indications of a severe illness, call a doctor. Describe all of the symptoms in detail, including the appearance of any rash and when it began.

Fever blisters
See COLD SORES.

Finger dislocation

EMERGENCY TREATMENT: Call a doctor and arrange for inspection and treatment of the injury. If a doctor is not immediately available, the finger dislocation may be reduced (put back in proper alignment) by grasping it firmly and carefully pulling it into normal position. Pull very slowly and avoid rough handling that might complicate the injury by damaging a tendon. If the dislocation cannot be reduced after the first try, go through the procedure once more. But do not try it more than twice.

Whether or not you are successful in reducing the finger dislocation, the finger should be immobilized after your efforts until a doctor can examine it. A clean flat wooden stick can be strapped along the palm side of the finger with adhesive tape or strips of bandage to hold it in place.

Fingernail injuries/hangnails

EMERGENCY TREATMENT: Wash the injured nail area thoroughly with warm water and soap. Trim off any torn bits of nail. Cover with a small adhesive dressing or bandage.

Apply petroleum jelly or cold cream to the injured nail area twice a day, morning and night, until it is healed. If redness or irritation develops in the adjoining skin area, indicating an infection, consult your doctor.

Fish poisoning

EMERGENCY TREATMENT: Induce vomiting in the victim to remove the bits of poisonous fish from the stomach. Vomiting usually can be started by pressing on the back of the throat with a finger or a spoon handle that is blunt and smooth, or by having the victim drink a solution of two tablespoons of salt in a glass of water.

Call a doctor as soon as possible. Describe the type of fish eaten and the symptoms, which may include nausea, diarrhea, abdominal pain, muscular weakness, and a numbness or tingling sensation that begins about the face and spreads to the extremities.

If breathing fails, administer mouth-to-mouth artificial respiration; a substance commonly found in poisonous fish causes respiratory failure. Also, be prepared to provide emergency treatment for convulsions.

Food poisoning

EMERGENCY TREATMENT: If the victim is not already vomiting, try to induce it to clear the stomach. Vomiting can be started in most cases by pressing gently on the back of the throat with a finger or a blunt smooth spoon handle, or by having the patient drink a glass of water containing two tablespoons of salt. If the victim has vomited, put him to bed.

Call a doctor and describe the food ingested and the symptoms which developed. If symptoms are severe, professional medical treatment with antibiotics and medications for cramps may be required. Special medications also may be needed for diarrhea caused by bacterial food poisoning.

Fractures

Any break in a bone is called a fracture. The break is called an *open* or *compound fracture* if one or both ends of the broken bone pierce the skin. A *closed* or *simple fracture* is one in which the broken bone doesn't come through the skin.

It is sometimes difficult to distinguish a strained muscle or a sprained ligament from a broken bone, since sprains and strains can be extremely painful even though they are less serious than breaks. However, when there is any doubt, the injury should be treated as though it were a simple fracture.

EMERGENCY TREATMENT: Don't try to help the injured person move around or get up unless he has slowly tested out the injured part of his body and is sure that nothing has been broken. If he is in extreme pain, or if the injured part has begun to swell, or if by running the finger lightly along the affected bone a break can be felt, *do not* move him. Under no circumstances should he be crowded into a car if his legs, hip, ribs, or back are involved in the accident. Call for an ambulance immediately, and until it arrives, treat the person for shock.

SPLINTING: In a situation where it is imperative to move someone who may have a fracture, the first step is to apply a splint so that the broken bone ends are immobilized.

Splints can be improvised from anything rigid enough and of the right length to support the fractured part of the body: a metal rod, board, long cardboard tube, tightly rolled newspaper or blanket. If the object being used has to be padded for softness, use a small blanket or any other soft material, such as a jacket.

The splint should be long enough so that it can be tied with a bandage, torn sheet, or neckties beyond the joint above and below the fracture as well as at the site of the break. If a leg is involved, it should be elevated with pillows or any other firm support after the splint has been applied. If the victim has to wait a considerable length of time before receiving professional attention, the splint bandaging should be checked from time to time to make sure it isn't too tight.

In the case of an open or compound fracture, additional steps must be taken. Remove that part of the victim's clothing which is covering the wound. Do not wash or probe into the wound, but control bleeding by applying pressure over the wound through a sterile or clean dressing.

Frostbite

EMERGENCY TREATMENT: Begin rapid rewarming of the affected tissues as soon as possible. If possible, immerse the victim in a warm bath, but avoid scalding. (The temperature should be between 102° and 105° F.) Warm wet towels also will help if changed frequently and applied gently. Do not massage, rub, or even touch the frostbitten flesh. If warm water or a warming fire is not available, place the patient in a sleeping bag or cover him with coats and blankets. Hot liquids can be offered if available to help raise the body temperature.

For any true frostbite case, prompt medical attention is important. The depth and degree of the frozen tissue cannot be determined without a careful examination by a physician.

Gall bladder attacks

Although gallstones can affect a wide variety of individuals, the most common victims are overweight persons who enjoy rich foods. The actual attack of spasms caused by gallstones passing through the duct leading from the gall bladder to the digestive tract usually is preceded by periods of stomach distress including belching. X rays usually will reveal the presence of gallstones when the early warning signs are noted, and measures can be taken to reduce the threat of a gall-bladder attack.

EMERGENCY TREATMENT: Call a doctor and describe in detail the symptoms, which may include colic high in the abdomen and pain extending to the right shoulder; the pain may be accompanied by nausea, vomiting, and sweating. Hot water bottles may be applied to the abdomen to help relieve distress while waiting for professional medical care. If the doctor permits, the victim may be allowed to sip certain fluids such as fruit juices, but do not offer him solid food.

Gas poisoning

Before attempting to revive someone overcome by toxic gas poisoning, the most important thing to do is to remove him to the fresh air. If this isn't feasible, all windows and doors should be opened to let in as much fresh air as possible.

Any interior with a dangerous concentration of carbon monoxide or other toxic gases is apt to be highly explosive. Therefore, gas and electricity should be shut off as quickly as possible. *Under no circumstances should any matches be lighted in an interior where there are noxious fumes.*

The rescuer needn't waste time covering his face with a handkerchief or other cloth. He should hold his breath instead, or take only a few quick, shallow breaths while bringing the victim to the out-of-doors or to an open window.

EMERGENCY TREATMENT: Administer artificial respiration if the victim is suffering respiratory arrest. Arrange for medical help as soon as possible, requesting that oxygen be brought to the scene.

Head injuries

Accidents involving the head can result in concussion, skull fracture, or brain injury. Symptoms of head injury include loss of consciousness, discharge of a watery or blood-tinged fluid from the ears, nose, or mouth, and a difference in size of the pupils of the eyes. Head injuries must be thought of as serious; they demand immediate medical assistance.

EMERGENCY TREATMENT: Place the victim in a supine position, and, if there is no evidence of injury to his neck, arrange for a slight elevation of his head *and* shoulders. Make certain that he has a clear airway and administer artificial respiration if necessary. If vomitus, blood, or other fluids appear to flow from the victim's mouth, turn his head gently to one side. Control bleeding and treat for shock. Do not administer stimulants or fluids of any kind.

Heart attack

A heart attack is caused by interference with the blood supply to the heart muscle. When the attack is brought on because of a blood clot in the coronary artery, it is known as *coronary occlusion* or *coronary thrombosis.*

The most dramatic symptom of a serious heart attack is a crushing chest pain that usually travels down the left arm into the hand or into the neck and back. The pain may bring on dizziness, cold sweat, complete collapse, and loss of consciousness. The face has an ashen pallor, and there may be vomiting.

EMERGENCY TREATMENT: The victim *must not be moved* unless he has fallen in a dangerous place. If no doctor is immediately available, an ambulance should be called at once. No attempt should be made to get the victim of a heart attack into an automobile.

Until help arrives, give the victim every reassurance that he will get prompt treatment, and keep him as calm and quiet as possible. Don't give him any medicine or stimulants. If oxygen is available, start administering it to the victim immediately, either by mask or nasal catheter, depending on which is available.

If the victim is suffering from respiratory arrest, begin artificial respiration. If he is suffering from cardiac arrest, begin cardiac massage.

Heat exhaustion

Heat exhaustion occurs when the body is exposed to high temperatures and large amounts of blood accumulate in the skin as a way of cooling it. As a result, there is a marked decrease in the amount of blood that circulates through the heart and to the brain. The victim becomes markedly pale and is covered with cold perspiration. Breathing is increasingly shallow and the pulse weakens. In acute cases, fainting occurs. Medical aid should be summoned for anyone suffering from heat exhaustion.

EMERGENCY TREATMENT: Place the victim in a reclining position with his feet raised about 10 inches above his body. Loosen or remove his clothing, and apply cold, wet cloths to his wrists and forehead. If he has fainted and doesn't recover promptly, smelling salts or spirits of ammonia should be placed under his nose. When the victim is conscious, give him sips of salt water (approximately one teaspoon of salt per glass of water), the total intake to be about two glasses in an hour's time. If the victim vomits, discontinue the salt solution.

Heatstroke/sunstroke

Heatstroke is characterized by an acutely high body temperature caused by the cessation of perspiration. The victim's skin becomes hot, dry, and flushed, and he may suffer collapse. Should the skin turn ashen gray, a physician must be called immediately. Prompt hospital treatment is recommended for anyone showing signs of sunstroke who has previously had any kind of heart damage.

EMERGENCY TREATMENT: The following measures are designed to reduce the victim's body temperature as quickly as possible and prevent damage to the internal organs:

Place him in a tub of very cold water, or, if this is not possible, spray or sponge his body repeatedly with cold water or rubbing alcohol. Take his temperature by mouth, and when

it has dropped to about 100° F., remove him to a bed and wrap him in cold, wet sheets. If possible, expose him to an electric fan or an air conditioner.

Hiccups

EMERGENCY TREATMENT: Have the victim slowly drink a large glass of water. If cold water is not effective, have him drink warm water containing a teaspoonful of baking soda. Milk also can be employed. For babies and small children, offer sips of warm water. Do not offer carbonated beverages.

Another helpful measure is breathing into a large paper bag a number of times to raise the carbon dioxide level in the lungs. Rest and relaxation are recommended; have the victim lie down to read or watch television.

If the hiccups fail to go away, and continued spastic contractions of the diaphragm interfere with eating and sleeping, call your doctor.

Insect stings

Honeybees, wasps, hornets, and yellow jackets are the most common stinging insects and are most likely to attack on a hot summer day. Strongly scented perfumes or cosmetics and brightly colored, rough-finished clothing attract bees and should be avoided by persons working or playing in garden areas. It should also be noted that many commercial repellents do not protect against stinging insects.

EMERGENCY TREATMENT: If one is stung, the insect's stinger should be scraped gently but quickly from the skin; don't squeeze it. Apply Epsom salt solution to the sting area. Antihistamines are often helpful in reducing the patient's discomfort. If a severe reaction develops, call a doctor.

There are a few people who are critically allergic to the sting of wasps, bees, yellow jackets, or fire ants. This sensitivity causes the vocal cord tissue to swell to the point where breathing may become impossible. A single sting to a sensitive person may result in a dangerous drop in blood pressure, thus producing shock. Anyone with such a severe allergy who is stung should be rushed to a hospital immediately.

A person who becomes aware of having this type of allergy should consult with a physician about the kind of medicine to carry for use in a crisis.

Insulin shock

See DIABETIC COMA AND INSULIN SHOCK.

Jaw dislocation

The jaw can be dislocated during a physical attack or fight; from a blow on the jaw during sports activities; or from overextension of the joint during yawning, laughing, or attempting to eat a large mouthful of food. The jaw becomes literally locked open so the victim cannot explain his predicament.

EMERGENCY TREATMENT: Reducing a dislocated jaw will require that you insert your thumbs between the teeth of the victim. The jaw can be expected to snap into place quickly, and there is a danger that the teeth will clamp down on the thumbs when this happens, so the thumbs should be adequately padded with handkerchiefs or bandages. Once the thumbs are protected, insert them in the mouth and over the lower molars, as far back on the lower jaw as possible. While pressing down with the thumbs, lift the chin with the fingers outside the mouth. As the jaw begins to slip into normal position when it is pushed downward and backward with the chin lifted upward, quickly remove the thumbs from between the jaws.

Once the jaw is back in normal position, the mouth should remain closed for several hours while the ligaments recover from their displaced condition. If necessary, put a cravat bandage over the head to hold the mouth closed. If difficulty is experienced in reducing a jaw dislocation, the victim should be taken to a hospital where an anesthetic can be applied. A dislocated jaw can be extremely painful.

Jellyfish stings

EMERGENCY TREATMENT: Wash the area of the sting thoroughly with alcohol or fresh water. Be sure that any pieces of jellyfish tentacles have been removed from the skin. Aspirin or antihistamines can be administered to relieve pain and itching, but curtail the use of antihistamines if the victim has consumed alcoholic beverages. The leg or arm that received the sting can be soaked in hot water if the pain continues. Otherwise, apply calamine lotion.

If the victim appears to suffer a severe reaction from the sting, summon a doctor. The victim may experience shock, muscle cramps, convulsions, or loss of consciousness. Artificial respiration may be required while awaiting arrival of a doctor. The physician can administer drugs to relieve muscle cramps and provide sedatives or analgesics.

Kidney stones

EMERGENCY TREATMENT: Call a doctor if the victim experiences the agonizing cramps or colic associated with kidney stones. Discuss the symptoms in detail with the doctor to make sure the pain is caused by kidney stones rather than appendicitis.

Comforting heat may be applied to the back and the abdomen of the side affected by the spasms. Paregoric can be administered, if available, while waiting for medical care; about two teaspoonsful of paregoric in a half glass of water may help relieve symptoms.

Knee injuries

EMERGENCY TREATMENT: If the injury appears to be severe, including possible fracture of the kneecap, immobilize the knee. To immobilize the knee, place the injured leg on a board that is about four inches wide and three to four feet in length. Place padding between the board and the knee, and between the board and the back of the ankle. Then use four strips of bandage to fasten the leg to the padded board—one at the ankle, one at the thigh, and one each above and below the knee.

Summon a doctor or move the patient to a doctor's office. Keep the knee protected against cold or exposure to the elements, but otherwise do not apply a bandage or any type of pressure to the knee itself; any rapid swelling would be aggravated by unnecessary pressure in that area. Be prepared to treat the patient for shock.

Laryngitis

Laryngitis is associated with colds and influenza and may be accompanied by a fever. The ailment can be aggravated by smoking, and it is possible that the vocal cords can be damaged if the victim tries to force the use of his voice while the larynx is swollen by the infection.

EMERGENCY TREATMENT: Have the victim inhale the warm moist air of a steam kettle or vaporizer. A vaporizer can be improvised in an emergency by pouring boiling water into a bowl and forming a "tent" over the steaming bowl with a large towel or sheet, or by placing a large paper bag over the bowl and cutting an opening at the closed end of the bag so the face can be exposed to the steam. The hot water can contain a bit of camphor or menthol, if available, to make the warm moist air more soothing to the throat, but this is not necessary.

Continue the use of the vaporizer for several days, as needed. The victim should not use the vocal cords any more than absolutely necessary. If the infection does not subside within the first few days, a doctor should be consulted.

Leeches

EMERGENCY TREATMENT: Do not try to pull leeches off the skin. They will usually drop away from the skin if a heated object such as a lighted cigarette is held close to them. Leeches also are likely to let go if iodine is applied to their bodies. The wound caused by a leech should be washed carefully with soap and water and an antiseptic applied.

Lightning shock

EMERGENCY TREATMENT: If the victim is not breathing, apply artificial respiration. If a second person is available to help, have him summon a doctor while artificial respiration is administered. Continue artificial respiration until breathing resumes or the doctor arrives.

When the victim is breathing regularly, treat him for shock. Keep him lying down with his feet higher than his head, his clothing loosened around the neck, and his body covered with a blanket or coat for warmth. If the victim shows signs of vomiting, turn his head to one side so he will not swallow the vomitus.

If the victim is breathing regularly and does not show signs of shock, he may be given a few sips of a stimulating beverage such as coffee, tea, or brandy.

Motion sickness

EMERGENCY TREATMENT: Have the victim lie down in a position that is most comfortable to him. The head should be fixed so that any view of motion is avoided. Reading or other use of the eyes should be prohibited. Food or fluids should be restricted to very small amounts. If traveling by car, stop at a rest area; in an airplane or ship, place the victim in an area where motion is least noticeable.

Drugs, such as Dramamine, are helpful for control of the symptoms of motion sickness; they are most effective when started about 90 minutes before travel begins and repeated at regular intervals thereafter.

Muscle cramps

EMERGENCY TREATMENT: Gently massage the affected muscle, sometimes stretching it to help relieve the painful contraction. Then relax the muscle by using a hot water bottle or an electric heating pad, or by soaking the affected area in a warm bath.

A repetition of cramps may require medical attention.

Nosebleeds

EMERGENCY TREATMENT: Have the victim sit erect but with the head tilted slightly forward to prevent blood from running down the throat. Apply pressure by pinching the nostrils; if bleeding is from just one nostril, use pressure on that side. A small wedge of absorbent cotton or gauze can be inserted into the bleeding nostril. Make sure that the cotton or gauze extends out of the nostril to aid in its removal when the bleeding has stopped. Encourage the victim to breathe through the mouth while the nose is bleeding. After five minutes, release pressure on the nose to see if the bleeding has stopped. If the bleeding continues, repeat pressure on the nostril for an additional five minutes. Cold compresses applied to the nose can help stop the bleeding.

If bleeding continues after the second five-minute period of pressure treatment, get the victim to a doctor's office or a hospital emergency room.

Poison ivy/poison oak/poison sumac

EMERGENCY TREATMENT: The poison of these three plants is the same and the treatment is identical. Bathe the skin area exposed to poison ivy, poison oak, or poison sumac with soap and water or with alcohol within 15 minutes after contact. If exposure is not discovered until a rash appears, apply cool wet dressings. Dressings can be made of old bed sheets or soft linens soaked in a solution of one teaspoon of salt per pint of water. Dressings should be applied four times a day for periods of 15 to 60 minutes each time; during these periods, dressings can be removed and reapplied every few minutes. The itching that often accompanies the rash can be relieved by taking antihistamine tablets.

Creams or lotions may be prescribed by a doctor or supplied by a pharmacist. Do not use such folk remedies as ammonia or turpentine; do not use skin lotions not approved by a doctor or druggist. Haphazard application of medications on poison ivy blisters and rashes can result in complications including skin irritation, infection, or pigmented lesions of the skin.

Rabies

See ANIMAL BITES.

Sciatica/lower back pain

Although lower back pain is frequently triggered by fatigue, anxiety, or by strained muscles or tendons, it may be a symptom of a slipped or ruptured disk between the vertebrae, or of a similar disorder requiring extensive medical attention.

EMERGENCY TREATMENT: Reduce the pressure on the lower back by having the victim lie down on a hard flat surface; if a bed is used there should be a board or sheet of plywood between the springs and mattress. Pillows should be placed under the knees instead of under the head, to help keep the back flat. Give aspirin to relieve the pain, and apply heat to the back. Call a doctor if the symptoms do not subside overnight.

Scorpion stings

EMERGENCY TREATMENT: Apply ice to the region of the sting, except in the case of an arm or leg, in which event the limb may be immersed in ice water. Continue the ice or ice-water treatment for at least one hour. Try to keep the area of the sting at a position lower than the heart. No tourniquet is required. Should the breathing of a scorpion sting victim becomes depressed, administer artificial respiration. If symptoms fail to subside within a couple of hours, notify a physician, or transfer the victim to a doctor's office or hospital.

For children under six, call a physician in the event of any scorpion sting. Children stung by scorpions may become convulsive, and this condition can result in fatal exhaustion unless it receives prompt medical treatment.

Snakebites

Of the many varieties of snakes found in the United States, only four kinds are poisonous: copperheads, rattlesnakes, moccasins, and coral snakes. The first three belong to the category of pit vipers and are known as *hemotoxic* because their poison enters the bloodstream. The coral snake, which is comparatively rare, is related to the cobra and is the most dangerous of all because its venom is *neurotoxic*. This means that the poison transmitted by its bite goes directly to the nervous system and the brain.

HOW TO DIFFERENTIATE BETWEEN SNAKEBITES: Snakes of the pit viper family have a fang on each side of the head. These fangs leave characteristic puncture wounds on the skin in addition to two rows of tiny bites or scratches left by the teeth. A bite from a nonpoisonous snake leaves six rows—four upper and two lower—of very small bite marks or scratches and no puncture wounds.

The marks left by the bite of a coral snake do not leave any puncture wounds either, but this snake bites with a chewing motion, hanging on to the victim rather than attacking quickly. The coral snake is very easy to recognize because of its distinctive markings: wide horizontal bands of red and black separated by narrow bands of yellow.

SYMPTOMS: A bite from any of the pit vipers produces immediate and severe pain and darkening of the skin, followed by weakness, blurred vision, quickened pulse, nausea, and vomiting. The bite of a coral snake produces somewhat the same symptoms, although there is less local pain and considerable drowsiness leading to unconsciousness.

If a doctor or a hospital is a short distance away, the patient should receive professional help *immediately.* He should be transported lying down, either on an improvised stretcher or carried by his companions—with the wounded part lower than his heart. He should be advised to move as little as possible.

EMERGENCY TREATMENT: If several hours must elapse before a doctor or a hospital can be reached, the following procedures should be applied promptly:

1. Keep the victim lying down and as still as possible.

2. Tie a constricting band *above* the wound between it and the heart and tight enough to slow but not stop blood circulation. A handkerchief, necktie, sock, or piece of torn shirt will serve.

3. If a snakebite kit is available, use the knife it contains; otherwise, sterilize a knife or razor blade in a flame. Carefully make small cuts in the skin where the swelling has developed. Make the cuts along the length of the limb, not across or at right angles to it. The incisions should be shallow because of the danger of severing nerves, blood vessels, or muscles.

4. Use the suction cups in the snakebite kit, if available, to draw out as much of the venom as possible. If suction cups are not available, the venom can be removed by sucking it out with the mouth. Although snake venom is not a stomach poison, it should not be swallowed but should be rinsed from the mouth.

5. This procedure should be continued for from 30 to 60 minutes or until the swelling subsides and the other symptoms decrease.

6. You may apply cold compresses to the bite area while waiting for professional assistance.

7. Treat the victim for shock.

8. Give artificial respiration if necessary.

Splinters

EMERGENCY TREATMENT: Clean the area about the splinter with soap and water or an antiseptic. Next, sterilize a needle by holding it over an open flame. After it cools, insert the needle above the splinter so it will tear a line in the skin, making the splinter lie loose in the wound. Then, gently lift the splinter out, using a pair of tweezers or the point of the needle. If tweezers are used, they should be sterilized first.

Wash the wound area again with soap and water, or apply an antiseptic. It is best to cover the wound with an adhesive bandage. If redness or irritation develops around the splinter wound, consult a doctor.

Sprains

A sprain occurs when a joint is wrenched or twisted in such a way that the ligaments holding it in position are ruptured, possibly damaging the surrounding blood vessels, tendons, nerves, and muscles. This type of injury is more serious than a strain and is usually accompanied by pain, sometimes severe, soreness, swelling, and discoloration of the affected area. Most sprains occur as a result of falls, athletic accidents, or improper handling of heavy weights.

EMERGENCY TREATMENT: This consists of prompt rest, the application of cold compresses to relieve swelling and any internal bleeding in the joint, and elevation of the affected area. Aspirin is recommended to reduce discomfort. If the swelling and soreness increase after such treatment, a physician should be consulted to make sure that the injury is not a fracture or a bone dislocation.

Sting ray

EMERGENCY TREATMENT: If an arm or leg is the target of a sting ray, wash the area thoroughly with salt water. Quickly remove any pieces of the stinger imbedded in the skin or flesh; poison can still be discharged into the victim from the sting-ray sheath. After initial cleansing of an arm or leg sting, soak the wound with hot water for up to an hour. Apply antiseptic or a sterile dressing after the soak.

Consult a physician after a sting-ray attack. The doctor will make a thorough examination of the wound to determine whether stitches or antibiotics are required. Fever, vomiting, or muscular twitching also may result from an apparently simple leg or arm wound by a sting ray.

If the sting occurs in the chest or abdomen, the victim should be rushed to a hospital as soon as possible because such a wound can produce convulsions or loss of consciousness.

Strains

When a muscle is stretched because of misuse or overuse, the interior bundles of tissue may tear, or the tendon which connects it to the bone may be stretched. This condition is known as strain. It occurs most commonly to the muscles of the lower back when heavy weights are improperly lifted, or in the area of the calf or ankle as the result of a sudden, violent twist or undue pressure.

EMERGENCY TREATMENT: Bed rest, the application of heat, and gentle massage are recommended for back strain. If the strain is in the leg, elevate the limb to help reduce pain and swelling, and apply cold compresses or an ice bag to the area. Aspirin may be taken to reduce discomfort.

In severe cases of strained back muscles, a physician may have to be consulted for strapping. For a strained ankle, a flexible elastic bandage can be helpful in providing the necessary support until the injured muscle heals.

Stroke

Stroke, or apoplexy, is caused by a disruption of normal blood flow to the brain, either by rupture of a blood vessel within the brain or by blockage of an artery supplying the brain. The condition is enhanced by hardening of the arteries and high blood pressure, and is most likely to occur in older persons. A stroke usually occurs with little or no warning and the onset may be marked by a variety of manifestations ranging from headache, slurred speech, or blurred vision, to sudden collapse and unconsciousness.

EMERGENCY TREATMENT: Try to place the victim in a semi-reclining position, or, if he is lying down, be sure there is a pillow under his head. Avoid conditions that might increase the flow of blood toward the head. Summon a doctor immediately. Loosen any clothing that may be

tight. If the patient wears dentures, remove them.

Before professional medical assistance is available, the victim may vomit or go into shock or convulsions. If he vomits, try to prevent a backflow of vomitus into the breathing passages. If shock occurs, do not place the victim in the shock position but do keep him warm and comfortable. If convulsions develop, place a handkerchief or similar soft object between the jaws to prevent tongue biting.

Sty on eyelid

Sties usually develop around hair follicles because of a bacterial infection. Like cold sores, they are most likely to develop in association with poor health and lowered resistance to infection.

EMERGENCY TREATMENT: Apply warm, moist packs or compresses to the sty for periods of 15 to 20 minutes at intervals of three or four hours. Moist heat generally is more penetrating than dry heat.

The sty should eventually rupture and the pus should then be washed carefully away from the eye area. If the sty does not rupture or is very painful, consult a doctor. Do not squeeze or otherwise handle the sty except to apply the warm moist compresses.

Sunburn

EMERGENCY TREATMENT: Apply cold wet compresses to help relieve the pain. Compresses can be soaked in whole milk, salt water, or a solution of corn starch mixed with water. The victim also may get some relief by soaking in a bathtub filled with plain water. Soothing lotions, such as baby oil or a bland cold cream, can be applied after carefully drying the skin. Don't rub the burn area while drying. Avoid the use of "shake" lotions, like calamine, which may aggravate the burn by a drying action. The victim should, of course, avoid further exposure to sunlight.

If pain is excessive, or extensive

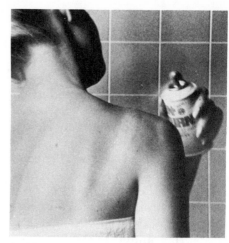

Avoid using topical anesthetics on sunburnt skin. They may cause allergic reactions. Use a soothing lotion such as baby oil.

blistering is present, consult a physician. Avoid application of over-the-counter topical anesthetics that may cause allergic skin reactions.

A severe or extensive sunburn is comparable to a second-degree thermal burn and may be accompanied by symptoms of shock; if such symptoms are present the victim should be treated for shock. See also BURNS, THERMAL.

Sunstroke

See HEATSTROKE.

Tick bites

EMERGENCY TREATMENT: Do not try to scrape or rub the insect off the skin with your fingers; scraping, rubbing, or pulling may break off only part of the insect body, leaving the head firmly attached to the skin. Rubbing also can smear disease organisms from the tick into the bite. To make the tick drop away from the skin cover it with a heavy oil, such as salad, mineral, or lubricating oil. Oil usually will block the insect's breathing pores, suffocating it. If oil is not readily available, carefully place a heated object against the tick's body; a lighted cigarette or a match that has been ignited and snuffed out can serve as a hot object.

Carefully inspect the bite area to be sure that all parts of the tick have been removed. Use a pair of tweezers to remove any tick parts found.

Then carefully wash the bite and surrounding area with soap and water and apply an antiseptic. Also, wash your hands and any equipment that may have come in contact with the tick. Consult a physician if symptoms of tick fever or tularemia, such as unexplained muscular weakness, occur following a bite.

Toothaches

EMERGENCY TREATMENT: Give an adult one or two aspirin tablets; a young child should be given no more than one-half of an adult tablet. The aspirin should be swallowed with plenty of water. Do not let it dissolve in the mouth or be held near the aching tooth. Aspirin becomes effective as a pain-killer only after it has gone through the digestive tract and into the bloodstream; if aspirin is held in the mouth, it may irritate the gums.

Oil of cloves can be applied to the aching tooth. Dip a small wad of cotton into the oil of cloves, then gently pack the oil-soaked cotton into the tooth cavity with a pair of tweezers. Do not let the tweezers touch the tooth.

If the jaw is swollen, apply an ice bag for periods of 15 minutes at a time, at intermittent intervals. Never apply heat to a swollen jaw when treating a toothache. Arrange to see your dentist as soon as possible.

Tooth, broken

EMERGENCY TREATMENT: Apply a few drops of oil of cloves to the injured tooth to help relieve pain. If oil of cloves is not available, give an adult one to two regular aspirin tablets. One-half of a regular tablet can be given to a young child.

Make an emergency filling from a wad of cotton containing a few drops of oil of cloves. An emergency filling also can be made from powdered chalk; it is important to protect the cavity from infection while providing pain relief.

If the tooth has been knocked out of the socket, retrieve the tooth, because it can be restored in some cases. Do not wash the tooth; ordinary washing can damage dental tissues. A dentist will take care of cleaning it properly. Wrap the tooth in a damp clean handkerchief or tissue or place the tooth in a container of slightly salty warm water for the trip to the dentist.

Unconsciousness

Unconsciousness is the condition which has the appearance of sleep, but is usually the result of injury, shock, or serious physical disturbance. A brief loss of consciousness followed by spontaneous recovery is called *fainting*. A prolonged episode of unconsciousness is a *coma*.

EMERGENCY TREATMENT: Call a doctor at once. If none is available, get the victim to the nearest hospital. If the loss of consciousness is accompanied by loss of breathing, begin mouth-to-mouth respiration. If the victim is suffering cardiac arrest, administer cardiac massage. Don't try to revive the victim with any kind of stimulant unless told to do so by a doctor.

Vertigo

See DIZZINESS.

CHAPTER 35

100 Commonly Prescribed Generic Drugs

The table that follows gives the names of 100 commonly prescribed generic drugs. These drugs are not patented, or the patents on them have expired. For that reason any drug company may manufacture and sell them under their generic names or under completely new brand names. The generic names are also called the "official" or "non-proprietary" names. They usually describe the chemical makeup or the class of the drug.

With each drug included in the table, several types of information are given. The table shows, for example, what the drug does, what its medical description is (anti-emetic, diuretic, and so on), and what illnesses, diseases, or disorders it is usually used to treat. Some, but not all, of each generic drug's trade-name equivalents are also shown.

It should be remembered that the list of 100 includes only some of the most commonly prescribed generic drugs. Hundreds of others, less widely used, might be listed. To save money, it's generally wise to ask your doctor when he writes a prescription whether the drug is available generically.

Name	Action	Prescribed for	Trade Names (CD = comb. drug)
ACETAMINOPHEN (Paracetamol)	Believed to reduce concentration of chemicals involved in production of pain, fever, and inflammation (analgesic; antipyretic)	Relief of mild to moderate pain; reduction of fever	Datril Tylenol Co-Tylenol (CD) Excedrin (CD) Sinarest (CD) Sinutab (CD)
AMITRIPTYLINE	Believed to restore to normal levels the constituents of brain tissue that transmit nerve impulses (antidepressant)	Relief of emotional depression; gradual improvement of mood	Elamil Etrafon (CD) Triavil (CD)
AMPICILLIN	Interferes with ability of susceptible bacteria to produce new protective cell walls as they grow and multiply (antibiotic)	Elimination of infections responsive to action of this drug	Amcill Pensyn Polycillin Principen
ANTACIDS (Aluminum Hydroxide) (Calcium Carbonate) (Sodium Bicarbonate)	Neutralizes stomach acid; reduces action of digestive enzyme pepsin (relief from gastric hyperacidity)	Relief of heartburn, sour stomach, acid indigestion, and discomfort associated with peptic ulcer, gastritis, esophagitis, hiatal hernia	Absorbable: Sodium bicarbonate: Alka-Seltzer Brioschi Bromo-Seltzer Less absorbable: Aluminum hydroxide: Amphojel Calcium carbonate: Alka-2 Amitone
ASPIRIN (Acetylsalicylic Acid)	Dilates blood vessels in skin, thus hastening loss of body heat (antipyretic); reduces tissue concentration of chemicals involved in production of inflammation and pain (analgesic; antirheumatic)	Reduction of fever; relief of mild to moderate pain and inflammation; prevention of blood clots, as in phlebitis, heart attack, stroke	Bayer Aspirin St. Joseph Children's Aspirin Preparations containing aspirin: (all CD) Alka-Seltzer Anacin A.P.C. Tablets Bufferin Empirin Compound 4-Way Tablets Vanquish
ATROPINE (Belladonna, Hyoscyamine)	Prevents stimulation of muscular contractions and glandular secretion in organ involved (antispasmodic [anticholinergic])	Relief of discomfort associated with excessive activity and spasm of digestive tract; irritation and spasm of lower urinary tract; painful menstruation	Donna Extendtabs Bellergal (CD) Donnagel-PG (CD) Donnatal (CD) Nembu-donna (CD)
BENDROFLUMETHIAZIDE	Increases elimination of salt and water (diuretic); relaxes walls of smaller arteries, allowing them to expand; combined effect lowers blood pressure (antihypertensive)	Elimination of excessive fluid retention (edema); reduction of high blood pressure	Naturetin Rautrax-N (CD) Rauzide (CD)
BROMPHENIRAMINE	Blocks action of histamine after release from sensitized tissue cells, thus reducing intensity of allergic response (antihistamine)	Relief of symptoms of hayfever (allergic rhinitis) and of allergic reactions of skin (itching, swelling, hives, rash)	Dimetane Veltane Dimetapp (CD)
BUTABARBITAL	Believed to block transmission of nerve impulses (hypnotic; sedative)	Low dosage: relief of moderate anxiety or tension (sedative effect); higher dosage: at bedtime to induce sleep (hypnotic effect)	Buticaps Butisol Butte Quiebar
CAFFEINE	Constricts blood vessel walls; increases energy level of chemical systems responsible for nerve tissue activity (cardiac, respiratory, psychic stimulant)	Prevention and early relief of vascular headaches such as migraine; relief of drowsiness and mental fatigue	Nodoz Cafergot (CD) Cafermine (CD)
CARISOPRODOL	Believed to block transmission of nerve impulses and/or to produce a sedative effect (muscle relaxant)	Relief of discomfort caused by spasms of voluntary muscles	Rela Soma (CD) Soma Compound (CD)
CHLORAL HYDRATE	Believed to affect wake-sleep centers of brain (hypnotic)	Low dosage: relief of mild to moderate anxiety or tension (sedative effect); higher dosage: at bedtime to relieve insomnia (hypnotic effect)	Noctec Oradrate Somnos
CHLORAMPHENICOL	Prevents growth and multiplication of susceptible bacteria by interfering with formation of their essential proteins (antibiotic)	Elimination of infections responsive to action of this drug	Amphicol Chloromycetin Ophthochlor
CHLORDIAZEPOXIDE	Believed to reduce activity of some parts of limbic system (tranquilizer)	Relief of mild to moderate anxiety and tension without significant sedation	Libritabs Librium
CHLOROTHIAZIDE	Increases elimination of salt and water (diuretic); relaxes walls of smaller arteries, allowing them to expand; combined effect lowers blood pressure (antihypertensive)	Elimination of excessive fluid retention (edema); reduction of high blood pressure	Diuril Aldoclor (CD) Diupres (CD)
CHLORPHENIRAMINE	Blocks action of histamine after release from sensitized tissue cells, thus reducing intensity of allergic response (antihistamine)	Relief of symptoms of hayfever (allergic rhinitis) and of allergic reactions of skin (itching, swelling, hives, rash)	Chlor-Trimeton Polaramine Teldrin

Name	Action	Prescribed for	Trade Names (CD = comb. drug)
CHLORPROMAZINE	Believed to inhibit action of dopamine, thus correcting an imbalance of nerve impulse transmissions thought to be responsible for certain mental disorders (antiemetic; tranquilizer)	Relief of severe anxiety, agitation, and psychotic behavior	Klorazine Promapar Thorazine
CODEINE	Believed to affect tissue sites that react specifically with opium and its derivatives (antitussive; narcotic analgesic)	Relief of moderate pain; control of coughing	None as a single entity—many for combination products
DEXAMETHASONE	Believed to inhibit several tissue mechanisms that induce inflammation (adrenocortical steroid [anti-inflammatory])	Symptomatic relief of inflammation (swelling, redness, heat, pain)	Decadron Dexameth Hexadrol
DEXTROAMPHETAMINE (d-Amphetamine)	Increases release of nerve impulse transmitter (central stimulant); this may also improve concentration and attention span of hyperactive child (primary calming action unknown); alters chemical control of nerve impulse transmission in appetite control center of brain (appetite suppressant [anorexiant])	Reduction or prevention of sleep epilepsy (narcolepsy); reduction of symptoms of abnormal hyperactivity (as in minimal brain dysfunction); suppression of appetite in management of weight reduction	Dexedrine Bamadex (CD) Biphetamine (CD) Dexamyl (CD)
DIAZEPAM	Believed to reduce activity of some parts of limbic system (tranquilizer)	Relief of mild to moderate anxiety and tension without significant sedation	Valium
DICYCLOMINE	Believed to produce a local anesthetic action that blocks reflex activity responsible for spasm (antispasmodic)	Relief of discomfort from muscle spasm of the gastrointestinal tract	Bentyl Dispas Triactin (CD)
DIGITOXIN	Increases availability of calcium within the heart muscle, thus improving conversion of chemical energy to mechanical energy; slows pacemaker and delays transmission of electrical impulses (digitalis preparations [cardiotonic])	Improvement of heart muscle contraction force (as in congestive heart failure); correction of certain heart rhythm disorders	Crystodigin Digitaline Purodigin
DIGOXIN	Same as above	Same as above	Davoxin Lanoxin Thegitoxin
DIPHENHYDRAMINE	Blocks action of histamine after release from sensitized tissue cells, thus reducing intensity of allergic response (antihistamine)	Relief of symptoms of hayfever (allergic rhinitis) and of allergic reactions of skin (itching, swelling, hives, rash)	Benadryl Ambenyl (CD) Benylin (CD)
DOXYLAMINE	Same as above	Same as above	Decapryn Bendectin (CD) Nyquil (CD)
EPHEDRINE	Blocks release of certain chemicals from sensitized tissue cells undergoing allergic reaction; relaxes bronchial muscles; shrinks tissue mass (decongestion) by contracting arteriole walls in lining of respiratory passages (adrenergic [bronchodilator])	Prevention and symptomatic relief of bronchial asthma; relief of congestion of respiratory passages	Bronkaid (CD) Bronkotabs (CD) Marax (CD) Nyquil (CD) Quelidrine (CD) Quibron Plus (CD) Tedral (CD)
ERGOTAMINE	Constricts blood vessel walls, thus relieving excessive dilation that causes pain of vascular headaches (migraine analgesic [vasoconstrictor])	Prevention and early relief of vascular headaches such as migraine or histamine headaches	Ergomar Bellergal (CD) Cafergot (CD) Migral (CD)
ERYTHRITYL TETRANITRATE	Acts directly on muscle cells to produce relaxation which permits expansion of blood vessels, thus increasing supply of blood and oxygen to heart	Management of pain associated with angina pectoris (coronary insufficiency)	Anginar Cardilate
ERYTHROMYCIN	Prevents growth and multiplication of susceptible bacteria by interfering with formation of their essential proteins (antibiotic)	Elimination of infections responsive to action of this drug	Bristamycin E-Mycin Erythrocin Ethril Pfizer-E
ESTROGEN (Estrogenic Substances) Conjugated Estrogens, Esterified Estrogens (Estrone and Equilin)	Prepares uterus for pregnancy or induces menstruation by cyclic increase and decrease in tissue stimulation; when taken regularly, blood and tissue levels increase to resemble those during pregnancy, thus preventing pituitary gland from producing hormones that induce ovulation; reduces frequency and intensity of menopausal symptoms (female sex hormone)	Regulation of menstrual cycle; prevention of pregnancy; relief of symptoms of menopause	Amnestrogen Femogen Menotabs Menrium (CD) Milprem (CD)
GRISEOFULVIN	Believed to prevent growth and multiplication of susceptible fungus strains by interfering with their metabolic activities (antibiotic; antifungal)	Elimination of fungus infections responsive to action of this drug	Fulvicin-U/F Grifulvin V
HYDRALAZINE	Lowers pressure of blood in vessels by causing direct relaxation and expansion of vessel walls—mechanism unknown (antihypertensive)	Reduction of high blood pressure	Apresoline Dralserp (CD) Ser-Ap-Es (CD)
HYDROCHLOROTHIAZIDE	Increases elimination of salt and water (diuretic); relaxes walls of smaller arteries, allowing them to expand; combined effect lowers blood pressure (antihypertensive)	Elimination of excessive fluid retention (edema); reduction of high blood pressure	Esidrix HydroDiuril Oretic Thiuretic

Name	Action	Prescribed for	Trade Names (CD = comb. drug)
HYDROCORTISONE (CORTISOL)	Believed to inhibit several tissue mechanisms that induce inflammation (adrenocortical steroid [anti-inflammatory])	Symptomatic relief of inflammation (swelling, redness, heat, pain)	Cortef Cortril Hydrocortone
HYDROXYZINE	Believed to reduce excessive activity in areas of brain that influence emotional health (antihistamine; tranquilizer)	Relief of anxiety, tension, apprehension, and agitation	Atarax Vistaril Marax (CD)
INSULIN	Facilitates passage of sugar through cell wall to interior of cell (hypoglycemic)	Control of diabetes	Iletin Preparations Insulin Preparations: Lente Insulin NPH Insulin Regular Insulin Semilente Insulin Ultralente Insulin
ISONIAZID	Believed to interfere with several metabolic activities of susceptible tuberculosis organisms (antibacterial; tuberculostatic)	Prevention and treatment of tuberculosis	Laniazid Niconyl Nydrazid
ISOPROPAMIDE	Prevents stimulation of muscular contraction and glandular secretion in organ involved (antispasmodic [anticholinergic])	Relief of discomfort from excessive activity and spasm of digestive tract	Darbid Combid (CD) Ornade (CD)
ISOPROTERENOL/ ISOPRENALINE	Dilates bronchial tubes by stimulating sympathetic nerve terminals (Isoproterenol: adrenergic [bronchodilator]; Isoprenaline: sympathomimetic)	Management of acute bronchial asthma, bronchitis, and emphysema	Isuprel Norisodrine Brondilate (CD) Isuprel Compound (CD)
ISOSORBIDE DINITRATE	Acts directly on muscle cells to produce relaxation which permits expansion of blood vessels, thus increasing supply of blood and oxygen to heart (coronary vasodilator)	Management of pain associated with angina pectoris (coronary insufficiency)	Isordil Sorbitrate Sorquad
LEVODOPA	Believed to be converted to dopamine in brain tissue, thus correcting a dopamine deficiency and restoring more normal balance of chemicals responsible for transmission of nerve impulses (anti Parkinsonism)	Management of Parkinson's disease	Larodopa Parda Sinemet
LIOTHYRONINE (T-3)	Increases rate of cellular metabolism and makes more energy available for biochemical activity (thyroid hormone)	Correction of thyroid hormone deficiency (hypothyroidism)	Cytomel Euthroid (CD) Thyrolar (CD)
LITHIUM	Believed to correct chemical imbalance in certain nerve impulse transmitters that influence emotional behavior (antidepressant)	Improvement of mood and behavior in chronic manic-depression	Eskalith Lithane Lithotabs
MECLIZINE	Blocks transmission of excessive nerve impulses to vomiting center (antiemetic)	Management of nausea, vomiting, and dizziness associated with motion sickness	Antivert Bonine Vertrol
MEPERIDINE/PETHIDINE	Believed to increase chemicals that transmit nerve impulses (narcotic analgesic)	Relief of moderate to severe pain	Demerol
MEPROBAMATE	Not known (tranquilizer)	Relief of mild to moderate anxiety and tension (sedative effect); relief of insomnia due to anxiety and tension (hypnotic effect)	Equanil Kalmm Miltown SK-Bamate Tranmep
METHACYCLINE	Prevents growth and multiplication of susceptible bacteria by interfering with formation of their essential proteins (antibiotic)	Elimination of infections responsive to action of this drug	Rondomycin
METHADONE	Believed to increase chemicals that transmit nerve impulses (narcotic analgesic)	Relief of moderate to severe pain	Dolophine
METHAQUALONE	Not known (hypnotic)	Low dosage: relief of mild to moderate anxiety or tension (sedative effect); higher dosage: at bedtime to relieve insomnia (hypnotic effect)	Quaalude Sopor Somnafac
METHYCLOTHIAZIDE	Increases elimination of salt and water (diuretic); relaxes walls of smaller arteries, allowing them to expand; combined effect lowers blood pressure (antihypertensive)	Elimination of excess fluid retention (edema); reduction of high blood pressure	Enduron Diutensen (CD) Enduronyl (CD)
METHYLPHENIDATE	Believed to increase release of nerve impulse transmitter, which may also improve concentration and attention span of hyperactive child (primary action unknown) (central stimulant)	Management of fatigue and depression; reduction of symptoms of abnormal hyperactivity (as in minimal brain dysfunction)	Ritalin
NICOTINIC ACID/NIACIN	Corrects a deficiency of nicotinic acid in tissues; dilation of blood vessels is believed limited to skin—increased blood flow within head has not been demonstrated; reduces initial production of cholesterol and prevents conversion of fatty tissue to cholesterol and triglycerides (vitamin B-complex component; cholesterol reducer)	Management of pellagra; treatment of vertigo, ringing in ears, premenstrual headache; reduction of blood levels of cholesterol and triglycerides	Niacin Nicobid Nicotinex Elixir

Name	Action	Prescribed for	Trade Names (CD = comb. drug)
NITROFURANTOIN	Believed to prevent growth and multiplication of susceptible bacteria by interfering with function of their essential enzyme systems (antibacterial)	Elimination of infections responsive to action of this drug	Furadantin Macrodantin Parfuran Trantoin
NITROGLYCERIN	Acts directly on muscle cells to produce relaxation which permits expansion of blood vessels, thus increasing supply of blood and oxygen to heart (coronary vasodilator)	Management of pain associated with angina pectoris (coronary insufficiency)	Nitrobid Nitroglyn Nitrostat
NYSTATIN	Prevents growth and multiplication of susceptible fungus strains by attacking their walls and causing leakage of internal components (antibiotic; antifungal)	Elimination of fungus infections responsive to action of this drug	Mycostatin Nilstat Declostatin (CD) Mycolog (CD)
ORAL CONTRACEPTIVES	Suppresses the two pituitary gland hormones that produce ovulation (oral contraceptives)	Prevention of pregnancy	Combination type: Enovid-E Ortho-Novum 2mg. Ovulen Zorane "Mini-Pill" type: Micronor 0.35mg. Ovrette
OXYCODONE	Believed to affect tissue sites that react specifically with opium and its derivatives (narcotic analgesic)	Relief of moderate pain; control of coughing	Percobarb (CD) Percodan (CD)
OXYTETRACYCLINE	Prevents growth and multiplication of susceptible bacteria by interfering with their formation of essential proteins (antibiotic)	Elimination of infections responsive to action of this drug	Oxlopar Terramycin Urobiotic (CD)
PAPAVERINE	Causes direct relaxation and expansion of blood vessel walls, thus increasing volume of blood which increases oxygen and nutrients (smooth muscle relaxant; vasodilator)	Relief of symptoms associated with impaired circulation in extremities and within brain	Cerespan Pavabid Vasopan
PARA-AMINOSALICYLIC ACID (PAS)	Prevents growth and multiplication of susceptible tuberculosis organisms and makes them vulnerable to more potent drugs (antibacterial; tuberculostatic)	To increase effectiveness of other drugs used in management of tuberculosis	Pamisyl P.A.S. Rezipas
PAREGORIC (Camphorated Tincture of Opium)	Believed to affect tissue sites that react specifically with opium and its derivatives to relieve pain; its active ingredient, morphine, acts as a local anesthetic and blocks release of chemical that transmits nerve impulses to muscle walls of intestine (antiperistaltic)	Relief of mild to moderate pain; relief of intestinal cramping and diarrhea	Donnagel-PG (CD) Kaoparin (CD) Parepectolin (CD)
PENICILLIN G	Interferes with ability of susceptible bacteria to produce new protective cell walls as they grow and multiply (antibiotic)	Elimination of infections responsive to action of this drug	Pentids Pfizerpen G Sugracillin
PENICILLIN V	Same as above	Same as above	Ledercillin Pfizerpen VK Robicillin-VK V-Cillin Veetids
PENTAERYTHRITOL TETRANITRATE	Acts directly on muscle cells to produce relaxation which permits expansion of blood vessels, thus increasing supply of blood and oxygen to heart (coronary vasodilator)	Management of pain associated with angina pectoris (coronary insufficiency)	Peritrate SK-Petn. Miltrate (CD)
PENTOBARBITAL	Believed to block transmission of nerve impulses (hypnotic; sedative)	Low dosage: relief of mild to moderate anxiety or tension (sedative effect); higher dosage: at bedtime to induce sleep (hypnotic effect)	Nembutal Night-Caps Carbrital (CD)
PHENACETIN (Acetophenetidin)	Believed to reduce concentration of chemicals involved in production of pain, fever, and inflammation (analgesic; antipyretic)	Relief of mild to moderate pain; reduction of fever	Bromo-Seltzer (CD) Empirin Compound (CD) Percodan (CD) Sinubid (CD)
PHENAZOPYRIDINE	Acts as local anesthetic on lining of lower urinary tract (urinary-analgesic)	Relief of pain and discomfort associated with acute irritation of lower urinary tract as in cystitis, urethritis, and prostatitis	Pyridium Azo Gantano (CD) Thiosulfil-A (CD) Urobiotic (CD)
PHENIRAMINE	Blocks action of histamine after release from sensitized tissue cells, thus reducing intensity of allergic response (antihistamine)	Relief of symptoms of hayfever (allergic rhinitis) and of allergic reactions of skin (itching, swelling, hives, and rash)	Inhiston Robitussin-AC (CD) Triaminicin (CD) Tussagesic (CD)
PHENOBARBITAL/ PHENOBARBITONE	Believed to block transmission of nerve impulses (anticonvulsant; hypnotic; sedative)	Low dosage: relief of mild to moderate anxiety or tension (sedative effect); higher dosage: at bedtime to induce sleep (hypnotic effect); continuous dosage: prevention of epileptic seizures (anticonvulsant effect)	Barbipil Bar-15, -25, -100 Eskabarb Stental

Name	Action	Prescribed for	Trade Names (CD = comb. drug)
PHENTERMINE	Believed to alter chemical control of nerve impulse transmitter in appetite center of brain (appetite suppressant [anorexiant])	Suppression of appetite in management of weight reduction	Fastin Ionamin Tora Wilpo
PHENYLBUTAZONE	Believed to suppress formation of chemical involved in production of inflammation (analgesic; anti-inflammatory; antipyretic)	Symptomatic relief of inflammation, swelling, pain, and tenderness associated with arthritis, tendinitis, bursitis, superficial phlebitis	Azolid Butazolidin Azolid-A (CD) Sterazolidin (CD)
PHENYLEPHRINE	Shrinks tissue mass (decongestion) by contracting arteriole walls in lining of nasal passages, sinuses, and throat, thus decreasing volume of blood (decongestant [sympathomimetic])	Relief of congestion of nose, sinuses, and throat associated with allergy	Neo-Synephrine Sinarest Nasal Spray Chlor-Trimeton Expectorant (CD) Co-Tylenol (CD) 4-Way Tablets, Nasal Spray (CD) Sinex (CD)
PHENYL PROPANOLAMINE	Same as above	Same as above	Allerest (CD) Contac (CD) Ornacol (CD) Sinutab (CD) Triaminicin (CD)
PHENYTOIN (formerly Diphenylhydantoin)	Believed to promote loss of sodium from nerve fibers, thus lowering their excitability and inhibiting spread of electrical impulse along nerve pathways (anticonvulsant)	Prevention of epileptic seizures	Dilantin Di-Phen Diphenylan Ekko
PILOCARPINE	Lowers internal eye pressure (antiglaucoma [miotic])	Management of glaucoma	Almocarpine Isopto-Carpine Pilocar
POTASSIUM	Maintains and replenishes potassium content of cells (potassium preparations)	Management of potassium deficiency	Kaon Kay Ciel Pfiklor Potassium Triplex
PREDNISOLONE	Believed to inhibit several mechanisms that induce inflammation (adrenocortical steroid [anti-inflammatory])	Symptomatic relief of inflammation (swelling, redness, heat, and pain)	Delta-Cortef Hydeltra Prednis Sterane
PREDNISONE	Same as above	Same as above	Deltasone Delta Paracort Servisone
PROBENECID	Reduces level of uric acid in blood and tissues; prolongs presence of penicillin in blood (antigout [uricosuric])	Management of gout	Benemid Probalan Colbenemid (CD)
PROMETHAZINE	Blocks action of histamine after release from sensitized tissue cells, thus reducing intensity of allergic response (antihistamine); blocks transmission of excessive nerve impulses to vomiting center (antiemetic); action producing sedation and sleep is unknown (sedative)	Relief of symptoms of hayfever (allergic rhinitis) and of allergic reactions of skin (itching, swelling, hives, rash); prevention and management of nausea, vomiting, and dizziness associated with motion sickness; production of mild sedation and light sleep	Phenergan Prosedin Remsed Synalgos-DC (CD)
PROPANTHELINE	Prevents stimulation of muscular contraction and glandular secretion within organ involved (antispasmodic [anticholinergic])	Relief of discomfort associated with excessive activity and spasm of digestive tract	Norpanth Pro-Banthine Ropanth Probital (CD)
PROPOXYPHENE	Increases chemicals that transmit nerve impulses, somehow contributing to the analgesic effect (analgesic)	Relief of mild to moderate pain	Darvon Darvon-N Darvon Compound (CD) Proproxychel
PSEUDOEPHEDRINE (Isoephedrine)	Shrinks tissue mass (decongestion) by contracting arteriole walls in lining of nasal passages, sinuses, and throat, thus decreasing volume of blood (decongestant [sympathomimetic])	Relief of congestion of nose, sinuses, and throat associated with allergy	Sudafed Actifed (CD) Dimacol (CD) Emprazil (CD) Phenergan (CD)
PYRILAMINE/ MEPYRAMINE	Blocks action of histamine after release from sensitized tissue cells, thus reducing intensity of allergic response (antihistamine)	Relief of symptoms of hayfever (allergic rhinitis) and of allergic reactions of skin (itching, swelling, hives, and rash)	Triaminic (CD) Triaminicin (CD) Triaminicol (CD)
QUINIDINE	Slows pacemaker and delays transmission of electrical impulses (cardiac depressant)	Correction of certain heart rhythm disorders	Cardioquin Cin-Quin Quinidex Quinidine M.B. (CD)
RAFAMPIN	Prevents growth and multiplication of susceptible tuberculosis organisms by interfering with enzyme systems involved in formation of essential proteins (antibiotic; tuberculostatic)	Treatment of tuberculosis	Rifadin Rifomycin Rimactane

Name	Action	Prescribed for	Trade Names (CD = comb. drug)
RESERPINE	Relaxes blood vessel walls by reducing availability of norepinephrine (antihypertensive; tranquilizer)	Reduction of high blood pressure	Rau-Sed Reserpoid Sandril Serp Serpasil
SECOBARBITAL	Believed to block transmission of nerve impúlses (hypnotic; sedative)	Low dosage: relief of mild to moderate anxiety or tension (sedative effect); higher dosage: at bedtime to induce sleep (hypnotic effect)	Seco-8 Seconal Tuinal (CD)
SULFAMETHOXAZOLE	Prevents growth and multiplication of susceptible bacteria by interfering with their formation of folic acid (antibacterial)	Elimination of infections responsive to action of this drug	Gantanol Azo Gantanol (CD) Bactrium (CD) Septra (CD)
SULFISOXAZOLE	Same as above	Same as above	Gantrisin G-Sox SK-Soxazole Soxomide Sulfalar
TETRACYCLINE	Prevents growth and multiplication of susceptible bacteria by interfering with their formation of essential proteins (antibiotic)	Elimination of infections responsive to action of this drug	Achromycin V Cycline-250 Cyclopar Panmycin Robitet Sumycin Tetracyn Tetrex Achrostatin V (CD)
THEOPHYLLINE (Aminophylline, Oxtriphylline)	Reverses constriction by increasing activity of chemical system within muscle cell that causes relaxation of bronchial tube (bronchodilator)	Symptomatic relief of bronchial asthma	Amesec (CD) Brondecon (CD) Bronkotabs (CD) Elixophyllin (CD) Marax (CD) Quadrinal (CD) Quibron (CD)
THYROID (Thyroid Preparations)	Makes more energy available for biochemical activity and increases rate of cellular metabolism by altering processes of cellular chemicals that store energy (thyroid hormones)	Correction of thyroid hormone deficiency (hypothyroidism)	Armour Thyroid Proloid S-P-T Thyrobrom
THYROXINE (T-4)	Same as above	Same as above	Levothroid Synthroid Thyrolar (CD)
TOLBUTAMIDE	Stimulates secretion of insulin by pancreas (hypoglycemic)	Correction of insulin deficiency in adult diabetes	Orinase
TRIDIHEXETHYL	Prevents stimulation of muscular contraction and glandular secretion in organ involved (antispasmodic [anticholinergic])	Relief of discomfort from excessive activity and spasm of digestive tract	Pathilon Milpath (CD) Pathibamate (CD)
TRIMETHOPRIM	Prevents growth and multiplication of susceptible organisms by interfering with formation of proteins (antibacterial)	Elimination of infections responsive to action of this drug	Syraprim Bactrim (CD) Septra (CD)
TRIPROLIDINE	Blocks action of histamine after release from sensitized tissue cells, thus reducing intensity of allergic response (antihistamine)	Relief of symptoms of hayfever (allergic rhinitis) and of allergic reactions of skin (itching, swelling, hives, and rash)	Actidil Actifed (CD) Actifed-C (CD)
VITAMIN C (Ascorbic Acid)	Believed to be essential to enzyme activity involved in formation of collagen; increases absorption of iron from intestine and helps formation of hemoglobin and red blood cells in bone marrow; inhibits growth of certain bacteria in urinary tract; enhances effects of some antibiotics (vitamin)	Prevention and treatment of scurvy; treatment of some types of anemia; maintenance of an acid urine	Ascorbicap Cetane Cevalin Synchro-C

Index

612